GW01458442

# MANU

# SMALL ANIMAL INTERNAL MEDICINE

**Second Edition**

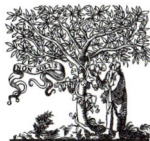

## ELSEVIER
## MOSBY

# MANUAL OF

# $\int$ MALL ANIMAL INTERNAL MEDICINE

**Second Edition**

**RICHARD W. NELSON, DVM, Dipl ACVIM**
Professor, Department of Medicine and Epidemiology
School of Veterinary Medicine
University of California, Davis
Davis, California

**C. GUILLERMO COUTO, DVM, Dipl ACVIM**
Professor, Department of Veterinary Clinical Sciences
College of Veterinary Medicine
Chief, Oncology/Hematology Service
Veterinary Teaching Hospital
The Ohio State University
Columbus, Ohio

Prepared by
**CHRISTINE KING, BVSc, MACVSc, MVetClinStud**
**KAREN ASHBY, DVM**

# ELSEVIER
# MOSBY

11830 Westline Industrial Drive
St. Louis, Missouri 63146

MANUAL OF SMALL ANIMAL INTERNAL MEDICINE          0-323-02600-1
**Copyright © 2005, 1999 by Mosby, Inc.**

---

### NOTICE

---

**International Standard Book Number 0-323-02600-1**

*Publishing Director:* Linda L. Duncan
*Senior Editor:* Liz Fathman
*Developmental Editor:* John Dedeke
*Publishing Services Manager:* Patricia Tannian
*Project Manager:* Sarah Wunderly
*Design Manager:* Mark Bernard

Printed in United States
Last digit is the print number:    9   8   7   6   5   4   3   2   1

# CONTRIBUTORS

**Susan E. Bunch,** DVM, PhD, Dipl ACVIM
Professor of Medicine
Department of Clinical Sciences
College of Veterinary Medicine
North Carolina State University
Raleigh, North Carolina

**C. Guillermo Couto,** DVM, Dipl ACVIM
Professor
Department of Veterinary Clinical Sciences
College of Veterinary Medicine
The Ohio State University
Columbus, Ohio

**Denise A. Elliot,** BVSc, PhD, Dipl ACVIM, ACVN
Communications Manager
Waltham, USA
Vernon, California

**Gregory F. Grauer,** DVM, MS, Dipl ACVIM
Professor and Head
Department of Clinical Sciences
College of Veterinary Medicine
Kansas State University
Manhattan, Kansas

**Eleanor C. Hawkins,** DVM, Dipl ACVIM
Professor
Department of Clinical Sciences
College of Veterinary Medicine
North Carolina State University
Raleigh, North Carolina

**Cheri A. Johnson,** DVM, MS, Dipl ACVIM
Professor and Chief of Medicine
Department of Small Animal Clinical Sciences
College of Veterinary Medicine
Michigan State University
East Lansing, Michigan

**Michael R. Lappin,** DVM, PhD, Dipl ACVIM
Professor and Section Head of Small Animal Internal Medicine
College of Veterinary Medicine and Biomedical Sciences
Colorado State University
Fort Collins, Colorado

**Richard W. Nelson,** DVM, Dipl ACVIM
Professor
Department of Medicine and Epidemiology
School of Veterinary Medicine
University of California, Davis
Davis, California

**Susan M. Taylor,** DVM, Dipl ACVIM
Professor and Chief of Small Animal Medicine
Department of Small Animal Clinical Sciences
Western College of Veterinary Medicine
University of Saskatchewan
Saskatoon, Saskatchewan

**Wendy A. Ware,** DVM, MS, Dipl ACVIM
Professor
Departments of Veterinary Clinical Sciences and Biomedical Sciences
Iowa State University
Ames, Iowa

**Michael D. Willard,** DVM, MS, Dipl ACVIM
Professor
Department of Veterinary Small Animal Medicine and Surgery
Texas A&M University
College Station, Texas

# PREFACE

*Manual of Small Animal Internal Medicine, Second Edition,* is designed as a handy, current reference for use by veterinarians, veterinary students, veterinary technicians, and other clinic staff. The goal of this manual is to provide readers with fast, helpful information on assessment, diagnosis, and treatment of the most common problems encountered in dogs and cats. In no way is it an exhaustive work; it is best used in conjunction with the third edition of *Small Animal Internal Medicine,* in which the reader will find more detailed discussions of relevant anatomy and physiology, pathophysiology, diagnostic testing, procedures, and underlying rationales for treatment options, as well as hundreds of supporting illustrations and extensive reference lists. Helpful page cross-references to the parent text have been provided throughout the *Manual* to direct readers to more detailed information.

Features of the *Manual* include a focus on key information related to assessment, diagnosis, and treatment of common medical conditions in dogs and cats; material organized by body system, with important sections on hematology, oncology, and immunology; nearly 300 tables highlighting important points on etiology, clinical signs, treatment regimens, and much more; and extensive drug tables at the end of each part display common drugs used for that particular system

New material added to this second edition includes a new chapter on therapeutic diets; thorough updating of all diagnostic tools, treatment modalities, references, and so on, reflecting revisions to the third edition of *Small Animal Internal Medicine*; and a new glossary of key terms for quick identification of major abbreviations used throughout the text.

It is our belief that this second edition of *Manual of Small Animal Internal Medicine* serves as both a useful companion to the third edition of *Small Animal Internal Medicine* and an effective stand-alone quick reference for veterinary students and practitioners.

**RICHARD W. NELSON**
**C. GUILLERMO COUTO**

# CONTENTS

# PART IX: Neuromuscular Disorders

# PART X: Joint Disorders

# PART XI: Oncology

# PART XII: Hematology and Immunology

# PART XIII: Infectious Diseases

Michael R. Lappin

# GLOSSARY OF ABBREVIATIONS

| | |
|---|---|
| Ab | antibody |
| ACEI | angiotensin-converting enzyme inhibitor |
| ACHR | acetylcholine receptor |
| ACT | activated clotting time |
| ACTH | adrenocorticotropic hormone |
| AE | acanthomatous epulis |
| Ag | antigen |
| AGID | agar gel immunodiffusion |
| AHA | acetohydroxamic acid |
| AI | artificial insemination |
| ALL | acute lymphoid leukemia |
| ALT | alanine aminotransferase |
| AML | acute myeloid leukemia |
| ANA | antinuclear antibody |
| AP | alkaline phosphatase |
| ARD | anemia of renal disease |
| ARDS | acute respiratory distress syndrome |
| ARE | antibiotic-responsive enteropathy |
| ARF | acute renal failure |
| ASD | atrial septal defect |
| AT | adrenocortical tumor |
| ATLS | acute tumor lysis syndrome |
| AV | atrioventricular |
| BAER | brainstem-auditory evoked response |
| BAL | bronchoalveolar lavage |
| BCS | body condition score |
| BP | arterial blood pressure |
| BPH | benign prostatic hyperplasia |
| BSA | body surface area |
| BUN | blood urea nitrogen |
| CaVC | caudal vena cava |
| CBC | complete blood count |
| CDI | central diabetes insipidus |
| CDV | canine distemper virus |
| CEH | cystic endometrial hyperplasia |
| CFU | colony-forming units |
| CHF | congestive heart failure |
| CHV | canine herpes virus |
| CK | creatine kinase |
| CK-MB | myocardial-bound creatine kinase |
| CL | corpus luteum |
| CLL | chronic lymphocytic leukemia |
| CR | complete remission |
| CNS | central nervous system |
| CPR | cardiopulmonary resuscitation |
| CRF | chronic renal failure |
| CRI | constant rate infusion |
| CRT | capillary refill time |
| CSF | cerebrospinal fluid |
| CT | computerized tomography |

| | |
|---|---|
| CTX | cyclophosphamide |
| cTSH | canine thyroid-stimulating hormone |
| CVP | central venous pressure |
| CW | continuous wave |
| DAT | direct antibody test |
| DC | direct current |
| DCM | dilated cardiomyopathy |
| DDAVP | desmopressin acetate |
| DEA | dog erythrocyte antigen |
| DEC | diethylcarbamazine |
| DES | diethylstilbestrol |
| DIC | disseminated intravascular coagulation |
| DIF | direct immunofluorescence |
| DJD | degenerative joint disease |
| DKA | diabetic ketoacidosis |
| DM | diabetes mellitus |
| DMSO | dimethyl sulfoxide |
| DOCP | desoxycorticosterone pivalate |
| DTIC | dacarbazine |
| DV | dorsoventral |
| ECG | electrocardiography |
| echo | echocardiography |
| EEG | electroencephalogram |
| EGE | eosinophilic gastroenterocolitis |
| EHEC | enterohemorrhagic *E. coli* |
| ELISA | enzyme-linked immunosorbent assay |
| EMH | extramedullary hematopoiesis |
| EMG | electromyography |
| EPI | exocrine pancreatic insufficiency |
| ERG | electroretinography |
| FBMI | Feline Body Mass Index |
| FC | fractional clearance |
| FCE | fibrocartilaginous embolism |
| FCV | feline calicivirus |
| FeLV | feline leukemia virus |
| FeSFV | feline syncytia-forming virus |
| FECV | feline enteric coronavirus |
| FHV | feline herpes virus |
| FIE | feline ischemic encephalopathy |
| FIP | feline infectious peritonitis |
| FIV | feline immunodeficiency virus |
| FLUTD | feline lower urinary tract disease |
| FLUTI | feline lower urinary tract inflammation |
| FNA | fine-needle aspiration |
| FS | fractional shortening |
| FSA | fibrosarcoma |
| FUO | fever of undetermined (unknown) origin |
| G-CSF | granulocyte colony-stimulating factor |
| GDV | gastric dilatation/volvulus |
| GFR | glomerular filtration rate |
| GH | growth hormone |
| GI | gastrointestinal |
| GME | granulomatous meningoencephalitis |
| GN | glomerulonephritis |
| GnRH | gonadotropin-releasing hormone |
| GUE | gastroduodenal ulceration/erosion |

| | |
|---|---|
| hCG | human chorionic gonadotropin |
| HCM | hypertrophic cardiomyopathy |
| HCT | histiocytoma |
| HDDS | high-dose dexamethasone suppression |
| HE | hepatic encephalopathy |
| HES | hypereosinophilic syndrome |
| HHM | humoral hypercalcemia of malignancy |
| HRV | heart rate variability |
| HSA | hemangiosarcoma |
| HWD | heartworm disease |
| IBD | inflammatory bowel disease |
| IBO | intestinal bacterial overgrowth |
| IBS | irritable bowel syndrome |
| IDDM | insulin-dependent diabetes mellitus |
| IFA | indirect fluorescent antibody |
| IHA | immune hemolytic anemia |
| IGF-I | insulin-like growth factor I |
| IL | intestinal lymphangiectasia |
| IM | intramuscularly |
| IMD | immune mediated disease |
| IMT | immune mediated thrombocytopenia |
| INR | international normalization ratio |
| IO | intraosseously |
| IT | intratracheally |
| IV | intravenously |
| KCl | potassium chloride |
| LA | latex agglutination |
| LAE | left atrial enlargement |
| LAFB | left anterior fascicular block |
| LBBB | left bundle branch block |
| LCAT | latex agglutination capsular antigen test |
| LDDS | low-dose dexamethasone suppression |
| LE | lupus erythematosus |
| LG | lymphomatoid granulomatosis |
| LGL | large granular lymphocyte |
| LH | luteinizing hormone |
| LIM | leg index measurement |
| LMN | lower motor neuron |
| LMWH | low molecular weight heparin |
| LPC | lymphocytic-plasmacytic colitis |
| LPE | lymphocytic-plasmacytic enteritis |
| LPFB | left posterior fascicular block |
| LRS | lactated Ringer's solution |
| LRT | lower respiratory tract |
| LSA | lymphosarcoma/lymphoma |
| LV | left ventricular/ventricle |
| LVE | left ventricular enlargement |
| M dys | mitral dysplasia |
| MAT | microscopic agglutination test |
| MCT | medium-chain triglyceride |
| MD | muscular dystrophy |
| MDI | metered-dose inhaler |
| ME | metabolizable energy |
| MEA | mean electrical axis |
| MED | modified equilibrium dialysis |
| MG | myasthenia gravis |

| | |
|---|---|
| MIC | minimum inhibitory concentrations |
| MM | malignant melanoma |
| MMM | masticatory muscle myositis |
| MR | magnetic resonance |
| MRI | magnetic resonance imaging |
| NB-BAL | nonbronchoscopic bronchoalveolar lavage |
| NCV | nerve conduction velocity |
| NDI | nephrogenic diabetes insipidus |
| NIDDM | non–insulin-dependent diabetes mellitus |
| NMB | new methylene blue |
| NSAID | nonsteroidal antiinflammatory drug |
| OSA | osteosarcoma |
| PAS | periodic acid-Schiff |
| PCR | polymerase chain reaction |
| PCV | packed cell volume |
| PCWP | pulmonary capillary wedge pressure |
| PCT | plasma cell tumor |
| PD | polydipsia |
| PDA | patent ductus arteriosus |
| PDH | pituitary-dependent hyperadrenocorticism |
| PIE | pulmonary infiltrates with eosinophils |
| PIV | parainfluenza virus |
| PLE | protein-losing enteropathy |
| PLO | pluronic lecithin organogel |
| PLR | pupillary light reflex |
| PMA | pituitary macroadenoma |
| PMI | point of maximal intensity |
| PMN | polymorphonuclear neutrophil |
| PPA | phenylpropanolamine |
| PPDH | peritoneopericardial diaphragmatic hernia |
| PR | partial remission |
| PRAA | persistent right aortic arch |
| PRCA | pure red cell aplasia |
| PS | pulmonic stenosis |
| PSS | portosystemic shunt |
| PT | prothrombin time |
| PTE | pulmonary thromboembolism |
| PTH | parathyroid hormone |
| PTHrp | parathyroid hormone-related protein |
| PTT | partial thromboplastin time |
| PU | polyuria |
| PU/PD | polyuria/polydipsia |
| PW | pulsed wave |
| PZI | protamine-zinc insulin |
| RA | rheumatoid arthritis |
| RAE | right atrial enlargement |
| RBBB | right bundle branch block |
| RBC | red blood cell |
| RCM | restrictive cardiomyopathy |
| RCT | round cell tumor |
| RF | rheumatoid factor |
| RI | reticulocyte index |
| RIA | radioimmunoassay |
| RMSF | Rocky Mountain spotted fever |
| RPLA | reversed passive latex agglutination |
| RSAT | rapid slide agglutination |

| | |
|---|---|
| RV | right ventricle |
| RVE | right ventricular enlargement |
| S | solute |
| SA | sinoatrial |
| SAECG | signal-averaged electrocardiography |
| SAP | serum alkaline phosphatase |
| SARD | sudden acquired retinal degeneration |
| SAS | subaortic stenosis |
| SBA | serum bile acids |
| SC | subcutaneous |
| SCC | squamous cell carcinoma |
| SD | stable disease |
| SG | specific gravity |
| SIRS | subinvolution of placental sites |
| SLE | systemic lupus erythematosus |
| SQ | subcutaneously |
| ST | sulfa-trimethroprim |
| SVT | supraventricular tachycardia |
| T dys | tricuspid dysplasia |
| TAT | tube agglutination |
| TCC | transitional cell carciroma |
| TICM | tachycardia-induced cardiomyopathy |
| TLI | trypsin-like immunoreactivity |
| T of F | tetralogy of Fallot |
| TPN | total parenteral nutrition |
| TRH | thyrotropin-releasing hormone |
| TSH | thyroid-stimulating hcrmone |
| TVT | transmissible venereal tumor |
| UMN | upper motor neuron |
| UPP | urethral pressure profile |
| URI | upper respiratory infection |
| UTI | urinary tract infection |
| US | ultrasonography |
| USMI | urethral sphincter mechanism incompetence |
| UTI | urinary tract infection |
| V/Q | ventilation/perfusion |
| VAS | vaccine-associated sarcomas |
| VD | ventrodorsal |
| VHS | vertebral heart score |
| VLDL | very low density lipoprotein |
| VPC | ventricular premature contractions or complex |
| VSD | ventricular septal defect |
| VWD | von Willebrand disease |
| VWF | von Willebrand factor |
| WBC | white blood cell |
| WPW | Wolff-Parkinson-White |

# PART I

# Cardiovascular System Disorders

WENDY A. WARE

# 1

# Cardiovascular Examination

## (Text pp 1-11)

## HISTORY AND CLINICAL SIGNS

### Signs of Heart Disease and Heart Failure

Signs of heart disease may be present even if the animal is not in "heart failure." Objective signs include murmurs, rhythm disturbances, jugular pulsations, and cardiac enlargement. Other signs are listed in Table 1-1.

#### Weakness and syncope

In animals with heart disease cardiac output may become inadequate, resulting in episodes of weakness or collapse, especially during activity. Syncope is an abrupt and transient loss of consciousness and postural tone caused by inadequate oxygen or glucose delivery to the brain. It is a sign of underlying disease. Cardiovascular causes of intermittent weakness or syncope include the following:

- bradyarrhythmia (e.g., second- or third-degree atrioventricular [AV] block, sinus arrest, sick sinus syndrome, atrial standstill)
- tachyarrhythmia (e.g., paroxysmal atrial or ventricular tachycardia, reentrant supraventricular tachycardia, atrial fibrillation)
- congenital ventricular outflow obstruction (e.g., pulmonic or subaortic stenosis)
- acquired ventricular outflow obstruction (e.g., heartworm disease, hypertrophic obstructive cardiomyopathy, thrombus, tumor)
- cyanotic heart disease (e.g., tetralogy of Fallot, right-to-left shunts)
- impaired forward cardiac output (e.g., valvular insufficiency, dilated cardiomyopathy, myocardial infarction)
- cardiac tamponade or constrictive pericarditis
- excessive doses of cardiovascular drugs (e.g., diuretics, vasodilators)
- activation of vasodepressor reflexes

Noncardiac causes include the following:

- pulmonary diseases that cause hypoxemia
- cough-syncope ("cough-drop") in dogs with respiratory disease or bronchial compression from marked left atrial enlargement
- pulmonary hypertension
- metabolic disturbances (e.g., hypoglycemia, electrolyte imbalances [$K^+$, $Ca^{2+}$])
- hypoadrenocorticism
- anemia or sudden hemorrhage
- seizures
- neuromuscular disease
- cerebrovascular accident
- narcolepsy, cataplexy

A description of the animal's behavior or activity before, during, and after collapse and the drug history help to differentiate among syncopal attacks, episodic weakness,

**Table 1-1**

## Clinical Signs of Left- and Right-Sided Heart Failure

| Low output signs | Congestive signs—left side | Congestive signs—right side |
|---|---|---|
| Tiring | Pulmonary congestion and | Systemic venous congestion |
| Exertional weakness | edema (resulting in cough, | (high central venous |
| Syncope | tachypnea, dyspnea, | pressure, jugular vein |
| Prerenal azotemia | orthopnea, pulmonary | distention) |
| Cyanosis (from poor | crackles, tiring, hemoptysis, | Hepatic ± splenic congestion |
| cutaneous circulation) | cyanosis) | Pleural effusion (resulting in |
| Cardiac arrhythmias | Secondary right-sided heart | dyspnea, orthopnea, ascites, |
| | failure | cyanosis) |
| | Cardiac arrhythmias | Small pericardial effusion |
| | | Subcutaneous edema |
| | | Cardiac arrhythmias |

and true seizures. Syncope is often associated with exertion or excitement and may be characterized by rear limb weakness or by sudden collapse, lateral recumbency, stiffening of the forelimbs, opisthotonos, and micturition. Vocalization is common, but tonic-clonic motion, facial fits, and defecation are not. An "aura" before abnormal activity, postictal dementia, and neurologic deficits are generally not seen with cardiovascular syncope.

Diagnosis usually involves electrocardiography (ECG) (resting and during or after exercise or a vagal maneuver), complete blood count (CBC), serum biochemistry studies, neurologic examination, thoracic radiographs, heartworm testing, and echocardiography. Other studies performed to rule out neuromuscular or neurologic disease may also be valuable. Intermittent arrhythmias may be discovered by means of 24-hour ambulatory ECG (Holter monitor), event monitoring, or in-hospital continuous ECG monitoring.

### Cough

Congestive heart failure in dogs is often manifested by coughing, tachypnea, and dyspnea. These signs also occur in association with the pulmonary pathology of heartworm disease. The cough accompanying left-sided heart failure in dogs is often soft and moist but sometimes sounds like gagging. In contrast, cough is an unusual sign of pulmonary edema in cats. Compression of a mainstem bronchus caused by severe left atrial enlargement in dogs with chronic mitral insufficiency can stimulate a dry or "hacking" cough, even in the absence of pulmonary edema or congestion. In addition to respiratory diseases, other possible causes of cough include heartbase tumor or another mass that impinges on an airway, and pleural or pericardial effusion.

When respiratory signs are caused by heart disease, other evidence such as generalized cardiomegaly, left atrial enlargement, pulmonary venous congestion, diuretic-responsive lung infiltrates, or a positive heartworm test is usually present. Thorough physical examination, thoracic radiographs, echocardiography, and ECG facilitate differentiation of cardiac from noncardiac causes of cough and other respiratory signs.

## PHYSICAL EXAMINATION

Evaluation should involve a general physical examination, which includes observation of attitude, posture, body condition, level of anxiety, and respiratory pattern. In the absence of primary lung disease, hyperpnea is an early indicator of pulmonary edema; however, it can also be associated with excitement, fever, fear, or pain. Careful observation and physical examination are needed to identify the cause of hyperpnea.

Dyspneic animals usually appear anxious; increased respiratory effort, flared nostrils, and often hyperpnea are also evident. Pulmonary edema (and other lung infiltrates) cause rapid, shallow breathing. Prolonged, labored inspiration is usually associated with upper airway obstruction, whereas prolonged expiration occurs in association with lower airway obstruction or pulmonary infiltrative disease (including edema). Large-volume pleural effusion or other pleural space disease (e.g., pneumothorax) generally causes exaggerated respiratory motions in an effort to expand the collapsed lungs. Animals with severely compromised ventilation may refuse to lie down; they stand, sit, or crouch in a sternal position (cats) with elbows abducted, and they resist being positioned in lateral or dorsal recumbency. Open-mouth breathing is usually a sign of severe respiratory distress in cats.

The cardiovascular examination consists of evaluation of the peripheral circulation (mucous membranes), systemic veins (especially the jugular veins), arterial pulses, and precordium; palpation or percussion for abnormal fluid accumulation; and auscultation of the heart and lungs.

## Mucous Membranes

Mucous membrane color and capillary refill time (CRT) are used to estimate the adequacy of peripheral perfusion. Usually the oral membranes are assessed, but the ocular conjunctivae and caudal membranes (prepuce of vagina) can also be used.

Pale mucous membranes result from anemia or peripheral vasoconstriction. Injected, brick-red membranes occur with erythrocytosis, sepsis, excitement, and other causes of peripheral vasodilation. Icteric membranes are the result of hemolysis, hepatobiliary disease, or biliary obstruction.

Cyanotic mucous membranes can develop in animals with pulmonary parenchymal disease (including edema), airway obstruction, or pleural space disease. Congenital cardiac defects (with right-to-left shunting), hypoventilation, shock, cold exposure, and methemoglobinemia can also cause this discoloration. Differential (caudal) cyanosis is seen in patients with reversed patent ductus arteriosus (PDA) (see Chapter 9).

Normal CRT is less than 2 seconds. Slower refill times occur from dehydration and other causes of peripheral vasoconstriction. CRT is normal in anemic patients unless hypoperfusion is also present; however, it can be difficult to assess CRT in severely anemic animals because of lack of color contrast.

## Jugular Veins

The jugular veins should not be distended when the animal is standing with its head in a normal position. Persistent jugular vein distention occurs with right-sided congestive heart failure, external compression of the cranial vena cava, or thrombosis of the jugular vein or cranial vena cava. Specific causes include pericardial effusion and tamponade, right atrial mass or inflow obstruction, dilated cardiomyopathy, and cranial mediastinal mass.

Jugular pulsations extending higher than one third of the way up the neck are abnormal. Causes of jugular pulsations include tricuspid insufficiency, pulmonic stenosis, heartworm disease, and pulmonary hypertension. Arrhythmias such as ventricular premature contractions (VPCs) and complete (third-degree) heart block can also cause intermittent jugular pulsations. (Note: Sometimes the carotid pulse wave is transmitted through the adjacent soft tissues, mimicking a jugular pulse in thin or excited animals.)

### Hepatojugular reflux

Impaired right ventricular filling, reduced pulmonary blood flow, or tricuspid regurgitation can cause a positive hepatojugular reflux, even in the absence of jugular distension or pulsations. When firm pressure is applied to the cranial abdomen with the patient standing quietly, little or no change should occur in the jugular vein. Jugular distention that persists while abdominal pressure is applied constitutes a positive (abnormal) test.

## Arterial Pulses

The strength, regularity, and rate of the arterial pressure waves are assessed by palpation of the femoral or other peripheral arteries. (Note: Femoral pulses can be difficult to palpate in cats, even when normal.) Causes of abnormally strong (hyperkinetic) pulses include excitement, hypertrophic cardiomyopathy (cats), hyperthyroidism, and fever and sepsis. Very strong, bounding pulses may be found in patients with PDA, fever and sepsis, or severe aortic regurgitation. Abnormally weak (hypokinetic) pulses may be caused by dilated cardiomyopathy, (sub)aortic or pulmonic stenosis, shock, or dehydration.

Alternately weak then strong pulsations can result from severe myocardial failure or from a normal heartbeat alternating with a premature beat. A weaker arterial pulse strength might be detected during inspiration in patients with cardiac tamponade. Both femoral pulses should be palpated and compared; absence of pulse or a weaker pulse on one side may be a result of thromboembolism (see Chapter 7). The pulse rate should be evaluated simultaneously with the heart rate; fewer pulses than heartbeats constitutes a pulse deficit. Various cardiac arrhythmias cause pulse deficits.

## Precordium

Normally, the strongest cardiac impulse is felt during systole over the left apex (approximately the left fifth intercostal space, near the costochondral junction). Cardiomegaly or a space-occupying mass within the chest can shift the precordial impulse to an abnormal location. Decreased intensity of the precordial impulse can be caused by obesity, weak cardiac contractions, pericardial effusion, intrathoracic mass, pleural effusion, or pneumothorax. A stronger right precordial impulse can result from right ventricular hypertrophy or displacement of the heart into the right hemithorax, lung atelectasis, or chest deformity. Very loud cardiac murmurs cause palpable vibrations on the chest wall ("precordial thrill"), which is usually localized to the area of maximal murmur intensity (see text, Chapter 1).

## Evaluation for Fluid Accumulation

Congestive heart failure (especially if right sided) can promote abnormal fluid accumulation within body cavities or in the subcutis of dependent areas. Palpation and ballottement of the abdomen, percussion of the chest in the standing animal, and palpation of dependent areas are used to detect effusions and subcutaneous edema. Fluid accumulation is usually accompanied by abnormal jugular vein distention, pulsations, or both; hepatomegaly, splenomegaly, or both may also be found.

## Thoracic Auscultation
### Transient heart sounds

The heart sounds normally heard in dogs and cats are $S_1$ (closure and tensing of the AV valves and associated structures) and $S_2$ (closure of the aortic and pulmonic valves). The diastolic sounds ($S_3$ and $S_4$) are not audible in normal dogs and cats. The precordial impulse occurs just after $S_1$ (systole), with the arterial pulse between $S_1$ and $S_2$.

A loud $S_1$ may be heard in dogs and cats with a thin chest wall, high sympathetic tone, tachycardia, systemic arterial hypertension, or shortened PR intervals. A muffled $S_1$ can result from obesity, pericardial effusion, diaphragmatic hernia, dilated cardiomyopathy, hypovolemia or poor ventricular filling, or pleural effusion. A split or sloppy-sounding $S_1$ may be normal in large dogs, or it may result from VPCs or an intraventricular conduction delay. The intensity of $S_2$ is increased by pulmonary hypertension (e.g., with heartworm disease, congenital shunt with Eisenmenger's physiology, or cor pulmonale). Splitting of $S_2$ can result from VPCs, right bundle branch block, ventricular or atrial septal defect, or pulmonary hypertension. However, a physiologic splitting of $S_2$ with respiration is heard in some normal dogs.

*Gallop sounds.* The third ($S_3$) and fourth ($S_4$) heart sounds, when present, occur during diastole and cause a so-called "gallop rhythm." Gallop sounds are usually heard best using the bell of the stethoscope over the cardiac apex. At very fast heart rates differentiation of $S_3$ from $S_4$ is difficult. If both sounds are present, they may be superimposed (summation gallop).

An audible $S_3$ usually indicates ventricular dilation with myocardial failure. It may be the only auscultable abnormality in patients with dilated cardiomyopathy. An $S_3$

gallop may also be heard in dogs with advanced valvular heart disease and congestive failure. An audible $S_4$ is usually associated with increased ventricular stiffness and hypertrophy, as with hypertrophic cardiomyopathy.

***Other transient sounds.*** Systolic "clicks" are mid-to-late systolic sounds usually heard best over the mitral valve area. They can occur in patients with degenerative valvular disease (endocardiosis), mitral valve prolapse, or congenital mitral dysplasia. A concurrent mitral insufficiency murmur may be present. In dogs with degenerative valve disease, a mitral click may be the first abnormal sound noted, with a murmur developing over time. An early systolic, high-pitched "ejection sound" at the left base may occur in animals with pulmonic stenosis. Rarely, restrictive pericardial disease causes an audible "pericardial knock"; its timing is similar to $S_3$.

### Cardiac murmurs

The intensity of a murmur is graded on a I to VI scale (Table 1-2). The areas to which the murmur radiates can be extensive, so the entire thorax and the thoracic inlet and carotid arteries should be auscultated.

***Systolic murmurs.*** Systolic murmurs can be decrescendo, plateau-shaped (holosystolic), or crescendo-decrescendo (ejection) in configuration. It can be difficult to differentiate these murmurs by auscultation alone. However, establishing that a murmur occurs in systole, and determining its point of maximal intensity (PMI) and grade are the most important steps toward diagnosis.

Functional murmurs tend to be heard best over the left base. They are usually of soft-to-moderate intensity and are decrescendo (or crescendo-decrescendo) murmurs. These murmurs may have no apparent cause (e.g., "innocent" puppy murmurs), or they can result from an altered physiologic state (e.g., anemia, fever, high sympathetic tone, hyperthyroidism, peripheral arteriovenous fistulae, hypoproteinemia, and athletic hearts).

A mitral insufficiency murmur is heard best at the left apex, in the area of the mitral valve. It radiates dorsally and often to the left base and right chest wall. Mitral insufficiency typically causes a plateau or regurgitant murmur (holosystolic). However, in its early stages, the murmur may have a decrescendo configuration. Occasionally this murmur has a musical or "whoop-like" quality.

Systolic ejection murmurs are most often heard at the left base. They are caused by ventricular outflow obstruction, usually from a fixed narrowing (e.g., subaortic or pulmonic stenosis) or dynamic muscular obstruction. These murmurs become louder as cardiac output or contractile strength increases. The murmur of subaortic stenosis is heard well at the low left base and at the right base. The murmur of pulmonic stenosis is best heard high at the left base.

Most murmurs heard on the right side are holosystolic, plateau-shaped murmurs (except for subaortic stenosis). A tricuspid insufficiency murmur is loudest at the right apex, over the tricuspid valve. It may have a noticeably different pitch or quality from that of a concurrent mitral insufficiency murmur and often is accompanied by jugular pulsations.

### Table 1-2

#### Grading of Heart Murmurs

| Grade | Murmur |
|-------|--------|
| I | Very soft murmur; heard only in quiet surroundings after minutes of listening |
| II | Soft murmur but easily heard |
| III | Moderate-intensity murmur |
| IV | Loud murmur but not accompanied by a precordial thrill |
| V | Loud murmur with a palpable precordial thrill |
| VI | Very loud murmur that can be heard with the stethoscope off the chest wall; accompanied by a precordial thrill |

Ventricular septal defects also cause holosystolic murmurs. The PMI is usually at the right sternal border, reflecting the direction of the intracardiac shunt. A large ventricular septal defect may also cause a murmur of relative pulmonic stenosis.

**Diastolic murmurs.** Aortic insufficiency from bacterial endocarditis is the most common cause; congenital malformation or degenerative aortic valve disease occurs occasionally. Clinically relevant pulmonic insufficiency is rare but is more likely in the face of pulmonary hypertension. These murmurs are heard best at the left base. They begin at the time of $S_2$ then diminish in intensity (decrescendo) and extend a variable time into diastole. Some aortic insufficiency murmurs have a musical quality.

**Continuous murmurs.** Continuous ("machinery") murmurs occur throughout the cardiac cycle. No interruption of the murmur occurs at the time of $S_2$; rather, the intensity is often greater at that time. The murmur becomes softer toward the end of diastole, and at slow heart rates may even become inaudible. PDA is by far the most common cause. The murmur in PDA is loudest high at the left base, above the pulmonic valve area; it tends to radiate cranially, ventrally, and to the right. The systolic component is usually louder and heard well all over the chest, whereas the diastolic component is localized to the left base in many cases.

Continuous murmurs can be confused with concurrent systolic ejection and diastolic decrescendo murmurs. But in these so-called "to-and-fro murmurs," the ejection murmur tapers off in late systole, allowing $S_2$ to be heard as a distinct sound. The most common cause is the combination of subaortic stenosis and aortic insufficiency. Rarely, stenosis and insufficiency of the pulmonic valve cause this type of murmur.

# 2

# Diagnostic Tests for the Cardiovascular System

## *(Text pp 12–50)*

## ELECTROCARDIOGRAPHY

The electrocardiogram (ECG) waveforms P-QRS-T are generated as the heart muscle is depolarized and then repolarized (Fig. 2-1). For standard ECG recording the animal should be in right lateral recumbency with the proximal limbs parallel to each other and perpendicular to the torso.

### ECG Interpretation

The calibration used to record each lead, the paper speed, and the lead being evaluated must be known before waveform measurement and interpretation. A calibration square wave (1-mV amplitude) can be inscribed during recording of each lead. The heart rate, rhythm, and mean electrical axis (MEA) are then determined. Heart rhythm is evaluated by scanning the ECG for irregularities and identifying individual waveforms. The presence and relationships between the P waves and QRS-Ts are evaluated. Finally, individual waveforms are measured. Normal ECG values are given in Table 2-1.

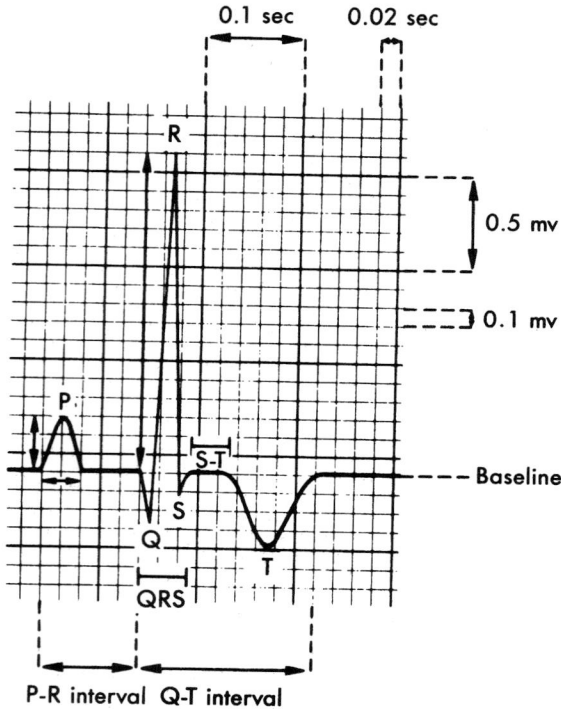

**FIG. 2-1** Normal canine P-QRS-T complex in lead II. Paper speed is 50 mm/sec, calibration is standard (1 cm = 1 mV). Time intervals (seconds) are measured from left to right; waveform amplitudes (millivolts) are measured as positive (upward) or negative (downward) motion from baseline. (From Tilley LE: *Essentials of canine and feline electrocardiography*, ed 3, Philadelphia, 1992, Lea & Febiger.)

The MEA describes the average direction of the ventricular depolarization process in the frontal plane. Estimating the MEA helps in identification of major intraventricular conduction disturbances and certain ventricular enlargement patterns. To estimate the MEA (using the six frontal leads), do either of the following:

1. Find the lead (I, II, III, $aV_R$, $aV_L$, or $aV_F$) with the largest R wave (positive deflection). The positive electrode of this lead is the approximate MEA orientation.
2. Find the lead with the most isoelectric QRS (approximately equal positive and negative deflections). Then identify the lead perpendicular to this on the hexaxial lead diagram (Fig. 2-2). If the QRS in this perpendicular lead is mostly positive, the MEA is toward the positive pole of this lead. If the QRS in the perpendicular lead is mostly negative, the MEA is oriented toward the negative pole.

### Common Artifacts

A good ECG recording has minimal artifacts and a clean baseline. Artifacts can be confused with arrhythmias. However, artifacts do not disturb the underlying cardiac rhythm. Careful examination usually allows differentiation between intermittent artifacts and arrhythmias. See text (pp 12-31) for more information on performing and interpreting an ECG.

Table 2-1

## Normal ECG Reference Ranges for Dogs and Cats

| Dogs | Cats |
|---|---|
| **HEART RATE** | |
| 70 to 160 beats/min (adults)*<br>to 220 beats/min (puppies) | 120 to 240 beats/min |
| **MEAN ELECTRICAL AXIS (FRONTAL PLANE)** | |
| +40 to +100 degrees | 0 to + 160 degrees |
| **MEASUREMENTS (LEAD II)**<br>**P-wave duration (maximum)** | |
| 0.04 sec (0.05 sec, giant breeds) | 0.035 to 0.04 sec |
| **P-wave height (maximum)** | |
| 0.4 mV | 0.2 mV |
| **PR interval** | |
| 0.06 to 0.13 sec | 0.05 to 0.09 sec |
| **QRS-complex duration (maximum)** | |
| 0.05 sec (small breeds)<br>0.06 sec (large breeds) | 0.04 sec |
| **R-wave height (maximum)** | |
| 2.5 mV (small breeds)<br>3 mV (large breeds)† | 0.9 mV; QRS total in any lead <1.2 mV |
| **ST-segment deviation** | |
| <0.2 mV depression<br><0.15 mV elevation | No marked deviation |
| **T wave** | |
| Normally <25% of R-wave height; can be positive, negative, or biphasic | Maximum 0.3 mV; can be positive (most common), negative, or biphasic |
| **QT-interval duration** | |
| 0.15 to 0.25 (to 0.27) sec; varies inversely with heart rate | 0.12 to 0.18 (range 0.07 to 0.2) sec; varies inversely with heart rate |
| **CHEST LEADS** | |
| $CV_5RL$ ($rV_2$): positive T wave<br>$CV_6LL$ ($V_2$): S wave 0.8 mV maximum; R wave 2.5 mV maximum†<br>$CV_6LU$ ($V_4$): S wave 0.7 mV maximum; R wave 3 mV maximum†<br>$V_{10}$: negative QRS; negative T wave (except Chihuahua) | R wave 1 mV maximum in chest leads<br><br><br>$V_{10}$: R/Q <1; negative T wave |

Each small box on the ECG paper grid is 0.02 second wide at 50 mm/sec paper speed, 0.04 second wide at 25 mm/sec, and 0.1 mV high at a calibration of 1 cm = 1 mV.

*Range may extend lower for large breeds and higher for toy breeds.

†May be greater in young (under 2 years old), thin, deep-chested dogs.

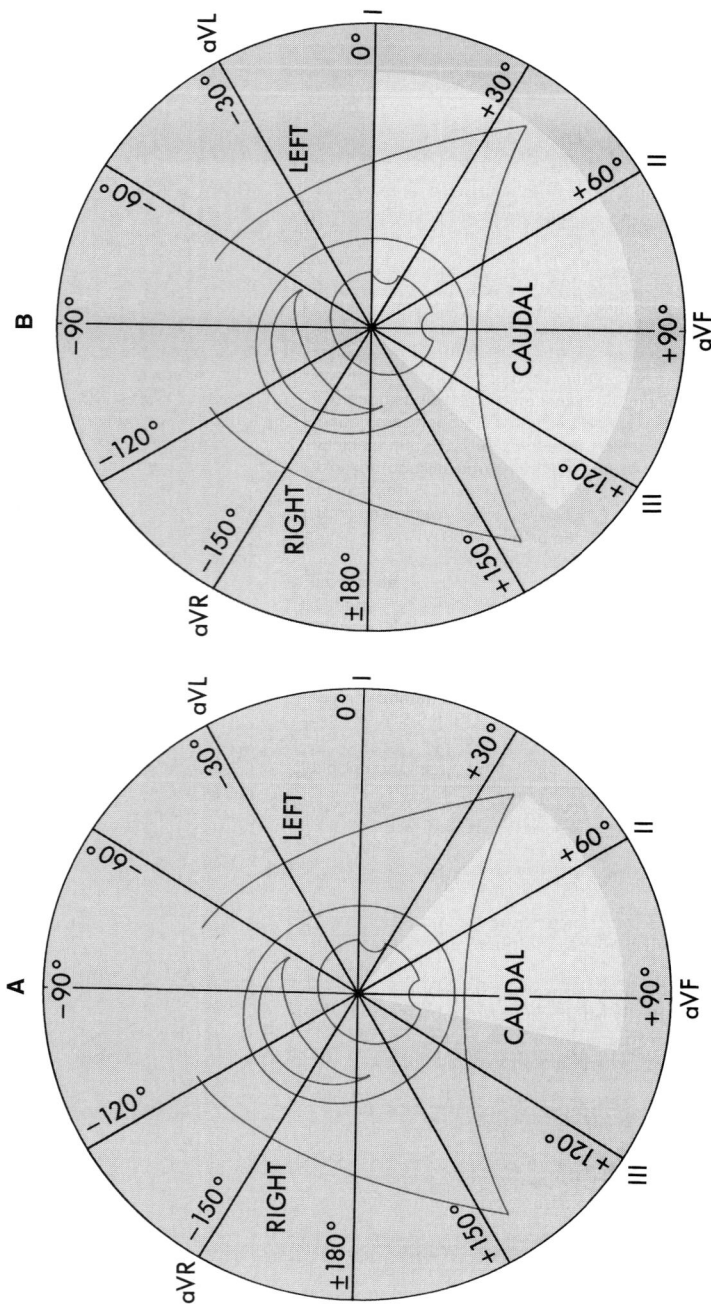

**FIG. 2-2** Frontal lead system: diagrams of six frontal leads over schematic of left and right ventricles within the thorax. Circular field is used for determining direction and magnitude of cardiac electrical activation. Each lead is labeled at its positive pole. Shaded area represents normal range for mean electrical axis. **A**, Dog. **B**, Cat.

## Chamber Enlargement and Bundle Branch Block Patterns

### Atrial enlargement

Widening of the P wave is seen with left atrial enlargement (p mitrale); sometimes the P wave is also notched. Causes include mitral insufficiency, cardiomyopathy, patent ductus arteriosus (PDA), subaortic stenosis, and ventricular septal defect. Right atrial enlargement may be manifested as tall, spiked P waves (p pulmonale). Causes include tricuspid insufficiency, chronic respiratory disease, atrial septal defect, and pulmonic stenosis. With atrial enlargement the atrial repolarization wave ($T_a$ wave) may be evident as a baseline shift in the opposite direction to the P wave.

### Ventricular enlargement

Right ventricular enlargement (dilation or hypertrophy) is usually pronounced if it is evident on ECG. Generally at least three of the criteria listed in Box 2-1 are present when right ventricular enlargement exists. Causes include pulmonic stenosis, tetralogy of Fallot, tricuspid insufficiency, severe heartworm disease, and pulmonary hypertension.

---

**Box 2-1**

### Ventricular Enlargement Patterns and Conduction Abnormalities

**NORMAL**

Normal mean electrical axis
No S wave in lead I
Lead II R wave taller than that in lead I
Lead $CV_6LL$ R wave larger than S wave

**RIGHT VENTRICULAR ENLARGEMENT**

Right-axis deviation
S wave present in lead I
S wave in $V_3$ ($CV_6LL$) deeper than R wave is tall or greater than 0.8 mV
Q-S (W shape) in $V_{10}$
Positive T wave in lead $V_{10}$ (except in Chihuahua breed)
Deep S wave in leads II, III, and $aV_F$

**RIGHT BUNDLE BRANCH BLOCK**

Same as right ventricular enlargement with the end of the QRS prolonged (wide, sloppy S wave)

**LEFT VENTRICULAR HYPERTROPHY**

Left-axis deviation
R wave in lead I taller than R wave in leads II or $aV_F$
No S wave in lead I

**LEFT ANTERIOR FASCICULAR BLOCK**

Same as left ventricular hypertrophy, possibly with wider QRS

**LEFT VENTRICULAR DILATION**

Normal frontal axis
Taller than normal R wave in leads II, $aV_F$, $CV_6LL$
Widened QRS; slurring and displacement of ST segment and enlargement of T wave may also occur

**LEFT BUNDLE BRANCH BLOCK**

Normal frontal axis
Very wide and sloppy QRS
Small Q wave may be present in leads II, III, and $aV_F$ (incomplete left bundle branch block)

Left ventricular dilation and eccentric hypertrophy often cause increased R wave voltages in the caudal leads (II and $aV_F$) and widening of the QRS. Left ventricular concentric hypertrophy is inconsistently accompanied by a left axis deviation. Causes of left ventricular dilation include mitral or aortic insufficiency, dilated cardiomyopathy, PDA, ventricular septal defect, and subaortic stenosis. Causes of left ventricular hypertrophy include hypertrophic cardiomyopathy and subaortic stenosis.

### Intraventricular conduction blocks

Abnormal intraventricular conduction alters QRS configuration, widening the QRS and orienting the terminal QRS forces toward the area of delayed activation. Box 2-1 and Fig. 2-3 summarize ECG patterns seen in association with ventricular enlargement or conduction delays.

### Decreased QRS amplitude

Small-voltage QRS complexes can be caused by pleural or pericardial effusion, obesity, intrathoracic masses, hypovolemia, or hypothyroidism. However, small complexes are occasionally seen in dogs without identifiable abnormalities.

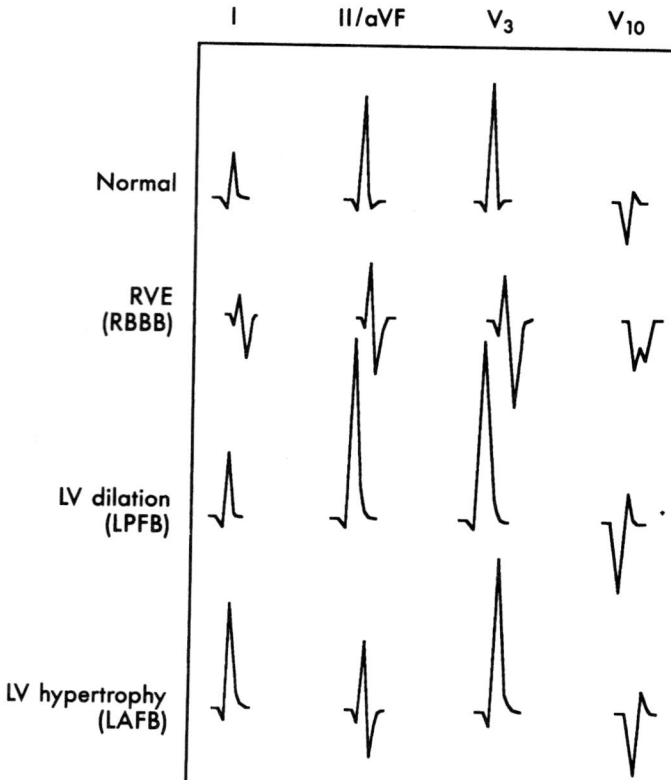

**FIG. 2-3** Schematic of common ventricular enlargement patterns and conduction abnormalities. ECG leads are listed across top. *LAFB,* Left anterior fascicular block; *LPFB,* left posterior fascicular block; *LV,* left ventricle; *RBBB,* right bundle branch block; *RVE,* right ventricular enlargement.

### Sinus rhythms

The normal cardiac rhythm begins in the sinus node and produces the waveforms shown in Fig. 2-1. Regular sinus rhythm occurs when the timing between QRS complexes is consistent. Sinus arrhythmia is characterized by a cyclic slowing and speeding of the sinus rate. It is usually associated with respiration; the sinus rate tends to increase on inspiration and decrease with expiration. A cyclic change also may occur in P-wave configuration ("wandering pacemaker"), with the P waves becoming taller and spiked during inspiration and flatter in expiration. Sinus arrhythmia is a common and normal rhythm variation, although it is not often seen clinically in cats. Pronounced sinus arrhythmia occurs in some animals with chronic pulmonary disease.

Sinus bradycardia and sinus tachycardia are rhythms that originate in the sinus node and are conducted normally. The rate of sinus bradycardia is slower than normal for the species, and that of sinus tachycardia is faster than normal. Causes are listed in Table 2-2.

Cessation of sinus activity lasting at least twice as long as the animal's longest expected R-R interval is called *sinus arrest*. Long pauses can cause fainting or weakness. Escape beats usually occur during prolonged sinus arrest.

## Ectopic Impulses

Impulses originating elsewhere than the sinus node (ectopic impulses) are abnormal and create an arrhythmia. Ectopic impulses are described on the basis of their general site of origin (atrial, junctional, supraventricular, ventricular) and their timing. *Timing* refers to whether the impulse occurs earlier than the next expected sinus impulse (premature) or after a longer pause (late or escape). Premature ectopic impulses or complexes occur singly or in multiples; groups of three or more constitute an episode of tachycardia. Episodes of tachycardia can be brief (paroxysmal) or prolonged (sustained). When one premature complex follows each normal QRS, a bigeminal pattern exists. The origin of the premature complexes (see following discussions) determines whether the rhythm is described as atrial or ventricular bigeminy. Fig. 2-4 shows examples of supraventricular and ventricular complexes.

### Supraventricular premature complexes

Supraventricular premature complexes are impulses that originate above the atrioventricular (AV) node, either in the atria or the AV junctional area. Because they are conducted into and through the ventricles via the normal conduction pathway, their QRS configuration is normal (unless an intraventricular conduction disturbance is also present).

**Table 2-2**

## Causes of Sinus Bradycardia and Sinus Tachycardia

| Sinus bradycardia | Sinus tachycardia |
|---|---|
| Hypothermia | Hyperthermia and fever |
| Hypothyroidism | Hyperthyroidism |
| Cardiac arrest (before or after) | Anemia or hypoxia |
| Drugs (e.g., tranquilizers, anesthetics, β-blockers, calcium entry blockers, digitalis) | Heart failure |
| | Shock |
| | Hypotension |
| Increased intracranial pressure | Sepsis |
| Brainstem lesions | Anxiety or fear |
| Severe metabolic disease (e.g., uremia) | Excitement |
| Ocular pressure | Exercise |
| Carotid sinus pressure | Pain |
| Other causes of high vagal tone | Drugs (anticholinergics, sympathomimetics) |
| Sinus node disease | Toxicities (e.g., chocolate, hexachlorophene) |
| Normal variation (athletic dog) | Electric shock |
| | Other causes of high sympathetic tone |

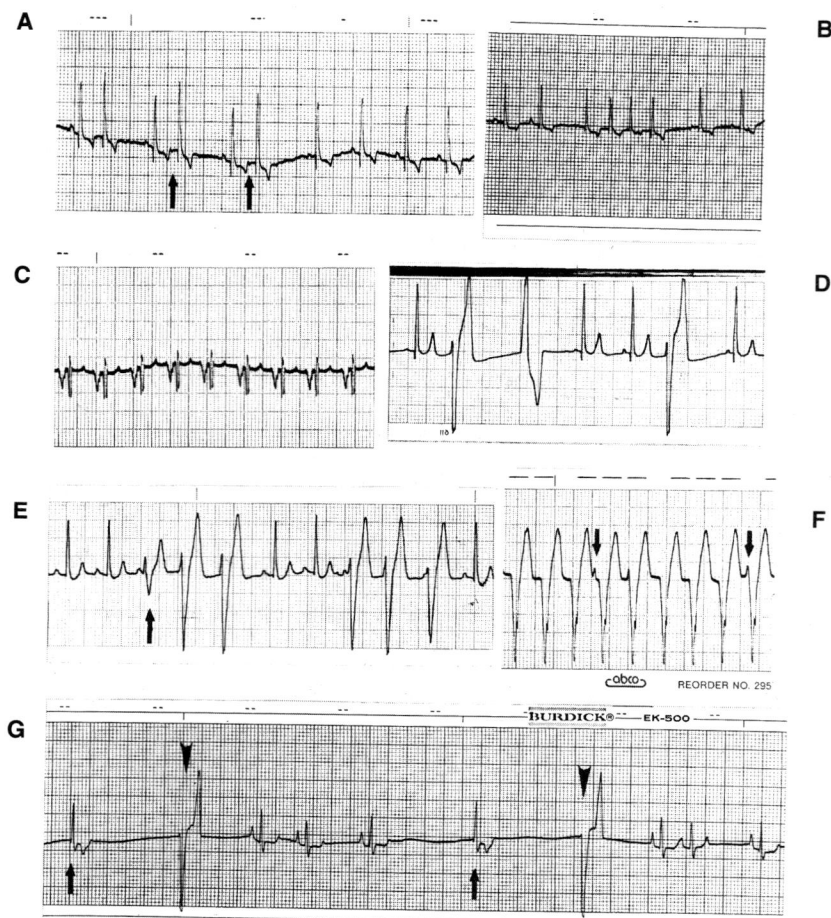

**FIG. 2-4** Ectopic complexes and rhythms. **A,** Atrial premature complexes in an old Cocker Spaniel with mitral insufficiency. Note small negative P waves *(arrows)* preceding early complexes. Slight increase in QRS size is thought to be related to minor intraventricular conduction delay with prematurity (lead III, 25 mm/sec). **B,** Short paroxysm of atrial tachycardia (lead II, 25 mm/sec, dog). **C,** Sustained atrial tachycardia in an Irish Setter with mitral stenosis. Note negative, abnormal P waves (lead II, 25 mm/sec). **D,** Multiform ventricular premature complexes (lead II, 25 mm/sec, dog). **E,** Intermittent paroxysms of ventricular tachycardia demonstrating fusion complex *(arrow)* (lead II, 25 mm/sec, dog). **F,** Sustained ventricular tachycardia with several nonconducted P waves *(arrows)* superimposed (lead aV$_F$, 25 mm/sec, dog). **G,** Sinus arrhythmia with periods of sinus arrest interrupted by junctional *(arrows)* and ventricular *(arrowheads)* escape complexes (lead II, 25 mm/sec, dog). Differentiation of escape and premature complexes is crucial.

Atrial premature complexes are usually preceded by an abnormal P wave (positive, negative, or biphasic) called a P′ wave. If a P′ wave occurs before the AV node has completely repolarized, the impulse may not be conducted into the ventricles (physiologic AV block). In some cases the premature impulse is conducted slowly (prolonged P′-Q interval) or with a bundle branch block pattern. Impulses originating in the AV junction are usually not preceded by a P' wave, although retrograde conduction of the impulse back through the atria may occur, causing a negative P' wave to precede, follow, or be superimposed on the QRS complex.

If it is unclear whether the ectopic complex is atrial or junctional in origin, the term *supraventricular premature complex* (or supraventricular tachycardia) is used. Clinically it is more important to distinguish whether an arrhythmia originates from above the AV node (supraventricular) or below it (ventricular) than to determine its specific location. Supraventricular premature complexes usually depolarize the sinus node, resetting the sinus rhythm and creating a "noncompensatory pause."

### Supraventricular tachycardia

Atrial tachycardia can be paroxysmal or sustained. A consistent ratio of atrial impulses to ventricular activation (e.g., 2:1 or 3:1) preserves the regularity of this arrhythmia. Sometimes the impulses traverse the AV node but are delayed within the ventricular conduction system, causing a bundle branch block pattern on ECG; differentiation from ventricular tachycardia may be difficult in these cases. Often, the P' waves are hidden in the QRS-T complexes.

### Atrial flutter

Atrial flutter is caused by a very rapid (usually >400 impulses/min) wave of electrical activation regularly cycling through the atria. The ventricular response may be irregular or regular, depending on the pattern of AV conduction. The ECG baseline consists of "sawtooth" flutter waves. Atrial flutter is not a stable rhythm; it often degenerates into atrial fibrillation or may convert back to sinus rhythm.

### Atrial fibrillation

This common arrhythmia is characterized by rapid, chaotic atrial activation. No P waves are present on the ECG; rather, the baseline usually shows irregular undulations (fibrillation waves). Atrial fibrillation causes an irregular heart rhythm that is usually quite rapid (Fig. 2-5). The heart (ventricular) rate is determined by AV conduction velocity and recovery time. Most often the QRS complexes are normal, although minor variations in height are common, and intermittent or sustained bundle branch blocks can occur. Atrial fibrillation tends to be a consequence of severe atrial disease and enlargement and is usually preceded by intermittent atrial tachyarrhythmias. However, atrial fibrillation sometimes occurs spontaneously in giant-breed dogs without evidence of underlying heart disease; the heart rate is generally normal in these dogs.

### Ventricular premature complexes

Ventricular premature complexes (VPCs or PVCs) have an abnormal and usually widened QRS configuration. The sinus rate continues undisturbed, so the VPC is followed by a "compensatory pause." When the configuration of multiple VPCs is consistent, the complexes are called *uniform, unifocal,* or *monomorphic;* VPCs of varying configurations are called *multiform* or *polymorphic.*

### Ventricular tachycardia

Ventricular tachycardia is a series of VPCs (usually >100 beats/min). The R-R interval generally is regular, although some variation can occur. Nonconducted sinus P waves may be superimposed on or between ventricular complexes. The term *capture beat* refers to the successful conduction of a P wave into the ventricles, uninterrupted by another VPC. If normal ventricular activation is interrupted by another VPC, a "fusion" complex, melding of the normal QRS and the VPC, can result (see Fig. 2-4, *E*). Fusion complexes are often observed at the onset or end of a paroxysm of ventricular tachycardia; they are preceded by a P wave and shortened P-R interval. Identification of P waves or fusion complexes helps differentiate ventricular tachycardia from supraventricular tachycardia with abnormal intraventricular conduction.

### Accelerated ventricular rhythm

Also called *idioventricular tachycardia,* this arrhythmia is an enhanced ventricular rhythm (rate of 60 to 100 beats/min in dogs; faster in cats). Because the rate is slower than true ventricular tachycardia, it is usually a less serious rhythm disturbance and may have no deleterious effects, although it could progress to ventricular tachycardia, particularly if the patient's clinical condition deteriorates.

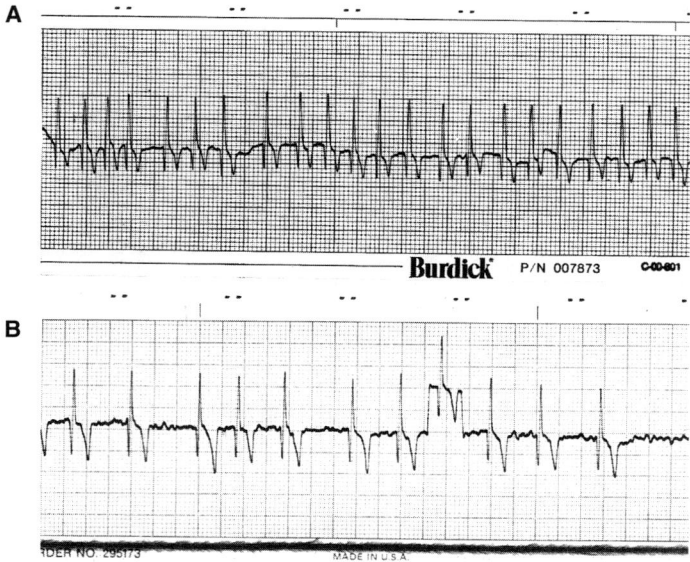

**FIG. 2-5** Atrial fibrillation. **A,** Uncontrolled atrial fibrillation (heart rate 220 beats/min) in a Doberman Pinscher with dilated cardiomyopathy (lead II, 25 mm/sec). **B,** Slower ventricular response rate after therapy in a different Doberman Pinscher with dilated cardiomyopathy showing baseline fibrillation waves. Note lack of P waves and irregular RR intervals. Eighth complex from left superimposed on calibration mark (lead II, 25 mm/sec).

### Ventricular fibrillation

This lethal rhythm is characterized by chaotic electrical activity in the ventricles; the ECG consists of an irregularly undulating baseline (Fig. 2-6). Ventricular flutter, appearing as rapid sine-wave activity on the ECG, may precede fibrillation. Ventricular fibrillation may be "coarse," with larger ECG oscillations, or "fine." Ventricular asystole is the absence of ventricular electrical (and mechanical) activity.

#### Escape complexes

An escape complex occurs after a pause in the dominant (usually sinus) rhythm. If the dominant rhythm does not resume, the escape focus continues to discharge at its own intrinsic rate. Escape rhythms are usually regular; the origin can be in the atria, the AV junction, or the ventricles (see Fig. 2-4, *G*). Ventricular escape rhythms (idioventricular rhythms) usually occur at less than 50 beats/min in dogs and 100 beats/min in cats, although rates in both species can be higher. Junctional escape rhythms usually range from 40 to 60 beats/min in dogs and faster in cats. It is important to differentiate escape from premature complexes because *escape activity should never be suppressed with antiarrhythmic drugs.*

### Conduction Disturbances

#### Atrial

Sinoatrial (SA) block and sinus arrest cannot reliably be differentiated on ECG, although with SA block the interval between P waves is a multiple of the normal P-P interval. An atrial, junctional, or ventricular escape rhythm should take over after prolonged sinus arrest or block. In atrial standstill, diseased atrial muscle results in the absence of P waves and a junctional or ventricular escape rhythm. Note: Hyperkalemia interferes with normal atrial function and can mimic atrial standstill.

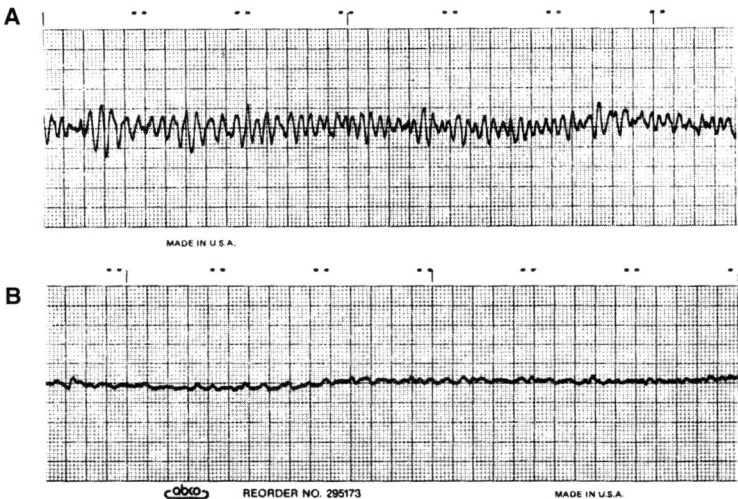

**FIG. 2-6** Ventricular fibrillation. Note chaotic baseline motion and absence of organized waveforms. **A,** Coarse fibrillation. **B,** Fine fibrillation (lead II, 25 mm/sec, dog).

#### AV nodal conduction disturbances

Abnormalities of AV conduction can be caused by excessive vagal tone, drugs (e.g., digoxin, xylazine, verapamil, anesthetic agents), and organic disease of the AV node, the intraventricular conduction system, or both. Three categories are described.

First-degree AV block occurs when conduction from the atria into the ventricles is prolonged, although all impulses are conducted (Fig. 2-7).

Second-degree AV block is characterized by intermittent AV conduction; some P waves are not followed by a QRS complex. When many P waves are not conducted, the patient has high-grade second-degree heart block. Mobitz type I (Wenckebach) block is characterized by progressive prolongation of the PR interval until a nonconducted P wave occurs; it is frequently associated with disorders within the AV node itself and high vagal tone. QRS configuration usually is normal and narrow. Mobitz type II is characterized by uniform PR intervals preceding the blocked impulse and is often associated with disease lower in the AV conduction system (e.g., His bundle or major bundle branches). Frequently, the QRS complexes are wide and abnormal. Supraventricular or ventricular escape complexes are common during long pauses in ventricular activation.

Third-degree or complete AV block is present when no sinus (or supraventricular) impulses are conducted into the ventricles. Often a regular sinus rhythm or sinus arrhythmia is evident; however, the P waves are not related to the QRS complexes, which result from a (usually) regular ventricular escape rhythm.

#### Intraventricular conduction disturbances

The QRS complexes appear wide and abnormal (see Fig. 2-3). Right bundle branch block is sometimes identified in otherwise normal dogs and cats, although it can result from disease or distention of the right ventricle. Left bundle branch block is usually related to disease of the left ventricle. The left anterior fascicular block pattern is common in cats with hypertrophic cardiomyopathy. A block in all three major bundle branches results in third-degree (complete) heart block.

#### Ventricular preexcitation

Early activation (preexcitation) of part of the ventricular myocardium can occur when an accessory conduction pathway bypasses the normal AV nodal pathway. Several

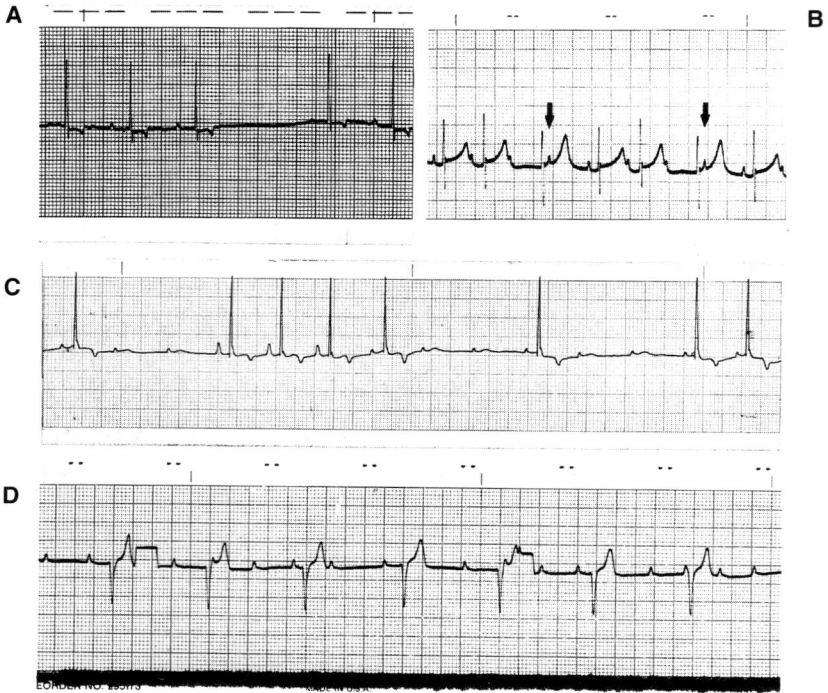

**FIG. 2-7** AV conduction abnormalities. **A,** First-degree AV block in a dog with digoxin toxicity (lead $aV_F$, 25 mm/sec). **B,** Second-degree AV block (Wenckebach) in an old cat under anesthesia. Note gradually prolonged PR interval with failed conduction of third (and seventh) P wave(s), followed by an escape complex. The fourth and eighth P waves *(arrows)* are not conducted because the ventricles are refractory (lead II, 25 mm/sec). **C,** Second-degree AV block in a comatose old dog with brainstem signs and seizures. Note the changing configuration of the P waves (wandering pacemaker) (lead II, 25 mm/sec). **D,** Complete (third-degree) heart block in a Poodle. An underlying sinus arrhythmia exists, but no P waves are conducted; a slow ventricular escape rhythm has resulted. Two calibration marks (half-standard, 0.5 cm = 1 mV) are seen (lead II, 25 mm/sec).

types have been described; most cause a shortened P-R interval. Wolff-Parkinson-White (WPW) preexcitation is also characterized by early widening and slurring of the QRS by a so-called delta wave. Preexcitation can be intermittent or concealed (not evident on ECG). A reentrant supraventricular tachycardia can occur using the accessory pathway and AV node (AV reciprocating tachycardia). Rapid AV reciprocating tachycardia can cause weakness, syncope, congestive heart failure, and death. The presence of the WPW pattern with reentrant supraventricular tachycardia that causes clinical signs characterizes the WPW syndrome.

## ST-T Abnormalities
### ST segment
Abnormal elevation (>0.15 mV in dogs, >0.1 mV in cats) or depression (>0.2 mV in dogs, >0.1 mV in cats) of the J point (end of the QRS complex) and ST segment in lead I, II, or $aV_F$ may be significant, as they can result from ischemia or other causes of myocardial injury. Atrial enlargement or tachycardia can cause pseudodepression of the ST segment because of prominent $T_a$ waves.

**T wave**

The T wave may be positive, negative, or biphasic in normal cats and dogs. Changes in size, shape, or polarity from previous recordings in a given animal are probably clinically important. T-wave abnormalities can be primary (unrelated to depolarization) or secondary (related to abnormalities of ventricular depolarization). Secondary ST-T changes tend to be in the opposite direction of the main QRS deflection. Box 2-2 lists some causes of ST-T abnormalities.

---

**Box 2-2**

## Causes of ST-Segment, T-Wave, and QT Abnormalities

**DEPRESSION OF J POINT or ST SEGMENT (>0.2 MV in caudal leads)**
Myocardial ischemia
Myocardial infarction or injury (subendocardial)
Hyperkalemia or hypokalemia
Cardiac trauma
Secondary change (ventricular hypertrophy, conduction disturbance, VPCs
Digitalis ("sagging" appearance)
Pseudodepression (prominent $T_a$)

**ELEVATION OF THE J POINT or ST SEGMENT (>0.15 MV in caudal leads)**
Pericarditis
Left ventricular epicardial injury
Myocardial infarction (transmural)
Myocardial hypoxia
Secondary change (ventricular hypertrophy, conduction disturbance, VPCs)
Digoxin toxicity

**PROLONGATION OF QT INTERVAL**
Hypocalcemia
Hypokalemia
Quinidine toxicity
Ethylene glycol poisoning
Secondary to prolonged QRS
Hypothermia
Central nervous system abnormalities

**SHORTENING OF QT INTERVAL**
Hypercalcemia
Hyperkalemia
Digitalis toxicity

**LARGE T WAVES**
Myocardial hypoxia
Ventricular enlargement
Intraventricular conduction abnormalities
Hyperkalemia
Metabolic or respiratory diseases and cardiac drug toxicities
Normal variation

**TENTED T WAVES**
Hyperkalemia

---

*VPC*, Ventricular premature complex.

### QT interval
The QT interval varies inversely with heart rate; faster rates have shorter QT intervals. Autonomic tone, various drugs, and electrolyte disorders influence the duration of the QT interval (see Box 2-2). Inappropriate prolongation of the QT interval may facilitate the development of serious reentrant arrhythmias when underlying nonuniformity in ventricular repolarization exists.

## Effects of Drug Toxicity and Electrolyte Imbalance
### Drugs
Digoxin, antiarrhythmic agents, and anesthetic drugs often alter heart rhythm and conduction, either by their direct electrophysiologic effects or by affecting autonomic tone. Box 2-3 summarizes common ECG manifestations of these drug effects.
### Hypokalemia
Abnormalities of potassium homeostasis have marked and complex influences on cardiac function and the ECG (Box 2-3). Hypokalemia may predispose to both supraventricular and ventricular arrhythmias. Severe hypokalemia can also increase QRS- and

---

**Box 2-3**

### ECG Changes Associated with Electrolyte Imbalances and Selected Drug Toxicities

**HYPERKALEMIA**
Large, spiked (± tented) T waves
QT interval abbreviation
Flat or absent P waves
Widened QRS
ST-segment depression

**HYPOKALEMIA**
ST-segment depression
Small, biphasic T waves
QT interval prolongation
Tachyarrhythmias

**HYPERCALCEMIA**
Few effects
Abbreviated QT interval
Prolonged conduction
Tachyarrhythmias

**HYPOCALCEMIA**
Prolonged QT interval
Tachyarrhythmias

**DIGOXIN**
PR prolongation
Second- (or third-) degree AV block
Sinus bradycardia or arrest
Accelerated junctional rhythm
Ventricular premature complexes
Ventricular tachycardia
Paroxysmal atrial tachycardia with block
Atrial fibrillation with slow ventricular rate

**QUINIDINE OR PROCAINAMIDE**
Atropine-like effects
QT prolongation
AV blocks
Ventricular tachyarrhythmias
QRS widening
Sinus arrest

**LIDOCAINE**
AV block
Ventricular tachycardia
Sinus arrest

**BARBITURATES OR THIOBARBITURATES**
Ventricular bigeminy

**HALOTHANE OR METHOXYFLURANE**
Sinus bradycardia
Ventricular arrhythmias (increased sensitivity to catecholamines, especially with halothane)

**XYLAZINE**
Sinus bradycardia
Sinus arrest or sinoatrial block
AV block
Ventricular tachyarrhythmias (especially with halothane or epinephrine)

---

*AV,* Atrioventricular.

P-wave amplitudes and durations. In addition, hypokalemia exacerbates digoxin toxicity and reduces the efficacy of class I antiarrhythmic agents (see Chapter 4). Hypernatremia and alkalosis worsen the cardiac effects of hypokalemia.

### Hyperkalemia

Moderate hyperkalemia actually has an antiarrhythmic effect; however, rapid or severe increases in serum potassium concentration are arrhythmogenic. The sinus node is relatively resistant to the effects of hyperkalemia and continues to function, although its rate often decreases. ECG manifestations of hyperkalemia are listed in Box 2-3. Hypocalcemia, hyponatremia, and acidosis accentuate the ECG changes caused by hyperkalemia, whereas hypercalcemia and hypernatremia tend to counteract them.

### Other electrolyte disturbances

Marked ECG changes caused by other electrolyte disturbances are uncommon. Severe hypercalcemia or hypocalcemia can have noticeable effects (see Box 2-3), but this situation is rarely seen clinically. Hypomagnesemia has no reported effects on the ECG, but it can predispose to digoxin toxicity and exaggerate the effects of hypocalcemia.

## Ambulatory ECG

### Holter monitoring

Holter monitoring allows continuous recording of cardiac electrical activity over a 24-hour period, during normal daily activities (except swimming), strenuous exercise, and sleep. It is useful for detecting and quantifying intermittent arrhythmias and therefore can help identify cardiac causes of syncope and episodic weakness. It is also used to assess the efficacy of antiarrhythmic drug therapy.

### Event recording

Cardiac event recorders are smaller than typical Holter units. They are used most often to determine if episodic weakness or syncope is caused by a cardiac arrhythmia. When an episode is observed, the owner activates the recorder, which then stores a short segment of the ECG recording for later analysis. Both methods of ambulatory ECG recording are described further in the text (pp 29).

## Other Methods of Assessment

Heart rate variability and signal-averaged ECG may be useful for identifying patients with myocardial dysfunction who may be at increased risk for sudden death. These techniques are described in the text (pp 29-31).

## THORACIC RADIOGRAPHY

Because of variations in chest conformation, as well as the influences of respiration, cardiac cycle, and positioning on apparent size of the cardiac shadow, mild cardiomegaly may be difficult to identify. Radiographic suggestion of abnormal cardiac size or shape should be considered within the context of the physical examination and other test results.

## Cardiomegaly

Generalized enlargement of the heart shadow on plain radiographs may indicate true cardiomegaly or distention of the pericardial sac. When the heart itself is enlarged, the contours of different chambers are usually still evident, although massive right ventricular and atrial dilation can make the heart appear round. Filling of the pericardial sac with fluid, fat, or viscera tends to obliterate these contours and create a globoid heart shadow. Box 2-4 lists the common causes of cardiac enlargement.

The vertebral heart score (VHS) can be used to identify and quantify cardiomegaly in dogs and cats. Measurements are obtained using the lateral view. The cardiac long axis is measured, and this distance is compared with the thoracic spine, beginning at the cranial edge of T4. The maximum perpendicular short axis is measured in the central third of the heart, then measured in number of vertebrae, beginning with T4. The two measurements are added to yield the VHS. A VHS of 8.5 to 10.5 vertebrae is considered normal for most breeds. An upper limit of 11 vertebrae may be normal in dogs with

---

**Box 2-4**

### Common Differential Diagnoses for Radiographic Signs of Cardiomegaly

**GENERALIZED ENLARGEMENT OF THE CARDIAC SHADOW**

Dilated cardiomyopathy
Mitral and tricuspid insufficiency
Pericardial effusion
Pericardioperitoneal diaphragmatic hernia
Tricuspid dysplasia
Ventricular septal defect
Patent ductus arteriosus

**LEFT ATRIAL ENLARGEMENT**

Early mitral insufficiency
Hypertrophic cardiomyopathy
Early dilated cardiomyopathy (especially Doberman Pinschers)
(Sub)aortic stenosis

**LEFT ATRIAL AND VENTRICULAR ENLARGEMENT**

Dilated cardiomyopathy
Hypertrophic cardiomyopathy
Mitral insufficiency (acquired or congenital)
Aortic insufficiency
Ventricular septal defect
Patent ductus arteriosus
(Sub)aortic stenosis

**RIGHT ATRIAL AND VENTRICULAR ENLARGEMENT**

Advanced heartworm disease
Chronic, severe pulmonary disease    *COR PULMONALE*
Tricuspid insufficiency (acquired or congenital)
Pulmonic stenosis
Tetralogy of Fallot
Atrial septal defect
Reversed shunting congenital defects (pulmonary hypertension)

---

a short thorax (e.g., Miniature Schnauzer), and an upper limit of 9.5 vertebrae may be appropriate in dogs with a long thorax (e.g., Dachshund).

### Cardiac Chamber Enlargement

Rarely is enlargement present in only one cardiac chamber. Most diseases that cause dilation or hypertrophy of the heart affect two or more chambers. Nevertheless, enlargement of specific chambers and great vessels is described individually.

#### Left atrium

On the lateral view, an enlarged left atrium bulges dorsally and caudally and elevates the left and possibly the right mainstem bronchi. Compression of the left mainstem bronchus occurs with severe left atrial enlargement. In cats, left atrial enlargement causes convexity of the normally straight dorsocaudal heart border, with elevation of the mainstem bronchi. On the dorsoventral (DV) or ventrodorsal (VD) view the mainstem bronchi are pushed laterally and curve slightly around the enlarged left atrium in both species. A bulge in the 2- to 3-o'clock position is common with concurrent left auricular enlargement. Massive left atrial enlargement sometimes appears as a large, rounded soft-tissue opacity superimposed over the central to caudal cardiac silhouette.

### Left ventricle

Left ventricular enlargement is manifested on the lateral view by an elevation of the carina and caudal vena cava (CaVC). The caudal heart border becomes convex. On DV or VD view, rounding and enlargement are visible in the 2- to 5-o'clock position.

### Right atrium

Right atrial enlargement causes a bulge of the cranial heart border and widening of the cardiac silhouette on the lateral view. Tracheal elevation may occur over the cranial portion of the heart shadow. Bulging on DV or VD view occurs in the 9- to 11-o'clock position. Because the right atrium is largely superimposed on the right ventricle, differentiation from right ventricular enlargement is difficult; however, concurrent enlargement of both chambers is common.

### Right ventricle

Right ventricular enlargement usually causes increased convexity of the cranio-ventral heart border and elevation of the trachea on the lateral view. With severe right ventricular enlargement and relatively normal left heart size, the apex is elevated off the sternum. The carina and CaVC are also elevated. On DV or VD view, the heart takes on a reverse-D configuration; the apex may be shifted leftward, and the right heart border bulges to the right.

## Intrathoracic Vessels

### Aorta and pulmonary trunk

Subaortic stenosis causes dilation of the ascending aorta. Dilation here is not easily detected, although widening and increased opacity of the dorsocranial heart shadow may be observed. PDA causes a localized dilation ("ductus bump") in the descending aorta just caudal to the arch on the DV or VD view. Severe dilation of the main pulmonary trunk can be seen as a bulge superimposed over the trachea on the lateral view. On the DV view in dogs, enlargement of the main pulmonary trunk causes a bulge in the vessel at the 1- to 2-o'clock position; pulmonic stenosis and pulmonary hypertension are the usual causes. In cats, the main pulmonary trunk is slightly more medial and is usually obscured within the mediastinum.

### Vena cava

The width of the CaVC is similar to that of the descending thoracic aorta, although its size varies with respiration. With enlargement of either ventricle the CaVC is pushed dorsally. Persistent widening of the CaVC could indicate right ventricular failure, cardiac tamponade, pericardial constriction, or other obstruction to right heart inflow. A narrow vena cava might indicate hypovolemia, poor venous return, or pulmonary overinflation.

### Pulmonary arteries

Pulmonary arteries are located dorsal and lateral to their accompanying veins and bronchi. An overcirculation pattern occurs when the lungs are hyperperfused, as in left-to-right shunts, overhydration, and other hyperdynamic states. Pulmonary arteries and veins are both prominent; the increased perfusion also gives a generally hazy appearance to the lungs. Pulmonary undercirculation is characterized by narrowed pulmonary arteries and veins, along with an increased lucency of the lung fields. Severe dehydration, hypovolemia, obstruction to right ventricular inflow, right-sided congestive failure, and tetralogy of Fallot can cause this pattern. Some animals with pulmonic stenosis also appear to have pulmonary undercirculation. Overinflation of the lungs or overexposure of the radiographs also minimizes the appearance of the pulmonary vessels.

Pulmonary arteries larger than their accompanying veins indicate pulmonary arterial hypertension; heartworm disease is a common cause (see Chapter 10). The pulmonary arteries become dilated, tortuous, and blunted, and visualization of the terminal portions is lost. In both dogs and cats the DV view is best for evaluating the caudal pulmonary arteries; they should be no wider than the ninth rib at their point of intersection.

### Pulmonary veins

Prominent pulmonary veins are a sign of pulmonary venous congestion, usually from left-sided congestive heart failure. On the lateral view the cranial lobar veins are larger and denser than their accompanying arteries and may sag ventrally. Dilated, tortuous pulmonary veins may be seen entering the dorsocaudal aspect of the enlarged left atrium in animals with chronic pulmonary venous hypertension. However, pulmonary venous dilation is not always seen in patients with left-sided heart failure. In cats with acute cardiogenic pulmonary edema, enlargement of both pulmonary veins and arteries can be seen.

### Pulmonary Edema

Pulmonary edema causes the lung parenchyma to appear hazy; pulmonary vessels become ill defined, and bronchial walls thicken. As the edema worsens, areas of fluffy or mottled fluid opacity progressively become more confluent, obscuring vessels and outer bronchial walls. The air-filled bronchi appear as lucent, branching lines surrounded by fluid density (air bronchograms). (Note: Phase of respiration and radiographic technique influence the apparent severity of interstitial infiltrates.)

Interstitial and alveolar patterns of pulmonary infiltration can be caused by many pulmonary diseases, as well as by cardiogenic edema. The distribution of pulmonary infiltrates is important, especially in dogs. Cardiogenic pulmonary edema in dogs is generally located in dorsal and perihilar areas and is often bilaterally symmetric. In contrast, the distribution of cardiogenic edema in cats is usually uneven and patchy, either throughout the lung fields or concentrated in the middle zones.

## ECHOCARDIOGRAPHY

Frequencies generally used for echocardiography range from 3.5 mHz (large dogs) to 7.5 mHz (cats and small dogs). The basic examination includes all standard 2-D imaging planes from both sides of the chest, M-mode measurements, and any other views needed to further evaluate specific lesions. Doppler evaluation, if available, can provide important additional information. Light tranquilization is helpful if the animal does not lie quietly. Buprenorphine (0.0075 to 0.01 mg/kg intravenous [IV]) with acepromazine (0.03 mg/kg IV) usually works well in dogs. Butorphanol (0.2 mg/kg intramuscular [IM]) with acepromazine (0.1 mg/kg IM) is adequate for many cats, although some require more sedation. Acepromazine (0.1 mg/kg IM) followed in 15 minutes by ketamine (2 mg/kg IV) can be used in cats, but this regimen can increase the heart rate. See text pp 35-47 for more detailed information on echocardiography.

### Two-Dimensional Echocardiography

Two-dimensional imaging allows an overall assessment of cardiac chamber size and wall thickness. Most standard views (see text pp 36-40) are obtained from either the right or left parasternal positions (directly over the heart and close to the sternum). The orientation, relative size, and wall thickness of the cardiac chambers; all valves and related structures; and the great vessels are systematically examined. Any suspected abnormality is scanned in multiple planes to verify and further delineate it.

### M-Mode Echocardiography

Measurements of cardiac dimensions and motion throughout the cardiac cycle are often more accurately obtained from M-mode tracings, which provide a one-dimensional view (depth) into the heart. Precise positioning of the ultrasound beam within the heart and clear endocardial edge images are essential for accurate M-mode measurements and calculations (see text pp 38-43 for measurement guidelines). Measurements may also be taken from the 2-D echocardiogram if the images are of high resolution and frames from the appropriate times in the cardiac cycle are used.

Echocardiographic measurements in dogs are greatly affected by body size, and some breed differences are reported. Endurance training also affects these measurements. Guidelines for commonly used echocardiographic measurements are given in Tables 2-3 and 2-4, but they should be regarded as approximate only. (See text pp 39-44 for detailed explanations.)

**Table 2-3**

## Approximate Echocardiographic Measurements in Dogs*

| | Weight (kg) | | | | | | | | | | |
|---|---|---|---|---|---|---|---|---|---|---|---|
| | 3 | 5 | 7 | 10 | 15 | 20 | 25 | 30 | 35 | 40 | 50 |
| $LVID_d$ (mm) | 24.6† | 27.4 | 30 | 32.7 | 37.1 | 41.4 | 44.8 | 48.3 | 51.7 | 54.8 | 60.7 |
| | (6.2) | (5.2) | (4.5) | (3.5) | (2.4) | (2.2) | (2.9) | (3.9) | (5) | (6.1) | (8.3) |
| $LVID_s$ (mm) | 13.6 | 16 | 17.9 | 20.6 | 24.3 | 28 | 31 | 33.9 | 36.9 | 39.6 | 44.6 |
| | (5.5) | (4.7) | (4) | (3.1) | (2.1) | (2) | (2.5) | (3.4) | (4.5) | (5.4) | (7.4) |
| $LVW_d$ (mm) | 5 | 5.4 | 5.7 | 6.2 | 6.8 | 7.4 | 7.9 | 8.4 | 8.9 | 9.3 | 10.2 |
| | (2.1) | (1.7) | (1.5) | (1.2) | (0.8) | (0.7) | (1) | (1.3) | (1.7) | (2) | (2.8) |
| $LVW_s$ (mm) | 7.2 | 7.9 | 8.4 | 9.2 | 10.2 | 11.3 | 12.1 | 13 | 13.8 | 14.5 | 16 |
| | (1.7) | (1.6) | (1.4) | (1.3) | (1.1) | (1.1) | (1.2) | (1.3) | (1.5) | (1.7) | (2.2) |
| $IVS_d$ (mm) | 5.8 | 6.2 | 6.5 | 7 | 7.6 | 8.2 | 8.7 | 9.2 | 9.7 | 10.2 | 11 |
| | (2.1) | (1.7) | (1.5) | (1.2) | (0.8) | (0.7) | (0.9) | (1.3) | (1.7) | (2) | (2.7) |
| $LVS_s$ (mm) | 9.8 | 10.2 | 10.4 | 10.9 | 11.5 | 12.3 | 13 | 13.9 | 14.6 | 15.4 | — |
| | (2.6) | (2.2) | (1.7) | (1.2) | (1.2) | (1.1) | (1.5) | (2.3) | (2.6) | (3.5) | |
| $LA^\ddagger$ (mm) | 12.7 | 14 | 15 | 16.3 | 18.3 | 20.2 | 21.8 | 23.3 | 24.8 | 26.2 | 28.8 |
| | (5.3) | (4.5) | (3.8) | (3) | (2) | (1.9) | (2.4) | (3.3) | (4.3) | (5.2) | (7.1) |
| $Ao$ (mm) | 13.8 | 15.3 | 16.4 | 18.1 | 20.4 | 22.8 | 24.6 | 26.4 | 28.3 | 30 | 33.1 |
| | (3.6) | (3) | (2.6) | (2) | (1.4) | (1.3) | (1.6) | (2.2) | (2.9) | (3.5) | (4.8) |

Measurements from Bonagura JD et al: Echocardiography: principles of interpretation, *Vet Clin North Am* 15:1177, 1985. (See Bibliography for additional references.) Some athletic normal dogs have a slightly lower fractional shortening (20% to 25%); normal Dobermans also may have FS values below the usual normal range.

*These are approximate guidelines only; values in normal dogs may be above or below these values, especially in dogs near the outer range of body weight.

†Mean value given; +/- standard deviation in parentheses below.

‡M-mode cursor position for LA measurement is often variable among animals; usually the maximal LA dimension is not represented by this dimension (see text for more information).

*Ao*, Aortic root; $IVS_d$, interventricular septum at end diastole; $IVS_s$, interventricular septum at end systole; *LA*, left atrium; $LVID_d$, left ventricular internal diameter at end diastole; $LVID_s$, left ventricular internal diameter at end systole; $LVW_d$, left ventricular wall at end diastole; $LVW_s$, left ventricular wall at end systole.

**Table 2-4**

## Echocardiographic Measurement Guidelines for Cats*

| LVID$_d$ (mm) | LVID$_s$ (mm) | LVW$_d$ (mm) | LVW$_s$ (mm) | IVS$_d$ (mm) | IVS$_s$ (mm) | LA† (mm) | Ao (mm) | FS | EPSS |
|---|---|---|---|---|---|---|---|---|---|
| 12-18 | 5-10 | ≤5.5 | ≤9 | ≤5.5 | ≤9 | 8-13 | 8-11 | 35%-65% | ≤4 mm |

*These values are based on my experience and compilation of published studies. Ketamine increases heart rate and decreases LVID$_d$. See Bibliography for additional references.

†M-mode cursor position for left at measurement is variable among animals. Maximal LA dimension is better assessed with 2-D imaging.

*Ao*, Aortic root; *FS*, fractional shortening; *EPSS*, mitral E-point septal separation; *IVS$_d$*, interventricular septum at end diastole; *IVS$_s$*, interventricular septum at end systole; *LA*, left atrium (systole); *LVID$_d$*, left ventricular internal diameter at end diastole; *LVID$_s$*, left ventricular internal diameter at end systole; *LVW$_d$*, left ventricular wall at end diastole; *LVW$_s$*, left ventricular wall at end systole.

## Doppler Echocardiography

Doppler echocardiography detects blood flow direction and velocity. Characteristic blood flow patterns are obtained from the different valve areas (see text pp 44-47 for details). Breed, age, and body weight appear to have little influence on normal Doppler measurements. Because blood flow patterns and velocity can be evaluated, detection and quantification of valvular insufficiency, obstructive lesions, and cardiac shunts are possible. Cardiac output and other indicators of systolic and diastolic function can also be assessed.

Several types of Doppler echocardiography are used clinically: pulsed wave (PW), continuous wave (CW), and color flow mapping (see text pp 44-47 for details). Semiquantification of valve regurgitation by determination of the size and shape of the regurgitant jet is sometimes done, especially with color flow Doppler. In general, wide and long regurgitant jets are associated with more severe regurgitation than are narrow jets.

## Transesophageal Echocardiography

Cardiac structures can be imaged through the esophageal wall with specialized transducers mounted on the tip of a flexible endoscope. This method can provide clearer images of cardiac structures at or above the AV junction. However, heavy sedation or general anesthesia is required.

## OTHER TECHNIQUES

See text pp 47-49 for further detail and additional techniques.

## Angiocardiography

When echocardiography is unavailable, nonselective angiocardiography can be useful for diagnosing several diseases, including cardiomyopathy and heartworm disease in cats; severe pulmonic, aortic, or subaortic stenosis; PDA; and tetralogy of Fallot. Although in most cases echocardiography can provide similar information more safely, evaluation of the pulmonary vasculature is better with nonselective angiocardiography.

Selective angiocardiography (performed by placing cardiac catheters into specific areas of the heart or great vessels) allows identification of anatomic abnormalities and the path of blood flow. Doppler echocardiography is now used more commonly, as it usually provides comparable information noninvasively with less expense, time, and risk.

## Cardiac Catheterization

Cardiac catheterization entails selective placement of specialized catheters into different areas of the heart and vasculature via the jugular vein, carotid artery, or femoral vessels. This allows measurement of pressures, cardiac output, and blood oxygen concentrations from specific areas.

### Pulmonary capillary wedge pressure

Pulmonary capillary wedge pressure is sometimes measured to monitor dogs with heart failure or to differentiate cardiogenic from noncardiogenic pulmonary edema, as it provides an estimate of left heart filling pressure (in the absence of left ventricular inflow obstruction).

### Central venous pressure

Measurement of central venous pressure (CVP) can be useful in the differentiation of high right-sided heart filling pressure (e.g., right-sided heart failure or pericardial disease) from other causes of pleural or peritoneal effusion and in the monitoring of critically ill patients receiving large-volume fluid infusions. (Note: Thoracocentesis should be performed before CVP is measured in patients with moderate-to-large volume pleural effusions.) CVP is not an accurate reflection of left-sided heart filling pressure and therefore should not be relied on in the monitoring of treatment of cardiogenic pulmonary edema. CVP in normal dogs and cats usually ranges from 0 to 8 (up to 10) cm $H_2O$; fluctuations that parallel intrapleural pressure changes occur during respiration.

Marked fluctuation associated with the heartbeat suggests either severe tricuspid insufficiency or placement of the catheter tip in the right ventricle.

**Biochemical markers of myocardial injury**

Circulating concentrations of cardiac troponin I (cTnI) and cardiac troponin T (cTnT) increase within several hours after acute myocardial injury or necrosis. One source has suggested that the normal plasma concentration of cTnI in dogs is <0.04 ng/ml and that concentrations >0.07 ng/ml may indicate cardiac pathology; concentrations >0.11 ng/ml appear to be abnormal in cats. Another source has suggested that the normal concentrations in both dogs and cats are <0.5 ng/ml for cTnI and <0.1 ng/ml for cTnT.

# 3

# Management of Congestive Heart Failure

## (Text pp 51-72)

### CAUSES OF HEART FAILURE

Causes of heart failure are diverse but can generally be grouped into the following categories:

*Myocardial failure*–characterized by poor ventricular contractility, with or without valvular insufficiency. Causes include drug toxicities (e.g., doxorubicin in dogs), myocardial ischemia or infarction, idiopathic dilated cardiomyopathy, and infective myocarditis. (Heart failure can also result from persistent cardiac arrhythmias.)

*Volume overload*–usually involves a leaky valve or abnormal systemic-to-pulmonary connection. Causes include valvular degeneration (endocardiosis), endocarditis, or dysplasia; ventricular septal defects; and patent ductus arteriosus. Chronic anemia and thyrotoxicosis can also cause this type of congestive heart failure (CHF).

*Pressure overload*–develops when higher than normal systolic pressure is needed to eject blood, resulting in ventricular hypertrophy and myocardial dysfunction. Causes include subaortic or pulmonic stenosis, systemic or pulmonary hypertension, and heartworm disease.

*Reduced ventricular compliance*–restricted ventricular filling leads to abnormal diastolic function, congestion, and diminished cardiac output. Causes include hypertrophic or restrictive cardiomyopathy, constrictive pericardial disease, and cardiac tamponade.

### PRINCIPLES OF TREATMENT (TEXT PP 56-71)

Therapy centers on (1) controlling edema and effusions, (2) improving cardiac output, (3) reducing cardiac workload, (4) supporting myocardial function, and (5) managing concurrent arrhythmias. Specific treatment varies somewhat with the underlying disease, particularly with those causing restriction to ventricular filling. Table 3-1 summarizes the treatment principles. The drugs listed are discussed later in this chapter.

**Table 3-1**

## Therapeutic Goals According to Pathophysiologic Group of Heart Failure

| Pathophysiologic group | Goal |
|---|---|
| Myocardial failure | Improve cardiac output (ACEI, digoxin, other positive inotropic drugs or vasodilators) |
| | Control edema and effusions (diuretics, vasodilators, diet) |
| | Improve myocardial function? (ACEI, digoxin, spironolactone?, other?) |
| | Reduce cardiac workload (rest, diuretics, vasodilators) |
| | Control arrhythmias and avoid complications |
| | Specific therapy if possible |
| Volume-flow overload | Control edema and effusions (diuretics, ACEI or other vasodilators, diet) |
| | Reduce valvular regurgitation if present (ACEI or arteriolar vasodilators) |
| | Improve forward cardiac output (ACEI, other arteriolar vasodilators, digoxin) |
| | Reduce cardiac workload (rest, diuretics, vasodilators) |
| | Control arrhythmias and avoid complications |
| | Specific therapy if possible |
| Pressure overload | Relieve stenosis or reduce arterial hypertension if possible |
| | Reduce cardiac workload (rest, diuretic; depending on cause: β-blocker, ACEI, other antihypertensives) |
| | Control edema or effusions (diuretic, diet; depending on cause: ACEI, other vasodilators) |
| | Support cardiac function (± digoxin) |
| | Control arrhythmias and avoid complications |
| Restricted ventricular filling–pericardial disease | Drain pericardial fluid |
| | Remove pericardium if necessary |
| | Treat underlying disease if possible |
| Restricted ventricular filling–hypertrophic cardiomyopathy | Enhance cardiac filling and slow heart rate (β-blocker or diltiazem) |
| | Reduce edema and effusions (diuretics, diet, ± ACEI) |
| | Reduce cardiac workload and stress (rest) |
| | Control arrhythmias and avoid complications (including thromboembolism) |
| | Seek and treat possible underlying disease (e.g., feline hyperthyroidism) |

*ACEI,* Angiotensin-converting enzyme inhibitor.

## Overview of Treatment

Restricting exercise and dietary sodium ($Na^+$) helps reduce cardiac workload. Regular, mild to moderate activity can be beneficial, however, as long as signs of excessive respiratory effort do not develop. Strenuous bursts of activity should be avoided.

## Diuretics

Diuretic therapy is indicated for treatment of cardiogenic pulmonary edema and effusions. Pleural effusion and large-volume ascites should first be drained to facilitate respiration; pericardial effusion that compromises cardiac filling also must be drained. Although aggressive furosemide therapy is indicated for acute, fulminant pulmonary edema (see below), the smallest effective doses are used for chronic heart failure. Note: Diuretic therapy is not recommended as the sole treatment for chronic heart failure.

## ACEIs and Digoxin

Angiotensin-converting enzyme inhibitors (ACEIs) have become the cornerstone of therapy for chronic heart failure resulting from most causes, especially myocardial contractile dysfunction and chronic valvular insufficiency. ACEIs improve the clinical status and survival in dogs with dilated cardiomyopathy or chronic mitral regurgitation and probably heart failure resulting from other causes. Digoxin is usually indicated for patients with myocardial failure or supraventricular tachyarrhythmias (except cats with hypertrophic cardiomyopathy). It is also often added to the therapy for advanced mitral regurgitation in dogs.

## Refractory Cases

Chronic heart failure that becomes refractory to initial furosemide and ACEI therapy, with or without digoxin, is usually managed by increasing the dose of furosemide, ACEI, or both. When doses approach the maximum recommended levels, another diuretic (e.g., spironolactone) or vasodilator can be cautiously added. Note: Arteriolar vasodilators are not recommended for cats with hypertrophic cardiomyopathy or dogs with fixed ventricular outflow obstruction (e.g., subaortic stenosis). Some animals benefit from the addition of a thiazide diuretic as failure becomes more refractory.

## Patient Monitoring

Periodic reevaluation is important. Medications and dosage schedules, problems with drug administration, and adverse effects or signs of toxicity should be reviewed with the owner at each visit. The animal's response to the medications, diet and appetite, activity level, and any other concerns should also be discussed.

A thorough physical examination with emphasis on the cardiovascular system is important at each evaluation. Clinical tests might include an electrocardiogram or ambulatory monitoring, thoracic radiographs, serum biochemistries (especially to evaluate renal function and electrolytes), echocardiogram, and serum digoxin concentration.

Many factors can exacerbate the signs of heart failure. Repeated episodes of acute, decompensated CHF that may require hospitalization and intensive diuresis are relatively common in patients with chronic progressive heart failure.

## Fulminant CHF

Therapy for fulminant CHF is aimed at rapidly reducing pulmonary edema, improving oxygenation, and optimizing cardiac output. Specific therapies are given in Box 3-1. More information is found in the text (pp 58-60).

### Vasodilators

Hydralazine is used for treating refractory pulmonary edema caused by mitral regurgitation (and sometimes dilated cardiomyopathy). An initial dose of 0.75 to 1 mg/kg orally (PO) is repeated every 2 to 3 hours until systolic blood pressure is 90 to 110 mm Hg or clinical improvement is seen. When blood pressure cannot be monitored, an initial dose of 1 mg/kg can be repeated in 2 to 4 hours if necessary. Addition of 2% nitroglycerine ointment promotes concurrent venodilation.

---

**Box 3-1**

## Therapy for Fulminant Congestive Heart Failure

### AVOID STRESS

Provide cage rest

Limit patient handling, including administration of oral medications

### ENHANCE OXYGENATION

Check airway patency

Give supplemental oxygen, preferably via oxygen ($O_2$) cage (6 to 10 L/min of 50% to 100% $O_2$; avoid using >50% $O_2$ for longer than 24 hr)

If frothing is evident, suction airways

Intubate and mechanically ventilate if needed (avoid overinflation and $O_2$ concentrations >70%)

Perform thoracocentesis if pleural effusion is suspected or present

### REMOVE ALVEOLAR FLUID
**Initiate Diuresis**

Furosemide (dogs: 2-5 mg/kg IV or IM q1-4h until respiratory rate decreases, then q6-12h*; cats: 1-2 mg/kg IV or IM q1-4h until respiratory rate decreases, then q6-12h*)

**Redistribute Blood Volume**

Vasodilators (2% nitroglycerin ointment—dogs: 1/2 to 1 1/2 inch cutaneously q6h; cats: 1/4 to 1/2 inch cutaneously q6h; *or* sodium nitroprusside 0.5-1 μg/kg/min CRI, titrate upward as needed)

Morphine *(dogs only):* 0.05-0.1 mg/kg IV boluses q2-3min until effective or 0.1-0.5 mg/kg single IM or SC dose)

± phlebotomy (6-10 ml/kg)

### REDUCE BRONCHOCONSTRICTION

Aminophylline (dogs: 6-10 mg/kg slow IV, IM, SC, PO[†] q6-8h; cats: 4-8 mg/kg IM, SC, PO[†] q8-12h) or similar drug

### MINIMIZE ANXIETY

Morphine *(dogs only):* dose given previously

Acepromazine (cats: 0.05-0.2 mg/kg SC) *or*

Diazepam (cats: 2-5 mg IV; dogs: 5-10 mg IV)

### REDUCE AFTERLOAD

Enalapril (0.5 mg/kg PO q12-24h) or other ACEI[‡] *or*

Hydralazine (dogs: 0.5-1 mg/kg PO repeated in 2-4 h; then q12h; see text)[‡] *or*

Amlodipine (dogs: 0.01-0.03 mg/kg PO q12-24h; see text)

### INCREASE CONTRACTILITY (*IF* MYOCARDIAL FAILURE PRESENT)

Digoxin (see text)

Dobutamine (1-10 μg/kg/min CRI; start low) *or*

Dopamine (dogs: 1-10 μg/kg/min CRI; cats: 1-5 μg/kg/min CRI; start low)

Amrinone (1-3 mg/kg IV; 10-100 μg/kg/min CRI)

### MONITOR AND MANAGE ABNORMALITIES AS POSSIBLE

Respiratory rate, heart rate and rhythm, pulse strength, body weight, urine output, hydration, attitude, serum biochemistry and blood gas analyses, arterial and pulmonary capillary wedge pressures

---

*Once diuresis has begun and respiration improves, reduce dose to prevent excessive volume contraction or electrolyte depletion.

[†]Oral therapy can be used once respiration improves.

[‡]Avoid nitroprusside concurrently.

*ACEI,* Angiotensin-converting enzyme inhibitor; *CRI,* constant-rate infusion; IM, intramuscular; *IV,* intravenous; *PO,* oral; *SC,* subcutaneous.

An alternative to hydralazine and nitroglycerine is infusion of sodium nitroprusside. However, blood pressure must be closely monitored and the dose titrated to maintain a systolic blood pressure of 90 to 100 mm Hg. Another option is an ACEI or amlodipine, with or without nitroglycerine ointment, although the onset of action is slower and effects are less pronounced.

### Positive inotropes

Patients with poor myocardial contractility (e.g., dilated cardiomyopathy) may benefit from positive inotropic therapy; however, it must be administered cautiously. Dobutamine is usually preferred over dopamine because it has less effect on heart rate and afterload. Amrinone or milrinone can also be used. Digoxin is usually not administered via the intravenous (IV) route, except for treatment of some supraventricular tachyarrhythmias (see Table 3-3 for doses). Note: Catecholamines can exacerbate interstitial fluid accumulation; they can also cause arrhythmias. Digoxin may induce arrhythmias in patients with severe pulmonary edema; monitoring electrolytes and acid-base balance is important in these patients.

## Cats with Hypertrophic Cardiomyopathy

For cats with hypertrophic cardiomyopathy, diuretic and oxygen therapy are given as outlined in Box 3-1. Diltiazem or a $\beta_1$-blocker (discussed later) is used after severe dyspnea has abated; IV esmolol could also be considered (see Table 4-3). Note: Arteriolar vasodilators may be detrimental if left ventricular outflow obstruction exists (see Chapter 7).

## Fluid Therapy

In very ill or anorectic animals, very conservative parenteral fluid therapy (e.g., 15 to 30 ml/kg/day) may be required. A 5% dextrose in water solution or a low-sodium fluid should be used. Arterial blood pressure and serum creatinine or blood urea nitrogen and electrolyte concentrations should be monitored to avoid excessive diuresis and hypotension.

## DIETARY MANAGEMENT

### Sodium restriction

Dietary salt restriction helps control fluid accumulation and reduces necessary drug therapy. The degree of salt restriction depends on the severity of the heart failure. Before signs of CHF develop, avoiding high-salt table scraps and treats may be sufficient. Moderate salt restriction ($Na^+$ of approximately 30 mg/kg/day [0.06% $Na^+$ for canned food, 210 to 240 mg/100 g for dry food]) is advised when clinical heart failure develops. Diets designed for geriatric animals or those with renal disease usually provide adequate salt restriction. Further restriction can be helpful in patients with advanced heart disease (see text).

### Caloric intake

A well-balanced diet and an adequate caloric and protein intake are important. Inappetence is common in dogs and cats with heart failure. Warming the food, adding small amounts of palatable low-salt human foods, using a salt substitute (KCl) or garlic powder, handfeeding, and feeding small quantities of the diet several times a day may encourage eating. Dietary supplementation with fish oils (which are high in n-3 fatty acids) may be beneficial in animals with cardiac cachexia. At the other extreme, obesity increases metabolic demands on the heart, predisposes to arrhythmias, and mechanically interferes with respiration. A weight-loss diet is indicated for grossly overweight patients.

### Specific nutrients

Prolonged taurine deficiency in cats causes myocardial failure. Most commercial and prescription cat foods contain adequate taurine, but some diets may still be deficient. Taurine-deficient cats should be given 250 to 500 mg taurine PO q12h. Some dogs with dilated cardiomyopathy appear to be deficient in taurine, L-carnitine, or both (see Chapter 6). Dogs fed protein-restricted diets can become taurine deficient, and some develop dilated cardiomyopathy. Oral supplementation with 1 to 2 g of L-carnitine q8-12h and 500 mg taurine twice daily (bid) is recommended for these dogs. Supplementation with antioxidants (e.g., vitamin C, coenzyme Q-10) may be beneficial in patients with heart failure.

## DRUG THERAPY

### Diuretics
Diuretics are fundamental to the management of CHF. However, when given in excess, they promote excessive volume contraction and activate the neurohormonal mechanisms involved in CHF. Diuretics must be used with caution, and at the lowest effective dose, in dehydrated or azotemic animals. Dosages are given in Table 3-2.

#### Furosemide
Furosemide is the loop diuretic used most widely in cats and dogs with heart failure. Diuresis begins within 5 minutes after IV injection; it peaks in approximately 30 minutes and lasts for approximately 2 hours. After oral administration diuresis begins within 1 hour, peaks in 1 to 2 hours, and may last for 6 hours. Dose varies with the clinical situation. Respiratory pattern, hydration, body weight, exercise tolerance, renal function, and serum electrolyte concentrations are used to monitor response to therapy. Adverse effects are usually related to excessive fluid or electrolyte losses. Cats are more sensitive than dogs, so lower doses should be used. Hypokalemia can occur, but it is unusual in animals that are eating.

#### Spironolactone and other $K^+$-sparing diuretics
Spironolactone, triamterene, and amiloride generally have only mild diuretic effects, but they can augment therapy for chronic, refractory heart failure when furosemide plus an ACEI is insufficient to control fluid accumulation (see text). Adverse effects relate to excess potassium ($K^+$) retention and gastrointestinal (GI) disturbances. These diuretics must be used with caution in patients receiving an ACEI or $K^+$ supplementation. They are absolutely contraindicated in patients with hyperkalemia.

#### Thiazides
Thiazide diuretics cause mild to moderate diuresis, but they also decrease renal blood flow and so should not be used in azotemic patients. Adverse effects are uncommon in nonazotemic animals, although hypokalemia, other electrolyte disturbances, and dehydration can occur with excessive use or in anorectic patients.

### Vasodilators
Vasodilator therapy improves cardiac output and reduces edema and effusions associated with heart failure. In most cases ACEIs are the agents of first choice because they have important effects in addition to vasodilation (see text). Arteriolar or mixed vasodilator therapy is generally begun with a low dose to avoid hypotension and reflex tachycardia. Reduction in concurrent diuretic dosage may be advisable. Monitoring for signs of hypotension (weakness, lethargy, tachycardia, poor peripheral perfusion) is important after initiating treatment. The dose can be titrated upward if necessary, monitoring for hypotension with each increase. Systolic pressures of <100 mm Hg should be avoided. Doses are given in Table 3-2.

#### ACEIs
ACEIs allow arteriolar and venous relaxation, reduce $Na^+$ and water retention, and otherwise moderate neurohormonal responses. Therefore, they have considerable advantages over other vasodilators. Adverse effects include hypotension, GI upset, deterioration of renal function, and hyperkalemia (especially when used with $K^+$-sparing diuretics or $K^+$ supplements).

Hypotension can usually be avoided with low initial doses. As long as cardiac output and renal perfusion improve with therapy, renal function is usually maintained. Decreasing the diuretic dose may restore renal function. If not, the ACEI dose is reduced or the drug is discontinued. Benazepril is eliminated equally in urine and bile in dogs, and in cats only 15% of the drug is excreted in the urine, so this ACEI may be a good choice in animals with renal disease. Specific pharmacokinetic information about this and other ACEIs is available in the text (pp 64-65).

**Table 3-2**

## Dosages of Diuretics and Vasodilators

| Drug | Dog | Cat |
|---|---|---|
| **DIURETICS** | | |
| Furosemide | 1-3 mg/kg q8-24h chronic PO; or 2-5 mg/kg q4-6h IV, IM, SC | 1-2 mg/kg q12h up to 4 mg/kg q8-12h IV, IM, SC, PO |
| Spironolactone | 2 mg/kg q12h PO | 1-2 mg/kg q12h PO |
| Chlorothiazide | 20-40 mg/kg q12h PO | same |
| Hydrochlorothiazide | 2-4 mg/kg q12h PO | 1-2 mg/kg q12h PO |
| Triamterene | 2 (to 4) mg/kg/day PO | — |
| **ACEI AND OTHER VASODILATORS** | | |
| Enalapril | 0.5 mg/kg q24(to 12)h PO | 0.25-0.5 mg/kg q24(to 12)h |
| Captopril | 0.5-2 mg/kg q8-12h PO (low initial dose) | 0.5-1.25 mg/kg q12-24h |
| Benazepril | 0.25-0.5 mg/kg q24h PO | Same |
| Lisinopril | 0.5 mg/kg q24h PO | 0.25-0.5 mg/kg q24h PO |
| Fosinopril | 0.25-0.5 mg/kg q24h PO | — |
| Hydralazine | 0.5-2 mg/kg q12h PO (to 1 mg/kg initial) | 2.5 (up to 10) mg/cat q12h PO |
| Amlodipine | 0.1-0.3 (0.05-0.5) mg/kg q24(to 12)h PO | 0.625 mg/cat q24(to 12)h PO |
| Prazosin | Small dogs (<5 kg): do not use; medium dogs: 1 mg q8-12h PO; large dogs: 2 mg q8h PO | — |
| Sodium nitroprusside | 0.5-1 µg/kg/min CRI (initial) to 5-15 µg/kg/min CRI | Same |
| Nitroglycerine ointment | 1/2-1 1/2 inch q4-6h cutaneously | 1/2-1/4 inch q4-6h cutaneously |
| Isosorbide dinitrate | 0.5-2 mg/kg q8h PO | — |

*ACEI*, Angiotensin-converting-enzyme inhibitor; *CRI*, Constant-rate infusion; *IM*, intramuscular; *IV*, intravenous; *PO*, oral; *SC*, subcutaneous.

### Hydralazine

Hydralazine directly relaxes arteriolar smooth muscle but has little effect on the venous system. The most common indication is acute, severe CHF from mitral regurgitation. Hydralazine reduces arterial blood pressure, improves pulmonary edema, and increases jugular venous partial pressure of oxygen ($PO_2$), presumably by increasing cardiac output. However, it causes reflex tachycardia in some animals; when this occurs, the dose should be reduced. Hydralazine is a less desirable vasodilator than ACEIs for chronic use, although it can be useful in animals that cannot tolerate ACEIs. Hypotension is the most common adverse effect; GI upset can occur, which may necessitate discontinuation of hydralazine therapy.

### Prazosin

Prazosin blocks vasoconstriction in both arteries and veins. Initial hemodynamic improvement may be followed by drug tolerance over time. For this reason and because of the inconvenient capsule size this drug is rarely used. Hypotension is the most common adverse effect, especially after the first dose.

### Sodium nitroprusside

Sodium nitroprusside is a potent arterial and venous dilator. It is given by IV infusion because of its short duration of action. Its major indication is fulminant CHF (see Box 3-1). Tolerance develops rapidly, necessitating careful monitoring and dose adjustment. Profound hypotension is the major adverse effect. Cyanide toxicity can result from excessive or prolonged use. Note: Because of the potential for severe hypotension, nitroprusside should be used only when hemodynamic monitoring is available.

### Venodilators

*Nitroglycerine* and other nitrates (e.g., isosorbide dinitrate) act mainly on venous smooth muscle. Their major indication is acute cardiogenic pulmonary edema. In some cases nitrates are used chronically in combination with hydralazine, especially if an ACEI is not tolerated. Excessive or inappropriate use of nitrates may cause hypotension. Large doses, frequent application, or long-acting formulations can result in drug tolerance.

Because of extensive first-pass hepatic metabolism after oral administration, the transcutaneous route is used most often, although nitroglycerine is also well absorbed sublingually. Nitroglycerine ointment (2%) is applied to the skin of the groin, axilla, or ear pinna. (Note: The person applying the ointment should use an application paper or gloves to avoid skin contact.) Dosage and absorption vary, but a lower dose is used initially in small dogs and in cats. Transdermal patches (5 mg), applied for 12 hr/day, have been used in large dogs.

## Positive Inotropic Drugs

### Digoxin

Digoxin has a modest positive inotropic effect, suppresses supraventricular arrhythmias, and sensitizes arterial baroreceptors (probably its most important effect in heart failure). Digoxin is indicated in heart failure caused by myocardial dysfunction, chronic mitral valve insufficiency, and other chronic volume or pressure overloads, although it may be ineffective in animals with myocardial disease. Its potential arrhythmogenic effects must be considered in patients with heart failure (see later discussion). Digoxin is usually contraindicated in patients with hypertrophic cardiomyopathy (especially those with ventricular outflow obstruction), pericardial disease, sinus or atrioventricular (AV) node disease, or serious ventricular arrhythmias.

***Pharmacokinetics.*** Dosages are given in Table 3-3. Digoxin is well absorbed orally in dogs; absorption is approximately 60% for tablets and 75% for the elixir, but bioavailability is reduced by the presence of food. Therapeutic concentrations are achieved in 2 to 4$^1$/$_2$ days with administration every 12 hours.

In cats the serum half-life ranges widely, from 25 hours to >78 hours; chronic oral administration increases the half-life. Administration of tablets with food can decrease serum concentrations by approximately 50%. The elixir, although poorly palatable, results in serum concentrations approximately 50% higher than those resulting from the tablet form. Digoxin administration every 48 hours results in effective serum concentrations; a steady state is achieved in approximately 10 days.

**Table 3-3**

## Dosage of Positive Inotropic Drugs

| Drug | Dog | Cat |
|---|---|---|
| Digoxin | PO: dogs <22 kg, 0.011 mg/kg q12h; dogs >22 kg, 0.22 mg/m² q12h or 0.005 mg/kg q12h; decrease by 10% for elixir Maximum: 0.5 mg/day (0.375 mg/day for Dobermans) IV loading: 0.01-0.02 mg/kg—give ¼ of this total dose in slow boluses over 2 to 4 hr until effective | PO: 0.007 mg/kg q48h IV loading: 0.005 mg/kg—give ½ of total, then 1 to 2 hr later give ¼-dose bolus(es) if needed |
| Digitoxin | 0.02-0.03 mg/kg q8h (small dogs) to q12h (large dogs) | Do not use |
| Dopamine | For CHF—1-10 µg/kg/min CRI; for shock—5-15 µg/kg/min CRI (40 mg of dopamine into 500 ml of fluid provides 80 µg/ml; infusion at 0.75 ml/kg/hr provides 1 µg of dopamine per kilogram per minute) | 1-5 µg/kg/min CRI |
| Dobutamine | 1-10 µg/kg/min CRI (250 mg of dobutamine into 500 ml of fluid yields 500 µg/ml; infusion at 0.6 ml/kg/hr provides 5 µg of dobutamine per kilogram per minute) | Same |
| Amrinone | 1-3 mg/kg initial bolus IV; 10-100 µg/kg/min CRI | Same? |
| Milrinone | 50 µg/kg IV over 10 min initially; 0.375-0.075 µg/kg/min CRI (human dose) | Same? |

*CHF,* Congestive heart failure; *CRI,* constant-rate infusion; *IV,* intravenous; *PO,* oral.

In dogs digoxin elimination is primarily via the kidney; renal and hepatic elimination are equally important in cats. Serum digoxin concentration (and risk of toxicity) increases with renal failure. No apparent correlation exists between the degree of azotemia and the serum digoxin concentration in dogs, but lower doses and close monitoring of serum digoxin concentration are recommended in animals with renal disease. Digitoxin might be preferable to digoxin in dogs with renal failure; digitoxin should not be used in cats. Digitoxin and other pharmacokinetic data for digoxin are discussed in the text (Chapter 3, pp 66-69).

*Initial therapy.* Digoxin therapy is started with a PO maintenance dose, because loading doses often result in toxic serum concentrations. When a more rapid therapeutic serum concentration is critical (e.g., for supraventricular tachyarrhythmia), the drug can be given at twice the PO maintenance dose for 1 or 2 doses or via the IV route with caution (slowly, over at least 15 min). Other IV therapy for supraventricular tachycardia is usually more effective (see Chapter 4). Other IV positive inotropes are safer and more effective for immediate support of myocardial contractility.

*Calculating dose.* The dose in dogs >22 kg is sometimes based on body surface area rather than on body weight. In obese animals the dose should be based on the calculated lean body weight. Animals with reduced muscle mass or cachexia and those with compromised renal function can easily enter a toxic state at the usual calculated doses. Conservative administration and measurement of serum digoxin concentration help prevent toxicity.

*Monitoring.* Measurement of serum digoxin concentration is recommended 7 to 10 days after initiating therapy or changing the dosage; the sample should be obtained 8 to 10 hours after the last dose. The therapeutic range is 1 to 2 (up to 2.4) ng/ml. If the concentration is <0.8 ng/ml, the dose can be increased by up to 30% and the serum concentration measured a week later. If serum concentrations cannot be measured and toxicity is suspected, the drug should be discontinued for 1 to 2 days and then reinstituted at half the original dose.

*Drug and other interactions.* Quinidine, verapamil, and amiodarone increase the serum digoxin concentration. When both quinidine and digoxin must be used, the digoxin dose should be reduced by 50% initially then guided by serum concentrations. Diltiazem, prazosin, spironolactone, and triamterene may also increase the serum digoxin concentration. Electrolyte disturbances (especially hypokalemia, but also hypercalcemia and hypernatremia) and thyroid disturbances can potentiate digoxin toxicity. Drugs that affect hepatic microsomal enzyme activity may also affect digoxin metabolism.

*Toxicity.* Myocardial and GI toxicity are the two major toxic effects of digoxin. Almost any cardiac rhythm disturbance can develop, including ventricular tachyarrhythmias, supraventricular premature complexes and tachycardia, sinus arrest, second-degree AV block, and junctional rhythms. Myocardial toxicity can occur before any other signs and can lead to collapse and death, especially in animals with myocardial failure; loading doses are therefore inadvisable in such patients. GI toxicity may be manifested as anorexia, depression, vomiting, borborygmi, or diarrhea.

Treatment depends on the manifestations. GI signs usually respond to drug withdrawal and correction of fluid and electrolyte disturbances. AV conduction abnormalities also resolve after drug withdrawal, but sometimes anticholinergic therapy is needed. Digoxin-induced ventricular tachycardia and frequent ventricular premature complexes should be vigorously treated with lidocaine or phenytoin (see Chapter 4).

IV $K^+$ supplementation is given if serum $K^+$ is <4 mEq/L. Magnesium sulfate at 25 to 40 mg/kg as a slow IV bolus, followed by infusion of the same dose over 12 to 24 hours, may also be effective in suppression of arrhythmias. Fluid therapy is indicated to correct dehydration and maximize renal function. Propranolol can help control ventricular tachyarrhythmias, but it is not used if an AV conduction block is present. *Quinidine should not be used.* Cholestyramine (a steroid-binding resin) is useful only very soon after accidental digoxin overdose; digoxin-specific antigen-binding fragments (digoxin-immune Fab) are occasionally used (see text p 69).

### Sympathomimetics

Sympathomimetic agents stimulate stronger myocardial contractions. Because of their very short half-life (<2 min) and extensive hepatic metabolism the catecholamines used clinically are administered IV by constant-rate infusion. $\beta_1$-Receptor downregulation develops with long-term use, so these drugs are generally used for <3 days. Doses are given in Table 3-3.

*Dopamine.* At low doses (<5 μg/kg/min IV infusion) dopamine causes vasodilation in the renal, mesenteric, coronary, and cerebral circulations. Peripheral vasoconstriction occurs at doses of 10 to 15 μg/kg/min, which can help maintain blood pressure after cardiac arrest or in cardiogenic shock. However, at the higher doses heart rate, myocardial $O_2$ demand, and the risk of induction of ventricular arrhythmias increase. In patients with acute myocardial failure, low to moderate doses are used to increase contractility and cardiac output. An initial dose of 1 μg/kg/min IV is titrated upward until effective. The infusion rate should be decreased if sinus tachycardia or other tachyarrhythmias develop. Note: By increasing renal blood flow, dopamine may enhance the renal clearance of other drugs.

*Dobutamine.* Dobutamine, a synthetic analog of dopamine, is used for short-term inotropic support in animals with severe myocardial failure. At lower infusion rates (3 to 7 μg/kg/min) it increases contractility with minimal effects on heart rate and blood pressure. It is less arrhythmogenic than other catecholamines, but it may precipitate arrhythmias at higher doses (10 to 20 μg/kg/min). The initial infusion rate should be low and gradually increased over hours to achieve greater inotropic effect. Heart rate and rhythm should be closely monitored. Note: Cats are more sensitive to dobutamine than are dogs and may develop seizures or other adverse effects at relatively low doses.

*Other catecholamines.* Epinephrine increases blood pressure, heart rate, and contractility. However, it is very arrhythmogenic, so it is unsuitable for inotropic support in patients with heart failure. It is the drug of choice for resuscitation after cardiac arrest (see Chapter 5).

Isoproterenol increases heart rate, contractility, and cardiac output. It also decreases blood pressure and is quite arrhythmogenic, so it should not be used in patients with heart failure or cardiac arrest. It has been used for symptomatic AV block that is refractory to atropine. Norepinephrine and methoxamine increase contractility but also increase blood pressure. They are sometimes used as pressor agents but are not indicated for treatment of heart failure.

### Phosphodiesterase inhibitors

Bipyridine compounds such as amrinone and milrinone increase contractility and induce vasodilation (probably their primary clinical benefit). However, higher doses can cause hypotension, tachycardia, and GI signs. Milrinone is much more potent. Doses are given in Table 3-3.

Amrinone and milrinone are relatively safe, although they can exacerbate ventricular arrhythmias. Their effects are short-lived (<30 minutes) after IV injection, so constant infusion is required for sustained effect. An initial slow IV bolus is followed by a constant infusion; with amrinone half the original bolus dose can be repeated after 20 to 30 minutes.

Amrinone is used only for short-term inotropic support in dogs and cats with myocardial failure. Milrinone is also an effective inotropic agent in dogs with heart failure. Clinical trials with oral administration (0.5 to 1 mg/kg) showed clinical, hemodynamic, and echocardiographic improvement in dogs with myocardial failure. However, milrinone is not currently available in oral form.

## Calcium Entry Blockers

Calcium entry blockers can cause coronary and systemic vasodilation, enhanced myocardial relaxation, and reduced cardiac contractility. Some also have antiarrhythmic effects (see Chapter 4). They are potentially useful for treating hypertrophic cardiomyopathy, hypertension, and myocardial ischemia. Diltiazem is used most often for feline hypertrophic cardiomyopathy (see Chapters 4 and 7). Amlodipine is also used in chronic heart failure as an adjunctive vasodilator.

# 4

# Cardiac Rhythm Disturbances and Antiarrhythmic Therapy

## (Text pp 73-97)

Cardiac arrhythmias occur for many reasons (Table 4-1). Although some arrhythmias are of no clinical consequence, others cause serious hemodynamic compromise and sudden death, especially in animals with underlying heart disease. Cardiac arrhythmias in a given animal often occur inconsistently and are influenced by drug therapy, prevailing autonomic tone, baroreceptor reflexes, and variations in heart rate. Treatment decisions are based on consideration of the origin (supraventricular or ventricular), timing (premature or escape), and severity of the rhythm disturbance, as well as the clinical context. Some rhythm abnormalities do not require therapy, whereas others demand immediate, aggressive treatment. Following is a general approach to management of cardiac rhythm disturbances.

1. Record and interpret an electrocardiogram (ECG) (see Chapter 2); identify and define any arrhythmias. An extended ECG recording (e.g., Holter monitor or prolonged in-hospital monitoring) may be needed.
2. Evaluate the patient as a whole, incorporating the history, physical examination, and clinical and laboratory tests. Are signs of hemodynamic impairment evident (e.g., episodic weakness, syncope, signs of congestive heart failure)? Are other signs of cardiac disease present (e.g., heart murmur, cardiomegaly)? Are additional abnormalities present (e.g., fever, abnormal blood chemistry values, respiratory or other extracardiac disease, trauma)? Is the animal receiving any medications? Correct what can be corrected.
3. Decide whether to use antiarrhythmic drug therapy. Consider the signalment, history, clinical signs, and underlying disease, as well as the potential benefits and risks of the drug(s) under consideration.
4. If an antiarrhythmic drug is to be used, define the goals of therapy for the patient. An immediate goal is to restore hemodynamic stability. Suppression of all abnormal beats is generally not a realistic goal. However, sufficient reduction in frequency (e.g., by 70%) or repetitive rate of ectopic beats to promote normal hemodynamics and eliminate clinical signs may constitute successful therapy.
5. Initiate treatment and determine drug effectiveness. Adjust dose or try alternate agents if needed.
6. Monitor patient status. Assess arrhythmia control (consider repeated Holter monitoring), manage underlying disease(s), and watch for adverse drug effects and other complications.

Table 4-1

## Factors Predisposing to Arrhythmias

| Cardiac | Extracardiac |
|---|---|
| **ATRIAL ARRHYTHMIAS** | |
| Mitral or tricuspid insufficiency | Catecholamines |
| Dilated, hypertrophic, or restrictive cardiomyopathy | |
| | Electrolyte imbalances |
| | Acidosis and alkalosis |
| Cardiac neoplasia | Hypoxia |
| Congenital malformation | Thyrotoxicosis |
| Accessory AV nodal bypass tract(s) | Severe anemia |
| Myocardial fibrosis | Electric shock |
| High sympathetic tone | Thoracic surgery |
| Digitalis glycosides | |
| Other drugs (anesthetic agents, bronchodilators) | |
| Ischemia | |
| Intraatrial catheter placement | |
| **VENTRICULAR ARRHYTHMIAS** | |
| Congestive heart failure | Hypoxia |
| Cardiomyopathy (especially Doberman Pinschers and Boxers) | Electrolyte imbalances (especially $K^+$) |
| | Acidosis/alkalosis |
| Myocarditis | Thyrotoxicosis |
| Pericarditis | Hypothermia |
| Degenerative valvular disease with myocardial fibrosis | Fever |
| | Sepsis or toxemia |
| Ischemia | Trauma (thoracic or abdominal) |
| Trauma | Gastric dilation and volvulus |
| Cardiac neoplasia | Splenic mass or splenectomy |
| Heartworm disease | Hemangiosarcoma |
| Congenital heart disease | Pulmonary disease |
| Ventricular dilation | Uremia |
| Mechanical stimulation (intracardiac catheter, pacing wire) | Pancreatitis |
| | Pheochromocytoma |
| Drugs (digitalis, sympathomimetics, anesthetics, tranquilizers, anticholinergics, antiarrhythmics) | Other endocrine diseases (diabetes mellitus, Addison's disease, hypothyroidism) |
| | High sympathetic tone (pain, anxiety, fever) |
| | Central nervous system disease (increases in sympathetic or vagal stimulation) |
| | Electric shock |

*AV*, Atrioventricular; $K^+$, potassium.

## COMMON HEART RHYTHM ABNORMALITIES (TEXT PP 74-86)

The more common rhythm disturbances found in dogs and cats are discussed in the following sections. Their ECG characteristics are described in Chapter 2. Classes and effects of the various antiarrhythmic drugs mentioned in this section are summarized in Table 4-2. Doses are given in Table 4-3. These drugs are discussed in more detail later in the chapter.

**Table 4-2**

## Classes and Effects of Antiarrhythmic Drugs

| Class | Drug | Mechanism and ECG effects |
|---|---|---|
| I | | Decrease fast inward $Na^+$ current; membrane-stabilizing effects (decreased conductivity, excitability, and automaticity) |
| IA | Quinidine Procainamide Disopyramide | Moderately decrease conductivity, increase action potential duration; can prolong QRS complex and QT interval |
| IB | Lidocaine Mexiletine Tocainide Phenytoin | Cause little change in conductivity, decrease action potential duration; QRS complex and QT interval unchanged |
| IC | Flecainide Encainide Propafenone | Markedly decrease conductivity without changing action potential duration |
| II | Propranolol Atenolol Esmolol Metoprolol Carvedilol Others | β-Adrenergic blockade—reduce effects of sympathetic stimulation (no direct myocardial effects at clinical doses) |
| III | Sotalol Amiodarone Bretylium Others | Selectively prolong action potential duration and refractory period; antiadrenergic effects; QT interval prolonged |
| IV | Verapamil Diltiazem Others | Decrease slow inward $Ca^{++}$ current (greatest effects on SA and AV nodes) |
| Others | Digoxin | Antiarrhythmic action results mainly from indirect autonomic effects (especially increased vagal tone) |
| | Atropine | Anticholinergic agents oppose vagal effects on SA and AV nodes (glycopyrrolate and other drugs also have this effect) |
| | Adenosine | Briefly opens $K^+$ channels and indirectly slows $Ca^{++}$ current (strongest effects on sinoatrial and AV nodes); can transiently block AV conduction |

*AV,* Atrioventricular; *ECG,* electrocardiogram; *SA,* sinoatrial.

### Irregular Tachyarrhythmias and Pulse Deficits

Irregular heart rhythms are common, and the ECG is important for differentiation of abnormal rhythms as well as sinus arrhythmia. Rapid atrial fibrillation and premature contractions of any origin often cause pulse deficits. Sustained, rapid arrhythmias lead to decreases in cardiac output, arterial blood pressure, and coronary perfusion; congestive and low-output heart failure can eventually result. Worsening of the rhythm disturbance and sudden death are possible consequences of heart failure.

#### Premature contractions and paroxysmal tachycardias

Frequent premature contractions and paroxysmal tachycardias can compromise ventricular filling, especially if underlying heart disease exists. Supraventricular tachyarrhythmias can result from various mechanisms; many are associated with atrial enlargement. Adverse hemodynamic effects may be clinically insignificant when ventricular premature contractions (VPCs) are infrequent or when underlying cardiac function is normal. However, hemodynamic impairment can be severe in animals with underlying heart

Table 4-3

## Doses of Antiarrhythmic Drugs

| Agent | Dose |
|---|---|
| **CLASS I** | |
| Lidocaine | Dog: Initial boluses of 2 mg/kg slowly IV, up to 8 mg/kg; or rapid IV infusion at 0.8 mg/kg/min; if effective, then 25-80 µg/kg/min CRI (see Box 4-1); can also be used intratracheally for CPR |
| | Cat: Initial bolus of 0.25-0.5 mg/kg slowly IV; can repeat at a dose of 0.15-0.25 mg/kg in 5-20 min; if effective, 10-20 µg/kg/min CRI |
| Procainamide | Dog: 6-10 (up to 20) mg/kg IV over 5-10 min; 10-50 µg/kg/min CRI; 6-20 (up to 30) mg/kg q4-6h IM; 10-25 mg/kg q6h PO (sustained release: q6-8h) |
| | Cat: 1-2 mg/kg slowly IV; 10-20 µg/kg/min CRI; 7.5-20 mg/kg q(6-)8h IM or PO |
| Quinidine | Dog: 6-20 mg/kg q6h IM (loading dose, 14-20 mg/kg); 6-16 mg/kg q6h PO; sustained action preparations, 8-20 mg/kg q8h PO |
| | Cat: 6-16 mg/kg q8h IM or PO |
| Tocainide | Dog: 10-25 mg/kg q8h PO |
| | Cat: — |
| Mexiletine | Dog: 4-10 mg/kg q8h PO |
| | Cat: — |
| Phenytoin | Dog: 10 mg/kg slowly IV; 30-50 mg/kg q8h PO |
| | Cat: Do not use |
| **CLASS II** | |
| Propranolol | Dog: 0.02 mg/kg initial bolus slowly IV (up to maximum of 0.1 mg/kg); initial dose, 0.1-0.2 mg/kg q8h PO, up to 1 mg/kg q8h |
| | Cat: Same IV instructions; 2.5 up to 10 mg/cat q8-12h PO |
| Atenolol | Dog: 0.2-1 mg/kg q12-24h PO |
| | Cat: 6.25-12.5 mg/cat q(12-)24h PO |
| Esmolol | Dog: 200-500 µg/kg IV over 1 min (loading dose), followed by infusion of 25-200 µg/kg/min |
| | Cat: Same |
| Metoprolol | Dog: Initial dose, 0.2 mg/kg q8h PO, up to 1 mg/kg q8h |
| | Cat: — |
| Nadolol | Dog: Initial dose, 0.2 mg/kg q8-12h PO, up to 1 mg/kg q8-12h |
| | Cat: — |
| **CLASS III** | |
| Sotalol | Dog: 1-3.5 mg/kg q12h PO |
| | Cat: — |
| Amiodarone | Dog: 10 mg/kg q12h PO for 7 days, then 8 mg/kg q24h PO (higher doses have been used); 3-5 mg/kg slowly IV (can repeat but do not give more than 10 mg/kg in 1 hr) |
| | Cat: — |
| Bretylium | Dog: 2-6 mg/kg IV; can repeat in 1-2 hr (human dose) |
| | Cat: — |
| **CLASS IV** | |
| Diltiazem | Dog: Initial dose, 0.5 mg/kg q8h PO up to 2 mg/kg; for atrial tachycardia, 0.15-0.25 mg/kg over 2-3 min IV (can repeat q15min until conversion or maximum dose of 0.75 mg/kg), or 0.5 mg/kg PO followed by 0.25 mg/kg PO q1h to a total of 1.5 (to 2) mg/kg or conversion |

*Continued.*

Table 4-3—cont'd

## Doses of Antiarrhythmic Drugs

| Agent | Dose |
|-------|------|
| **CLASS IV** | |
| Diltiazem | Cat: Same?; for hypertrophic cardiomyopathy, 1-2.5 mg/kg q8h; sustained-release preparations: Cardizem CD (Aventis Pharmaceutical, Inc., Kansas City, MO), 10 mg/kg/day (45 mg/cat is approximately 105 mg of Cardizem CD, or the amount that fits into small end of a no. 4 gelatin capsule); Dilacor XR (Watson Pharmaceuticals, Inc., Covona, CA), 30 mg/cat/day (one half of a 60-mg tablet contained within the 240-mg gelatin capsule) |
| Verapamil | Dog: Initial dose, 0.05 mg/kg slowly IV; can repeat q5min up to a total of 0.15(-0.2) mg/kg; 0.5-2 mg/kg q8h PO<br>Cat: Initial dose, 0.025 mg/kg slowly IV; can repeat q5min up to a total of 0.15(-0.2) mg/kg; 0.5-1 mg/kg q8h PO |
| **ANTICHOLINERGIC** | |
| Atropine | Dog: 0.02-0.04 mg/kg IV, IM, SC; can also be given intratracheally for CPR<br>Cat: Same |
| Glycopyrrolate | Dog: 0.005-0.01 mg/kg IV or IM; 0.01-0.02 mg/kg SC<br>Cat: Same |
| Propantheline Br | Dog: 3.73-7.5 mg q8-12h PO<br>Cat: unknown |
| **SYMPATHOMIMETIC** | |
| Isoproterenol | Dog: 0.045-0.09 μg/kg/min CRI<br>Cat: Same |
| Terbutaline | Dog: 2.5-5 mg/dog q8-12h PO<br>Cat: 1.25 mg/cat q12h PO |
| **OTHER AGENTS** | |
| Digoxin | See Table 3-3 |
| Adenosine | Dog: Up to 12 mg as rapid IV bolus<br>Cat: — |

*CRI,* Constant-rate infusion; *CPR,* cardiopulmonary resuscitation; *IM,* intramuscular; *IV,* intravenous; *PO,* oral; *SC,* subcutaneous; —, effective dosage not known.

disease, rapid ventricular rates, or myocardial depression resulting from a systemic disease. Correcting underlying hypoxia, electrolyte or acid-base imbalances, or abnormal hormone concentrations (e.g., thyroid) or discontinuing certain drugs may be important for arrhythmia control.

*Treatment of supraventricular arrhythmias.* Occasional premature beats do not require specific therapy, although predisposing factors should be minimized if possible. Digoxin (see text pp 66-69) is usually the initial drug of choice for treatment of frequent atrial premature contractions or paroxysmal atrial tachycardia in dogs with heart failure and cats with dilated cardiomyopathy. A β-blocker or diltiazem may be added if digoxin does not control the arrhythmia. Cats with hypertrophic cardiomyopathy or hyperthyroidism are usually given a β-blocker such as atenolol or propranolol; diltiazem is an alternative.

More aggressive initial therapy is warranted in patients with rapid and persistent supraventricular tachyarrhythmias, especially in the face of hemodynamic impairment.

Diltiazem (intravenous [IV] or oral [PO] loading) is preferred. Verapamil (IV) can be very effective but is not recommended for use in dogs with myocardial dysfunction or heart failure. A β-blocker (propranolol, esmolol) given slowly intravenously is an alternative, but such drugs have negative inotropic effects in animals with high underlying sympathetic tone. Digoxin IV generally is not recommended. Once the rhythm is better controlled, maintenance doses of PO digoxin, diltiazem, or both, or a β-blocker are options for chronic therapy. Amiodarone may be an alternative in cases refractory to these drugs.

Paroxysmal atrioventricular (AV) reciprocating tachycardia (see p 77) can be managed using β-blockers or diltiazem. High-dose procainamide, with or without a β-blocker or diltiazem, prevents recurrence of the tachycardia in some cases. Intracardiac electrophysiologic mapping and radiofrequency catheter ablation of accessory pathways is a therapeutic alternative in dogs with nonresponsive tachycardias and tachycardia-induced congestive heart failure (see text p 77).

**Acute treatment of VPCs and ventricular tachycardia.** Occasional VPCs in an otherwise asymptomatic animal usually are not treated. Moderately frequent (e.g., 20 to 40 per minute), single uniform VPCs also may not need treatment if underlying heart function is normal. Traditional indications for antiarrhythmic therapy include frequent VPCs (>30 per minute), paroxysmal or sustained ventricular tachycardia (e.g., rates >130 beats/min), multiform VPCs, or close coupling of the VPCs to preceding complexes (R-on-T phenomenon). However, consideration of underlying heart disease and whether signs of hypotension are related to the arrhythmia may be of greater importance. Animals thought to be hemodynamically unstable or that have a disease associated with sudden cardiac death should be treated earlier and more aggressively.

Lidocaine IV is usually the first-choice drug in dogs. Because IV boluses last only approximately 10 to 15 minutes, constant-rate infusion (CRI) is warranted if the drug is effective. Small supplemental IV boluses can be given in addition to CRI until steady state is achieved. IV infusions can be continued for several days if needed.

If lidocaine is ineffective, procainamide (IV, intramuscular [IM], or PO) or quinidine (IM or PO) is often tried next. The effects of a single IM or PO loading dose of either drug should occur within 2 hours. If the drug is effective, lower doses can be given every 4 to 6 hours IM or PO. If it is ineffective, the dose can be increased or another antiarrhythmic drug chosen.

If the arrhythmia has not been controlled, a β-blocker can be added. Alternative approaches include PO mexiletine or sotalol. Amiodarone IV may be effective for both ventricular and supraventricular tachyarrhythmias in dogs. Cats with frequent ventricular tachyarrhythmias are usually given a β-blocker first. Alternatively, very low doses of lidocaine can be administered. Procainamide may also be used.

Digoxin is not used for treatment of ventricular tachyarrhythmias specifically, although it may be a component of therapy for concurrent heart failure or supraventricular arrhythmias. Because digoxin can predispose to ventricular arrhythmias, simultaneous use of another antiarrhythmic drug may be necessary and should precede administration of digoxin if frequent or repetitive VPCs are present. Phenytoin is used in dogs only for the management of digitalis-induced ventricular arrhythmias refractory to lidocaine.

**Refractory cases.** If the ventricular tachyarrhythmia appears refractory to initial treatment, one or more of the following may be helpful:

1. Reevaluate the ECG. Could the initial diagnosis have been incorrect?
2. Reevaluate the serum potassium ($K^+$) and magnesium ($Mg^{++}$) concentrations. Hypokalemia reduces the efficacy of class I drugs and can predispose to arrhythmias. If serum $K^+$ is <3 mEq/L, KCl can be infused at 0.5 mEq/kg/hr; if serum $K^+$ is 3 to 3.5 mEq/L, KCl can be infused at 0.25 mEq/kg/hr. If serum $Mg^{++}$ is <1 mg/dl, give $MgSO_4$ or $MgCl_2$, diluted in 5% dextrose in water, at 0.75 to 1 mEq/kg/day by CRI.
3. Increase the dose of the antiarrhythmic drug having the greatest effect.

4. Administer a β-blocker in conjunction with a class I drug (e.g., propranolol, esmolol, or atenolol with procainamide) or a class IA with a class IB drug (e.g., procainamide with lidocaine or mexiletine), or try sotalol.
5. Consider the possibility that the drug therapy is exacerbating the rhythm disturbance. Polymorphous ventricular tachycardia has been associated with quinidine, procainamide, and other drug toxicities.
6. In animals with ventricular tachyarrhythmias associated with digoxin toxicity or with suspected polymorphous ventricular tachycardia, $MgSO_4$ can be effective at 25 to 40 mg/kg, diluted in 5% dextrose in water, by slow IV bolus, followed by an infusion of the same dose over 12 to 24 hours.
7. If the animal is tolerating the arrhythmia well, continue supportive care and close cardiovascular monitoring alone or with the most effective antiarrhythmic drug.
8. Try IV amiodarone, bretylium, or a newer or investigational antiarrhythmic agent (if available). Alternatively, consider referral for direct-current cardioversion or ventricular pacing.

*Chronic oral therapy.* Options currently used in dogs for the chronic management of ventricular tachyarrhythmias include (1) sustained-release procainamide or mexiletine (or possibly tocainide); (2) sustained-release procainamide or mexiletine combined with atenolol or propranolol; (3) sotalol; and (4) amiodarone. The last three options are favored, because they likely provide a greater antifibrillatory effect. Detailed discussion is provided in the text (pp 81-82).

Frequent reevaluation is important for animals on long-term antiarrhythmic therapy. Continuous 24- to 48-hr ambulatory ECG recordings can be used to document the frequency of arrhythmic events. The decision to continue or discontinue successful anti-arrhythmic therapy is based on consideration of the clinical situation and any underlying cardiac disease.

### Atrial fibrillation

Atrial fibrillation is a serious arrhythmia that most often occurs in association with marked atrial enlargement. Predisposing conditions include dilated cardiomyopathy, chronic degenerative AV valve disease, congenital malformations that cause atrial enlargement, and hypertrophic or restrictive cardiomyopathy in cats. Clinical heart failure is common in affected patients.

Long-lasting conversion to sinus rhythm is rare when clinically significant cardiac disease exists. Treatment is directed at reducing the ventricular response rate by slowing AV conduction, as a slower heart rate lessens the impact of atrial dysfunction. An in-hospital heart rate of <150 (<180 in cats) beats/min is desirable. Resting heart rate at home is a better indicator of drug effectiveness: rates of 70 to 120 beats/min in dogs and 80 to 140 beats/min in cats are acceptable, especially if the animal's activity level is good.

*Treatment options.* The initial drug of choice in most dogs is digoxin PO (see Table 3-3). If the heart rate exceeds 220 beats/min at rest, twice the eventual PO maintenance dose can be given for 1 to 2 days. For a more immediate decrease in heart rate, diltiazem IV can be used. When dobutamine or dopamine infusion is given to support myocardial function, IV diltiazem or an IV loading dose of digoxin can be used, but a β-blocker should be avoided.

Digoxin alone does not adequately reduce the heart rate in many animals. For chronic therapy, either a β-blocker or diltiazem can be added and titrated upward as needed. Because of their potential myocardial depressive effects, these drugs are usually added 1 to 2 days after PO digoxin is instituted in most dogs and in cats with dilated cardiomyopathy. Note: Digoxin should not be used in cats with hypertrophic cardiomyopathy that develop atrial fibrillation; a β-blocker or diltiazem is used instead.

*Large dogs.* Atrial fibrillation sometimes develops in large- or giant-breed dogs without evidence of heart disease, usually in association with trauma or surgery; it may also be an incidental finding. The arrhythmia may convert to sinus rhythm either spontaneously or with quinidine therapy (PO or IM). Diltiazem (PO) for 3 days may also be effective. Dogs that do not convert to sinus rhythm are either given digoxin (preferred) or monitored periodically without therapy if the ventricular rate is consistently low at rest.

### Rapid, Regular Rhythms

#### Sinus tachycardia

High sympathetic tone or drug-induced vagal blockade causes sinus tachycardia. Underlying causes include anxiety, pain, fever, thyrotoxicosis, heart failure, hypotension, shock, ingestion of stimulants or toxins (e.g., chocolate, caffeine), and various drugs (e.g., catecholamines, anticholinergics, theophylline and related agents). The heart rate is usually <300 beats/min, although it can be higher in animals with thyrotoxicosis or after ingestion of exogenous stimulants or drugs (particularly in cats). Correction of the cause and reversal of hypotension with IV fluids (if no edema is present) should decrease sympathetic tone and the sinus rate.

#### Sustained supraventricular tachycardia

It can be difficult to differentiate sustained supraventricular tachycardia (SVT) from sinus tachycardia. With SVT the heart rate is often >300 beats/min, whereas it is rare for the sinus rate to be so rapid. With both conditions the QRS configuration is normal. However, if an intraventricular conduction disturbance is present, SVT may look like ventricular tachycardia (see Chapter 2).

The initial approach to SVT includes performance of a vagal maneuver, which may transiently slow or intermittently block AV conduction, exposing abnormal atrial P′ waves and allowing an ectopic atrial focus to be identified. The maneuver is performed by massaging the area over the carotid sinuses (below the mandible in the jugular furrows) or by applying firm, bilateral ocular pressure for 15 to 20 seconds. Vagal maneuvers in dogs can be potentiated by administering morphine sulfate (0.2 mg/kg IM) or edrophonium chloride (1 to 4 mg IV; atropine and an endotracheal tube should be readily available). β-Blockers, calcium entry blockers, digoxin, and other agents may also increase the effectiveness of vagal maneuvers.

If the vagal maneuver does not terminate the SVT, drug therapy is used as described earlier for rapid paroxysmal SVT. Concurrently, IV fluids are administered to maintain blood pressure and enhance endogenous vagal tone. However, patients with known or suspected heart failure should receive a small volume slowly, if at all. Further cardiac diagnostic tests are indicated once conversion has been achieved or the ventricular rate has decreased to <200 beats/min. Refractory SVT might respond to sotalol, amiodarone, or a class IA or IC antiarrhythmic drug.

***Reentrant SVT.*** Reentrant SVT involving an accessory pathway and the AV node occurs in cats and dogs with ventricular preexcitation. When vagal maneuvers fail to interrupt the tachycardia, IV diltiazem or verapamil is tried. (Note: IV verapamil should not be used if atrial fibrillation is present.) An alternative is procainamide (slow IV). Vagal maneuvers can be repeated after these drugs are given. If these approaches are unsuccessful, an IV β-blocker or amiodarone may help.

#### Sustained ventricular tachycardia

Sustained ventricular tachycardia is treated aggressively, because it can result in marked decreases in arterial blood pressure, especially at faster rates. Lidocaine IV is usually the first-choice drug in dogs. Other options, including direct-current cardioversion, are discussed in the text (pp 84-86). In cats a β-blocker is usually the drug of choice. Lidocaine in small doses can be used instead; however, cats are sensitive to its neurotoxic effects, especially if not anesthetized. Procainamide and quinidine have also been used in cats.

Close electrocardiographic monitoring and further diagnostic testing should follow initial therapy. Total suppression of persistent ventricular tachyarrhythmias should not be expected. Consideration of the animal's clinical status and underlying disease, how well the drug has suppressed the arrhythmia, and the drug dose (e.g., can it be increased?) influence the decision to continue or discontinue current treatment or to use a different drug. Clinical status and the results of diagnostic testing also guide decisions about chronic PO therapy.

## Bradyarrhythmias

### Sinus bradycardia

Slow sinus rhythm (or arrhythmia) can be a normal finding, especially in athletic dogs. Sinus bradycardia may occur in a wide variety of circumstances, including administration of various drugs (e.g., xylazine, thorazine tranquilizers, anesthetic agents, digoxin, calcium entry blockers, β-blockers, parasympathomimetic drugs); trauma or diseases of the central nervous system (CNS); organic disease of the sinus node; hypothermia; hyperkalemia; hypothyroidism; and conditions that increase vagal tone (e.g., respiratory or gastrointestinal [GI] tract disease or a mass involving the vagosympathetic trunk). Chronic pulmonary disease is often associated with pronounced respiratory sinus arrhythmia.

In most cases the heart rate increases in response to exercise or atropine administration, and no clinical signs are associated with the slow heart rate. Symptomatic dogs usually have heart rates <50 beats/min, pronounced underlying disease, or both. Sinus bradycardia and sinus bradyarrhythmia are extremely rare in cats, so underlying cardiac or systemic disease (e.g., hyperkalemia) should be suspected in any cat with a slow heart rate.

*Treatment.* When sinus bradycardia is associated with signs of weakness, exercise intolerance, syncope, or worsening of the underlying disease, an anticholinergic (or adrenergic) agent is given (see Table 4-3). If sinus bradycardia is the result of a drug effect, discontinuation, dose reduction, or other therapy should be used as appropriate (e.g., reversal of anesthesia, calcium salts for calcium entry blocker overdose, dopamine or atropine for β-blocker toxicity). If acceleration of the heart rate is inadequate after medical therapy, temporary or permanent pacing is indicated.

### Sick sinus syndrome

Sick sinus syndrome is characterized by erratic sinoatrial function (episodes of marked sinus bradycardia with sinus arrest or sinoatrial block), resulting in episodic weakness, syncope, and Stokes-Adams seizures. Older female Miniature Schnauzers are most often affected, but the syndrome is also seen in Dachshunds, Pugs, and mixed-breed dogs. Sick sinus syndrome is extremely rare in cats.

Abnormalities of the AV conduction system may coexist, resulting in prolonged periods of asystole. Some affected dogs also have various paroxysmal supraventricular tachyarrhythmias, prompting the name *bradycardia-tachycardia syndrome.* Premature complexes may be followed by long pauses before sinus node activity resumes. Intermittent periods of accelerated junctional rhythms and variable junctional or ventricular escape rhythms may also occur. Degenerative AV valve disease also is often present. Some dogs have evidence of congestive heart failure, usually secondary to AV valve regurgitation, although the arrhythmias may be a complicating factor.

ECG abnormalities are frequently pronounced in dogs with long-standing sick sinus syndrome. Nevertheless, some dogs have one or more normal resting ECGs. Establishment of a definitive diagnosis is aided by 24-hour ambulatory or prolonged visual ECG monitoring. An atropine challenge test is done in dogs with persistent bradycardia (see text p 96). Dogs with sick sinus syndrome generally have a subnormal response.

*Treatment.* Therapy with an anticholinergic agent, methylxanthine bronchodilator, or terbutaline PO may temporarily help animals that have a positive response to atropine challenge; however, such therapy is often unrewarding. Anticholinergic or sympathomimetic drugs used to accelerate the sinus rate can also exacerbate any tachyarrhythmias that may already exist. Conversely, drugs used to suppress these supraventricular tachyarrhythmias can magnify the bradycardia, although digoxin or diltiazem is helpful in some dogs when used cautiously. Sick sinus syndrome with frequent or severe clinical signs is best managed by permanent artificial pacing.

### Atrial standstill

Persistent atrial standstill is rare in dogs and extremely rare in cats; most reported cases have occurred in English Springer Spaniels with fasciohumeral-type muscular dystrophy. Infiltrative and inflammatory diseases of the atrial myocardium can also result in atrial standstill. Persistent atrial standstill may indicate a serious and progressive cardiac disorder. On the other hand, apparent lack of atrial electrical and mechanical activity can be seen transiently ("silent atrium") in animals with hyperkalemia; once serum K$^+$ returns to normal, sinus node activity (and P waves) become evident.

Temporary acceleration of the escape rhythm can sometimes be achieved with an anticholinergic drug or infusion of dopamine (see Table 3-3) or isoproterenol (see Table 4-3), but medical treatment for persistent atrial standstill is rarely rewarding. If ventricular tachyarrhythmias result, the drug should be discontinued or the dose reduced. Terbutaline PO may have some beneficial effect. Antiarrhythmic agents are contraindicated, because they may suppress the escape focus, as well as the tachyarrhythmia. Permanent pacemaker implantation is the treatment of choice, although the prognosis is poor in patients with concurrent ventricular myocardial dysfunction.

### Second- and third-degree AV blocks

Second-degree, or intermittent, AV block usually causes an irregular heartbeat. In contrast, the ventricular escape rhythm resulting from a third-degree, or complete, AV block usually is regular. AV conduction disturbances may result from therapy with certain drugs (e.g., $\alpha_2$-agonists, opioids, digoxin), high vagal tone, or organic disease of the AV node (e.g., bacterial endocarditis of the aortic valve, hypertrophic cardiomyopathy, infiltrative myocardial disease, myocarditis). Idiopathic heart block may occur in middle-aged or older dogs; congenital third-degree heart block has also been reported. Symptomatic heart block is less common in cats; most cases have been associated with hypertrophic cardiomyopathy. Heart block is occasionally found in old cats without detectable organic heart disease.

In dogs type I second-degree block (see Chapter 2) and first-degree block are frequently associated with high vagal tone or drugs. Patients are often asymptomatic, and exercise or an anticholinergic drug (atropine or glycopyrrolate) usually abolishes the block. High-grade (many blocked P waves) second-degree block and complete heart block usually cause lethargy, exercise intolerance, weakness, syncope, and other signs of low cardiac output. Some dogs develop congestive heart failure from chronic bradycardia, especially when other cardiac disease is present.

*Treatment.*   An atropine challenge test (see text p 96) is used to determine the degree of vagal influence on the AV block. Long-term oral anticholinergic therapy (e.g., propantheline bromide) can be attempted in symptomatic animals that are atropine responsive. However, atropine and subsequent anticholinergic therapy is often ineffective, so artificial pacing is usually indicated (see text p 86). An emergency infusion of dopamine (see Table 3-3) or isoproterenol (see Table 4-3) may increase the ventricular escape rate in animals with high-grade second- or third-degree block, although ventricular tachyarrhythmias may be provoked.

## ANTIARRHYTHMIC DRUGS (TEXT P 86)

Drugs used to suppress arrhythmias have been grouped according to their electrophysiologic effects on cardiac cells (see Table 4-2). Class I agents slow conduction and decrease automaticity and excitability by means of their membrane-stabilizing effects; the "traditional" ventricular antiarrhythmic drugs belong to this class. Class II drugs include the β-adrenergic antagonists, which act by inhibiting the effects of catecholamines on the heart. Class III drugs prolong the effective refractory period of cardiac action potentials without decreasing conduction velocity; they may be most effective in suppressing reentrant arrhythmias or in preventing ventricular fibrillation. Class IV drugs are the calcium entry blockers; ventricular arrhythmias are usually not responsive to these agents. Established or suggested doses for the antiarrhythmic drugs used in dogs and cats are given in Table 4-3.

### Class I Antiarrhythmic Drugs

#### Lidocaine

Lidocaine (without epinephrine) is usually the agent of choice for treatment of ventricular arrhythmias in dogs, but it is generally ineffective for supraventricular arrhythmias. Lidocaine causes little or no depression of contractility at therapeutic doses when given slowly intravenously, making it the drug of choice in dogs with heart failure. It has greater effects on diseased and hypoxic cardiac cells and at faster stimulation rates. The drug is contraindicated in the presence of complete heart block and should be used cautiously in patients with sinus bradycardia, sick sinus syndrome, and first- or second-degree AV blocks. Hypokalemia may render the drug ineffective, whereas hyperkalemia intensifies its depressant effects on cardiac membranes.

***Dosage.*** Lidocaine is administered intravenously, usually as slow boluses followed by CRI (Box 4-1; see Table 4-3). An initial bolus of 2 mg/kg is used in dogs and can be repeated two to three times if necessary. Lower doses (0.25 to 0.5 mg/kg) should be used in cats to avoid toxicity.

***Toxicity.*** The most common toxic effect is CNS excitation: agitation, disorientation, muscle twitches, nystagmus, and seizures. Nausea can also occur. Worsening of arrhythmias (proarrhythmic effect) is seen occasionally. Cats are particularly sensitive and may suffer respiratory arrest along with seizures. Lidocaine should be discontinued until signs of toxicity disappear; a lower infusion rate may then be instituted. Diazepam (0.25 to 0.5 mg/kg IV) is used to control lidocaine-induced seizures. Propranolol, cimetidine, and other drugs that decrease liver blood flow slow the metabolism of lidocaine and predispose to toxicity. Animals with heart failure may also have reduced hepatic blood flow and may require a lower dose.

### Procainamide

Procainamide is indicated for premature ventricular (and sometimes atrial) depolarizations and tachycardias. It is less effective than quinidine for atrial arrhythmias and is ineffective in converting chronic atrial flutter or fibrillation to sinus rhythm. Procainamide should be used with caution in animals with sinus bradycardia, sick sinus syndrome, AV blocks, intraventricular conduction disturbances, or hypotensive states. It is contraindicated in animals with complete heart block.

---

**Box 4-1**

## Formulas to Calculate Constant-Rate Infusion

### METHOD 1

**Allows for "fine-tuning" fluid as well as drug administration rate**

- Determine desired drug infusion rate

  $\mu$g/kg/min × Body weight (kg) = $\mu$g/min                                    (A)

- Determine desired fluid infusion rate

  ml/hr ÷ 60 = ml/min                                                              (B)

  (A) ÷ (B) = mg/min ÷ ml/min = mg drug per milliliter of fluid

- Convert from $\mu$g to mg of drug needed (1 $\mu$g = 0.001 mg)

  mg drug/ml fluid × ml of fluid in bag (or bottle or burette) = mg of drug to add to fluid bag

### METHOD 2

**For total dose over a 6-hr period, must also calculate fluid volume and administration rate**

- *Total* dose in milligrams to infuse over a 6-hr period = Body weight (kg) × Dose ($\mu$g/kg/min) × 0.36

### METHOD 3 (FOR LIDOCAINE)

**Faster but less helpful if fluid rate is important or fine drug-dose adjustments are needed**

- For CRI of 44 $\mu$g/kg/min of lidocaine, add 25 ml of 2% lidocaine to 250 ml of $D_5W$
- Infuse at 0.25 ml/25 lb of body weight per minute

---

*CRI,* Constant-rate infusion; *$D_5W$,* 5% dextrose in water.

*Dosage.* Procainamide is well absorbed orally in dogs, but its half-life is short (2.5 to 4 hours). The sustained-release preparation has a slightly longer half-life (3 to 6 hours). Administration via the PO or IM route is not associated with marked hemo-dynamic effects; however, rapid IV injection can cause hypotension and cardiac depression. CRI may be used if the arrhythmia responds to an IV bolus; steady state is reached in 12 to 22 hours.

*Toxicity.* The toxic effects of procainamide are similar to those of quinidine (see next section) but usually milder. GI upset and prolongation of the QRS or QT intervals may occur. Procainamide can enhance the ventricular response rate to atrial fibrillation when used without digoxin or a β- or calcium entry blocker. More serious toxic effects include hypotension, depressed AV conduction (sometimes causing second- or third-degree heart block), and proarrhythmia (causing syncope or ventricular fibrillation). IV fluids, catecholamines, or calcium-containing solutions can be used to treat the hypotension. GI signs associated with oral therapy may respond to dosage reduction.

### Quinidine
Quinidine has been used for treatment of ventricular and, occasionally, supra-ventricular tachyarrhythmias. In large dogs with recent-onset atrial fibrillation and normal ventricular function, quinidine may cause conversion to sinus rhythm. The drug is contraindicated in animals with sinus bradycardia, sick sinus syndrome, high-grade second-degree AV block, or complete heart block. Quinidine should be used cautiously in animals with heart failure or hyperkalemia.

Quinidine causes dose-dependent ECG changes, including PR, QRS, and QT prolongation. At low doses it may increase the sinus rate or the ventricular response rate to atrial fibrillation. As with other class I agents, hypokalemia reduces its antiarrhythmic effectiveness.

*Dosage.* Quinidine is well absorbed orally, but it has fallen out of favor for chronic oral administration. IV administration is not recommended because of the potential for vasodilation, cardiac depression, and hypotension. The PO and IM routes are usually not associated with adverse hemodynamic effects, but close monitoring is warranted, especially in animals with underlying cardiac disease. Blood concentrations in the human therapeutic range (2.5 to 5 µg/ml) are usually reached within 12 to 24 hours. Slow-release sulfate, gluconate, and polygalacturonate salts of quinidine prolong the drug's absorption and elimination (see text p 90).

*Drug interactions.* Cimetidine may predispose to toxicity by slowing the drug's elimination. Quinidine can precipitate digoxin toxicity when the two drugs are used simultaneously. Anticonvulsants and other drugs that induce hepatic microsomal enzymes can speed the metabolism of quinidine, necessitating an increased dose.

*Toxicity.* Various conduction blocks, as well as ventricular tachyarrhythmias, can result from high blood concentrations of quinidine. The PR interval and QRS duration lengthen as the plasma concentration increases. Marked QT prolongation, development of right bundle branch block, or QRS widening exceeding 25% of the pretreatment value suggests toxicity. Lethargy, weakness, and congestive heart failure can result from the negative inotropic and vasodilatory effects of the drug and subsequent hypotension. Cardiotoxicity and hypotension may be partially reversed by administration of sodium bicarbonate (1 mEq/kg IV), which temporarily decreases the serum $K^+$ concentration and increases quinidine's protein binding. (Because quinidine is highly protein bound, severe hypoalbuminemia can predispose to quinidine toxicity.) GI signs such as nausea, vomiting, and diarrhea are common with PO quinidine therapy.

### Mexiletine
Mexiletine is similar in effect to lidocaine and effectively terminates or controls ventricular tachyarrhythmias in dogs. In some animals the combination of a β-blocker (or procainamide or quinidine) with mexiletine is more efficacious and associated with fewer adverse effects than mexiletine alone. The drug is readily absorbed orally. Mexiletine undergoes hepatic metabolism and some renal excretion; hepatic microsomal enzyme inducers may accelerate its clearance. Adverse effects include vomiting, anorexia, tremor, and disorientation; however, overall, mexiletine produces fewer adverse effects than tocainide. The effects of mexiletine in cats are unknown.

### Tocainide

Tocainide is effective against various ventricular tachyarrhythmias. It is similar to lidocaine in its effects but is administered orally; however, it is not favored for chronic PO therapy. Effective serum concentrations can be maintained for 6 to 8 hours after three doses. Loading can be achieved by administering two doses at a 2-hour interval and a third dose 6 hours later. Note: This regimen is not recommended for dogs concurrently receiving lidocaine.

Signs of toxicity can occur at therapeutic plasma concentrations. GI effects (anorexia and vomiting) are common; neurotoxic signs such as ataxia, disorientation, and twitching are seen occasionally. Administration of tocainide for >3 months causes ocular and renal toxicity in some dogs.

### Phenytoin

Phenytoin has effects similar to those of lidocaine. Its use in dogs is currently limited to the treatment of digitalis-induced ventricular arrhythmias that are unresponsive to lidocaine. Contraindications are as for lidocaine. Rapid IV injection should be avoided because the propylene glycol vehicle can depress myocardial contractility and cause vasodilation, hypotension, exacerbation of arrhythmias, and respiratory arrest. Slow IV infusion and PO administration do not cause relevant hemodynamic disturbances; however, oral bioavailability is poor.

IV administration has been associated with bradycardia, AV blocks, ventricular tachycardia, and cardiac arrest. CNS signs such as depression, nystagmus, disorientation, and ataxia can also occur. Phenytoin is metabolized in the liver; administration of cimetidine, chloramphenicol, and other drugs that inhibit microsomal enzymes can result in toxic serum concentrations of phenytoin. Note: Phenytoin is not recommended in cats because the half-life is >24 hours, and even low doses produce toxic serum concentrations.

## Class II Antiarrhythmic Drugs

The β-blockers are used to treat hypertrophic cardiomyopathy, certain ventricular outflow obstructions, systemic hypertension, hyperthyroid heart disease, supraventricular and ventricular tachyarrhythmias (especially those caused by enhanced sympathetic tone), and other diseases or toxicities that cause excessive sympathetic stimulation. These drugs slow the heart rate, reduce myocardial oxygen demand, and increase AV conduction time and refractoriness. A β-blocker is often used in conjunction with digoxin to slow the ventricular response rate in atrial fibrillation. These drugs are the first-line antiarrhythmic agents in cats with supraventricular or ventricular tachyarrhythmias.

β-Blockers must be used cautiously in animals with severe myocardial disease when cardiac output is being maintained by increased sympathetic drive. They are generally contraindicated in patients with sinus bradycardia, sick sinus syndrome, high-grade AV block, or severe congestive heart failure and in animals also receiving a calcium entry blocker.

β-Blockers enhance the depression of AV conduction by digitalis, class I drugs, and calcium entry blockers. Simultaneous use of a β-blocker and a calcium entry blocker is not recommended because it can lead to marked decreases in heart rate and myocardial contractility. Because of the possibility of β-receptor upregulation during long-term use, abrupt discontinuation of β-blocker therapy could result in serious arrhythmias.

Nonselective β-blockers (i.e., those with $\beta_1$- and $\beta_2$-receptor affinity) may increase peripheral vascular resistance and cause bronchoconstriction. β-Blockers may also prevent the appearance of early signs of acute hypoglycemia (e.g., tachycardia and blood pressure changes) in diabetics, and they also reduce the release of insulin in response to hyperglycemia.

### Propranolol

Propranolol is a nonselective β-blocker. In dogs the combination of propranolol with a class I agent often provides better ventricular tachyarrhythmia suppression than either drug alone. Propranolol may reduce arterial pressure in hypertensive dogs, especially when used in conjunction with a low-sodium diet (see Chapter 12). Propranolol should be used cautiously in patients with heart failure; if myocardial failure is present, prior digitalization is advised. Delay of propranolol therapy until after the resolution of pulmonary edema is suggested because of the potential for bronchoconstriction from $\beta_2$-receptor antagonism. (These effects also make propranolol relatively contraindicated in patients with asthma or chronic small airway disease.)

**Dosage.** The effects of propranolol depend on the level of sympathetic activation, so individual response is quite variable. Initial doses should be low and titrated upward as needed according to the patient's response. Some animals are unable to tolerate even small doses, so careful titration from an initial low dose is very important.

The IV form is used mainly in the treatment of refractory ventricular tachycardia (in conjunction with a class I drug) and in the emergency management of atrial or junctional tachycardia. Propranolol lowers hepatic blood flow, thereby prolonging its own elimination and that of certain drugs, including lidocaine. Feeding delays the rate of absorption via the PO route and increases the clearance of an IV dose.

**Toxicity.** Toxicity is usually related to excessive $\beta$-blockade. Bradycardia, heart failure, hypotension, and bronchospasm can occur. Infusion of a catecholamine (e.g., dopamine or dobutamine; see Table 3-3) will help reverse these effects. Propranolol can also cause depression and disorientation.

### Atenolol

Atenolol is a selective $\beta_1$-blocker. It is now used more often than propranolol to slow sinus rate and AV conduction and suppress VPCs in dogs and cats. $\beta$-Blocking effects are evident for 12 hours but are gone by 24 hours in normal animals. Atenolol is excreted in the urine, so renal impairment delays clearance. Atenolol does not readily cross the blood-brain barrier, so adverse CNS effects are unlikely. However, weakness or exacerbation of heart failure can occur.

### Other β-blockers

Several other $\beta$-blocking drugs are available. Their basic effects are similar, although their relative selectivity and pharmacologic characteristics vary. Some of these drugs are listed in Table 4-3. Esmolol has $\beta_1$-receptor selectivity but a very short half-life (<10 min). Although expensive, this drug has been used for the short-term treatment of tachyarrhythmias and feline hypertrophic obstructive cardiomyopathy.

Carvedilol and metoprolol have proved useful in the treatment of chronic, stable myocardial failure by improving cardiac function, promoting upregulation of cardiac $\beta$-receptors, and increasing survival time in people.

## Class III Antiarrhythmic Drugs

### Sotalol

Sotalol is a nonselective $\beta$-blocker that has class III effects. Although it has minimal hemodynamic effects, sotalol can cause proarrhythmia and may worsen heart failure in patients with serious myocardial disease. It has been associated with clinical deterioration in dogs with moderately to markedly reduced myocardial contractility. However, sotalol has been used successfully in large-breed dogs with persistent ventricular tachyarrhythmias and good myocardial function. Adverse effects include hypotension, depression, nausea, vomiting, diarrhea, and bradycardia.

### Amiodarone

Although considered a class III agent, amiodarone shares properties with drugs of all of the other antiarrhythmic drug classes. The $\beta$-blocking effects occur soon after administration, but maximal class III effects are not achieved for weeks with chronic administration. Therapeutic doses slow the sinus rate and decrease AV conduction velocity, with minimal depression of myocardial contractility and blood pressure. Veterinary experience with amiodarone is relatively limited, but it appears to be a promising drug for use in dogs. It has been used orally most often, although an IV form is available. The pharmacokinetics are complex; a suggested protocol is given in Table 4-3.

Amiodarone may have a proarrhythmic effect that is less than that of other agents and may reduce the risk of sudden death. However, the potential for profound cardiac depression and hypotension with IV amiodarone is of concern in dogs with myocardial disease. GI upset, hepatic dysfunction, and positive Coombs' test have been reported in dogs receiving PO amiodarone. This drug also reduces the clearance and increases the serum concentration of digoxin and diltiazem. Long-term therapy in humans is associated with numerous and potentially severe adverse effects (see text p 94).

### Bretylium tosylate

Bretylium increases the ventricular fibrillation threshold. It is indicated for the treatment of life-threatening ventricular arrhythmias that are unresponsive to conventional therapy and in patients at risk for development of ventricular fibrillation. It is not recommended as initial therapy for ventricular arrhythmias because the antifibrillatory effects can be delayed 4 to 6 hours. Extreme bradycardia or hypotension is a contraindication for its use.

Extremely poor PO absorption limits use to the IM or IV routes. Bretylium is eliminated through the kidneys, so renal disease reduces drug clearance. Adverse effects include ataxia, nausea, and vomiting after rapid IV injection. Aggravation of arrhythmias and tachycardia can also occur. Severe hypotension is uncommon and responds to fluid administration.

## Class IV Antiarrhythmic Drugs

The calcium entry blockers are a diverse group of drugs that can cause coronary and systemic vasodilation, enhance myocardial relaxation, and reduce cardiac contractility. Some have antiarrhythmic effects, especially on tissues dependent on the slow inward calcium ($Ca^{++}$) influx, such as the sinus and AV nodes. Other conditions for which calcium entry blockers are potentially useful include hypertrophic cardiomyopathy, myocardial ischemia, and hypertension.

### Diltiazem

Diltiazem slows AV conduction and causes potent coronary and mild peripheral vasodilation; it has a lesser negative inotropic effect than verapamil. Diltiazem is often combined with digoxin to further slow the ventricular response rate to atrial fibrillation in dogs. It is also used for other supraventricular tachyarrhythmias. Diltiazem is often used in cats with hypertrophic cardiomyopathy, where its beneficial effects can include enhancement of myocardial relaxation and perfusion, as well as mild reductions in heart rate, contractility, and myocardial oxygen demand; a decrease in left ventricular wall and septal thickness may also occur with chronic therapy.

*Dosage.* Initial doses should be low and increased as needed until effective or until the maximal recommended dose is reached. The sustained release preparation Cardizem CD (Aventis Pharmaceutical, Inc., Kansas City, MO) has been evaluated in cats at a dosage of 10 mg/kg daily. Peak plasma concentrations were reached in 6 hours, and therapeutic concentrations were maintained for 24 hours. Drugs that inhibit hepatic enzyme systems (e.g., cimetidine) decrease diltiazem's metabolism. Also, propranolol and diltiazem reduce each other's clearance when used simultaneously.

*Toxicity.* Adverse effects are uncommon at therapeutic doses, although anorexia, nausea, and bradycardia may occur. On rare occasions, other GI, cardiac, neurologic, and behavioral effects occur in cats. Overdose or exaggerated response is treated with supportive care: atropine for bradycardia or AV blocks; dopamine or dobutamine and furosemide for heart failure (see Chapter 3); and dopamine or IV calcium salts for hypotension.

### Verapamil

Verapamil is the most potent of the clinically used calcium entry blockers. It causes dose-related slowing of the sinus rate and AV conduction. The drug is effective in abolishing reentrant supraventricular tachycardia and slowing the ventricular response rate in atrial fibrillation. Verapamil is often effective against supraventricular and atrial tachycardias in animals without heart failure, but it has negative inotropic and vasodilatory effects that can cause serious decompensation, hypotension, and even death if underlying myocardial disease is present. Therefore verapamil is not recommended in animals with heart failure. Other contraindications include sick sinus syndrome, AV conduction disturbances, digitalis toxicity, and preexisting β-blocker therapy.

*Dosage.* An initial low dose is given very slowly intravenously; this can be repeated at 5-minute intervals if no adverse effects have occurred and the arrhythmia persists. Blood pressure monitoring is advisable because of the potential for hypotension. Verapamil is poorly absorbed orally.

*Toxicity.* Toxic effects include sinus bradycardia, AV block, hypotension, reduced myocardial contractility, and cardiogenic shock. The negative inotropic effects may be reversed with IV administration of calcium salts, sympathomimetic drugs, or amrinone (see Table 3-3). Atropine may also be required to treat bradycardia or conduction blocks.

### Amlodipine

Amlodipine is recommended as the first-line antihypertensive agent in cats and is also used in some hypertensive dogs (see Chapter 12). It is being incorporated into the therapy for chronic refractory heart failure in some dogs, beginning at lower doses (e.g., 0.05 to 0.1 mg/kg q24 or 12h).

Amlodipine besylate is a long-acting calcium entry blocker; in dogs maximal effects occur 4 to 7 days after initiation of therapy. Oral bioavailability is high (88%), and plasma concentrations increase with chronic therapy. The drug undergoes hepatic metabolism, so caution is warranted in animals with poor liver function. Excretion is via urine and feces. Pharmacokinetic data for cats are unavailable, but amlodipine's effects on blood pressure are thought to last at least 24 hours in cats.

## Anticholinergic Drugs

### Atropine and glycopyrrolate

Anticholinergic drugs can increase sinus node rate and AV conduction when vagal tone is excessive. Parenteral atropine or glycopyrrolate is indicated for bradycardia or AV block induced by anesthesia, CNS lesions, and certain other diseases or toxicities. Unlike atropine, glycopyrrolate does not produce centrally mediated effects, and it is longer lasting.

*Atropine challenge.* This test is used to determine the degree of vagal influence on sinus and AV nodal function. Although atropine given by any parenteral route can transiently exacerbate vagally mediated AV block, IV administration causes the fastest and most consistent onset and resolution of the exacerbated block as well as higher post-bradycardic heart rates. After a baseline ECG is recorded, atropine (0.02 to 0.04 mg/kg) is injected intravenously, and another ECG is recorded 5 to 10 minutes later. (Experimentally a dose rate of 0.04 mg/kg completely abolished parasympathetic tone, whereas 0.02 mg/kg did not.) If the heart rate has not increased by at least 150%, the ECG should be repeated 15 to 20 min after atropine injection. The normal sinus node response is an increase in rate to 150 to 160 beats/min. In animals with organic AV nodal disease, AV block may remain unchanged or worsen after anticholinergic administration.

### Oral anticholinergic drugs

Some animals that respond to parenteral atropine or glycopyrrolate will also respond to PO anticholinergics (e.g., propantheline bromide), at least transiently. However, animals with symptomatic bradyarrhythmias usually require permanent pacemaker implantation to effectively control the heart rate. Vagolytic drugs may aggravate paroxysmal supraventricular tachyarrhythmias (as occur in sick sinus syndrome) and should not be used as chronic therapy in such animals. Other adverse effects of anticholinergic therapy include vomiting, dry mouth, constipation, keratoconjunctivitis sicca, and drying of respiratory secretions.

## Sympathomimetic Drugs

Isoproterenol is a β-receptor agonist that has been used for treatment of symptomatic AV block and bradycardia that is refractory to atropine. However, it can cause hypotension, so it is not used for treatment of either heart failure or cardiac arrest. Isoproterenol can be arrhythmogenic, as can other catecholamines. The lowest effective dose should be used and the animal monitored closely for arrhythmias. PO administration is not effective because of marked first-pass hepatic metabolism. PO terbutaline may also have a mild stimulatory effect on heart rate. The methylxanthine bronchodilators (aminophylline and theophylline) increase the heart rate in some dogs with sick sinus syndrome when used at higher doses.

### Adenosine
Adenosine has been used for the acute termination of supraventricular tachycardias in humans, but veterinary experience with the drug is limited and not encouraging. It is rapidly degraded (the elimination half-life in humans is 1 to 6 seconds), so adenosine must be administered rapidly via the IV route, preferably into a central vein. Doses of 6 to 12 mg are used in humans. Transient sinus rate slowing or AV block occurs. Methylxanthine bronchodilators block the effects of adenosine.

# 5

# Cardiopulmonary Resuscitation

## *(Text pp 98-105)*

## SIGNS OF IMPENDING ARREST
Early recognition of cardiopulmonary deterioration helps prevent cardiac arrest, or at least allows a more rapid response. Any of the following signs should prompt immediate action:
- slowing of the heart or respiratory rate
- gasping or irregular respiration
- deteriorating consciousness
- progressive T-wave enlargement and ST-segment changes on electrocardiogram (ECG)
- cardiac arrhythmias

Animals in respiratory arrest may experience agonal gasps or apnea. They quickly become unconscious, with pale grayish or cyanotic mucous membranes, dilated pupils, and loss of muscle tone. Palpable pulse and heartbeat disappear when the systolic pressure drops below 60 mm Hg. Bleeding from surgical sites or wounds may also stop. Immediate cardiopulmonary resuscitation (CPR) is imperative.

## APPROACH TO CPR
The success rate of CPR in dogs and cats is reportedly less than 25%. Therefore the decision to begin or continue CPR should be based on the potential reversibility of the animal's underlying problems and on the owner's wishes. The immediate goal of CPR is restoration of ventilation and effective circulation to the heart and brain. Further goals are the restoration of normal heart rhythm and output and correction of tissue hypoxia and acidosis. The components of CPR should be addressed in the following order.

## Airway (A)

Establishing a patent airway is critical. Use a properly placed and securely cuffed endo-tracheal tube, and suction any mucus, fluid, or vomitus from the pharynx and trachea. Tracheostomy may be necessary in some animals.

## Breathing (B)

Intermittent positive-pressure ventilation can be accomplished using the reservoir bag on an anesthetic machine, a self-inflating resuscitation bag (e.g., Ambubag), or a mouth-to-tube technique. Prolonged use of 100% oxygen ($O_2$) may contribute to oxidative stress and delayed brain injury; use of room air may yield a better neurologic outcome. Give the patient two long (1- to 1.5-second) breaths; if spontaneous respiration does not resume, begin artificial ventilation. Ventilation rates vary with patient size but should be 20 to 24 breaths/min (higher for smaller animals). Give sufficient volume to approximate normal chest expansion. (Peak airway pressure should not exceed 20 cm $H_2O$.)

## Circulation (C)

### External cardiac massage

External (closed chest) cardiac massage is begun as soon as cardiac arrest is recognized, unless internal cardiac massage is indicated (see later). External massage is most effective in dogs weighing <15 kg and in cats.

*Technique.* Place small dogs and cats in lateral recumbency. Chest compression is accomplished with one hand placed on either side of the chest over the heart (fourth to fifth intercostal space). In very small dogs and cats one hand may provide effective massage if the thumb is placed on one side of the chest and the fingers on the other. Place large dogs (>15 kg) in dorsal recumbency and compress the chest over the caudal third of the sternum.

In small dogs and cats compress the chest abruptly 100 to 120 times per minute; in larger dogs compress 80 to 100 times per minute. The compression and relaxation phases should take the same amount of time, displacing the chest wall by 30% with each compression. If only one rescuer is present, alternate 15 chest compressions with 2 breaths.

Applying manual pressure or a compression bandage to the abdomen, wrapping the pelvic limbs, and performing abrupt abdominal compressions (performed between chest compressions) may improve coronary and cerebral blood flow.

*Evaluation.* Successful external massage and positive-pressure ventilation result in detectable arterial pulses and improved mucous membrane color. (Note: Return of normal pupillary size may be prevented by certain drugs used in CPR or by hypoxic injury to the retina.) If a response is not seen within 1 to 2 minutes, the CPR technique should be modified. Use of a pressor agent and an increase in intravenous (IV) fluid rate may help by improving venous return. If external massage is ineffective after 5 minutes, internal cardiac massage may be tried.

### Internal cardiac massage

Internal, or direct, cardiac massage is more effective than external massage. It is indicated when any of the following is true:

- External massage is ineffective after 5 minutes.
- The patient is a large or barrel-chested dog.
- Fractured ribs or other chest wall trauma is evident.
- Pneumothorax, pulmonary contusion, pleural or pericardial effusion, diaphragmatic hernia, or hypovolemia is suspected.

The patient's underlying condition and the owner's wishes must also be considered.

*Technique.* Make an incision in the left fifth or sixth intercostal space. Clipping a strip of hair over the incision site and swabbing the skin is ideal, but no more than a few seconds should be used for this. Incise down to the pleura rapidly but carefully, avoiding the intercostal vessels just caudal to the rib and the internal thoracic artery lateral to the sternum. Enter the pleural space bluntly while the animal is exhaling. Enlarge the opening in the pleural space with scissors, and use a self-retaining retractor to spread the ribs. (Pericardiotomy allows maximal diastolic filling and prevents development of cardiac tamponade if blood or transudate accumulates, but it may not be necessary in every case.)

Compress the heart between two fingers (small heart), the palm and flat portion of the fingers of one hand (mid-sized heart), or the palm and the opposite chest wall or both hands (large heart). Be careful not to rotate, traumatize, or perforate the heart. Apply enough compressive force to empty the ventricles (from apex to base), allowing time for ventricular filling before the next compression. The descending aorta can be compressed with a finger or a vascular clamp to maximize blood flow to the heart and brain. If used, aortic compression should be maintained until stable, spontaneous cardiac activity is restored; it should then be discontinued gradually over 10 to 20 minutes.

If cardiac massage is successful, thoroughly lavage the chest with sterile isotonic solution, and clean and disinfect the skin edges before closing the incision. If the pericardium was incised, leave it open. The chest should be carefully evacuated of air, and broad-spectrum antibiotic therapy initiated.

### Defibrillation

Ventricular fibrillation is treated by electrical defibrillation. Low energy levels are used initially; if unsuccessful, repeated shocks are given at progressively higher energy levels, paired in rapid succession, or both. Epinephrine may increase the chance of success when fine fibrillation waves are present on ECG. Chemical defibrillation is of little or no efficacy. A sharp precordial thump may occasionally convert ventricular fibrillation or tachycardia to sinus rhythm, but it can also precipitate fibrillation during ventricular tachycardia.

*External defibrillation.* Place the paddles firmly on both side of the chest, over the heart. Good skin contact with the entire face of the paddle is important. Use contact paste, ECG gel, pHisoHex soap, or KY jelly and salt to enhance conduction; alcohol should not be used. Take care that the paddles do not touch each other and that conductive material on the skin does not form a connection between the two paddles. Recommended initial energy settings are based on patient size: 2 watt-sec/kg for patients <7 kg; 5 watt-sec/kg for dogs weighing 8 to 40 kg; and up to 10 watt-sec/kg for very large dogs. Continue CPR between attempts.

*Internal defibrillation.* Place sterile, internal paddles on opposite sides of the heart so that their entire surface contacts the heart. Recommended energy settings are 0.2 to 0.4 watt-sec/kg (up to 2 watt-sec/kg).

## Drugs (D)

Routes for drug administration (Table 5-1) during CPR are as follows, in order of preference:

- central vein
- intratracheal, via a long flexible catheter inserted into the endotracheal tube (double the IV dose and dilute with 2 to 5 ml sterile water or saline; do not use this route for sodium bicarbonate)
- intraosseous, via bone marrow or spinal needle inserted into the intramedullary space of the proximal tibia, trochanteric fossa of the femur, or other site
- peripheral vein
- intralingual, under the dorsal mucosa of the tongue

Intracardiac injections are best avoided unless made under direct visualization with compression of the ascending aorta. The main goals of drug therapy for cardiac arrest are to (1) support the circulation, (2) minimize acidosis, and (3) stabilize the heart rhythm.

### Support circulation

*Epinephrine.* Epinephrine is usually indicated because of its cardiostimulatory and pressor effects. Resulting vasoconstriction helps maintain blood pressure and improve venous return, although it can worsen myocardial ischemia. Central venous administration is preferred, but intratracheal administration can also be used. Intranasal administration (14 mg epinephrine per nostril) may also be effective. Intracardiac injections can cause severe cardiac and pulmonary damage, and intramyocardial epinephrine can induce refractory ventricular fibrillation.

Table 5-1

## Drug Doses for CPR in Dogs and Cats

| Drug | Dose |
|---|---|
| Epinephrine | (0.1 to) 0.2 mg/kg IV or 0.4 mg/kg IT (diluted with 2-5 ml sterile water or saline) q(3-)5min as needed; also can use IO; 1:1000 = 1 mg/ml |
| Methoxamine | 0.1-0.2 mg/kg IV; can use IT |
| Metaraminol | 0.1-0.2 mg/kg IV |
| Mephentermine | 0.1-0.5 mg/kg IV |
| Phenylephrine | 0.01-0.1 mg/kg IV |
| Norepinephrine | 0.01-0.1 mg/average dog |
| Dopamine | Dogs: 5-15 µg/kg/min; cats: 1-5 µg/kg/min CRI; can use IO |
| Sodium bicarbonate | 0.5-1 mEq/kg initial dose; up to 8 mEq/mg if prolonged arrest or CPR; do *not* give IT; can use IO |
| Calcium chloride (10%) | 0.1-0.26 ml/kg IV (or 1.5-2 ml/dog) |
| Calcium gluconate (10%) | 0.1-0.3 ml/kg IV; can use IO |
| Dexamethasone SP | 4 mg/kg IV; can use IO |
| Atropine | 0.04 mg/kg IV, IM, IT, IO |
| Lidocaine | Dogs: 2 mg/kg, up to 8 mg/kg IV; can use IT or IO |
| | Cats: 0.25-0.5 mg/kg slowly IV; see Table 4-3; can use IT or IO |
| Bretylium tosylate | 10 mg/kg IV |

*CRI,* Constant-rate infusion (see Table 4-3); *IO,* intraosseously; *IT,* intratracheally; *IV,* intravenously.

Current recommendations are to use epinephrine undiluted (1:1000) every (3 to) 5 minutes as needed. (The hemodynamic effects of high-dose epinephrine during CPR appear to last >5 minutes, so longer intervals between injections could be used.) A 1:10,000 dilution can be made for very small animals.

**Dopamine.** Dopamine stimulates the heart during cardiac arrest; however, it may induce arrhythmias, including ventricular fibrillation. Hypoxia, acidosis, halothane or other anesthetics, and myocardial trauma encourage catecholamine-induced arrhythmias. Dobutamine is not effective in the initial treatment of cardiac arrest.

**Other drugs.** Norepinephrine, methoxamine, metaraminol, and phenylephrine may be as effective as epinephrine in treatment of cardiac arrest. Isoproterenol should not be used because it causes peripheral vasodilation. Drugs that block α-receptors (e.g., phenothiazine tranquilizers) also cause vasodilation and should not be used. Bradycardia may respond to atropine, glycopyrrolate, or dopamine.

**Calcium chloride.** Calcium is generally not recommended because it can cause ventricular arrhythmias, myocardial tetany and hyperpolarization, and postanoxic tissue damage. However, in some situations, including severe hyperkalemia, hypocalcemia, and overdose of calcium entry blocking drugs, calcium is indicated.

**Fluids.** Successful resuscitation may require both intravascular fluid administration and pressor agents to restore effective circulating blood volume and venous return. However, large loading doses of IV fluids may predispose to pulmonary edema, and fluid loading during cardiac arrest can impede coronary perfusion. Therefore, in animals that show an incomplete vasoconstrictor response to epinephrine or that are hypovolemic, initial fluid rates of only 10 to 20 ml/kg are recommended. After effective CPR the fluid rate and type are adjusted to maintain organ perfusion.

### Minimize acidosis

Both metabolic and respiratory acidosis develop after cardiac arrest and can worsen cardiac function. Immediate artificial ventilation and cardiac massage should prevent serious acidosis, making bicarbonate therapy unnecessary; but delayed or prolonged CPR may necessitate large doses of bicarbonate to reverse acidosis.

If CPR is delayed for more than 2 minutes or if preexisting metabolic acidosis is suspected, sodium bicarbonate may be helpful. Bicarbonate is indicated when the venous pH is <7.2. Initial doses of 0.5 to 1 mEq/kg are usually given; sometimes total doses of up to 8 mEq/kg are needed. If blood gases cannot be measured, 0.5 mEq/kg of bicarbonate is given, and repeated in 10 minutes. Adequate ventilation is necessary to eliminate generated carbon dioxide ($CO_2$). Note: Bicarbonate should not be combined with (or even given in the same IV line as) solutions containing calcium or catecholamines, and it should not be administered intratracheally.

### Stabilize heart rhythm
Animals in which cardiac arrest appears imminent may respond to antiarrhythmic therapy and other supportive care. Atropine or glycopyrrolate should be used for bradycardia. Frequent ventricular premature contractions or ventricular tachycardia may be suppressed by lidocaine or other antiarrhythmic agents (see Chapter 4).

ECG diagnosis of the heart rhythm is important for choosing appropriate therapy throughout CPR. After successful resuscitation, antiarrhythmic or anticholinergic agents may be useful to normalize the heart rhythm and prevent recurrence of arrest. Continued attention to blood pressure, venous return, oxygenation, and acid-base balance is important.

## Electrocardiogram (E)
As soon as possible after detection of cardiac arrest, an ECG monitor should be connected to the patient; accurate diagnosis of the cardiac rhythm facilitates successful CPR. Ventricular fibrillation should be treated with electrical defibrillation.

## Follow-up (F)
### Monitoring
After successful CPR the animal should be monitored closely, as recurrent cardiac arrest is common. General supportive measures include (1) maintenance of the partial pressure of arterial carbon dioxide ($PaCO_2$) at approximately 25 mm Hg and diastolic pressure >60 mm Hg; (2) provision of supplemental oxygen and adequate circulating volume; and (3) correction of acid-base, electrolyte, and other metabolic disturbances. Thoracic radiographs should be obtained to detect pulmonary contusions or edema, rib fractures, pneumothorax, or pleural effusion that may have resulted from resuscitation. A complete blood count, serum biochemical profile, and urinalysis may also be helpful. Underlying abnormalities that may have led to the arrest (e.g., acid-base or electrolyte disturbances, hypoxia, sepsis, toxicity, neurologic disease, anesthesia, hypovolemia, advanced metabolic disorders, primary lung or cardiac disease) should be addressed.

### Circulatory and ventilatory support
IV fluids are usually indicated to prevent hypovolemia and optimally perfuse previously ischemic tissue capillary beds. The fluid rate is guided by the animal's hemodynamic state and urinary output. Some animals also require continued ventilatory support. Artificial hyperventilation may be helpful in decreasing intracranial pressure.

It is important to manage cardiac arrhythmias and frequently assess hemodynamic state by checking mucous membrane color and perfusion, heart rate, femoral pulse quality, and, if possible, arterial blood pressure. The lungs and heart should also be auscultated periodically. Dopamine or dobutamine infusion may help offset the depressed ventricular function that frequently occurs after cardiac arrest. Continuous ECG monitoring is advisable. A constant infusion of lidocaine may prevent the recurrence of ventricular arrhythmias or fibrillation.

### Optimizing cerebral function
Brain injury can result from cardiac arrest and resuscitation. Cerebral edema can be assumed if consciousness has not improved by 15 to 30 minutes after successful CPR or if CPR was performed for >15 min. Corticosteroids, mannitol, and furosemide have been used to reduce postresuscitative cerebral edema. However, steroids may be of no

benefit in terms of survival or neurologic recovery. Experimentally, calcium antagonists, iron chelators, free-radical scavengers, antiprostaglandins, dimethylsulfoxide, mild hypothermia (to approximately 93° F or 34° C), and hyperventilation are variably helpful in minimizing postresuscitation neurologic damage. Deferoxamine mesylate (an iron chelator) has been advocated for postresuscitation reperfusion injury. IV or intramuscular doses of 10 mg/kg repeated in 2 hours, then every 8 hours for 24 hours have been used.

# 6

# Myocardial Diseases of the Dog

## *(Text pp 106-121)*

Myocardial disease resulting in poor contractile function and cardiac chamber enlargement is an important cause of heart failure in dogs. Most clinical cases are idiopathic dilated cardiomyopathy (DCM) and affect the larger breeds of dog and Cocker Spaniels. Other myocardial diseases are less common and have no particular breed predisposition.

## DILATED CARDIOMYOPATHY (TEXT PP 106-114)

### Causes

DCM is characterized by poor myocardial contractility, with or without arrhythmias. Most cases are primary or idiopathic, possibly representing the end stage of different pathologic processes or metabolic defects. Genetic factors probably play a role, especially in Doberman Pinschers, Boxers, and Cocker Spaniels. Poor myocardial function can also be secondary to a variety of insults, some of which are discussed in the subsequent sections.

*Cardiotoxins.* Doxorubicin causes both acute and chronic cardiotoxicity. Progressive myocardial damage and fibrosis have developed with cumulative doses as low as 100 mg/m$^2$, although clinical cardiotoxicity is uncommon until cumulative doses exceed 240 mg/m$^2$. Breeds with a higher prevalence of idiopathic DCM and dogs with underlying cardiac abnormalities are at greater risk. Use of prolonged infusion times and a low-dose weekly schedule reduces the risk. Measurement of circulating cardiac troponin concentrations (see text p 48) may be useful in monitoring dogs for doxorubicin-induced myocardial injury.

Ethyl alcohol can cause severe myocardial depression and death, so slow administration of a diluted (≤20%) solution is advised. Other cardiotoxins include plant toxins (e.g., *Taxus,* foxglove, black locust, buttercups, lily of the valley, gossypol), cocaine, anesthetic drugs, cobalt, catecholamines, and ionophores such as monensin.

*Nutritional deficiencies.* DCM has been associated with L-carnitine–linked defects in myocardial metabolism in some dogs. An underlying genetic or acquired metabolic defect is suspected, rather than simple L-carnitine deficiency, although DCM has been reported in dogs fed strictly vegetarian diets. An association may exist between DCM and carnitine deficiency in some families of Boxers, Doberman Pinschers, Great Danes, Irish Wolfhounds, Newfoundlands, and Cocker Spaniels.

Measurement of plasma carnitine concentration is not a sensitive indicator of myocardial carnitine concentration. Most dogs with myocardial carnitine deficiency, diagnosed by endomyocardial biopsy, have normal or high plasma carnitine concentrations. Furthermore, the response to oral carnitine supplementation is inconsistent, and few patients show echocardiographic evidence of improved function. L-Carnitine supplementation does not suppress arrhythmias or prevent sudden death.

Low plasma taurine (and sometimes carnitine) concentrations have been found in American Cocker Spaniels with DCM. Oral supplementation with these amino acids can improve left ventricular size and function and reduce the need for heart failure medications in this breed. The role of dietary taurine is less clear in other breeds with DCM that also have low plasma taurine concentrations (some Golden Retrievers, Labrador Retrievers, and Saint Bernards; see text).

*Tachycardia-induced cardiomyopathy.* Rapid, incessant tachycardia leads to progressive myocardial dysfunction, activation of neurohormonal compensatory mechanisms, and congestive heart failure (CHF), a condition known as *tachycardia-induced cardiomyopathy* (TICM). The myocardial failure is sometimes reversible if the heart rate can be normalized. TICM has been described in dogs with atrioventricular (AV) nodal reciprocating tachycardias associated with accessory conduction pathways bypassing the AV node (e.g., Wolff-Parkinson-White syndrome; see Chapter 2).

*Coronary artery disease.* Atherosclerosis of major coronary arteries is rare in dogs, but it can accompany severe hypothyroidism and lead to acute myocardial infarction. Hyalinization of small coronary vessels and intramural myocardial infarctions have been described in association with chronic degenerative AV valve disease and in older dogs without endocardiosis (see text).

Acute myocardial infarction resulting from coronary embolization is uncommon. Most cases have underlying disease that encourages embolus and thrombus formation, such as bacterial endocarditis, neoplasia, severe renal disease, immune-mediated hemolytic anemia, acute pancreatitis, disseminated intravascular coagulation, or corticosteroid use.

*Other diseases.* Reduced myocardial function has been associated with hypothyroidism, pheochromocytoma, and diabetes mellitus, but it is unusual for heart failure to occur in dogs secondary to these conditions alone. Excessive sympathetic stimulation stemming from brain or spinal cord injury results in myocardial hemorrhage, necrosis, and arrhythmias (brain-heart syndrome). Muscular dystrophy of the fasciohumeral type (reported in Springer Spaniels) can result in atrial standstill and heart failure. Canine X-linked (Duchenne's) muscular dystrophy in Golden Retrievers and other breeds also has been associated with myocardial fibrosis and mineralization. Rarely, nonneoplastic (e.g., glycogen storage disease) and neoplastic infiltrative myocardial diseases interfere with normal myocardial function. Immunologic mechanisms may also play an important role in the pathogenesis of myocardial dysfunction in some dogs with myocarditis.

### Clinical features

Idiopathic DCM is most common in large and giant breeds, such as Great Danes, Doberman Pinschers, Saint Bernards, Scottish Deerhounds, Irish Wolfhounds, Boxers, Newfoundlands, Afghan Hounds, and Dalmatians. It has been reported in English and American Cocker Spaniels, English Bulldogs, and other smaller breeds, but it is rare in dogs weighing <12 kg. Males may be affected more often than females. Most dogs with DCM manifest heart failure when they are between 4 and 10 years old. The disease probably develops slowly, with ventricular function declining gradually over at least 2 to 3 years before signs of heart failure are seen.

Signs can develop rapidly, especially in sedentary dogs, in which early signs may not be noticed. Presenting complaints can include weakness, lethargy, tachypnea or dyspnea, exercise intolerance, cough (gagging), anorexia, abdominal distention (ascites), and syncope. Loss of muscle mass (cardiac cachexia), accentuated along the dorsal midline, may be severe. Some giant-breed dogs with mild to moderate left ventricular dysfunction are relatively asymptomatic, even in the presence of atrial fibrillation.

Physical examination findings vary with the degree of cardiac decompensation. Poor cardiac output with high sympathetic tone causes pale mucous membranes and prolonged capillary refill time. Femoral arterial pulses and the precordial impulse are often weak and rapid. Signs of CHF (see Chapter 3) are usually present. Heart sounds can be muffled by pleural effusion or poor cardiac contractile strength. An audible $S_3$ gallop sound (see Chapter 1) is a classic finding, although it may be obscured by an irregular heart rhythm. Uncontrolled atrial fibrillation and frequent ventricular premature contractions (VPCs) cause a rapid and irregular heartbeat, with frequent pulse deficits and variable pulse strength. Soft-to-moderate intensity systolic murmurs of mitral or tricuspid regurgitation or both are common.

## Diagnosis
### Radiography
Generalized cardiomegaly is usually evident, although left atrial and ventricular enlargement may predominate. Cardiomegaly may be severe enough to mimic pericardial effusion. Dobermans and some Boxers appear to have mainly left atrial enlargement without marked cardiomegaly. Stage of disease, chest conformation, and hydration status influence the radiographic findings (see Chapter 2). Distended pulmonary veins and interstitial opacities, especially in the hilar and dorsocaudal regions, suggest left-sided heart failure and pulmonary edema. Pleural effusion, distention of the caudal vena cava, hepatomegaly, and ascites usually accompany right-sided heart failure.
### Electrocardiography
Electrocardiographic findings are variable. The QRS complexes may be tall (consistent with left ventricular dilation), normal sized, or smaller than usual. Myocardial disease can produce a widened QRS with sloppy R wave descent and slurred ST segment. Sometimes a bundle branch block pattern or other intraventricular conduction disturbance is present (see Chapter 2). The P waves frequently are widened and notched, suggesting left atrial enlargement. Premature atrial complexes, paroxysmal atrial tachycardia, and atrial fibrillation are common, especially in Great Danes and other giant breeds. VPCs and paroxysmal ventricular tachycardia may coexist with sinus rhythm or atrial fibrillation.
### Echocardiography
Dilated chambers and poor ventricular wall and septal motion are characteristic. All chambers are usually affected, but right atrial and ventricular dimensions may appear normal, especially in Dobermans and Boxers. Left ventricular systolic dimension is increased, and fractional shortening is decreased. Other common features are wide mitral valve E point–septal separation and reduced aortic root motion. Left ventricular free wall and septal thickness are normal or decreased. Mild to moderate AV valve regurgitation may be apparent with Doppler studies. Dobutamine stress testing may be useful in identification of early myocardial dysfunction in dogs at risk for DCM (see text).
### Clinical pathology
Prerenal azotemia and mildly increased serum liver enzyme activities may be present as a result of poor perfusion. Hypoproteinemia and dilutional hyponatremia can also be found in patients with severe heart failure, but serum biochemistry is unhelpful in many cases. Hypothyroidism with hypercholesterolemia occurs in some dogs. However, some dogs with DCM have decreased serum thyroid hormone concentrations without hypothyroidism (sick euthyroid), so thyroid-stimulating hormone (TSH) stimulation or free-$T_4$ determination may be useful. High serum cardiac troponin (cTnT or cTnI; see Chapter 2) concentrations are present in some dogs with DCM.
### Treatment
Therapy is aimed at controlling signs of CHF, optimizing cardiac output, managing arrhythmias, improving the quality of life, and prolonging survival. Digoxin, an angiotensin-converting enzyme inhibitor (ACEI), and furosemide form the core treatments for most dogs (Table 6-1). A stronger inotropic agent and other therapy may be needed for dogs with fulminant heart failure (see Chapter 3). Antiarrhythmic agents and other drugs are used as needed in individual patients (see Chapter 4). Exercise and dietary salt restriction help decrease cardiac workload and water retention (see Chapter 3).

**Table 6-1**

## Treatment Outline for Dogs with Dilated Cardiomyopathy

| Therapy | Drug |
| --- | --- |
| **INITIAL THERAPY OF ACUTE FAILURE** | |
| Diuretic | Furosemide |
| Inotropic support | Digoxin |
| | + Dobutamine or dopamine |
| | + Amrinone (or milrinone) |
| ACEI | Enalapril or other |
| **and/or** | |
| Other vasodilator | Nitroprusside or hydralazine-nitroglycerine, or amlodipine |
| Oxygen | — |
| Bronchodilator | + Theophylline or aminophylline |
| Cage confinement | — |
| Other therapy | + Morphine |
| | ± Fluids |
| Antiarrhythmic drugs, as needed | (see Chapter 4 and Table 4-3) |
| **CHRONIC THERAPY** | |
| Diuretic | Furosemide and spironolactone |
| Inotropic support | Digoxin |
| ACEI | Enalapril or other |
| + Other vasodilator | Amlodipine or hydralazine (+ nitrate) |
| Exercise restriction | — |
| Sodium restriction | — |
| Other therapy | + Trial of L-carnitine, taurine, other (see text) |
| Antiarrhythmic drugs, as needed | (see Chapter 4 and Table 4-3) |
| **THERAPY FOR ATRIAL FIBRILLATION IF HEART RATE INADEQUATELY CONTROLLED WITH DIGOXIN** | |
| β-Blocker | Atenolol, propranolol, or other |
| **or** | |
| $Ca^+$ entry blocker | Diltiazem |

See Tables 3-2, 3-3, and 4-3 for dosages and Chapters 3 and 4 for further information.
*ACEI,* Angiotensin-converting enzyme inhibitor; *$Ca^+$,* calcium.

Most dogs with DCM are presented with some degree of CHF. The severity of failure generally determines the aggressiveness of therapy. Because clinical status can deteriorate rapidly, frequent reevaluation is important. Cardiogenic shock can result from the markedly decreased ventricular contractility of severe DCM, especially after excessive diuresis and vasodilation.

*Inotropic support.* Therapy usually includes oral digoxin. If necessary, stronger inotropic support can be temporarily provided by IV infusion of dobutamine or dopamine for 2 (to 3) days, with or without the addition of amrinone or milrinone. However, long-term use of strong positive inotropes can have detrimental effects on the myocardium. During infusion the animal must be closely observed for worsening tachycardia or arrhythmias. If VPCs or other arrhythmias develop, the drug is discontinued or infused at up to half the original rate. If atrial fibrillation is present, catecholamines can be harmful.

When dopamine or dobutamine is necessary, digoxin should first be given either by mouth (PO) or by cautious intravenous (IV) loading. Diltiazem (rapid PO or cautious IV administration) is an alternative to IV digoxin. Amrinone or milrinone can be helpful for short-term stabilization of some dogs and can be used concurrently with digoxin and a catecholamine. Dose rates and regimens for these drugs are given in Chapter 3.

Some dogs, especially Dobermans, develop digoxin toxicity at relatively low doses. An upper limit of 0.5 mg/day is generally used for larger and giant breed dogs, except for Dobermans, which are given a total maximum dose of 0.25 to 0.375 mg/day.

*Antiarrhythmic agents.* Dogs with atrial fibrillation and a ventricular rate >200 beats/min can be cautiously given IV digoxin (see Table 3-3), or twice the PO maintenance dose on the first day, to more rapidly achieve effective blood concentrations. However, diltiazem (IV or rapid PO) is probably safer. Serum electrolyte, creatinine, and blood urea nitrogen (BUN) concentrations should be monitored, as hypokalemia and azotemia predispose to digoxin toxicity.

If digoxin alone has not significantly reduced the heart rate after 36 to 48 hours, a β-blocker or diltiazem can be added (see Table 4-3). Because these agents can have negative inotropic effects, a low initial dose and gradual dosage titration until effective or until maximum recommended level is reached are advised. Heart rate control in dogs with atrial fibrillation is very important. An in-hospital maximum ventricular rate of 150 beats/min is the recommended target; heart rates <100 beats/min are the goal at home.

The electrocardiogram (ECG) should be monitored for ventricular arrhythmias. If frequent or repetitive VPCs are present initially, digoxin should be used only at low doses or withheld until the VPCs are controlled with antiarrhythmic therapy (see Chapter 4). Quinidine should be avoided.

*Diuretics.* Furosemide is the most commonly used diuretic. High doses (3 to 5 mg/kg, up to 8 mg/kg) can initially be used parenterally if needed. For chronic therapy the lowest effective dose given PO at consistent time intervals is best; dose and frequency can be increased as necessary. Hypokalemia and alkalosis are uncommon unless anorexia or vomiting occurs. Potassium supplements may be given if hypokalemia is documented, but they must be used cautiously if an ACEI or spironolactone is also being administered.

Spironolactone, in combination with ACEIs and loop diuretics, can reduce mortality in humans with moderate to severe heart failure. In addition to the ACEIs, furosemide, and digoxin used for chronic therapy of DCM, simultaneous use of spironolactone is gaining favor.

*Vasodilators.* An ACEI should be used in the treatment of DCM. These drugs minimize clinical signs, increase exercise tolerance, and improve survival in dogs with myocardial failure. Therapy with an ACEI may also benefit dogs with subclinical myocardial dysfunction.

Hydralazine can also improve cardiac output and exercise tolerance and help reduce congestion. However, it can precipitate hypotension and reflex tachycardia and tends to increase the neurohormonal activation of heart failure. In dogs that do not tolerate an ACEI, hydralazine can be used in combination with a nitrate. Amlodipine could also be useful as adjunct therapy for dogs with refractory heart failure, although it is necessary to carefully monitor arterial blood pressure in such animals.

Any vasodilator must be used judiciously in dogs with low cardiac reserve because of the increased potential for hypotension. Therapy is initiated with a low dose; if this is well tolerated, the next dose is increased to a low maintenance level. The animal should be evaluated for several hours after each incremental dose (see Chapter 3).

*Fluid therapy.* Fluid administration (subcutaneous [SC] or IV) may be needed, especially after aggressive diuretic therapy. High cardiac filling pressures are often necessary to maintain cardiac output in these dogs. Dextrose (5%) in water with KCl added (12 mEq/500 ml), or 0.45% NaCl and 2.5% dextrose with KCl added can be used at conservative rates, such as 20 to 40 ml/kg/day. Careful monitoring is essential, as overhydration and pulmonary edema may develop rapidly.

*Bronchodilators.* Bronchodilator therapy may be beneficial in dogs with severe acute pulmonary edema and bronchoconstriction. Aminophylline also has transient diuretic properties and a mild positive inotropic effect. It can be given via the IV or IM (4 to 8 mg/kg) route or PO (6 to 10 mg/kg) q8h. Chronic bronchodilator administration is not recommended.

*Monitoring.* Owners should be instructed to monitor the dog's resting respiratory and heart rates at home. Periodic reevaluation, once or twice a week at first, is advised. Serum electrolyte and creatinine (or BUN) concentrations, ECG, pulmonary status, serum digoxin concentration, body weight, and other appropriate parameters can be evaluated, and treatment adjusted as needed.

*Dietary supplementation.* Oral L-carnitine supplementation improves survival times in some dogs. Doses of 50 to 200 mg/kg every 8 hours or 1 g (Cocker Spaniels) to 2 g (large or giant breeds) every 8 to 12 hours have been used. A small percentage of dogs show marked improvement, but it is doubtful that high doses of L-carnitine in the absence of myocardial carnitine deficiency are beneficial. Nevertheless, as carnitine supplementation appears to be safe, a 3- to 6-month trial of supplementation is reasonable. Dogs that respond exhibit improved activity within 1 to 4 weeks and echocardiographic improvement after 2 to 3 months of supplementation. However, a response plateau is reached in 6 to 8 months.

Supplemental taurine (500 mg PO q8h) can be given to dogs with plasma taurine concentrations <25 nmol/ml. Empiric supplementation of taurine and carnitine may be beneficial in American Cocker Spaniels with DCM. Supplementation with antioxidant vitamins and fish oil (a source of ω-3 fatty acids) may be of value in dogs with myocardial dysfunction (see text).

*Chronic β-blocker therapy.* Long-term, low-dose β-blocker therapy with carvedilol or metoprolol may be beneficial if the dog can tolerate it. Note: This approach is only for dogs with chronic, stable DCM. β-Blockers can acutely worsen myocardial function and cause clinical deterioration. Definitive recommendations await further study and clinical experience.

*Other therapies.* Pimobendan (a phosphodiesterase III inhibitor) improves cardiac function and can cause marked clinical improvement when added to conventional therapy. This drug is now available in the United States for clinical trials. Dynamic cardiomyoplasty has been described for the treatment of DCM. Although results in some dogs are encouraging, this is unlikely to become a widely used treatment.

### Prognosis

The prognosis is guarded to poor. Sudden death can occur, even in the occult stage. Most dogs do not survive longer than 3 months after clinical manifestations of heart failure, although 25% to 40% live longer than 6 months if the initial response to therapy is good. The probability of survival for 2 years is estimated at 7.5% to 28%. Pleural effusion (and possibly ascites) and pulmonary edema are independent indicators of poor prognosis. Doberman Pinschers have especially short survival times. In each case, however, it is reasonable to assess response to initial treatment before pronouncing an unequivocally dismal prognosis.

## Cardiomyopathy in Boxers

Boxers with cardiomyopathy have a high prevalence of ventricular arrhythmias and syncope. Clinical features vary, and three disease categories have been described: (1) asymptomatic dogs that have ventricular tachyarrhythmia; (2) dogs that have normal heart size and left ventricular function but signs of syncope and weakness resulting from paroxysmal or sustained ventricular tachycardia; and (3) less prevalent, dogs with poor myocardial function and CHF, as well as ventricular arrhythmias. Histologic myocardial changes are more extensive than those in other breeds with cardiomyopathy.

### Clinical features

Clinical signs can appear at any age, although the mean age is 8.5 years. The disease is more prevalent in some bloodlines. The most consistent clinical finding is arrhythmia. When CHF occurs, left-sided signs are more common than ascites or other signs of right-sided heart failure. Many affected Boxers also develop a mitral insufficiency murmur.

#### Diagnosis
*ECG findings.* The ECG usually documents an underlying sinus rhythm, although atrial fibrillation, supraventricular tachycardia, conduction abnormalities, and evidence of chamber enlargement sometimes occur. The characteristic finding is ventricular ectopy. VPCs occur singly, in pairs, in short runs, or as sustained ventricular tachycardia. Most ectopic ventricular complexes appear upright in leads II and $aV_F$; some Boxers have multiform VPCs.

Twenty-four–hour Holter monitoring is often recommended as a screening test for Boxer cardiomyopathy, as well as a means of evaluating the efficacy of antiarrhythmic drug therapy. Frequent VPCs and complex ventricular arrhythmias are characteristic findings in affected dogs. Dogs with very frequent VPCs or episodes of ventricular tachycardia are at increased risk for syncope and sudden death.

*Diagnostic imaging.* Radiographic findings are variable; many Boxers have no visible abnormalities. Those with signs of CHF usually have evidence of cardiomegaly and pulmonary edema. Echocardiographic findings vary, from normal cardiac size and function to chamber dilation with poor fractional shortening. Dogs with mild echocardiographic changes and those with syncope or weakness may develop CHF at a later time.

#### Treatment
Therapy for symptomatic Boxers with normal heart size and left ventricular function is usually limited to antiarrhythmic drugs. However, antiarrhythmic therapy that reduces the number of VPCs may still not prevent sudden death. The focus now is on drugs or drug combinations that also increase the ventricular fibrillation threshold, such as sotalol, amiodarone, or atenolol with either procainamide or mexiletine (see Chapter 4). The class III agents (sotalol, amiodarone) are gaining favor. Suppression of persistent supraventricular tachyarrhythmias is sometimes necessary.

Therapy for CHF is similar to that described for dogs with DCM; however, digoxin is used sparingly or not at all if frequent ventricular tachyarrhythmias are present. Myocardial carnitine deficiency has been documented in some Boxers with DCM and heart failure; some of these dogs responded to L-carnitine supplementation (see text p 114).

#### Prognosis
The prognosis for affected Boxers is guarded to poor. If heart failure is present, death usually occurs within 6 months. Asymptomatic dogs may have a more optimistic future, but the likelihood of development of serious, refractory arrhythmias and CHF is high. Many Boxers with cardiomyopathy die suddenly, presumably from VPCs that lead to ventricular fibrillation.

### Cardiomyopathy in Doberman Pinschers
This breed appears to have the highest prevalence of DCM; a genetic basis is believed to exist. The prevalence of subclinical (occult) disease in adult Dobermans may be as high as 44%. The disease evolves over years before clinical signs become evident. (Most symptomatic dogs are between 5 and 10 years old at the time of death.) Males generally become symptomatic at an earlier age than females. Sudden death before the onset of CHF is common.

#### Clinical features
The disease is clinically similar to idiopathic DCM in other large-breed dogs. However, the combination of ventricular tachyarrhythmias and severely compromised left ventricular contractility is very common in Dobermans. The history often includes episodic weakness or syncope. Sudden death from ventricular tachycardia–fibrillation is common, although some Dobermans exhibit syncope resulting from bradycardia associated with excitement or exertion, rather than from ventricular tachycardia. Fulminant pulmonary edema often appears acutely, and cardiogenic shock can result from poor cardiac output and CHF.

#### Diagnosis
*ECG findings.* The ECG often documents an underlying sinus rhythm, although atrial fibrillation is relatively common. Ventricular tachyarrhythmias occur frequently in Dobermans with DCM. Once left ventricular function begins to deteriorate, the

frequency of tachyarrhythmias increases. Paroxysmal or sustained ventricular tachycardia, fusion complexes, and multiform VPCs are common, and the QRS complexes often appear wide and sloppy. Twenty-four–hour Holter monitoring usually documents frequent ventricular ectopy.

*Diagnostic imaging.* Radiographically the heart may not appear greatly enlarged, with the exception of the left atrium. Severe and diffuse infiltrates of pulmonary edema occur in dogs with CHF. On echocardiography, Dobermans with fulminant CHF typically have prominent left ventricular dilation and extremely low fractional shortening (often <10%).

### Treatment and prognosis

Therapy is as described for DCM in large and giant breeds (see Table 6-1), with specific antiarrhythmic therapy frequently indicated, as for Boxers. The prognosis in most cases is guarded to grave, depending on the severity of heart failure and response to initial therapy. Sudden death occurs in 20% to 40% of affected dogs, often before the onset of clinical CHF. Dogs with mild DCM diagnosed before clinical signs appear do well for a time, but their condition usually deteriorates within 6 to 12 months. Dogs in overt CHF when first seen generally do not live long (median, <7 weeks). The prognosis is worse if atrial fibrillation is present in dogs with CHF.

### Screening

Early diagnosis may help prolong life. Cardiac evaluation is indicated in dogs with a history of reduced exercise tolerance, weakness, or syncope or in which an arrhythmia, murmur, or gallop sound is detected. Ambulatory (Holter) ECG monitoring for 24 to 48 hours is useful for screening. A finding of >50 VPCs in 24 hours or any couplets or triplets is thought to be predictive of future DCM. However, many dogs with <50 VPCs in 24 hours on initial evaluation have developed cardiomyopathy several years later. Signal-averaged electrocardiography may be useful if available (see text).

The following echocardiographic criteria may indicate a high risk for overt DCM within 2 to 3 years in asymptomatic dogs: left ventricular internal diameter at end diastole ($LVID_d$) >46 mm; left ventricular internal diameter at end systole ($LVID_s$) >38 mm; or VPCs during initial examination (see Table 2-3). Occult DCM in clinically normal Dobermans may be suggested by the following indices: $LVID_d$ >45 mm (dogs <38 kg) or >49 mm (dogs >37 kg); fractional shortening <25%; and mitral valve E point–septal separation >8 mm.

## HYPERTROPHIC CARDIOMYOPATHY (TEXT PP 115-116)

Hypertrophic cardiomyopathy (HCM) is uncommon in dogs. The cause is unknown, although a genetic basis is suspected. Several disease processes may produce similar ventricular changes.

### Clinical features

Young to middle-aged, large-breed dogs are most commonly diagnosed with HCM; there may be a higher incidence in males. Clinical signs of heart failure, episodic weakness, and syncope occur in some dogs; however, sudden death can occur before other cardiac signs, probably as a result of ventricular arrhythmias. A systolic murmur of left ventricular outflow obstruction or mitral insufficiency may be heard on auscultation. The ejection murmur is accentuated when contractility is increased (e.g., by exercise or in beats after VPCs) or when systemic arterial pressure is decreased by a vasodilator. An atrial gallop sound ($S_4$) is heard in some dogs.

### Diagnosis

Echocardiography is the best diagnostic tool. An abnormally thick left ventricle, with or without narrowing of the left ventricular outflow area or asymmetric septal hypertrophy, and left atrial enlargement are characteristic. Mitral regurgitation may be evident on Doppler echocardiography. Severe outflow obstruction causes systolic anterior motion of the mitral valve and partial systolic aortic valve closure. Other causes of left ventricular hypertrophy include congenital subaortic stenosis, hypertensive renal disease, thyrotoxicosis, and pheochromocytoma.

Thoracic radiographs may be normal or may indicate left atrial and ventricular enlargement, with or without pulmonary congestion or edema. Ventricular tachyarrhythmias and conduction abnormalities are common on ECG. Criteria for left ventricular enlargement are variably present.

### Treatment

The goals are to enhance myocardial relaxation and ventricular filling, control pulmonary edema, and suppress arrhythmias. A β-blocker or calcium entry blocker may lower the heart rate, prolong ventricular filling time, and reduce ventricular contractility and myocardial oxygen ($O_2$) demand (see Chapter 4). β-Blockers may also increase the threshold for arrhythmias, and the mild negative inotropic effects of these agents and of verapamil reduce dynamic outflow obstruction. However, both classes of drugs may worsen AV conduction abnormalities, so they may be contraindicated in certain patients. Diuretics are indicated if signs of CHF are present. Digoxin should not be used, because it may increase myocardial $O_2$ demand, worsen outflow obstruction, and predispose to ventricular arrhythmias. Marked exercise restriction is advised in dogs with HCM.

## ARRHYTHMOGENIC RIGHT VENTRICULAR CARDIOMYOPATHY (TEXT P 116)

A rare form of cardiomyopathy limited mainly to the right ventricle has been observed in dogs. It appears to be similar to right ventricular cardiomyopathy in cats (see Chapter 7). Pathologic changes are characterized by widespread replacement of the right ventricular myocardium by fibrous and fatty tissue. Trypanosomiasis may be a differential diagnosis in certain geographic areas. Clinical manifestations are largely related to right-sided CHF with marked right heart dilation and severe ventricular tachyarrhythmias. Sudden death is a common outcome.

## MYOCARDITIS (TEXT PP 116-118)

### Infective Myocarditis

The heart can be injured by direct invasion of the infective agent, by toxins it elaborates, or by the host's immune response. Myocarditis can cause persistent cardiac arrhythmias and progressive impairment of myocardial function.

#### Etiology and clinical features

*Viral.* Parvovirus can cause a fatal, peracute necrotizing myocarditis in puppies 4 to 8 weeks old that are not protected by maternal antibodies; this condition is now uncommon. Parvovirus can also cause a form of DCM in young dogs that survive neonatal infection. Canine distemper virus can cause myocarditis in young puppies, although multisystemic signs usually predominate.

*Bacterial.* Bacteremia and bacterial endocarditis or pericarditis can cause focal or multifocal suppurative myocardial inflammation or abscess formation. Localized infections elsewhere in the body may be the source of the organisms. Clinical signs include malaise, weight loss, and, inconsistently, fever. Arrhythmias and cardiac conduction abnormalities are common, but murmurs are rare unless valvular endocarditis or another underlying cardiac defect is present. Serial blood cultures may allow identification of the organism. Recently, *Bartonella vinsonii* spp. have been associated with cardiac arrhythmias, myocarditis, and endocarditis in dogs.

*Lyme disease.* Lyme carditis is recognized more frequently in the northeastern, western coastal, and north central United States. It can cause third-degree (complete) or high-grade second-degree heart block. Syncope, CHF, impaired myocardial contractility, and ventricular arrhythmias have also been identified in affected dogs. A presumptive diagnosis is made by positive (or increasing) serum titers and concurrent signs of myocarditis, with or without other systemic signs. Endomyocardial biopsy, if available, may help in confirming the diagnosis. Treatment with an appropriate antibiotic should be instituted (see Chapter 98), although antimicrobial therapy may not resolve AV conduction disturbances. Cardiac drugs are used as needed.

*Trypanosoma cruzi.* Trypanosomiasis (Chagas' disease) occurs mainly in young dogs in Texas, Louisiana, and other southern states. Acute, latent, and chronic phases of Chagas' myocarditis have been described. Lethargy, depression, and other systemic signs, as well as tachyarrhythmias, AV conduction defects, and sudden death have been reported with acute infection, although clinical signs can be subtle. Diagnosis in the acute stage is by identification of trypomastigotes in thick peripheral blood smears. Isolation of the organism can be done in cell culture or by mouse inoculation. Animals that survive enter a latent phase of variable duration, during which parasitemia resolves and antibodies against the organism develop.

Chronic Chagas' disease is characterized by progressive, right-sided or generalized cardiomegaly and arrhythmias (most notably ventricular, but sometimes supraventricular, tachyarrhythmias). Ventricular dilation and reduced myocardial function are usually evident on echocardiogram, and clinical signs of biventricular failure are common. Serologic testing may allow antemortem diagnosis in chronic cases. Therapy for the acute stage is aimed at eliminating the organisms and minimizing myocardial inflammation. Therapy for chronic Chagas' disease is directed at supporting myocardial function, controlling signs of CHF, and suppressing arrhythmias.

*Other protozoa.* Myocardial involvement with *Hepatozoon canis* has been reported in dogs along the Texas coast. Clinical signs include stiffness, anorexia, fever, neutrophilia, and periosteal new bone reaction.

*Miscellaneous causes.* In rare instances myocarditis is caused by fungi *(Aspergillus, Cryptococcus, Coccidioides, Histoplasma, Paecilomyces);* rickettsiae *(Rickettsia rickettsii, Ehrlichia canis, Bartonella elizabethae);* algaelike organisms *(Prototheca);* and nematode larval migration *(Toxocara* spp.) Affected animals are usually immunosuppressed and have systemic signs of disease. Rocky Mountain spotted fever *(R. rickettsii)* occasionally causes fatal ventricular arrhythmias, along with necrotizing vasculitis, myocardial thrombosis, and ischemia.

### Diagnosis

The classic clinical presentation of acute myocarditis involves the unexplained onset of arrhythmias or heart failure after a recent episode of infectious disease or drug exposure. The diagnosis may be equivocal, however, because no clinical or clinicopathologic findings specific for myocarditis are present. In addition to complete blood count, serum biochemical profile, thoracic and abdominal radiographs, and urinalysis, serum cardiac troponin concentrations (see Chapter 2) may be useful.

Nonspecific electrocardiographic changes include ST segment shifts, T-wave or QRS voltage changes, and AV conduction abnormalities. Echocardiographic signs of poor regional or global wall motion, altered myocardial echogenicity, or pericardial effusion may also be found but are fairly nonspecific. In dogs with persistent fever, serial bacterial (or fungal) blood cultures may be rewarding. Serologic screening for known infectious causes may also be helpful. However, endomyocardial biopsy is presently the only means of obtaining a definitive antemortem diagnosis, although it may not provide diagnostic tissue samples when the lesions are focal.

### Treatment

Unless a specific cause can be identified and treated, therapy for suspected myocarditis is largely supportive: strict rest, antiarrhythmic therapy as needed (see Chapter 4), an ACEI with or without digoxin, a diuretic, and other support as needed (see Chapter 3). Corticosteroids have not proved to be beneficial in dogs with myocarditis, and considering the possible infective cause, they are not recommended as nonspecific therapy.

## Noninfective Myocarditis

Myocardial inflammation can result from the effects of drugs, toxins, or immunologic responses. Potential causes include heavy metals (e.g., arsenic, lead, mercury), antineoplastic drugs (doxorubicin, cyclophosphamide, 5-fluorouracil, interleukin-2, interferon-$\alpha$), other drugs (e.g., catecholamines, thyroid hormone, cocaine, amphetamines, lithium), and toxins (wasp or scorpion stings, snake venom, spider bites). Immune-mediated diseases and pheochromocytoma can also cause myocarditis.

## Traumatic Myocarditis

Blunt trauma to the chest can cause arrhythmias that appear 24 to 48 hours after trauma. VPCs, ventricular tachycardia, and accelerated idioventricular rhythms (60 to 100 beats/min) occur most often. Accelerated idioventricular rhythms usually are manifested only when the sinus rate slows or pauses. They are benign in most dogs with normal underlying heart function and generally disappear within a week. Antiarrhythmic therapy is usually unnecessary, although the animal should be closely monitored. More serious arrhythmias (e.g., faster rate or multiform configuration) and hemodynamic deterioration are indications for antiarrhythmic therapy (see Chapter 4).

Traumatic avulsion of AV valve papillary muscles, septal perforation, and rupture of the heart or pericardium may also result from chest trauma. Acute low-output failure and shock, as well as arrhythmias, can develop quickly in such animals. Traumatic papillary muscle avulsion causes acute volume overload and rapid onset of CHF. Chest radiographs, serum biochemistries, and ECG are recommended in the assessment of patients with chest trauma. Echocardiography may be indicated to define preexisting heart disease or unexpected cardiovascular findings, but it is not a sensitive tool for identifying small areas of myocardial injury. Measurement of serum cardiac troponin concentrations may be more useful.

## CARDIOGENIC SHOCK (TEXT PP 118-120)

Cardiogenic shock results from profound impairment of cardiac pumping ability. Possible causes are listed in Box 6-1. Severe DCM is the most common cause of cardiogenic shock in dogs.

### Clinical features

Tachycardia (unless shock is caused by a bradyarrhythmia), weak pulses, pallor, prolonged capillary refill time, cyanosis, hyperventilation, oliguria, and depression are common. Arrhythmias, a murmur or gallop sound, decreased-intensity heart sounds, acute pulmonary edema, and systemic venous distention (with right-sided heart failure or cardiac tamponade) can also occur.

### Treatment

Therapy is aimed at restoring organ perfusion; support of arterial blood pressure, forward cardiac output, and vascular volume is crucial. The underlying abnormality must also be identified and corrected for optimal treatment. Glucocorticoids are unlikely to be of benefit in animals with cardiogenic shock.

*Renal perfusion.* Acute renal failure is a major sequela of prolonged hypotension and renal hypoperfusion. Dopamine, infused at low doses (see Table 3-3), promotes renal vasodilation; however, at higher doses it can cause peripheral vasoconstriction. Fluid therapy is important but must be administered cautiously to patients in heart failure.

*Acidosis.* Severe metabolic acidosis frequently occurs in patients in shock. Ideally, bicarbonate therapy is guided by evaluation of venous blood gases. Measurement of total carbon dioxide can be used to estimate acid-base status, as long as pulmonary function is relatively normal. Clinical evaluation of peripheral perfusion can also help guide bicarbonate therapy. Mild, moderate, and severe impairments of perfusion are treated with IV sodium bicarbonate at 1, 3, or 5 mEq/kg, respectively. Complications of rapid or excessive bicarbonate administration include alkalosis, hypotension, paradoxic CSF acidosis, cerebral edema, hypercapnia, and vomiting.

*Ventilation support.* Supplemental $O_2$ is indicated for animals with pulmonary edema. Thoracocentesis should be performed when pleural effusion is present. Assisted ventilation, with positive end-expiratory pressure, may be of benefit in dogs with severe edema or other pulmonary complications (see Chapter 3).

*Monitoring.* Frequent reassessment is important, particularly indirect or direct measurement of arterial blood pressure. A mean arterial pressure consistently >60 mm Hg or systolic pressure >80 mm Hg is desirable. Indirect measures of organ perfusion (CRT, mucous membrane color, urine output, toe-web temperature, and improved mentation) are also helpful. Reversal of severe peripheral vasoconstriction, combined

---

**Box 6-1**

## Causes of Cardiogenic Shock

**MYOPATHIC**

Dilated cardiomyopathy
Myocarditis
Myocardial infarction

**VALVULAR**

Rupture of chordae tendineae
Papillary muscle avulsion
Acute aortic regurgitation

**INTRACARDIAC OBSTRUCTION**

Intracardiac tumor
Hypertrophic obstructive cardiomyopathy
Aortic stenosis

**ARRHYTHMIAS**

Sustained ventricular tachycardia
Sustained atrial or supraventricular tachycardia
Uncontrolled atrial fibrillation or flutter
Complete heart block or atrial standstill with slow escape rhythm
Severe sinus bradycardia

**DRUG OVERDOSE**

Vasodilators
β-Adrenergic blockers
Calcium entry blockers

**EXTRACARDIAC OBSTRUCTION**

Cardiac tamponade
Heartworm disease
Massive pulmonary thromboembolism
Other causes of pulmonary hypertension

---

with strong femoral pulses, often indicates effective therapy. However, arterial blood pressure and femoral pulse strength are not always associated with adequate tissue perfusion or volume replacement.

Measurement of pulmonary arterial and capillary wedge pressures is useful and also provides access to mixed venous blood samples. Maintaining pulmonary wedge pressure in the high-normal range (10 to 15 mm Hg) is desirable. Electrolyte balance and renal function should also be monitored. A serum potassium concentration maintained in the mid- to high-normal range is especially important in animals with arrhythmias.

# 7

# Myocardial Diseases of the Cat

## (Text pp 122-138)

Diseases that cause myocardial hypertrophy are most common in cats and lead to abnormal ventricular stiffness and impaired cardiac filling. Restrictive pathophysiology is also common, but dilated cardiomyopathy (DCM) is rare. Myocardial disease in some cats is considered indeterminate or unclassified.

## HYPERTROPHIC CARDIOMYOPATHY (TEXT PP 122-129)

### Etiology

The cause of primary or idiopathic hypertrophic cardiomyopathy (HCM) in cats is unknown, although a genetic basis is thought to underlie some cases. The prevalence is high in several breeds, including Maine Coon, Persian, Ragdoll, and American Shorthair. Viral myocarditis may play a role in some cases.

Myocardial (ventricular) hypertrophy can also develop as a compensatory response to certain stresses or diseases, including hyperthyroidism, systemic arterial hypertension, fixed (e.g., subaortic stenosis) or dynamic left ventricular outflow obstruction, and hypersomatotropism (acromegaly). Increased myocardial thickness occasionally results from infiltrative myocardial disease (e.g., lymphoma). Secondary causes should be ruled out when left ventricular hypertrophy is identified.

### Clinical features

HCM is most common in middle-aged male cats, but clinical signs can occur in cats of any age. Cats with milder disease may be asymptomatic for years. Symptomatic cats are most often presented for respiratory signs (caused by pulmonary edema, pleural effusion, or both) or signs caused by acute thromboembolism (see later).

Respiratory signs include tachypnea, panting associated with activity, dyspnea, or, rarely, coughing (which can be misinterpreted as gagging). Disease onset may seem acute in sedentary cats. Syncope or sudden death is the only sign in some cats. Occasionally lethargy or anorexia is the only evidence of disease. Asymptomatic HCM is sometimes discovered by a murmur or gallop sound heard on auscultation. Stresses such as anesthesia, surgery, fluid administration, systemic illnesses (e.g., fever or anemia), and even boarding can precipitate heart failure.

Systolic murmurs of either mitral regurgitation or dynamic left ventricular outflow obstruction (functional subaortic stenosis) are common. However, some cats do not have an audible murmur, even with marked ventricular hypertrophy. A diastolic gallop sound (usually $S_4$) may be heard, especially if heart failure is evident or imminent. Cardiac arrhythmias are relatively common. Femoral pulses are usually strong, unless aortic thromboembolism has occurred. A vigorous precordial impulse is often palpable. Prominent lung sounds, pulmonary crackles, and sometimes cyanosis accompany severe pulmonary edema; pleural effusion attenuates pulmonary sounds ventrally. However, physical examination findings can be normal.

Note: Testing for hyperthyroidism (see Chapter 51) is indicated in cats >6 years of age with myocardial hypertrophy. Cardiovascular signs often include a systolic murmur, hyperdynamic precordial beat and arterial pulses, tachycardia and arrhythmias, and evidence of left ventricular enlargement or hypertrophy. Signs of congestive heart failure (CHF) develop in approximately 15% of hyperthyroid cats.

### Diagnosis

*Radiography.* Radiographic features of HCM include a prominent left atrium and variable left ventricular enlargement (see Chapter 2). The classic valentine-shaped appearance of the heart on dorsoventral or ventrodorsal view is not always present, although usually the point of the left ventricular apex is maintained. The cardiac silhouette appears normal in most cats with mild HCM. Enlarged and tortuous pulmonary veins may be seen. Variable degrees of patchy pulmonary edema develop in cats with left-sided heart failure. Pleural effusion suggests biventricular failure; hepatomegaly may also be noted in cats with right-sided failure.

*Electrocardiography.* Many cats with HCM (up to 70%) have abnormalities on the electrocardiogram (ECG). These often include criteria for left atrial and ventricular enlargement, ventricular or (less often) supraventricular tachyarrhythmias or both, or a left anterior fascicular block pattern (see Chapter 2). Occasionally, atrioventricular (AV) conduction delay, complete AV block, or sinus bradycardia is found.

*Echocardiography.* Echocardiography is the best diagnostic tool. Because the distribution of hypertrophy is variable, the entire ventricle should be carefully scanned (see text, p 124). The diagnosis may be questionable in cats with mild or only focal thickening. Cats with severe HCM have diastolic left ventricular or septal thicknesses (or both) >8 mm (normal value is 5 mm), although the degree of hypertrophy is not necessarily correlated with the severity of clinical signs. Left ventricular fractional shortening is generally normal or increased. However, some cats have mild-to-moderate left ventricular dilation and reduced contractility. Right ventricular enlargement and pericardial or pleural effusion are occasionally detected.

Cats with dynamic left ventricular outflow obstruction also often have systolic anterior motion of the mitral valve or premature closure of the aortic valve leaflets; mitral regurgitation and left ventricular outflow turbulence may be evident on Doppler scan. Left atrial enlargement may be mild to marked. Spontaneous contrast (swirling, smoky echoes) is visible within the enlarged left atrium of some cats and is thought to result from blood stasis and to be a harbinger of thromboembolism. A thrombus is occasionally seen within the left atrium, usually in the auricle.

Other causes of myocardial hypertrophy should be excluded before a diagnosis of idiopathic HCM is made. Myocardial thickening can also result from infiltrative disease; variation in myocardial echogenicity or wall irregularities may be noted in such cases.

### Treatment

The main therapeutic goals are to facilitate ventricular filling, relieve congestion, control arrhythmias, minimize ischemia, and prevent thromboembolism (Table 7-1). Stress and activity should be minimized. Diltiazem or a β-blocker (see Chapter 4 and Table 4-3) is the foundation of long-term oral therapy. Note: In general, digoxin, other positive inotropic agents, and arterial vasodilators are contraindicated in cats with HCM.

*Asymptomatic cats.* Debate exists regarding whether (and how) asymptomatic cats with HCM should be treated. It is unclear whether disease progression can be slowed or survival prolonged by instituting drug therapy before clinical signs develop. Nevertheless, some cats show an increased activity level or improved attitude with diltiazem or a β-blocker.

*β-Blockers.* The β-blockers can produce greater decreases in heart rate than diltiazem. They are also useful in controlling tachyarrhythmias and reducing systolic outflow obstruction and myocardial oxygen ($O_2$) demand through their negative inotropic

Table 7-1

## Outline of Therapy for Hypertrophic Cardiomyopathy

| Therapy | Drug |
|---|---|
| **INITIAL THERAPY OF ACUTE FAILURE** | |
| Diuretic | Furosemide |
| Oxygen | — |
| Vasodilator | Nitroglycerine, possibly ACEI |
| Bronchodilator | Aminophylline or theophylline |
| Cage confinement | — |
| Calcium entry blocker | Diltiazem |
| *or* | |
| β-blocker | Atenolol, propranolol (avoid with pulmonary edema or thromboembolism), or esmolol |
| ± Anticoagulants | Aspirin |
| | Heparin |
| | ± Others (see text) |
| Other therapy | ± Acepromazine |
| | ± Fluids |
| Antiarrhythmic drugs | β-blocker (or diltiazem) |
| | ± Lidocaine |
| | ± Procainamide |
| **CHRONIC Therapy** | |
| Diuretics (±) | Furosemide |
| | ± Other |
| Calcium entry blocker | Diltiazem |
| *or* | |
| β-blocker | Atenolol or propranolol |
| ± Anticoagulants | Aspirin, warfarin, LMWH |
| Exercise restriction | — |
| Sodium restriction | — |
| Antiarrhythmic (±) | β-blocker or other |

See text, Box 3-1 and Tables 3-2, and 4-3 for doses and Chapters 3 and 4 for further information.

*ACEI,* Angiotensin-converting enzyme inhibitor; *LMWH,* low–molecular-weight heparin.

effects. These effects can be especially important in cats with severe outflow obstruction, paroxysmal arrhythmias, or myocardial infarction. Atenolol is favored over diltiazem for cats with these problems.

Because propranolol is a nonselective β-blocker, it can cause bronchoconstriction. If propranolol is used in cats with CHF, its administration is usually delayed until after pulmonary edema is largely resolved. Some cats do not tolerate propranolol well (e.g., lethargy, anorexia). In these cases, atenolol or another β-blocker may be better tolerated, or diltiazem can be used.

**Diltiazem.** Diltiazem is well tolerated and effective in many cases. It promotes coronary vasodilation, enhances ventricular relaxation, causes mild decreases in heart rate and contractility, and may decrease systolic outflow gradients if peripheral vasodilation does not enhance ventricular shortening. However, it is generally less effective than the β-blockers in decreasing heart rate. Longer-acting diltiazem products are more convenient for chronic use (see Table 4-3).

Calcium entry blockers that have primarily vasodilatory effects (e.g., nifedipine, nicardipine) can cause reflex tachycardia and worsen systolic outflow gradients, so they are not used for cats with HCM. Verapamil has a greater negative inotropic effect than diltiazem, so it should be better for reducing ventricular outflow obstruction. However, it is not recommended because of its variable bioavailability and risk of toxicity in cats.

*Acute CHF.* Treatment of fulminant CHF is discussed in Chapter 3 and summarized in Box 3-1. After initial medications have been given, the cat should be allowed to rest, preferably while receiving $O_2$. Other manipulations should be delayed until the cat is more stable. Aminophylline could be helpful in cats with severe pulmonary edema, although it may increase the heart rate. Acepromazine can be used to reduce anxiety and promote peripheral redistribution of blood.

*Diuretic therapy.* Once respiratory distress has been alleviated, furosemide (approximately 1 mg/kg) can be continued q8-12h, guided by the cat's respiratory rate and effort. Once pulmonary edema has been controlled, furosemide is gradually reduced to the lowest effective oral dose and administration interval. Some cats do well with administration a couple of times per week, whereas others require it several times per day.

Complications of excessive diuresis include azotemia, anorexia, electrolyte disturbances, and suboptimal left ventricular filling pressure. Cautious fluid administration may be needed after excessive diuresis (e.g., 15 to 20 ml/kg/day of half-strength saline, 5% dextrose in water, or other low-sodium fluid). Some cats that have had an episode of CHF but are responding well to long-term therapy with diltiazem or a β-blocker can be weaned from furosemide therapy, but close monitoring for recurrence of pulmonary edema is necessary.

*Refractory heart failure.* Enalapril (and other angiotensin-converting enzyme inhibitors [ACEIs]) may be beneficial, especially in cats with refractory heart failure. Occasionally a β-blocker is added to diltiazem therapy (or vice versa) in cats in which failure is hard to control or in order to further reduce heart rate in cats with atrial fibrillation. However, care must be taken to prevent bradycardia or hypotension in animals receiving this combination.

Refractory pulmonary edema or pleural effusion is difficult to manage. Moderate- to large-volume pleural effusions should be drained. Other therapeutic strategies to consider include increasing the dose of furosemide (up to 4 mg/kg q8h), adding an ACEI, maximizing the dose of diltiazem or β-blocker, or adding another diuretic such as spironolactone, with or without hydrochlorothiazide (see Table 3-2). Frequent monitoring for azotemia or electrolyte disturbances is warranted. Digoxin can also be considered for the treatment of refractory right-sided heart failure in the absence of outflow obstruction.

Progressive development of left ventricular dilation and myocardial systolic failure is difficult to manage successfully. An ACEI, digoxin, and cautious β-blocker therapy along with diuretics are suggested. The blood taurine concentration should be measured, and oral supplementation initiated if needed (see discussion of DCM later in this chapter).

*Chronic therapy.* In addition to diltiazem or a β-blocker, long-term therapy for HCM usually includes a drug to decrease the likelihood of thromboembolism, such as aspirin or warfarin (see later). Exercise and dietary sodium restrictions are also recommended.

*Hyperthyroid cats.* Cardiac complications of hyperthyroidism may require specific therapy in addition to antithyroid treatment. β-Blockers can temporarily control many of the cardiac effects of excess thyroid hormone, especially tachyarrhythmias. Diltiazem is another option. Treatment for CHF is as described for HCM. The rare case of hypodynamic (dilated) cardiac failure is treated as for DCM (see later). Note: β-Blocker or other cardiac therapy is not a substitute for antithyroid treatment.

### Complications

A major complication of hypertrophic and other forms of cardiomyopathy in cats is arterial thromboembolism (see later). Atrial fibrillation and other tachyarrhythmias further impair diastolic filling and exacerbate venous congestion. Ventricular tachycardia or other arrhythmias may lead to syncope or sudden death. Development of refractory biventricular failure is another potential serious complication.

### Prognosis

The prognosis is quite variable and depends on the response to therapy, occurrence of thromboembolism, disease progression, and the presence of arrhythmias. Asymptomatic cats with only mild to moderate left ventricular hypertrophy and atrial enlargement often live well for several years. Cats with more severe hypertrophy and atrial enlargement are at greater risk for heart failure, thromboembolism, and sudden death.

Cats with CHF may live for several days to several years, but the median survival time is 1 to 2 years. Atrial fibrillation or refractory right-sided heart failure worsens the prognosis. Cats presented with thromboembolism and CHF generally have a guarded prognosis (median survival of 2 to 6 months), although some do well if congestive signs can be controlled and vital organs have not been infarcted. Recurrence of thromboembolism is common.

## RESTRICTIVE CARDIOMYOPATHY (TEXT PP 129-130)

### Etiology

Restrictive cardiomyopathy (RCM) is associated with extensive endocardial or myocardial fibrosis. The cause is unclear and probably is multifactorial. The disease may be a sequela of endomyocarditis or possibly the end stage of HCM. Occasionally, secondary RCM results from neoplastic or other infiltrative or infectious diseases.

### Clinical features

RCM occurs most often in middle-aged or older cats. Clinical signs are variable but usually reflect the presence of left- or right-sided CHF or both. Signs are often precipitated by stress or concurrent disease that increases cardiovascular demands; signs develop or worsen suddenly. Thromboembolism is common. Inactivity, poor appetite, vomiting, and weight loss may be part of the cat's recent history. Sometimes an asymptomatic cat is diagnosed based on auscultation abnormalities or radiographic evidence of cardiomegaly.

Common findings can include asystolic murmur (of mitral or tricuspid regurgitation), a gallop sound, and arrhythmias. Abnormal pulmonary sounds may accompany pulmonary edema or pleural effusion. Femoral arterial pulses are normal or slightly weak. Jugular vein distention and pulsation are associated with right-sided heart failure. Signs of thromboembolism may be the cause for presentation.

### Diagnosis

Diagnostic test results are often similar to those in cats with HCM. Radiographs show left atrial enlargement, which can be massive, and left ventricular or generalized heart enlargement. Pericardial effusion exacerbates the cardiomegaly. Dilated, tortuous proximal pulmonary veins may be noted; infiltrates of pulmonary edema or pleural effusion and sometimes hepatomegaly are seen in cats with heart failure. The ECG is often abnormal; wide QRS complexes, tall R waves, intraventricular conduction disturbances, wide P waves, and atrial tachyarrhythmias or fibrillation are common.

Echocardiographic features include marked left (and sometimes right) atrial enlargement, variable left ventricular free wall and septal thickening, and often normal to somewhat depressed wall motion. Hyperechoic areas of fibrosis may appear within the left ventricular wall, endocardial areas, or both. Endocardial scarring can be extensive and bridge to the septum. Excess moderator bands are occasionally seen. Right ventricular dilation is frequently identified. Sometimes an intracardiac thrombus is found, usually in the left auricle or atrium, but occasionally in the left ventricle. Doppler evaluation may show mild mitral or tricuspid regurgitation.

Clinicopathologic findings are nonspecific. Plasma taurine concentration is low in some affected cats and should be measured if decreased contractility is identified.

### Treatment

Therapy for acute CHF is as described for HCM. Treatment for thromboembolism is outlined later. Chronic therapy for heart failure includes furosemide as needed; enalapril is also used, starting with very low doses and increasing to the usual maintenance dose of 0.25 to 0.5 mg/kg/day. Twice-daily administration can be helpful in refractory cases. Ideally, blood pressure should be monitored when ACEI therapy is initiated or adjusted. The doses of furosemide and enalapril should be reduced if hypotension or azotemia occurs.

A β-blocker is usually used for tachyarrhythmias or if myocardial infarction is suspected. Alternatively, diltiazem could be used, although its value in the face of significant fibrosis is questioned. Cats with refractory failure or reduced systolic function are also given digoxin (see Table 3-3). Prophylaxis against thromboembolism (aspirin or warfarin) is recommended, and a low-sodium diet is fed, if accepted.

Refractory failure with pleural effusion is difficult to manage. In addition to repeated thoracocentesis, dosages of enalapril or furosemide can be cautiously increased, and hydrochlorothiazide and spironolactone (2 to 3 mg/kg of the combination per day) or nitroglycerine ointment can be added.

### Prognosis
The overall prognosis for cats with RCM heart failure is guarded to poor, although some cats live well for over a year after diagnosis. Thromboembolism and refractory pleural effusion are common.

## DILATED CARDIOMYOPATHY (TEXT PP 130-133)

### Etiology
DCM has been linked to taurine deficiency in cats. However, since this association has been discovered and diets corrected, the incidence of feline DCM has markedly decreased. The relatively few cases identified now usually are not related to taurine deficiency and may instead be the end stage of another myocardial metabolic abnormality, toxicity, or infection. Doxorubicin causes characteristic myocardial lesions, although cats are fairly resistant to clinical dilated myocardial failure. Some cats show echocardiographic changes after cumulative doses of 170 to 240 mg/m$^2$.

### Clinical features
DCM occurs in cats of all ages, with no breed or gender predilection. Clinical signs are frequently vague and include acute onset of anorexia, lethargy, and/or dyspnea. Increased respiratory effort, depression, dehydration, and hypothermia are frequent findings. Jugular venous distention, an attenuated precordial impulse, weak femoral pulses, a gallop sound (usually $S_3$), and a left and/or right apical systolic murmur (of mitral or tricuspid regurgitation) are common. Bradycardia and arrhythmias occur often, although many cats have a normal rhythm. Increased lung sounds and pulmonary crackles can be auscultated in some cats, or pleural effusion may muffle ventral lung sounds. Clinical signs of arterial thromboembolism may also be present.

### Diagnosis
Generalized cardiomegaly with rounding of the cardiac apex is a common radiographic finding. Pleural effusion is also common and tends to obscure the heart shadow and evidence of pulmonary edema or venous congestion. Hepatomegaly and ascites might be seen. A left ventricular enlargement pattern, AV conduction disturbances, and arrhythmias are frequent findings on the ECG .

Definitive diagnosis is best made by echocardiography. Findings are similar to those in dogs with DCM (see Chapter 6). A thrombus may be identified within the left atrium. Nonselective angiocardiography is a more risky alternative to echocardiography (see text).

The pleural effusion is usually a modified transudate, although true chylous effusions occur. Prerenal azotemia, mild increases in liver enzyme activities, and a stress leukogram are other common clinicopathologic abnormalities. Elevated serum muscle enzyme activities, an abnormal blood-clotting profile, and disseminated intravascular coagulation (DIC) can occur in cats with thromboembolism.

A plasma taurine concentration of <20 nmol/ml is diagnostic for taurine deficiency in a cat with DCM. Nonanorectic cats with plasma taurine concentrations <60 nmol/ml should receive taurine supplementation or a different diet.

### Treatment

The goals of treatment are to increase cardiac output and improve pulmonary function. Pleural fluid is removed by thoracocentesis. In cases of acute failure furosemide is used to promote diuresis, as described previously for HCM. However, excessive diuresis can significantly reduce cardiac output in cats with poor systolic function. Supplemental $O_2$ may be needed in cats with severe pulmonary edema; nitroglycerine may also be helpful. Vasodilators (e.g., hydralazine, an ACEI, or amlodipine) may help maximize cardiac output, but with the risk of hypotension. Blood pressure, hydration, renal function, electrolyte balance, and peripheral perfusion should be monitored closely. Hypothermia is common in cats with decompensated DCM, so external warming should be provided as needed. Once pulmonary edema is controlled, furosemide is tapered to the lowest effective oral dosage.

*Positive inotropes.* Positive inotropic support is indicated. Dobutamine or dopamine (see Table 3-3) can be used for critical cases. Oral digoxin (see Table 3-3) is the drug of choice for maintenance therapy. Toxicity easily occurs, especially with concurrent use of other drugs, so periodic evaluation of serum digoxin concentration is recommended (see Chapter 3).

*Fluid therapy.* Furosemide and vasodilators can reduce cardiac filling and predispose to cardiogenic shock in cats with DCM. Half-strength saline solution with 2.5% dextrose or other low-sodium fluids can be used intravenously (IV) at 15 to 35 ml/kg/day in several divided doses or by constant infusion. Potassium supplementation may also be needed. Subcutaneous fluid administration can be used if necessary, although absorption may be impaired.

*Chronic therapy.* Chronic treatment includes oral furosemide, an ACEI, digoxin, aspirin (or warfarin), and (if cat is taurine deficient) taurine supplementation (250 to 500 mg orally [PO] q12h). Supportive therapy for cats with thromboembolism is described later.

Clinical improvement generally is not seen until after 1 to 2 weeks of taurine supplementation, so supportive cardiac care is vital. Echocardiographic evidence of improved systolic function is seen in most taurine-deficient cats within 6 weeks of initiation of taurine supplementation. Addition of taurine can then be decreased and eventually discontinued, as long as the cat continues to eat a diet containing adequate amounts of taurine.

Reevaluation of plasma taurine concentration 2 to 4 weeks after discontinuation of supplementation is advised. After 6 to 12 weeks drug therapy may become unnecessary in some cats, although it is advised that resolution of pleural effusion and pulmonary edema be radiographically confirmed before the cat is weaned from medications.

### Prognosis

Taurine-deficient cats that survive a month after initial diagnosis have approximately a 50% chance for 1-year survival. Survival in cats not supplemented with taurine or those that are unresponsive to taurine is guarded to poor. Thromboembolism in a cat with DCM is a grave sign.

## ARRHYTHMOGENIC RIGHT VENTRICULAR CARDIOMYOPATHY (TEXT P 133)

An idiopathic cardiomyopathy mainly involving the right ventricle (RV) has been reported in cats. Moderate-to-severe dilation of the RV with either focal or diffuse RV wall thinning is characteristic; RV wall aneurysm is also common. Right, and less often left, atrial dilation may occur.

### Clinical features

The clinical presentation is usually that of right-sided CHF, with labored respirations, jugular venous distension, ascites or hepatosplenomegaly, and occasionally syncope. However, some affected cats show only lethargy and inappetence.

### Diagnosis

Thoracic radiography demonstrates right-sided heart and sometimes left atrial enlargement. Pleural effusion is common; ascites, caudal vena caval distention, and evidence for pericardial effusion may also be noted. Various arrhythmias may be found on ECG, including ventricular premature complexes, ventricular tachycardia, atrial fibrillation, and supraventricular tachyarrhythmias. A right bundle branch block pattern is common, and some cats have first-degree AV block.

Severe right atrial and RV enlargement is found on echocardiography. Other echocardiographic findings can include abnormal muscular trabeculation, aneurysmal dilation, areas of dyskinesias, and paradoxic septal motion. Tricuspid regurgitation appears to be a consistent finding on Doppler examination.

### Treatment and prognosis

Recommended therapy includes diuretics as necessary, digoxin, and an ACEI. Additional therapy for specific arrhythmias may be needed (see Chapter 4). The prognosis is guarded once signs of heart failure appear.

## MYOCARDITIS (TEXT PP 133-134)

Acute and chronic cases of suspected viral myocarditis (e.g., feline coronavirus–associated pericarditis or epicarditis) have been described in cats. CHF or fatal arrhythmias may result from severe, widespread myocarditis, but cats with focal myocardial inflammation may remain asymptomatic. Endomyocarditis has been identified mostly in younger cats. Sudden death with or without signs of pulmonary edema is the most common presentation. Therapy involves management of CHF and arrhythmias and supportive care.

Bacterial myocarditis may result from sepsis or from bacterial endocarditis or pericarditis, as in dogs. Myocarditis caused by *Toxoplasma gondii* also occurs occasionally, usually in immunosuppressed cats as part of a generalized disease process. Traumatic myocarditis is infrequently recognized in cats.

## ARTERIAL THROMBOEMBOLISM (TEXT PP 134-137)

Thromboembolism can occur with any form of feline cardiomyopathy. Poor intracardiac blood flow, especially within the left atrium, may result in blood stasis and clot formation. The most common site of embolization is the distal aortic trifurcation ("saddle thrombus"). Thromboemboli can also lodge in a brachial artery, various organs, and the heart itself.

### Clinical features

Middle-aged male cats appear to be at higher risk for thromboembolism. Clinical signs occur acutely and are usually dramatic. Often there exists no history of cardiac disease. Clinical findings depend on the area embolized as well as on the extent and duration of arterial blockage.

Acute distal aortic embolization is manifested by hindlimb paresis. The femoral pulses are absent, the limbs cool, the nailbeds cyanotic, and the affected muscles firm and painful. The cat is usually able to flex and extend the hips but drags the lower legs; sensation to the lower legs is poor. One side may show greater neurologic deficits than the other; occasionally only distal embolization of one limb occurs, resulting in paresis of the lower limb only.

Embolization of a brachial artery (usually the right) causes forelimb monoparesis; intermittent claudication occurs occasionally. Thromboembolism of the renal, mesenteric, or pulmonary arterial circulation may result in failure of those organs and death. Emboli that lodge in the central nervous system can cause seizures and various neurologic deficits.

Respiratory distress, a cardiac murmur, or an arrhythmia is often noted on presentation. Other signs of heart failure include anorexia, lethargy and weakness, gallop sounds, and effusions.

### Diagnosis

*Clinicopathologic abnormalities.* Azotemia is common and may result from dehydration, poor cardiac output, and/or embolization of the renal arteries. Skeletal muscle damage and necrosis are accompanied by elevations of alanine aminotransferase and aspartate aminotransferase activities, beginning within 12 hours and peaking by 36 hours. Widespread muscle injury causes increased lactate dehydrogenase and creatine kinase activities soon after the event; these enzymes may remain elevated for weeks. Metabolic acidosis, DIC, and hyperkalemia may be present; stress hyperglycemia is also common.

*Diagnostic imaging.* Echocardiography delineates the type of myocardial disease and may reveal the presence of an intracardiac thrombus. Most cats have prominent left atrial enlargement. If echocardiography is unavailable, nonselective angiocardiography can define the cardiac disease and reveal the location and extent of the embolus; however, angiocardiography should be delayed until the patient's condition is stabilized.

*Differential diagnoses.* The absence of palpable femoral pulses, in conjunction with other physical and radiographic findings, is often diagnostic. However, the presence of a cardiac murmur, gallop sound, or arrhythmia is inconsistent, and a few affected cats have no radiographic evidence of cardiomegaly. Other possible causes of acute posterior paresis include intervertebral disk disease, spinal neoplasia, trauma, fibrocartilaginous infarction, diabetic neuropathy, and myasthenia gravis.

### Treatment

No treatment for thromboembolism has been proved best. The goals of treatment are to manage concurrent CHF and arrhythmias (if present), prevent extension of the embolus and formation of additional thrombi, promote collateral circulation, and provide supportive care. Treatment of heart failure is outlined in Table 7-1. Unless DCM is identified, digoxin is not used. Propranolol is also avoided, as it may lead to peripheral vasoconstriction.

*Supportive care.* Supportive care should be given to allow time for establishment of collateral circulation (2 to 5 days). An analgesic is recommended for pain. Butorphanol (0.15 to 0.5 mg/kg intramuscularly [IM] into the cranial lumbar area, or subcutaneously [SC] q1-3h) is given for the first 24 to 36 hours. Low-dose morphine (0.1 to 0.3 mg/kg q3-6h IM or SC) could be considered, but it causes dysphoria in some cats. A fentanyl patch (25-μg/hr size) could be used for up to 3 days. However, it takes approximately 12 hours to become effective, so another analgesic is used simultaneously during this initial period. Respiratory depression and reduced gastrointestinal motility are potential side effects.

Acepromazine is no longer recommended. It has not been documented to improve collateral flow, and it (as well as other vasodilators) could worsen cardiac function by causing hypotension or exacerbating a preexisting outflow tract obstruction.

Other supportive therapy includes general nursing care, correction of hypothermia, treatment of dehydration, and monitoring of renal function and serum electrolyte concentrations daily. Continuous electrocardiographic monitoring during the first several days can help in detection of acute hyperkalemia. Nutritional support and loose bandaging of the affected limb(s) to prevent self-mutilation may be needed in some cats. Surgical removal of the clot is not advised (except, perhaps, for a suprarenal thrombus). The surgical risk is high in most cases because of decompensated heart failure, arrhythmias, DIC, and hypothermia. Also, significant neuromuscular ischemic injury has probably already occurred.

*Heparin.* Sodium heparin (200 IU/kg IV, then 150 to 200 IU/kg SC q6-8h) is often used for 2 to 4 days to prevent further thrombus formation, although its efficacy is unclear. Heparin does not affect existing thromboemboli. Adjustments in the subcutaneous dose are made to prolong the cat's thromboplastin time or activated coagulation time to 1.5 to 2.5 times the pretreatment level (see Chapter 89).

The coagulation tests should be monitored daily. If bleeding occurs, protamine sulfate may be given; however, overdose of protamine can cause irreversible hemorrhage. Dosage guidelines for protamine sulfate are 1 mg/100 U of heparin if the heparin was given within the previous 60 min; 0.5 mg/100 U heparin if the heparin was given 1 to 2 hours previously; and 0.25 mg/100 U heparin if >2 hours have elapsed since the heparin was administered.

Low–molecular-weight heparins (LMWHs) may be a safer alternative to unfractionated heparin. Initial experience in cats has been variable but appears promising. Current doses are based on human recommendations: enoxaparin, 1 mg/kg q12(to 24)h SC, and dalteparin, 100 U/kg q24h SC.

*Streptokinase.* The reported protocol for streptokinase is 90,000 IU/cat, infused IV over 30 min, then 45,000 IU/hr for 3 to 8 hours. However, the mortality rate in treated cats is very high. It is unclear if lower doses would be effective with fewer complications. Streptokinase therapy should not even be considered if heparin has already been administered, the cat is anuric, or serum potassium and the ECG cannot be monitored continuously.

### Prognosis

If concurrent CHF can be controlled and other complications avoided, return of function in the affected limbs should begin within 7 to 14 days. Some cats become clinically normal in 1 to 2 months, although residual deficits may persist; occasionally, amputation is necessary.

In general, though, the prognosis is guarded. About two thirds of affected cats die or are euthanized soon after the thromboembolic event. Some cats survive well over a year, although repeated events are common and worsen the long-term prognosis. Embolization of the kidneys, intestines, or other organs carries a grave prognosis. Other poor prognostic signs include refractory heart failure or arrhythmias, progressive hyperkalemia or azotemia, progressive limb injury (continued muscle contracture after 2 to 3 days, necrosis), persistent hypothermia, severe left atrial enlargement, presence of intracardiac thrombi or spontaneous contrast on echocardiogram, DIC, and previous thromboembolism.

### Prevention

The risk of thromboembolism is thought to be greater in cats with marked left atrial enlargement, echocardiographic evidence of intracardiac spontaneous contrast, visible intracardiac thrombi, and/or a prior thromboembolic event. Unfortunately, thromboembolism is not consistently prevented with any current therapeutic strategy.

*Aspirin.* Aspirin can inhibit platelet aggregation and improve collateral circulation when administered orally at 10 to 25 mg/kg (1.25 grains/cat) once every 2 to 3 days. It has been used widely with little risk but does not consistently prevent initial or recurrent thromboembolism. Nevertheless, aspirin is still often recommended in cats with at least moderate left atrial enlargement, especially if the closer monitoring needed for warfarin is problematic. Vomiting and inappetence are seen in some cats and necessitate discontinuation of therapy. The aspirin-Maalox combination (Ascriptin) may be better tolerated. More aggressive preventative therapy (e.g., warfarin, LMWH) may be prudent in cats that have survived an episode of thromboembolism.

*Warfarin.* Chronic therapy with warfarin has been advocated for cats that survive an acute thromboembolic event or are otherwise at high risk for thromboembolism. It may give better protection than aspirin, but recurrent thromboembolism still occurs. Furthermore, warfarin has greater potential for serious adverse effects, even with close monitoring. A transient hypercoagulable state occurs, so heparin is usually given for the first few days of warfarin therapy.

A baseline coagulation profile and platelet count should be obtained. Aspirin, if previously given, should be discontinued. The usual initial warfarin dose is 0.1 mg/kg/day orally (or 1/4 to 1/2 of a 1-mg warfarin tablet), although 1/4 of a tablet q48h may be sufficient in some cats. Heparin (100 IU/kg SC q8h) is administered for 3 to 4 days if not already being used for a prior thromboembolic event. It is preferable to keep medication and blood sampling times consistent. The prothrombin time (PT) is evaluated daily (several hours after warfarin administration) for 5 to 6 days. Subsequent PT evaluation can be at progressively increasing time intervals, as long as the cat's condition appears stable. Clinical signs of bleeding may include weakness, lethargy, or pallor, rather than overt hemorrhage.

The initial warfarin dose is adjusted to maintain a PT value of 1.3 to 2 times baseline at 8 to 10 hours after administration. A more precise method is to use a standardized

PT by means of the international normalization ratio (INR; see text for details). If the PT or INR is excessively increased, warfarin should be discontinued and vitamin $K_1$ (1 to 2 mg/kg/day, PO or SC) administered and continued until the PT is normal and the packed cell volume is stable. Some cats with severe bleeding need fresh-frozen plasma, packed red blood cells, or whole fresh blood transfusions. Warfarin therapy can then be resumed at half the original dose, along with heparin for several days.

The combination of aspirin and warfarin seems to be no more effective than either alone in prevention of recurrent thromboembolism. Low–molecular-weight heparin is another option for chronic therapy, although it must be given by injection.

*Supplementation.* Some cats with thromboembolism have decreased plasma concentrations of arginine and vitamins $B_6$ and $B_{12}$, risk factors for thromboembolism in humans. It is not yet known whether B vitamin or arginine supplementation would be helpful in reducing the risk of thromboembolism in cats with cardiomyopathy.

# 8

# Acquired Valvular and Endocardial Diseases

## *(Text pp 139-150)*

### DEGENERATIVE MITRAL AND TRICUSPID VALVE DISEASE (TEXT PP 139-145)

Chronic degenerative atrioventricular (AV) valve disease, or endocardiosis, is the most common cause of heart failure in dogs. Lesions most often involve the mitral valve, although both AV valves are affected in many dogs. Clinically important degenerative valve lesions are extremely rare in cats.

#### Etiology

The etiology is unknown, but a hereditary basis is likely. Mitral valve prolapse may be important in the pathogenesis in some predisposed breeds. Pathologic valve changes develop gradually with age. Early lesions consist of small nodules on the free margins of the valve; over time, large, coalescing plaques thicken and distort the valve. Redundant tissue often bulges (prolapses) toward the atrium, and the valve gradually begins to leak. The chordae tendineae are also affected, becoming thickened and weak. As the lesions progress, the valve insufficiency becomes clinically evident. In advanced cases grossly deformed, thickened, and possibly shrunken leaflets are found.

Compensatory increases in blood volume and cardiac size (atrial and ventricular dilation, eccentric myocardial hypertrophy) allow most dogs to remain asymptomatic for a prolonged period. Left atrial enlargement may be massive before any signs of heart failure appear; some affected dogs never show clinical signs of heart failure. The rate at which regurgitation worsens, as well as atrial distensibility and ventricular contractility, influences how well the disease is tolerated.

### Complicating factors

Although endocardiosis usually progresses slowly, various complicating events can cause the acute onset of clinical signs. Decompensation is generally related to the development of pulmonary edema, decreased cardiac output, or both.

Specific causes include arrhythmias (especially atrial or supraventricular), drug toxicity (e.g., digoxin), ruptured chordae tendineae, iatrogenic volume overload (e.g., excessive volumes of intravenous fluids or blood, high-sodium fluids or diet), erratic or improper medication administration, insufficient medication for the stage of disease, increased cardiac workload (e.g., physical exertion, anemia, infection and sepsis, hypertension), disease of other organ systems (e.g., pulmonary, renal, hepatic, endocrine), environmental stress (e.g., hot, humid conditions or excessive cold), cough-syncope (secondary to massive left atrial enlargement and bronchial compression), left atrial tear (with intrapericardial bleeding), secondary right-sided heart failure, and myocardial degeneration with poor contractility.

Atrial wall rupture usually causes acute cardiac tamponade. There appears to be a higher prevalence of this complication in male Miniature Poodles, Cocker Spaniels, and Dachshunds. In most cases severe valve disease, marked atrial enlargement, atrial jet lesions, and, often, ruptured chordae tendineae are present.

### Epidemiology

The prevalence and severity of chronic, degenerative AV valve disease increases with age. Clinical evidence of the condition is found most commonly in middle-aged and older dogs of small to mid-size breeds. A higher prevalence is reported in Poodles, Miniature Schnauzers, Chihuahuas, Fox Terriers, Cocker Spaniels, and Boston Terriers. An especially high incidence and early onset have been reported in Cavalier King Charles Spaniels; >50% of these dogs older than 4 years have characteristic murmurs. The overall prevalence of mitral regurgitation murmurs and degenerative valve disease is similar in males and females of this breed, but progression, severity, and prevalence of congestive heart failure (CHF) are greater in males.

### Clinical features

In many cases the accompanying murmur of mitral (or tricuspid) insufficiency is an incidental finding. Diminished exercise capacity and cough or tachypnea with exertion are common initial complaints in symptomatic dogs. As pulmonary congestion and edema worsen, resting respiratory rate also increases. Coughing occurs at night and in the early morning, as well as with activity. Severe edema results in obvious respiratory distress, often with a moist cough; signs can develop gradually or acutely. Intermittent episodes of pulmonary edema between periods of compensated heart failure over months or years are also common. Episodes of transient weakness or syncope may occur secondary to arrhythmias, coughing, or atrial tear.

Capillary refill and arterial pulse strength are usually good, although pulse deficits accompany some tachyarrhythmias. A palpable precordial thrill accompanies loud (grade V to VI) murmurs. With tricuspid regurgitation, jugular distention and pulsations are more evident after exercise, with excitement, or with cranial abdominal compression (hepatojugular reflux; see Chapter 1). Signs from decompensated tricuspid regurgitation, often overshadowed by those from mitral disease, can include hepatomegaly, ascites, respiratory distress from pleural effusion, and rarely, peripheral tissue edema. Gastrointestinal signs may accompany splanchnic congestion.

*Auscultation.* Mitral regurgitation is generally accompanied by a holosystolic murmur heard best over the left apex (see Chapter 1). However, mild regurgitation may cause a murmur heard only in early systole. Exercise and excitement often increase the intensity of soft mitral regurgitation murmurs. Louder murmurs have been associated with more advanced disease; however, the murmur can be soft or even inaudible in dogs with massive regurgitation and severe heart failure. Occasionally the murmur sounds like a musical tone or whoop. Some dogs have an audible mid- to late-systolic click, with or without a murmur. An $S_3$ gallop at the left apex may be audible in dogs with advanced disease.

Tricuspid regurgitation causes a murmur similar to that of mitral regurgitation, but it is heard best at the right apex. Radiation of a mitral murmur to the right chest wall may mimic or mask a tricuspid murmur. Jugular vein pulsations, a precordial thrill over the right apex, and a different quality to the murmur heard over the tricuspid region help in identifying tricuspid insufficiency.

Normal breath sounds are heard in the absence of CHF or with mild pulmonary edema. Accentuated, harsh breath sounds and end-inspiratory crackles (especially in ventral lung fields) develop as edema worsens. Fulminant pulmonary edema causes widespread inspiratory and expiratory crackles and wheezes. Some dogs with chronic mitral regurgitation also have abnormal lung sounds associated with pulmonary or airway disease, rather than heart failure. Dogs with CHF tend to have sinus tachycardia, whereas those with chronic pulmonary disease frequently have marked sinus arrhythmia and a normal heart rate. Pleural effusion causes diminished pulmonary sounds ventrally.

### Diagnosis

*Radiography.* Thoracic radiographs typically show some degree of left atrial and ventricular enlargement, which progresses over months to years. Extreme dilation of the left atrium can develop, even in the absence of clinical heart failure. Variable right heart enlargement occurs with chronic tricuspid regurgitation, but this may be masked by left heart and pulmonary changes from concurrent mitral disease. Elevation of the left and sometimes the right mainstem bronchi, with compression of the left mainstem bronchus, occurs in dogs with severe left atrial enlargement (see Chapter 2).

Pulmonary venous congestion and interstitial edema occur with left-sided CHF. However, the presence and severity of pulmonary edema are not necessarily correlated with the degree of cardiomegaly. Acute, severe mitral regurgitation (e.g., with rupture of chordae tendineae) can cause cardiogenic edema with minimal left atrial enlargement, whereas slowly developing regurgitation can produce massive left atrial enlargement with no evidence of CHF. Early signs of right-sided heart failure include caudal vena cava distention, pleural fissure lines, and hepatomegaly. Overt pleural effusion and ascites occur in dogs with advanced failure.

*Electrocardiography.* The electrocardiogram (ECG) may suggest left atrial or biatrial enlargement and left ventricular dilation, although it is often normal. Right ventricular enlargement indices (see Chapter 2) are occasionally seen in dogs with severe tricuspid regurgitation. Arrhythmias (especially sinus tachycardia, supraventricular tachyarrhythmias, ventricular premature contractions, and atrial fibrillation) are common in dogs with advanced disease.

*Echocardiography.* Atrial and ventricular dilation secondary to chronic AV valve insufficiency is evident on echocardiograms. Depending on the degree of volume overload, this enlargement can be severe. With mitral regurgitation, left ventricular wall and septal motion are accentuated when contractility is normal. The diastolic ventricular dimension is increased, but the systolic dimension is normal until the myocardium begins to fail. Ventricular wall thickness typically is normal. Right ventricular and atrial enlargement is seen in dogs with severe tricuspid disease; volume overload of the right ventricle may cause paradoxic septal motion. Pericardial fluid is evident with a left atrial tear.

The affected valve cusps are thicker than normal and may appear knobby. Exaggerated motion and thick mitral echoes are commonly seen on M-mode examinations. Smooth thickening is characteristic of degenerative disease (endocardiosis), whereas bacterial endocarditis tends to cause rough and irregular vegetative valve lesions. However, differentiation between degenerative changes and infective endocarditis is often impossible on echocardiogram.

Systolic prolapse or ballooning of a portion of one or both valve leaflets into the atrium is common. Sometimes a ruptured chorda tendineae or leaflet tip flails into the atrium during systole. The direction and extent of disturbed flow in the atrium can be seen with color-flow Doppler scanning.

***Differential diagnosis.*** Clinicopathalogic data may be normal or may reflect changes compatible with CHF or concurrent extracardiac disease. Other diseases that may be confused with symptomatic degenerative mitral or tricuspid valve disease include tracheal collapse, chronic bronchitis, bronchiectasis, pulmonary fibrosis, pulmonary neoplasia, pneumonia, pharyngitis, heartworm disease, dilated cardiomyopathy, and bacterial endocarditis.

**Treatment**

Surgical procedures such as mitral annuloplasty, other valve repair techniques, and mitral valve replacement are available at some referral centers, but most cases are treated medically. The main goals of medical therapy are to (1) control signs of CHF (see Box 3-1), (2) enhance forward blood flow (using arteriolar vasodilators), (3) reduce regurgitant volume (using diuretics, vasodilators, and positive inotropes), and (4) modulate the excessive neurohormonal activation.

Many dogs with advanced mitral regurgitation (or tricuspid regurgitation) can maintain clinical compensation for months to years with appropriate therapy, although frequent reevaluation and medication adjustment become necessary as the disease progresses. Although congestive signs appear gradually in some dogs, severe pulmonary edema or episodes of syncope develop rapidly in others. Many dogs on long-term therapy for heart failure have intermittent episodes of decompensation that can be successfully managed.

***Asymptomatic regurgitation.*** Dogs that are asymptomatic do not require drug therapy. Convincing evidence of the benefit of angiotensin-converting enzyme inhibitor (ACEI) therapy in these dogs is lacking. Client education is important so that owners recognize the early signs of heart failure. It is wise to pursue weight reduction in obese dogs, advise moderate exercise restriction, and remove high-salt foods from the dog's diet. Moderate dietary sodium restriction may be helpful (see Chapter 3).

***Mild to moderate CHF.*** The severity of heart failure and any complicating factors influence the aggressiveness of therapy. An ACEI is generally prescribed for dogs with early signs of failure (see Chapter 3). Long-term enalapril (or other ACEI) therapy may improve exercise tolerance, cough, and respiratory effort, but whether it enhances survival is unclear.

In dogs with respiratory signs that could be caused by either heart failure or a noncardiac cause, an initial therapeutic trial of furosemide (1 to 2 mg/kg orally [PO] q8-12h) is indicated; cardiogenic pulmonary edema usually responds rapidly. Dogs with radiographic evidence of pulmonary edema or more severe clinical signs are also treated with furosemide (see Table 3-2). Higher and more frequent doses are used for more severe edema. When signs of failure are controlled, the dose and frequency are reduced to the lowest effective levels for long-term therapy.

Digoxin is advocated for the chronic treatment of failure resulting from advanced AV valve regurgitation. Digoxin is usually added after ACEI and furosemide therapy has been initiated, especially if marked left ventricular enlargement is present. Indications for digoxin therapy include frequent atrial premature beats or tachycardia, atrial fibrillation, and recurrent episodes of pulmonary edema despite furosemide and ACEI. Conservative doses and monitoring of serum concentrations are used to avoid toxicity (see Chapter 3).

Exercise restriction is enforced until signs of failure abate. Mild to moderate regular activity can be beneficial during chronic, compensated disease, but strenuous exercise is best avoided. Dogs with persistent cough caused by mainstem bronchus compression may require antitussive therapy (see Chapter 21).

***Severe CHF.*** Dogs with severe pulmonary edema and dyspnea at rest constitute true emergencies (see Chapter 3). Aggressive treatment but gentle handling are crucial, as any added stress can lead to death. Cage rest, supplemental oxygen, high-dose parenteral furosemide, and vasodilator therapy are indicated (see Box 3-1). Hydralazine is recommended for acute therapy; a reduced dose is used in patients already receiving an ACEI. Topical nitroglycerine can also be used. Intravenous nitroprusside can be used instead of other vasodilators; however, blood pressure must be closely monitored to avoid hypotension. Doses for these drugs are given in Table 3-2. Thoracocentesis is indicated in dogs with moderate- to large-volume pleural effusion. Ascites severe enough to impede respiration should also be drained.

Digoxin therapy (see Table 3-3) can be initiated (or continued if previously prescribed) once dyspnea has subsided. Paroxysmal atrial tachycardia or atrial fibrillation may respond to digoxin, but intravenous digitalization should be avoided unless the arrhythmia appears to be life threatening. Diltiazem or a β-blocker (Table 4-3) can be used instead of, or in addition to, digoxin for supraventricular tachyarrhythmias. If poor contractility is documented, other, more potent inotropic agents (e.g., dobutamine, dopamine, amrinone) can be given intravenously [IV] (Table 3-3), or pimobendan used, if available. Occasionally, therapy for ventricular tachyarrhythmias is warranted. However, it is important to watch for drug toxicities and adverse effects (e.g., azotemia, electrolyte abnormalities, arrhythmias).

After the patient is stabilized, medications are adjusted over several days or weeks to determine the best regimen for long-term treatment. Furosemide is titrated to the lowest dose (and longest interval) that controls signs of CHF. If hydralazine or nitro-prusside is the vasodilator used initially, changing to an ACEI for ongoing therapy is recommended. If hydralazine is used initially, the first dose of ACEI should be $1/2$ the usual dose (e.g., 0.25 mg/kg for enalapril); this precaution is not necessary after nitroprusside administration.

***Chronic refractory CHF.*** When CHF becomes decompensated, therapy is inten-sified as needed. Some dogs respond to rest and an increased furosemide dose for a few days; they can then return to their previous or a slightly higher dose. Increasing the frequency of ACEI administration (e.g., enalapril q12h instead of q24h) can also be effective. Digoxin can be added if not already being used; the dose is not titrated upward unless subtherapeutic serum concentrations are documented (see Chapter 3). Dietary sodium restriction can be intensified.

If ACEI and furosemide doses are already maximized, low-dose hydralazine (0.25 to 0.5 mg/kg PO q12h) or amlodipine (0.05 to 0.2 mg/kg PO q24h) can be added, although blood pressure should be monitored. Adding another diuretic, such as spironolactone alone (1 to 2 mg/kg PO q12-24h) or in combination with hydrochlorothiazide (1 to 2 mg/kg of the combination 25 mg/25 mg product), may reduce chronic refractory pulmonary edema or effusions.

### Patient monitoring and reevaluation

Client education regarding the disease process, clinical signs of failure, and the drugs prescribed is essential for successful long-term therapy. At-home monitoring by the owner is important, because decompensation often occurs unexpectedly. Respiratory and heart rates should be noted when the dog is quietly resting or sleeping. A persistent increase in either can signal early decompensation.

Reevaluation of asymptomatic dogs is recommended at least yearly. Dogs with recently diagnosed or decompensated heart failure should be checked frequently (at least weekly) until stable. Those with chronic heart failure that appears well controlled can be reevaluated several times per year. Medication supply, administration compliance, drugs and doses being given, and diet should be reviewed with the owner at each visit. ECG, thoracic radiographs, and/or echocardiography may be indicated depending on concerns reported by the owner and physical examination findings. Frequent monitoring of serum electrolyte concentrations and renal function is impor-tant. Dogs receiving digoxin should have a serum concentration measured 7 to 10 days after initiation or change in dosage (see Chapter 3).

### Prognosis

The prognosis in symptomatic dogs is quite variable. With appropriate therapy and attentive management of complications, some dogs live well for >4 years after signs of heart failure first appear. Some dogs die during an initial episode of fulminant pulmo-nary edema. The survival time for most symptomatic dogs ranges from several months to a few years.

## INFECTIVE ENDOCARDITIS (TEXT PP 145-150)

Endocarditis is an infection involving the cardiac valves or endocardial tissues. The mitral and aortic valves are most often affected in dogs and cats. Common sites for resulting vegetative lesions include the ventricular side of the aortic valve with subaortic stenosis, the atrial surface of a regurgitant mitral valve, and the right ventricular side of a ventricular septal defect. The prevalence is fairly low in dogs and even lower in cats.

### Etiology

Bacteremia is necessary for endocardial infection. Dentistry procedures, endoscopy, urethral catheterization, anal surgery, and other "dirty" procedures can cause transient bacteremia. Recurrent bacteremia can result from infections of the skin, mouth, urinary tract, prostate gland, lungs, and other organs. The most common organisms identified in dogs and cats with endocarditis are *Streptococcus* spp., *Staphylococcus* spp., and *Escherichia coli.* Less common organisms include *Corynebacterium (Arcanobacterium)* spp., *Pasteurella* spp., *Pseudomonas aeruginosa, Erysipelothrix rhusiopathiae (Erysipelothrix tonsillaris)*, and *Bartonella vinsonii* ssp. *berkhoffi.* Culture-negative endocarditis may be caused by fastidious organisms.

Microbial colonization results in ulceration of the valve endothelium, which leads to the formation of vegetations consisting of aggregated platelets, fibrin, blood cells, and bacteria. Vegetations cause valve deformity and result in valvular insufficiency, which in turn can lead to CHF (most often left sided). Arrhythmias may develop and cause weakness, syncope, and sudden death or contribute to the development of CHF. Fragments of vegetative lesions often break loose; embolization of other body sites causes infarction or metastatic infection, which results in diverse clinical signs. Septic arthritis, diskospondylitis, urinary tract infections, and renal and splenic infarctions are common in affected animals. Circulating immune complexes also contribute to the disease syndrome. Sterile polyarthritis, glomerulonephritis, and other immune-mediated organ damage are common. Rheumatoid factor and antinuclear antibody test results may be positive.

### Clinical features

Male dogs are affected more commonly than females, and the prevalence of endocarditis increases with age. German Shepherd and other large-breed dogs may be at greater risk. Subaortic stenosis is a known risk factor for aortic valve endocarditis.

Clinical signs are quite variable. Cardiac signs (e.g., those resulting from left-sided congestion or arrhythmias) may be the reason for presentation. However, cardiac signs may be overshadowed by systemic signs resulting from infarction, infection, or immune-mediated damage (Box 8-1). Nonspecific signs of lethargy, weight loss, inappetence, recurrent fever, and weakness may predominate.

It is important to maintain an index of suspicion for this disease, which has been nicknamed "the great imitator." Infective endocarditis often mimics immune-mediated disease, and dogs with endocarditis are commonly evaluated for "fever of unknown origin" (see Chapter 95). Many affected animals have evidence of past or concurrent infections, but often a clear history of predisposing factors is absent.

### Diagnosis

Definitive antemortem diagnosis is difficult. Presumptive diagnosis is based on two or more positive blood cultures *in addition to* either (1) echocardiographic evidence of vegetations or valve destruction or (2) recent appearance of a regurgitant murmur. Endocarditis is likely even when blood culture results are negative or intermittently positive if there exists echocardiographic evidence of vegetations or valve destruction along with supporting clinical evidence, such as a predisposing heart condition (e.g., subaortic stenosis), fever, vascular phenomena (e.g., major arterial emboli, septic infarcts), or immunologic phenomena (e.g., glomerulonephritis, positive antinuclear antibody or rheumatoid factor tests). For example, the combination of a new diastolic murmur at the left heart base, hyperkinetic pulses, and fever is strongly suggestive of aortic valve endocarditis.

Signs of heart failure occurring in an unexpected clinical setting or in an animal with a murmur of recent onset could indicate the existence of infected valve damage,

---

**Box 8-1**

## Potential Sequelae of Infective Endocarditis

### HEART
Valve insufficiency or stenosis
Murmur
Congestive heart failure
Coronary embolization (aortic valve*)
Myocardial infarction
Myocardial abscess
Myocarditis
Decreased contractility (segmental or global)
Myocarditis (direct invasion by microorganisms)
Arrhythmias
Atrioventricular conduction abnormalities (aortic valve*)
Decreased contractility
Pericarditis (direct invasion by microorganisms)
Pericardial effusion
Cardiac tamponade (?)

### KIDNEY
Infarction
Reduced renal function
Abscess formation and pyelonephritis
Reduced renal function
Urinary tract infection
Renal pain
Glomerulonephritis (immune mediated)
Proteinuria
Reduced renal function

### MUSCULOSKELETAL
Septic arthritis
Joint swelling and pain
Lameness

Immune-mediated polyarthritis
Shifting leg lameness
Septic osteomyelitis
Bone pain
Myositis
Muscle pain

### BRAIN AND MENINGES
Abscesses
Associated neurologic signs
Encephalitis and meningitis

### VASCULAR SYSTEM (GENERAL)
Vasculitis
Thrombosis
Petechiae and small hemorrhages (e.g., eye, skin)
Obstruction
Ischemia of tissues served, with associated signs

### LUNG
Pulmonary emboli (tricuspid or pulmonic valves, rare*)
Pneumonia (tricuspid or pulmonic valves, rare*)

### NONSPECIFIC
Sepsis
Fever
Anorexia
Malaise and depression
Shaking
Vague pain
Inflammatory leukogram
Mild anemia
± Positive antinuclear antibody test
± Positive blood cultures

*Diseased valve most commonly associated with abnormality.

---

especially if other suggestive signs are present. However, such a murmur could be caused by noninfective acquired disease (e.g., degenerative valve disease, cardiomyopathy), previously undiagnosed congenital disease, or physiologic alterations (e.g., fever, anemia). Conversely, endocarditis may develop in an animal with a known murmur resulting from another cardiac disease.

*Blood cultures.* Several samples of at least 10 ml of blood should be aseptically collected over a 24-hour period, with >1 hour elapsing between collections. Different venipuncture sites should be used for each sample. Large sample volumes (e.g., 20 to

30 ml) increase culture sensitivity. Both aerobic and anaerobic cultures have been recommended, although the value of routine anaerobic culture is questionable. Prolonged incubation (3 weeks) is recommended, as some bacteria are slow growing.

Blood cultures are positive in many dogs with infective endocarditis, but negative results do not rule out this condition. Chronic endocarditis, recent antibiotic therapy, intermittent bacteremia, and fastidious or slow-growing organisms, as well as noninfective endocarditis, can cause negative culture results. Serologic and polymerase chain reaction tests are available for *Bartonella* spp.

**Echocardiography.** Echocardiography is especially supportive if oscillating vegetative lesions and abnormal valve motion are identified. However, false-negative and false-positive findings can occur, so cautious interpretation is important. Differentiation of mitral vegetations from degenerative thickening may be impossible; but classically, vegetative endocarditis has a rough, ragged appearance in contrast to the smooth valvular thickenings of degenerative disease.

Cardiac sequelae of valve dysfunction include chamber enlargement and abnormal valve leaflet motion. Aortic insufficiency can cause a high-frequency flutter of the anterior mitral valve leaflet during diastole as the regurgitant jet hits this leaflet. Aortic valve regurgitation appears as a diastolic "flame" of color extending from the valve on color-flow Doppler examination. Myocardial dysfunction and arrhythmias might also be identified with echocardiography.

**Other tests.** The ECG may be normal or may document premature beats, tachycardia, conduction disturbances, or evidence of myocardial ischemia. Radiographs may be unremarkable or may show evidence of left-sided heart failure. Radiography may also indicate other organ involvement (e.g., diskospondylitis).

Clinicopathologic findings usually reflect an inflammatory process and variable biochemical abnormalities. Neutrophilia with a left shift is typical of acute endocarditis, whereas mature neutrophilia with or without monocytosis usually develops with chronicity. Nonregenerative anemia is seen in approximately 50% of cases in dogs. Azotemia, hyperglobulinemia, hematuria, pyuria, and proteinuria are also relatively common. Rheumatoid factor and antinuclear antibody tests may be positive in dogs with subacute or chronic bacterial endocarditis.

### Treatment

Aggressive therapy with bactericidal antibiotics and supportive care are indicated. Ideally, drug choice is guided by positive culture results and in vitro susceptibility. Broad-spectrum combination therapy is usually begun immediately after blood culture samples have been obtained; therapy is altered as necessary when culture results are available. Patients with negative culture results should be continued on the broad-spectrum regimen.

An initial combination of a cephalosporin, penicillin, or synthetic penicillin (e.g., ampicillin) with an aminoglycoside (gentamicin or amikacin) or a fluoroquinolone (e.g., enrofloxacin) is often effective (see Chapter 98 for doses). Antibiotics are administered IV (preferable) or intramuscularly (IM) for at least the first week. Oral therapy is often used thereafter, although parenteral administration is probably better. Antimicrobial therapy should continue for at least 4 weeks, although therapy for 6 to 8 weeks is often recommended. Aminoglycosides are discontinued after 2 to 3 weeks, or sooner if renal toxicity develops (see Chapter 44).

Supportive care includes treatment of CHF (see Chapter 3) and, when present, arrhythmias (see Chapter 4), in addition to treatment of any complications related to the primary source of infection, embolic events, or immune responses. Attention to hydration status, nutritional support, and general nursing care is important. Corticosteroids are contraindicated. It is unclear whether aspirin is of benefit in reducing the incidence of embolic events.

### Prognosis

Long-term prognosis is generally guarded to poor. Evidence of vegetations and volume overload on echocardiogram suggests a poor prognosis. Aggressive therapy may be successful if valve dysfunction is not severe and large vegetations are not present.

CHF is the most common cause of death, although sepsis, systemic embolization, arrhythmias, or renal failure may be the cause. Aortic valve involvement and gram-negative organisms independently worsen the prognosis.

**Prevention**

Antimicrobial prophylaxis is recommended before dental or other dirty procedures (e.g., those involving the oral cavity or the intestinal or urogenital tract) in dogs with high-risk cardiovascular conditions (e.g., subaortic stenosis, ventricular septal defect, patent ductus arteriosus, cyanotic congenital heart disease), an implanted pacemaker, a history of endocarditis, or immunocompromise. Administration of high-dose ampicillin or amoxicillin (plus an aminoglycoside, depending on the procedure) 1 hour before and 6 hours after the procedure is suggested.

# 9

# Common Congenital Cardiac Anomalies

## (Text pp 151-168)

Most congenital cardiac anomalies are accompanied by an audible murmur, although some serious malformations are not. A murmur, especially if loud, in a young puppy or kitten may be an indication of congenital disease. However, clinically insignificant "innocent" murmurs are relatively common in young animals. Innocent murmurs are usually soft systolic ejection-type murmurs heard best at the left heart base; their intensity may vary with heart rate or body position. These murmurs tend to get softer and usually disappear by approximately 4 months of age. Murmurs associated with congenital disease usually persist and may get louder with time.

Patent ductus arteriosus (PDA) and subaortic stenosis (SAS) are the most common anomalies in dogs; pulmonic stenosis (PS) is also quite common. The most common malformations in cats are atrioventricular valve dysplasias, atrial or ventricular septal defects (VSDs), and endocardial fibroelastosis (mainly in Burmese and Siamese cats).

Congenital malformations in both species can occur as isolated defects (most often) or in various combinations. Purebred animals have a higher prevalence of congenital defects; Table 9-1 lists recognized breed predispositions. Other breeds and mixed-breed animals can be affected with any defect. In cats congenital malformations are more prevalent in males than in females.

## EXTRACARDIAC ARTERIOVENOUS SHUNTS (TEXT PP 153-155)

### Patent Ductus Arteriosus

Functional closure of the ductus arteriosus normally occurs within hours after birth. In animals with inherited PDA the ductus fails to close, both structurally and functionally. Consequently, blood shunts from the descending aorta into the pulmonary

### Table 9-1
### Breed Predispositions for Congenital Heart Disease

| Disease | Breed |
|---|---|
| Patent ductus arteriosus | Maltese, Pomeranian, Shetland Sheepdog, English Springer Spaniel, Keeshond, Bichon Frise, Toy and Miniature Poodles, Yorkshire Terrier, Collie, Cocker Spaniel, German Shepherd Dog, Chihuahua, Kerry Blue Terrier, Labrador Retriever, Newfoundland; female > male |
| Subaortic stenosis | Newfoundland, Golden Retriever, Rottweiler, Boxer, German Shepherd Dog, English Bulldog, Great Dane, German Short-Haired Pointer, Bouvier des Flandres, Samoyed(?) |
| Pulmonic stenosis | English Bulldog (male > female), Mastiff, Samoyed, Miniature Schnauzer, West Highland White Terrier, Cocker Spaniel, Beagle, Airedale Terrier, Boykin Spaniel, Chihuahua, Scottish Terrier, Boxer, Fox Terrier(?) |
| Ventricular septal defect | English Bulldog, English Springer Spaniel, Keeshond; cats |
| Atrial septal defect | Samoyed, Doberman Pinscher, Boxer |
| Tricuspid dysplasia | Labrador Retriever, German Shepherd Dog, Boxer, Weimaraner, Great Dane, Old English Sheepdog, Golden Retriever; other large breeds; (male > female?) |
| Mitral dysplasia | Bull Terrier, German Shepherd Dog, Great Dane, Golden Retriever, Newfoundland, Mastiff, Rottweiler(?); cats; (male > female?) |
| Tetralogy of Fallot | Keeshond, English Bulldog |
| Persistent right aortic arch | German Shepherd Dog, Great Dane, Irish Setter |

artery, during both systole and diastole. This left-to-right shunt causes volume overload of the pulmonary circulation and the left atrium and ventricle.

Occasionally the excess pulmonary blood flow leads to pulmonary hypertension. If the pulmonary pressure rises to equal the aortic pressure, very little blood shunting occurs. If the pulmonary artery pressure exceeds the aortic pressure, reverse shunting (right-to-left flow) occurs. Reversed shunt is reported in 15% of dogs with inherited PDA; female Cocker Spaniels may be at increased risk.

#### Clinical features
Certain dog breeds have a higher prevalence of PDA (see Table 9-1); the prevalence is approximately three times greater in females than in males. Left-to-right shunting PDA is by far the most common presentation. Many affected animals are asymptomatic when first diagnosed, although a history of reduced exercise capacity, tachypnea, or cough is present in some cases. Characteristic findings include a continuous murmur heard best high at the left base, often with a precordial thrill, hyperkinetic (bounding or "waterhammer") arterial pulses, and pink mucous membranes.

#### Diagnosis
Radiographic findings are summarized in Table 9-2. A triad of bulges (pulmonary trunk, aorta, and left auricle) in the 1 o'clock to 3 o'clock positions on a dorsoventral radiograph is classic but not always seen. Evidence of pulmonary edema accompanies left-sided heart failure. Characteristic findings on the electrocardiogram (ECG) include wide P waves, tall R waves, and deep Q waves in leads II, $aV_F$, and $CV_6LL$. Changes secondary to left ventricular enlargement may occur in the ST-T segment.

**Table 9-2**

## Radiographic Findings in Common Congenital Heart Defects

| Defect | Heart | Pulmonary vessels | Other |
|---|---|---|---|
| PDA | LAE, LVE; L auricular bulge; ± increased cardiac width | Overcirculated | Bulge in descending aorta + pulmonary trunk; ± pulmonary edema |
| SAS | ± LAE, LVE | Normal | Wide cranial waist (ascending aorta dilation) |
| PS | RAE, RVE; reverse D | Normal to undercirculated | Pulmonary trunk bulge |
| VSD | LAE, LVE; ± RVE | Overcirculated | ± Pulmonary edema; ± pulmonary trunk bulge (large shunts) |
| ASD | RAE, RVE | ± Overcirculated | ± Pulmonary trunk bulge |
| T dys | RAE, RVE; ± globoid shape | Normal | Caudal cava dilation; ± pleural effusion, ascites, hepatomegaly |
| M dys | LAE, LVE | ± Venous hypertension | ± Pulmonary edema |
| T of F | RVE, RAE; reverse D | Undercirculated; ± prominent bronchial vessels | Normal to small pulmonary trunk; ± cranial aortic bulge on lateral view |

*ASD,* Atrial septal defect; *L,* left; *LAE,* left atrial enlargement; *LVE,* left ventricular enlargement; *M dys,* mitral dysplasia; *PDA,* patent ductus arteriosus; *PS,* pulmonic stenosis; *RAE,* right atrial enlargement; *RVE,* right ventricular enlargement; *SAS,* subaortic stenosis; *T dys,* tricuspid dysplasia; *T of F,* tetralogy of Fallot; *VSD,* ventricular septal defect.

*Echocardiography.* Left heart enlargement and dilation of the pulmonary trunk are found on echocardiogram. Fractional shortening may be normal or decreased. Although the ductus itself may be difficult to visualize, Doppler studies document continuous, turbulent flow in the pulmonary artery and allow estimation of the aortic-to-pulmonary artery pressure gradient.

### Treatment

Closure of the left-to-right PDA is recommended as early as feasible. Surgical ligation is successful in most cases (perioperative mortality is approximately 11%). Transcatheter PDA occlusion is a much less invasive alternative; however, not all cases are suitable for nonsurgical PDA closure. A normal lifespan can be expected after uncomplicated ductal closure. The concurrent mitral regurgitation usually resolves after ductus ligation or occlusion if the valve is structurally normal.

Animals with congestive heart failure (CHF) are treated with furosemide, an angiotensin-converting enzyme inhibitor, rest, and dietary sodium restriction (see Chapter 3). Digoxin is often used, as contractility tends to decline with time. Arrhythmias are treated as necessary (see Chapter 4).

### Prognosis

If the ductus is not closed, the prognosis depends on the ductus size and the amount of pulmonary vascular resistance; CHF is the eventual outcome in most cases, with >50% of affected dogs dying within the first year. In animals with pulmonary hypertension and shunt reversal, ductal closure is contraindicated because the ductus acts as a "pop-off" valve for the high right-sided pressures in these cases. Ductal ligation in animals with reversed PDA produces no improvement and promotes right ventricular failure.

## VENTRICULAR OUTFLOW OBSTRUCTIONS (TEXT PP 155-160)

Obstruction to ventricular outflow can occur at the semilunar valve, just below the valve, or above the valve in the proximal great vessel. Stenosis below the aortic valve (subaortic) is the most common left-sided defect. On the right, malformations of the pulmonary valve itself (often with narrowing below the valve from muscular hypertrophy) are most common.

Stenotic lesions induce pressure overload of the affected ventricle. Concentric myocardial hypertrophy is the typical response, but some dilation of the affected ventricle may also occur. Ventricular hypertrophy can impede diastolic filling or lead to secondary AV valve regurgitation. Heart failure results from high ventricular diastolic and atrial pressures. Arrhythmias also cause or contribute to the development of CHF. The combination of an outflow obstruction, paroxysmal arrhythmias, and inappropriate bradycardia secondary to ventricular baroreceptor stimulation can result in signs of low cardiac output, including exercise intolerance, syncope, or sudden death.

### Subaortic Stenosis

#### Epidemiology

Subvalvular narrowing caused by a fibrous or fibromuscular ring is the most common type of aortic stenosis in dogs. SAS is thought to be inherited as an autosomal dominant trait with modifying genes that influence its phenotypic expression. SAS also occurs in cats, as does supravalvular stenosis.

In Newfoundland dogs three grades of SAS have been described. The mildest (grade I) causes no clinical signs or murmur. Dogs with moderate (grade II) stenosis have only mild clinical and hemodynamic evidence of the disease. Dogs with grade III SAS have severe disease and a complete fibrous ring around the outflow tract; malformations of the mitral valve apparatus may also be present.

Outflow tract narrowing and dynamic obstruction (plus a discrete subvalvular ridge) have also been reported in Golden Retrievers. Dynamic left ventricular outflow tract obstruction may also be important in other dogs (see Table 9-1).

The obstructive lesion of SAS develops during the first several months of life, so no audible murmur may exist at an early age. In some dogs no murmur is detected until

1 to 2 years of age. Therefore identification of subclinical and mildly affected carriers in the breeding population is a major challenge.

### Clinical features

Fatigue, exercise intolerance or exertional weakness, syncope, or sudden death occurs in approximately $^1/_3$ of dogs with SAS. With severe outflow obstruction, tachyarrhythmias or sudden reflex bradycardia and hypotension cause low-output signs. Left-sided CHF can develop, usually with concurrent mitral or aortic regurgitation, other cardiac malformations, or acquired endocarditis. Dyspnea is the most commonly reported sign of SAS in cats.

Moderate to severe SAS typically causes weak and late-rising femoral pulses, a precordial thrill low on the left heart base, and absence of a jugular pulse. Evidence of pulmonary edema or arrhythmias may be found. A harsh systolic ejection murmur is heard at or below the aortic valve area on the left hemithorax. This murmur often radiates equally or more loudly to the right heartbase, following the course of the aortic arch. Often the murmur is also heard over the carotid arteries, and it may even radiate to the calvarium.

In mild cases a soft, poorly radiating ejection murmur at the left, and sometimes, right heartbase may be the only abnormality found. Exercise or excitement generally increases the intensity of the murmur. Aortic regurgitation may produce a diastolic murmur at the left base and may increase the arterial pulse strength.

### Diagnosis

Radiographic abnormalities (see Table 9-2) may be subtle, especially in animals with mild SAS. The ECG is often normal, although evidence of left ventricular hypertrophy or enlargement can occur (see Chapter 2), and depression of the ST segment can be present in leads II and $aV_F$. Ventricular tachyarrhythmias are common.

*Echocardiography.* Echocardiography reveals the extent of left ventricular hypertrophy and subaortic narrowing. A discrete ridge of tissue below the aortic valve is evident in many animals with moderate to severe disease. Systolic turbulence originating below the aortic valve and extending into the aorta, as well as high peak systolic outflow velocities, can be identified during Doppler studies. Many cases also have some degree of aortic or mitral regurgitation or both evident on color-flow and spectral Doppler (see text).

### Treatment

Various surgical techniques involving open-heart surgery have been used to reduce the outflow obstruction. Although surgical resection of the stenotic membrane can significantly reduce the left ventricular systolic pressure gradient and possibly improve exercise ability, it does not appear to improve long-term survival. Transcatheter balloon dilation of the stenotic area may reduce the measured gradient, although partial stenosis may redevelop with time, and no survival benefit has been documented with this procedure.

Animals with a high pressure gradient, marked ST-segment depression, frequent ventricular premature contractions, or a history of syncope may benefit from β-blocker therapy (see Chapter 4). Exercise should be restricted in animals with moderate to severe SAS. Prophylactic antibiotic therapy is indicated before procedures that may cause bacteremia (see Chapter 8).

### Prognosis

Prognosis in dogs and cats with severe stenosis is guarded. In one study >50% of severely affected dogs died suddenly before 3 years of age, although the overall prevalence of sudden death in dogs with SAS is just over 20%. Dogs with mild stenosis are more likely to be asymptomatic and live longer. However, infective endocarditis and CHF may develop later. Arrhythmias and worsened mitral regurgitation are complicating factors.

## Pulmonic Stenosis

Some cases of PS result from simple fusion of the valve cusps, but dysplasia of the pulmonic valve (variably thickened, asymmetric, and partially fused valve leaflets with a hypoplastic valve annulus) is more common. Right ventricular hypertrophy and secondary dilation result.

### Clinical features

PS is more common in smaller breeds of dog (see Table 9-1). Many dogs are asymptomatic at the time of diagnosis. Signs of right-sided CHF or a history of exercise intolerance or syncope may be present, but even with considerable stenosis these signs may not develop until the animal is several years old.

Findings characteristic of moderate to severe stenosis include a prominent right precordial impulse, a thrill high at the left base, normal to slightly diminished femoral pulses, pink mucous membranes, and, occasionally, jugular pulses. On auscultation, a systolic ejection murmur is heard best high at the left base. The murmur may radiate cranioventrally and to the right, but usually it is not heard over the carotid arteries. An early systolic click is sometimes identified. The murmur of secondary tricuspid insufficiency may also be heard, and arrhythmias are present in some cases.

### Diagnosis

Radiographic findings are summarized in Table 9-2. Dilation of the caudal vena cava is also seen in some animals. Electrocardiographic features include a right ventricular hypertrophy pattern, right axis deviation, and sometimes a right atrial enlargement pattern (P pulmonale) and/or tachyarrhythmias (see Chapter 2).

*Echocardiography.* Right ventricular hypertrophy and enlargement are found, and right atrial enlargement is frequently seen. A thickened, asymmetric, or otherwise malformed pulmonic valve usually can be visualized, although the outflow area may be narrow and difficult to see clearly. Poststenotic dilation of the main pulmonary trunk may be detected. Pleural effusion and prominent right heart dilation often accompany secondary CHF; paradoxic septal motion may be noted in such cases. Doppler evaluation provides an estimate of lesion severity; PS is considered mild if the estimated systolic pressure gradient is <50 mm Hg and severe if it is >(80 to) 100 mm Hg.

### Treatment

Palliation of the defect by balloon valvuloplasty is recommended, especially if infundibular hypertrophy is not excessive. This procedure can reduce or eliminate clinical signs in severely affected animals, but it is unclear whether long-term survival is improved. Balloon valvuloplasty is more likely to be successful in dogs with simple fusion of the valve cusps; however, most dogs with PS have dysplastic valves, which are more difficult to dilate effectively. Various surgical procedures have also been used to palliate moderate to severe PS in dogs.

Exercise restriction is generally recommended, especially for animals with moderate to severe stenosis. β-Blocker therapy may be helpful if infundibular hypertrophy is prominent. Signs of CHF are managed medically (see Chapter 3).

### Prognosis

Prognosis depends on the severity of the stenosis. Patients with mild PS may have a normal life span, but animals with severe stenosis often die within 3 years of diagnosis. Sudden death or onset of CHF is common. Concurrent tricuspid regurgitation, atrial fibrillation or other tachyarrhythmias, and CHF significantly worsen the prognosis.

## INTRACARDIAC SHUNTS (TEXT PP 160-162)

### Ventricular Septal Defect

Most VSDs are located just below the aortic valve on the left and under the septal tricuspid leaflet on the right. In cats a VSD may be part of an endocardial cushion defect (combination of a high VSD, low atrial septal defect (ASD), and AV valve malformation).

### Clinical features

Clinical sequelae depend on the size of the defect and the pressure gradient. Exercise intolerance or evidence of left-sided CHF are the most common manifestations, although many animals are asymptomatic at the time of diagnosis. Characteristic findings include a holosystolic murmur loudest at the cranial right sternal border (the direction of shunt flow). A large shunt volume can cause relative or functional PS with a systolic ejection murmur at the left base. When the VSD is associated with aortic regurgitation, a corresponding diastolic decrescendo murmur may be heard at the left base.

### Diagnosis

Radiographic findings are variable (see Table 9-2) and depend on the size of the shunt. The ECG may be normal or may suggest left atrial and/or ventricular enlargement; in some cases, disturbed intraventricular conduction is apparent (fractionated or splintered QRS complexes). A right ventricular enlargement pattern usually indicates a very large defect, pulmonary hypertension, right ventricular outflow obstruction, or endocardial cushion defect, although it may result from a right bundle branch block (see Chapter 2).

*Echocardiography.* Left-sided heart (plus right ventricular) dilation is found in patients with large shunts. Larger defects usually can be seen just below the aortic valve in the right parasternal long axis plane, optimized for the left ventricular outflow tract. Doppler studies demonstrate the shunt flow.

### Treatment

Definitive therapy requires intracardiac surgery. Palliation of large left-to-right shunts is sometimes accomplished by placement of a constrictive band around the pulmonary trunk to create mild supravalvular PS. Note: Palliative surgery should not be attempted in the presence of pulmonary hypertension and shunt reversal. Animals that develop left-sided heart failure are managed medically (see Chapter 3).

### Prognosis

Animals with moderate-size defects can have a fairly normal life span. Occasionally, spontaneous closure occurs within the first 2 years of life. Those with a large septal defect are likely to develop left-sided CHF; some develop pulmonary hypertension with shunt reversal, usually at an early age.

## Atrial Septal Defect

High ASDs are more common in dogs; in cats defects low in the interatrial septum are likely to be part of the endocardial cushion defect complex. ASDs are often associated with other cardiac anomalies. In most cases, blood shunts from the left to right atrium, resulting in volume overload of the right heart. If PS or pulmonary hypertension is also present, right-to-left shunting and cyanosis may occur.

### Clinical features

The clinical history is usually nonspecific. Physical examination may be unremarkable with an isolated ASD. Large left-to-right shunts are associated with a murmur of relative PS and splitting of $S_2$. Rarely a soft diastolic murmur of relative tricuspid stenosis is audible.

### Diagnosis

Radiographic findings are summarized in Table 9-2. The left heart is not enlarged unless another defect such as mitral insufficiency is present. ECG may be normal or may reveal right ventricular and atrial enlargement patterns. Cats with an endocardial cushion defect may have right ventricular enlargement and a left axis deviation (see Chapter 2).

*Echocardiography.* Right atrial and ventricular dilation may be found, with or without paradoxic interventricular septal motion. Large ASDs can be visualized, although the thinner fossa ovalis region of the interatrial septum can be confused with a septal defect. Doppler echocardiography may allow identification of smaller shunts that cannot be visualized on 2-D examination.

### Treatment and prognosis

Large shunts can be treated surgically, similarly to VSDs. Otherwise, medical management is used if CHF develops (see Chapter 3). The prognosis is variable and depends on the shunt size, presence of other defects, and pulmonary vascular resistance in the patient.

## ATRIOVENTRICULAR VALVE MALFORMATIONS (TEXT PP 162-163)

### Mitral Dysplasia

Congenital malformations of the mitral valve apparatus include shortened or overly elongated chordae tendineae; direct attachment of the valve cusp to a papillary muscle; thickened, cleft, or shortened valve cusps; prolapse of valve leaflets; upwardly displaced or malformed papillary muscles; and excessive dilation of the valve annulus. Mitral valve dysplasia is more common in large-breed dogs (see Table 9-1); it also occurs in cats. Valvular regurgitation is the predominant functional abnormality and may be severe. Stenosis of the mitral valve orifice is uncommon and coexists with regurgitation; obstruction to ventricular filling increases left atrial pressure and can precipitate pulmonary edema.

#### Clinical features and diagnosis

Except for the young age of the animal, clinical features are similar to those of severe degenerative mitral valve disease in older dogs (see Chapter 8). Exercise intolerance, respiratory signs of left-sided CHF, anorexia, and atrial arrhythmias (especially atrial fibrillation) commonly develop. The systolic murmur of mitral regurgitation is heard at the left apex. Radiographic, electrocardiographic, echocardiographic, and catheterization findings are similar to those in animals with severe acquired mitral insufficiency. Specific malformations of the mitral apparatus can be identified with echocardiography.

#### Treatment and prognosis

Therapy consists of medical management for signs of CHF (see Chapter 3). Prognosis is poor. Surgical valve reconstruction or replacement might be possible.

### Tricuspid Dysplasia

Malformations of the tricuspid valve and its support structures are similar to those of mitral valve dysplasia. In some cases the tricuspid valve is displaced ventrally into the ventricle (Ebstein-like anomaly). Tricuspid dysplasia is most frequently diagnosed in large-breed dogs (see Table 9-1), perhaps more often in males than in females.

#### Clinical features

Historical signs and clinical findings are similar to those of advanced degenerative tricuspid valve disease (see Chapter 8). Initially the animal may be asymptomatic or only mildly exercise intolerant. However, exercise intolerance, ascites, dyspnea (pleural effusion), anorexia, and cardiac cachexia frequently develop. Physical examination features include a tricuspid regurgitation murmur (not always audible) and jugular vein pulsations. Jugular vein distention, muffled heart and lung sounds, and ballottable abdominal fluid occur in patients with CHF.

#### Diagnosis

Radiographic findings are summarized in Table 9-2. The ECG usually shows right ventricular and occasionally right atrial enlargement patterns; a splintered QRS complex is common (see Chapter 2). Atrial arrhythmias, including atrial fibrillation, may also be noted. Evidence for ventricular preexcitation is sometimes seen. Echocardiography depicts the often massive right heart dilation. Malformations of the valve apparatus can also be seen.

#### Treatment and prognosis

Medical management is provided for CHF and arrhythmias (see Chapters 3 and 4). Periodic thoracocentesis is helpful when heart failure and pleural effusion cannot be controlled with medication and diet. Prognosis is guarded to poor, especially in patients with marked cardiomegaly. However, some affected dogs survive for several years.

## CARDIAC ANOMALIES CAUSING CYANOSIS (TEXT PP 163-166)

Cardiac malformations that allow unoxygenated blood to reach the systemic circulation result in hypoxemia and, when severe, cyanosis and polycythemia. Severe polycythemia (packed cell volume [PCV] >65%) can cause microvascular sludging and poor tissue oxygenation, intravascular thrombosis, hemorrhage, stroke, and cardiac arrhythmias.

The possibility that a venous embolus will cross the shunt to the systemic circulation poses another danger in these cases.

The anomalies that most commonly cause cyanosis in dogs and cats are Tetralogy of Fallot (T of F) and pulmonary arterial hypertension secondary to a large PDA, VSD, or ASD. Despite the pressure overload of the right side of the heart, CHF is rare because the shunt provides a pop-off valve.

## Tetralogy of Fallot

The anomalies associated with this defect are VSD, PS, dextropositioning of the aorta, and right ventricular hypertrophy. The VSD is often quite large. Sometimes the pulmonary artery is hypoplastic or atretic. A polygenic inheritance pattern has been identified in Keeshonds.

### Clinical features

A history of syncope, exertional weakness, dyspnea, cyanosis, and stunted growth is common; findings vary with the severity of the disease components. Cyanosis is detected at rest in some animals, but others have pink mucous membranes until exercised. The precordial impulse on the right chest wall may be of equal or greater intensity than that on the left. A precordial thrill is sometimes palpable at the right sternal border or left basilar area. Jugular pulsation may be noted. Auscultation may reveal a holosystolic murmur at the right sternal border (VSD) and/or a systolic ejection murmur at the left base (PS). However, polycythemia renders the murmur(s) inaudible in some patients.

### Diagnosis

Radiographic findings are summarized in Table 9-2. The thick right ventricle displaces the left side of the heart dorsally, simulating left heart enlargement. The ECG typically suggests right ventricular hypertrophy, although a left axis deviation is occasionally present in cats. Echocardiography allows visualization of the VSD, a large aortic root shifted rightward and overriding the ventricular septum, some degree of PS, and right ventricular hypertrophy. Doppler studies demonstrate the right-to-left shunt and high-velocity stenotic pulmonary outflow jet. An echocontrast study will document the right-to-left shunt.

### Treatment

Definitive surgical repair requires open-heart surgery. Palliative procedures can increase pulmonary blood flow by surgically creating a left-to-right vascular shunt. Some dogs are helped by β-blocker therapy. Exercise restriction is also important. Systemic vasodilators should be avoided.

*Phlebotomy.* Periodic phlebotomy is recommended in patients with severe polycythemia and clinical signs of hyperviscosity (e.g., weakness, shortness of breath, seizures). A sufficient volume of blood is withdrawn (and sometimes replaced with isotonic fluid) to maintain the PCV at a level at which clinical signs are minimal. Further reduction in the PCV can exacerbate signs of hypoxemia. Alternatively, hydroxyurea may be tried to manage the polycythemia (see later).

### Prognosis

Prognosis depends on the degree of PS and polycythemia. Mildly affected animals or those with successful palliative surgical shunts may live for 4 to 7 years. However, progressive hypoxemia, polycythemia, and sudden death at an earlier age are common.

## Pulmonary Hypertension with Shunt Reversal

A small percentage of dogs and cats with shunts (e.g., PDA, VSD) develop pulmonary hypertension. It is unclear why pulmonary hypertension develops in some animals and not in others, but when it occurs the associated defect is usually large. When pulmonary artery pressure exceeds aortic pressure, unoxygenated blood shunts into the aorta.

### Clinical features

The history and clinical presentation are similar to those associated with T of F. Exercise intolerance, shortness of breath, syncope, seizures, and sudden death are common. Cough and hemoptysis may also occur. Cyanosis may be evident with exercise or excitement. Reversed PDA causes cyanosis of the caudal mucous membranes only (differential cyanosis); rear limb weakness is seen in these animals. Intracardiac shunts cause equally intense cyanosis throughout the body.

A murmur typical of the underlying defect(s) may be present. However, often no murmur or only a very soft systolic murmur is heard because of the polycythemia. With pulmonary hypertension, $S_2$ may be loud and "snapping" or split. A gallop sound is occasionally heard. Other findings include a pronounced right precordial impulse and jugular pulsations.

### Diagnosis

Thoracic radiographs often reveal heart enlargement, a prominent pulmonary trunk, and tortuous, proximally widened pulmonary arteries. A bulge in the descending aorta may be seen in dogs with reversed PDA; the left side of the heart may also be enlarged in patients with reversed PDA or VSD. ECG usually indicates right ventricular and sometimes right atrial enlargement, with a right axis deviation.

*Echocardiography.* Echocardiography substantiates right ventricular hypertrophy and may reveal the anatomic defect and a widened pulmonary trunk. Doppler scan or an echocontrast study can confirm an intracardiac right-to-left shunt. Reversed PDA flow can be shown by imaging the abdominal aorta during venous echocontrast injection. Measurement of the peak velocity of a tricuspid regurgitation jet, if present, allows estimation of right ventricular (and pulmonary artery) systolic pressures.

### Treatment and prognosis

Treatment is limited to exercise restriction and either periodic phlebotomy (as described for T of F) or hydroxyurea therapy to minimize the signs of hyperviscosity. Surgical closure of the shunt is contraindicated. Vasodilators are of little benefit and may be detrimental. Prognosis is generally poor, although some patients have done well for years with periodic phlebotomy.

*Hydroxyurea.* Chronic hydroxyurea therapy (40 to 50 mg/kg orally [PO] q48h or three times a week) may be a useful alternative to periodic phlebotomy. Complete blood count and platelet count should be monitored weekly or biweekly to start. A target PCV between 54% and 60% is suggested. Possible adverse effects include anorexia, vomiting, bone marrow hypoplasia, alopecia, and pruritus. Depending on the patient's response, the dose can be divided and given twice a day on treatment days, administered twice a week, or given at a dose of <40 mg/kg (see Chapter 86).

## OTHER CARDIOVASCULAR ANOMALIES (TEXT PP 166-167)

### Vascular Ring Anomalies

Various malformation of vessels arising from the embryonic aortic arches can occur. These may entrap the esophagus, and sometimes the trachea, within a vascular ring over the heartbase. The most common vascular ring anomaly in dogs is persistent right aortic arch. Other anomalies, such as a left cranial vena cava or PDA, may also be found in these patients. Vascular ring anomalies are rare in cats.

### Clinical features

Clinical signs of regurgitation and stunted growth commonly develop within 6 months of weaning. The esophagus dilates cranial to the ring and may retain food; occasionally it also dilates caudal to the stricture, suggesting altered esophageal motility as well. Respiratory signs such as cough, wheezing, stridor, and cyanosis occur in animals with a double aortic arch or in association with secondary aspiration pneumonia. The animal may appear clinically normal (although thin), but progressive debilitation generally occurs. In some animals a dilated cervical esophagus (containing food or gas) can be palpated at the thoracic inlet.

### Diagnosis

Thoracic radiographs usually reveal a widened cranial mediastinum and ventral displacement of the trachea, with or without evidence of aspiration pneumonia. A barium swallow allows visualization of the esophageal stricture over the heartbase and esophageal dilation.

### Treatment

Therapy involves surgical division of the ligamentum arteriosum (or other anomalous vessel). Medical management involves the feeding of frequent, small, semisolid or liquid meals, fed with the animal in an upright position. Some dogs experience persistent regurgitation despite successful surgery, which suggests a permanent esophageal motility disorder.

## Cor Triatrium

Cor triatrium is an uncommon malformation caused by division of the right or left atrium into two chambers by an abnormal membrane. There are several reports of this defect in dogs, but it is rarely described in cats. Obstruction to venous flow through the opening in the abnormal membrane results in higher pressures within the caudal vena cava and the structures that it drains.

### Clinical features

Large and medium-size dogs are most often affected. Development of persistent ascites at an early age is the most prominent clinical sign. Exercise intolerance, lethargy, distended cutaneous abdominal veins, and sometimes diarrhea have also been reported. Neither cardiac murmur nor jugular venous distention is a feature of this anomaly.

### Diagnosis

Radiographs show a distended caudal vena cava without generalized cardiomegaly. The diaphragm may be displaced cranially by massive ascites. The ECG is generally normal. Echocardiography reveals the abnormal membrane with a prominent caudal right atrial chamber and vena cava. Doppler studies allow estimation of the pressure gradient within the right atrium and visualization of the flow disturbance.

### Treatment and prognosis

Successful therapy requires enlargement of the membrane orifice or excision of the abnormal membrane to remove flow obstruction. Surgical techniques and percutaneous balloon dilation have been described.

## Endocardial Fibroelastosis

Endocardial fibroelastosis is a congenital abnormality characterized by diffuse fibrosis and elastic thickening of the endocardium. It is reported more commonly in cats, especially Burmese and Siamese. Left-sided or biventricular heart failure commonly develops early in life. The murmur of mitral regurgitation may be present. Criteria for left ventricular and left atrial enlargement are seen on radiographs, ECG, and echocardiogram. Evidence of reduced left ventricular myocardial function and increased stiffness may be present. Nevertheless, definitive antemortem diagnosis can be difficult.

# 10

# Heartworm Disease

## *(Text pp 169-184)*

Heartworm disease (HWD) is an important cause of pulmonary hypertension (cor pulmonale). The adult worms live mainly in the pulmonary arteries, where their presence incites reactive vascular lesions that result in pulmonary hypertension. Occasionally, mechanical occlusion of the right ventricular outflow tract, tricuspid valve, vena cavae, or pulmonary arteries occurs when a massive number of worms is present (caval syndrome).

## DIAGNOSTIC TESTING
### Serologic Tests
#### Heartworm antigen tests
Adult heartworm antigen (Ag) tests are the primary method of screening in dogs. Commercial test kits are quite accurate and are more sensitive than microfilaria tests, especially in dogs on monthly heartworm preventive drugs (which virtually eliminate microfilaremia). Circulating Ag is generally detectable by 7 months after infection, so no reason exists to test puppies younger than 7 months of age.

Positive results are consistently obtained if the animal has at least three female worms that are at least 7 months old; most kits can often detect infections with only one live adult female. However, most cannot detect infections <5 months old, nor male unisex infections.

False-positive results are usually caused by technical error; false-negative results usually occur from a low worm burden, presence of only immature females, male unisex infections, or a cold test kit. Animals with weak-positive results should be further evaluated using a repeat test or a different Ag test kit, a microfilaria test, and/or thoracic radiographs.

Enzyme-linked immunosorbent assay (ELISA)–based Ag tests are highly specific for detecting adult heartworms in cats, but their sensitivity depends on the gender, age, and number of worms. As the adult heartworm burden is low in cats and there exists a greater probability of male unisex infections, false-negative results are more likely in this species. Also, a longer time is required for cats to become Ag positive.

#### Heartworm antibody tests for cats
ELISA-based antibody (Ab) test kits are commercially available to screen for HWD in cats. The Ab tests are more sensitive than Ag tests in cats, as larvae of either gender can provoke an immune response. However, the specificity of the Ab tests is of some concern, because serum Ab to both immature and adult worms is detected as early as 60 days after infection. As some immature larvae never develop into adults, all a positive Ab test indicates is exposure to larval or adult heartworms.

A positive Ab test should be supported by other evidence of HWD before a definitive diagnosis is made. The concentration of Ab does not appear to correlate with the number of worms present, nor with severity of clinical disease or radiographic signs. It is also unclear how long circulating Abs remain after elimination of heartworm infection.

False-negative results occur in an estimated 3% to 14% of cats, usually in association with a single worm. If clinical findings suggest HWD but the Ab test is negative, testing should be repeated using a different Ab test and a heartworm Ag test. Thoracic radiographs and 2-D echocardiogram are also recommended. The Ab test can be repeated in a few months.

### Detection of Microfilaria

Tests for circulating microfilaria are no longer recommended for routine screening. However, they may be used for confirmation in some Ag-positive cases and to determine if microfilaricidal therapy is needed. Microfilaria testing is still important if diethylcarbamazine (DEC) is used as a heartworm preventive. Circulating microfilaria are rarely found in cats with HWD.

Concentration tests using at least 1 ml of blood are recommended to detect microfilaria in peripheral blood. Nonconcentration tests (fresh blood smear or buffy coat examination) are not recommended, because low numbers of microfilaria are likely to be missed. An occasional false-positive result occurs when microfilaria are present in the absence of live adult worms. Concentration tests are done using either a millipore filter or the modified Knott's technique (see text). Microfilaria of *Dirofilaria immitis* (heartworm) must be differentiated from those of *Dipetalonema reconditum*.

## HWD IN DOGS (TEXT PP 171-180)

HWD in dogs has no specific age or breed predilection. Most affected dogs are between 4 and 8 years old, although HWD is often diagnosed in dogs <1 year of age (but >6 months) and geriatric animals. Males are affected two to four times as often as females. Large-breed dogs and those primarily living outdoors are at much greater risk of infection.

### Clinical features

Many dogs are asymptomatic when the disease is diagnosed by routine screening. Dogs with occult disease or those that have not been routinely tested are more likely to have advanced pulmonary arterial disease and clinical signs. Symptomatic dogs often have a history that includes exertional dyspnea, fatigue, syncope, cough, hemoptysis, shortness of breath, weight loss, and/or signs of right-sided congestive heart failure (CHF).

Physical examination may be normal in early or mild cases. Severe disease is frequently associated with poor body condition, tachypnea or dyspnea, jugular vein distention and/or pulsations, and ascites. Increased or abnormal lung sounds (wheezes, crackles), a loud and often split $S_2$, an ejection click or murmur at the left base, a murmur of tricuspid insufficiency, or cardiac arrhythmias are variably heard on auscultation. Severe pulmonary arterial disease and thromboembolism can lead to epistaxis, disseminated intravascular coagulation (DIC), thrombocytopenia, and possibly hemoglobinuria (also a sign of caval syndrome).

Occasionally, aberrant worms migrate to the central nervous system, eye, femoral arteries, subcutis, peritoneal cavity, and other sites and cause related signs. Several cases of systemic arterial migration, causing hindlimb lameness, paresthesia, and ischemic necrosis, have been described.

### Diagnosis

*Radiography.* Thoracic radiographs may be normal early in the disease, although marked changes develop rapidly in dogs with heavy worm burdens. Characteristic findings include right ventricular enlargement, a pulmonary trunk bulge, and centrally enlarged and tortuous lobar pulmonary arteries with peripheral blunting and no associated venous distention. The caudal lobar arteries, usually the most severely affected, are best evaluated on a dorsoventral view; the width of these vessels as they cross the ninth rib is normally no larger than that rib. An enlarged caudal vena cava ($>3/4$ the length of the fifth thoracic vertebra) may also be present. Patchy pulmonary interstitial or alveolar infiltrates are common.

*Electrocardiography.* The electrocardiogram (ECG) is usually normal, but advanced disease may cause a right axis deviation or an arrhythmia. Dogs with heartworm-induced CHF almost always have ECG criteria for right ventricular enlargement (see Chapter 2). Tall P waves occasionally occur, suggesting right atrial enlargement.

*Echocardiography.* Echocardiographic findings in dogs with advanced HWD include right ventricular and atrial dilation, right ventricular hypertrophy, paradoxic septal motion, a small left side of the heart, and pulmonary artery dilation. Heartworms within the heart, main pulmonary artery and its bifurcation, and the venae cavae appear as small, bright, parallel echoes. Suspected caval syndrome can be quickly confirmed by echocardiography. Secondary right-sided heart failure can be evidenced by pleural or pericardial effusion or ascites.

*Clinicopathologic findings.* Eosinophilia, basophilia, and/or monocytosis are inconsistent findings; <50% of dogs with HWD have eosinophilia. Mild regenerative anemia is present in <30% of cases and likely results from hemolysis. Platelet counts may be decreased after adulticidal treatment; DIC can also occur in dogs with advanced disease. The immune response to the heartworms results in a polyclonal gammopathy. Azotemia and mild to moderate serum liver enzyme elevations can occur; proteinuria and hypoalbuminemia may also develop in severely affected animals.

### Pretreatment evaluation

A thorough history and physical examination are indicated in all cases. Thoracic radiographs provide the best overall assessment of pulmonary arterial and parenchymal disease and are useful for determining prognosis. The risk of postadulticidal pulmonary thromboembolism is increased in dogs with preexisting clinical and radiographic signs of severe pulmonary vascular disease, especially in those with right-sided heart failure or a high worm burden.

In young, asymptomatic dogs the addition of a complete blood count (CBC), blood urea nitrogen or creatinine concentration, and urinalysis provides a sufficient database. For middle-aged or older dogs and those with clinical signs, a more complete serum chemistry profile is also recommended. A platelet count is advised when severe pulmonary arterial disease is present. When hypoalbuminemia or proteinuria is detected, urine protein loss should be quantified.

### Adulticidal therapy in dogs

Melarsomine and thiacetarsamide are the only effective heartworm adulticides. Melarsomine is the drug of choice. It causes less systemic toxicity and is a more effective adulticide, with no greater risk for thromboembolism and pulmonary hypertension than thiacetarsamide. Furthermore, thiacetarsamide is no longer being manufactured.

Strict rest should be enforced for 4 to 6 weeks after adulticidal therapy, and longer in working dogs. Heartworm Ag testing should be repeated 3 to 4 months after therapy. The test should be negative if therapy was completely successful. The decision to repeat treatment in a dog with persistent antigenemia is guided by the animal's overall health, performance expectations, and age. Complete worm kill is probably not necessary; even if some adult worms survive, pulmonary arterial disease improves considerably after adulticidal therapy.

In asymptomatic dogs, the decision to withhold adulticidal therapy is controversial. The presence of concurrent disease and the dog's age and activity level are all important considerations. If adulticidal therapy is not provided, the dog should at least receive a macrolide preventive agent to stop further worm development and disease transmission.

*Melarsomine.* Melarsomine (Immiticide) is effective against immature and mature heartworms. A classification system of disease severity is useful in guiding therapy (Table 10-1). Dogs with mild to moderate disease are given the standard protocol. Dogs with severe disease or those in which a more conservative approach is desired are given the alternate dose regimen. Note: *Dogs with caval syndrome should not be given adulticidal treatment* until the worms have been surgically removed.

*Protocol.* Standard melarsomine therapy is summarized in Box 10-1. The manufacturer's recommendations should be followed exactly. If the dog is still Ag positive

Table 10-1

## Classification of Heartworm Disease Severity in Dogs

| Class | Clinical signs | Radiographic signs | Clinicopathologic abnormalities |
|---|---|---|---|
| 1 (mild) | None; or occasional cough, fatigue on exercise, or mild loss of condition | None | None |
| 2 (moderate) | None; or occasional cough, fatigue on exercise, or mild to moderate loss of condition | Right ventricular enlargement and/or some pulmonary artery enlargement; ± perivascular and mixed alveolar or interstitial opacities | ± Mild anemia (PCV 20% to 30%); ± proteinuria (2+ on dipstick) |
| 3 (severe) | General loss of condition or cachexia; fatigue on exercise or mild activity; occasional or persistent cough; ± dyspnea; ± right-sided heart failure | Right ventricular ± atrial enlargement; moderate to severe pulmonary artery enlargement; perivascular or diffuse mixed alveolar or interstitial opacities; ± evidence of thromboembolism | ± Anemia (PCV <30%); ± proteinuria (≥2+ on dipstick) |
| 4 (very severe) | Caval syndrome (see text) | | |

*PCV,* Packed cell volume.

| Box 10-1 |
| --- |

## Checklist for Melarsomine (Immiticide) Adulticide Therapy

### BEFORE INITIATING TREATMENT

Confirm diagnosis.
Perform pretreatment evaluation and management.
Determine class (severity) of disease (see Table 10-1).
Determine melarsomine treatment regimen.

### STANDARD TREATMENT REGIMEN (FOR CLASS 1 AND MOST CLASS 2 DOGS)

1. Draw melarsomine, 2.5 mg/kg, into a syringe; attach a fresh, sterile 23-gauge needle: 1 in (2.5 cm) long for dogs <10 kg or 1.5 in (3.75 cm) long for dogs >10 kg.
2. Give by deep intramuscular injection into lumbar (epaxial) musculature in the L3 to L5 region; avoid subcutaneous leakage.
3. Repeat steps 1 and 2 24 hr after first dose; use opposite side for injection.
4. Enforce rest for 4 to 6 weeks minimum; administer symptomatic treatment as needed.

### ALTERNATE TREATMENT REGIMEN (FOR CLASS 3 AND SOME CLASS 2 DOGS)

1. Administer symptomatic treatment as needed; enforce rest.
2. When condition is stable, administer one dose of 2.5 mg/kg as described above in the standard treatment regimen.
3. Continue enforced rest and symptomatic treatment as needed.
4. One month later, administer two more doses, 24 hr apart, according to the standard treatment regimen.

after 4 months, treatment can be repeated. In dogs that receive the alternate protocol the standard regimen is given 1 month later.

*Adverse effects.* Adverse effects at recommended doses are generally mild. Most signs in treated dogs are behavioral (tremors, lethargy, unsteadiness or ataxia, restlessness), respiratory (panting, shallow or labored breathing, crackles), or related to the injection site (edema, redness, tenderness, vocalization, increased muscle enzyme activities).

Lethargy, depression, and anorexia occur infrequently (approximately 15%); fever, vomiting, and diarrhea occur occasionally. At recommended dose rates, coughing or gagging and (less often) dyspnea after treatment are most likely related to HWD itself. Melarsomine causes a local reaction at the injection site that is clinically noticeable in approximately 1/3 of treated dogs. Injection site reactions are generally mild to moderate and resolve completely in 4 to 12 weeks; occasionally these reactions are severe.

*Overdose.* Overdose of melarsomine can cause pulmonary inflammation, edema, and death. Some clinical reversal of toxicity can be achieved with BAL (British Anti-Lewisite, dimercaprol) at 3 mg/kg given intramuscularly (IM), but this will decrease adulticidal activity.

*Thiacetarsamide.* Thiacetarsamide (Caparsolate) is an older agent that may still be available, although it is no longer manufactured. The drug is extremely caustic, so meticulous intravenous injection, preferably using a butterfly catheter and saline flush, is required. The usual treatment protocol is 2.2 mg/kg (0.22 ml/kg) given intravenously (IV) twice a day for 2 days. During and after treatment the dog should be carefully monitored for signs of toxicity (acute depression, anorexia, repeated emesis, icterus, fever, diarrhea, death). Vomiting after administration is relatively common, but treatment can continue if no other adverse signs occur and the patient's appetite is good. Complete anorexia, icterus, and persistent vomiting are indications that treatment should be halted.

***Pulmonary thromboembolic complications.*** Worsening of pulmonary arterial disease can occur 5 to 30 days after adulticidal therapy; severe pulmonary thrombo-embolization is most likely to occur 7 to 17 days after adulticidal therapy. Signs include depression, fever, tachycardia, tachypnea or dyspnea, cough, hemoptysis, and sometimes right-sided heart failure, collapse, or death. Pulmonary crackles and muffled lung sounds may be heard on auscultation. Patchy alveolar infiltrates with air bronchograms may appear on thoracic radiographs, especially near the caudal lobar arteries. CBC may show thrombocytopenia or a regenerative left shift.

### Treatment

Treatment includes strict cage confinement and glucocorticoid therapy (prednisone, 1 to 2 mg/kg/day initially, then tapered down). Supplemental oxygen ($O_2$) is recommended; a bronchodilator (e.g., aminophylline, 10 mg/kg q8h given orally [PO], IM, or IV; or theophylline, 9 mg/kg q6-8h PO), judicious fluid therapy, and cough suppressants may also be helpful. Unless evidence of concurrent bacterial infection is present, antibiotics are of questionable benefit. Hydralazine (see Table 3-2) or diltiazem (see Table 4-3) may improve the respiratory signs, but systemic hypotension and tachycardia must be avoided.

In severe cases heparin therapy can be considered, either as sodium heparin (200 to 400 U/kg given subcutaneously [SC] q8h) or calcium heparin (50 to 100 U/kg SC q8-12h). Excessive bleeding is a serious potential effect. Low–molecular-weight heparin might be a safer alternative than unfractionated heparin (see text, p 176).

### Treatment of dogs with complicated HWD
#### Pulmonary complications.

*Pneumonitis.* Allergic or eosinophilic pneumonitis has been reported in 10% to 15% of dogs with occult HWD. Clinical manifestations include a progressively worsening cough, crackles on auscultation, tachypnea or dyspnea, and sometimes cyanosis, weight loss, and anorexia.

Eosinophilia, basophilia, and hyperglobulinemia are inconsistent findings. Serologic tests for adult heartworm are usually positive. Diffuse interstitial and alveolar infiltrates, especially in the caudal lobes, are common on radiographs. Frequently no clinically relevant cardiomegaly or pulmonary lobar artery enlargement is present. A sterile eosinophilic exudate with variable numbers of well-preserved neutrophils and macrophages is typical on tracheal wash cytology.

Therapy with glucocorticoids (prednisone, 1 to 2 mg/kg/day initially) usually results in rapid and marked improvement. Gradually tapered prednisone doses (to 0.5 mg/kg every other day) can be continued as needed and probably do not adversely affect melarsomine adulticidal efficacy.

*Eosinophilic granulomatosis.* Pulmonary eosinophilic granulomatosis is an uncommon syndrome associated with HWD. Clinical signs are similar to those of eosinophilic pneumonitis. Variable clinicopathologic findings include leukocytosis, neutrophilia, eosinophilia, basophilia, monocytosis, and hyperglobulinemia. In some cases an exudative, primarily eosinophilic pleural effusion develops. Radiographic findings include multiple pulmonary nodules of varying size with mixed alveolar and interstitial pulmonary infiltrates; hilar and mediastinal lymphadenopathy may also be present.

The condition is treated initially with prednisone (1 to 2 mg/kg q12h); additional cytotoxic therapy may also be needed. Not all dogs respond completely; relapse is common, especially when therapy is reduced or discontinued. Adulticidal therapy can be administered when pulmonary disease abates.

*Severe pulmonary arterial disease.* Severe pulmonary arterial disease is likely in dogs with long-standing heartworm infections, those with many adult worms, and active dogs. Clinical signs include severe cough, exercise intolerance, tachypnea or dyspnea, episodic weakness, syncope, weight loss, ascites, and death. Thrombocytopenia may occur in dogs with concurrent thromboembolism; some dogs develop DIC. Radiographically, affected pulmonary arteries are markedly enlarged, tortuous, and blunt. Supportive therapy includes supplemental $O_2$, prednisone, and a bronchodilator. After initial stabilization, the alternate melarsomine protocol can be started (see Box 10-1). Aspirin should be avoided if hemoptysis is present. Prophylactic antibiotics are sometimes recommended.

*Right-sided CHF.* Severe pulmonary arterial disease and pulmonary hypertension can cause right ventricular failure. Typical signs include jugular venous distention and/or pulsation, ascites, syncope, exercise intolerance, or arrhythmias. Pleural or pericardial effusion can develop, and other signs secondary to pulmonary arterial and parenchymal disease may also be present. Treatment is as for dogs with severe pulmonary arterial disease, with the addition of furosemide (1 to 2 mg/kg/day), an angiotensin-converting enzyme inhibitor (e.g., enalapril), and a sodium-restricted diet. CHF is discussed in detail in Chapter 3.

*Caval syndrome.* This shocklike condition occurs when venous inflow to the heart is obstructed by a mass of worms. It has been estimated that this complication develops in 15% to 20% of dogs with HWD; it is more likely to occur in geographic areas in which HWD is endemic.

*Clinical features.* Most dogs with caval syndrome have no history of heartworm-related signs. Acute collapse is common, often with anorexia, weakness, tachypnea or dyspnea, pallor, hemoglobinuria, and bilirubinuria. A tricuspid insufficiency murmur, jugular distention and pulsation, weak pulse, loud and possibly split $S_2$, or a cardiac gallop rhythm is often found. Sometimes coughing or hemoptysis and ascites occur. Unless treated, most dogs die within 24 to 72 hours from cardiogenic shock complicated by metabolic acidosis, DIC, and anemia.

*Diagnosis.* Clinicopathologic findings can include microfilaremia, Coombs' negative hemolytic anemia, hemoglobinemia and hemoglobinuria, azotemia, increased liver enzyme activities, and DIC. Right-sided heart and pulmonary artery enlargement are evident on thoracic radiographs. ECG usually indicates right ventricular enlargement. Echocardiography reveals a mass of worms entangled at the tricuspid valve and in the right atrium and cavae. Right ventricular dilation and hypertrophy, paradoxic septal motion, and a small left ventricle are other features.

*Treatment.* The only effective therapy is surgical removal of the worms via right jugular venotomy or right auricular cannulation (during thoracotomy). Survival rates of 50% to 80% are reported for removal via jugular venotomy. Supportive care, including cautious intravenous fluid administration, is given during and after surgical worm removal. A broad-spectrum antibiotic is recommended. Platelet counts should be monitored, and thrombocytopenia managed as discussed in Chapter 89. Adulticidal therapy to eliminate the remaining worms can be given a few weeks after the dog's condition is stabilized.

*Other complications.* Azotemia, severe proteinuria, or both develop in some dogs with HWD. Prerenal azotemia should be corrected with fluid therapy before adulticidal treatment. Mild to moderate azotemia and proteinuria without hypoalbuminemia may not adversely affect the outcome of adulticidal therapy, but dogs with nephrotic syndrome or severe azotemia with proteinuria are poor candidates for thiacetarsamide therapy. Melarsomine should not adversely affect compromised renal function. Severe pulmonary thromboembolism and renal or hepatic failure are associated with a poor outcome.

### Microfilaricidal therapy

Ivermectin and milbemycin have been used effectively as microfilaricidal drugs, although neither is federally approved for this purpose in the United States. Treatment is administered 3 to 4 weeks after adulticidal therapy. Rapid death of many microfilaria within 3 to 8 hours of the first dose can cause lethargy, inappetence, salivation, retching, defecation, pallor, and tachycardia. Usually, adverse effects are mild. However, dogs with high numbers of circulating microfilaria occasionally experience circulatory collapse that is responsive to glucocorticoids (e.g., prednisolone sodium succinate 10 mg/kg or dexamethasone 1 mg/kg IV) and intravenous fluids (e.g., 80 ml/kg over

2 hours). Close observation is recommended for 8 to 12 hours after initial microfilaria treatment.

The microfilaricidal dose for ivermectin is a single dose of 0.05 mg/kg (50 μg/kg) PO. This dose is safe for Collies. If the concentrated livestock product is used, 1 ml of ivermectin (10 mg/ml) is diluted in 9 ml of propylene glycol and given PO at a dose of 1 ml/20 kg of body weight.

The standard preventive dose of milbemycin oxime (Interceptor; 0.5 to 1 mg/kg) is an alternative to ivermectin. Adverse reactions from rapid microfilaria death occasionally occur with milbemycin in dogs with high numbers of microfilaria. Treatment with either drug can be repeated every 2 weeks until microfilaria are no longer found; usually 1 or 2 doses are sufficient.

### Heartworm prevention

Heartworm prophylaxis is indicated for all dogs living in endemic areas. For most of the United States, monthly preventive therapy is necessary only from June through October or November, and in the southern third of the country from April through November or December. Year-long monthly preventive therapy is prudent in the southernmost areas of the United States. Preventive therapy can begin at 6 to 8 weeks of age. Before starting prophylaxis for the first time, dogs older than 6 months should be tested for circulating Ag and, if DEC is to be used, microfilaria. Retesting for circulating Ag should be done periodically; usually every 2 to 3 years is adequate.

*Ivermectin.* Ivermectin (Heartgard 30) is effective at monthly doses of 6 to 12 μg/kg PO and is safe in Collies. Ivermectin can be given to microfilaria-positive dogs. The drug is completely effective against larvae acquired 2 to 3 months before the drug is administered, and is somewhat effective in preventing heartworm development in dogs infected 4 months before monthly treatment begins. Prolonged monthly administration (for at least 16 months) is moderately effective against adult heartworms.

*Milbemycin oxime.* Milbemycin oxime (Interceptor) at 0.5 to 1 mg/kg PO monthly provides complete protection if the drug is started within 2 to 3 months of potential exposure to infected mosquitoes. There is no contraindication to its use in Collies. It is not effective against adult heartworms. A shocklike reaction has occurred in a small percent of dogs with high circulating microfilaria counts.

*Selamectin.* Selamectin (Revolution) effectively prevents heartworm infection. It is applied topically at a recommended dose of 6 mg/kg. In heartworm-positive dogs microfilaremia disappears within 4 months, and the adult worm burden is reduced by at least 39% within 18 months after treatment is initiated. At the dose range of 6 to 12 mg/kg the drug is safe in ivermectin-sensitive Collies, heartworm-positive dogs and cats, and breeding animals.

*Moxidectin.* Moxidectin (ProHeart) is also a safe and effective monthly heartworm preventive for dogs. The recommended minimum dose in dogs >8 weeks of age is 3 μg/kg. The manufacturer recommends its use only in heartworm-negative dogs. Sustained-release moxidectin (ProHeart 6) is available as an SC-injected suspension. Its protective effects last at least 6 months at the recommended dose (0.05 ml/kg of reconstituted suspension, or 0.17 mg/kg of moxidectin). This product is recommended for use in dogs >6 months of age. Transient, localized inflammatory reactions occur at the injection site in some animals. Other adverse effects may include vomiting, diarrhea, lethargy, weight loss, and seizures. At recommended dose rates, moxidectin in either formulation (monthly oral or semiannual subcutaneous injection) is safe in ivermectin-sensitive Collies.

*Diethylcarbamazine.* DEC (Filaribits, Nemacide) is given at 3 mg/kg (6.6 mg/kg of the 50% citrate) PO once a day. In areas with cold winters the drug can be discontinued 2 months after a killing frost and reinstituted 1 month before mosquito season in the spring. Before beginning or restarting DEC, dogs must be negative for microfilaria. Even in areas in which the drug is given year round, annual microfilaria tests are strongly recommended.

*Adverse reactions.* Microfilaremic dogs can develop adverse reactions of variable severity when given DEC. Reactions usually begin within 1 hour after administration.

Depression, lethargy, and reduced responsiveness are variably followed by vomiting, diarrhea, or defecation. Later, bradycardia, weak femoral pulse, and diminished heart sounds occur. Finally shock develops; recumbency, hepatomegaly, hypersalivation, and death usually follow. Therapy with high doses of dexamethasone (at least 2 mg/kg IV), fluids, and other supportive measures are used; atropine is given for severe bradycardia. Dogs experiencing this reaction either show clinical improvement within 3 to 5 hours or die.

Dogs with occult HWD may be given DEC. Dogs receiving DEC prophylaxis that are subsequently discovered to have circulating microfilariae should be continued on the drug during adulticidal and microfilaricidal therapy to prevent reinfection. The combination of DEC and oxibendazole (Filaribits-Plus) has been associated with acute and chronic periportal hepatitis, which may be fatal. Concurrent phenobarbital administration may increase the toxic potential of this drug combination.

*Retesting.* Periodic retesting is an important part of heartworm prophylaxis. After the first year of monthly prophylaxis, a heartworm Ag test should be done to confirm the dog's negative status. When DEC is used, yearly microfilaria testing is important; supplemental Ag testing is also recommended.

## HWD IN CATS

The overall prevalence of HWD in cats is 5% to 20% of that in dogs from the same area. Reported prevalence ranges from 0% to >15%. Infected cats generally have fewer adult worms than infected dogs (only one or two worms in most infected cats), and most cats have no or only a brief period of microfilaremia. Unisex infections are common. Even one adult worm can cause death in cats. Aberrant worm migration is more common in cats.

Pathophysiologic changes occur in two stages. Immature worms (4 to 6 months after infection) cause acute inflammation in the pulmonary arteries and lung tissue; this phase is fatal in some cats. Lesions tend to be focal, so clinically relevant pulmonary hypertension usually does not develop. Dead and degenerating worms cause recrudescence of pulmonary inflammation and thromboembolism. Although some cats recover, sudden death can occur, usually associated with degenerating worms in the pulmonary arteries. Pulmonary hypertension may be present, but secondary right ventricular hypertrophy and right-sided CHF are uncommon.

### Clinical features

Most reported cases have been in cats 3 to 6 years of age, although cats of any age are susceptible. Domestic Shorthair cats seem to be overrepresented. Strictly indoor housing is not protective; in some reports approximately 1/3 of infected cats lived only indoors. Severe clinical signs usually develop 5 to 6 months after infection (as worms arrive in the pulmonary arteries) and with thromboembolism after the death of one or more worms.

Signs are variable and may be transient or nonspecific. Respiratory signs (especially dyspnea and/or paroxysmal cough) occur in >50% of symptomatic cats. Other complaints include lethargy, anorexia, vomiting, syncope, neurologic signs, and sudden death. However, HWD is sometimes an incidental finding. Auscultation may reveal pulmonary crackles, muffled lung sounds, tachycardia, or occasionally a cardiac gallop sound or murmur.

Chronic vomiting is the only sign in some cats; others have vomiting and respiratory or other signs. Pleural effusion from right-sided CHF as well as syncope is less common than in dogs. Other uncommon sequelae include chylothorax, ascites, and caval syndrome. Sudden onset of neurologic signs, often in association with anorexia and lethargy, is common with aberrant worm migration. Only rarely do cardiopulmonary and neurologic signs coexist.

### Diagnosis

HWD is more difficult to diagnose in cats. Serology, thoracic radiographs, echocardiography, and occasionally microfilaria testing are helpful, but are not uniformly definitive. Serologic test results may be negative early in the infection, yet the cat may have clinical signs. Postmortem diagnosis can be difficult if the worms are located in distal pulmonary arteries or aberrant sites.

*Radiography.* Radiographic findings often suggest the presence of HWD but may not correlate with clinical signs or serologic results. Findings may include pulmonary artery enlargement (plus tortuosity and pruning), right ventricular or generalized cardiac enlargement, and diffuse or focal pulmonary bronchointerstitial infiltrates. Pulmonary hyperinflation is sometimes evident. Changes in the pulmonary artery and right heart typically are more subtle than in dogs.

The dorsoventral view is best for evaluating the caudal lobar arteries, which are more frequently abnormal. Enlargement of the left caudal pulmonary artery (>1.6 times the width of the ninth rib at that level) may be the most discriminating finding. Note: The main pulmonary artery segment is not usually visible on dorsoventral or ventrodorsal views in cats.

Right heart enlargement is more likely when signs of right-sided CHF (e.g., pleural effusion) exist. Radiographs are normal in a small percentage of cats with HWD. Pulmonary arteriography may confirm a suspected diagnosis of HWD when an Ag test is negative and echocardiogram is normal.

*Echocardiography.* Echocardiography allows visualization of worms in 40% to 78% of heartworm-positive cats. However, findings may be normal unless worms are located in the heart, main pulmonary artery segment, or proximal left and right pulmonary arteries. Worms are seen in the pulmonary arteries more often than in right-sided heart chambers.

*Clinicopathologic data.* Only 33% to 43% of infected cats have eosinophilia; in most cases the eosinophil count is normal. A similar proportion have mild nonregenerative anemia. Basophilia is uncommon but is suggestive when seen. Advanced pulmonary arterial disease and thromboembolism may be accompanied by neutrophilia (sometimes with a left shift), monocytosis, thrombocytopenia, and DIC. Hyperglobulinemia, the most common biochemical abnormality, occurs inconsistently.

Tracheal wash or bronchoalveolar lavage cytology may yield an eosinophilic exudate suggestive of allergic or parasitic disease, similar to that found with feline asthma and pulmonary parasites. However, the absence of an eosinophilic exudate does not exclude a diagnosis of HWD.

*Other tests.* The ECG is often normal, although most infected cats with right-sided heart failure have changes suggesting right ventricular enlargement. Congenital heart disease or a right bundle branch block with or without cardiomyopathy should also be considered. Arrhythmias are uncommon, although advanced pulmonary arterial disease and CHF can cause ventricular tachyarrhythmias.

A low and transient (1 to 2 month) microfilaremia occurs in approximately 50% of infected cats $6^{1}/_{2}$ to 7 months after infection. Therefore microfilaria concentration tests are usually negative. More than 1 ml (e.g., 3 to 5 ml) of blood should be used to increase the probability of detection of microfilaria.

### Treatment of cats with HWD

*Medical therapy and complications.* Adulticidal therapy is not recommended in cats. The incidence of severe complications is high; cats are not significant reservoirs for heartworm transmission; the shorter life span of heartworms (2 to 3 years) in cats makes spontaneous cure possible; and survival is not improved by adulticidal therapy.

A more conservative approach is to use prednisone as needed, along with a monthly heartworm preventive drug. Interstitial infiltrates usually respond to diminishing doses of prednisone (e.g., 2 mg/kg/day, declining gradually over 2 weeks to 0.5 mg/kg q48h, then discontinuing after 2 more weeks). Treatment can be repeated periodically if respiratory signs recur. Serologic tests should be repeated every 6 to 12 months to monitor infection status. Ag-positive cats usually become negative within 4 to 5 months of worm death. Serial thoracic radiographs and echocardiograms are also useful for monitoring cats in which results of these tests have been abnormal.

*Supportive care.* Supportive care for acutely ill cats can include IV glucocorticoids, fluid therapy, bronchodilator therapy, and supplemental $O_2$. Diuretics are not indicated.

Aspirin and other nonsteroidal antiinflammatory drugs have not been shown to be beneficial and may exacerbate the pulmonary disease.

*Congestive heart failure.* Right-sided CHF develops in some cats with severe pulmonary arterial disease. Cough, pulmonary parenchymal disease, or thromboembolic events occur inconsistently. Dyspnea (pleural fluid accumulation) and jugular venous distention or pulsation are common. Evidence of right ventricular enlargement is usually found on radiographs and ECG. Therapy directed at controlling the signs of heart failure includes thoracocentesis as needed, cage confinement, and cautious furosemide therapy (e.g., 1 mg/kg q12-24h). An angiotensin-converting enzyme inhibitor may be helpful. Digoxin therapy is generally not recommended.

*Caval syndrome.* Although rare, caval syndrome has been reported in cats. Successful removal of adult worms via jugular venotomy has also been reported.

*Adulticidal therapy.* Adulticidal therapy is a last medical resort for cats in a stable condition that continue to manifest clinical signs despite prednisone treatment. Potentially fatal thromboembolism is possible even when only one worm is present. Approximately 1/3 of treated cats can be expected to have thromboembolic complications. Thiacetarsamide has been used in combination with prednisone and extremely close monitoring (see text). Very little clinical experience with melarsomine in cats has been reported.

*Surgical therapy.* Several surgical approaches have been described for removal of adult heartworms in cats. Options include right jugular venotomy and atriotomy or pulmonary arteriotomy via thoracotomy (see text).

*Microfilaricidal and preventive therapy.* Microfilaricidal therapy is usually not necessary as microfilaremia is brief, but ivermectin and milbemycin should be effective. Preventive medication is recommended in endemic areas. Selamectin, ivermectin, and milbemycin oxime are all marketed in the United States for heartworm prevention in cats. Selamectin is used at the same dose as in dogs (6 to 12 mg/kg topically); ivermectin is given at 24 µg/kg PO monthly. The minimum recommended dose for milbemycin oxime is 2 mg/kg. An Ag test is recommended before initiation of prophylaxis if infection could have occurred >8 months before. DEC has been used at doses similar to those in dogs with no apparent adverse effects.

# 11

# Pericardial Diseases and Cardiac Tumors

## *(Text pp 185-197)*

### PERICARDIAL EFFUSION (TEXT PP 185-192)

#### Etiology

Most pericardial effusions in dogs are serosanguineous or hemorrhagic and of neoplastic or idiopathic origin. Transudates, modified transudates, and exudates are found occasionally in dogs and cats.

*Hemorrhagic effusion.* In dogs >7 years of age, hemorrhagic pericardial effusion is likely to have a neoplastic cause. Hemangiosarcoma is by far the most common tumor in dogs (uncommon in cats). Less common neoplasms include heartbase tumors, lymphoma, pericardial mesotheliomas, and (rarely) metastatic carcinomas.

Idiopathic (benign) pericardial effusion is sometimes seen in medium and large breed dogs; Golden Retrievers, German Shepherd Dogs, Great Danes, and Saint Bernards may be predisposed. Dogs of any age can be affected, but most are 6 to 7 years old. More cases are diagnosed in males than in females. The pericarditis typically is mild, with diffuse fibrosis and focal hemorrhage. Constrictive pericardial disease is a potential sequela.

Less common causes of intrapericardial hemorrhage include left atrial rupture secondary to severe mitral insufficiency; coagulopathy (e.g., warfarin-type rodenticides); penetrating trauma (including coronary artery laceration during pericardiocentesis); and uremic pericarditis.

*Transudates.* Transudative effusions can be caused by congestive heart failure (CHF), pericardioperitoneal diaphragmatic hernias (PPDH), hypoalbuminemia, pericardial cysts, or toxemias that increase vascular permeability (including uremia). Usually these conditions are associated with small volumes of pericardial effusion; cardiac tamponade rarely develops.

*Exudates.* Exudative pericardial effusions are rare in small animals. Infectious pericarditis has been reported, usually related to plant awn migration, bite wounds, or extension of pleural or mediastinal infections. Sterile exudative effusions can occur in association with leptospirosis, canine distemper, and idiopathic pericardial effusion in dogs and with feline infectious peritonitis or toxoplasmosis in cats. Chronic uremia occasionally causes a sterile, serofibrinous or hemorrhagic effusion.

### Cardiac tamponade

Cardiac tamponade develops when pericardial fluid accumulation raises intrapericardial pressure above normal cardiac diastolic pressure; the external cardiac compression progressively limits filling, and cardiac output falls. Cardiogenic shock and death can result. Tamponade is relatively common in dogs and rare in cats. Very large pericardial effusions occasionally cause clinical signs, even in the absence of cardiac tamponade. Lung and/or tracheal compression can cause dyspnea and cough; and esophageal compression can cause dysphagia or regurgitation.

### Clinical features

Clinical findings reflect poor cardiac output and usually right-sided CHF. Signs may be nonspecific (e.g., lethargy, weakness, poor exercise tolerance, inappetence) before obvious ascites develops. Rapid accumulation of even small volumes of fluid can cause acute tamponade, shock, and death. In such cases jugular venous distention, hypotension, and pulmonary edema may be evident without radiographic evidence of cardiomegaly or pleural and peritoneal effusions.

Gradual accumulation of larger pericardial fluid volumes can also culminate in CHF. Signs of right-sided failure predominate, although biventricular failure may occur (see Chapter 3). A palpable decrease in arterial pulse strength during inspiration may be discernible. The precordial impulse is attenuated by large pericardial fluid volumes. Auscultation reveals muffled heart and ventral lung sounds; concurrent cardiac disease could cause a murmur. Fever may be associated with infectious pericarditis; rarely, a pericardial friction rub may be heard.

### Diagnosis

*Radiography.* Massive pericardial effusion causes a classic globoid-shaped cardiac shadow. However, smaller fluid accumulations allow various cardiac contours to be identified, especially dorsally. Tamponade may be accompanied by pleural effusion, caudal vena cava distention, hepatomegaly, and ascites. Pulmonary opacities (edema) and distended pulmonary veins are noted less frequently. Some heartbase tumors cause deviation of the trachea or a soft-tissue mass effect; metastatic lung lesions are common in dogs with hemangiosarcoma.

### Electrocardiography.

No pathognomonic findings are present on the electrocardiogram (ECG), although the following abnormalities are suggestive of pericardial effusion: diminished QRS amplitude (<1 mV in dogs), recurring alteration in QRS amplitude (electrical alternans), and ST-segment elevation. Electrical alternans is most evident at heart rates of 90 to 140 beats/min and/or in the standing position. Sinus tachycardia is common in association with cardiac tamponade. Atrial or ventricular tachyarrhythmias may also occur.

### Echocardiography.

Pericardial effusion appears as an echo-free space between the bright parietal pericardium and the epicardium. Abnormal cardiac wall motion and chamber shape, and intrapericardial or intracardiac masses can also be imaged. Tamponade is manifested by diastolic compression and collapse of the right atrium and sometimes right ventricle. Better visualization of the heartbase and mass lesions is generally obtained before pericardiocentesis is performed.

### Pericardiocentesis

*Procedure.* Pericardiocentesis is relatively safe when performed with care. Performing the procedure from the right side minimizes the risk of trauma to the lungs and major coronary vessels. The need for sedation depends on the clinical status and temperament of the patient. The animal is usually placed in left lateral or sternal recumbency. Echo guidance can be used but is not necessary unless the effusion is of very small volume or appears compartmentalized. An ECG monitor should be in place because needle or catheter contact with the heart commonly induces ventricular arrhythmias.

A butterfly catheter (19 to 21 gauge) or appropriately long hypodermic or spinal needle with extension tubing attached is adequate in emergency situations. An over-the-needle catheter (12 to 16 gauge, 4 to 6 in for large dogs; 20 gauge, 1.5 to 2 in for small dogs or cats) reduces the risk of cardiopulmonary laceration during fluid aspiration.

The puncture site is located by palpating the place at which the cardiac impulse is strongest (usually between the fourth and sixth ribs, just lateral to the sternum). The skin is shaved and surgically prepared; sterile gloves and aseptic technique are used. Local anesthesia is necessary when large catheters are used and is recommended for needle pericardiocentesis. Intercostal vessels just caudal to each rib must be avoided when the chest is entered.

Once the needle has penetrated the skin, the operator's assistant should apply gentle negative pressure to the attached syringe as the operator slowly advances the needle toward the heart. It sometimes helps to aim the tip of the needle toward the animal's opposite elbow. Pleural fluid (usually straw colored) may enter the tubing first. The pericardium creates increased resistance to needle advancement and may produce a subtle scratching sensation. Gentle pressure is used to advance the needle through the pericardium; a loss of resistance may be noted with needle penetration.

If the needle contacts the heart, a marked scratching or tapping sensation is usually felt, the needle may move with the heartbeat, and ventricular premature complexes are provoked; the needle should be retracted slightly if cardiac contact occurs. Pericardial effusion usually appears quite hemorrhagic (which can be disconcerting). Initial fluid samples are saved for cytology and microbiologic culture, and then as much fluid as possible is aspirated.

*Fluid analysis.* Samples should be submitted for cytology and saved for possible bacterial (or fungal) culture. Neoplastic lymphoid cells are easily identified in dogs and cats with lymphoma. In other cases differentiation of neoplastic effusions from benign hemorrhagic pericarditis is usually impossible on the basis of cytology. Reactive mesothelial cells in the effusion may closely resemble neoplastic cells; and chemodectomas and hemangiosarcomas may not shed cells into the effusion.

Many neoplastic (and other noninflammatory) effusions have a pH of >7, whereas inflammatory effusions tend to have a lower pH. However, too much overlap exists for pericardial pH to be a reliable discriminator. Culture should be done if cytology suggests an infectious or inflammatory cause. In some patients fungal titers (e.g., coccidiomycosis) or other serologic tests are helpful.

*Hemorrhagic effusions.* With hemorrhagic effusions, the fluid is dark red, with a packed cell volume of >7%, specific gravity >1.015, and protein concentration of 3 to 6 g/dl. The fluid does not clot unless hemorrhage was very recent. Mostly red blood cells are found on cytology, but reactive mesothelial, neoplastic, or other cells may be seen.

*Transudates and exudates.* Pure transudates are clear, with a low cell count (<1500 cells/μl), specific gravity (<1.012), and protein content (<2.5 g/dl). Modified transudates may appear slightly cloudy or pink tinged; cellularity (1500 to 5000 cells/μl) and total protein concentration (approximately 3 g/dl) are higher than those of a pure transudate. Exudates appear cloudy or opaque, and serofibrinous or serosanguineous. They are characterized by a high nucleated cell count (usually >7000 cells/μl), protein concentration (usually >3 g/dl), and specific gravity (>1.015).

**Treatment and prognosis**

Pericardiocentesis is the initial treatment of choice for cardiac tamponade. Most signs of CHF resolve after pericardial fluid is removed, although a diuretic may be of value in some animals. Pericardial effusion secondary to other diseases that cause CHF or to congenital malformations or hypoalbuminemia does not usually cause tamponade and often resolves with management of the underlying condition.

*Idiopathic effusion.* Dogs with idiopathic pericardial effusion are treated conservatively with pericardiocentesis and sometimes a 1- to 2-week course of antibiotics. After an infectious cause is ruled out, a glucocorticoid is often used (e.g., prednisone, 1 mg/kg/day orally [PO], tapering down over 2 to 4 weeks). Periodic reevaluation by radiography or echocardiography is advised. Apparent recovery occurs after one or two pericardial taps in approximately 50% of dogs; tamponade recurs after a variable time span (days to years) in other cases. Recurrent effusion that does not respond to repeated pericardiocentesis and antiinflammatory therapy is usually treated by surgical subtotal pericardiectomy (via thoracotomy or thoracoscopy) or transcutaneous balloon pericardiotomy (see text).

*Neoplastic effusion.* Neoplastic pericardial effusions are drained to relieve cardiac tamponade. Therapy may involve attempted surgical resection or surgical biopsy, a trial of chemotherapy, or conservative therapy until episodes of cardiac tamponade become unmanageable (see later).

*Infectious pericarditis.* Infectious pericarditis should be treated aggressively with appropriate antimicrobial drugs, as determined by microbial culture and sensitivity testing. Surgical therapy is likely to be more effective than drainage with an indwelling pericardial catheter, and it also allows removal of any foreign bodies. Prognosis is guarded; even with successful elimination of infection, fibrin deposition may lead to constrictive pericardial disease.

*Intrapericardial hemorrhage.* Hemorrhage into the pericardial space, whether from trauma, left atrial rupture, or a systemic coagulopathy, should be drained if signs of cardiac tamponade result. Only enough blood to control signs of tamponade should be removed, as continued drainage may predispose to further bleeding. Surgery may be needed to stop continued bleeding or remove large clots. Dogs that survive an initial episode of left atrial rupture still have a guarded to poor prognosis. Animals with intrapericardial hemorrhage of undetermined cause should be evaluated for a coagulation disorder (see Chapter 89).

**Complications**

Complications relate to (1) compression of surrounding structures (cardiac tamponade), (2) effects of associated inflammation (e.g., arrhythmias, local and systemic effects of infectious agents, and further fluid formation), (3) pericardial fibrosis and subsequent constrictive pericarditis, and (4) sequelae of neoplastic processes (e.g., further bleeding, metastases, local invasion and obstruction, seeding of the pleura, loss of function).

Pericardiocentesis itself can cause (1) cardiac injury or puncture, resulting in arrhythmias (common, but usually self-limiting when the needle is withdrawn), (2) coronary artery laceration with myocardial infarction or further pericardial bleeding, (3) lung laceration causing pneumothorax and/or hemorrhage, and (4) dissemination of infection or neoplastic cells into the pleural space.

## CONGENITAL PERICARDIAL DISORDERS (TEXT PP 192-194)
### Peritoneopericardial Diaphragmatic Hernia
Peritoneopericardial diaphragmatic hernia occurs when abnormal embryonic development allows persistent communication between the pericardial and peritoneal cavities at the ventral midline. Abdominal contents herniate into the pericardial space and cause associated clinical signs. Trauma can facilitate movement of abdominal contents through the defect.
#### Clinical features
Clinical signs can appear at any age, but most cases are diagnosed during the first 4 years of life, usually within the first year; some animals never develop signs. Males appear to be affected more frequently than females, and Weimaraners may be predisposed. This malformation is also relatively common in cats. Gastrointestinal (GI) or respiratory signs are most common. Vomiting, diarrhea, anorexia, weight loss, abdominal pain, cough, dyspnea, and wheezing are most often reported; shock and collapse can also occur. Physical examination findings may include muffled heart sounds on one or both sides, displacement or attenuation of the apical precordial impulse, and empty feel on abdominal palpation (with herniation of many organs); rarely, signs of cardiac tamponade are found.
#### Diagnosis
Thoracic radiography is often diagnostic or highly suggestive of PPDH. Characteristic findings include enlargement of the cardiac silhouette, dorsal tracheal displacement, overlap of the diaphragmatic and caudal heart borders, and abnormal fat and/or gas densities within the cardiac silhouette. A pleural fold is usually evident extending between the caudal heart shadow and the diaphragm ventral to the caudal vena cava. Gas-filled loops of bowel crossing the diaphragm into the pericardial sac, a small liver, or few organs within the abdominal cavity may also be seen. Echocardiography is useful in confirming the diagnosis. A GI barium study is diagnostic if stomach and/or intestines are in the pericardial cavity.
#### Treatment and prognosis
Therapy involves surgical closure of the defect after the viable organs have been returned to their normal locations. The presence of other congenital abnormalities and the animal's clinical signs may influence the decision to operate. The prognosis in uncomplicated cases is excellent. Older animals without clinical signs may do well without surgery, especially because organs adhered to the heart or pericardium may be traumatized during attempted repositioning.

### Pericardial Cysts
Pericardial cysts are rare. The clinical presentation is similar to that of pericardial effusion. The cardiac shadow may appear enlarged and deformed radiographically. Diagnosis may be made with echocardiography or pneumopericardiography. Surgical removal of the cyst, in conjunction with partial pericardiectomy, usually is curative.

## CONSTRICTIVE PERICARDIAL DISEASE (TEXT PP 194)
Constrictive pericardial disease occurs occasionally in dogs, but rarely in cats. Sometimes a small amount of pericardial effusion is present (constrictive-effusive pericarditis). The cause is often unknown. Specific causes include recurrent idiopathic hemorrhagic effusion, infectious pericarditis, metallic foreign bodies in the pericardium, tumors, and idiopathic osseous metaplasia and/or fibrosis of the pericardium.
#### Clinical features
Large to medium-sized, middle-aged dogs are most often affected; males and German Shepherd Dogs may be at higher risk. Clinical signs of right-sided CHF predominate. Historical complaints include abdominal distention (ascites), dyspnea or tachypnea, tiring, syncope, weakness, and weight loss. Signs can develop over weeks or months. Occasionally, the animal has a history of pericardial effusion. Ascites and jugular venous distention are the most consistent clinical findings; weakened femoral pulses and muffled heart sounds are also found. An audible diastolic pericardial knock has been

described, but it is not common. A systolic murmur or click (probably caused by valve disease unassociated with the pericardial pathology) or a diastolic gallop sound may also be heard.

### Diagnosis

Diagnosis can be difficult. Typical radiographic findings include mild to moderate cardiomegaly, pleural effusion, and caudal vena cava distention. Constrictive pericardial disease can produce subtle but suggestive echocardiographic changes, such as flattening of the left ventricular free wall in diastole and abnormal septal motion. The pericardium may appear thickened and intensely echogenic, but differentiation from normal pericardial echogenicity may be difficult. ECG abnormalities include sinus tachycardia, P wave prolongation, and small QRS complexes. Invasive hemodynamic studies are the most diagnostic (see text).

### Treatment and prognosis

Surgical pericardiectomy is successful if only the parietal pericardium is involved. Epicardial stripping is required when visceral pericardial disease contributes to the constriction. Pulmonary thrombosis (sometimes massive) is a relatively common post-operative complication; tachyarrhythmias are another complication of surgery. Without surgical intervention the disease is progressive and ultimately fatal.


## CARDIAC TUMORS (TEXT PP 194-196)

Cardiac tumors are uncommon (<0.2% in dogs and <0.03% in cats). These tumors can cause severe clinical signs (typically associated with pericardial effusion and cardiac tamponade), although some are diagnosed fortuitously. Approximately 85% of affected dogs are between 7 and 15 years of age; the risk is lowest in intact females. Approximately 30% of affected cats are <7 years of age.

Hemangiosarcoma is by far the most common cardiac tumor in dogs. Most are located in the right atrium and/or auricle; some also infiltrate the ventricular wall. Metastases have frequently occurred by the time of diagnosis. Golden Retrievers, German Shepherd Dogs, Afghan Hounds, Cocker Spaniels, English Setters, and Labrador Retrievers are at higher risk for this tumor.

Masses at the heartbase are the second most common cardiac tumor in dogs. Heartbase tumors tend to be locally invasive around the root of the aorta and surrounding structures; metastases to other organs are rare. Chemodectomas occur more frequently in brachycephalic dogs (e.g., Boxer, Boston Terrier, English Bulldog). Other primary tumors and metastatic tumors, including lymphoma, other sarcomas, and various carcinomas, may also involve the heart. The most common cardiac tumors in cats are lymphoma and metastatic carcinomas.

### Clinical features

Cardiac tumors in dogs commonly affect the right side of the heart. Signs of right-sided CHF, as well as syncope and exertional weakness, can result from cardiac tamponade, blood flow obstruction, arrhythmias, or impaired myocardial function. Tachyarrhythmias and conduction disturbances can result from tumor infiltration into the conduction system. Lethargy or collapse can occur with bleeding tumors (e.g., hemangiosarcoma). Auscultation may reveal a murmur (caused by intracardiac blood flow obstruction or an unrelated disease such as degenerative mitral regurgitation), an arrhythmia, or muffled heart sounds (marked pericardial effusion). However, auscultation is normal in some cases.

### Diagnosis

*Radiography and electrocardiography.* Radiographic findings can range from a normal cardiac silhouette to unusual cardiac bulge(s), a mass effect adjacent to the heart, or a "globoid" cardiac silhouette (pericardial effusion). Other radiographic findings may relate to impaired cardiac filling (see Chapter 2). Dorsal deviation of the trachea and increased perihilar opacity are seen with some heartbase tumors. Evidence of pulmonary metastases may be seen in dogs and cats with some primary or metastatic cardiac neoplasms. ECG may be normal or may show abnormalities reflective of the location and sequelae of the underlying disease.

*Echocardiography.* Echocardiography can identify cardiac masses and any pericardial effusion. Secondary changes in cardiac chamber size, shape, and ventricular function can also be detected. Assessment of the location, size, attachment (pedunculated or broad based), and extent (superficial or invading the myocardium) of the tumor is valuable in determining whether surgical resection or biopsy is possible.

*Pericardiocentesis.* Cytologic analysis of any pericardial fluid is recommended; however, definitive diagnosis of neoplasia usually cannot be made based on cytology alone. Visualization of a cardiac mass using echocardiography, computed tomography, pneumopericardiography, or another modality is usually necessary for definitive diagnosis of neoplasia.

### Treatment and prognosis

Few good long-term options exist for most patients with cardiac tumors. Management of cardiac tamponade was described previously; most signs of CHF resolve once the pericardial fluid is removed. Conservative therapy (pericardiocentesis as needed, plus glucocorticoid therapy) is used in some patients. Effusion secondary to myocardial lymphoma often responds to pericardiocentesis and chemotherapy.

In dogs with cardiac hemangiosarcoma or mesothelioma, partial pericardiectomy should avert recurrence of tamponade. Although it may facilitate tumor dissemination throughout the thoracic cavity, survival time is the same as for pericardiocentesis alone. Prognosis is poor for dogs with these tumors (median, 2 to 3 weeks for hemangiosarcoma, longer for mesothelioma), although chemotherapy is effective in some patients. Partial pericardiectomy is also recommended for dogs with heartbase tumors and may prolong survival for years. Percutaneous balloon pericardiotomy may also be an effective palliative procedure.

Surgical resection may be possible, depending on tumor location, size, and invasiveness. Tumors involving only the tip of the right auricle and pedunculated masses in surgically accessible locations are more likely to be resectable. However, attempts at aggressive resection are often met with severe bleeding and death. Surgical biopsy of a nonresectable mass may be helpful if chemotherapy is being contemplated. Many cardiac tumors are fairly unresponsive to chemotherapy, but some are treated with good short-term success (see Chapters 82 and 84).

# 12

# Systemic Arterial Hypertension

## (Text pp 198-205)

Hypertension is defined as abnormally high blood pressure, although the level at which arterial pressure becomes "abnormally high" is not clear-cut. Various factors can influence arterial blood pressure in healthy animals, and although some dogs and cats clearly have clinical disease caused by hypertension, many animals with "abnormally high" blood pressure have no evidence of related pathology (although a predisposing disease may be present). Therefore careful clinical evaluation and repeated blood pressure measurements over time are indicated before a diagnosis of hypertension is made. Direct and indirect methods of blood pressure measurement are discussed in the text.

In general, blood pressures in normal, untrained, unanesthetized dogs and cats do not exceed 160/100 mm Hg (systolic/diastolic), although normal pressures may be above this range in sight hounds and cats. Some normal animals have systolic pressures >180 mm Hg when stressed or anxious, but pressures of 180 to 200/110 mm Hg are generally considered borderline or mildly increased. Arterial pressures >200/110 mm Hg are considered in the hypertensive range.

### Etiology

Hypertension in dogs and cats is usually secondary to another disease process. Primary (essential) hypertension is a diagnosis of exclusion. It is infrequently diagnosed in animals, although inherited essential hypertension has been documented in dogs.

Secondary hypertension may be associated with renal disease (tubular, glomerular, or vascular), hyperadrenocorticism, hyperthyroidism (cats) or hypothyroidism (dogs), pheochromocytoma, chronic anemia (cats), high-salt diet, diabetes mellitus, liver disease, or obesity. A high prevalence of hypertension exists in cats with renal disease or hyperthyroidism. In dogs renal disease (especially that involving glomerular function) and hyperadrenocorticism are commonly associated with hypertension. Transient hypertension can occur with administration of vasoconstrictive agents, including topical ocular phenylephrine.

### Clinical features

Most dogs and cats with clinical hypertension are middle-aged or older, presumably because of their associated disease conditions. Male dogs may be at higher risk than females. Signs relate either to the associated disease process or to organ damage caused by the hypertension. Organs that are particularly sensitive are the eye, kidney, heart, and brain.

Blindness is the most common presenting complaint and usually results from acute retinal hemorrhage or detachment; sight does not return in most cases. Other ocular fundic changes include evidence of old retinal hemorrhages; hyperreflective scars; papilledema; perivasculitis; and retinal edema, atrophy, or arteriolar tortuosity. Vitreal or anterior chamber hemorrhage, closed-angle glaucoma, and corneal ulceration can also occur.

Another common complaint is polyuria-polydipsia, usually caused by renal disease, hyperadrenocorticism (dogs), or hyperthyroidism (cats). Other common findings include a soft systolic murmur, a gallop sound (especially in cats), and epistaxis (resulting from vascular rupture in the nasal mucosa). Seizures, paresis, syncope, collapse, or other neurologic signs can be manifestations of cerebrovascular accidents ("strokes") resulting from hypertensive arteriolar spasm or hemorrhage.

### Diagnosis

Blood pressure measurement should be obtained whenever signs compatible with hypertension are found, and also when a disease associated with hypertension is diagnosed. It is important to confirm a diagnosis of hypertension by measuring blood pressure multiple times and on different days. Routine complete blood count, serum biochemical profile, and urinalysis are indicated in all patients. Other tests are submitted as needed to rule out possible underlying diseases or complications (e.g., endocrine tests, radiographs, ultrasonography, echocardiography, electrocardiogram, ocular examination, serologic tests).

Thoracic radiographs often reveal some degree of cardiomegaly in dogs and cats with chronic hypertension. Other findings in cats include a prominent aortic arch and an undulating aorta, although these are not pathognomonic for hypertension. Left ventricular hypertrophy or aortic root dilation may be identified on echocardiogram.

### Treatment

Animals with severe hypertension (>200/110 mm Hg) and those with clinical signs presumed to be caused by hypertension should be treated. Whether every dog and cat with mild hypertension (repeatable systolic pressures of 170 to 200 mm Hg) would benefit from specific antihypertensive therapy is unclear. The expense and time commitment required for long-term management, as well as potential adverse medication effects, must be considered.

The approach to managing the hypertensive patient is summarized in Box 12-1. The goal of therapy is to reduce blood pressure to below 170/100 mm Hg, as restoration of normal pressure is unlikely. Underlying or concurrent diseases should be addressed in all patients.

*General measures.* High sodium ($Na^+$) loads should be avoided in both foods and medications. Reduced dietary sodium intake (e.g., <0.25% $Na^+$ on a dry-matter basis) is advised for all cases. Weight reduction is recommended for obese animals. Drugs that can potentiate vasoconstriction (e.g., phenylpropanolamine and other $\alpha_1$-adrenergic agonists), as well as glucocorticoids and progesterone derivatives, should be avoided.

A diuretic (thiazide or furosemide; see Chapter 3) may help, but diuretic therapy alone is rarely effective. Diuretics should be avoided or used only with caution in azotemic animals. Serum potassium should be monitored, especially in cats with chronic renal disease.

*Antihypertensive agents.* Several drugs have been used as antihypertensive agents in dogs and cats. Most commonly prescribed are angiotensin-converting enzyme inhibitors (ACEIs), amlodipine (a calcium entry blocker), and β-adrenergic blockers. Doses are given in Table 12-1; these drugs are discussed further in Chapters 3 and 4. Drugs used for treatment of cardiovascular disorders are summarized in the table at the end of this section.

Usually, one drug is used at a time and the animal is monitored; it may take at least 2 weeks before blood pressure decreases significantly. In some cases therapy with one agent is effective; combination therapy may be needed for adequate blood pressure control in other animals. An ACEI is recommended as the initial agent in dogs. Amlodipine is recommended as first-line treatment in hypertensive cats unless hyperthyroidism is the cause, in which case atenolol or another β-blocker is used first.

*Cats with renal disease.* β-Blockers are often ineffective as monotherapy in cats with renal disease. Hypertensive cats with chronic renal failure are often unresponsive to ACEIs. Nevertheless, ACEIs may help protect against hypertensive renal damage; they reduce proteinuria and slow the progression of renal disease. Amlodipine has been used successfully and with minimal adverse effects as a single agent in cats. It generally

---

**Box 12-1**

## Approach to the Hypertensive Patient

### SUSPECTED HYPERTENSION OR DISEASE ASSOCIATED WITH HYPERTENSION

Measure BP
- Use quiet environment; allow 5-10 min for patient to acclimate; if animal is easily stressed, have owner present when possible
- Use appropriate-size cuff (use same cuff size for subsequent measurements); use consistent measurement technique
- Take at least five BP readings; discard highest and lowest, average the remaining readings

Repeat BP measurements at other (one to three) times, preferably on different days, except when the following is true:
- Acute, hypertension-induced clinical signs are present (e.g., ocular hemorrhage, retinal detachment, neurologic signs); in this case begin therapy immediately (see text)

Screen for underlying disease(s)
- CBC, serum biochemistry tests, and urinalysis in every patient
- Depending on individual presentation, also consider endocrine testing, thoracic and abdominal radiographs, ocular examination, ECG, echocardiography, other tests as indicated

### CONFIRMED HYPERTENSION

Manage underlying disease(s)
Use reduced-sodium diet
Begin initial antihypertensive drug therapy (see text and Table 12-1)
- Dogs: enalapril or other ACEI (unless hypertension is pheochromocytoma induced)
- Nonhyperthyroid cats: amlodipine
- Hyperthyroid cats: atenolol or other β-blocker
- Emergent therapy if needed (see text)

Client education (patient's disease, potential complications, medication and reevaluation schedules, potential adverse effects of medications, diet)

### PATIENT REEVALUATION

Recheck BP in 1-2 weeks in clinically stable patients and sooner in unstable patients (although full effects of antihypertensive drugs may not yet be realized)
Repeat or perform other tests as indicated
Decide whether to continue therapy as before or adjust dose (up or down)
Continue weekly or biweekly BP monitoring and management of underlying disease
- If BP control not achieved even with maximized dosage of initial agent, try alternative drug or piggyback two agents

When BP (and underlying disease) controlled, gradually increase time between recheck examinations
- Recheck at least every 2-3 months, because medication requirements may change

---

*ACEI,* Angiotensin-converting enzyme inhibitor; *BP,* arterial blood pressure; *CBC,* complete blood count; *ECG,* electrocardiogram.

does not have significant effects on serum creatinine concentration or body weight in cats with chronic renal failure. Mild reduction in serum potassium concentration can be successfully treated with oral potassium supplementation.

***Adverse effects.*** Adverse effects of antihypertensive therapy such as lethargy or ataxia and reduced appetite are usually related to hypotension. The ability to monitor blood pressure is important when antihypertensive drugs are prescribed. Serial measurements are needed to assess treatment efficacy and avoid hypotension.

***Emergency care.*** Emergency antihypertensive therapy is indicated in patients with acute retinal detachment and hemorrhage, encephalopathy or other evidence of intracranial hemorrhage, acute renal failure, or acute heart failure. Vasodilators such as hydralazine or nitroprusside can be used for acute hypertensive crises, provided constant-rate infusion and adequate monitoring are available. Intravenous (IV) propranolol or acepromazine may also be used (see Table 12-1).

Oral therapy with a calcium entry blocker, prazosin, or an ACEI may be effective for acute clinical hypertension of various causes, although parenteral therapy (or oral hydralazine) is advised in patients with severe hypertension.

***Pheochromocytoma.*** $\alpha_1$-Adrenergic antagonists (e.g., prazosin, phenoxybenzamine) are especially useful for the treatment of hypertension caused by pheochromocytoma. In a hypertensive crisis phentolamine (Regitine) is used as an IV bolus, followed by an infusion titrated until effective (see Table 12-1). A $\beta$-blocker may also be indicated for pheochromocytoma-induced tachyarrhythmias but should not be used alone or before an $\alpha$-blocker is used.

***Periodic monitoring.*** Periodic monitoring of dogs and cats with hypertension is important; some animals respond initially but become refractory to the same therapy later. In nonemergency cases blood pressure monitoring is initially done every 1 to 2 weeks. When satisfactory blood pressure control is attained (which may take several weeks), monitoring every 2 to 3 months is usually adequate.

### Prognosis

Because most cases of hypertension are associated with severe underlying disease, the long-term prognosis is often guarded, despite apparent response to antihypertensive drugs. Some treatments for underlying disease (e.g., fluid therapy, corticosteroids, erythropoietin) can exacerbate hypertension.

**Table 12-1**

## Drugs Used to Treat Hypertension

| Drug | Dog | Cat |
|---|---|---|
| **DIURETICS (see also Chapter 3 and Table 3-2)** | | |
| Furosemide | 1-3 mg/kg q8-24h PO | 1-2 mg/kg q12-24h PO |
| Hydrochlorothiazide | 2-4 mg/kg q12h PO | 1-2 mg/kg q12h PO |
| **β-ADRENERGIC BLOCKERS (see also Chapter 4 and Table 4-3)** | | |
| Atenolol | 0.2-1 mg/kg q12-24h PO (start low) | 6.25-12.5 mg/cat q(12-)24h PO |
| Propranolol | 0.1-1 mg/kg q8h PO (start low) | 2.5-10 mg/cat q8-12h PO |
| **ACEIs (see also Chapter 3 and Table 3-2)** | | |
| Enalapril | 0.5 mg/kg q24(-12)h PO | 0.25-0.5 mg/kg q24(-12)h PO |
| Captopril | 0.5-2 mg/kg q8-12h PO | 0.5-1.25 mg/kg q12-24h PO |
| **CALCIUM ENTRY BLOCKER** | | |
| Amlodipine besylate | 0.1-0.3 (0.5) mg/kg q24(-12)h PO | 0.625 mg/cat q24(-12)h PO |
| **α₁-ADRENERGIC BLOCKERS (see also Chapter 3)** | | |
| Prazosin | Large dog: 1 mg q8-12h PO | Do not use |
| Phenoxybenzamine | 0.25-1.5 mg/kg q12h PO | 0.25-1 mg/kg q12h PO |
| **AGENTS USED FOR HYPERTENSIVE CRISIS** | | |
| Hydralazine (see also Chapter 3) | 0.5-0.2 mg/kg q12h PO | 2.5-10 mg/cat q12h PO |
| Nitroprusside (see also Chapter 3) | 0.5-1 µg/kg/min CRI (initially), to 5-15 µg/kg/min CRI | Same |
| Acepromazine | 0.05-0.1 mg/kg (up to 3 mg total) IV | Same |
| Propranolol | 0.02 mg/kg initially, slowly IV (to maximum 1 mg/kg) | Same |
| Esmolol | 200-500 µg/kg IV over 1 min, then 25-200 µg/kg/min CRI | Same |
| Phentolamine | 0.02-0.1 mg/kg IV bolus, followed by CRI until effective | Same |

*ACEI,* Angiotensin-converting enzyme inhibitor; *CRI,* constant-rate infusion; *IV,* intravenously; *PO,* orally.

## Drugs Used to Treat Cardiovascular Disorders

| Generic name | Trade name | Dog | Cat |
|---|---|---|---|
| **DIURETICS** | | | |
| Furosemide | Lasix Distal Furotabs Diuride | 1-3 mg/kg q8-24h chronic PO; or 2-5 mg/kg q4-6h IV, IM, SC | 1-2 mg/kg q12h up to 4 mg/kg 18-12h IV, IM, SC, PO |
| Chlorothiazide | Diuril | 20-40 mg/kg q12h PO | — |
| Hydrochlorothiazides | Hydrodiuril Esidrix | 2-4 mg/kg q12h PO | 1-2 mg/kg q12h PO |
| Spironolactone | Aldactone | 2 mg/kg q12h PO | — |
| Triamterene | Dyrenium | 2(-4) mg/kg/day PO | — |
| **VASODILATORS** | | | |
| Enalapril | Enacard Vasotec | 0.5 mg/kg q(12-)24h PO | 0.25-0.5 mg/kg q(12-)24h PO |
| Captopril | Capoten | 0.5-2 mg/kg q8-12h PO (0.25-0.5 mg/kg initial dose) | 0.5-1.25 mg/kg q12-24h PO |
| Benazepril | Lotensin | 0.25-0.5 mg/kg q24h PO | — |
| Lisinopril | Prinivil Zestril | 0.5 mg/kg q24h PO | — |
| Hydralazine | Apresoline | 0.5-2 mg/kg q12h PO (to 1 mg/kg initial) For decompensated CHF: 0.5-1 mg/kg PO, repeat in 2-4h, then q12h | 2.5 (up to 10) mg/cat q12h PO |
| Prazosin | Minipress | Small dogs (<5 kg): do not use Medium dogs: 1 mg q8-12h PO Large dogs: 2 mg q8h PO | Do not use |
| Na$^+$ nitroprusside | Nitropress Nipride | 0.5-1 µg/kg/min CRI (initial), to 5 to 15 µg/kg/min CRI | Same |

*Continued.*

## Drugs Used to Treat Cardiovascular Disorders—cont'd

| Generic name | Trade name | Dog | Cat |
|---|---|---|---|
| Nitroglycerine ointment 2% | Nitrobid<br>Nitrol | 1/2-11/2 inch q4-6h cutaneously | 1/4-1/2 inch q4-6h cutaneously |
| Isosorbide dinitrate | Isordil Titradose<br>Sorbitrate | 0.5-2 mg/kg q8h PO | — |
| Amlodipine besylate | Norvasc | ? | 0.625 mg/cat PO |
| Phenoxybenzamine | Dibenzyline | 0.25(-1.5) mg/kg q12h PO | 0.25-0.5 mg/kg q12h PO |
| Phentolamine | Regitine | 0.02-0.1 mg/kg IV bolus, followed<br>by CRI until effective | Same |
| Acepromazine | | 0.05-0.1 mg/kg (up to 3 mg total) IV | 0.05-0.2 mg/kg SC |
| **POSITIVE INOTROPIC DRUGS** | | | |
| Digoxin | Cardoxin<br>Cardoxin LS<br>Lanoxin | Oral: dogs <22 kg: 0.011 mg/kg q12h; dogs >22 kg:<br>0.22 mg/m$^2$ q12h; or 0.005 mg/kg q12h; decrease<br>by 10% for elixir; max. 0.5 mg/day or 0.375 mg/day<br>for Dobermans<br>IV loading: 0.01-0.02 mg/kg; give 1/4 of total dose<br>in slow boluses over 2-4h until effective<br>IV loading: 0.005 mg/kg—give 1/2 of total,<br>then 1-2h later give 1/4-dose bolus as needed | Oral: 0.007 mg/kg q48h |
| Digitoxin | Crystodigin | 0.02-0.03 mg/kg q8h (small dogs)-q12h (large dogs) | Do not use |
| Dopamine | Intropin | For CHF: 1-10 µg/kg/min CRI (start low)<br>For shock: 5-15 µg/kg/min CRI | 1-5 µg/kg/min CRI (start low) |
| Dobutamine | Dobutrex | 1-10 µg/kg/min CRI (start low) | Same |
| Amrinone | Inocor | 1-3 mg/kg initial bolus, IV; 10-100 µg/kg/min CRI | Same? |
| Milrinone | Primacor | 50 µg/kg IV over 10 min initially;<br>0.375-0.75 µg/kg/min CRI (humans) | Same? |

## ANTIARRHYTHMIC DRUGS

### Class I

| Drug | Trade name | Dog | Cat |
|---|---|---|---|
| Lidocaine | Xylocaine | Initial boluses of 2 mg/kg slowly IV, up to 8 mg/kg; or rapid IV infusion at 0.8 mg/kg/min; if effective, then 25-80 µg/kg/min CRI (can also be used intratracheally for CPR) | Initial bolus of 0.25-0.5 mg/kg slowly IV; can repeat at 0.15-0.25 mg/kg in 5-20 min; if effective, 10-20 µg/kg/min CRI |
| Procainamide | Pronestyl | 6-20 mg/kg IV over 5-10 min; 10-50 µg/kg/min CRI; 6-30 mg/kg q4-6h IM, 10-20 mg/kg q6h PO (sustained release: q6-8h) | 1-2 mg/kg slow IV; 10-20 µg/kg/min CRI; 7.5-20 mg/kg q(6 to)8h IM, PO |
| Quinidine | Quinalan Quinidex Extentabs Quinaglute Dura-Tabs Cardioquin | 6-20 mg/kg q6h IM (loading dose 14-20 mg/kg); 6-16 mg/kg q6h PO; sustained action preparations 8-20mg/kg q8h PO | 6-16 mg/kg q8h IM, PO |
| Tocainide | Tonocard | 10-25 mg/kg q8h PO | — |
| Phenytoin | Dilantin | 10 mg/kg slow IV; 30-50 mg/kg q8h PO | Do not use |
| Mexiletine | Mexitil | 4-10 mg/kg q8h PO | — |

### Class II

| Drug | Trade name | Dog | Cat |
|---|---|---|---|
| Propranolol | Inderal Inderal LA | IV: initial bolus of 0.02 mg/kg slowly; up to max. of 0.1 mg/kg 12h; PO: initial dose of 0.1-0.2 mg/kg q8h, up to max. of 1 mg/kg q8h | IV: Same PO: 2.5 up to 10 mg/cat q8-12h |
| Atenolol | Tenormin | 0.2-1 mg/kg q12-24h PO (start low) | 6.25-12.5 mg/cat q(12-)24h PO |
| Esmolol | Brevibloc | 200-500 µg/kg IV over 1 min, followed by infusion of 25-200 µg/kg/min | Same |
| Metoprolol | Lopressor | 0.2 mg/kg initial dose q8h PO; up to 1 mg/kg q8h | — |
| Nadolol | Corgard | 0.2 mg/kg initial dose q8-12h PO; up to 1 mg/kg q8-12h | — |

*Continued.*

## Drugs Used to Treat Cardiovascular Disorders—cont'd

| Generic name | Trade name | Dog | Cat |
|---|---|---|---|
| **Class III** | | | |
| Bretylium | Bretylol | 2-6 mg/kg IV; may repeat in 1-2h (humans) | — |
| Amiodarone | Cordarone | ?10-15 mg/kg q12h PO for 7 days; then 5-7.5 mg/kg q12h PO for 14 days; then 7.5 mg/kg q24h PO for maintenance | — |
| Sotalol | Betapace | Large dogs: 40-80 mg (approximately 1-2 mg/kg) q12h PO | — |
| **Class IV** | | | |
| Verapamil | Calan<br>Isoptin | Initial dose: 0.05 mg/kg slowly IV; can repeat q5 min, up to total of 0.15 (to 0.2) mg/kg; 0.5-2 mg/kg q8h PO | Initial dose 0.025 mg/kg slowly IV; can repeat q5min, up to total of 0.15(-0.2) mg/kg; 0.5-1 mg/kg q8h PO |
| Diltiazem | Cardizem<br>Cardizem-CD<br>Dilacor XR | Initial dose 0.5 mg/kg q8h PO, up to 2 mg/kg; for atrial tachycardia, 0.5 mg/kg PO, followed by 0.25 mg/kg q1h to total of 1.5(-2) mg/kg or conversion; or 0.15-0.25 mg/kg over 2-3 min IV | Same?<br>For hypertrophic cardiomyopathy, 1-2.5 mg/kg q8h PO; sustained release Cardizem-CD: 10 mg/kg/day; Dilacor XR: 30 mg/cat/day |
| **ANTICHOLINERGICS** | | | |
| Atropine | | 0.01-0.02 mg/kg IV, IM; 0.02-0.04 mg/kg SC; can also be used intratracheally for CPR | Same |
| Glycopyrrolate | Robinul | 0.005-0.01 mg/kg IV, IM; 0.01-0.02 mg/kg SC | Same |
| Propantheline Br | Pro-Banthine | 3.73-7.5 mg q8-12h PO | — |

## SYMPATHOMIMETICS

| Drug | | Dog | Cat |
|---|---|---|---|
| Isoproterenol | Isuprel | 0.045-0.09 µg/kg/min CRI | Same |
| Terbutaline | Brethine<br>Bricanyl | 2.5-5 mg/dog q8-12h PO | 1.25 mg/cat q12h PO |

## OTHER ANTIARRHYTHMIC AGENT

| Drug | | Dog | Cat |
|---|---|---|---|
| Adenosine | Adenocard | Up to 12 mg rapid IV bolus | — |

## CPR DRUGS

| Drug | | Dog | Cat |
|---|---|---|---|
| Epinephrine | Adrenaline Cl | 0.2 mg/kg IV; 0.4 mg/kg IT (diluted with equal volume saline), q3-5 min as needed; also can use IO (previously recommended: 0.1-0.5 mg/10 kg); 1:1000 = 1 mg/ml | Same |
| Methoxamine | Vasoxyl | 0.1-0.2 mg/kg IV; can use IT | Same |
| Metaraminol | | 0.1-0.2 mg/kg IV | Same |
| Mephentermine | | 0.1-0.5 mg/kg IV | Same |
| Phenylephrine | | 0.01-0.1 mg/kg IV | Same |
| Norepinephrine | Levophed | 0.01-0.1 mg/average dog | — |
| Dopamine | | 5-15 µg/kg/min CRI; can also use IO | 1-5 µg/kg/min CRI; can also use IO |
| Sodium bicarbonate | | 0.5-1 mEq/kg initial; up to 8 mEq/kg if prolonged arrest and/or CPR<br>Do *not* give IT; can use IO | Same |
| Calcium chloride (10%) | | 0.1-0.26 mg/kg IV (or 1.5-2 ml/dog) | Same |
| Calcium gluconate (10%) | | 0.1-0.3 mg/kg IV; can use IO | Same |
| Dexamethasone SP | | 4 mg/kg IV; can use IO | Same |
| Atropine | | 0.01-0.02 mg/kg IV, IM, IT, IO | Same |
| Lidocaine | | 2 mg/kg up to 8 mg/kg IV; see Table 4-2; can also use IT or IO | 0.25-0.5 mg/kg slowly IV; see Table 4-2; can also use IT or IO |

*Continued.*

## Drugs Used to Treat Cardiovascular Disorders—cont'd

| Generic name | Trade name | Dog | Cat |
|---|---|---|---|
| **DRUGS FOR ADULT HEARTWORM INFECTIONS** | | | |
| Melarsomine | Immiticide | Follow manufacturer's instructions carefully; 2.5 mg/kg deep into lumbar muscles q24h for two doses | — |
| Thiacetarsamide | Caparsolate | 2.2 mg/kg IV (0.22 ml/kg) q12h for 2 days | Same |
| **MICROFILARICIDAL THERAPY** | | | |
| Ivermectin | Ivomec Heartgard-30 | One dose (0.05 mg/kg) orally 3-4 weeks after adulticidal therapy; can repeat in 2 weeks | Same |
| Milbemycin oxime | Interceptor | One dose of 0.5 mg/kg PO; can repeat in 2 weeks | Same |
| Levamisole | Levasol | 10-11 mg/kg/day for 7-14 days; if necessary, repeat for 5-7 days | 10 mg/kg/day for 7 days |
| Fenthion | Spotton | 15 mg/kg applied cutaneously once a week for up to 3 weeks; 15 mg/kg topically once a week for 3 weeks (4-6 weeks after adulticidal therapy) | — |
| **HEARTWORM PREVENTION** | | | |
| Ivermectin | Heartgard-30 | 0.006-0.012 mg/kg PO once a month | 0.024 mg/kg PO once a month |
| Milbemycin oxime | Interceptor | 0.5-(0.9) mg/kg PO once a month | 0.5 mg/kg PO once a month |
| Moxidectin | Proheart | 0.001-0.003 mg/kg PO once a month | |
| Diethylcarbamazine | Filaribits Nemacide Caricide | 2.5-3 mg/kg (5-6 mg/kg of 50% citrate) PO once a day | Same |

*CPR, Cardiopulmonary resuscitation; IM, intramuscularly; IO, intraosseously; IT, intratracheally; IV, intravenously; max., maximum; PO, orally; SC, subcutaneously.*

# PART II

# Respiratory System Disorders

ELEANOR C. HAWKINS

# 13

## Clinical Manifestations of Nasal Disease

### (Text pp 210-216)

Diseases of the nasal cavity and paranasal sinuses can cause nasal discharge, sneezing, stertor (snoring or snorting sounds), facial deformity, systemic signs of illness (e.g., lethargy, inappetence, weight loss), and rarely, central nervous system signs.

## NASAL DISCHARGE (TEXT PP 210-214)

Nasal discharge is the most common sign of nasal disease. It is most often the result of localized disease in the nasal cavity and/or paranasal sinuses, but it can also develop with lower respiratory tract disorders such as bacterial pneumonia and infectious tracheo-bronchitis and systemic disorders such as coagulopathies and systemic hypertension. Specific causes are listed in Box 13-1.

### Etiology and Clinical Presentation

#### Serous discharge

Serous nasal discharge has a clear, watery consistency. Depending on the quantity and duration, a serous discharge may be normal or it may be indicative of viral upper respiratory infection or impending mucopurulent discharge.

#### Mucopurulent discharge

Mucopurulent nasal discharge has a thick, ropy consistency and a white, yellow, or green tint. It is a common presenting sign in animals with intranasal disease, and it implies inflammation, possibly with secondary bacterial infection. If mucopurulent discharge is present with signs of lower respiratory tract disease (e.g., cough, respiratory distress, auscultable crackles), the diagnostic emphasis should be on evaluation of the lower airways and pulmonary parenchyma. Bleeding with mucopurulent discharge is usually suggestive of neoplasia or mycotic infection.

#### Epistaxis

Pure hemorrhage (epistaxis) can result from trauma, locally aggressive neoplasia or mycotic infection, systemic hypertension, or bleeding disorders. Systemic hemostatic disorders that can cause epistaxis include thrombocytopenia, thrombocytopathies, Von Willebrand's disease, rodenticide toxicity, and vasculitis. Ehrlichiosis and Rocky Mountain spotted fever can also cause epistaxis. Nasal foreign bodies can cause hemorrhage, but the bleeding tends to subside quickly. Epistaxis can also result from vigorous or paroxysmal sneezing.

### Diagnostic Approach

The general diagnostic approach to nasal discharge is given in Box 13-2. A complete history and physical examination are used to prioritize the differential diagnoses. Acute processes, such as foreign bodies or acute feline viral infections, often result in a sudden

**Box 13-1**

## Differential Diagnoses for Nasal Discharge in Dogs and Cats

### SEROUS DISCHARGE
Normal
Viral infection
Early sign of condition that causes mucopurulent discharge

### MUCOPURULENT DISCHARGE WITH OR WITHOUT HEMORRHAGE
Viral infection
    Feline herpesvirus (rhinotracheitis virus)
    Feline calicivirus
Bacterial infection
Fungal infection
    *Aspergillus*
    *Cryptococcus*
    *Penicillium*
    *Rhinosporidium*
Nasal parasites
Foreign body
Neoplasia
    Carcinoma
    Sarcoma
    Malignant lymphoma
Nasopharyngeal polyp
Lymphocytic plasmacytic rhinitis
Allergic rhinitis
Extension of oral disease
    Tooth root abscess
    Oronasal fistula
    Deformed palate

### PURE HEMORRHAGIC DISCHARGE (EPISTAXIS)
Nasal disease
    Acute trauma
    Acute foreign body
    Neoplasia
    Fungal infection
Systemic disease
Coagulopathy
    Systemic hypertension
    Polycythemia
    Hyperviscosity syndrome
    Vasculitis

onset of signs. In chronic processes, such as mycotic infections or neoplasia, signs are present for longer, and the animal may begin to lose weight. A history of gagging or retching can indicate a mass or foreign body in the caudal nasopharynx.

#### Physical examination
Thorough examination of the head, including facial symmetry, teeth, gingiva, hard and soft palate, mandibular lymph nodes, and eyes, should be performed. Ulceration of the nasal plane often occurs in dogs with nasal aspergillosis. Polyps protruding from

---

**Box 13-2**

## General Diagnostic Approach to Dogs and Cats with Chronic Nasal Discharge

### PHASE I (NONINVASIVE TESTING)

| All patients | Dogs and cats with hemorrhage | Cats |
|---|---|---|
| History | Complete blood count | Nasal swab cytologic |
| Physical examination | Platelet count | evaluation (cryptococcosis) |
| Thoracic radiographs | Coagulation times | Cryptococcal antigen titer |
| *Aspergillus* titer (dogs) | Buccal mucosal bleeding | Viral testing |
| | times | Feline leukemia virus |
| | Rickettsial titers | Feline immunodeficiency |
| | Arterial blood pressure | virus |
| | Von Willebrand's factor | ± Herpesvirus |
| | assay | ± Calicivirus |

### PHASE II (GENERAL ANESTHESIA REQUIRED)
Nasal radiography or computed tomography
Oral examination
Rhinoscopy: external nares and nasopharynx
Nasal biopsy and histologic examination
Deep nasal culture
    Fungal
    Bacterial

### PHASE III (REFERRAL USUALLY REQUIRED)
Computed tomography (if not previously performed)

### PHASE IV (CONSIDER REFERRAL)
Repeat phase II using computed tomography
Exploratory rhinotomy with turbinectomy

---

the external nares are typical of rhinosporidiosis in dogs and cryptococcosis in cats. Pain on palpation of the nasal bones is typical of aspergillosis. Gingivitis, dental calculi, loose teeth, or pus in the gingival sulcus can indicate oronasal fistulas or a tooth root abscess, especially if unilateral nasal discharge is present. Foci of inflammation and folds of hyperplastic gingiva in the dorsum of the mouth should be probed for oronasal fistulas. The hard and soft palates are examined for deformation, erosions, and congenital defects such as clefts and hypoplasia.

Mandibular lymph node enlargement suggests active inflammation or neoplasia; fine needle aspirates of enlarged or firm nodes should be evaluated for organisms such as *Cryptococcus* spp. and for neoplastic cells. With epistaxis, the presence of petechiae or hemorrhage in other mucous membranes, skin, ocular fundus, feces, or urine suggests a systemic bleeding disorder. (Note: Melena may be present as a result of swallowing blood from the nasal cavity.)

*Unilateral versus bilateral discharge.* Systemic disorders and infectious diseases tend to involve both sides of the nasal cavity, whereas foreign bodies, polyps, and tooth root abscesses usually cause unilateral discharge. Neoplasia causes unilateral discharge initially but may progress to bilateral discharge after destruction of the nasal septum. When nasal discharge is apparently unilateral, a cold microscope slide can be held close to the external nares to determine the patency of the side without discharge.

Condensation will not be visible in front of the naris if airflow is obstructed, implying that the disease is actually bilateral.

**Laboratory tests**

A complete blood count with platelet count, coagulation panel, buccal mucosal bleeding time, and arterial blood pressure should be evaluated in dogs and cats with epistaxis. Von Willebrand's factor assays are also performed in purebred dogs and dogs with prolonged mucosal bleeding times.

*Serology.* *Ehrlichia* and Rocky Mountain spotted fever titers are indicated in endemic areas. Tests for feline immunodeficiency virus and leukemia virus should be performed in cats with potential exposure and chronic nasal discharge.

Fungal titers are available for aspergillosis in dogs and cryptococcosis in dogs and cats. A single positive titer for aspergillosis suggests active infection; however, a negative titer does not rule out the disease. The result must be interpreted in conjunction with nasal imaging, rhinoscopy, histology, and culture. In the case of cryptococcosis the organism is usually identifiable in specimens from infected organs. A latex agglutination capsular antigen test (LCAT) is performed if cryptococcosis is suspected but the organism is not found. LCAT can also be used to monitor response to therapy.

**Further evaluation**

Signalment, history, and physical examination findings dictate in part which other tests may be needed. When acute viral infection is not a consideration, nasal imaging, rhinoscopy, and biopsy or deep nasal culture are often required for definitive diagnosis. These tests are discussed in Chapter 14. When a diagnosis cannot be made, nasal imaging (preferably computed tomography), rhinoscopy, and biopsy can be repeated in 1 to 2 months.

## SNEEZING (TEXT P 215)

Intermittent, occasional sneezing is considered normal; persistent, paroxysmal sneezing is abnormal. Disorders commonly associated with acute-onset, persistent sneezing include nasal foreign body and feline upper respiratory infection. The canine nasal mite, *Pneumonyssoides caninum*, and exposure to irritating aerosols are less common causes of sneezing. The various causes of nasal discharge (see Box 13-1) can also cause sneezing, although nasal discharge generally is the primary complaint.

### Diagnostic Approach

Owners should be questioned carefully about possible exposure of the pet to foreign bodies (e.g., grass awns), powders, aerosols, or, in cats, exposure to new cats or kittens. The presence of a foreign body should not be excluded just because sneezing subsides. In dogs a history of acute sneezing followed by development of nasal discharge is suggestive of a foreign body. Other supportive findings include pawing at the nose, unilateral serosanguineous or mucopurulent nasal discharge, and gagging, retching, or reverse sneezing (if the object is in the caudal nasopharynx). Dogs that develop acute, paroxysmal sneezing should undergo prompt rhinoscopic examination.

Cats sneeze more often as a result of acute viral infection than from foreign bodies, so immediate rhinoscopic examination is usually not indicated. Other signs of upper respiratory infection, such as conjunctivitis and fever, may be present, as well as a history of exposure to other cats or kittens.

## REVERSE SNEEZING (TEXT P 216)

Reverse sneezing is a paroxysm of noisy, labored inspiration initiated by nasopharyngeal irritation. Such irritation can be the result of a foreign body or viral infection; epiglottic entrapment of the soft palate is another proposed cause. Most cases are idiopathic and affect small-breed dogs. Signs are commonly associated with excitement or drinking. Although reverse sneezing may persist throughout the animal's life, the problem rarely progresses.

The diagnosis is generally based on thorough history and physical examination findings. Generally, no treatment is needed. Some owners report that massaging the neck shortens an ongoing episode, and that antihistamines decrease the frequency and severity. Further evaluation for nasal or pharyngeal disorders is indicated if syncope, exercise intolerance, or other signs of respiratory compromise are reported, or if reverse sneezing is severe or progressive.

## STERTOR (TEXT P 216)

Stertor indicates upper airway obstruction, most often the result of pharyngeal disease (see Chapter 16). Intranasal causes include obstruction from congenital deformities, masses, exudate, or blood clots.

## FACIAL DEFORMITY (TEXT P 216)

The most common causes of facial deformity adjacent to the nasal cavity are neoplasia and, in cats, cryptococcosis. Visible swellings can often be evaluated with fine-needle aspiration or punch biopsy. If such an approach is not possible or is unsuccessful, other diagnostic tests are required (see Chapter 14).

# 14

# Diagnostic Tests for the Nasal Cavity and Paranasal Sinuses

## *(Text pp 217-227)*

The following diagnostic tests are performed with the animal under general anesthesia, except for nasal swab. Nasal radiography or computed tomography (CT) is usually performed first, followed by rhinoscopic examination and specimen collection.

## RADIOGRAPHY (TEXT PP 217-221)

### Views

At least four radiographic views should be taken: lateral, ventrodorsal, intraoral, and frontal sinus (skyline). Lateral-oblique views or dental films are also indicated for possible tooth root abscess, and radiographs of the tympanic bullae are obtained in cats with suspected nasopharyngeal polyps. The intraoral view is particularly helpful for detection of subtle asymmetry between the left and right nasal cavities. The frontal sinus view is useful in animals with aspergillosis or neoplasia, as the frontal sinuses may be the only area of disease involvement.

Most animals with intranasal disease have normal thoracic radiographs. However, thoracic radiographs can be useful in identification of primary bronchopulmonary disease, pulmonary involvement with cryptococcosis, and rare metastases from neoplastic disease.

### Interpretation

Nasal radiographs are evaluated for increased fluid density, loss of turbinates, lysis of facial bones, radiolucency at the tips of the tooth roots, and the presence of radiodense foreign bodies (Box 14-1). Nasal radiographs rarely provide a definitive diagnosis and generally must be followed by rhinoscopy and nasal biopsy.

Increased fluid density can be caused by mucus, exudate, blood, or soft-tissue masses such as polyps, tumors, or granulomas. Fluid density within the frontal sinuses may represent mucous accumulation caused by obstruction of drainage into the nasal cavity, extension of disease into the frontal sinuses, or primary frontal sinus disease.

Loss of the normal turbinate pattern with increased fluid density in the nasal cavity occurs with chronic inflammation of various causes; it can also be an early neoplastic change. Multiple, well-defined lytic zones within the nasal cavity and increased radiolucency in the rostral portion of the nasal cavity suggest aspergillosis.

## COMPUTED TOMOGRAPHY (TEXT P 221)

CT provides excellent visualization of the nasal turbinates, nasal septum, hard palate, and cribriform plate. It is more accurate than radiography in assessing the extent of neoplasia; therefore it allows more accurate localization of mass lesions for subsequent biopsy and for radiotherapy planning. It may also reveal lesions in animals with undiagnosed nasal disease when other techniques have failed.

## RHINOSCOPY (TEXT P 221-224)

Rhinoscopy is used to visualize and remove foreign bodies; to grossly assess the nasal mucosa for inflammation, turbinate erosion, mass lesions, fungal plaques, and parasites; and to aid in collection of specimens for histopathology and culture. Rhinoscopy is usually performed after nasal radiography or CT unless a foreign body is strongly suspected.

The oral cavity and caudal nasopharynx should be assessed first. The hard and soft palates are examined and palpated for deformation, erosions, and other defects; and the gingival sulci are probed for fistulas. The caudal nasopharynx is examined for polyps, neoplasia, and foreign bodies (particularly grass or plant material). It is best visualized with a flexible fiberoptic endoscope that is passed into the oral cavity and retroflexed around the soft palate.

### Rostral nasal cavity

Inflammation (mucosal swelling, hyperemia, excess mucus, exudate) is a nonspecific finding. Potential causes are similar to those of mucopurulent nasal discharge (see Box 13-1). Other abnormal rhinoscopic findings and possible causes include the following:

- masses—neoplasia, nasopharyngeal polyp, cryptococcosis, mat of fungal hyphae or fungal granuloma (aspergillosis, penicilliosis, rhinosporidiosis)
- mild turbinate erosion—feline herpesvirus, chronic inflammatory process
- marked turbinate erosion—neoplasia, aspergillosis, penicilliosis, cryptococcosis
- parasites—nasal mites *(Pneumonyssoides caninum),* worms *(Capillaria [Eucoleus] boehmi)*
- foreign bodies

Lesions and foreign bodies can be missed if only the smaller recesses of the nasal cavity are involved. Swollen and inflamed nasal mucosa, hemorrhage caused by the procedure, and accumulation of exudate and mucus can also interfere with complete evaluation of the nasal cavity.

## NASAL BIOPSY (TEXT PP 224-226)

The various nasal biopsy techniques are briefly described in the following sections. The more aggressive collection methods (e.g., pinch biopsy and core biopsy) are more

---

**Box 14-1**

## Radiographic Signs of Common Nasal Diseases*

### CHRONIC VIRAL RHINITIS (FELINE)
Soft-tissue opacity within nasal cavity, may be asymmetric
Mild turbinate lysis
Soft-tissue opacity in frontal sinus(es)

### NASOPHARYNGEAL POLYP
Soft-tissue opacity above soft palate
Soft-tissue opacity within nasal cavity, usually unilateral
Mild turbinate lysis possible
Bulla osteitis: soft-tissue opacity within bulla, thickening of bone

### NASAL NEOPLASIA
Soft-tissue opacity, may be asymmetric
Turbinate destruction
Vomer bone and/or facial bone destruction
Soft-tissue mass external to facial bones

### NASAL ASPERGILLOSIS
Well-defined lucent areas within the nasal cavity
Increased radiolucency rostrally
Increased soft-tissue opacity may also be present
No destruction of vomer or facial bones, although signs often bilateral
Vomer bone may be roughened
Fluid density within the frontal sinus; frontal bones may be thickened or motheaten

### CRYPTOCOCCOSIS
Soft-tissue opacity, may be asymmetric
Turbinate lysis
Facial bone destruction
Soft-tissue mass external to facial bones

### LYMPHOPLASMACYTIC RHINITIS
Soft-tissue opacity
Lysis of nasal turbinates, especially rostrally

### ALLERGIC RHINITIS
Increased soft-tissue opacity
Mild turbinate lysis possible

### TOOTH ROOT ABSCESS
Radiolucency adjacent to tooth root, commonly apically

### FOREIGN BODIES
Mineral and metallic dense foreign bodies readily identified
Plant foreign bodies: focal, ill-defined, increased soft-tissue opacity
Lucent rim around abnormal tissue (rare)

---

*These descriptions represent typical cases and are not specific findings.

likely to provide pieces of tissue that extend beneath the superficial inflammation common to many nasal disorders. Fine-needle aspirates can also be obtained from mass lesions. Blood-clotting capabilities should be assessed before the more aggressive biopsy techniques are performed if the animal has a history of hemorrhagic exudate or epistaxis or if any other indication of coagulopathy is present.

## Techniques

### Nasal swab

Nasal swabs can be collected from a conscious animal. They are useful for identification of cryptococcal organisms and should be collected early in the evaluation of cats with chronic rhinitis. Routine cytologic stains are used, although India ink can be applied to demonstrate cryptococcal organisms. Other findings are generally nonspecific.

### Nasal flush

Nasal flush is a minimally invasive technique. A soft catheter is positioned in the caudal nasal cavity via the oral cavity, with the tip of the catheter pointing rostrally. The fluid exiting the external nares can be examined cytologically; large particles can be submitted for histopathologic examination. However, these specimens are usually insufficient to permit a definitive diagnosis.

### Pinch biopsy

Alligator-cup biopsy forceps are used to obtain full-thickness pieces of nasal mucosa for histologic evaluation. The technique is best performed under endoscopic guidance. If no localizable lesion is identified radiographically or rhinoscopically, biopsies are obtained from several sites on both sides of the nasal cavity.

### Core biopsy

Core biopsy is an excellent method of tissue collection when a mass lesion is present. A polypropylene dog urinary catheter or the plastic sleeve of a spinal needle can be used. A 12-ml syringe is used to aspirate a dislodged core of tissue from the mass. The tissue is submitted for histologic evaluation.

### Turbinectomy

Turbinectomy provides the best tissue specimens for histologic examination and allows identification and removal of abnormal tissue and placement of drains for topical nasal therapy. It is performed through a rhinotomy incision and should be considered only when less invasive techniques have failed to establish a diagnosis. Potential complications include pain, excessive hemorrhage, inadvertent entry into the cranial vault, and recurrent nasal infections. Cats may be anorectic postoperatively; placement of a gastrostomy tube can be considered in these patients.

## Complications

The major complication of nasal biopsy is hemorrhage. The severity depends on the biopsy method, but even with aggressive techniques the hemorrhage is rarely life-threatening. For minor hemorrhage, the rate of intravenous (IV) fluid administration should be increased and manipulations within the nasal cavity stopped until the bleeding subsides. Cold saline solution, with or without diluted epinephrine (1:100,000), can be gently infused into the nasal cavity.

Persistent, severe hemorrhage can be controlled by packing the nasal cavity with umbilical tape. The tape must be packed through the nasopharynx as well as through the external nares. In the rare event of uncontrolled hemorrhage the external carotid artery on the involved side can be ligated. Rhinotomy should not be attempted. In the vast majority of patients, time and/or cold saline infusions will control hemorrhage.

Brain injury is avoided by never passing any object into the nasal cavity beyond the level of the medial canthus of the eye without visual guidance. Aspiration of blood, saline, or exudate into the lungs is avoided by placement of a cuffed endotracheal tube before the procedure and packing of the caudal pharynx with gauze. Pointing the animal's nose toward the floor over the end of the table also helps once the procedure is completed. The pharynx should be examined for continued fluid accumulation after the gauze is removed and before extubation.

## NASAL CULTURES (TEXT PP 226-227)

Aerobic and anaerobic bacterial cultures and fungal cultures can be performed on material obtained by swab, nasal flush, or tissue biopsy. Normal nasal flora can include *Staphylococcus, Streptococcus, Escherichia coli, Pseudomonas, Pasteurella, Aspergillus,* and a variety of other aerobic and anaerobic bacteria and fungi. Therefore bacterial or fungal growth from nasal specimens does not necessarily indicate disease. A diagnosis of nasal aspergillosis or penicilliosis requires supporting signs and results of other tests, such as radiography, rhinoscopy, and serology, in addition to fungal culture.

### Interpreting bacterial growth

It is difficult, if not impossible, to distinguish between normal growth and abnormal overgrowth of normal flora on the basis of culture alone. Samples for culture should be collected from deep within the nasal cavity, using a guarded catheter swab, a sterile swab carefully inserted deep into the nasal cavity (accepting some contamination with this option), or sterile biopsy forceps.

Abundant growth of one or two types of bacteria more likely reflects abnormal growth, whereas growth of many different organisms represents normal flora. The presence of septic inflammation (based on cytology) and a positive response to antibiotic therapy supports a diagnosis of bacterial infection.

Although bacterial rhinitis is rarely, if ever, a primary disease, improvement in nasal discharge may be seen if the bacterial component of the problem is treated. Improvement is generally transient, unless the underlying disease process is corrected. However, some patients in which a primary disease is never identified or cannot be corrected respond well to long-term antibiotic therapy. Sensitivity data from bacterial cultures considered to represent significant infection help in antibiotic selection.

# 15

# Disorders of the Nasal Cavity

## *(Text pp 228-240)*

## FELINE UPPER RESPIRATORY INFECTION (TEXT PP 228-232)

### Etiology

Upper respiratory infections (URIs) are common in cats. Feline herpesvirus (FHV), also called *feline rhinotracheitis virus,* and feline calicivirus (FCV) cause nearly 90% of these infections. *Bordetella bronchiseptica* and *Chlamydophila felis* (previously *Chlamydia psittaci*) are less commonly involved. Other viruses and *Mycoplasma* spp. may play a primary or secondary role. Cats become infected through contact with actively infected cats, carrier cats, and fomites. Cats that are young, stressed, or immunosuppressed are most likely to develop clinical signs.

### Clinical features

Clinical manifestations can be acute, chronic and intermittent, or chronic and persistent. Acute disease is the most common; signs include fever, sneezing, serous or mucopurulent nasal discharge, conjunctivitis and ocular discharge, hypersalivation, anorexia, and dehydration. FHV can also cause corneal ulceration, abortion, and neonatal death; FCV can cause oral ulcerations, mild interstitial pneumonia, and polyarthritis. *Bordetella* can cause cough and, in young kittens, pneumonia. Signs of *Chlamydophila* infection are usually limited to conjunctivitis.

Periodic recurrence may occur in association with stressful or immunosuppressive events. Other cats may have chronic, persistent signs, most notably a serous to mucopurulent nasal discharge.

### Diagnosis

Acute URI is usually diagnosed by typical historic and physical examination findings; chronic URI is diagnosed by eliminating other causes of nasal discharge.

*Laboratory tests.* Specific tests to identify FHV, FCV, *Bordetella,* and *Chlamydophila* include fluorescent antibody testing, virus isolation or bacterial culture, and serum antibody titers. Tests for specific agents are particularly useful in cattery outbreaks. Several cats, with and without clinical signs, should be tested.

Fluorescent antibody tests for FHV and FCV are performed on smears from conjunctival scrapings or pharyngeal or tonsillar swabs or on impression smears from tonsillar biopsies. Virus isolation can be performed on pharyngeal, conjunctival, and nasal swabs and on tissue specimens such as tonsillar biopsies. Finding intracytoplasmic inclusion bodies on cytologic examination of conjunctival smears is suggestive of *Chlamydophila* infection. Bacterial culture of the oropharynx can be used to identify *Bordetella,* but this organism may be found in healthy cats.

### Treatment for acute infection

In most cats URI is a self-limiting disease. Appropriate supportive care, especially adequate hydration and nutrition, should be provided when necessary. Dried mucus and exudate should be cleaned from the face and nares. The cat can be placed in a steamy bathroom for 15 to 20 minutes two or three times a day or in a small room with a vaporizer overnight to help clear excess secretions.

*Decongestants.* Severe nasal congestion is treated with pediatric topical decongestants, such as 0.25% phenylephrine or 0.025% oxymetazoline. A drop is gently placed in each nostril daily for up to 3 days. If longer therapy is necessary, the decongestant is withheld for 3 days before beginning another 3-day course. Another option is to alternate the naris treated each day.

*Antibiotics.* Antibiotic therapy is indicated in cats with severe clinical signs. The initial antibiotic of choice is ampicillin (22 mg/kg q8h) or amoxicillin (22 mg/kg q8-12h). If *Bordetella, Chlamydophila,* or *Mycoplasma* infection is suspected, doxycycline (5 to 10 mg/kg q12h) or chloramphenicol (10 to 15 mg/kg q12h) should be used. Azithromycin (5 to 10 mg/kg q24h for 3 days, then q72h) can be prescribed for cats that are difficult to medicate.

*Chlamydophila* infection should be suspected when conjunctivitis is the primary problem and in catteries in which the disease is endemic. Oral antibiotics are administered for 3 weeks. In addition, chloramphenicol or tetracycline ophthalmic ointment should be applied at least three times a day for at least 14 days beyond resolution of signs.

*Corneal ulcers.* Corneal ulcers resulting from FHV infection are treated with topical antiviral drugs, such as trifluridine, idoxuridine, or adenine arabinoside. One drop should be applied to each affected eye five to six times a day for up to 3 weeks. Routine ulcer management is also indicated (tetracycline or chloramphenicol ophthalmic ointment two to four times a day, and topical atropine as needed). Treatment is continued for 1 to 2 weeks after reepithelialization has occurred.

*Glucocorticoids.* Topical or systemic glucocorticoids are *contraindicated* in cats with acute URI or ocular manifestations of FHV infection, because they can prolong signs and increase viral shedding.

### Treatment for chronic infection

Cats with chronic, persistent signs of URI often require management for years. Treatment strategies include facilitating drainage of discharge, controlling secondary bacterial infections, treating possible herpesvirus infection, reducing inflammation, and, as a last resort, turbinectomy and frontal sinus ablation.

*Facilitating drainage.* Keeping secretions moist, performing intermittent nasal flushes, and using topical decongestants judiciously facilitate drainage. Keeping the cat in a room with a vaporizer at night can provide symptomatic relief. Alternatively, drops of sterile saline can be placed into the nares. Some cats have marked improvement in clinical signs for weeks after flushing of the nasal cavity with copious amounts of saline or dilute Betadine solution. Topical decongestants also provide relief during episodes of severe congestion.

*Antibiotics.* Chronic antibiotic therapy may be required to manage secondary bacterial infections. Broad-spectrum antibiotics such as amoxicillin (22 mg/kg q12h) or trimethoprim-sulfadiazine (15 mg/kg q12h) are often successful. Chloramphenicol (10 to 15 mg/kg q12h) or doxycycline (5 to 10 mg/kg q12h) can be effective when other drugs have failed. Fluoroquinolones should be reserved for cats with documented resistant gram-negative infections. If a beneficial response is seen within 1 week, the antibiotic should be continued for at least 4 to 6 weeks.

Cats that respond well during the prolonged course of antibiotics but suffer relapse shortly after discontinuation of the drug are candidates for continuous long-term antibiotic therapy. Success can often be achieved with twice-daily amoxicillin.

*Lysine.* Treatment with lysine (250 mg given orally [PO] q12h) may be effective in cats with active FHV infections. A trial of at least 4 weeks is necessary to assess treatment efficacy.

*Glucocorticoids.* Cats with severe, persistent signs despite supportive care may benefit from glucocorticoids; however, these drugs should be prescribed only after a complete diagnostic evaluation has been performed to rule out other diseases. Prednisone is administered at 0.5 mg/kg q12h. If a beneficial response is seen within 1 week, the dose is gradually decreased to the lowest effective level. If a clinical response is not seen within 1 week, the drug should be discontinued.

*Surgery.* Cats with severe or deteriorating signs despite conscientious care are candidates for turbinectomy and frontal sinus ablation, provided a thorough evaluation to eliminate other causes of chronic nasal discharge has been performed. Complete elimination of respiratory signs is unlikely, but signs may be more easily managed. Anorexia can be a postoperative problem and may require placement of a gastrostomy tube.

### Prognosis

The prognosis for cats with acute URI is good. Most cats do not develop chronic disease, and nearly all of those that do have good quality of life with appropriate care.

### Prevention in individual cats

Prevention of URI in all cats is based on avoiding exposure to infectious agents and strengthening immunity against infection. In most household cats, routine health care and regular vaccination is adequate. Although vaccination does not prevent infection, it decreases the severity of clinical signs resulting from URI. Owners should be discouraged from allowing cats to roam freely outdoors.

*Vaccination.* Modified-live vaccines for FHV and FCV are used in most cats. These vaccines provide adequate protection for cats that are not heavily exposed to these viruses, but they are not effective in kittens while maternal immunity persists. Kittens are usually vaccinated at 8 to 10 weeks of age and again 3 to 4 weeks later. At least two vaccines must be given initially, with the final vaccine given after the kitten is 12 weeks old. Thereafter, booster vaccinations are recommended every 1 to 3 years. Queens should be vaccinated before breeding.

Modified-live vaccines should not be used in pregnant queens; killed FHV and FCV vaccines are available for use in these cats. Killed vaccines are also recommended for cats with feline leukemia virus (FeLV) or feline immunodeficiency virus (FIV) infection.

Intranasal *Bordetella* and injectable *Chlamydophila* vaccines are available, but these infections are uncommon in household cats and they can be effectively treated with antibiotics. These vaccines are recommended for use only in catteries or shelters in which *Bordetella* or *Chlamydophila* is endemic.

### Prevention in multiple-cat households

Control of URI in multiple-cat households is based on the same principles as defined for the individual pet cat: avoiding exposure to the infectious agents and strengthening immunity against infection.

*Minimizing exposure.* Ideally, all cats with a history of URI should be eliminated from the cattery, as they may be carriers. Cats must be segregated to limit the extent of outbreaks and to facilitate identification of carrier cats. Kittens are kept separated, along with their queens before weaning, until 1 to 2 weeks after completion of the vaccination series.

Animals new to the household should be isolated and observed for at least 3 weeks. Ideally, new cats are already quarantined for several months as part of an FeLV prevention program. Clinically ill cats are maintained in separate isolation facilities for at least 3 weeks after resolution of clinical signs. Overcrowding should be avoided. Good hygiene and good ventilation are also very important.

Cats should be handled in order of susceptibility: kittens first, healthy adults second, quarantined cats third, and clinically ill cats last. Hands must be carefully washed between groups, and cleaning and feeding supplies kept separate or disinfected between groups. Interactions with cats in the reverse order for any reason is strictly avoided.

In breeding facilities, litters should be staggered to avoid having large numbers of kittens at the same time. In queens with a history of recrudescent infection associated with pregnancy, disease in young kittens may be avoided through early weaning (at 5 to 6 weeks of age).

*Strengthening immunity.* Selective breeding for healthy kittens, maintenance of excellent nutrition, and eradication of controllable infections (e.g., FeLV, FIV, parasites) increase overall resistance to disease. Specific immunity is strengthened through vaccination. Households without major URI problems are advised to use routine vaccination protocols, as described for individual cats. Intensified vaccination schedules are useful in controlling outbreaks of disease, but chronic use should not be necessary.

Households experiencing outbreaks among young kittens can begin vaccinations with a killed product when the kittens are 4 to 5 weeks of age and repeat when they are 6 to 7 weeks of age. Routine vaccination with an injectable modified-live product is begun at 9 weeks of age. Use of the intranasal *Bordetella* or injectable *Chlamydophila* vaccine is indicated if one of these agents has been identified.

*Intranasal viral vaccines.* Intranasal modified-live vaccines for FHV and FCV can be considered when injectable products are inadequate. However, upper respiratory signs can occur after vaccination; they tend to be self-limiting but are unacceptable to many owners. For humane organizations, new admissions should be vaccinated intranasally at the time of entry. In young kittens vaccination is repeated after 12 weeks of age and at least 2 weeks after initial intranasal vaccination.

Households with uncontrollable outbreaks in young kittens can begin vaccination intranasally when the kittens are as young as 4 to 5 weeks of age. When kittens are affected at an even younger age, intranasal vaccines can be administered as early as 8 to 10 days of age at a reduced dose (one drop in each nostril). The series is completed with either intranasal vaccination at 9 and 12 weeks of age or subcutaneous vaccinations beginning at 6 to 7 weeks of age.

## NASOPHARYNGEAL POLYPS (TEXT PP 232-233)

Nasopharyngeal polyps are benign growths that occur in kittens and young adult cats. They are often attached to the base of the eustachian tube and can extend into the external ear canal, middle ear, pharynx, or nasal cavity. Their gross appearance can be mistaken for neoplasia. Signs include stertorous breathing, upper airway obstruction, and serous to mucopurulent nasal discharge. Signs of otitis externa or media and interna, such as head tilt, nystagmus, or Horner's syndrome, can also occur.

### Diagnosis

Visualization of a mass in the nasopharynx, nasal cavity, or external ear canal, as well as radiographic identification of a soft-tissue opacity above the soft palate, support a tentative diagnosis of nasopharyngeal polyp. Complete evaluation also includes a deep otoscopic examination and radiographs of the osseous bullae. Most cats with polyps have otitis media, detectable radiographically as thickened bone or increased soft-tissue opacity of the bullae. Definitive diagnosis is made by histopathologic analysis of tissue biopsy, usually obtained during surgical excision.

### Treatment and prognosis

Treatment consists of surgical excision, usually performed through the oral cavity. Bulla osteotomy should be performed in cats with radiographic involvement of the osseous bullae. Rarely, rhinotomy is required for complete removal. The prognosis is excellent. Regrowth occurs at the same site if the abnormal tissue was not removed completely, with signs usually recurring within 1 year.

## NASAL TUMORS (TEXT PP 233-235)

Most nasal tumors in dogs and cats are malignant. Adenocarcinoma, squamous cell carcinoma, and undifferentiated carcinoma are common nasal tumors in dogs. Lymphoma and adenocarcinoma are common in cats. Fibrosarcomas and other sarcomas also occur in both species. Benign tumors can include adenomas, fibromas, papillomas, and transmissible venereal tumors (dogs).

### Clinical features

Nasal tumors usually occur in aged animals, but they may be found in young animals. Clinical features (usually chronic) reflect the locally invasive nature of these tumors. Nasal discharge (serous, mucoid, mucopurulent, or hemorrhagic) is the most common complaint. One or both nostrils may be involved. With bilateral involvement, the discharge is often worse from one nostril. For many animals, the discharge was initially unilateral and progressed to become bilateral. Sneezing may also be reported.

Deformation of the facial bones, hard palate, or maxillary dental arcade may be seen. Tumor growth may also result in neurologic signs or exophthalmos, although these signs are rarely the primary complaint. Weight loss and anorexia may accompany respiratory signs but are often absent.

### Diagnosis

A diagnosis of neoplasia is based on clinical findings, radiography, computed tomography (CT), and/or rhinoscopy. Definitive diagnosis requires histopathologic examination of a biopsy specimen, although fine-needle aspirates may yield conclusive results.

Not all cases of neoplasia are diagnosed on initial evaluation. Radiography, rhinoscopy, and biopsy may need to be repeated in 1 to 3 months. Repeated evaluation is particularly indicated in dogs with chronic nasal discharge because, unlike cats, they do not develop chronic viral rhinitis.

Determining the extent of the disease is important when one is selecting the appropriate therapy. CT is more sensitive than radiography for evaluating the extent of abnormal tissue. Aspirates of mandibular lymph nodes should be examined cytologically for evidence of local spread. Thoracic radiographs should also be evaluated, although pulmonary metastases are uncommon. Cytologic evaluation of bone marrow aspirates and abdominal radiographs or ultrasound are indicated for patients with lymphoma. Cats with lymphoma should also be tested for FeLV and FIV.

### Treatment

Benign tumors should be surgically excised. Malignant nasal tumors can be treated with radiation therapy (plus surgery), chemotherapy, or both. Cats with nasal lymphoma are best treated with either radiation therapy or chemotherapy using standard lymphoma protocols (see Chapter 82). Radiation therapy is the treatment of choice for most other malignant nasal tumors. Surgical debulking before radiation is recommended if orthovoltage radiation is used. Carcinomas may be responsive to cisplatin, carboplatin, or multiagent chemotherapy.

Treatment with piroxicam can be considered for carcinomas in dogs when radiation therapy is not elected. Potential side effects include gastrointestinal ulceration (can be severe) and kidney damage. In dogs with other types of tumors and in cats, improvement of clinical signs may be seen with antiinflammatory doses of prednisone (0.5 to 1 mg/kg/day, tapered to lowest effective dose). Note: Prednisone should not be given in conjunction with piroxicam.

### Prognosis

The prognosis for untreated malignant nasal tumors is poor. Survival after diagnosis is usually only a few months. Radiation therapy can prolong survival and improve quality of life in some patients. The therapy is well tolerated by most animals, and in those that achieve remission the quality of life is usually excellent.

## NASAL MYCOSES (TEXT PP 235-237)

### Cryptococcosis

*Cryptococcus neoformans* is a fungal agent that infects cats and, less commonly, dogs. In cats clinical signs usually reflect infection of the nasal cavity, central nervous system (CNS), eyes, or skin and subcutaneous tissues. In dogs signs of CNS involvement are most common. The lungs are commonly infected in both species, but clinical signs of lung involvement (e.g., cough, dyspnea) are rare. Clinical features, diagnosis, and treatment of cryptococcosis are discussed in Chapter 103.

### Aspergillosis

*Aspergillus fumigatis* is a normal inhabitant of the nasal cavity in many animals. In some dogs and rarely in cats it becomes a pathogen, invading the nasal mucosa and creating visible fungal plaques ("fungal mats"). Animals that develop aspergillosis may have another nasal disease, such as neoplasia, foreign body, traumatic injury, or immune deficiency that predisposes to secondary fungal infection.

#### Clinical features

Aspergillosis can cause chronic nasal disease in any dog, but it is most common in young male dogs. Nasal discharge can be mucoid, mucopurulent, or hemorrhagic and may be unilateral or bilateral. Sneezing is sometimes reported. Sensitivity to palpation of the face or depigmentation and ulceration of the external nares is highly suggestive of aspergillosis. The lungs are rarely involved.

#### Diagnosis

No single test result is diagnostic for aspergillosis. Diagnosis is based on the cumulative findings of a comprehensive evaluation. Aspergillosis can be an opportunistic infection, so underlying nasal disease must always be considered.

Radiographic signs include well-defined lucent areas within the nasal cavity and increased radiolucency rostrally. Other signs are listed in Box 14-1. In some patients the frontal sinus is the only site of infection. Rhinoscopic abnormalities include erosion of nasal turbinates and white to green fungal plaques on the nasal mucosa, but absence of such lesions does not rule out aspergillosis. If affected tissue is sampled, the organisms can generally be seen histologically after routine staining of nasal mucosal biopsies. Invasion of fungal organisms into the nasal mucosa is indicative of aspergillosis. Multiple biopsies should be obtained, ideally of grossly abnormal tissue, because the disease is usually multifocal rather than diffuse.

Results of fungal culture are difficult to interpret. The organism can be found in the nasal cavity of normal animals, and false-negative culture results can also occur. A positive culture, in conjunction with other clinical and diagnostic findings, supports the diagnosis. Positive serum antibody titers also support a diagnosis of aspergillosis. Animals in which the organism is a normal nasal inhabitant usually do not develop measurable titers. However, both false-positive and false-negative results can occur.

#### Treatment and prognosis

Current treatments of choice are topical clotrimazole (success rate 85% to 90%) and oral itraconazole (success rate 60% to 70%). Oral therapy is simpler to administer but is somewhat less successful, requires prolonged treatment, and is relatively expensive. Itraconazole is administered at a dose of 5 mg/kg PO q12h for 60 to 90 days, and possibly longer.

Topical clotrimazole therapy is administered with the patient under general anesthesia (see text). Clinical signs generally resolve in 1 to 2 weeks. A second treatment is performed if signs persist after 2 weeks. Trephination of the affected sinus, debulking of fungal granulomas, and intranasal administration of clotrimazole is recommended if a frontal sinus granuloma is suspected.

With the use of these newer antifungal agents the prognosis for most patients with nasal aspergillosis is fair to good.

## BACTERIAL RHINITIS (TEXT P 238)

In the vast majority of cases, bacterial rhinitis is a secondary complication, not a primary disease process. Bacterial rhinitis occurs secondarily with almost all diseases of the nasal cavity and typically involves overgrowth of normal inhabitants of the nasal cavity. Antibiotic therapy often leads to clinical improvement, but the response is usually temporary. Therefore management of dogs and cats with suspected bacterial rhinitis should include a thorough diagnostic evaluation for underlying disease.

### Clinical findings and diagnosis

Most dogs and cats with bacterial rhinitis have mucopurulent nasal discharge. No clinical signs are pathognomonic for bacterial rhinitis, and it is difficult to make a definitive diagnosis because of the diverse flora in the normal nasal cavity (see Chapter 14). Beneficial response to antibiotic therapy is often used to support a diagnosis of bacterial involvement.

### Treatment

The bacterial component of nasal disease is treated with antibiotic therapy. If growth on bacterial culture is believed to be significant, sensitivity data can be used in selecting antibiotics. Effective broad-spectrum antibiotics include amoxicillin (22 mg/kg q8-12h), trimethoprim-sulfadiazine (15 mg/kg q12h), chloramphenicol (50 mg/kg q8h for dogs, 10 to 15 mg/kg q12h for cats), or clindamycin (5.5 to 11 mg/kg q12h). Doxycycline (5 to 10 mg/kg q12h) or chloramphenicol is often effective against *Bordetella* and *Mycoplasma*.

For acute infection or in cases in which the primary cause has been eliminated (e.g., foreign body, diseased tooth root), antibiotics are administered for 7 to 10 days. Chronic infections require prolonged treatment. Antibiotics are administered for 1 week; if a beneficial response is seen, the drug is continued for a minimum of 4 to 6 weeks. If signs recur after discontinuation of the drug, the same antibiotic is reinstituted for even longer.

If no response is seen after the first week of treatment, the drug should be discontinued. Another antibiotic can be tried, although further evaluation for an underlying disorder should be pursued, particularly in dogs. Frequent stopping and starting of different antibiotics every 7 to 14 days is not recommended and may predispose to growth of resistant gram-negative infections.

### Prognosis

Bacterial rhinitis is usually responsive to antibiotic therapy. Long-term resolution of signs depends on the identification and correction of any underlying disease processes.

## NASAL PARASITES (TEXT PP 238-239)

### Nasal Mites

*Pneumonyssoides caninum* is a small, white mite approximately 1 mm in size. Most infestations are clinically silent, but some dogs have moderate to severe clinical signs. A common clinical feature is sneezing, which is often violent. Head shaking, pawing at the nose, reverse sneezing, chronic nasal discharge, and epistaxis can also occur. These signs are similar to those caused by nasal foreign bodies.

### Diagnosis

The mites are often located in the frontal sinuses and caudal nasal cavity. Diagnosis generally requires rhinoscopy or retrograde nasal flushing (see Chapter 14). The mites are easily overlooked in the retrieved solution without the use of slight magnification or dark material behind the specimen. Flushing the nasal cavities with halothane in oxygen is also effective; the mites migrate to the caudal nasopharynx, where they can be seen with an endoscope.

### Treatment and prognosis
Treatment with milbemycin oxime (0.5 to 1 mg/kg PO every 7 to 10 days for three treatments) or ivermectin (0.2 mg/kg given subcutaneously [SC], repeated in 3 weeks) is effective. Any dogs in direct contact with the patient should also be treated. The prognosis is excellent.

## Nasal Capillariasis
Nasal capillariasis is caused by the nematode *Capillaria (Eucoleus) boehmi.* The small, thin, white adult worm lives on the mucosa of the nasal cavity and frontal sinuses of dogs. Clinical signs include sneezing and mucopurulent nasal discharge, sometimes with hemorrhage. The diagnosis is based on identification of double-operculated *Capillaria* eggs on routine fecal flotation or visualization of adult worms during rhinoscopy.

### Treatment
Treatment involves ivermectin (0.2 mg/kg PO, once) or fenbendazole (25 to 50 mg/kg q12h for 10 to 14 days). In addition to resolution of clinical signs, treatment success should be confirmed with repeated fecal examinations. Repeated treatments may be necessary, and reinfection is possible if exposure to contaminated soil continues.

## LYMPHOPLASMACYTIC RHINITIS (TEXT P 239)
Lymphoplasmacytic rhinitis is an uncommon cause of nasal disease. Infectious or neoplastic diseases of the nasal cavity, particularly aspergillosis or penicilliosis, can result in lymphoid reactivity and must be ruled out before initiation of treatment for lympho-plasmacytic rhinitis. Signs are typical of most nasal diseases and include sneezing and nasal discharge (serous, mucopurulent, or hemorrhagic). Improvement is not seen with antibiotic therapy.

### Diagnosis
Diagnosis is based on histologic examination of nasal biopsy specimens after other diseases are ruled out by extensive diagnostic evaluation. Histologic examination reveals infiltration of the mucosa and submucosa with mature lymphocytes and plasma cells. Nonspecific abnormalities attributable to chronic inflammation (e.g., epithelial hyperplasia, fibrosis) can also be seen. Increased soft-tissue opacity and turbinate lysis in the rostral nasal cavity can be evident radiographically.

### Treatment and prognosis
Treatment involves immunosuppressive doses of prednisone (1 mg/kg q12h). A positive response is expected within 2 weeks, at which time the dose is gradually decreased to the lowest effective level. If no response is seen, the dose of prednisone can be doubled or other immunosuppressive drugs, such as azathioprine, can be added (see Chapter 93). If clinical signs worsen during treatment, therapy should be discontinued and the dog carefully reevaluated for other diseases. The prognosis is unknown.

## ALLERGIC RHINITIS (TEXT PP 239-240)
Allergic rhinitis is generally considered a hypersensitivity response to airborne antigens. Other antigens are capable of inducing this response, so the differential diagnoses must include parasites, other infectious diseases, and neoplasia. Clinical signs include sneezing and/or serous or mucopurulent nasal discharge. Signs may be acute or chronic. Careful questioning of the owner may reveal a relationship between signs and potential allergens. Debilitation of the animal is not expected.

### Diagnosis
Allergic rhinitis is best diagnosed by identifying a relationship between signs and a particular allergen and the resolution of signs after removal of the suspected agent.

When this approach is not possible or successful, a thorough diagnostic evaluation of the nasal cavity is indicated. Nasal radiographs reveal increased soft-tissue opacity with minimal or no turbinate destruction. Nasal biopsy reveals eosinophilic inflammation. No diagnostic tests indicate an aggressive disease process, parasites or other active infection, or neoplasia.

### Treatment

Allergic rhinitis is best treated by removing the offending allergen from the animal's environment. When this is not possible, a beneficial response may be seen with antihistamines (e.g., chlorpheniramine, 4 to 8 mg/dog or 2 mg/cat, PO q8 to 12h). Glucocorticoids can be used if antihistamines are unsuccessful. Prednisone is initiated at 0.25 mg/kg q12h until signs resolve; the dose is then tapered to the lowest effective level. If treatment is effective, signs generally resolve within a few days. Drugs are continued only as long as needed to control signs.

### Prognosis

Prognosis is excellent if the allergen can be eliminated. Otherwise, the prognosis for control is good, but a cure is unlikely.

# 16

# Clinical Manifestations of Laryngeal and Pharyngeal Disease

## (Text pp 241-242)

### LARYNX (TEXT P 241)

Diseases of the larynx result in respiratory distress and stridor. Voice change is specific for laryngeal disease but is not always volunteered by the owner; specific questioning may be necessary to obtain this important information. Localization of disease to the larynx can generally be achieved with a thorough history and physical examination.

#### Respiratory distress

Respiratory distress with laryngeal disease results from airway obstruction, which can be severe and ultimately fatal. Although most laryngeal diseases are progressive over several weeks or months, animals typically are presented in acute distress, having compensated for the disease for a time through self-imposed exercise restriction. Often an exacerbating event (e.g., exercise, excitement, high ambient temperature) is described.

A characteristic breathing pattern can often be identified in patients with upper airway obstruction. The respiratory rate is normal or only slightly elevated (often 30 to 40 breaths/min), despite overt distress, and inspiratory efforts are prolonged and labored relative to expiratory efforts. On auscultation, referred upper airway sounds are heard; lung sounds are normal or increased.

### Stridor

Stridor (a high-pitched, audible wheezing sound) may be heard during inspiration. It is audible without a stethoscope, although auscultation of the neck may aid in identifying mild disease. Stridor is caused by air turbulence through a narrowed laryngeal opening or, less often, extrathoracic trachea. In patients that are not presented for respiratory distress, it may be necessary to exercise the animal to identify the characteristic breathing pattern and stridor associated with laryngeal disease.

### Other findings

Some patients with laryngeal disease have subclinical or overt aspiration pneumonia. Findings may include cough, lethargy, anorexia, fever, tachypnea, and abnormal lung sounds (see Chapter 19).

## PHARYNX (TEXT PP 241-242)

Space-occupying lesions of the pharynx can cause signs of upper airway obstruction, but overt respiratory distress occurs only with advanced disease. More typical presenting signs are stertor (a loud, coarse, snoring or snorting sound), reverse sneezing, gagging, retching, and dysphagia.

## DIFFERENTIAL DIAGNOSES FOR LARYNGEAL SIGNS (TEXT P 242)

Differential considerations for dogs and cats with laryngeal disease are summarized in Box 16-1; respiratory distress is discussed further in Chapter 26. Laryngeal disease, and particularly laryngeal paralysis, is more common in dogs than in cats. Acute laryngitis is not well characterized in dogs or cats, but presumably it could result from viral or other infectious agents or from excessive barking.

## DIFFERENTIAL DIAGNOSES FOR PHARYNGEAL SIGNS (TEXT P 242)

The most common pharyngeal disorders in dogs are brachycephalic airway syndrome and elongated soft palate (see Chapter 18). The most common pharyngeal disorders in cats are lymphosarcoma and nasopharyngeal polyps. Other differential diagnoses in dogs and cats with signs of pharyngeal disease include foreign body, abscess or granuloma, other neoplasms, and extraluminal mass.

---

**Box 16-1**

**Differential Diagnoses for Laryngeal Disease in Dogs and Cats**

Laryngeal paralysis
Laryngeal neoplasia
Obstructive laryngitis
Laryngeal collapse
Web formation (adhesions or fibrotic tissue across the laryngeal opening, usually as a complication of surgery)
Trauma
Foreign body
Extraluminal mass
Acute laryngitis

# 17

# Diagnostic Tests for the Larynx and Pharynx

## (Text pp 243-245)

### RADIOGRAPHY AND ULTRASONOGRAPHY (TEXT P 243)

Radiographs of the pharynx and larynx should be evaluated in animals with suspected upper airway disease. A lateral view, including the caudal nasopharynx and cranial trachea, is usually obtained. Oblique views may be helpful in some cases.

Soft-tissue masses within or distorting the airway are apparent in some animals with neoplasia, granulomas, abscesses, or polyps; elongated soft palate is sometimes detectable. Foreign bodies may also be identified; however, opacities are often misleading, particularly if rotation of the head and neck is present, and overt abnormalities are not often identified. Abnormal soft-tissue opacities or narrowing of the airway lumen must be confirmed with endoscopy.

Ultrasonography is another noninvasive imaging modality for evaluating the pharynx and larynx, assessing laryngeal motion, localizing mass lesions, and guiding needle aspiration. However, accurate assessment of this area can be difficult.

### LARYNGOSCOPY AND PHARYNGOSCOPY (TEXT PP 243-245)

Laryngoscopy and pharyngoscopy allow visualization of the larynx and pharynx for assessment of structural abnormalities and function of the arytenoid cartilages and vocal cords. These procedures are indicated whenever clinical signs suggest upper airway obstruction or laryngeal or pharyngeal disease. Techniques are described in the text.

Note: Patients with increased respiratory effort resulting from upper airway obstruction may have difficulty during recovery from anesthesia. Laryngoscopy should not be undertaken in these patients unless the clinician is prepared to perform whatever surgical treatments may be indicated during the same anesthetic period.

#### Laryngeal dysfunction

The motion of the arytenoid cartilages is evaluated while the patient takes several deep breaths. Normally the cartilages abduct symmetrically and widely with each inspiration and close on expiration. Laryngeal paralysis that results in clinical signs is usually bilateral. The cartilages are not abducted during inspiration but may be passively forced outward during expiration (paradoxic motion). If normal motion is not present, observation of the cartilages should be continued as long as possible while the animal recovers from anesthesia. Effects of anesthesia and shallow breathing are the most common causes for an erroneous diagnosis of laryngeal paralysis.

#### Other abnormalities

After evaluation of laryngeal function, the pharynx, larynx, and caudal nasopharynx are thoroughly evaluated for structural abnormalities, masses, and foreign bodies. Biopsy specimens for histologic examination should be obtained from any lesions. The normal diverse flora of the pharynx makes culture results difficult or impossible to interpret, although bacterial growth from abscesses or granulomatous lesions may be useful.

Eversion of the laryngeal saccules, thickening and elongation of the soft palate, and inflammation with thickening of the pharyngeal mucosa can result from prolonged upper airway obstruction. Obliteration of most of the airway lumen by the surrounding mucosa is known as *laryngeal collapse.* The laryngeal cartilages can become soft and deformed, unable to support the soft tissues of the pharynx. This chondromalacia may be a concurrent or secondary component of laryngeal collapse. Collapse most often occurs in dogs with brachycephalic airway syndrome but can occur with any chronic obstructive disorder.

The length of the soft palate should be assessed; an elongated soft palate can contribute to signs of upper airway obstruction. The trachea should be examined endoscopically if no abnormalities are identified on laryngoscopy.

# 18

# Disorders of the Larynx and Pharynx

## (Text pp 246-249)

### LARYNGEAL PARALYSIS (TEXT PP 246-247)

Failure of the arytenoid cartilages to abduct during inspiration creates an extrathoracic (upper) airway obstruction. When clinical signs develop, both arytenoid cartilages are usually affected.

#### Etiology

Potential causes are listed in Box 18-1. Laryngeal paralysis is most often idiopathic. Congenital laryngeal paralysis is reported in Bouviers des Flandres and suspected in Siberian Huskies and Bull Terriers. Dogs with polyneuropathy-myopathy can be presented with laryngeal paralysis as the predominant clinical sign. A laryngeal paralysis-polyneuropathy complex has been described in young Dalmatians and Rottweilers. Laryngeal paralysis is uncommon in cats.

#### Clinical features

Laryngeal paralysis can occur at any age and in any breed, although the idiopathic form is most common in older, large-breed dogs. There may be an increased incidence of idiopathic laryngeal paralysis in older Golden and Labrador Retrievers.

Clinical signs include respiratory distress and stridor. The owner may also note a change in voice (bark or meow). Most patients are presented for acute respiratory distress, despite the chronic, progressive nature of this disease (see Chapter 16). Cyanosis, syncope, and death can occur. Dogs with respiratory distress require immediate emergency therapy.

Some dogs with laryngeal paralysis exhibit gagging or coughing when eating or have overt aspiration pneumonia, presumably resulting from concurrent pharyngeal dysfunction or a more generalized polyneuropathy-polymyopathy.

---

**Box 18-1**

### Potential Causes of Laryngeal Paralysis

**IDIOPATHIC**

**VENTRAL CERVICAL LESION**
Trauma to nerves
   Direct trauma
   Inflammation
   Fibrosis
Neoplasia
Other inflammatory or mass lesion

**ANTERIOR THORACIC LESION**
Neoplasia
Trauma
   Postoperative
   Other
Other inflammatory or mass lesion

**POLYNEUROPATHY AND POLYMYOPATHY**
Idiopathic
Immune mediated
Endocrinopathy
   Hypothyroidism
   Hypoadrenocorticism
Other systemic disorder
   Toxicity
Congenital disease

---

### Diagnosis

Definitive diagnosis requires laryngoscopy (see Chapter 17). With laryngeal paralysis, the arytenoid cartilages and vocal folds remain closed during inspiration and open slightly during expiration. The vocal folds may vibrate during inspiration and expiration. Pharyngeal edema and inflammation may also be found. The larynx and pharynx should be examined for laryngeal collapse and for neoplasia, foreign bodies, or other diseases that might interfere with normal function.

Once a diagnosis of laryngeal paralysis is established, additional tests should be considered to identify underlying or associated diseases and to rule out concurrent pulmonary problems (such as aspiration pneumonia) or pharyngeal or esophageal motility problems (Box 18-2). The latter is especially important if surgical correction for laryngeal paralysis is being considered. If a cause cannot be identified, idiopathic laryngeal paralysis is diagnosed.

### Treatment

Emergency medical therapy is indicated for animals in respiratory distress (see Chapter 26). After stabilization and thorough diagnostic evaluation, surgery is usually the treatment of choice. Even when specific therapy can be directed at an associated disease (e.g., hypothyroidism), complete resolution of laryngeal signs rarely occurs. Also, most cases are idiopathic, and signs are generally progressive.

Various laryngoplasty techniques have been described. The recommended initial procedure in most dogs and cats is unilateral arytenoid lateralization. If surgery is not an option, medical management consisting of glucocorticoid therapy (e.g., prednisone, 0.5 mg/kg q12h initially) and cage rest may provide symptomatic relief.

---

**Box 18-2**

## Diagnostic Evaluation of Dogs and Cats with Confirmed Laryngeal Paralysis

**UNDERLYING CAUSE**
Thoracic radiographs
Cervical radiographs
Serum biochemical panel
Thyroid hormone evaluation
    Baseline $T_4$, free $T_4$, cTSH
    TSH stimulation test
Ancillary tests in select cases
    Evaluation for diffuse neuropathy-myopathy
    Electromyography
    Nerve conduction measurements
Antinuclear antibody test
Antiacetylcholine receptor antibody test
Cortisol evaluation
    ACTH stimulation test

**CONCURRENT PULMONARY DISEASE**
Thoracic radiographs

**CONCURRENT PHARYNGEAL DYSFUNCTION**
Evaluation of gag reflex
Observation of swallowing of food and water
Fluoroscopic observation of barium swallow

**CONCURRENT ESOPHAGEAL DYSFUNCTION**
Thoracic radiographs
Contrast-enhanced esophagram
Fluoroscopic observation of barium swallow

---

*ACTH*, Adrenocorticotropic hormone; *cTSH*, canine thyroid-stimulating hormone; *TSH*, thyroid-stimulating hormone.

### Prognosis

The overall prognosis for dogs with surgically treated laryngeal paralysis is fair to good. The most common complication is aspiration pneumonia. A guarded prognosis is warranted for patients with signs of aspiration, dysphagia, megaesophagus, or systemic polyneuropathy or myopathy. Dogs with laryngeal paralysis as an early manifestation of generalized polymyopathy or polyneuropathy may experience progression of signs.

## BRACHYCEPHALIC AIRWAY SYNDROME (TEXT PP 248-249)

Brachycephalic airway syndrome refers to the multiple anatomic abnormalities commonly found in brachycephalic dogs and, to a lesser extent, short-faced cats (e.g., Himalayans). Abnormalities include the following:

- stenotic nares
- elongated soft palate
- everted laryngeal saccules
- laryngeal collapse
- hypoplastic trachea (English Bulldogs)

The severity of these abnormalities is variable, and one or any combination may be present in any given brachycephalic dog or short-faced cat.

### Clinical features

The abnormalities cause signs of extrathoracic airway obstruction: loud breathing sounds, stertor, increased inspiratory effort, cyanosis, and syncope. Signs are exacerbated by exercise, excitement, and high ambient temperature. The increased inspiratory effort may cause inflammation and edema of the laryngeal and pharyngeal mucosa and enhance eversion of the laryngeal saccules, further narrowing the glottis and therefore exacerbating clinical signs and creating a vicious cycle. As a result, some dogs are presented in life-threatening respiratory distress and require emergency therapy.

### Diagnosis

A tentative diagnosis is made on the basis of breed, clinical signs, and appearance of the external nares. Stenotic nares are generally bilaterally symmetric, and the alar folds may be sucked inward during inspiration. Definitive diagnosis and assessment of the number and severity of abnormalities requires laryngoscopy and radiographic evaluation of the trachea.

### Treatment

Therapy should be designed to minimize the factors that exacerbate the clinical signs (e.g., exercise, excitement, overheating) and to enhance the passage of air through the upper airways. Surgical correction of the anatomic defects is the treatment of choice.

The specific surgical procedure(s) depends on the existing problems and can include widening of the external nares and removal of excessive soft palate and everted laryngeal saccules. Correction of stenotic nares is a simple procedure and can dramatically improve clinical signs. In puppies and kittens stenotic nares can be safely corrected during routine ovariohysterectomy or castration, ideally before clinical signs develop. The soft palate should be evaluated at the same time and corrected if elongated.

Medical management consisting of glucocorticoid therapy (e.g., prednisone, 0.5 mg/kg q12h initially) and cage rest can reduce pharyngeal and laryngeal inflammation and edema, but it will not eliminate the problem. Emergency therapy may be required in animals presented in respiratory distress (see Chapter 26).

### Prognosis

The prognosis depends on the severity of the abnormalities and the ability to surgically correct them. In many patients the prognosis is good after early surgical correction. Laryngeal collapse carries a poor prognosis. Hypoplastic trachea is not surgically correctable, but no clear relationship exists between the degree of hypoplasia and morbidity or mortality.

## OBSTRUCTIVE LARYNGITIS (TEXT P 249)

Nonneoplastic infiltration with inflammatory cells can cause irregular proliferation, hyperemia, and swelling of the larynx. Clinical signs of extrathoracic airway obstruction result. The larynx appears neoplastic on laryngoscopic examination, but histopathologic evaluation of biopsy specimens reveals inflammatory infiltrates (either granulomatous, pyogranulomatous, or lymphocytic-plasmacytic). Etiologic agents have not been identified.

Some animals respond to glucocorticoid therapy (e.g., prednisone, 1 mg/kg orally [PO] q12h initially). Once clinical signs have resolved, the dose can be tapered to the lowest effective level. With severe signs or large granulomatous masses, excision of the obstructing tissue may be necessary. The prognosis is variable, depending on the size of the lesion, severity of laryngeal damage, and response to glucocorticoid therapy.

## LARYNGEAL NEOPLASIA (TEXT P 249)

Tumors involving the larynx include carcinoma (squamous cell, undifferentiated, adenocarcinoma), lymphoma, melanoma, mast cell tumors and other sarcomas, and benign neoplasia. Lymphoma is the most common tumor in cats. Neoplasms originating in the larynx are uncommon. More often, tumors originating in tissues adjacent to the larynx, such as thyroid carcinoma or lymphoma, compress or invade the larynx and cause distortion of normal laryngeal structures. Clinical signs of extrathoracic airway obstruction result.

### Clinical features

Clinical signs are similar to those of other laryngeal diseases and include noisy respiration, stridor, increased inspiratory effort, cyanosis, syncope, and change in bark or meow. Mass lesions can also cause concurrent dysphagia, aspiration pneumonia, or a visible or palpable mass in the ventral neck.

### Diagnosis

Extralaryngeal masses are often identified by palpation. Primary laryngeal tumors are rarely palpable and are best identified by laryngoscopy. Laryngeal radiography, ultrasonography, or computed tomography can be useful in assessing the extent of disease. Differential diagnoses include obstructive laryngitis, nasopharyngeal polyp, foreign body, traumatic granuloma, and abscess. Definitive diagnosis requires histologic or cytologic examination of a biopsy specimen; a diagnosis of malignant neoplasia should not be made on gross appearance alone.

### Treatment and prognosis

Treatment depends on the type of tumor involved. Benign tumors should be surgically excised, if possible. Complete surgical excision of malignant tumors is rarely possible, although ventilation may be improved and time may be gained to allow other treatments (e.g., radiation, chemotherapy) to become effective. Complete laryngectomy and permanent tracheostomy can be considered in select patients. Prognosis for patients with benign tumors is excellent if they can be totally resected. Malignant neoplasms carry a poor prognosis.

# 19

# Clinical Manifestations of Lower Respiratory Tract Disorders

## *(Text pp 250-254)*

## CLINICAL SIGNS (TEXT PP 250-252)

Dogs and cats with lower respiratory tract (LRT) diseases are commonly presented for evaluation of cough. LRT disease can also result in respiratory distress, exercise intolerance, weakness, cyanosis, or syncope. Nonspecific signs such as fever, anorexia, weight loss, and depression also occur and in some patients are the only presenting signs. In rare instances misleading signs such as vomiting are seen. Auscultation and thoracic radiography help to localize the disease to the LRT in these animals.

## Cough

Cough is generally a protective reflex to expel material from the airways; inflammation or compression of the airways can also stimulate a cough. Differential diagnoses (Box 19-1) can often be prioritized by characterizing the cough (productive or nonproductive, intensity, associated sounds) and noting any temporal associations.

### Productive versus nonproductive

A productive cough results in the delivery of mucus, exudate, edema fluid, or blood from the airways into the oral cavity. A moist sound can often be heard during the cough. Animals rarely expectorate the fluid, but swallowing can be seen after a coughing episode. If expectoration occurs, clients may confuse the cough with vomiting. Recognition of a productive cough is more difficult in veterinary than in human patients. Not hearing or seeing evidence of productivity does not rule out a productive cough. The most common causes of productive cough are inflammatory or infectious diseases of the airways or alveoli and heart failure.

#### Hemoptysis.

Blood-tinged saliva may be seen within the oral cavity or dripping from the commissures of the mouth after a cough. Hemoptysis is an unusual sign; it most commonly occurs with heartworm disease or pulmonary neoplasia. Other possible causes are listed in Box 19-1.

### Intensity

Intensity of the cough is another quality that may be useful in prioritizing the differential diagnoses. Cough associated with airway inflammation (e.g., bronchitis) or airway collapse is often loud, harsh, and paroxysmal. The cough associated with tracheal collapse is often described as a "goose honk." Cough resulting from tracheal disease can usually be induced by palpation of the trachea, although concurrent involvement

---

**Box 19-1**

#### Differential Diagnoses for Productive Cough* in Dogs and Cats

**EDEMA**
  Heart failure
  Noncardiogenic pulmonary edema

**MUCUS OR EXUDATE**
  Canine infectious tracheobronchitis
  Chronic bronchitis
  Allergic bronchitis
  Bacterial infection (bronchitis or pneumonia)
  Parasitic disease
  Aspiration pneumonia
  Fungal pneumonia (severe)

**BLOOD (HEMOPTYSIS)**
  Heartworm disease
  Neoplasia
  Fungal pneumonia
  Thromboembolism
  Severe heart failure
  Foreign body
  Lung lobe torsion
  Systemic bleeding disorder

---

*These differential diagnoses should also be considered in patients with nonproductive cough.

of deeper airways is possible. The cough associated with pneumonia or pulmonary edema is usually soft.

### Temporal associations

The association of coughing with temporal events can be helpful. Cough resulting from tracheal disease is exacerbated by pressure on the neck, such as pulling on the animal's collar. Cough caused by heart failure tends to occur more frequently at night, whereas cough caused by airway disease tends to occur more often on rising from sleep or during and after exercise or exposure to cold air.

## Exercise Intolerance and Respiratory Distress

Diseases of the LRT (Box 19-2) can compromise oxygenation of the blood. Clinical signs of such compromise begin as mildly increased respirations and subtle decrease in activity; these early signs are missed by most owners. Signs progress through exercise intolerance (reluctance to exercise or respiratory distress with exertion) to overt respiratory distress at rest. Respiratory effort in cats normally is minimally visible. Cats showing noticeable chest excursions or open-mouth breathing are severely compromised.

Cyanosis is a sign of severe hypoxemia. Pallor is a more common sign of acute hypoxemia resulting from respiratory disease. Many veterinary patients with compromised lung function arrive in overt respiratory distress. These patients require rapid physical assessment and immediate stabilization (see Chapter 26) before further diagnostic testing.

## DIAGNOSTIC APPROACH (TEXT PP 252-254)

The initial diagnostic approach includes a complete history, physical examination, thoracic radiographs, and complete blood count (CBC). Further diagnostic tests are then selected.

---

**Box 19-2**

### Differential Diagnoses for Lower Respiratory Tract Disease in Dogs and Cats

#### DISORDERS OF THE TRACHEA AND BRONCHI

Canine infectious tracheobronchitis
Collapsing trachea
Feline bronchitis
Allergic bronchitis
Canine chronic bronchitis
Bronchiectasis

*Oslerus osleri* infection
Bronchial compression
Left atrial enlargement
Hilar lymphadenopathy
Tracheal tear
Neoplasia

#### DISORDERS OF THE PULMONARY PARENCHYMA

Infectious diseases
  Viral pneumonia
  Canine distemper
  Bacterial pneumonia
  Protozoal pneumonia
  Toxoplasmosis
  Fungal pneumonia
  Blastomycosis
  Histoplasmosis
  Coccidioidomycosis
Parasitic diseases
  Heartworm disease

Pulmonary parasites
*Paragonimus* infection
*Aelurostrongylus* infection
*Capillaria* infection
*Crenosoma* infection
Infiltrative or inflammatory diseases
  Aspiration pneumonia
  Pulmonary neoplasia
Pulmonary contusions
Pulmonary thromboembolism
Pulmonary edema

## Physical Examination

Findings that assist in localizing the cause of compromise to the LRT include rapid and often shallow respirations, increased inspiratory and/or expiratory effort, and abnormal lung sounds on auscultation. Intrathoracic large airway obstruction generally results in normal to slightly increased respiratory rate, prolonged and labored expiration, and audible or auscultable expiratory sounds.

A complete physical examination, including fundic examination, is warranted to identify signs of disease that may be concurrently or secondarily affecting the lungs (e.g., systemic mycosis, metastatic neoplasia, megaesophagus). The cardiovascular system should be carefully evaluated (see Chapter 1).

Mitral insufficiency murmurs are frequently auscultated in older, small-breed dogs with the primary complaint of cough. Mitral insufficiency is often an incidental finding, but both cardiac and respiratory tract diseases must be considered. Mitral insufficiency can lead to left atrial enlargement with compression of the mainstem bronchi (causing cough) or it can lead to congestive heart failure (CHF). Dogs with CHF are nearly always tachycardic. Other signs of heart disease are discussed in Chapter 1. Thoracic radiographs and occasionally echocardiography may be needed before cardiac problems can be comfortably ruled out as a cause of LRT signs.

### Thoracic auscultation

Careful auscultation of the upper airways and lungs is a critical component of the physical examination. Decreased lung sounds over one or both sides of the thorax occur with pleural effusion, pneumothorax, diaphragmatic hernia, and intrathoracic masses. Consolidated lung lobes and mass lesions can result in enhanced lung sounds (improved transmission of sounds from adjacent lobes).

Abnormal lung sounds are described as increased breath sounds (or harsh lung sounds), crackles (nonmusical, discontinuous noises that sound like paper being crumpled or bubbles popping), or wheezes (musical, continuous sounds). Increased breath sounds are common in patients with pulmonary edema or pneumonia. Crackles can be heard with diseases that result in formation of edema or exudate within the airways and with some interstitial lung diseases (particularly interstitial fibrosis).

Wheezes are indicative of airway narrowing, whether as a result of bronchoconstriction, bronchial wall thickening, exudate or fluid within the bronchial lumen, masses, or external airway compression. They are most commonly heard in cats with bronchitis. Wheezes caused by intrathoracic airway obstruction are loudest during early expiration. Sudden snapping at the end of expiration can be heard in some dogs with intrathoracic tracheal collapse.

## Radiography

Thoracic radiographs are indicated in dogs and cats with LRT signs. Neck radiographs should also be obtained in animals with suspected tracheal disease. Radiography helps localize the problem to an organ system (cardiac, pulmonary, mediastinal, pleural), identify the area of involvement within the LRT (vascular, bronchial, alveolar, interstitial), narrow the list of differential diagnoses, and establish a diagnostic plan. Additional tests are necessary in most patients to make a definitive diagnosis. Radiography is discussed further in Chapter 20.

## Complete Blood Count

In patients with LRT disease the CBC may show an anemia of inflammatory disease, polycythemia secondary to chronic hypoxia, or a white blood cell response characteristic of an inflammatory process. However, these hematologic changes are nonspecific and insensitive, and absence of abnormalities cannot be used to rule out inflammatory lung disease.

## Further Diagnostic Evaluation

Based on the history, physical examination, thoracic radiographs, and CBC a prioritized list of differential diagnoses is developed. Additional tests are nearly always required for definitive diagnosis, which is necessary for optimal therapy and outcome. Selection of appropriate tests is based on the most likely differential diagnoses, localization of disease within the LRT (e.g., diffuse bronchial disease, single mass lesion), degree of respiratory compromise, and the client's motivation for optimal care.

In most patients with LRT disease, collection of a pulmonary specimen for microscopic and microbiologic analysis is required. Techniques include tracheal wash, bronchoalveolar lavage, bronchoscopy, transthoracic lung aspiration, and lung biopsy (see Chapter 20). Noninvasive tests include serology for pulmonary pathogens, fecal examination for parasites, and specialized radiographic techniques such as fluoroscopy, angiography, computed tomography, ultrasonography, and nuclear imaging.

Valuable information can also be obtained from arterial blood gas analysis. Results are rarely helpful in making a final diagnosis, but they are useful in determining degree of compromise and in monitoring response to therapy. Pulse oximetry is particularly valuable in monitoring patients with respiratory compromise during anesthetic procedures or respiratory crises.

# 20

# Diagnostic Tests for the Lower Respiratory Tract

## (Text pp 255-286)

### THORACIC RADIOGRAPHY (TEXT PP 255-261)

A minimum of two views of the thorax should be taken; usually, right-lateral and ventrodorsal (VD) views are preferred. Evaluating both right- and left-lateral views improves sensitivity if disease of the right middle lung lobe, metastatic disease, or other condition that causes subtle changes is suspected. Dorsoventral (DV) views are taken to evaluate the dorsal pulmonary arteries in animals with suspected heartworm disease and in animals with respiratory distress. Horizontal-beam lateral radiographs, taken with the patient standing, can be used in animals with suspected cavitary lesions or pleural effusion.

### Trachea

When one is evaluating the trachea in patients with suspected airway obstruction or primary tracheal disease, it is important to take radiographs of the cervical portion during inspiration and the thoracic portion during both inspiration and expiration.

#### Abnormal appearance or position

Only the inner wall of the trachea should be visible; identification of the outer wall suggests pneumomediastinum. The trachea may appear elevated near the carina as a result of heart enlargement or pleural effusion. Flexion or extension of the neck may cause bowing of the trachea. On VD views the trachea deviates to the right of midline in some dogs. Calcification of tracheal cartilage occurs in some older dogs and chondrodystrophic breeds.

### Abnormal dimensions

The normal tracheal lumen is nearly as wide as the laryngeal lumen. With hypoplastic trachea the lumen is less than half normal size. Strictures and fractured cartilage rings can cause an abrupt, localized narrowing of the air stripe. Masses adjacent to the trachea can compress it, causing a more gradual, localized narrowing of the air stripe. In animals with intrathoracic tracheal collapse, the air stripe is narrowed in the cervical region during inspiration. In animals with intrathoracic tracheal collapse, the air stripe is narrowed during expiration. Fluoroscopy provides a more sensitive assessment of tracheal collapse.

The air contrast sometimes allows visualization of foreign bodies or masses within the trachea. Most foreign bodies lodge at the carina or within the bronchi, but inability to identify a foreign body does not rule out the diagnosis.

## Lungs

The lungs are examined for four major abnormal patterns: vascular, bronchial, alveolar, and interstitial. Animals with severe respiratory distress and normal thoracic radiographs usually have thromboembolic disease or a very recent insult to the lungs, such as trauma or aspiration.

### Vascular pattern

The pulmonary vasculature is assessed by evaluating the vessels to the cranial lung lobes on the lateral view and the vessels to the caudal lung lobes on the VD/DV view. Abnormal vascular patterns generally involve an increase or decrease in the size of arteries or veins. The basic patterns and possible causes are as follows:

- enlarged arteries—heartworm disease, thromboembolism, pulmonary hypertension
- enlarged veins—left-sided heart failure
- enlarged arteries and veins—pulmonary overcirculation caused by left-to-right shunts (e.g., patent ductus arteriosus, atrial or ventricular septal defect)
- small arteries and veins—pulmonary undercirculation (e.g., severe hypovolemia, hypoadrenocorticism, pulmonic stenosis) or hyperinflation (e.g., feline or allergic bronchitis)

### Bronchial pattern

Bronchial structures are not normally visible in the peripheral regions of the lungs. In older dogs and chondrodystrophic breeds the cartilage may be calcified, making the walls more prominent.

A bronchial pattern occurs with thickening of the bronchial walls or bronchial dilation. Thickening may result from accumulation of mucus or exudates, infiltration of inflammatory cells, muscular hypertrophy, epithelial hyperplasia, or a combination of these changes. Possible causes of a bronchial pattern include the following:

- bronchitis (feline, allergic, bacterial, or canine chronic bronchitis)
- bronchiectasis (see following discussion)
- pulmonary parasites

When bronchial disease occurs in conjunction with parenchymal disease, a mixed pattern results.

*Bronchiectasis.* Bronchiectasis is irreversible dilation of the airways caused by chronic bronchial disease. It is identified by the presence of widened, nontapering airways and is described as either cylindric (tubular) or saccular (cystic). Cylindric bronchiectasis is characterized by fairly uniform airway dilation. The saccular form has localized dilations peripherally that can lead to a honeycomb appearance. Usually, all major bronchi are affected.

### Alveolar pattern

Alveolar patterns occur when alveoli fill with fluid-dense material, whether edema fluid, blood, or cellular infiltrates. If the fluid continues to accumulate, the airway lumen eventually becomes fluid-filled, resulting in solid areas of fluid opacity, or consolidation (see later). Possible causes of an alveolar pattern include the following:

- pulmonary edema (see following discussion)
- severe inflammatory disease (e.g., bacterial, aspiration, or fungal pneumonia)

- hemorrhage (e.g., pulmonary contusion, thromboembolic disease, neoplasia, fungal pneumonia, systemic coagulopathy)
- neoplasia

Any of the differential diagnoses for interstitial patterns can cause an alveolar pattern if associated with severe inflammation, edema, or hemorrhage.

*Edema.* Edema is most often the result of left-sided heart failure (see Chapter 3). In dogs the fluid initially accumulates in the perihilar region; eventually the entire lung is affected. Enlargement of pulmonary veins supports the cardiac origin.

*Inflammatory infiltrates.* Inflammatory infiltrates can be caused by infectious agents, noninfectious inflammatory disease, or neoplasia. The location can often help establish a tentative diagnosis. Most bacterial and aspiration pneumonias primarily affect the dependent lung lobes, whereas dirofilariasis and thromboemboli primarily affect the caudal lung lobes. Localized processes involving only one lung lobe suggest foreign body, neoplasia, abscess, granuloma, or lung lobe torsion.

*Hemorrhage.* Hemorrhage most often results from trauma. It is a common cause of a predominant alveolar pattern.

### Interstitial pattern

Abnormal interstitial patterns are described as reticular (unstructured), nodular, or reticulonodular.

*Nodular interstitial pattern.* The nodular interstitial pattern is characterized by roughly circular, fluid-dense lesions in one or more lung lobes. (Note: Nodules must be nearly 1 cm in diameter to be detected.) Possible causes include the following:

- mycotic infection—blastomycosis, histoplasmosis, coccidioidomycosis
- neoplasia
- pulmonary parasites—*Aelurostrongylus, Paragonimus*
- abscesses—bacterial pneumonia, foreign body
- pulmonary infiltrates with eosinophils
- miscellaneous inflammatory diseases
- inactive lesions

Active inflammatory nodules often have poorly defined borders. Mycotic infections typically result in multiple, diffuse nodules. The nodules may be small (miliary) or large and coalescing. Parasitic granulomas are often multiple, although paragonimiasis can result in a single pulmonary nodule.

Inflammatory nodules can persist as inactive lesions once clinical disease has resolved. The borders of inactive nodules are often well demarcated. Mineralization can occur in animals with some conditions, such as histoplasmosis. Well-defined, small, inactive nodules are sometimes seen in healthy older dogs with no history of disease.

No radiographic pattern is diagnostic for neoplasia. Neoplastic nodules may be single or multiple; they are often well defined, although secondary inflammation, edema, or hemorrhage can obscure the margins. Lesions caused by parasites, fungal infection, and noninfectious inflammatory diseases may be indistinguishable from neoplasia.

*Reticular interstitial pattern.* A diffuse, unstructured, "lacy" increase in the opacity of the pulmonary interstitium characterizes the reticular interstitial pattern. The opacity partially obscures normal vascular and airway markings. Possible causes include the following:

- pulmonary edema (mild)
- infection—viral, bacterial, or mycotic pneumonia; toxoplasmosis; other parasites (which more often cause a bronchial or nodular interstitial pattern)
- neoplasia
- pulmonary fibrosis
- pulmonary infiltrates with eosinophils
- miscellaneous inflammatory diseases
- hemorrhage (mild)

With continued accumulation of fluid or cells, flooding of the alveoli can occur, resulting in an alveolar pattern. Focal interstitial accumulations of cells (i.e., nodules) can also develop with time, causing a reticulonodular pattern. This pattern is often seen in older dogs with no clinically apparent disease, presumably as a result of pulmonary fibrosis.

### Lung lobe consolidation

Lung lobe consolidation is characterized by a lobe that is entirely of soft-tissue opacity. It occurs when an alveolar or interstitial disease progresses to the point where the entire lobe is filled with fluid or cells. Common causes include severe bacterial or aspiration pneumonia, neoplasia, lung lobe torsion, and hemorrhage.

### Atelectasis

Atelectasis is also characterized by a lobe that is entirely of soft-tissue opacity. In this instance the lobe is collapsed as a result of airway obstruction. It is distinguished from consolidation by the small size of the lobe and the resultant shift of the heart toward the atelectatic lobe. Atelectasis most often involves the right middle lung lobe in cats with bronchitis.

### Cavitary lesions

Cavitary lung diseases include cysts and bullae. Cysts may be apparent as localized accumulations of air or fluid, often with a partially visible wall. An air-fluid interface may be seen on standing horizontal-beam views. Cysts may be congenital, acquired, or idiopathic. They can be caused by *Paragonimus* infection, trauma, abscess, neoplasia, lung infarction (from thromboembolism), and granulomas. Bullae are most often a result of chronic airway disease (emphysema) and are rarely apparent radiographically.

Cavitary lesions may be found in dogs and cats with spontaneous pneumothorax or they may be incidental findings. If pneumothorax is present, surgical excision is usually indicated. If inflammatory or neoplastic disease is suspected, further diagnostic testing is indicated. If the lesion is found incidentally, the animal can be periodically reevaluated to determine whether the lesion is progressing or resolving. If the lesion does not resolve within 1 to 3 months, surgical removal is considered for diagnostic purposes and to avoid potentially life-threatening spontaneous pneumothorax.

### Lung lobe torsion

Lung lobe torsion can develop spontaneously in deep-chested dogs or in other dogs and cats as a complication of pleural effusion or lobectomy. The right middle and left cranial lobes are most commonly involved. Torsion is difficult to identify radiographically. Consolidation from severe bacterial or aspiration pneumonia results in similar changes and is far more common. Pulmonary vessels or bronchi traveling in an abnormal direction strongly suggest torsion, but pleural fluid often develops and obscures assessment of the affected lobe. Ultrasonography is often useful, although bronchoscopy, bronchography, or thoracotomy is necessary to confirm the diagnosis in some patients.

## OTHER IMAGING MODALITIES (TEXT P 262)

### Angiography

Angiography is used to confirm presumptive dirofilariasis in cats with negative antigen blood tests and echocardiographic findings (see Chapter 10). Angiography is also used to confirm thromboembolism. If several days have elapsed since embolization occurred, lesions may no longer be identifiable. Therefore angiography should be performed as soon as the disorder is suspected and the patient is stabilized.

### Ultrasonography

Ultrasonography is used to evaluate pulmonary masses adjacent to the body wall, diaphragm, or heart, and consolidated lung lobes. Biopsy instruments can be guided by ultrasound for specimen collection. Ultrasonography is also useful for evaluating the heart when clinical signs cannot be readily localized to either the cardiac or respiratory systems. Use of ultrasonography to evaluate animals with pleural disorders is discussed in Chapter 24.

## Computed Tomography and Magnetic Resonance Imaging

Computed tomography and magnetic resonance imaging can be useful in evaluation of lung disease. The extent and location of disease and the potential involvement of other structures, such as major vessels, can be assessed more accurately than with routine radiography.

## Nuclear Imaging

Nuclear imaging can be used for evaluation of pulmonary perfusion and ventilation. Restrictions for handling radioisotopes and the need for specialized recording equipment limit availability to specialty centers.

## PARASITOLOGIC EVALUATION (TEXT PP 262-264)

### Bronchoscopy and Bronchial Washing

*Oslerus osleri* resides in nodules near the carina, which can be identified bronchoscopically. Other parasites are rarely visualized. Parasites that may be found in tracheal or bronchial washings include *O. osleri* (larvae), *Aelurostrongylus abstrusus* (larvae), *Crenosoma vulpis* (larvae or larvated eggs), *Capillaria aerophila* (eggs), and *Paragonimus kellicotti* (eggs).

### Fecal Flotation and Sedimentation

Routine fecal flotation can be used to concentrate eggs from *C. aerophila*. High-density fecal flotation can be used to concentrate *P. kellicotti* eggs, but sedimentation techniques are preferred, particularly if few eggs are present. Migrating intestinal parasites can cause transient pulmonary signs in young animals. As migration primarily occurs during the prepatent period, eggs may not be found in the feces.

Parasitic larvae are identified using the Baermann technique. Zinc sulfate flotation is recommended for identification of *O. osleri* larvae, as they are not sufficiently motile for reliable identification with the Baermann technique.

Because shedding is intermittent, parasitic disease cannot be excluded solely on the basis of negative fecal examination findings. At least three examinations should be performed if parasitic disease is highly suspected.

### Toxoplasma

*Toxoplasma gondii* occasionally causes pneumonia in dogs and cats. Dogs do not shed *Toxoplasma* organisms in the feces, but cats may. Infection is therefore diagnosed by finding tachyzoites in pulmonary specimens or by positive serologic tests.

## SEROLOGIC TESTS (TEXT P 264)

Antibody tests provide indirect evidence of infection; in general, they should be used only to confirm a diagnosis. Common pulmonary pathogens for which tests are available include *Histoplasma, Blastomyces, Coccidioidomyces, Toxoplasma,* and feline coronavirus (FIP). These tests are discussed in Chapter 97. Antibody tests are also available for dirofilariasis (see Chapter 10). Serum antigen tests are available for *Cryptococcus* (see Chapter 103) and adult heartworms (see Chapter 10).

## LOWER RESPIRATORY TRACT SAMPLING TECHNIQUES (TEXT PP 264-281)

Techniques for sampling the lower respiratory tract (airways and pulmonary parenchyma) include tracheal wash, bronchoalveolar lavage (BAL), transthoracic lung aspiration, bronchoscopy, and lung biopsy via thoracotomy or thoracoscopy. The advantages and disadvantages of and indications for these techniques are summarized in Table 20-1.

**Table 20-1**

## Comparisons of Techniques for Collecting Specimens from the Lower Respiratory Tract

| Technique | Site of collection | Specimen size | Advantages | Disadvantages | Indications |
|---|---|---|---|---|---|
| Tracheal wash | Large airways | Moderate | Simple technique; minimal expense; no special equipment; complications rare; volume adequate for cytology and culture | Airway must be involved for specimen to represent disease | Bronchial and alveolar disease; because of safety and ease, consider for any lung disease; less likely to be representative of interstitial or small focal processes |
| BAL | Small airways, alveoli, sometimes interstitium | Large | Simple technique; NB-BAL requires no special equipment and minimal expense; bronchoscopic BAL allows airway evaluation and direct sampling; resultant hypoxemia is transient and responsive to $O_2$ supplementation; safe for animals in stable condition; large volume of lung sampled; high cytologic quality; large volume for analysis | General anesthesia required; special equipment and expertise required for bronchoscopic collection; not recommended for animals in respiratory distress; capability to provide oxygen supplementation is required | Small airway, alveolar, or interstitial disease; routine during bronchoscopy |
| Lung aspirate | Interstitium, alveoli when flooded | Small | Simple technique; minimal expense; no special equipment; solid masses adjacent to body wall; excellent representation with minimal risk | Potential for complications (pneumothorax, hemothorax, pulmonary hemorrhage); relatively small area of lung sampled; specimen adequate only for cytology; specimen blood contaminated | Solid masses adjacent to chest wall (for solitary or localized disease; see also thoracotomy and lung biopsy); diffuse interstitial disease |
| Thoracotomy and lung biopsy | Small airways, alveoli, interstitium | Large | Ideal specimen; allows histologic examination in addition to culture | Relatively expensive; requires expertise; requires general anesthesia; major surgical procedure | Localized process where excision may also be therapeutic; any progressive disease not diagnosed by less invasive methods |

*BAL,* Bronchoalveolar lavage; *NB-BAL,* nonbronchoscopic bronchoalveolar lavage; $O_2$, oxygen.

## Tracheal Wash

Tracheal wash can provide valuable information in animals with cough, respiratory distress, or radiographic abnormalities resulting from lower respiratory tract (LRT) disease. Interstitial or focal disease processes are less likely to be identified than are bronchial or diffuse alveolar diseases. Complications are rare and include tracheal laceration, subcutaneous emphysema, and pneumomediastinum. Cats with bronchitis can be treated with bronchodilators before the procedure to decrease the risk of bronchospasm.

Techniques and sample handling are described in the text. The fluid is evaluated cytologically and microbiologically, so it should be collected before antibiotic therapy whenever possible. Fungal cultures are performed if mycotic disease is a consideration; *Mycoplasma* culture may be worthwhile in cats and dogs with bronchitis.

### Interpretation

Normal tracheal wash fluid primarily contains respiratory epithelial cells; few inflammatory cells are present. Occasionally, macrophages are retrieved from the small airways and alveoli. Oral contamination is indicated by the presence of numerous squamous epithelial cells, often coated with bacteria, and *Simonsiella* organisms (large, basophilic rods frequently found in stacks). Specimens with overt oral contamination generally do not provide accurate information about the airways, particularly with regard to bacterial infection.

**Neutrophilic inflammation.** Neutrophilic (suppurative) inflammation is common with bacterial infections. Before antibiotic therapy the neutrophils may be degenerate and organisms are often seen. Neutrophilic inflammation can also be caused by other infectious agents, chronic bronchitis, miscellaneous noninfectious inflammatory diseases, and even neoplasia. Some cats with bronchitis have neutrophilic rather than eosinophilic inflammation.

**Eosinophilic inflammation.** Eosinophilic inflammation reflects a hypersensitivity response. Common causes include allergic bronchitis, parasitic disease (lung worms or flukes, migrating intestinal parasites, heartworms), and eosinophilic lung diseases. Over time, mixed inflammation can occur in parasitized patients. Nonparasitic infection or neoplasia occasionally causes eosinophilia, usually as part of a mixed inflammatory response.

**Macrophagic inflammation.** Macrophagic or granulomatous inflammation is characterized by increased numbers of activated (vacuolated) macrophages, along with increased numbers of other inflammatory cells. This response is often nonspecific; infectious and allergic diseases, neoplastic processes, thromboembolism, and aspiration of lipids or particles can each cause macrophagic inflammation.

**Lymphocytic inflammation.** Lymphocytic inflammation alone is uncommon. Viral or rickettsial infection, noninfectious inflammatory disease, and lymphoma are considerations.

**Hemorrhage.** True hemorrhage can be differentiated from traumatic specimen collection by the presence of erythrophagocytosis and hemosiderin-laden macrophages; usually, an inflammatory response is also present. Causes include neoplasia, mycotic infection, heartworm disease, thromboembolism, foreign body, lung lobe torsion, and coagulopathies. A small amount of hemorrhage is seen in some patients with congestive heart failure.

**Neoplasia.** An interpretation of neoplasia must be made with extreme caution. For definitive diagnosis, overt characteristics of malignancy must be present in many cells without concurrent inflammation.

**Microorganisms.** Bacteria can be present in the large airways of healthy animals in low numbers. As a general guide, bacteria identified cytologically (in the absence of oral contamination) or grown in culture without enrichment broth are significant. Growth of systemic mycotic agents in culture is also clinically significant.

## Nonbronchoscopic BAL

BAL is considered in patients that have lung disease involving the small airways, alveoli, or interstitium and that are not in respiratory distress. Collected specimens are of large volume, providing adequate material for cytology (routine and special stains), multiple types of culture (bacterial, fungal, mycoplasmal), and other specific tests that may be indicated (e.g., flow cytometry, polymerase chain reaction).

Although general anesthesia is required, complications are uncommon. The primary complication is transient hypoxemia, which can generally be corrected with oxygen supplementation. Patients in respiratory distress in room air are not good candidates for BAL. For patients with bacterial or aspiration pneumonia, tracheal washing routinely results in an adequate specimen for cytologic and microbiologic analysis and avoids the need for general anesthesia.

Nonbronchoscopic techniques (NB-BAL) have been developed that allow BAL to be performed in cats and dogs with minimal expense in routine practice settings (see text). Visual guidance is not possible using these methods, so they are used primarily for patients with diffuse disease. The technique described for cats probably samples the cranial and middle regions of the lung on the side of the cat placed against the table, whereas the technique described for dogs consistently samples one of the caudal lung lobes.

### Interpretation

In general, total nucleated cell counts in normal animals are <500/μl. Differential cell counts for normal dogs and cats are given in Table 20-2. The same types of abnormal responses described for tracheal wash specimens may be seen in BAL specimens and are suggestive of similar diseases, although the specimens are from the deep lung rather than the airways. The normal population of pulmonary macrophages must not be misinterpreted as macrophagic or chronic inflammation.

Definitive diagnosis is made through the identification of organisms or abnormal cell populations. Fungal, protozoal, or parasitic organisms may be present in extremely low numbers in BAL specimens, so the entire concentrated slide preparation must be carefully scanned. Profound epithelial hyperplasia can occur in the presence of an inflammatory response and should not be confused with neoplasia.

### Bacterial culture

If quantitative bacterial culture is available, infection is suggested by $>1.7 \times 10^3$ colony-forming units (CFU)/ml. In the absence of quantitative numbers, growth of

**Table 20-2**

## Differential Cell Counts in Bronchoalveolar Lavage Fluid from Normal Animals

|  | Bronchoscopic BAL | | Nonbronchoscopic BAL | |
|---|---|---|---|---|
| Cell type | Dog (%)* | Cat (%)[†] | Dog (%)[‡] | Cat (%)[§] |
| Macrophages | 70 ± 11 | 71 ± 10 | 81 ± 11 | 78 ± 15 |
| Lymphocytes | 7 ± 5 | 5 ± 3 | 2 ± 5 | 0.4 ± 0.6 |
| Neutrophils | 5 ± 5 | 7 ± 4 | 15 ± 12 | 5 ± 5 |
| Eosinophils | 6 ± 6 | 16 ± 70 | 2 ± 3 | 16 ± 14 |
| Epithelial cells | 1 ± 1 | — | — | — |
| Mast cells | 1 ± 1 | — | — | — |

*Mean ± SD, six clinically and histologically normal dogs. (From Kuehn NF: *Canine bronchoalveolar lavage profile* [master's thesis], West Lafayette, Ind, 1987, Purdue University.)

[†]Mean ± SE, 11 clinically normal cats. (From King RR et al: Bronchoalveolar lavage cell populations in dogs and cats with eosinophilic pneumonitis. In *Proceedings of the Seventh Veterinary Respiratory Symposium*, Chicago, 1988, Comparative Respiratory Society.)

[‡]Mean ± SD, 9 clinically normal dogs. (From Hawkins EC et al: Use of a modified stomach tube for bronchoalveolar lavage in dogs, *J Am Vet Med Assoc* 215:1635, 1999.)

[§]Mean + SD, 34 specific-pathogen-free cats. (From Hawkins EC et al: Cytologic characterization of bronchoalveolar lavage fluid collected through an endotracheal tube in cats, *Am J Vet Res* 55:795, 1994.)

*BAL,* Bronchoalveolar lavage.

organisms on a plate directly inoculated with BAL fluid is considered significant, whereas growth from fluid that occurs only after multiplication in enrichment broth may be a result of normal inhabitants or contamination. Patients who are already receiving antibiotics at the time of specimen collection may have significant infection with few or no bacteria by culture.

## Transthoracic Lung Aspiration and Biopsy

Pulmonary parenchymal specimens can be obtained by transthoracic needle aspiration or biopsy. Techniques are described in the text. Only a small region of lung is sampled, but collection can be guided by radiographic findings or ultrasonography. Potential complications include pneumothorax, hemothorax, and pulmonary hemorrhage. These procedures are not performed in animals with suspected cysts, abscesses, pulmonary hypertension, or coagulopathies, and they should not be performed unless the clinician is prepared to place a chest tube and provide other support as necessary.

Transthoracic lung aspiration can be performed in animals with diffuse interstitial pulmonary disease when other procedures have failed to provide a diagnosis. However, BAL should be considered before lung aspiration in animals that can tolerate it; tracheal wash generally is indicated before lung aspiration in patients that cannot tolerate BAL.

These procedures are also indicated for nonsurgical diagnosis of intrathoracic mass lesions adjacent to the thoracic wall. If a solitary, localized mass lesion is present, thoracotomy and biopsy should be considered instead, because they allow both diagnosis and the potentially therapeutic benefits of complete excision during the same procedure.

### Interpretation

Slides are evaluated cytologically. Increased numbers of inflammatory cells, infectious agents, or neoplastic cell populations are potential abnormalities. Alveolar macrophages are normal findings in parenchymal specimens; they should be examined carefully for signs of activation and for phagocytosis of bacteria, fungi, or red blood cells. Epithelial hyperplasia can occur with inflammation and should not be confused with neoplasia. Sometimes, particularly in deep-chested dogs, the liver is aspirated inadvertently, yielding a population of cells resembling those of adenocarcinoma. Bacterial culture is indicated in some patients, although the specimen size is quite small.

## Bronchoscopy

Bronchoscopy is indicated in patients with suspected structural abnormalities, for visual assessment of airway inflammation or pulmonary hemorrhage, and for specimen collection. Bronchoscopy requires general anesthesia, and the presence of the scope in the airway compromises ventilation. It is therefore contraindicated in animals with severe respiratory compromise unless the procedure is likely to be therapeutic (e.g., foreign body removal). The technique is described in the text.

Abnormalities that may be observed during bronchoscopy and their common clinical correlations are listed in Table 20-3. A definitive diagnosis is rarely possible on the basis of gross examination alone. Bronchial specimens are obtained by bronchial washing or brushing or by pinch biopsy. Material for bacterial culture can be collected with guarded culture swabs. Foreign bodies are removed with retrieval forceps. Deeper lung tissue is sampled by BAL or transbronchial biopsy.

### Bronchoscopic BAL

BAL is performed as a routine part of diagnostic bronchoscopy after thorough visual examination of the airways. The technique is described in the text. Interpretation is the same as described for NB-BAL. Differential cell counts for bronchoscopic BAL fluid from normal dogs and cats are given in Table 20-2.

Several lobes are lavaged in each patient to maximize the likelihood of identification of active disease. Specific lobes are selected on the basis of abnormal radiographic or bronchoscopic findings. Because nearly half of the dogs with radiographically diffuse lung disease have cytologic differences in the BAL fluid collected from different lobes, ideally BAL fluid collected from different lobes is analyzed separately. Specimens from

Table 20-3

### Bronchoscopic Abnormalities

| Abnormality | Clinical correlation |
|---|---|
| **TRACHEA** | |
| Hyperemia, loss of normal vascular pattern, excess mucus, exudate | Inflammation |
| Redundant tracheal membrane | Tracheal collapse |
| Flattened cartilage rings | Tracheal collapse |
| Uniform narrowing | Hypoplastic trachea |
| Strictures | Prior trauma |
| Mass lesions | Fractured rings, foreign body granuloma, neoplasia |
| Tears | Usually a result of excessive endotracheal tube cuff pressure |
| **CARINA** | |
| Widened | Hilar lymphadenopathy, extraluminal mass |
| Multiple raised nodules | *Oslerus osleri* |
| Foreign body | Foreign body |
| **BRONCHI** | |
| Hyperemia, excess mucus, exudate | Inflammation |
| Collapse of airways during expiration | Chronic inflammation, weakened airway walls |
| Collapse of airway, inspiration and expiration, able to pass scope through narrowed airway | Chronic inflammation, weakened airway walls |
| Collapse of airway, inspiration and expiration, unable to pass scope through narrowed airway | Extraluminal mass lesions (neoplasia, granuloma, abscess) |
| Collapse of airway with "puckering" of mucosa | Lung lobe torsion |
| Hemorrhage | Neoplasia, fungal infection, heartworm, thromboembolic disease, coagulopathy, trauma (including foreign body related) |
| Single mass lesion | Neoplasia |
| Multiple polypoid masses | Usually chronic bronchitis; at carina, *Oslerus* |
| Foreign body | Foreign body |

different lobes can be combined for the purpose of bacterial, fungal, or mycoplasmal culture.

### Transbronchial Lung Biopsy
Collection of pinch biopsy specimens through the bronchial wall is most valuable for sampling intraluminal masses. Bronchial wall and a small amount of parenchymal tissue can be obtained from sites of small airway division. The specimens are extremely small and fragile, so multiple biopsy specimens should be collected for histopathologic evaluation. Primary complications are pulmonary hemorrhage and problems associated with general anesthesia. Pneumothorax can occur, but less frequently than with transthoracic techniques.

### Open-Chest Lung Biopsy and Thoracoscopy
Thoracotomy and surgical biopsy are performed in animals with progressive clinical signs of LRT disease that has not been diagnosed using less invasive means. Surgical

biopsy provides excellent specimens for histologic analysis and culture. Abnormal lung tissue and accessible lymph nodes are biopsied. In animals with localized disease, excisional biopsy of abnormal tissue can be therapeutic; removal of localized neoplasms, abscesses, cysts, and foreign bodies can be curative. Removal of large, localized lesions can improve ventilation and perfusion, and therefore clinical signs, even in patients with evidence of diffuse lung involvement.

Thoracoscopy is a less invasive technique that can be used for initial assessment of intrathoracic disease. Similarly, a "minithoracotomy" through a relatively small incision can be performed. If disease is obviously disseminated throughout the lungs such that surgical intervention would not be therapeutic, biopsies of abnormal tissue can be obtained. For patients with questionable findings or apparently localized disease, a full thoracotomy can be performed during the same anesthesia.

## BLOOD GAS ANALYSIS (TEXT PP 281-285)

Arterial blood gas measurements can be used to document pulmonary failure, differentiate hypoventilation from other causes of hypoxemia, help determine the need for supportive therapy, and assist in monitoring response to therapy. Arterial blood gas values for normal dogs and cats breathing room air are as follows:

| | |
|---|---|
| $Pao_2$ | 85 to 100 mm Hg |
| $Paco_2$ | 35 to 45 mm Hg |
| Bicarbonate ($HCO_3$) | 21 to 27 mmol/L |
| pH | 7.35 to 7.45 |

### Hypoxemia

Hypoxemia is defined as a $Pao_2$ below the normal range. Clinical signs are unlikely if the $Pao_2$ is >80 mm Hg. Treatment for hypoxemia is indicated when the value drops below 60 mm Hg and in all cyanotic animals. In general, animals become cyanotic when the $Pao_2$ reaches 50 mm Hg; polycythemic animals develop cyanosis more quickly than those with anemia, and acute hypoxemia resulting from lung disease produces pallor more often than cyanosis.

*Mechanisms of hypoxemia.* Determining the mechanism of hypoxemia is useful in selection of appropriate supportive therapy. Mechanisms include hypoventilation, diffusion abnormality, and inequality of ventilation and perfusion ($\dot{V}/\dot{Q}$ mismatch). Hypoventilation results in both hypercapnia and hypoxemia; causes are listed in Box 20-1. Diffusion abnormalities alone do not result in clinically significant hypoxemia.

*$\dot{V}/\dot{Q}$ mismatch.* Poorly ventilated portions of lung with normal blood flow have low $\dot{V}/\dot{Q}$ ratios. Regionally decreased ventilation occurs in most pulmonary diseases. Except where shunts (blood flow past nonaerated tissue) are present, the $Pao_2$ can be improved by provision of supplemental oxygen. In some cases positive-pressure ventilation is necessary to combat atelectasis. Normal ventilation of areas with decreased circulation (high $\dot{V}/\dot{Q}$ ratio) occurs with thromboembolism, although subsequent changes result in a net decrease in $\dot{V}/\dot{Q}$ ratio.

*A-a gradient.* Hypoventilation is associated with hypoxemia and hypercapnia, whereas $\dot{V}/\dot{Q}$ abnormalities are generally associated with hypoxemia and normocapnia or hypocapnia. Quantitative evaluation is possible by calculating the alveolar-arterial *(A-a)* oxygen gradient as follows:

$$A\text{-}a = P_{A}O_2 - Pao_2$$

where $P_{A}O_2 = 150$ mm Hg $- (Paco_2/0.8)$ in patients at sea level breathing room air.

The normal *A-a* gradient is <10 mm Hg in room air. Low $Pao_2$ with a normal *A-a* gradient indicates hypoventilation alone. Low $Pao_2$ with a wide *A-a* gradient (>15 mm Hg in room air) indicates a component of $\dot{V}/\dot{Q}$ mismatch.

### Acid-base status

Retention of $CO_2$ (hypercapnia) as a result of hypoventilation leads to respiratory acidosis, whereas hyperventilation (and the resulting hypocapnia) results in respiratory

---

**Box 20-1**

## Clinical Correlations of Blood Gas Abnormalities

**DECREASED Pao$_2$ AND INCREASED Paco$_2$ (NORMAL *A-a* GRADIENT)**
Venous specimen
Hypoventilation
Airway obstruction
Decreased ventilatory muscle function
    Anesthesia
    Central nervous system disease
    Polyneuropathy
    Polymyopathy
    Neuromuscular junction disorders (myasthenia gravis)
    Extreme fatigue (prolonged distress)
Restriction of lung expansion
    Thoracic wall abnormality
    Excessive thoracic bandage
    Pneumothorax
    Pleural effusion
Increased dead space (low alveolar ventilation)
    Severe chronic obstructive pulmonary disease or emphysema
End-stage severe pulmonary parenchymal disease
Severe pulmonary thromboembolism

**DECREASED Pao$_2$ AND NORMAL OR DECREASED Paco$_2$ (WIDE *A-a* GRADIENT)**
$\dot{V}/\dot{Q}$ abnormality
    Pulmonary parenchymal disease (see Box 19-2)
    Lung lobe collapse
    Pulmonary thromboembolism

---

*A-a,* Alveolar-arterial oxygen; $\dot{V}/\dot{Q}$, ventilation/perfusion.

alkalosis. Actual pH depends on metabolic (HCO$_3$) status. Hyperventilation is usually an acute phenomenon, potentially caused by shock, sepsis, severe anemia, anxiety, or pain.

The respiratory system partially compensates for metabolic acid-base disorders: hyperventilation (and hypocapnia) occurs in response to metabolic acidosis; hypoventilation (and hypercapnia) occurs in response to metabolic alkalosis.

*Interpretation.* In most cases acid-base disturbances can be identified as primarily respiratory or metabolic based on the pH. The body's compensatory responses do not alter the pH beyond normal limits. An animal with acidosis (pH <7.35) has a primary respiratory acidosis if the Paco$_2$ is increased and a compensatory respiratory response if the Paco$_2$ is decreased. An animal with alkalosis (pH >7.45) has a primary respiratory alkalosis if the Paco$_2$ is decreased and a compensatory respiratory response if the Paco$_2$ is increased. If both the Paco$_2$ and the HCO$_3$ concentration are abnormal, such that both contribute to the same alteration in pH, a mixed disturbance is present.

## PULSE OXIMETRY (TEXT PP 285-286)

Pulse oximetry is used to monitor blood oxygen saturation. Methodology is discussed in the text. Common problems that can interfere with accurate detection of pulses include position of the probe, patient motion (e.g., respiration, shivering), and weak or irregular pulse pressures (e.g., as with tachycardia, hypovolemia, hypothermia, arrhythmias).

The measured value indicates saturation of hemoglobin (Hb) in the local circulation. This value can be affected by factors other than pulmonary function, such as vasoconstriction, low cardiac output, and local blood stasis. Other intrinsic factors that can affect oximetry readings include anemia, hyperbilirubinemia, carboxyhemoglobinemia, and methemoglobinemia. External lights and probe location can also influence results.

### Interpretation

Normal dogs and cats with $PaO_2$ values >85 mm Hg have Hb saturation of >95%. When $PaO_2$ values decrease to 60 mm Hg, Hb saturation is approximately 90%. Any further decrease in $PaO_2$ results in a precipitous decrease in Hb saturation. Pulse oximetry readings of oxygen saturation are less accurate below values of 80%. Ideally, Hb saturation should be maintained above 90% through oxygen supplementation or ventilatory support and specific treatment of the underlying disease.

Because of the many variables associated with pulse oximetry, such strict guidelines are not always valid. In practice a baseline measurement of Hb saturation is made. Subsequent changes in that measurement are used to assess improvement or deterioration in oxygenation.

# 21

# Disorders of the Trachea and Bronchi

## *(Text pp 287-298)*

### CANINE INFECTIOUS TRACHEOBRONCHITIS (TEXT PP 287-289)

Canine infectious tracheobronchitis ("kennel cough") is a highly contagious, acute disease localized to the airways. It is caused by one or more of the following infectious agents: canine adenovirus 2 (CAV-2), parainfluenza virus (PIV), and *Bordetella bronchiseptica.* Other organisms may also be involved as secondary pathogens. In nearly all dogs the disease is self-limiting, with clinical signs resolving in approximately 2 weeks.

### Clinical features

The presenting sign in affected dogs is severe cough of sudden onset that is often exacerbated by exercise, excitement, or pressure from the collar. Palpating the trachea easily induces the cough. Gagging, retching, or nasal discharge can also occur. A recent history of boarding, hospitalization, or exposure to a puppy or dog with similar signs is common.

In uncomplicated cases the patients do not show signs of systemic illness. Dogs with weight loss, persistent anorexia, or signs of other organ involvement (e.g., diarrhea, chorioretinitis, seizures) likely have a more serious disease, such as canine distemper or mycotic infection. Although uncommon, respiratory complications can occur. Very young puppies, immunocompromised dogs, and dogs with preexisting lung abnormalities can develop secondary bacterial pneumonia. Dogs with chronic airway disease or tracheal collapse can experience acute, severe exacerbation of their problem.

### Diagnosis

Diagnosis is usually based on presenting signs. Complete blood count (CBC), thoracic radiographs, and tracheal wash are indicated when signs suggest more serious disease or when signs do not resolve. CBC and thoracic radiographs are unremarkable in uncomplicated cases, and often tracheal wash fluid simply indicates acute inflammation. Bacterial culture of the fluid can be useful for identification of any bacteria involved, and determination of antibiotic sensitivity is helpful in selection of antibiotics.

### Treatment and prognosis

Uncomplicated kennel cough is self-limiting. Rest for at least 7 days, with avoidance of exercise and excitement, is indicated to minimize continual airway irritation by excessive coughing. Cough suppressants are useful but should not be used if the cough is productive or if fluid accumulation in the lungs is suspected after auscultation or thoracic radiographs. Glucocorticoids should not be used.

*Cough suppressants.* A variety of cough suppressants can be used in dogs (Table 21-1). With butorphanol or hydrocodone, sedation can occur at high doses. Cold remedies with additional ingredients, such as antihistamines and decongestants, should be avoided.

*Antibiotics.* Antibiotics are not indicated in most cases, but they are often prescribed because of the potential role of *Bordetella*. Antibiotics effective against most *Bordetella* isolates include doxycycline (5 to 10 mg/kg q12h), chloramphenicol (50 mg/kg q8h), and amoxicillin with clavulanate (20 to 25 mg/kg q8h). Bacterial susceptibility data from tracheal wash is useful in the selection of an appropriate antibiotic. Antibiotics are administered for 5 days beyond the resolution of clinical signs, or for at least 10 days. If clinical signs have not resolved within 2 weeks, further diagnostic evaluation is indicated.

### Prognosis

Prognosis for complete recovery from uncomplicated infectious tracheobronchitis is excellent.

### Prevention

Canine infectious tracheobronchitis can be prevented by minimizing exposure to organisms and by vaccination. Excellent nutrition, routine deworming, and avoidance of stress improve the dog's ability to respond to infection without developing serious signs.

*Minimizing exposure.* Dogs should be kept isolated from puppies or dogs that have recently been boarded. Careful sanitation should be practiced in kennel facilities. Adequate air exchange and humidity control are necessary in rooms housing several dogs. An isolation area is essential for dogs with clinical signs of kennel cough.

*Vaccination.* Injectable and intranasal vaccines are available for the three major pathogens (CAV-2, PIV, *B. bronchiseptica).* Injectable modified-live vaccines against CAV-2 and PIV are adequate for most pet dogs. Maternal antibodies interfere with the response to the vaccine, so puppies must be vaccinated every 2 to 4 weeks, beginning at 6 to 8 weeks of age, until 14 to 16 weeks of age. In any dog at least two vaccines must

**Table 21-1**

## Common Cough Suppressants for Use in Dogs*

| Agent | Dose |
| --- | --- |
| Dextromethorphan | 1 to 2 mg/kg orally (PO) q6-8h |
| Butorphanol | 0.5 mg/kg PO q6-12h |
| Hydrocodone bitartrate | 0.25 mg/kg PO q8-12h |

*Centrally acting cough suppressants are rarely, if ever, indicated for use in cats and can result in adverse reactions. The listed doses are for dogs only.

be given initially. Frequency of booster vaccination has traditionally been every year, but such frequent vaccination may not be necessary in most healthy pet dogs.

Dogs at high risk, such as those in endemic kennels or those that are frequently boarded, may benefit from vaccines incorporating *B. bronchiseptica.* These vaccines do not prevent infection but aim to decrease clinical signs if infection occurs. Both the parenteral and intranasal vaccines afford similar protection. Greatest benefit may be achieved by administering both forms of vaccine sequentially at a 2-week interval. Intranasal *Bordetella* vaccines occasionally cause clinical signs (particularly cough); signs are generally self-limiting but can be disturbing to owners.

## COLLAPSING TRACHEA (TEXT PP 289-291)

### Etiology

With tracheal collapse the tracheal lumen is narrowed by flattening of the cartilaginous rings and/or redundancy of the dorsal tracheal membrane. The condition can affect the extrathoracic trachea, the intrathoracic trachea, or both. Chronic bronchitis with collapse of the mainstem bronchi coexists in many dogs with intrathoracic tracheal collapse.

Certain dogs may be predisposed to tracheal collapse because of inherent abnormalities in the tracheal cartilage, but they are initially asymptomatic. These dogs develop cough when an exacerbating problem develops. Once the cough begins, a cycle is started involving chronic tracheal inflammation, changes in the tracheal mucosa, and perpetuation of the cough.

### Clinical features

Tracheal collapse is common in middle-aged toy and miniature dogs, although it can occur early in life and in large-breed dogs. Tracheal collapse is rare in cats; generally it results from tracheal obstruction caused by a tumor or traumatic injury.

Signs may occur acutely, then slowly progress over months to years. The primary clinical feature is a nonproductive cough, described as a "goose honk." The cough is worse during excitement, exercise, or with pressure from the collar. Eventually (usually after years of chronic cough), respiratory distress may be brought on by exercise, overheating, or excitement. Systemic signs such as weight loss, anorexia, and depression are uncommon.

Cough can often be elicited by palpation of the trachea. An end-expiratory snap or click may be heard during auscultation with intrathoracic collapse. In advanced cases or after exercise, increased inspiratory effort is observed in dogs with extrathoracic collapse, and increased expiratory effort in those with intrathoracic collapse.

History and physical examination should also emphasize a search for exacerbating or complicating disease, such as cardiac disease causing left atrial enlargement and bronchial compression or pulmonary edema; airway inflammation caused by bacterial infection, allergic bronchitis, exposure to smoke, chronic bronchitis, or recent intubation; upper airway obstruction caused by elongated soft palate, stenotic nares, or laryngeal paralysis; and systemic disorders such as obesity or hyperadrenocorticism.

### Diagnosis

Tracheal collapse is most often diagnosed on the basis of clinical signs and cervical and thoracic radiography. Radiographically, narrowing caused by collapse of the extrathoracic trachea is more evident during inspiration. Intrathoracic collapse is more apparent during expiration, but inspiratory radiographs of the thorax should also be taken to check for bronchial or parenchymal abnormalities.

Fluoroscopy and bronchoscopy are more sensitive than routine radiography. Tracheal wash or bronchoscopy with bronchoalveolar lavage (BAL) should be performed to identify airway inflammation and infection. Fluid samples are submitted for cytologic analysis and bacterial culture.

### Treatment

Medical therapy is adequate for most animals. Dogs that are overweight are placed on a weight-reducing diet. The collar should be replaced by a harness, and owners counseled to keep their dogs from becoming overheated. Excessive excitement should also be avoided. In some patients sedatives such as phenobarbital are prescribed, to be given before known stressful events.

*Medications.* In the absence of pneumonia, cough suppressants are used to control signs and disrupt the cough cycle (see Table 21-1). Cough suppressants can often be given with decreasing frequency and then discontinued if the cough resolves. Bronchodilators (Table 21-2) may be beneficial in dogs with signs of chronic bronchitis. Antiinflammatory doses of glucocorticoids can be given for a short period during exacerbation of signs (e.g., prednisone, 0.5 to 1 mg/kg q12h for 3 to 5 days, then tapered down and discontinued over 3 to 4 weeks). Dogs with signs referable to mitral insufficiency are managed for this disease (see Chapter 8). Dogs with abnormalities causing upper airway obstruction are treated with corrective surgical procedures. Management of dogs in acute respiratory distress is discussed in Chapter 26.

Antibiotics are not routinely indicated. Dogs with evidence of infection should be treated with appropriate antibiotics (based on results of sensitivity testing). Relatively high doses should be used for several weeks, as described later for canine chronic bronchitis.

*Surgery.* Surgical treatment should be considered for patients that are no longer responsive to medical management. The most common method of correction involves support of the trachea with an external splint (see text). Dogs with extrathoracic collapse are better surgical candidates than those with intrathoracic collapse.

### Prognosis

In most dogs clinical signs can be controlled with conscientious medical management and reevaluation during exacerbation for secondary infection or concurrent disease. Animals that develop severe signs despite appropriate medical care have a guarded prognosis.

## FELINE BRONCHITIS (TEXT PP 291-295)

Bronchitis is a common cause of respiratory signs (cough, wheeze, episodic respiratory distress) in cats. However, the term *feline bronchitis* or *feline asthma,* as applied to all cats

**Table 21-2**

### Common Bronchodilators for Use in Dogs and Cats

| Bronchodilator | Dose |
|---|---|
| **METHYLXANTHINES** | |
| Aminophylline | Cats: 5 mg/kg orally (PO) q12h |
| | Dogs: 11 mg/kg PO q8h |
| Oxtriphylline elixir (Choledyl, Parke-Davis) | Cats: None |
| | Dogs: 14 mg/kg PO q8h |
| Long-acting theophylline* | Cats: 25 mg/kg q24h, in evening |
| | Dogs: 10 mg/kg q12h† |
| **SYMPATHOMIMETIC** | |
| Terbutaline | Cats: 1/8-1/4 of 2.5-mg tablet/cat PO q12h to start; or 0.01 mg/kg subcutaneously (SC); can repeat once |
| | Dogs: 1.25-5 mg/dog PO q8-12h |

From Bach JF et al: *JAVMA* 224:1113-1119, 2004.

*Absorption of currently available products is unpredictable in dogs and cats. Monitoring of plasma concentrations is recommended.

†Theophylline SR, Inwood Laboratories, Inwood, NY.

with bronchial disease, belies the wide variety of pathologic processes that can affect individual cats and the wide range in severity of clinical signs and response to therapy.

### Etiology

Feline bronchitis is not a specific disease, but rather a descriptive diagnosis. In many cats, the bronchitis is idiopathic. However, treatable diseases that can be associated with feline bronchitis should be considered in the diagnostic evaluation. These include allergic bronchitis, pulmonary parasites *(Aelurostrongylus abstrusus, Capillaria aerophila, Paragonimus kellicotti)*, heartworm disease, and bacterial or mycoplasmal infection.

Small airway obstruction is a consistent feature of feline bronchial disease. Possible causes are many and varied, and different combinations are present in each animal. They include the following:

- bronchoconstriction
- bronchial smooth muscle hypertrophy
- increased mucous production
- decreased mucous clearance
- inflammatory exudate in airway lumens
- inflammatory infiltrate in airway walls
- epithelial hyperplasia
- glandular hypertrophy
- fibrosis
- emphysema

Some of these factors are reversible (e.g., bronchospasm, inflammation), but others are permanent (e.g., fibrosis, emphysema).

*Classification.* The following classification system better defines bronchial disease for the purpose of treatment and prognosis in individual cats:

- bronchial asthma—reversible airway obstruction caused by bronchoconstriction; common features are smooth muscle hypertrophy, increased mucous production, and eosinophilic inflammation
- acute bronchitis—reversible airway inflammation of short duration (<3 months); common features are increased mucous production and neutrophilic or macrophagic inflammation
- chronic bronchitis—chronic airway inflammation (>3 months) resulting in irreversible damage (e.g., fibrosis); common features are increased mucous production, airway inflammation (neutrophilic, eosinophilic, or mixed), isolation of bacteria or *Mycoplasma* (either causal or nonpathogenic inhabitants), and concurrent bronchial asthma
- emphysema—destruction of bronchiolar and alveolar walls, resulting in enlarged peripheral airspaces; caused by, or concurrent with, chronic bronchitis; cavitary lesions (bullae) are common

A cat can have more than one type of bronchitis. Although it is not always possible to absolutely determine the type(s) of bronchial disease present without sophisticated pulmonary function testing, routine clinical data (history and physical examination findings, thoracic radiographs, analysis of airway specimens, progression of signs) can be used to classify the disease in most cats.

### Clinical features

Cats of any age can develop bronchitis, although it most often develops in young adult and middle-aged cats. The major clinical features are cough, episodic respiratory distress, or both. Owners may report wheezing that occurs during an episode. Signs are often slowly progressive. Weight loss, anorexia, depression, and other systemic signs are not present. Owners should be questioned carefully for association with potential allergens or irritants, such as seasonal exacerbations, new cat litter (usually perfumed), cigarette or fireplace smoke, carpet cleaners, household items that contain perfumes, recent remodeling, or any other change in the cat's environment.

Physical examination findings indicate small airway obstruction. Tachypnea with increased expiratory effort is found in cats in respiratory distress. Auscultation reveals expiratory wheezes, particularly during such episodes. Crackles are occasionally present. Physical examination may be unremarkable between episodes.

### Diagnosis

Presumptive diagnosis is based on historical, physical, and radiographic findings. Tracheal wash or BAL fluid analysis can confirm airway inflammation; one of these procedures should be performed, along with tests for heartworm disease and pulmonary parasitism. Peripheral eosinophilia is neither specific nor sensitive and cannot be used to rule out or definitively diagnose feline bronchitis.

*Radiography.* A bronchial pattern is generally present on thoracic radiographs. Increased reticular interstitial markings and patchy alveolar opacities may also be seen (see Chapter 20). Overinflation of the lungs may be evident, and occasionally collapse (atelectasis) of the right middle lung lobe is seen. However, clinical signs can precede radiographic changes, and radiographs cannot detect mild airway changes, so radiographs may be normal in cats with bronchitis. Radiographs should also be examined for evidence of specific diseases, such as heartworm disease or pulmonary parasites.

*Tracheal wash or BAL.* Typical findings on fluid analysis include increased numbers of inflammatory cells and increased amounts of mucus; inflammation may be eosinophilic, neutrophilic, or mixed (see Chapter 20). Although not a specific finding, eosinophilic inflammation is suggestive of a hypersensitivity response to allergens or parasites. Neutrophils should be evaluated for signs of degeneration suggesting bacterial infection, and slides carefully examined for the presence of organisms, particularly bacteria and parasitic larvae or ova. The fluid should be cultured for bacteria, although growth may or may not represent true infection. Mycoplasmal cultures can be helpful.

*Other tests.* Tests for feline heartworm disease should also be performed (see Chapter 10). Young cats and cats with airway eosinophilia should be evaluated further for pulmonary parasites by multiple fecal examinations (see Chapter 20).

### Treatment

*Acute respiratory distress.* Cats in acute respiratory distress should be stabilized before diagnostic tests are performed. Effective treatment includes administration of a bronchodilator (see Table 21-2), rapid-acting glucocorticoids (e.g., prednisolone sodium succinate, 10 to 20 mg/kg given intravenously [IV] or intramuscularly [IM]), and supplemental oxygen. Terbutaline can be administered subcutaneously to avoid stress. After treatment is administered, the cat is placed in a cool, stress-free, oxygen-enriched environment. Management of respiratory distress is discussed further in Chapter 26.

*Antibiotics.* Because of the difficulty in documenting *Mycoplasma* infection, a therapeutic trial of antibiotics should be considered. Doxycycline (5 to 10 mg/kg q12h) or chloramphenicol (10 to 15 mg/kg q12h) is given for 14 days. In cats that are difficult to medicate, azithromycin (5 to 10 mg/kg q24h for 3 days, then q72h) can be tried.

*Environmental control.* Therapeutic trials to eliminate inhaled allergens from the cat's environment should be performed, particularly in cats with eosinophilic airway inflammation. Potential reactions to smoke and litter perfumes should be tested even in patients with no obvious association. The condition of indoor cats may improve when measures are taken to decrease the level of dust, molds, and mildew in the home. Any beneficial response to environmental change is usually seen within 1 to 2 weeks.

*Glucocorticoids.* Glucocorticoids, with or without bronchodilators, are necessary in most cats. Results can be quite dramatic. Drug therapy can interfere with environmental testing, so the ability of the cat to tolerate delay of drug therapy must be assessed on an individual basis. Short-acting products such as prednisone are recommended; a dose of 0.5 mg/kg is administered q8 to 12h initially and doubled if signs are not controlled within 1 week. Once the signs are controlled, the dose is tapered down. A reasonable goal is <0.5 mg/kg every other day. Outdoor cats that cannot be treated frequently can be treated with depot steroid products, such as methylprednisolone acetate (10 mg/cat IM).

*Bronchodilators.* Cats that require relatively large amounts of glucocorticoids to control clinical signs, those that react unfavorably to glucocorticoid therapy, and those that suffer from periodic exacerbation of signs can benefit from bronchodilator therapy. Recommended drugs and doses are listed in Table 21-2.

*Methylxanthines.* Methylxanthines are preferred. Long-acting theophyllines are the most convenient for owners; however, absorption is unpredictable with currently available formulations. Individual metabolism of all methylxanthines is variable, so plasma theophylline concentrations should be monitored in patients that respond poorly and those receiving long-acting theophylline (see text).

The immediate-release forms are rapidly absorbed orally (PO). If IV administration is required, the drug should be injected slowly. Potential adverse effects of methylxanthines include gastrointestinal signs, cardiac arrhythmias, nervousness, and seizures. Serious adverse effects are extremely rare at therapeutic concentrations.

*Sympathomimetics.* Sympathomimetic drugs such as terbutaline are also effective bronchodilators (see Table 21-2). Potential adverse effects include nervousness, tremors, hypotension, and tachycardia. Terbutaline can be administered subcutaneously for the treatment of respiratory emergencies.

*Metered-dose inhaler therapy.* Glucocorticoids such as fluticasone propionate (Flovent) and bronchodilators such as albuterol can be administered to cats, either in the clinic or at home, using a metered-dose inhaler. Advantages, disadvantages, and practical considerations are discussed in the text.

*Other drugs.* Antihistamines are not recommended for treatment of feline bronchitis. Cyproheptadine (2 mg/cat PO q12h) can be attempted when signs cannot be controlled with bronchodilators and glucocorticoids. Oral leukotriene inhibitors (e.g., Accolate, Singulair, Zyflo) are not currently advocated for use in cats.

### Prognosis
Prognosis for control of clinical signs is good in most cats. Complete cure is unlikely unless an underlying cause can be eliminated; most cats require continued medication. Cats that have severe, acute asthmatic attacks are at risk for sudden death. Cats with persistent, untreated airway inflammation can develop the permanent changes of chronic bronchitis and emphysema.

## ALLERGIC BRONCHITIS (TEXT P 295)

Allergic bronchitis is an inflammatory airway response, usually to an inhaled antigen. It is less common in dogs than in cats. The inflammatory response is typically eosinophilic, as demonstrated in tracheal wash or BAL specimens. Long-standing allergic bronchitis can result in the permanent changes described for chronic bronchitis. Allergic bronchitis in cats is discussed in the preceding section on feline bronchitis.

### Clinical features and diagnosis
Young to middle-aged dogs are most often affected. The disease can result in acute or chronic cough. Rarely, respiratory distress and wheezing occur. Physical examination and radiographic findings reflect bronchial disease. Heartworm tests and fecal examinations for pulmonary parasites should be performed to eliminate parasitism as the cause. In dogs <1 year of age, bronchoscopic examination for *Oslerus osleri* should also be considered.

### Treatment and prognosis
Treatment consists of an attempt to identify and remove potential allergens from the environment (as discussed for feline bronchitis) and administration of glucocorticoids and bronchodilators (as discussed below for canine chronic bronchitis). Animals with allergic bronchitis should be treated aggressively to minimize long-term airway inflammation and chronic bronchial changes. Response to therapy is often excellent, but continued treatment is usually necessary unless inciting allergens can be identified and eliminated.

## CANINE CHRONIC BRONCHITIS (TEXT PP 295-297)

### Etiology
Chronic bronchitis is long-term airway inflammation, generally with a component of irreversible damage. Histologic changes include fibrosis, epithelial hyperplasia, glandular hypertrophy, and inflammatory infiltrates. Excessive mucus is present within

the airways, and small airway obstruction and collapse occur. Another potential complication is bronchiectasis (permanent dilation of the airways). The dilation generally involves all major airways, but occasionally it is localized. Recurrent infections and overt pneumonia are common.

The cause is often unknown, but long-standing inflammatory processes resulting from infections, allergies, or inhaled irritants can be responsible. Infections can also occur secondary to chronic bronchitis, making a cause-and-effect relationship difficult to determine.

Chronic bronchitis occurs most often in middle-aged or older small-breed dogs. These breeds are also predisposed to tracheal collapse and mitral insufficiency with left atrial enlargement that causes compression of mainstem bronchi. These diseases must be differentiated and their contribution to the current clinical picture determined for appropriate management.

### Clinical features

Dogs with chronic bronchitis are presented with a cough. The cough may be productive or nonproductive. Usually it is slowly progressive over months or years, with no systemic signs of illness. With disease progression, exercise intolerance develops; incessant coughing or overt respiratory distress is then seen.

The breathing pattern is characterized by marked expiratory effort. Presentation is often attributable to a sudden exacerbation in signs. The change in signs may result from (1) transient worsening of the chronic bronchitis, perhaps because of a period of excitement, stress, or exposure to irritants or allergens; (2) a secondary complication, such as bacterial infection; or (3) concurrent disease. Exacerbating and concurrent disorders that contribute to worsening of the cough are the same as those described for collapsing trachea.

Increased breath sounds, wheezes, or crackles are auscultated. End-expiratory clicks may be heard in advanced cases and result from collapse of mainstem bronchi or the intrathoracic trachea. A prominent or split second heart sound occurs with secondary pulmonary hypertension.

### Diagnosis

Diagnosis is based on clinical signs and on the ruling out of other diseases using various diagnostic tests.

*Radiography.* A bronchial pattern with increased interstitial markings is typically present on thoracic radiographs, although thoracic radiographs may be normal. Bronchiectasis is observed in some patients. An alveolar pattern, particularly with a dependent distribution, suggests a complicating disease, such as bacterial pneumonia (see Chapter 20).

*Tracheal wash or BAL.* Tracheal wash or BAL fluid should be collected on initial presentation and after acute exacerbation of signs. Neutrophilic or mixed inflammation and increased mucus are usually present. Degenerative neutrophils suggest bacterial infection. Although not a specific finding, eosinophils suggest a hypersensitivity reaction, as can occur with allergy, parasites, or heartworm disease. Slides should be carefully examined for microorganisms. Bacterial cultures are performed and interpreted as discussed in Chapter 20. Although the role of mycoplasmal infections is unknown, mycoplasmal cultures should also be considered.

*Bronchoscopy.* Bronchoscopy, with specimen collection, is performed in selected cases, primarily to help rule out other diseases. Maximum benefit is obtained early in the course of disease, before severe permanent damage has occurred and while the risk of the procedure is minimal (see Chapter 20).

*Other tests.* Further diagnostic procedures may be necessary to rule out other potential causes of chronic cough. Considerations include heartworm tests, fecal examinations for pulmonary parasites, echocardiography, and systemic evaluation (CBC, serum biochemistries, urinalysis).

*Ciliary dyskinesia.* Abnormal ciliary motion is uncommon but should be considered in dogs with bronchiectasis or recurrent infection. Abnormalities exist in all ciliated tissues, and situs inversus (lateral transposition of the abdominal and thoracic organs) occurs in 50% of dogs. Dextrocardia with chronic bronchitis is extremely suggestive of this disease. Sperm motility can be evaluated in intact male dogs; normal sperm motility rules out a diagnosis of ciliary dyskinesia. The disease is diagnosed by measuring the clearance of radioisotopes deposited at the carina and electron microscopic examination of bronchial or nasal biopsies or sperm.

### Treatment

Chronic bronchitis is managed symptomatically, with specific treatment possible only for identified underlying or complicating diseases. Each dog must be managed as an individual. Ideally, medications are initiated one at a time to assess the most effective combination. Treatment modification is often necessary over time. Commonly used medications include bronchodilators, glucocorticoids, antibiotics, and cough suppressants. Airway hydration is maintained, and stimuli that exacerbate signs are avoided.

*Bronchodilators.* Bronchodilators are discussed in the section on Feline Bronchitis; dose recommendations for dogs are given in Table 21-2. The response in dogs may be less dramatic than that in cats.

*Glucocorticoids.* Glucocorticoids are often effective in controlling signs and may slow development of permanent airway damage. They are particularly helpful in dogs with eosinophilic airway inflammation. Because of the potential for negative effects, short-acting products are used, and if they are effective the dose is tapered to the lowest effective level (<0.5 mg/kg q48h); the drug is discontinued if no beneficial effect is seen. Prednisone is initially given at 0.5 to 1 mg/kg q12h, with a positive response expected within 1 week.

*Antibiotics.* Antibiotics are prescribed for dogs with infection, ideally documented by culture of tracheal or BAL fluid with accompanying sensitivity data. *Bordetella* is most commonly recovered, but a variety of gram-positive and gram-negative organisms can be found, making antibiotic susceptibility difficult to predict. Antibiotics that are likely to reach adequate concentrations against susceptible organisms include doxycycline, chloramphenicol, fluoroquinolones, or amoxicillin with clavulanate. Fluoroquinolones should be reserved for resistant infections.

If an antibiotic is effective, a positive response is generally seen within 1 week. Treatment is continued for at least 1 week beyond stabilization of clinical signs. (Complete resolution is unlikely.) Usually 3 to 4 weeks is necessary, and longer if bronchiectasis or overt pneumonia is present.

*Cough suppressants.* Cough suppressants are used cautiously because cough is an important mechanism to clear airway secretions. In some dogs, however, the cough is incessant and exhausting, or ineffective because of marked bronchial collapse. In such patients, cough suppressants can provide some relief and may even aid ventilation and decrease anxiety. Although the doses provided in Table 21-1 can give prolonged relief, less frequent administration (e.g., only when coughing is most severe) may preserve some beneficial effect of coughing.

*Airway hydration.* Maintaining airway hydration is critical for facilitating mucociliary clearance. Systemic hydration must be maintained, and diuretic therapy should be avoided. Placing the animal in a steamy bathroom or a room with a vaporizer can provide relief, although the moisture does not reach far into the airways. Nebulization allows the moisture to reach deeper areas in the lungs (see Chapter 22).

*Controlling exacerbating factors.* Irritants, such as smoke and perfumed products, should be avoided. Short-term administration of acepromazine or phenobarbital can be helpful for patients in which excitement or stress acutely worsens the signs. Weight loss should be attempted in obese patients. Routine dental prophylaxis may help maintain a healthy oral flora, some of which is normally aspirated into the airways.

Animals with localized bronchiectasis benefit from surgical removal of the affected lung lobe if signs are severe or if infections recur. In most patients, however, the problem is generalized; these animals are particularly predisposed to infection from decreased airway clearance. Glucocorticoids should be avoided or used in low doses.

### Prognosis

Chronic bronchitis is irreversible. Prognosis for control of signs and a satisfactory quality of life is good if the owner is conscientious with regard to medical management and is willing to adjust treatment over time and treat secondary problems as they occur.

## *O. OSLERI* (TEXT PP 297-298)

*O. osleri* is an uncommon parasite of young dogs (usually <2 years of age). The adult worms live at the carina and mainstem bronchi and cause a local, nodular inflammatory reaction with fibrosis. Most affected dogs become infected as puppies through intimate contact with their dams.

### Clinical features and diagnosis

Acute, nonproductive cough occasionally accompanied by wheezing is the primary complaint. Affected dogs appear otherwise healthy, making initial presentation indistinguishable from that of canine infectious tracheobronchitis. However, the cough persists, and eventually airway obstruction results from the formation of reactive nodules.

Nodules at the carina can occasionally be recognized radiographically, but the most sensitive diagnostic method is bronchoscopy. The nodules are readily seen, and immediate microscopic examination of brushings reveals the larvae. If a definitive diagnosis is not obtained through brushing, biopsies are taken. Cytologic examination of tracheal wash fluid may show characteristic ova or larvae, providing a definitive diagnosis. Rarely, larvae are found in fecal specimens (see Chapter 20).

### Treatment and prognosis

Treatment with ivermectin (400 µg/kg PO or subcutaneously [SQ]) is recommended. The dose is repeated every 3 weeks for four treatments. Note: This protocol has not been extensively investigated and is not an approved use of this drug; *it should not be used in Collies*. The prognosis is good.

# 22

# Disorders of the Pulmonary Parenchyma

## *(Text pp 299-314)*

## VIRAL PNEUMONIA (TEXT P 299)

Several viruses can infect the lungs, including canine adenovirus 1, parainfluenza virus, and canine distemper virus in dogs and calicivirus and feline infectious peritonitis virus in cats. Rarely do signs of viral pneumonia predominate; clinical signs of pneumonia usually result from secondary bacterial infection.

## BACTERIAL PNEUMONIA (TEXT PP 299-302)

### Etiology

A wide variety of bacteria can infect the lungs. Common isolates include *Pasteurella* spp., *Klebsiella* spp., *Escherichia coli, Pseudomonas* spp., staphylococci, streptococci, and *Bordetella bronchiseptica.* Anaerobes may be present as part of a mixed infection, particularly in animals with aspiration pneumonia or lung lobe consolidation. *Mycoplasma* spp. have also been isolated from dogs and cats with pneumonia.

In most cases bacteria enter via the airways, causing bronchopneumonia primarily in the cranial and ventral lobes. Hematogenous spread usually causes pneumonia with a caudal or diffuse pattern and marked interstitial involvement.

A predisposing abnormality usually exists. Such conditions include (1) decreased clearance of normally inhaled debris from the lungs (e.g., chronic bronchitis, ciliary dyskinesia, bronchiectasis); (2) immunosuppression from drugs, malnutrition, stress, endocrinopathies, or viral infections; (3) aspiration of ingested material or gastric contents; and (4) fungal or parasitic infections. Cats, particularly kittens, from stressful housing situations (e.g., overcrowding) appear predisposed to develop pneumonia from *Bordetella* infections.

### Clinical features

Dogs and cats with bacterial pneumonia are presented for respiratory signs, systemic signs, or both. Respiratory signs can include cough (usually productive and soft), bilateral mucopurulent nasal discharge, exercise intolerance, and respiratory distress. Cough is rare in cats with pneumonia. Affected cats may have a history of chronic airway disease or regurgitation. Systemic signs include lethargy, anorexia, fever, and weight loss, although fever is present in only approximately 50% of patients. Crackles and occasionally expiratory wheezes may be auscultated, particularly over the cranioventral lung fields.

### Diagnosis

Diagnosis is based on complete blood count (CBC), thoracic radiographs, and tracheal wash cytology and culture. A finding of neutrophilic leukocytosis with a left shift, neutropenia with a degenerative left shift, or moderate to marked neutrophil toxicity is supportive of bacterial pneumonia. However, a normal or stress leukogram is just as likely to be found.

Abnormal radiographic patterns vary. An alveolar pattern is typical, possibly with consolidation that is most severe in the dependent lobes. Increased bronchial and interstitial markings are often present. A bronchial pattern alone may be present in animals with primarily bronchial infection; an interstitial pattern may be all that is seen in early or mild disease or in animals with infections of hematogenous origin. Radiographs should also be evaluated for megaesophagus.

In most cases tracheal wash is sufficient for diagnosis. Septic neutrophilic inflammation is seen, and growth on bacterial culture is expected (see Chapter 20). Further diagnostic tests (e.g., bronchoscopy, conjunctival scrapings for distemper virus, serology for fungal infections, hormonal assays for hyperadrenocorticism) are sometimes indicated.

### Treatment

Effective treatment involves antibiotic therapy, airway hydration, and physiotherapy.

*Antibiotics.* Infections with gram-negative organisms or with multiple organisms occur in the majority of cases, making antibiotic susceptibility difficult to predict. Therefore antibiotics should be selected on the basis of susceptibility data from culture of pulmonary specimens. Cytologic characteristics (e.g., gram-staining characteristics and morphology) provide some initial guidance while culture results are pending.

Antibiotics that can be initiated before susceptibility results are available include amoxicillin-clavulanate (20 to 25 mg/kg q8h), cephalexin (20 to 40 mg/kg q8h), or chloramphenicol (50 mg/kg q8h for dogs; 10 to 15 mg/kg q12h for cats). Fluoroquinolones are reserved for animals with resistant gram-negative infections.

Animals with severe clinical signs or possible sepsis should be treated initially with intravenous antibiotics. For life-threatening infections, broad-spectrum coverage can be achieved with imipenem (2 to 5 mg/kg q6 to 8h) or a combination of ampicillin-sulbactam (50 mg/kg of combined drugs q8h) and either a fluoroquinolone or an aminoglycoside (e.g., amikacin, 5 to 10 mg/kg q8h).

Kittens from stressful environments suspected of having *Bordetella*-induced pneumonia should be treated with doxycycline (5 to 10 mg/kg q12h), a fluoroquinolone, or amoxicillin-clavulanate while culture results are awaited. If *Toxoplasma* or *Neospora* infection is a possibility, the combination of a fluoroquinolone and either clindamycin or azithromycin can be used.

***Airway hydration.*** Dehydrated animals should receive fluid therapy. Diuretics are contraindicated. Airway moisture can be increased with humidification or nebulization. Such therapy is especially beneficial in animals with areas of consolidation or decreased airway clearance (e.g., bronchiectasis). Humidification can be achieved simply by placing the animal in a steamy bathroom or small room with a vaporizer.

Nebulization (using sterile saline) is necessary to provide moisture deeper in the airways. Nebulized oxygen can be delivered through a face mask or into an enclosed cage. Nebulization is recommended two to six times per day for 10 to 30 min each time. It should be followed immediately by physiotherapy to encourage expectoration.

***Physiotherapy.*** Recumbent animals should be turned at least every 2 hours. Mild exercise is used when possible. Otherwise, coupage is performed. Coupage involves repeatedly striking the patient's chest over the lung fields with cupped hands. The action should be forceful but not painful, and should be continued for 5 to 10 minutes if tolerated by the patient.

***Other therapies.*** Bronchodilators may be used in animals with increased respiratory effort, particularly if expiratory wheezes are auscultated. They are discontinued if clinical signs worsen or do not improve. Bronchodilators are discussed in Chapter 21. Expectorants are of questionable value, and glucocorticoids are contraindicated. Oxygen therapy (see Chapter 27) is provided as indicated by clinical signs, partial pressure of arterial oxygen ($PaO_2$), or pulse oximetry.

***Monitoring.*** Patients should be closely monitored for deterioration of pulmonary function. If signs do not improve within 72 hours, alteration of treatment or reevaluation of a pulmonary specimen may be necessary. Animals with improving signs can be sent home and reevaluated in 2 weeks. Once clinical and radiographic signs have resolved, antibiotics are continued for an additional week. In patients with recurrent infection or suspected localized disease, radiographs should be reevaluated 1 week after antibiotics have been discontinued. Persistence of localized disease after long-term antibiotic therapy is an indication for bronchoscopy or thoracotomy.

***Pulmonary abscess.*** Pulmonary abscess is a potential complication. Abscesses are identified radiographically as focal lesions, although entire lobes may be involved. Horizontal-beam radiographs are useful in determining whether the lesions are fluid filled. Ultrasonography can also be helpful in characterizing areas of consolidation. Abscesses resolve with prolonged medical therapy in some patients, but if improvement is not seen or if radiographic evidence of disease recurs after therapy is discontinued, surgical excision (lobectomy) is indicated.

### Prognosis

Bacterial pneumonia responds readily to appropriate therapy. The prognosis is more guarded in animals with underlying problems that predispose to infection. The likelihood of correcting these problems must be considered.

## TOXOPLASMOSIS (TEXT P 302)

The lungs are a common site of involvement in cats with toxoplasmosis. Thoracic radiographs typically show fluffy alveolar and interstitial opacities throughout the lungs. Less often, nodular or diffuse interstitial patterns, lung lobe consolidation, or pleural effusion is seen. Organisms are rarely recovered with tracheal wash; bronchoalveolar lavage (BAL) is more likely to be diagnostic. Toxoplasmosis is discussed further in Chapter 104.

## FUNGAL PNEUMONIA (TEXT P 302)

The common fungal diseases that involve the lungs are blastomycosis, histoplasmosis, and coccidiomycosis. The animal may successfully eliminate the infection without clinical signs or with only transient respiratory signs. In other cases infection can progress to cause disease involving the lungs alone, to spread systemically to other organs, or both. Cryptococcal organisms can also infect the lungs, particularly in cats, although presenting signs in cats generally reflect nasal infection (see Chapter 103). Pulmonary signs are most often the primary presenting complaint in dogs with blastomycosis and cats with histoplasmosis.

### Clinical features

Pulmonary mycoses should be considered in dogs and cats with progressive signs of lower respiratory tract (LRT) disease, especially when in conjunction with weight loss, fever, lymphadenopathy, chorioretinitis, or other evidence of multisystemic involvement.

### Diagnosis

Thoracic radiographs typically show a diffuse, nodular interstitial pulmonary pattern; the nodules are often miliary. This pattern in dogs with suspicious clinical signs supports a diagnosis of mycotic infection, although other diseases can cause a similar pattern, including neoplasia, parasitic or atypical bacterial (e.g., mycobacterial) infections, and eosinophilic lung disease. Other potential radiographic abnormalities include alveolar or bronchointerstitial patterns and consolidated regions. Hilar lymphadenopathy can occur, most commonly in animals with histoplasmosis; lesions caused by histoplasmosis can also be calcified.

Organisms can occasionally be retrieved by tracheal wash. BAL or lung aspirates are more likely to be successful because of the interstitial nature of these diseases. Fungal culture is probably more sensitive than cytology alone, although an inability to find organisms in a pulmonary specimen does not rule out the diagnosis of mycotic disease.

### Treatment

Treatment of systemic mycosis is discussed in Chapter 103.

## PULMONARY PARASITES (TEXT PP 302-303)

Certain intestinal parasites, especially *Toxocara canis,* can cause a transient pneumonia in young animals as they migrate through the lungs. Infestation with *Dirofilaria immitis* can result in severe pulmonary disease (see Chapter 10). *Oslerus osleri* resides at the carina and mainstem bronchi of dogs (see Chapter 21).

The other primary lung parasites that are most commonly diagnosed are *Capillaria aerophila* and *Paragonimus kellicotti* in dogs and cats and *Aelurostrongylus abstrusus* in cats. An eosinophilic inflammatory response often occurs in the lungs, resulting in clinical signs in some animals. When present, signs are similar to those of allergic bronchitis (see Chapter 21). Definitive diagnosis is made by identifying characteristic eggs or larvae in respiratory or fecal specimens (see Chapter 20).

### *C. aerophila*

*C. aerophila* is a small nematode. Adult worms reside beneath the epithelium of the large airways. Very few animals develop clinical signs; the disease is most often identified when characteristic eggs are found on routine fecal examination. Thoracic radiographs are generally normal, although a bronchial or bronchointerstitial pattern may be seen. Tracheal wash fluid can show eosinophilic inflammation.

Fenbendazole (25 to 50 mg/kg q12h for 2 weeks) is the treatment of choice in symptomatic animals. In dogs levamisole may be used at 8 mg/kg for 10 to 20 days. Ivermectin has been suggested for treatment, but an effective dosage has not been established. The prognosis is excellent.

### *P. kellicotti*

*P. kellicotti* is a small fluke that causes disease in animals living near the Great Lakes and in the midwestern and southern United States. Adult flukes are walled off by fibrous tissue, with a connection to an airway. A local granulomatous reaction can develop around the adults, or a generalized inflammatory response may result from the eggs.

### Clinical features and diagnosis

Infestation is more common in cats than in dogs. Some animals have no clinical signs. When clinical signs are present, they can be the same as those in animals with allergic bronchitis. Alternatively, signs of spontaneous pneumothorax can result from cyst rupture.

The classic radiographic abnormality is a solid or cavitary mass, most often in the right caudal lobe. Other abnormal patterns include bronchial, interstitial (reticular or nodular), and alveolar patterns, depending on the severity of the inflammatory response. Pneumothorax is possible from ruptured cysts. Definitive diagnosis is made through identification of ova in fecal specimens or tracheal wash or other pulmonary specimens. Eggs are not always present, and a presumptive diagnosis is necessary in some cases.

### Treatment and prognosis

Fenbendazole is used at the same dosage recommended for capillariasis. Alternatively, praziquantel can be used at 23 mg/kg q8h for 3 days. Animals with pneumothorax should be stabilized by thoracocentesis. If air continues to accumulate within the pleural space, chest tube placement and suction may be necessary until the leak has been sealed. Surgical intervention is rarely required. Response to treatment is monitored by thoracic radiography and periodic fecal examination. Treatment may need to be repeated in some cases. The prognosis is excellent.

### A. abstrusus

*A. abstrusus* infests the small airways and pulmonary parenchyma of cats. Most infected cats show no clinical signs; those that do are usually young. The clinical signs are those of feline bronchitis (see Chapter 21). Radiographic abnormalities can also mimic feline bronchitis, although in some patients a diffuse miliary or nodular interstitial pattern is present. Eosinophilic inflammation may be apparent in peripheral blood and airway specimens. Definitive diagnosis is made by identification of larvae in fecal or airway specimens. In suspected cases multiple fecal specimens should be examined, because larvae are not always present.

Patients with clinical signs should be treated with fenbendazole as described for capillariasis. Ivermectin at 0.4 mg/kg subcutaneously may be effective. Glucocorticoids often resolve the clinical signs, but they may interfere with success of antiparasitic therapy. Bronchodilators may provide symptomatic relief without interfering with antiparasitic drugs. The prognosis is excellent.

## EOSINOPHILIC LUNG DISEASE (TEXT PP 303-304)

Eosinophilic inflammation can primarily involve the airways or the interstitium. When airway signs predominate, the disease is called *allergic bronchitis* (see Chapter 21). Bronchitis is by far the most common eosinophilic lung disease seen in cats.

Interstitial infiltration, with or without concurrent bronchitis, is sometimes referred to as *pulmonary infiltrates with eosinophils* (PIE) or *eosinophilic bronchopneumopathy*. Eosinophilic pulmonary granulomatosis is a severe type of PIE in dogs that is characterized by pulmonary nodules, with or without hilar lymphadenopathy. It is strongly associated with heartworm disease.

### Etiology

Eosinophilic inflammation is a hypersensitivity response. Potential antigens include heartworms, pulmonary parasites, drugs, and inhaled allergens. Bacteria, fungi, or neoplasia can also induce a hypersensitivity response but not usually as a predominant finding. In many cases no underlying cause can be found.

### Clinical features

Dogs are presented with slowly progressive respiratory signs: cough, increased respiratory effort, and exercise intolerance. Systemic signs such as anorexia and weight loss are usually mild. Lung sounds are often normal, although crackles or expiratory wheezes may be heard.

### Diagnosis

A diffuse interstitial pattern is present on thoracic radiographs. Eosinophilic pulmonary granulomatosis results in nodules (sometimes quite large), usually with indistinct borders; hilar lymphadenopathy may also be present. Patchy alveolar opacity and consolidation can occur. Mycotic infection and neoplasia can cause similar radiographic signs.

Pulmonary specimens must be examined to establish a diagnosis of PIE. In some cases tracheal wash indicates eosinophilic inflammation. In other cases more invasive techniques such as BAL, lung aspiration, or lung biopsy are required to identify the eosinophilic response. Other inflammatory cell populations are frequently present in lesser numbers.

Potential antigen sources should be considered. Pulmonary specimens should be carefully examined for infectious agents and malignancy. Heartworm tests and fecal examinations for pulmonary parasites are indicated in all cases.

### Treatment

Identified primary diseases are treated directly. Eliminating the source of antigen that is triggering the excessive immune response results in a cure in some cases.

***Glucocorticoids.*** Glucocorticoids are indicated when an antigen source cannot be identified and when PIE causes respiratory compromise in dogs with heartworm disease (see Chapter 10). Dogs may be treated with prednisone at an initial dose of 1 to 2 mg/kg q12h. Clinical signs and thoracic radiographs should be reevaluated every week initially. Once signs have resolved, the dosage is decreased to the lowest effective level. If signs have remained suppressed for 3 months, therapy can usually be discontinued. If signs are exacerbated by glucocorticoid therapy, immediate reevaluation for underlying infectious agents is indicated.

***Cytotoxic agents.*** Dogs with large nodular (mass) lesions (i.e., eosinophilic granulomatosis) should be treated with a combination of glucocorticoids and a cytotoxic agent. Prednisone is administered at 1 mg/kg q12h along with cyclophosphamide at 50 mg/m$^2$ q48h (see Chapter 93). Clinical signs and thoracic radiographs are evaluated every 1 to 2 weeks until remission is achieved. CBC is also performed every 1 to 2 weeks and the findings assessed for excessive bone marrow suppression. Attempts to discontinue therapy can be made after several months of remission. Cyclophosphamide may need to be discontinued earlier if sterile hemorrhagic cystitis develops.

### Prognosis

The prognosis is generally fair to good, although it is guarded in dogs with severe eosinophilic pulmonary granulomatosis.

## ASPIRATION PNEUMONIA (TEXT PP 304-307)

### Etiology

Aspiration pneumonia generally results from inhalation of solid or liquid material, typically stomach contents or food. It often indicates an underlying abnormality, such as one of the following:

- esophageal disorders—megaesophagus, reflux esophagitis, esophageal obstruction, myasthenia gravis (localized), bronchoesophageal fistula
- localized oropharyngeal abnormalities—cleft palate, cricopharyngeal motor dysfunction, laryngoplasty, brachycephalic airway syndrome
- systemic neuromuscular disorders—myasthenia gravis, polyneuropathy, polymyopathy
- decreased mentation—general anesthesia, sedation, postictal state, head trauma, severe metabolic disease
- iatrogenic—overzealous feeding, incorrect stomach tube placement or loss of lower esophageal sphincter competence because of the presence of the tube
- vomiting—in combination with other predisposing factors

### Clinical features

Animals with aspiration pneumonia are frequently presented because of acute, severe respiratory signs. The animal may be in shock. Vomiting, regurgitation, or eating may have preceded the onset of distress by a few hours. Other patients are seen because of chronic, intermittent or progressive respiratory signs (cough, increased respiratory effort) or with signs of the predisposing disease. Crackles and wheezes are often auscultated, particularly over the dependent lung lobes. Systemic signs such as fever, anorexia, and depression are common. A thorough neuromuscular examination should be performed once the animal is stable.

Inhalation of mineral oil elicits a chronic inflammatory response. Clinical signs are often mild, but in rare instances they can be severe. Radiographic abnormalities persist and can be erroneously interpreted as neoplastic lesions.

### Diagnosis

Aspiration pneumonia is usually diagnosed on the basis of suggestive radiographic findings, along with evidence of a predisposing condition or history. Radiographs typically show diffuse interstitial opacities with alveolar flooding and consolidation of dependent lung lobes. However, radiographic abnormalities may not be apparent until 12 to 24 hours after aspiration.

Nodular interstitial patterns can be seen in chronic cases. Large nodules may develop around solids; miliary nodules often form with aspiration of mineral oil. Localized abnormalities or soft-tissue masses within large airways suggest large airway obstruction, but these are unusual findings. A marked, diffuse alveolar pattern can be seen in dogs that develop severe, secondary pulmonary edema.

*Complete blood count.* The peripheral blood count may reflect the pulmonary inflammatory process, but it can be normal. Neutrophils are examined for toxic changes indicative of sepsis.

*LRT specimens.* Tracheal wash is indicated in all patients that can tolerate the procedure. Cytology reveals a marked inflammatory response characterized by a predominance of neutrophils. In acute aspiration, hemorrhage may also be present. Bacteria may be seen; regardless, bacterial culture should always be performed. Bronchoscopy can be used to detect and remove large solids, but the procedure is performed only if clear signs of large airway obstruction are present or if the patient is unconscious.

*Other tests.* Blood gas analysis can be helpful in differentiating hypoventilation from ventilation-perfusion abnormalities (see Chapter 20), although in most cases of aspiration pneumonia a combination of abnormalities exists. Animals with profound hypoventilation may have large airway obstruction or muscle weakness secondary to an underlying neuromuscular disorder (e.g., myasthenia gravis). Blood gas analysis also assists in management and can be used to monitor response to therapy.

Diagnostic evaluation is indicated to identify any underlying disease. A thorough oral and pharyngeal examination, contrast studies of the esophagus, and specific neuromuscular tests may be necessary.

### Treatment

Suctioning the airways is helpful only in animals that aspirate in the hospital while already anesthetized or unconscious. If a bronchoscope is available, suctioning can be performed through the biopsy channel with visual guidance. Alternatively, a sterile soft rubber tube attached to a suction pump can be passed blindly into the airways through an endotracheal tube. Low pressure should be used to prevent lung lobe collapse. Airway lavage is contraindicated. Animals with large airway obstruction can benefit from bronchoscopy and foreign body removal.

*Severe respiratory distress.* Animals with severe respiratory distress should be treated with fluid therapy, supplemental oxygen, bronchodilators, and glucocorticoids. Fluids are initially administered intravenously (IV) at shock rates; they should be continued after the animal's condition is stabilized, although overhydration must be avoided. Oxygen supplementation (see Chapter 27) is initiated immediately; positive-pressure ventilation may be required in patients that are unresponsive to supplemental oxygen.

Bronchodilators (see Chapter 21) can be administered to decrease bronchospasm and ventilatory muscle fatigue. They are most likely to be effective in cats. Bronchodilators are discontinued if no improvement is seen or if clinical signs worsen after administration.

Rapid-acting glucocorticoids are administered for the treatment of shock. Low doses of a short-acting drug (e.g., prednisone at 0.25 to 0.5 mg/kg q12h) can be used during the first 24 hours to control severe clinical signs but should then be discontinued.

*Antibiotics.* Intravenous antibiotics are administered immediately in animals with overt systemic signs of sepsis. Broad-spectrum antibiotics, such as imipenem or a combination of ampicillin-sulbactam and either a fluoroquinolone or an aminoglycoside, are recommended (see discussion of bacterial pneumonia).

In animals without sepsis, tracheal wash is performed as soon as the patient's condition is stable, to document infection and obtain antibiotic susceptibility data. This step is important, as assumptions regarding antibiotic susceptibility are prone to error. Pending culture results it is reasonable to initiate treatment with amoxicillin-clavulanate or ampicillin-sulbactam.

Frequent monitoring by means of physical examination, CBC, and radiography is necessary to detect deterioration consistent with secondary infection. If infection is suspected, tracheal wash is repeated.

### Prognosis

Animals with mild signs and a correctable underlying problem have an excellent prognosis. The prognosis is worse in animals with more severe disease or uncorrectable underlying problems.

## PULMONARY NEOPLASIA (TEXT PP 307-309)

Most primary lung tumors are malignant. Carcinomas predominate and include adenocarcinoma, bronchoalveolar carcinoma, and squamous cell carcinoma. Small-cell carcinoma, or oat cell tumor, is rare in dogs and cats, as are sarcomas and benign tumors. Metastatic or multicentric neoplasms can also involve the lungs. Multicentric tumors that more often invade the lungs include lymphoma, malignant histiocytosis, and mastocytoma.

### Clinical features

Neoplasia is most common in older animals but does occur in young adults. Tumors involving the lungs can result in a wide spectrum of clinical signs. Signs are usually chronic and slowly progressive, but peracute manifestations such as pneumothorax or hemorrhage can occur. Infiltration of the lungs can cause increased respiratory effort and exercise intolerance. Masses can compress airways, stimulating cough and interfering with ventilation. Pleural effusion of nearly any character can occur.

Nonspecific signs can include weight loss, anorexia, depression, and fever. Gastrointestinal signs may be the primary complaint; cats are often presented because of vomiting or regurgitation. Hypertrophic osteopathy occurs in some animals secondary to thoracic masses; the presenting sign often is lameness. Animals with metastatic or multicentric pulmonary neoplasia may be presented because of signs of other organ involvement. Some patients have no clinical signs, and the tumor is discovered as an incidental finding.

Lung sounds may be normal, decreased, or increased. They are decreased over all lung fields in patients with pneumothorax or pleural effusion. Localized decrease or increase in lung sounds can occur over consolidated regions. Crackles and wheezes may be caused by infiltration, inflammation, or airway obstruction.

### Diagnosis

Thoracic radiographs can allow a tentative diagnosis of neoplasia and define the disease location for specimen collection. Good radiographs are needed, including both left and right lateral views. Primary lung tumors can appear as localized masses or consolidation of entire lobes. Margins are often distinct but can be indistinct because of inflammation and edema; cavitation may also be evident.

In cats, primary lung tumors are often multifocal or diffuse, and the radiographic pattern may be suggestive of edema or pneumonia. Metastatic or multicentric disease results in a diffuse reticular interstitial pattern, nodular interstitial pattern, or both. Hemorrhage, edema, inflammation, infection, and airway occlusion can result in alveolar patterns and consolidation. Lymphadenopathy, pleural effusion, or pneumothorax may also be seen.

Confirmation of malignant neoplasia in other organs, in conjunction with typical thoracic radiographic abnormalities, is often adequate for a presumptive diagnosis of pulmonary metastasis. Overinterpretation of subtle radiographic lesions should be avoided, however. The absence of radiographic changes does not eliminate the possibility of metastatic disease.

*Pulmonary specimens.* Nonneoplastic diseases, including fungal infection, lung parasites, aspiration of mineral oil, eosinophilic granulomatosis, atypical bacterial infections, and inactive lesions, can result in similar radiographic abnormalities. Definitive diagnosis therefore requires cytologic or histologic evaluation of pulmonary specimens. Tracheal wash rarely results in a definitive diagnosis. It is generally necessary to evaluate lung aspirates, BAL fluid, or lung biopsy specimens to make a definitive diagnosis.

In asymptomatic patients with multifocal disease or in those with significant unrelated problems, it may be appropriate to delay pulmonary specimen collection. Rather, radiographs are repeated in 4 to 6 weeks to check for lesion progression; however, such a delay is never recommended in dogs or cats with potentially resectable disease.

### Treatment
Solitary pulmonary tumors are treated by surgical resection. For clear margins to be obtained, usually the entire lung lobe must be excised. Biopsies of lymph nodes and any grossly abnormal lung are obtained for histologic analysis. In animals with large masses respiratory signs may improve after excision, even if metastases are present throughout the lungs.

If the lesions cannot be surgically removed, chemotherapy may be attempted (see Chapter 79). However, no protocol is uniformly effective for primary lung tumors. Metastatic neoplasms are also treated with chemotherapy. In most patients the initial protocol is based on expected sensitivity of the primary tumor. Unfortunately, metastatic neoplasms do not always have the same response to specific agents as the primary tumor. Multicentric tumors are treated with standard chemotherapeutic protocols regardless of whether the lungs are involved (see Chapter 79).

### Prognosis
The prognosis for patients with benign neoplasia is excellent, but these tumors are rare. The prognosis for animals with malignant neoplasia depends on tumor histologic score, presence of regional lymph node involvement, and clinical signs. Survival times of several years are possible after surgical excision. Animals with unresectable primary malignant or metastatic tumors have a grave prognosis.

## LYMPHOMATOID GRANULOMATOSIS (TEXT P 309)
Lymphomatoid granulomatosis (LG) is characterized by accumulation of pleomorphic lymphoreticular and plasmacytoid cells within and around blood vessel walls. Eosinophils, neutrophils, lymphocytes, and plasma cells may also accumulate in the affected area. Presenting signs are similar to those of diffuse pulmonary neoplasms.

### Diagnosis
Thoracic radiographs reveal increased interstitial opacities, often coalescing to form nodules of various sizes. Hilar lymphadenopathy is common. Cytologic examination of tracheal wash fluid and other pulmonary specimens demonstrates a nonspecific mixed inflammatory response, often including lymphocytes, plasma cells, eosinophils, and mast cells. The radiographic and cytologic findings are similar to those found in patients with eosinophilic pulmonary granulomatosis, metastatic or multicentric neoplasia, fungal infection, and mycobacterial infection. Heartworm tests, fungal titers, and cultures of pulmonary specimens are indicated.

Definitive diagnosis of LG is made from tissue biopsy of specimens collected via thoracotomy. Biopsies reveal infiltration of atypical lymphoreticular cells, centered around and invading blood vessels and accompanied by eosinophils, lymphocytes, and plasma cells.

### Treatment and prognosis

Dogs with LG are treated as for lymphoma, with combination chemotherapy (Chapter 82). Thoracic radiographs are monitored every 1 to 2 weeks for resolution of lesions. Although not all dogs respond well to treatment, >50% may remain in remission for months to years after treatment.

## PULMONARY CONTUSION (TEXT PP 309-310)

Pulmonary contusion occurs with blunt trauma and is a common finding in animals that have been hit by cars. Hemorrhage into the interstitium and alveoli is usually localized. Concurrent pneumothorax, hemothorax, and rib fractures can occur. Chest involvement should be considered in all animals with evidence of severe trauma, even if external signs do not suggest thoracic damage.

### Clinical features and diagnosis

Historical or physical evidence of trauma is generally present. Increased respiratory effort may be noted, although pneumothorax, pain from rib fractures, cardiovascular shock, or neurologic damage may affect the breathing pattern. Crackles may be auscultated over contused areas.

Diagnosis is based on evidence of trauma and typical radiographic signs, although radiographic abnormalities may not be present until a day after trauma. Large, localized areas of alveolar and interstitial opacities are seen. The pleura, skeleton, and diaphragm should also be scrutinized for abnormalities.

### Treatment

Animals with pulmonary contusions should be supported for trauma-related problems as indicated by clinical signs. The contusions themselves are not treated. Antibiotics have been recommended to prevent infection in damaged tissue, but they are more effectively used to treat animals that have developed signs of infection.

Potential complications include secondary bacterial infection, abscess, lung lobe consolidation, and formation of cavitary lesions. Periodic radiographic evaluation is recommended to monitor recovery. Consolidated lung lobes are monitored radiographically for several months unless clinical signs of respiratory compromise persist, in which case lobectomy is performed. Cavitary lesions are also monitored for several months, unless pneumothorax occurs. Most traumatic cysts resolve during that time without surgical excision.

### Prognosis

The prognosis is excellent, provided the animal can be stabilized after the traumatic episode. Complications are rare.

## PULMONARY THROMBOEMBOLISM (TEXT PP 310-312)

Thromboemboli in the lung generally form as a result of disease in other organs, so a search for the underlying cause of clot formation is essential. Emboli can also consist of bacteria, parasites, neoplasia, or fat. Abnormalities that predispose to clot formation include venous stasis, turbulent blood flow, endothelial damage, and hypercoagulation. Specific conditions potentially associated with pulmonary thromboembolism (PTE) include the following:

- surgery
- severe trauma
- hyperadrenocorticism
- immune-mediated hemolytic anemia
- hyperlipidemia
- glomerulopathies

- dirofilariasis and adulticidal therapy
- cardiomyopathy
- endocarditis
- pancreatitis
- disseminated intravascular coagulation
- hyperviscosity syndromes
- neoplasia

**Clinical features**

Animals with PTE may have historical or physical findings related to the underlying disease process. In many instances the predominant sign is peracute tachypnea with respiratory distress, which may be fatal. Other common signs include labored breathing and lethargy or depression. Cardiovascular shock can also develop. Milder or more chronic signs are possible. Crackles or wheezes may be heard on auscultation. A prominent or split second heart sound may be heard if pulmonary hypertension develops.

**Diagnosis**

Routine diagnostic methods do not provide sufficient information to make a definitive diagnosis of PTE. A high index of suspicion must be maintained, as this disease is frequently overlooked. The diagnosis is suspected on the basis of clinical signs, thoracic radiography, arterial blood gas analysis, echocardiography, and clinicopathologic data. Confirmation requires angiography or nuclear imaging.

*Radiography.* PTE is suspected in patients with acute-onset, severe dyspnea, particularly if radiographic signs of respiratory disease are minimal or nonexistent. In many cases the lungs appear normal on radiographs, despite severe LRT signs. When radiographic lesions occur, the caudal lobes are most often involved. Blunted pulmonary arteries, in some cases ending with focal or wedge-shaped areas of interstitial or alveolar opacities (blood or edema), may be present. Areas of lung without blood supply can appear hyperlucent. Diffuse interstitial and alveolar opacities and right-sided heart enlargement can also occur. Pleural effusion is present in some cases but is usually mild.

*Other tests.* Echocardiography may show secondary changes (e.g., right ventricular enlargement, increased pulmonary artery pressures), underlying disease (e.g., heartworm, primary cardiac disease), or residual thrombi. Arterial blood gas analysis may show mild or profound hypoxemia. Tachypnea leads to hypocapnia, except in severe cases, and the abnormal *A-a* gradient supports the presence of a ventilation-perfusion disorder (see Chapter 20). A poor response to oxygen supplementation supports a diagnosis of PTE. Clinicopathologic evidence of a predisposing disease further heightens suspicion for this disorder. Measurement of clotting parameters is not helpful in making the diagnosis.

*Angiography.* Definitive diagnosis is obtained by angiography. Sudden pruning of pulmonary arteries or intravascular filling defects, as well as extravasation of dye, are seen. Because these changes may be apparent only for a few days after the event, the decision to perform this test must be made early. Nuclear perfusion scans are also useful, but availability is limited.

**Treatment**

Acutely animals are treated for cardiovascular shock with high doses of rapid-acting glucocorticoids (e.g., prednisolone sodium succinate, 10 to 20 mg/kg IV) and oxygen therapy (see Chapter 27).

*Anticoagulant therapy.* Animals with suspected hypercoagulability may benefit from anticoagulant therapy, although it should be reserved for animals with a high probability of PTE. Dogs with heartworm disease suffering from postadulticide reactions are not usually treated with anticoagulants. Potential surgical candidates should be treated with great caution. Clotting times must be monitored frequently to minimize the risk of severe hemorrhage.

General guidelines for anticoagulant therapy are provided here. A current pharmacology text should be consulted before anticoagulants are used.

*Heparin.* Initially heparin is administered at 200 to 300 U/kg subcutaneously (SC) q8h. The goal is to maintain the partial thromboplastin time at 1.5 to 2.5 times normal (an increase of 1.2 to 1.4 times the normal activated clotting time). Clotting times are evaluated before and 2 hours after administration of heparin, and the dose is adjusted accordingly. Low–molecular-weight heparin (see Chapter 7) may be easier and safer to use, but it has not been extensively studied in dogs and cats with clinical disease.

Hemorrhage is a potential complication of heparin therapy. Protamine sulfate is a heparin antagonist that can be used to control bleeding (see Chapter 7). When heparin therapy is to be discontinued, tapering the dose over several days may prevent rebound hypercoagulable effects.

*Warfarin.* Long-term anticoagulation can also be maintained with oral warfarin. Frequent monitoring is necessary, and dosage adjustments are common. The potential for drug interactions with all concurrent medications must be investigated. An initial dose of 0.1 to 0.2 mg/kg orally (PO) q24h is prescribed for dogs, and 0.5 mg total PO q24h for most cats. The goal is to maintain a prothrombin time (PT) of 1.5 to 2 times normal or, preferably, an international normalization ratio of 2 to 3 (see text). Once the desired prolongation has been reached, heparin can be discontinued. It may be possible to decrease the frequency of oral warfarin to q48h after several days.

Until the PT has stabilized (which takes at least 5 days), clotting times are assessed daily. Subsequent examination and evaluation of clotting times are performed at least every 5 days, with the interval gradually increasing to every 4 to 6 weeks if results are consistent and favorable.

Excessive hemorrhage is the primary complication of warfarin therapy. Plasma or vitamin $K_1$ (2 to 5 mg/kg/day, divided) can be used to treat uncontrollable hemorrhage, but vitamin K interferes with further attempts at anticoagulation for several weeks.

**Other drugs.** Aspirin is controversial for the treatment of PTE. Unpredictable increases in bleeding tendency can occur when aspirin is used in combination with other anticoagulant drugs. Use of fibrinolytic agents for PTE in animals has not been well established. Recombinant tissue plasminogen activator shows promise.

### Prognosis

The prognosis depends on the severity of respiratory signs and the ability to eliminate the underlying process. Because of the serious problems associated with anticoagulant therapy, eliminating the predisposing problem must be a major priority. In general a guarded prognosis is warranted.

## PULMONARY EDEMA (TEXT PP 312-313)

Potential causes of pulmonary edema are listed in Box 22-1.

### Clinical features

Animals with pulmonary edema are presented with cough, tachypnea, respiratory distress, or signs of inciting disease. Crackles are heard on auscultation, except in animals with mild or early disease. Immediately preceding death from pulmonary edema, blood-tinged froth may appear at the nares. Respiratory signs can be peracute (acute respiratory distress syndrome, or ARDS) or subacute (as with hypoalbuminemia). A prolonged history of respiratory signs (e.g., months) is not consistent with a diagnosis of pulmonary edema.

### Diagnosis

In most cases pulmonary edema is diagnosed by typical radiographic changes in conjunction with clinical evidence (history, physical examination, radiography, echocardiography, serum biochemical analysis) of a disease associated with pulmonary edema.

*Radiography.* Early pulmonary edema causes an interstitial pattern that progresses to become an alveolar pattern. In dogs edema caused by heart failure is generally more severe in the hilar region. In cats the opacities are more often patchy. Edema from increased vascular permeability tends to be most severe in the dorsocaudal lung regions. Radiographs should be carefully examined for signs of heart disease, venous congestion, PTE, pleural effusion, and mass lesions.

*Other tests.* Echocardiography is helpful in identification of primary cardiac disease when signs and radiographic findings are ambiguous. Plasma protein quantitation using

---

**Box 22-1**

## Possible Causes of Pulmonary Edema

**DECREASED PLASMA ONCOTIC PRESSURE**
Hypoalbuminemia
    Gastrointestinal loss
    Glomerulopathy
    Liver disease
    Iatrogenic overhydration
    Starvation

**VASCULAR OVERLOAD**
Cardiogenic
    Left-sided heart failure
    Left-to-right shunts
Overhydration

**LYMPHATIC OBSTRUCTION (RARE)**
Neoplasia

**INCREASED VASCULAR PERMEABILITY**
Inhaled toxins
    Smoke inhalation
    Gastric acid aspiration
    Oxygen toxicity
Drugs or toxins
    Snake venoms
    Cisplatin in cats
Electrocution
Trauma
    Pulmonary
    Multisystemic
Sepsis
Pancreatitis
Uremia
Disseminated intravascular coagulation
Inflammation (infectious or noninfectious)*

**MISCELLANEOUS CAUSES**
Thromboembolism
Upper airway obstruction
Near drowning
Neurogenic edema
Seizures
Head trauma

*Inflammation is usually the prominent clinical abnormality, not edema.

a refractometer can provide indirect measurement of albumin concentration in emergency situations. Serum albumin concentrations <1 g/dl are usually required before decreased oncotic pressure alone causes pulmonary edema. Arterial blood gas analysis and pulse oximetry are useful for selection and monitoring of therapy. Hypoxemia is present, usually with hypocapnia and a widened alveolar-arterial *(A-a)* oxygen gradient (see Chapter 20).

*Acute respiratory distress syndrome.* Vascular permeability edema, or non-cardiogenic pulmonary edema, can result in the full range of compromise, from minimal clinical signs that spontaneously resolve, to the frequently fatal, fulminant process of ARDS—a syndrome of acute, rapidly progressive pulmonary edema. Pulmonary specimens from patients with vascular permeability edema are not cytologically unique, showing a predominantly neutrophilic response.

### Treatment

Initial management should be aggressive. In all patients with pulmonary edema, cage rest with minimal stress is essential. Those with significant hypoxemia should receive oxygen therapy (see Chapter 27). Positive-pressure ventilation is required in severe cases. Methylxanthine bronchodilators (see Chapter 21) may be beneficial in some patients. As soon as the patient is stabilized, any active, underlying problem should be identified and corrected. Treatment of cardiogenic edema is discussed in Chapter 3.

*Diuretics.* Diuretics are indicated for most forms of edema, except in hypovolemic animals, which require conservative fluid therapy. If fluids are necessary in patients with cardiac impairment or decreased oncotic pressure, then positive inotropic agents or plasma infusions, respectively, are necessary.

Overhydration is treated by discontinuing fluid therapy; furosemide is administered if respiratory compromise is present. If excessive fluid administration is not the cause of overhydration, a search for the cause of fluid intolerance, such as oliguric renal failure, heart failure, or increased vascular permeability, is indicated.

*Colloids.* Edema caused by hypoalbuminemia is treated with plasma or colloid infusions. Plasma protein concentrations do not need to reach normal levels to decrease edema formation. Furosemide can be administered to more quickly mobilize the fluid from the lungs, but hypovolemia and dehydration must be avoided. Diagnostic and therapeutic efforts are directed at the underlying disease.

*Acute respiratory distress syndrome.* Edema caused by increased vascular permeability is difficult to treat. In some cases pulmonary compromise is mild and the edema is transient; routine supportive care with oxygen supplementation may be sufficient. Any active, underlying problem should be identified and corrected.

ARDS responds poorly to treatment. Ventilator therapy with positive end-expiratory pressure is indicated, but even with such aggressive support the mortality rate is high. Furosemide is generally ineffective, but it is reasonable to include this drug in the initial management of affected patients. Glucocorticoids are of no clear benefit. Many novel therapies for ARDS have been studied in people. To date, none has been consistently effective.

### Prognosis

The prognosis depends on the severity of the edema and the ability to eliminate or control the underlying problem. Aggressive management early in the course of edema formation improves the prognosis. Animals with ARDS have a guarded to grave prognosis.

# 23

# Clinical Manifestations of Pleural Cavity and Mediastinal Disease

## (Text pp 315-319)

Respiratory signs caused by pleural disease result from interference with normal lung expansion. Exercise intolerance is an early sign; ultimately, overt respiratory distress occurs. Physical examination findings that assist in localizing the cause of respiratory compromise to the pleural space include tachypnea, increased inspiratory effort relative to expiratory effort, increased abdominal excursions, and decreased lung sounds on auscultation. In cats with mediastinal masses, decreased compressibility of the cranial thorax may be noted on palpation. Thoracic radiography, thoracocentesis, or both are used to confirm the presence of pleural space disease (see Chapter 24).

## PLEURAL EFFUSION (TEXT PP 315-318)

### Diagnostic Approach

The presence of pleural effusion in a dog or cat is usually confirmed by radiography or thoracocentesis. In animals presented in respiratory distress and suspected of having pleural effusion, thoracocentesis is performed immediately to stabilize the patient before radiographs are made. Patients that are stable at presentation can be evaluated radiographically first. Radiographic features are discussed in Chapter 24.

Ultrasonography is a valuable tool for evaluation of patients with pleural effusion, particularly those in critical condition. It can be used to confirm the presence of fluid and to direct needle placement for thoracocentesis. Ultrasonography is also useful in evaluation of the thorax for mass lesions (those adjacent to the chest wall, heart, or diaphragm), hernias, and primary cardiac or pericardial disease. If the patient is stable, it is best to evaluate the thorax ultrasonographically before the pleural fluid is removed.

Cytologic analysis of the fluid is indicated for all patients with pleural effusion. Measurement of protein concentration and total nucleated cell count and qualitative assessment of individual cells are essential for classification of the effusion, formulation of a diagnostic plan, and initiation of appropriate therapy.

Pulmonary thromboembolism (PTE) can cause pleural effusion (exudate or modified transudate). The effusion is generally mild, so PTE should be a strong consideration in patients in which respiratory efforts seem excessive relative to the volume of effusion. PTE is discussed in Chapter 22.

### Classification

Pleural effusion is classified as a transudate (pure or modified), an exudate (septic or nonseptic), chylous, or hemorrhagic. In addition to the various inflammatory cell types, mesothelial cells are generally present and are often reactive. Effusions may also contain neoplastic cells. The diseases commonly associated with the specific types of effusion and the recommended diagnostic tests are listed in Table 23-1.

### Transudates

Pure transudates are fluids with low protein concentration (<3 g/dl) and low nucleated cell count (<1000/μl). The primary cell types are macrophages, lymphocytes, and mesothelial cells. Modified transudates have a slightly higher protein concentration (up to 3.5 g/dl) and nucleated cell count (up to 5000 μl); the primary cell types include neutrophils and mononuclear cells.

### Exudates

Exudates have a high protein concentration (>3 g/dl) and high nucleated cell count (>5000/μl).

*Nonseptic exudates.* Cell types in nonseptic exudates can include neutrophils, macrophages, eosinophils, and lymphocytes. The macrophages and lymphocytes may be activated, but the neutrophils are nondegenerative and no organisms are present. Note: In animals with septic effusions, treatment with antibiotics can alter the characteristics of the neutrophils in the fluid (making them appear nondegenerative) and decrease the number of organisms in the fluid to an undetectable level. Pleural fluid analysis should therefore be performed before antibiotics are initiated.

*Septic exudates.* Septic exudates often have extremely high nucleated cell counts (e.g., 50,000 to 100,000/μl); degenerate neutrophils are the predominant cells. Bacteria are often observed within neutrophils and macrophages and extracellularly. The fluid may have a foul odor. Gram stains, aerobic and anaerobic bacterial cultures, and antibiotic susceptibility testing should be performed on the fluid, as mixed bacterial infections are common, and not all septic exudates result in bacterial growth in culture. Gram stains also provide immediate information to assist in antibiotic selection.

### Chylous effusions

Chylous effusions result from leakage of the thoracic duct and are categorized as congenital, traumatic, nontraumatic, or idiopathic (see Chapter 25). Chyle is usually grossly white and turbid; occasionally it is blood tinged. Clear, colorless fluid is possible, particularly in anorectic patients, but it is uncommon.

Chyle must be differentiated from other types of pleural effusion, especially nonseptic exudates. Chyle has a moderate protein concentration (usually >2.5 g/dl) and a low to moderate nucleated cell count (400 to 10,000/μl). Early in the disease the predominant cell type is the small lymphocyte, with a few neutrophils present. With time, nondegenerative neutrophils predominate; macrophages increase in number, and plasma cells may appear. Chylothorax is confirmed by measuring the concentration of triglycerides in the pleural fluid and serum; chyle is higher in triglycerides.

### Hemorrhagic effusions

Hemorrhagic effusions are grossly red and have >3 g/dl protein and >1000 nucleated cells/μl, with a distribution similar to that of peripheral blood. Over time neutrophils and macrophages increase in number. Except for samples collected immediately after bleeding into the thorax, hemorrhagic effusions are readily distinguished from peripheral blood (e.g., traumatic thoracocentesis) by several features: erythrophagocytosis, inflammatory response on cytologic evaluation, lack of clot formation, and lower packed cell volume than peripheral blood. Hemangiosarcoma of the heart or lungs is a common neoplastic cause of hemorrhagic effusion, but malignant cells are rarely identified cytologically.

### Effusions caused by neoplasia

Neoplasia within the thoracic cavity can result in almost any type of effusion (modified transudate, exudate, chylous, or hemorrhagic). In some cases neoplastic cells exfoliate into the effusion, allowing a diagnosis to be made cytologically. Mediastinal lymphoma is often diagnosed in this way. With most other tumors, neoplastic cells are not present in the fluid, so it is not possible to establish a definitive diagnosis on the basis of pleural fluid cytology alone.

Inflammation can result in considerable hyperplastic changes in mesothelial cells that are easily confused with neoplasia. Therefore a cytologic diagnosis of neoplasia other than lymphoma should be made with extreme caution.

**Table 23-1**

## Diagnostic Approach in Dogs and Cats with Pleural Effusion, Based on Fluid Type

| Fluid type | Common diseases | Diagnostic tests |
|---|---|---|
| Pure and modified transudates | Right-sided heart failure | Evaluation of pulses, auscultation, ECG, thor rad, echo |
| | Pericardial disease | See right-sided heart failure |
| | Hypoalbuminemia (pure transudate) | Serum albumin concentration |
| | Neoplasia | Thor rad and US, CT, thoracoscopy, thoracotomy |
| | Diaphragmatic hernia | Thor rad and US |
| Nonseptic exudates | Feline infectious peritonitis | Pleural fluid cytology is generally sufficient; in questionable cases consider systemic evaluation, ophthalmoscopic examination, serum or fluid electrophoresis, coronavirus antibody titer, PCR assay of tissues or effusion (see Chapter 102) |
| | Neoplasia | As for pure and modified transudates |
| | Diaphragmatic hernia | As for pure and modified transudates |
| | Lung lobe torsion | Thor rad and US, bronchoscopy, thoracotomy |
| Septic exudates | Pyothorax | Gram staining, aerobic anaerobic culture, serial thor rad |
| Chylous effusion | Chylothorax | See Box 25-1 |
| | Trauma | History |
| Hemorrhagic effusion | Bleeding disorder | Systemic examination, coagulation tests (ACT, PT, PTT), platelet count |
| | Neoplasia | As for pure and modified transudates |
| | Lung lobe torsion | As for nonseptic exudates |

*ACT,* Activated, clotting time; *CT,* computed tomography; *ECG,* electrocardiography; *echo,* echocardiography; *PCR,* polymerase chain reaction; *PT,* prothrombin time; *PTT,* partial thromboplastin time; *thor rad,* thoracic radiography; *US,* ultrasonography.

## PNEUMOTHORAX (TEXT P 318)

Air leakage through the thoracic wall can occur after a traumatic injury or from a faulty pleural drainage system. Air can also enter the thorax during abdominal surgery through a previously undetected diaphragmatic hernia. These causes are readily identifiable. Pneumothorax from pulmonary air can occur after blunt trauma to the chest (traumatic pneumothorax) or as a result of existing pulmonary lesions (spontaneous pneumothorax). Traumatic pneumothorax occurs frequently and is often accompanied by pulmonary contusions.

### Traumatic Pneumothorax

Traumatic pneumothorax is readily diagnosed on the basis of the history and physical examination findings. Dogs and cats with pneumothorax and a recent history of trauma are managed conservatively. Cage rest, removal of accumulating air by periodic thoracocentesis or chest tube, and radiographic monitoring are indicated. If abnormal radiographic opacities persist without improvement for more than several days, further diagnostic tests should be performed (see Chapter 25).

### Spontaneous Pneumothorax

Cavitary lung diseases that can lead to spontaneous pneumothorax include blebs, bullae, and cysts. They may be congenital, idiopathic, or the result of trauma, chronic airway disease, or *Paragonimus* infestation. Neoplasms, thromboembolic regions, abscesses, and granulomas involving airways can develop necrotic centers and rupture, allowing air to escape into the pleural space. Radiographs are used to identify cavitary lesions in animals with spontaneous pneumothorax, although these lesions are not always apparent.

## MEDIASTINAL MASSES (TEXT PP 318-319)

Mediastinal masses can cause respiratory distress. Coughing, regurgitation, or facial edema may also be present. Neoplasia is the primary diagnostic consideration. Lymphoma involving the mediastinum is common, particularly in cats. Other types of neoplasia include thymoma, thyroid carcinoma, parathyroid carcinoma, and chemodectoma. Nonneoplastic masses such as abscesses, granulomas, hematomas, and cysts also occur.

### Approach to diagnosis

In cats, mediastinal masses are often palpable by gentle compression of the cranial thorax. Radiographically, mediastinal masses appear as a soft-tissue opacity in the cranial mediastinum. Pleural fluid can make accurate identification difficult by either mimicking a mass or obscuring the borders of a mass. Ultrasonography before fluid removal is helpful in identifying a mass and determining the extent of involvement with surrounding structures.

Thoracocentesis and fluid analysis should be performed in patients with pleural effusion. Lymphoma can frequently be diagnosed by identifying malignant cells in the effusion. Transthoracic fine-needle aspirates or biopsies can be performed to obtain specimens for cytologic evaluation of the mass itself. Ultrasonography can be helpful in determination of the consistency of the mass and can also be used to guide biopsy attempts. Alternatively, sampling sites can be estimated using two radiographic views of the thorax. Surgical exploration may be necessary to perform biopsy of small lesions, cavitary lesions, or lesions adjacent to the heart or major vessels. Complete excision of the mass should be attempted at that time unless lymphoma is diagnosed.

## PNEUMOMEDIASTINUM (TEXT P 319)

Mediastinal air usually originates from rupture or tears of the trachea, bronchi, or alveoli. These leaks can result from bite wounds in the neck or sudden changes in intrathoracic pressure with coughing, blunt trauma, or excessive respiratory effort against obstructed airways. Air can also enter the mediastinum from esophageal tears (e.g., caused by foreign bodies). Potential iatrogenic causes include tracheal wash, tracheostomy, and endotracheal tube placement (usually because of excessive cuff pressure). Subcutaneous emphysema or pneumothorax can occur concurrently or secondarily.

Pneumomediastinum is identified radiographically. Strict cage rest is indicated to facilitate natural sealing of the tear. If air continues to accumulate and causes respiratory compromise, bronchoscopy is performed to identify tracheal or bronchial lacerations for possible surgical correction.

# 24

# Diagnostic Tests for the Pleural Cavity and Mediastinum

## *(Text pp 320-326)*

### RADIOGRAPHY (TEXT PP 320-322)

#### Pleural Cavity

Abnormalities of the pleural cavity include pleural thickening, effusion, and pneumothorax. In dogs and cats, the mediastinum is not an effective barrier, so effusion or pneumothorax is usually bilateral. To improve the sensitivity of detection of masses, both left and right lateral views in addition to a ventrodorsal view should be evaluated.

##### Pleural thickening

Pleural thickening results in a thin, fluid-dense line between lung lobes, arcing from the periphery toward the hilar region. Pleural fissure lines can indicate prior pleural disease and subsequent fibrosis, mild active pleuritis, or small-volume pleural effusion. They may be an incidental finding in older dogs.

##### Pleural effusion

Pleural effusion is visible radiographically once 50 to 100 ml have accumulated. Early effusion results in pleural fissure lines and can be confused with pleural thickening. As fluid accumulates, the lung lobes retract and the borders become rounded, especially at the caudodorsal angles of the caudal lobes. The fluid obscures the borders of the heart and diaphragm. The lungs float on top of the fluid, displacing the trachea dorsally and causing the illusion of a mediastinal mass or cardiomegaly.

The lung parenchyma appears abnormally dense as a result of incomplete expansion, and eventually lung lobe collapse can occur. Collapsed lobes should be examined carefully for evidence of torsion (see Chapter 20). The presence of pockets of fluid accumulation or unilateral effusion suggests pleural adhesions.

Critical evaluation of the lungs, heart, diaphragm, and mediastinum cannot be performed until the fluid has been removed. An exception to this rule is the presence of gas-filled intestinal loops in the thorax, which is diagnostic for diaphragmatic hernia.

### Pneumothorax

Air opacity without vessels or airways can be identified between the lung lobes and chest wall. The lung parenchyma is often more dense than the pleural air because of incomplete expansion. The heart may be elevated off the sternum. Radiographs should be examined carefully for cavitary lesions (not always apparent radiographically) or rib fractures. For accurate evaluation of the pulmonary parenchyma, the air must be removed and the lungs allowed to expand.

## Mediastinum

Radiographic abnormalities include pneumomediastinum, alterations in size, displacement, and abnormalities involving the structures within the mediastinum.

### Pneumomediastinum

Pneumomediastinum allows visualization of the outer wall of the trachea and other cranial mediastinal structures (esophagus, major branches of the aortic arch, cranial vena cava).

### Alterations in size

Abnormal soft-tissue opacities can be found in the cranial mediastinum, although concurrent pleural effusion often obscures them. Localized lesions can represent neoplasia, abscesses, granulomas, or cysts. Less discrete disease can cause general widening of the mediastinum, greater than the width of the vertebrae on dorsoventral/ventrodorsal (DV/VD) view. Exudates, edema, hemorrhage, tumor infiltration, and fat can cause mediastinal widening. Megaesophagus can often be observed in the cranial mediastinum, especially on the lateral view.

In the caudal mediastinum the most common abnormalities are megaesophagus and diaphragmatic hernia. Megaesophagus is an important consideration in patients with respiratory signs because it is a common cause of aspiration pneumonia (see Chapter 22).

### Displacement

The mediastinum can be shifted to one side, identified by displacement of the heart on DV/VD view. Lung lobe collapse, lobectomy, or adhesions between the mediastinum and chest wall can cause shifting in the same direction. Space-occupying lesions can shift the mediastinum in the opposite direction.

### Abnormalities of mediastinal structures

Enlargement of the sternal lymph nodes is seen on the lateral view as discrete mass lesions. Enlargement of the hilar nodes results in generalized soft-tissue opacity in the perihilar region, most easily seen on the lateral view. Common differential diagnoses for hilar lymphadenopathy are lymphoma and fungal infections (especially histoplasmosis). Other differential diagnoses include metastatic neoplasia, eosinophilic pulmonary granulomatosis, and mycobacterial infections. Any inflammatory disease can result in lymphadenopathy. Other considerations for increased perihilar opacity include atrial enlargement and heartbase tumors.

## ULTRASONOGRAPHY (TEXT P 322)

Ultrasonography is indicated in animals with pleural effusion to identify masses, diaphragmatic hernia, lung lobe torsion, and cardiac disease. Mediastinal masses, masses involving the pulmonary parenchyma adjacent to the body wall, and masses extending into the thorax from the body wall may be identified and evaluated. Ultrasonography is also used to direct biopsy instruments and thoracocentesis, although biopsies can be safely done only on solid masses.

## THORACOCENTESIS (TEXT PP 322-323)

Thoracocentesis is indicated for specimen collection and for removal of pleural fluid or air to improve ventilation and/or aid radiographic evaluation. Possible complications include pneumothorax (caused by lung laceration), hemothorax, and pyothorax. Complications are rare if careful technique is used.

### Technique

Thoracocentesis is performed with the animal in lateral or sternal recumbency, whichever is least stressful. Fluid or air can be retrieved from the seventh intercostal space (approximately two thirds of the way between the costochondral junction and the spine). If initial attempts are unsuccessful, other sites are tried or the animal's position changed. Fluid may be more successfully retrieved from gravity-dependent sites, and air from nondependent sites. Thoracic radiography and ultrasonography are useful in guiding needle placement.

Local anesthetic can be used; sedation is rarely required but may be useful for decreasing patient stress. The site is shaved and surgically prepared, and the procedure is performed using sterile technique. Most often a 21-gauge butterfly catheter, three-way stopcock, and syringe are used. A larger catheter may be required to collect extremely viscous fluids.

With the syringe snugly attached and the stopcock open between the catheter and syringe (closed to room air), the needle is advanced through the skin only. The needle and skin are then moved approximately two rib spaces to the actual collection site. This technique prevents air from entering the chest through the needle tract after the procedure. The needle is then advanced into the thorax immediately in front of the rib to avoid the intercostal vessels and nerves.

The needle is held with a hand resting on the chest wall so that the needle will not move with patient respirations or movement. Slight negative pressure can be applied by the syringe so that entry into the pleural space is immediately identified by recovery of fluid or air.

Fluid specimens are saved for cytologic and microbiologic analysis (see Chapter 23). As much fluid or air as possible is then removed, except in cases of hemothorax (see Chapter 26).

## CHEST TUBES (TEXT PP 323-326)

Chest tubes are indicated for patients with pyothorax and those with pneumothorax when air continues to accumulate despite repeated evacuation by needle thoracocentesis. If possible, patients in critical condition are stabilized by needle thoracocentesis and treated for shock before chest tubes are placed.

The major complication is pneumothorax caused by a leak in the apparatus. Animals with chest tubes must be carefully monitored at all times to ensure that they do not disrupt the tubing connections, pull the tube partway out, or bite through the tubing. Leaks can result in life-threatening pneumothorax within minutes. Hemothorax, pyothorax, and pneumothorax caused by lung laceration can also occur with improper technique. Proper technique is described in the text.

Thoracic radiographs are taken to evaluate tube position and effectiveness. Ideally the tube extends along the floor of the pleural space to the thoracic inlet. The most important sign of adequate tube placement is the absence of fluid or air. If areas of fluid or air persist, the tube may need to be replaced or a second tube placed in the opposite side. Position and effectiveness are reassessed radiographically every 24 to 48 hours. Maintenance of the chest tube and drainage system is discussed in the text.

## THORACOSCOPY AND THORACOTOMY (TEXT P 326)

Definitive diagnosis of the cause of pleural effusion sometimes requires thoracoscopy or thoracotomy. These procedures allow visual assessment of the thoracic cavity and collection of specimens for histologic and bacteriologic analysis.

# 25

# Disorders of the Pleural Cavity

## (Text pp 327-332)

### PYOTHORAX (TEXT PP 327-329)

#### Etiology

Septic exudate in the pleural cavity (pyothorax) is most often idiopathic in origin, particularly in cats. It can result from foreign bodies (e.g., migrating grass awns), puncture wounds through the chest wall, esophageal tears (usually from ingested foreign bodies), or extension of pulmonary infection.

#### Clinical Features

Signs are referable to pleural effusion and abscess and may be acute or chronic. Tachypnea, decreased lung sounds, and increased abdominal excursions are typical of pleural effusion. In addition, fever, lethargy, anorexia, and weight loss are common. Animals may be presented in septic shock.

#### Diagnosis

Pyothorax is diagnosed on the basis of thoracic radiographs and cytologic evaluation of pleural fluid. Radiographs are used to confirm the presence of pleural effusion and to determine if the disease is localized, unilateral, or bilateral. In most patients fluid is present throughout the pleural space. Localized accumulation suggests pleural fibrosis, mass lesions, or lung lobe torsion. Radiographs are taken again after fluid removal for investigation of underlying disease (e.g., bacterial pneumonia, foreign body) that may have caused the pyothorax.

*Fluid analysis.* Cytologic evaluation of pleural fluid shows septic suppurative inflammation, except in animals that are receiving antibiotics (see Chapter 23). Pleural fluid is always evaluated by gram stain and aerobic and anaerobic bacterial cultures. Anaerobes are usually present. In many dogs and cats more than one type of bacteria is present; however, not all of the involved bacteria may grow on culture. *Actinomyces* and *Nocardia*, in particular, do not grow well using routine culture procedures. Lack of bacterial growth does not rule out a diagnosis of pyothorax.

#### Treatment

Medical therapy includes antibiotics, pleural drainage, and supportive care. Exploratory thoracotomy is indicated for removal of a suspected nidus of infection and in patients that do not respond to medical therapy. Surgery may be necessary to remove fibrotic and diseased tissue or a foreign body. Lack of response is evidenced by the continued need for a chest tube for >1 week after appropriate antibiotic treatment and drainage are begun.

*Antibiotics.* Antibiotics are initially administered intravenously. Results of gram staining and of culture and sensitivity testing are helpful in selection of antibiotics. Generally, anaerobes and *Pasteurella* (a common isolate in cats with pyothorax) are susceptible to amoxicillin-clavulanate. Other gram-negative organisms are often, but unpredictably, susceptible to this combination. Ampicillin with sulbactam is an excellent substitute for intravenous use (50 mg/kg of combined drug q8h).

Other drugs with good activity against anaerobes are chloramphenicol, metronidazole, and clindamycin. If metronidazole or clindamycin is used, or in patients who are receiving other drugs but fail to improve within the first few days of treatment, additional gram-negative coverage is necessary (e.g., a fluoroquinolone or an aminoglycoside).

Oral antibiotics are used once significant improvement is seen, usually about the time of chest tube removal. Amoxicillin-clavulanate (20 to 25 mg/kg administered orally [PO] q8h) is used in patients that have responded to ampicillin-sulbactam. Oral antibiotic therapy is continued for an additional 4 to 6 weeks.

*Drainage.* Drainage of the septic exudate is essential. Indwelling chest tubes provide the best drainage and can keep the exudate from accumulating during the initial days of antibiotic therapy. Response to therapy is most rapid with constant suction (using a suction pump), although intermittent suction is certainly adequate and often more feasible. When intermittent suction is used, fluid should be removed every 2 hours during the first few days of treatment.

*Lavage.* Lavage is performed twice daily. Any fluid within the chest is removed, and warm sterile saline (approximately 10 ml/kg) is slowly infused into the chest. Fluid infusion is discontinued if any distress is noted. The animal is gently rolled from side to side, then the fluid is removed. Sterile technique is necessary throughout the procedure. The volume recovered should be approximately 75% of the volume infused. If less fluid is retrieved, the chest tube may no longer be providing adequate drainage.

*Initial monitoring.* Thoracic radiographs should be taken every 24 to 48 hours to ensure complete drainage. Serum electrolyte concentrations are also monitored. Many animals with pyothorax are dehydrated and anorectic on presentation and require intravenous fluid therapy. Addition of potassium to the fluids may be necessary.

The decision to discontinue drainage and remove the chest tube is based on fluid volume and cytologic characteristics. The volume of fluid recovered should decrease to <2 ml/kg/day. Slides of the fluid are prepared daily and evaluated cytologically. Bacteria should no longer be visible intracellularly or extracellularly. Neutrophils will persist, but should no longer appear degenerative. When these criteria have been met and no pockets of fluid are present on radiographs, the chest tube can be removed and the animal monitored clinically for at least 24 hours for pneumothorax or recurrence of effusion. Thoracic radiographs can be taken for more sensitive evaluation.

*Subsequent monitoring.* Thoracic radiographs are evaluated 1 week after removal of the chest tube and 1 week and 1 month after discontinuation of antibiotics. The purpose is to identify any localized nidus of disease, such as a foreign body or abscess, and recurrence of pyothorax before large volumes of fluid accumulate.

### Prognosis

The prognosis for animals with idiopathic pyothorax is good when it is recognized early and treated aggressively. Long-term complications such as pleural fibrosis and restrictive lung disease are uncommon. The prognosis for pyothorax secondary to foreign bodies is more guarded, as radiolucent foreign bodies can be difficult to find.

## CHYLOTHORAX (TEXT PP 330-332)

### Etiology

Chylothorax can be categorized as congenital, traumatic, or nontraumatic. Congenital chylothorax occurs in Afghan Hounds. Traumatic chylothorax can be caused by thoracic duct rupture subsequent to overt trauma, such as being hit by a car, or damage during thoracotomy. Traumatic chylothorax is unusual and generally self-limiting.

Nontraumatic processes that can cause leakage of lymph include generalized lymphangiectasia, inflammation, increased venous pressure, and lymphatic obstruction. Neoplasia, particularly mediastinal lymphoma in cats, is a major cause of thoracic duct obstruction and chylothorax. Other specific causes of chylothorax include cardiomyopathy, dirofilariasis, pericardial disease, right-sided heart failure, lung lobe torsion, diaphragmatic hernia, and systemic lymphangiectasia. In most patients, however, no underlying disease can be identified and a diagnosis of idiopathic chylothorax is made.

### Clinical features

Chylothorax can occur in dogs or cats of any age. The primary clinical sign is respiratory distress, typical of pleural effusion. Although distress is often acute in onset, more subtle signs have generally been present for over a month. Lethargy, anorexia, weight loss, and exercise intolerance are common. Cough can also occur.

### Diagnosis

Chylothorax is diagnosed when pleural fluid is seen on thoracic radiographs and chyle is identified by thoracocentesis (see Chapter 23). Lymphopenia and hypoproteinemia may be present in peripheral blood. Further testing is required to identify potential underlying disease (Box 25-1).

### Treatment

Animals with chylothorax are stabilized as needed with thoracocentesis and appropriate fluid therapy. A concerted effort is made to identify the cause, as correction of

---

**Box 25-1**

**Diagnostic Tests to Identify Underlying Diseases in Dogs and Cats with Chylothorax**

**COMPLETE BLOOD COUNT, SERUM BIOCHEMICAL PANEL, URINALYSIS**
Evaluate systemic status

**CYTOLOGIC EXAMINATION OF FLUID**
Infectious agents
Neoplastic cells (especially lymphoma)

**THORACIC RADIOGRAPHS (AFTER FLUID REMOVAL)**
Cranial mediastinal masses
Other neoplasia
Cardiac disease
Heartworm disease
Pericardial disease

**ULTRASONOGRAPHY (IDEALLY, IN THE PRESENCE OF FLUID)**
**Cranial mediastinum**
Mass
**Heart (echocardiography)**
Cardiomyopathy
Heartworm disease
Pericardial disease
Congenital heart disease
**Other fluid densities adjacent to body wall**
Neoplasia
Lung lobe torsion

**HEARTWORM ANTIBODY AND ANTIGEN TESTS**
Heartworm disease

**LYMPHANGIOGRAPHY**
Preoperative and postoperative assessment of thoracic duct

the underlying problem can resolve the chylothorax. Medical management for idiopathic chylothorax is generally required for several weeks, or even months. Chylothorax of traumatic origin generally resolves in 1 to 2 weeks.

*Medical management.* Thoracocentesis is performed as needed, based on observation of increased respiratory rate or effort or on decreased activity or appetite. Initially, thoracocentesis may need to be performed every 5 to 15 days. Ultrasound guidance is helpful in removing pockets of chyle from the pleural cavity, and, by increasing the effectiveness of drainage, it can prolong the interval between thoracocenteses.

A low-fat, nutritionally complete diet is fed, such as Hill's Prescription Diet w/d. Medium-chain triglyceride oil can be fed if additional calories are needed, although these triglycerides enter the thoracic duct in dogs. Medical management may be facilitated by administration of rutin (50 mg/kg PO q8h). Rutin's effectiveness has not yet been proven in clinical studies, and the dosage is merely extrapolated from that in humans; however, no adverse reactions have been noted.

*Surgical management.* If clinical signs have not improved within 2 to 3 months of medical therapy or if signs are intolerable, surgery is considered. Surgical management involves thoracic duct ligation and placement of drains (pleuroperitoneal or pleurovenous shunts, or mesh inserted in the diaphragm to allow drainage into the abdominal cavity). However, thoracic duct ligation is successful in only approximately half of the cases, and drains commonly become nonfunctional within months of placement. If surgery is elected, multiple ligations of the thoracic duct and its collaterals are performed. Lymphangiography is necessary before surgery to identify the ducts and must be repeated after surgery to assess the success of ligation.

### Prognosis

The prognosis is guarded, unless the chylothorax was traumatically induced or is the result of a reversible condition. Long-standing chylothorax can result in pleural fibrosis, which can lead to pocketing of fluid, precluding adequate drainage and ultimately preventing lung expansion. Surgical decortication can be attempted, but the prognosis is poor.

## SPONTANEOUS PNEUMOTHORAX (TEXT P 332)

Mechanisms and diagnosis of spontaneous pneumothorax are discussed in Chapter 23. Sudden, profound respiratory distress occurs in patients that develop tension pneumothorax.

### Management

Thoracocentesis is useful for initial stabilization of the animal's condition. If frequent thoracocentesis is needed to control the pneumothorax, a chest tube is placed and continuous suction or a one-way Heimlich valve used. The animal is evaluated for underlying disease with thoracic radiographs (repeated after full lung expansion), multiple fecal examinations for *Paragonimus* ova (see Chapter 20), heartworm tests, and possibly tracheal wash or bronchoscopy.

Patients with *Paragonimus* infections generally respond to medical treatment (see Chapter 22). Otherwise, surgical therapy is indicated. Most dogs with spontaneous pneumothorax that is managed medically (cage rest, chest tube) ultimately require surgery to resolve the problem. Because unobserved recurrence of spontaneous pneumothorax can be fatal, conservative treatment may carry more risk than surgery. Recurrence and mortality rates are lower in dogs that undergo surgery than in dogs managed medically. A median sternotomy is generally recommended to allow exposure of all lung lobes. Abnormal tissue is evaluated histologically and microbiologically for definitive diagnosis.

### Prognosis

Regardless of the treatment used, recurrence is a possibility. Accurate diagnosis of the underlying lung disease and determination of the extent of involvement assist in determination of the prognosis.

## NEOPLASTIC EFFUSION (TEXT P 332)

Neoplastic effusions resulting from mediastinal lymphoma are treated with radiation or chemotherapy (see Chapter 81). Effusions caused by mesothelioma or carcinoma of the pleural surfaces may respond to palliative therapy with intracavitary infusions of cisplatin or carboplatin. Placement of pleuroperitoneal shunts or intermittent thoracocentesis to alleviate respiratory compromise can be considered to prolong the life of patients with no clinical signs beyond those of pleural effusion.

# 26

# Emergency Management of Respiratory Distress

## *(Text pp 333-336)*

Respiratory distress caused by respiratory tract disease most commonly develops as a result of large airway obstruction, severe pulmonary parenchymal disease (including pulmonary thromboembolism), pleural effusion, or pneumothorax. Respiratory distress can also occur as a result of primary cardiac disease. Noncardiopulmonary causes include severe anemia, hypovolemia, acidosis, hyperthermia, and neurologic disease. Normal breath sounds may be increased in dogs and cats with these diseases, but crackles or wheezes are not expected.

Physical examination should be performed quickly, with particular attention paid to breathing pattern, auscultatory abnormalities of the thorax and trachea, pulses, and mucous membrane color and perfusion. Attempts at stabilizing the patient should then be performed before further diagnostic testing.

Animals in respiratory distress at rest should be managed aggressively, and their clinical status frequently reassessed. These patients benefit from rest, decreased stress, a cool environment, and oxygen supplementation. Cage rest is extremely important, and the least stressful method of oxygen supplementation should be selected (see Chapter 27). Sedation may also be beneficial (Table 26-1). More specific therapy depends on the location and cause of the respiratory distress.

## LARGE AIRWAY DISEASE (TEXT PP 333-335)

Animals presented in respiratory distress caused by large airway obstruction typically have a markedly increased respiratory effort with a minimally increased respiratory rate (Table 26-2). Chest excursions may be increased (i.e., deep breaths are taken), and breath sounds are often increased.

### Extrathoracic (Upper) Airway Obstruction

Patients with upper airway obstruction typically have the greatest breathing effort during inspiration, which is generally prolonged relative to expiration. Stridor or stertor is usually heard, generally during inspiration. A history of voice change may be present

**Table 26-1**

## Drugs Used to Decrease Stress in Animals with Respiratory Distress

| Drug | Animal | Dose |
|---|---|---|
| **UPPER AIRWAY OBSTRUCTION** | | |
| **Decrease anxiety and lessen respiratory efforts, decreasing negative pressure within upper airways** | | |
| Acepromazine | Dogs and cats | 0.05 mg/kg IV, SC |
| Morphine | Dogs only, particularly brachycephalic dogs | 0.1 mg/kg IV; repeat q3min until effective; duration 1-4 hr |
| **PULMONARY EDEMA** | | |
| **Decrease anxiety; morphine reduces pulmonary venous pressure** | | |
| Morphine | Dogs only | 0.1 mg/kg IV; repeat q3min until effective; duration 1-4 hr |
| Acepromazine | Dogs and cats | 0.05 mg/kg IV, SC; duration 3-6 hr |
| **RIB FRACTURES, AFTER THORACOTOMY OR OTHER TRAUMA** | | |
| **Pain relief** | | |
| Hydromorphone | Dogs | 0.05 mg/kg IV, IM; can repeat IV q3min until effective; duration 2-4 hr |
| | Cats | 0.025-0.05 mg/kg IV, IM; can repeat IV q3min until effective, but stop if mydriasis occurs; duration 2-4 hr |
| Butorphanol | Cats | 0.1 mg/kg IV, IM, SC; can repeat IV q3min until effective; duration 1-6 hr |
| Buprenorphine | Dogs and cats | 0.005 mg/kg IV, IM; repeat until effective; duration 4-8 hr |

*IM,* Intramuscularly; *IV,* Intravenously; *SC,* subcutaneously.

**Table 26-2**

**Localization of Respiratory Tract Disease by Physical Examination Findings in Dogs and Cats with Severe Respiratory Distress**

| | Respiratory rate | Relative effort | Audible sounds | Auscultatable sounds |
|---|---|---|---|---|
| **Pleural space disease** | Markedly increased | Slightly increased on inspiration | None | Decreased breath sounds |
| **Large airway disease** | | | | |
| Extrathoracic (upper) | Normal or slightly increased | Markedly increased on inspiration | Inspiratory stridor, stertor | Referred upper airway sounds; increased breath sounds |
| Intrathoracic | Normal or slightly increased | Increased on expiration | Expiratory cough, wheezes | Referred upper airway sounds; increased breath sounds |
| **Pulmonary parenchymal disease** | | | | |
| Obstructive | Markedly increased | Slightly increased on expiration | Rarely, expiratory wheezes | Expiratory wheezes or increased breath sounds; rarely, decreased breath sounds with air trapping |
| Restrictive | Markedly increased | Increased on inspiration | none | Increased breath sounds; ± crackles |
| Obstructive and restrictive | Markedly increased | No difference between inspiration and expiration | none | Increased breath sounds, crackles, and/or wheezes |

Normal respiratory rates for dogs and cats at rest are ≤20/min. In the hospital setting, rates of ≤30/min are generally accepted as normal.

with laryngeal disease. Laryngeal paralysis and brachycephalic airway syndrome are the most common causes.

### Emergency treatment

Patients with upper airway obstruction usually are presented in acute distress. Initial management involves sedation and a cool, oxygen-rich environment (oxygen cage). Morphine is given to dogs with pharyngeal disease, especially brachycephalic airway syndrome (see Table 26-1). Otherwise, acepromazine is used. Short-acting glucocorticoids (e.g., dexamethasone, 0.1 mg/kg intravenously [IV] or prednisolone sodium succinate, 10 to 20 mg/kg IV) may be effective in decreasing local inflammation.

Rarely, sedation and oxygen supplementation do not resolve the respiratory distress, and the obstruction must be physically bypassed. Placement of an endotracheal tube is generally effective. If an endotracheal tube cannot be placed, a transtracheal catheter can be inserted distal to the obstruction (see Chapter 27). If a tracheostomy tube is needed, it can then be placed under controlled, sterile conditions. Rarely is it necessary to perform a nonsterile emergency tracheostomy.

## Intrathoracic Large Airway Obstruction

Respiratory distress caused by intrathoracic large airway obstruction is rare. Patients with intrathoracic obstruction typically have the greatest breathing effort during expiration, which is prolonged relative to inspiration. The most common cause of intrathoracic large airway obstruction is collapse of the mainstem bronchi and/or intrathoracic trachea as a result of chronic bronchitis. A high-pitched, wheezing, coughlike sound is often heard during expiration, and crackles or wheezes may be auscultated in these patients.

### Emergency treatment

Sedation, oxygen supplementation, and minimizing stress are often effective in stabilizing patients with intrathoracic airway obstruction. Dogs with end-stage bronchitis may benefit from bronchodilators and glucocorticoids; high doses of butorphanol or hydrocodone provide cough suppression and sedation (see Chapter 21).

## PULMONARY PARENCHYMAL DISEASE (TEXT PP 335-336)

Animals presented in respiratory distress caused by pulmonary parenchymal disease typically have a markedly increased respiratory rate (see Table 26-2). Patients with primarily obstructive disease (e.g., cats with bronchial disease) may have prolonged expiration relative to inspiration with increased expiratory efforts. Expiratory wheezes are commonly auscultated.

Patients with primarily restrictive disease (e.g., dogs with pulmonary fibrosis) may have prolonged inspiration relative to expiration, and effortless expiration. Crackles are commonly auscultated. Patients with a combination of these processes have increased efforts during both phases of respiration, shallow breathing, and crackles, wheezes, or increased breath sounds on auscultation. Differential diagnoses for pulmonary disease are provided in Box 19-2.

### Emergency treatment

Oxygen therapy is the treatment of choice for respiratory distress caused by pulmonary disease (see Chapter 27). Bronchodilators, diuretics, or glucocorticoids can be considered if oxygen therapy alone is inadequate.

*Bronchodilators.* Bronchodilators, such as short-acting theophyllines or β-agonists, are used if obstructive lung disease is suspected (see Table 21-2). In combination with oxygen they are the treatment of choice for cats with signs of bronchial disease (see Chapter 21). Terbutaline (0.01 mg/kg subcutaneously [SC]; repeated in 5 to 10 minutes if necessary) is most often used in emergency situations.

*Diuretics.* Diuretics, such as furosemide (2 mg/kg IV), are indicated for pulmonary edema (see Chapter 22). Potential complications caused by volume contraction and dehydration should be considered. Prolonged use of diuretics is contraindicated in patients with exudative lung disease or bronchitis.

*Glucocorticoids.* Rapid-acting glucocorticoids, such as prednisolone sodium succinate (10 to 20 mg/kg IV), are indicated for animals in respiratory distress caused by acute allergic bronchitis, feline bronchial disease, thromboembolism after adulticidal heartworm treatment, or respiratory failure during initial treatment for pulmonary mycosis. Animals with other inflammatory diseases or acute respiratory distress syndrome may also respond favorably to glucocorticoids.

Potential negative effects must be considered before glucocorticoid use. Immunosuppressive effects can exacerbate infectious disease. Short-acting corticosteroids for initial stabilization probably do not greatly interfere with antimicrobial therapy; however, long-acting agents or prolonged administration should be avoided. Glucocorticoids may also interfere with future diagnostic tests, particularly if lymphoma is a differential diagnosis. Appropriate tests should be performed as soon as the patient can tolerate the stress.

*Antibiotics.* Broad-spectrum antibiotics are administered if there exists evidence of sepsis (e.g., fever, neutrophilic leukocytosis with left shift and moderate to marked toxicity of neutrophils) or a high degree of suspicion of bacterial or aspiration pneumonia (see Chapter 22). Airway specimens (usually tracheal wash) should be obtained for culture if at all possible before antibiotic therapy is initiated. If sepsis is suspected, blood and urine cultures may also be useful.

*Ventilatory support.* If the patient does not respond to this management, it may be necessary to provide positive-pressure ventilation (with intubation performed after administration of a short-acting anesthetic agent) until a diagnosis can be established and specific therapy initiated. Ventilatory support is discussed further in Chapter 27.

## PLEURAL SPACE DISEASE (TEXT P 336)

Pleural space diseases cause respiratory distress by preventing normal lung expansion. Animals presented in respiratory distress typically have a markedly increased respiratory rate (see Table 26-2). Relatively increased inspiratory efforts may be noted but are not always obvious. In tachypneic patients, decreased lung sounds on auscultation distinguish pleural space disease from pulmonary parenchymal disease. Increased abdominal excursions during breathing may be noted.

### Emergency treatment

Most patients in respiratory distress from pleural space disease have pleural effusion or pneumothorax (see Chapter 23). If either condition is suspected, needle thoracocentesis should be performed immediately (see Chapter 24). Oxygen can be provided by mask while the procedure is performed, but successful drainage of the pleural space will quickly improve the animal's condition. Occasionally, emergency placement of a chest tube is necessary to evacuate rapidly accumulating air.

As much fluid or air should be removed as possible, except in animals with hemothorax. The respiratory distress associated with hemothorax is often the result of acute blood loss, rather than an inability to expand the lungs. In this situation as little volume as is needed to stabilize the animal's condition is removed. The remainder will be reabsorbed (autotransfusion), to the benefit of the animal. Aggressive fluid therapy is indicated.

# 27

# Ancillary Therapy: Oxygen Supplementation and Ventilation

## *(Text pp 337-340)*

### OXYGEN SUPPLEMENTATION (TEXT PP 337-340)

Oxygen supplementation is generally indicated to maintain arterial blood oxygen pressures ($PaO_2$) above 60 mm Hg. Oxygen supplementation is indicated in every dog or cat with signs of respiratory distress, labored breathing, or cyanosis. Whenever possible the cause of hypoxemia should be identified, and specific treatment initiated. Assisted ventilation is indicated in animals with inadequate $PaO_2$ despite supplementation and for animals with arterial blood carbon dioxide pressures ($PaCO_2$) >60 mm Hg.

All patients with respiratory diseases should be systemically hydrated. Moisture should be added to the airways of animals receiving oxygen supplementation for longer than a few hours, particularly when the nasal cavity has been completely bypassed. Humidifiers or humidity filters can be incorporated into ventilation systems. Nebulization can also be used to increase airway moisture. Less effective methods include instillation of sterile 0.9% sodium chloride (NaCl) directly into tubes or catheters and addition of water vapor with pass-over or bubble humidifiers.

Oxygen concentrations >50% should not be provided for longer than 12 hours. If higher concentrations are necessary to maintain adequate arterial oxygen concentrations, ventilatory support is initiated.

### Methods

#### Oxygen masks

Oxygen masks are useful for short-term supplementation. The animal experiences minimal stress, and manipulations such as venous catheter placement and thoracocentesis can be performed. A snug fit is desirable to decrease the volume of dead space. Sterile eye ointment is applied to avoid corneal desiccation. A relatively high flow rate is necessary (Table 27-1).

#### Oxygen hoods

An oxygen hood can be placed over the animal's head during recovery from anesthesia or when the patient is severely depressed or heavily sedated. A means of escape for the exhaled air must be provided to prevent buildup of $CO_2$ within the hood.

#### Nasal catheters

Nasal catheters are useful for long-term oxygen supplementation. The animal is relatively free to move and is accessible for evaluation and treatment. Most animals tolerate the catheter well, although catheters can become obstructed by nasal secretions. Soft red rubber or infant feeding tubes or polyurethane catheters can be used. Tube size is based on patient size. In general, a 2.5 to 5 French tube is used for cats, and a 5 to 8 French tube is used for dogs. Catheter placement and maintenance are discussed in the text.

**Table 27-1**

## Maximum Achievable Oxygen Concentrations and Associated Flow Rates for Various Methods of Supplementation

| Method of administration | Maximum oxygen concentration (%) | Flow rate (L/min)* |
|---|:---:|:---:|
| Mask | 50-60 | 8-12 |
| Nasal catheter | 50 | 6-8 |
| Transtracheal catheter | 30-40 | 1-2 |
| Endotracheal tube | 100 | 0.2 L/kg/min |
| Tracheal tube | 100 | 0.2 L/kg/min |
| Oxygen cage | 60 | 2-3* |

From Court MH et al: Inhalation therapy: oxygen administration, humidification, and aerosol therapy, *Vet Clin North Am Small Anim Pract* 15:1041, 1985.
*After cage is filled, flow is adjusted based on oxygen concentration as measured by oxygen sensor.

**Transtracheal catheters**
Oxygen can be administered through a jugular catheter placed aseptically into the trachea. This technique is particularly useful for emergency stabilization of animals with upper airway obstruction. A large jugular catheter is placed as described for transtracheal wash (see text).

**Endotracheal tubes**
Endotracheal tubes are used for the administration of oxygen during surgical procedures and cardiopulmonary resuscitation. They can also be used to bypass most upper airway obstructions for emergency stabilization. Conscious animals must be given sedatives, analgesics, paralyzing agents, or a combination of these drugs for intubation. The combination of ketamine and diazepam (Valium) may be safer than other protocols for initial intubation in hypoxemic patients.

Pure oxygen can be administered for short periods. Longer supplementation requires mixing of oxygen with room air. Unless positive-pressure ventilation is being used, the cuff can remain deflated, thereby minimizing the potential for trauma to the trachea.

**Tracheal tubes**
Tracheal tubes are generally used for management of animals with upper airway obstruction. Room air often contains sufficient oxygen for these patients once the obstruction has been bypassed. Tracheal tubes are placed through the tracheal rings and are readily tolerated by conscious animals. Nearly all patients can be stabilized by other means, allowing tracheal tube placement to be performed using careful, sterile, surgical technique. The procedure is described in the text, as is tube maintenance.

**Oxygen cages**
Oxygen cages can provide an oxygen-enriched environment with minimal stress. The animal is isolated from direct contact, which can be a disadvantage. Other environmental factors, such as humidity, temperature, and $CO_2$ concentration, must be controlled or extreme stress and even death can occur. The animal is totally dependent on proper cage function.

## VENTILATORY SUPPORT (TEXT P 340)

Animals with severe lung disease may be unable to maintain adequate oxygenation without ventilatory support. Positive-pressure ventilation is routinely necessary for patients with acute respiratory distress syndrome (see Chapter 22). Ventilatory support is labor intensive and associated with complications (see text). The extensive nursing care and monitoring required limit the use of long-term ventilatory support to large referral hospitals.

## Drugs Used in Dogs and Cats with Respiratory Disorders

| Generic name | Trade name | Dogs (mg/kg*) | Cats (mg/kg*) |
|---|---|---|---|
| Acepromazine | — | 0.05 IV, IM, SC (maximum 4 mg) | 0.05 IV, IM, SC (maximum, 1 mg) |
| Amikacin | Amiglyde | 5-10 IV, SC q8h | Same |
| Aminophylline | — | 11 PO, IV, IM q8h | Same |
| Amoxicillin | Amoxi-tabs, Amoxi-drops | 22 PO q8-12h | 5 PO, IV, IM q12h |
| Ampicillin | — | 22 PO, IV, SC q8h | Same |
| Amoxicillin-clavulanate | Clavamox | 20-25 PO q8h | Same |
| Ampicillin-sulbactam | Unasyn | 50 mg/kg (combined) IV q8h | Same |
| Atropine | — | 0.05 SC | Same |
| Azithromycin | Zithromax | 5-10 mg/kg PO q24h for 3 days, then q48-72h | 5-10 mg/kg PO q24h for 3 days, then q72h |
| Butorphanol | Torbutrol | 0.5 PO q6-12h (antitussive) | Not recommended |
| Cefazolin | — | 20-25 IM, IV q8h | Same |
| Cephalexin | Keflex | 20-40 PO q8h | Same |
| Chloramphenicol | — | 50 PO, IV, SC q8h | 10-15 PO, IV, SC q12h |
| Chlorpheniramine | Chlor-Trimeton | 4-8 mg/dog q8-12h | 2 mg/cat q8-12h |
| Clindamycin | Antirobe | 5.5-11 PO, IV, SC q12h | Same |
| Cyclophosphamide | Cytoxan | 50 mg/m² PO q48h | Same |
| Cyproheptadine | Periactin | — | 2 mg/cat PO q12h |
| Dexamethasone | Azium | 0.1-0.2 IV q12h | Same |
| Dextromethorphan | — | 1-2 PO q6-8h | Not recommended |
| Diazepam | Valium | 0.2-0.5 IV | — |
| Diphenhydramine | Benadryl | 1 IM; 2-4 PO | Same |
| Doxycycline | — | 5-10 PO, IV q12h | Same |
| Enrofloxacin | Baytril | 10-20 PO, IV, SC q24h | — |
| Fenbendazole (for lungworm) | Panacur | 25-50 PO q12h for 14 days | Same |
| Furosemide | Lasix | 2 PO, IV, IM q8-12h | Same |
| Glycopyrrolate | — | 0.005 IV, SC | Same |
| Heparin | — | 200-300 U/kg SC q8h | Same |
| Hydrocodone bitartrate | Hycodan | 0.25 PO q8-12h | Not recommended |
| Hydromorphone | — | 0.05 IV, IM; can repeat IV q3min until effective; duration 2-4h | 0.025-0.05 IV, IM; can repeat IV q3min until effective; stop if mydriasis occurs |

| | | Dog | Cat |
| --- | --- | --- | --- |
| Imipenem-cilastin | Primaxin | 3-10 IV, q6-8h | Same |
| Itraconazole (for aspergillosis) | Sporanox | 5 PO q12h with food | See text for specific parasites |
| Ivermectin | — | See text for specific parasites | 2-5 IV |
| Ketamine | Ketaset, Vetalar | — | 250 mg/cat PO q12h |
| Lysine | — | — | Same |
| Marbofloxacin | Zeniquin | 3-5.5 PO q24h | 10 mg/cat IM q2-4wk |
| Methylprednisolone acetate | Depo Medrol | — | 10 PO q12h |
| Metronidazole | Flagyl | 10 PO q8h | — |
| Milbemycin (for nasal mites) | Interceptor | 0.5-1 PO q7-10d for three treatments | — |
| Morphine | — | 0.1 IV; repeat q3min to effect; duration 1-4h | 1 drop/nostril q24h for 3 days, then withhold for 3 days |
| Oxtriphylline | Choledyl | 14 PO q8h | 1 drop/nostril q24h for 3 days, then withhold for 3 days |
| Oxymetazoline 0.025% | Afrin (0.025%) | — | Same |
| Phenylephrine 0.25% | Neo-Synephrine (0.25%) | — | Same |
| Praziquantel (for *Paragonimus*) | Droncit | 23 PO q8h for 3 days | Same |
| Prednisone | Prednisone | 0.25-2 PO q12h | $1/8$-$1/4$ of 2.5-mg tablet/cat q12h PO, to start; 0.01 mg/kg SC, repeat once in 5-10 min if necessary |
| Prednisolone sodium succinate | Solu-Delta-Cortef | 10-20 IV | Same |
| Terbutaline | Brethine | 1.25-5 mg/dog PO q8-12h | q4-8h |
| Tetracycline | — | 22 PO q8h | 25 PO q24h, in evening |
| Tetracycline ophthalmic ointment | — | — | 25 PO q24h, in evening |
| Theophylline (long-acting formulations)† | Slo-BID | 10 PO q12h‡ | Same |
| Trimethoprim-sulfadiazine | Tribrissen | 25-30 PO q12h | Same |
| Vitamin K$_1$ | Mephyton, Aquamephyton | 15-30 PO q12h | 0.5 mg/cat |
| Warfarin | Coumadin | 2-5 PO, SC divided daily | |
| | | 0.1-0.2 PO q24h | |

From Bach JF et al: Proceedings of the Twentieth Symposium of the Veterinary Comparative Respiratory Society, Boston, 2002.

*Unless otherwise noted.

†Because of differences in available products, appropriate doses are uncertain and therapeutic monitoring of animals should be performed (see text).

‡Dog dose is of theophylline SR (Inwood Laboratories, Inwood, NY).

*IM,* Intramuscularly; *IV,* intravenously; *PO,* orally; *SC,* subcutaneously.

# PART III

# Digestive System Disorders

MICHAEL D. WILLARD

# 28

## Clinical Manifestations of Gastrointestinal Disorders

### *(Text pp 343-364)*

#### DYSPHAGIA, HALITOSIS, AND DROOLING (TEXT PP 343-345)

**Causes**

Dysphagia, halitosis, and/or drooling occur in many animals with oral disease. Dysphagia usually results from oral pain, masses, foreign objects, trauma, and/or neuromuscular dysfunction. Specific causes are listed in Box 28-1.

---

**Box 28-1**

### Causes of Dysphagia

**ORAL PAIN**

Fractured bones or teeth
Trauma
Periodontitis or caries (especially in cats)
Osteomyelitis
Other causes
  Retrobulbar abscess or inflammation
  Various other abscesses or
    granulomas of the oral cavity
  Temporal-masseter myositis
Stomatitis, glossitis, pharyngitis,
  gingivitis, tonsillitis, or sialoadenitis
Immune-mediated disease
Feline viral rhinotracheitis, calicivirus,
  leukemia virus, or
  immunodeficiency virus
Lingual foreign objects, other foreign
  objects, or granulomas
Tooth root abscess
Uremia
Miscellaneous causes
  Thallium
  Caustics
Pain associated with swallowing
  Esophageal stricture or esophagitis

**ORAL MASS**

Tumor (malignant or benign)
Eosinophilic granuloma
Foreign object (oral, pharyngeal, or
  laryngeal)
Sialocele

**ORAL TRAUMA**

Fractured bones
Soft-tissue laceration
Hematoma

**NEUROMUSCULAR DISEASE**

Oral, pharyngeal, or cricopharyngeal
  dysfunction
Various cranial nerve dysfunctions
Rabies
Tetanus
Localized myasthenia
Temporal-masseter myositis
Temporomandibular joint disease

---

## Halitosis

Halitosis typically signifies bacterial proliferation in the mouth, the esophagus, or both. Specific causes include the following:
- retention of food in the mouth—anatomic defect (e.g., exposed tooth roots, tumor, large ulcer) or neuromuscular defect (e.g., pharyngeal dysphagia) that allows retention
- retention of food in the esophagus
- tartar or periodontal disease
- damaged oral tissues
- neoplasia or granuloma of the mouth or esophagus
- severe stomatitis or glossitis
- ingestion of noxious substances—necrotic or odoriferous food or feces

## Ptyalism

Drooling occurs because patients are unable or in too much pain to swallow; rarely do animals produce excess saliva. Major causes of ptyalism include the following:
- nausea
- hepatic encephalopathy (especially in cats)
- seizure activity
- chemical or toxic stimulation—e.g., organophosphates, caustic substances, bitter drugs (such as atropine)
- behavior
- hyperthermia
- salivary gland hypersecretion

### Pseudoptyalism

Causes of pseudoptyalism include the following:
- oral pain, especially stomatitis, glossitis, gingivitis, pharyngitis, tonsillitis, or sialoadenitis (see Box 28-1)
- oral or pharyngeal dysphagia (see Box 28-1)
- facial nerve paralysis

## Diagnostic Approach

When dysphagia is acute in onset, foreign objects or trauma should be considered first. The environment and vaccination history should also be assessed for the possibility of rabies.

### Physical examination

Most problems that produce oral pain can be partially or completely defined after thorough oral, laryngeal, and cranial examinations. If oral pain cannot be localized, then retrobulbar lesions, temporomandibular joint disease, or posterior pharyngeal lesions should be considered. Clinicopathologic evaluation may be useful, especially if oral examination suggests systemic disease (e.g., lingual necrosis from uremia). When the history and oral examination reveal little except mild to moderate tartar accumulation, the teeth should be cleaned.

*Neurologic examination.* Neurogenic dysphagia is caused by disorders in the oral, pharyngeal, and/or cricopharyngeal phases of swallowing. Rabies is always a consideration; once it is ruled out, cranial nerve deficits (especially V, VII, IX, and XII) should be considered. Clinical signs vary depending on the nerve(s) affected. Careful neurologic examination is needed.

### Biopsy

Mucosal lesions and painful masticatory muscles should undergo biopsy. Any vesicles should be removed intact for histopathology and immunofluorescence. If vesicles are not found, at least two tissue samples of both new and old lesions should be submitted.

*Neuromuscular dysfunction.* Dysphagic patients with no demonstrable lesions or pain may have neuromuscular disease. Dysphagia of muscular origin is usually a result of atrophic myositis. Finding swollen, painful temporal muscles suggests acute myositis. Severe temporomasseter muscle atrophy and difficulty opening the mouth even when the patient is anesthetized suggests chronic temporomasseter myositis. Biopsy of affected muscles is indicated. Finding serum antibodies against type 2M muscle fibers is also consistent with masticatory myositis (see Chapter 66).

### Culture
Oral cultures are rarely useful because the normal flora makes interpretation difficult. Even in patients with severe bacterial stomatitis, bacterial culture is rarely helpful unless a draining tract or abscess is present.

### Diagnostic imaging
If oral examination is unhelpful, plain oral and laryngeal radiographs should be taken. Halitosis not attributable to an oropharyngeal lesion or ingestion of malodorous material may be originating from the esophagus. Contrast radiographs or esophagoscopy may reveal tumors or food retention secondary to stricture or weakness.

Dysphagia may be noticeable in dogs and cats with pharyngeal and cricopharyngeal dysfunction, but regurgitation is often the more prominent sign. Dynamic contrast studies (e.g., fluoroscopy) are best for detecting and defining neuromuscular dysphagia. When neuromuscular problems are ruled out, anatomic lesions and occult causes of pain (e.g., soft-tissue inflammation or infection) must be reconsidered.

## REGURGITATION (TEXT PP 345-347)

### Distinguishing Regurgitation from Vomiting
Regurgitation is expulsion of material from the mouth, pharynx, or esophagus, whereas vomiting is expulsion of material from the stomach or intestines. (Expectoration is expulsion of material from the respiratory tract and is generally associated with coughing. Animals that regurgitate, and occasionally those that vomit, may cough as a result of aspiration, but oral expulsion is not consistently associated with coughing.)

### Behavior and material produced
Some animals that appear to be regurgitating are vomiting, and vice versa. Vomiting is usually associated with prodromal nausea and retching (forceful, vigorous abdominal contractions or dry heaves). Signs of prodromal nausea may include salivation, licking of the lips, pacing, and an anxious expression. Neither prodromal nausea nor retching is seen with regurgitation.

Food may be expelled during vomiting or regurgitation. With vomiting the expelled material may contain bile and/or blood (either digested or undigested), whereas regurgitated material does not contain bile, and if it contains blood it is undigested. The amount of material expelled and the timing relative to eating are not helpful in differentiating regurgitation and vomiting. Distention of the cervical esophagus may be associated with regurgitation, but not with vomiting.

*pH and bilirubin.* For further clarification a urine dipstick can be used to determine the pH and presence or absence of bilirubin in the material. If the pH is 5, the material originated from the stomach and probably resulted from vomiting. A pH of >7 and absence of bilirubin is consistent with regurgitation. The presence of bilirubin indicates duodenal contents (i.e., vomiting), as does a pH >8.

### General Diagnostic Approach
Once regurgitation is confirmed, the disease should be localized to the oral cavity, pharynx, or esophagus. If the patient is dysphagic, an oral, pharyngeal, or cricopharyngeal problem should be considered. Dysphagia can be detected by watching the animal eat. Some animals with neuromuscular disorders have more difficulty swallowing liquids than solid foods; attempts to swallow water often produce coughing. Cinefluoroscopic or fluoroscopic evaluation of swallowing during a barium meal is needed to differentiate pharyngeal from cricopharyngeal dysfunction.

### Esophageal dysfunction
If the patient is not dysphagic, esophageal dysfunction is tentatively diagnosed. The two main causes are obstruction and muscular weakness (see below). Plain and barium

contrast-enhanced esophageal radiographs are used initially. If the patient seems to be regurgitating but contrast radiographs fail to reveal esophageal dysfunction, either the assessment of regurgitation is wrong or occult disease is present (e.g., partial stricture, esophagitis, gastroesophageal reflux). Repeating the contrast esophagogram using barium plus food or performing esophagoscopy is recommended.

### Esophageal obstruction

Esophageal obstruction is characterized as congenital or acquired and intraluminal, intramural, or extraesophageal. Congenital obstructions are usually extraesophageal vascular ring anomalies, such as persistent fourth right aortic arch.

*Acquired causes.* Causes of acquired esophageal obstruction include the following:
- foreign object
- cicatrix or stricture
- esophageal neoplasia—e.g., carcinoma, sarcoma caused by *Spirocerca lupi,* leiomyoma of the lower esophageal sphincter
- extraesophageal neoplasia—e.g., thyroid or pulmonary carcinoma
- achalasia of the lower esophageal sphincter (rare)
- gastroesophageal intussusception (rare)

Acquired intraluminal obstructions are usually foreign objects. However, patients with esophageal foreign objects may have a partial stricture that predisposes them to obstruction. Endoscopy may be both diagnostic and therapeutic in such patients.

### Esophageal weakness

Esophageal weakness may be congenital or acquired. Congenital weakness is generally idiopathic and is not pursued diagnostically.

*Acquired causes.* Acquired esophageal weakness is most likely the result of an underlying neuromuscular problem. Causes include the following:
- myasthenia (generalized or localized)
- hypoadrenocorticism
- esophagitis—e.g., persistent vomiting, hiatal hernia, gastroesophageal reflux, caustic ingestion
- *S. lupi*
- myopathies or neuropathies—e.g., hypothyroidism (rare), systemic lupus erythematosus
- miscellaneous conditions—e.g., lead poisoning, Chagas' disease, canine distemper, dermatomyositis (Collies), dysautonomia
- an idiopathic condition

*Laboratory tests.* Complete blood count (CBC), serum biochemistry profile, urinalysis, serum antibody titers to acetylcholine receptors, thyroid function tests (free $T_4$ and endogenous thyroid-stimulating hormone levels), adrenocorticotropic hormone (ACTH)–stimulation test, fecal examination for *S. lupi* ova, and/or serum antinuclear antibody titers may be used to identify the cause. Investigation of lead intoxication (nucleated red cells and basophilic stippling, serum and urine lead concentrations), canine distemper (retinal lesions), Chagas' disease (serum antibody titer), or neuropathy or myopathy (electromyography, nerve or muscle biopsy) may also be indicated.

### Diagnostic imaging

Esophagoscopy may be used to detect esophagitis or small lesions (e.g., partial strictures) that contrast esophagograms do not reveal. The stomach and lower esophageal sphincter should be examined for leiomyomas. Gastroduodenoscopy is also performed to look for gastric and duodenal reasons for gastroesophageal reflux or vomiting. If fluoroscopy is available, the lower esophageal sphincter can be observed for several minutes to note the frequency and severity of gastroesophageal reflux.

## VOMITING (TEXT PP 347-350)

Differentiating regurgitation from vomiting is discussed in the preceding section. Causes of vomiting are many and varied (Box 28-2).

---

**Box 28-2**

## Causes of Vomiting

### EMETOGENIC SUBSTANCES (ACUTE)
Drugs: almost any drug can cause vomiting (especially drugs administered orally), but the following drugs most often seem to cause vomiting:
Digoxin
Cyclophosphamide
Cisplatin
Dacarbazine
Adriamycin
Erythromycin
Tetracycline or doxycycline
Amoxicillin + clavulanic acid
Nonsteroidal antiinflammatory drugs
Toxic chemicals

### GASTROINTESTINAL TRACT OBSTRUCTION (ACUTE OR CHRONIC)
Gastric outflow obstruction
Benign pyloric stenosis
Foreign object
Gastric antral mucosal hypertrophy
Neoplasia
Nonneoplastic infiltrative disease
(e.g., pythiosis)
Gastric malpositioning
Gastric dilatation or volvulus (primarily see nonproductive retching)
Partial gastric dilatation and volvulus
Intestinal obstruction
Foreign object
Nonlinear objects
Linear objects
Neoplasia
Cicatrix
Torsion and volvulus
Intussusception

### GASTROINTESTINAL/ABDOMINAL INFLAMMATION (ACUTE OR CHRONIC)
Inflammatory bowel disease (usually chronic)
Gastritis with or without ulceration or erosion (acute or chronic)
Enteritis (acute)
Parvovirus
Hemorrhagic gastroenteritis
Parasites (acute or chronic), especially *Physaloptera*
Colitis (acute or chronic)

### EXTRAALIMENTARY TRACT DISEASES (ACUTE OR CHRONIC)
Uremia
Adrenal insufficiency
Hypercalcemia
Hepatic insufficiency or disease
Cholecystitis
Diabetic ketoacidosis
Pyometra
Peritonitis (acute or chronic)
Pancreatitis (acute or chronic)

### MISCELLANEOUS CAUSES (ACUTE OR CHRONIC)
Motion sickness (acute)
Dysautonomia
Feline hyperthyroidism
Feline heartworm disease (?)
Postoperative nausea
Overeating
Idiopathic hypomotility
Central nervous system disease
Limbic epilepsy
Tumor
Meningitis
Increased intracranial pressure
Sialoadenitis or sialoadenosis
Behavior

## Diagnostic Approach

In patients with acute vomiting without hematemesis, obvious causes (e.g., foreign body, intoxication, organ failure, parvovirus) should be investigated. Conditions requiring prompt, specific therapy (e.g., fluid, electrolyte, or acid-base abnormalities; sepsis) also warrant thorough investigation. If the patient seems stable and no cause is obvious, symptomatic treatment is often used for 1 to 3 days. If the patient is very ill or if vomiting persists for 2 to 4 days despite symptomatic therapy, then more aggressive diagnostic testing is usually indicated.

### Physical examination

Physical examination may identify abdominal pain or masses, linear foreign objects caught under the tongue (especially in cats), and evidence of extraabdominal disease (e.g., uremia, hyperthyroidism). If a cause cannot be found and the patient is not ill, a therapeutic trial (e.g., pyrantel and dietary change) may be used to rule out certain conditions.

### Laboratory tests

CBC, serum biochemistry profile, and urinalysis are indicated in animals with acute vomiting that are severely ill and in those with chronic vomiting. Fecal examination for parasites may also be worthwhile. It may be necessary to measure serum bile acids or perform an ACTH-stimulation test to identify hepatic or adrenal insufficiency. Cats should be tested for feline leukemia virus (FeLV), feline immunodeficiency virus (FIV), and heartworm infection and for hyperthyroidism.

### Diagnostic imaging

Plain abdominal radiographs or ultrasonography may reveal intestinal obstruction, foreign objects, masses, pancreatitis, peritonitis, or other abnormalities. Abdominal ultrasound is often more revealing than plain radiography.

### Endoscopy and biopsy

If the procedures already noted are not diagnostic, the best next step is endoscopy with biopsy. During endoscopy the stomach and duodenum should undergo biopsy, regardless of gross mucosal appearance. In cats endoscopic biopsy of the ileum and ascending colon may also be helpful. If laparotomy is performed, the entire abdomen should be examined, and the stomach, duodenum, jejunum, ileum, mesenteric lymph nodes, liver, and pancreas (in cats) should undergo biopsy.

### Reevaluation

If the cause of vomiting remains undiagnosed after biopsy, the basis for previous elimination of the different diseases should be reviewed. Inflammatory bowel disease may be localized to one area of the stomach or intestine; hyperthyroid cats may have normal serum thyroxin concentrations; dogs and cats with hepatic failure may have normal serum alanine aminotransferase (ALT) and alkaline phosphatase (AP); animals with pancreatitis often have normal serum amylase and lipase activities; and *Physaloptera* infestation is rarely diagnosed by fecal examination. Finally, less common diseases that are more difficult to eliminate (e.g., idiopathic gastric hypomotility, occult central nervous system [CNS] disease, limbic epilepsy) may have to be considered.

## HEMATEMESIS (TEXT PP 351-352)

Causes of hematemesis are listed in Box 28-3. The first priority is to check for shock (hypovolemic or septic) and acute abdomen. Hematocrit and plasma total protein concentration are evaluated to determine whether blood transfusion is necessary. The next step is to narrow the list of possible causes to coagulopathy, ingestion of blood from another site (e.g., respiratory tract), or gastroduodenal ulceration and erosion (GUE). The most common cause is GUE.

### Diagnostic approach

Historical and physical findings help eliminate coagulopathy and oral or respiratory tract disease as causes of hematemesis. Platelet numbers and clotting capability (e.g., one-stage prothrombin time, partial thromboplastin time, buccal mucosal bleeding time) are more precise tests for coagulopathy. Obvious causes of GUE (e.g., acute gastritis, hemorrhagic gastroenteritis, use of nonsteroidal antiinflammatory drugs [NSAIDs]) should then be investigated.

If acute gastritis, NSAID-induced GUE, or shock is strongly suspected, symptomatic treatment for 3 to 5 days is reasonable. However, if the cause is unknown, and especially if vomiting and blood loss are severe or chronic, further diagnostics are indicated.

### Further evaluation

CBC, serum biochemistry profile, urinalysis, and abdominal imaging should be performed. In particular, renal and hepatic failure should be investigated. The stomach and duodenum are imaged with radiographs or preferably ultrasonography to look for

---

**Box 28-3**

## Causes of Hematemesis

### COAGULOPATHY (UNCOMMON CAUSE)
Thrombocytopenia and platelet dysfunction
Clotting factor deficiency
Disseminated intravascular coagulation

### ALIMENTARY TRACT LESION
Gastrointestinal tract ulceration and erosion
  Infiltrative disease
    Neoplasia (especially older dogs)
    Pythiosis (younger dogs in the southeastern United States)
    Inflammatory bowel disease
  Stress ulceration
    Hypovolemic shock (common cause)
    Septic shock (i.e., systemic inflammatory response syndrome)
    After gastric dilatation or volvulus
    Neurogenic shock
  Hyperacidity
    Mast cell tumor
    Gastrinoma (rare)
  Iatrogenic causes
    Nonsteroidal antiinflammatory drugs (very common cause)
    Corticosteroids (high-dose dexamethasone or any steroid that is combined with
      nonsteroidal antiinflammatory drugs)
  Other causes
    Hepatic disease
    Renal disease (not common)
    Hypoadrenocorticism
    Inflammatory diseases
  Foreign objects (rarely a primary cause but will worsen preexisting ulceration or
    erosion)
Gastritis
  Acute gastritis (very common cause)
  Hemorrhagic gastroenteritis
  Chronic gastritis
  *Helicobacter*-associated disease (questionable association with hematemesis
    in dogs and cats)
Esophageal disease (uncommon cause)
  Tumor
  Inflammatory disease (e.g., severe esophagitis)
  Trauma
Bleeding oral lesion
Gallbladder disease (rare)

### EXTRAALIMENTARY TRACT LESION (RARE CAUSE)
Respiratory tract disorders
  Lung lobe torsion
  Pulmonary tumor
  Posterior nares lesion

alimentary tract infiltration, foreign objects, and masses. Endoscopy is the best means of finding and evaluating gastroduodenal ulcers and erosions and allows biopsy of ulcers to rule out neoplasia or inflammatory bowel disease.

Exploratory surgery can be performed instead of endoscopy, but it is easy to miss mucosal lesions at surgery. Intraoperative endoscopy (i.e., endoscopic examination of the mucosal surfaces of the stomach and duodenum during laparotomy) may allow identification of lesions that can then be resected.

If gastroduodenoscopy does not reveal the source of bleeding, other considerations are as follows: (1) bleeding from a site beyond the reach of the endoscope, (2) blood swallowed from a lesion in the mouth, caudal nares, trachea, or lungs, (3) hemorrhage from the gall bladder, and (4) an intermittently bleeding gastric or duodenal lesion.

## DIARRHEA (TEXT PP 352-355)

### Acute Diarrhea

Acute diarrhea is usually caused by diet, parasites, and/or infectious diseases (Box 28-4). Dietary problems are often detected by history; parasites are detected by history and fecal examination; and infectious diseases are detected by history, CBC, fecal enzyme-linked immunosorbent assay for canine parvoviral antigen, and elimination of other causes. If acute diarrhea is severe or persistent, additional diagnostic tests are recommended.

---

**Box 28-4**

### Causes of Acute Diarrhea

**DIET**

Intolerance or allergy
Poor-quality food
Rapid dietary change (especially in puppies and kittens)
Bacterial food poisoning

**PARASITES**

Helminths
Protozoa
  *Giardia*
  *Tritrichomonas*
  *Coccidia*

**INFECTIOUS CAUSES**

Viral causes
  Parvovirus (canine, feline)
  Coronavirus (canine, feline)
  Feline leukemia virus (including infections secondary to it)
  Feline immunodeficiency virus (specifically infections secondary to it )
  Various other viruses (e.g., rotavirus, canine distemper virus)

Bacterial causes
  *Salmonella* spp.
  *Clostridium perfringens*
  Verotoxin-producing *Escherichia coli*
  *Campylobacter jejuni*
  *Yersinia enterocolitica*
  Various other bacteria
Rickettsial infection
  Salmon poisoning

**OTHER CAUSES**

Hemorrhagic gastroenteritis
Intussusception
Irritable bowel syndrome
Ingestion of toxins
  "Garbage can" intoxication (spoiled foods)
  Chemicals
  Heavy metals
  Various drugs (antibiotics, antineoplastics, anthelmintics, antiinflammatories, digitalis, lactulose)
Acute pancreatitis (diarrhea usually modest component of clinical signs)
Hypoadrenocorticism

**Table 28-1**

## Differentiation of Chronic Small Intestinal from Large Intestinal Diarrheas

| Sign | Small intestinal disease | Large intestinal disease |
|---|---|---|
| Weight loss | Expected | Rare* |
| Polyphagia | Sometimes | Rare or absent |
| Frequency of bowel movements | Often near normal | Sometimes very increased |
| Volume of feces | Often increased | Sometimes decreased (because of the increased frequency) |
| Blood in feces | Melena (rare) | Hematochezia (sometimes†) |
| Mucus in feces | Uncommon | Sometimes |
| Tenesmus | Uncommon (but may occur later in chronic cases) | Sometimes |
| Vomiting | May be seen | May be seen |

*Failure to lose weight or condition is the most reliable indication that an animal has large bowel disease. However, animals with colonic histoplasmosis, pythiosis, lymphoma, or similar infiltrative diseases may have weight loss despite large bowel involvement.

†Hematochezia becomes much more important as a differentiating feature in animals that are losing weight. Its presence in such animals confirms large bowel involvement (either by itself or in combination with small bowel disease) despite weight loss.

## Chronic Diarrhea

Animals with chronic diarrhea should first be examined for parasites; multiple fecal examinations for nematodes, *Giardia*, and *Tritrichomonas* are indicated. Next, it should be determined if the diarrhea originates in the small or large intestine (Table 28-1). Absence of weight loss almost always indicates large bowel disease, although some large bowel diseases (e.g., pythiosis, histoplasmosis, malignancy) can cause weight loss. Patients with these latter problems usually have obvious indications of colonic involvement (e.g., fecal mucus, marked tenesmus, hematochezia).

Chronic small intestinal diarrhea can be separated into that caused by maldigestion and that caused by malabsorption (either the non–protein-losing or protein-losing type). These problems are discussed separately in the following sections.

## Maldigestion

Maldigestion is principally caused by exocrine pancreatic insufficiency (EPI) and rarely causes hypoalbuminemia. The most sensitive and specific test for EPI is serum trypsinlike immunoreactivity (TLI) concentration (see Chapter 40). This test is indicated in any dog with chronic small intestinal diarrhea. Diagnosing EPI by evaluating response to therapy is not recommended. EPI is rare in cats, but if it is suspected, feline serum TLI measurement is recommended.

## Malabsorption

Malabsorptive intestinal disease (enteropathy) may be protein-losing enteropathy (PLE) or non–protein-losing enteropathy. Serum albumin usually is markedly decreased ($\beta$2.1 g/dl) in the former but not in the latter; hypoglobulinemia may also occur. Diarrhea is seen only if the absorptive capacity of the colon is exceeded. Therefore a dog or cat can lose weight because of small intestinal malabsorption yet not have diarrhea (see discussion of weight loss, later). When marked hypoproteinemia is not attributable to nephropathy or hepatic insufficiency, PLE is the main consideration.

### Causes of malabsorption in dogs

Major causes of malabsorption in dogs are as follows:
- food intolerance or allergy
- parasitism–giardiasis

- antibiotic-responsive enteropathy (ARE; formerly called *small intestinal bacterial overgrowth*, or IBO)
- inflammatory bowel disease–lymphocytic-plasmacytic, eosinophilic, or purulent enteritis and idiopathic villous atrophy
- neoplastic bowel disease–lymphoma
- pythiosis

ARE may be idiopathic or it may be caused by immunoglobulin A deficiency, partial obstruction or blind loops, EPI, underlying intestinal disease that affects motility, or deficient gastric acid secretion.

### Protein-losing enteropathy

Major causes of PLE in dogs include the following:

- severe inflammatory bowel disease (common)
- alimentary tract lymphoma (very common)
- alimentary tract histoplasmosis
- intestinal lymphangiectasia
- chronic intussusception (young dogs)
- alimentary hemorrhage–e.g., ulceration or erosion, neoplasia, parasites
- unusual enteropathies–e.g., chronic purulent enteropathy, severe ectasia of mucosal crypts, severe mucosal edema
- massive hookworm or whipworm infestation

Except for lymphangiectasia, these diseases do not consistently produce PLE; when PLE is present, however, they are the most common causes.

### Causes of malabsorption in cats

Major causes of malabsorption in cats are as follows:

- food intolerance or allergy
- giardiasis
- lymphocytic-plasmacytic enteritis
- alimentary tract lymphoma

### Protein-losing enteropathy

Major causes of PLE in cats are as follows:

- alimentary tract lymphoma
- severe inflammatory bowel disease–lymphocytic-plasmacytic enteritis
- alimentary tract hemorrhage (e.g., neoplasia)

### Diagnostic approach to malabsorption

If non–protein-losing malabsorptive disease is suspected, diagnostic tests and/or therapeutic trials (e.g., elimination diet for dietary intolerance, treatment for occult giardiasis, antibiotics for ARE) are reasonable if the animal is not too debilitated. If PLE is suspected, ultrasonography and intestinal biopsy are recommended because PLE usually requires prompt, appropriate therapy.

*Antibiotic-responsive enteropathy.* Treatment is indicated when ARE is found; however, definitive diagnosis is difficult. This condition cannot reliably be diagnosed by quantitative duodenal culture. Alterations in serum concentrations of vitamin $B_{12}$ (decreased) and folate (increased) are probably specific for ARE, but they are of questionable sensitivity. Duodenal mucosal cytology and histology are rarely diagnostic.

*Biopsy.* The final diagnostic step is usually intestinal biopsy. Absorption tests and barium contrast radiography are rarely helpful and do not eliminate the need for biopsy. Biopsy specimens are typically obtained by laparotomy or endoscopy. If biopsy does not reveal a cause, the main possibilities are that (1) the samples are inadequate, (2) the lesion was beyond the scope's reach, (3) the patient has occult giardiasis, or (4) the patient has ARE or dietary intolerance. Lymphadenopathy or intestinal masses may be identified on ultrasonography and aspirated percutaneously.

## Chronic Large Intestinal Diarrhea

### Causes in dogs

Major causes of chronic large intestinal diarrhea in dogs include the following:

- food intolerance or allergy
- parasitism–e.g., whipworms, *Giardia, Tritrichomonas*

- clostridial colitis
- irritable bowel syndrome
- histoplasmosis
- pythiosis
- inflammatory bowel disease—lymphocytic-plasmacytic, eosinophilic, chronic ulcerative, or histiocytic ulcerative (in Boxers) colitis

**Causes in cats**

Major causes of chronic large intestinal diarrhea in cats are as follows:

- food intolerance or allergy
- lymphocytic-plasmacytic colitis
- irritable bowel syndrome
- FeLV and secondary infections
- infections secondary to FIV

**Diagnostic approach**

Patients with chronic large intestinal diarrhea or fecal mucus should first undergo a digital rectal examination to search for mucosal thickening or proliferation. The rectum is the most common site of canine colonic neoplasia, and obvious mucosal lesions indicate the need for biopsy.

*Therapeutic trials.* If the rectal mucosa seems normal and the patient has not lost weight or become hypoalbuminemic, therapeutic trials may be tried. However, multiple fecal examinations for whipworms and *Giardia* are always indicated. Therapeutic trials usually consist of high-fiber diets, hypoallergenic diets, antibiotics to control clostridial colitis, and/or treatment for whipworms.

*Diagnostic tests.* Additional tests that may be performed instead of therapeutic trials include colonic mucosal biopsies (via colonoscopy), fecal cultures, and assays for clostridial toxins. Fecal cultures for specific pathogens (e.g., *Salmonella* spp.) should be submitted if the history suggests an infectious disorder or if the patient is not responding to therapy.

If mucosal biopsies are not diagnostic, three main possibilities exist: (1) the samples may not be representative of the entire colonic mucosa, (2) the pathologist may not have recognized the lesions, or (3) mucosal infiltrates may not be present. The latter commonly occurs in dogs with dietary intolerance or allergy, clostridial colitis, chronic giardiasis, or irritable bowel syndrome.

## HEMATOCHEZIA (TEXT PP 355-356)

Hematochezia is defined as fresh blood in the feces. Streaks of blood on the outside of otherwise normal feces suggest an anal or rectal lesion, whereas blood mixed into the feces or diarrheic stools implies bleeding higher in the colon. Specific causes are listed subsequently. A thorough digital rectal examination is indicated, even if anesthesia is necessary. Each anal sac should be expressed and its contents examined. If the problem is chronic and these tests are uninformative, colonoscopy and biopsy are usually indicated. Biopsies should include submucosa.

**Causes**

*Dogs.* Causes of hematochezia in dogs include the following:

- parasites—e.g., whipworms, hookworms (severe infection)
- food intolerance or allergy
- clostridial colitis
- histoplasmosis
- pythiosis
- neoplasia—e.g., rectal adenocarcinoma or polyps, colorectal leiomyoma or leiomyosarcoma
- intussusception (ileocolic or cecocolic)
- hemorrhagic gastroenteritis
- parvoviral enteritis

- inflammatory bowel disease
- colonic trauma—e.g., foreign objects, automobile-associated trauma
- anal sacculitis
- coagulopathy (rarely a cause of rectal bleeding only)

These diseases do not consistently cause hematochezia; when hematochezia is present, however, they are the most common causes.

*Cats.* The major causes of hematochezia in cats are as follows:
- food intolerance or allergy
- lymphocytic-plasmacytic colitis
- coccidiosis

## MELENA (TEXT P 356)

Melena (coal-tar black feces) is often absent in animals with alimentary tract hemorrhage. When it is present, it strongly suggests upper alimentary bleeding or ingestion of blood.

### Causes

Major causes of melena in dogs include the following:
- hookworms
- GUE
- gastric or small intestinal tumor—e.g., lymphoma, adenocarcinoma, leiomyoma or leiomyosarcoma
- ingested blood—e.g., oral, nasopharyngeal, or pulmonary lesions; diet
- coagulopathy

These diseases do not consistently cause melena; when melena is present, however, they are the most common causes.

### Causes in cats

Melena is rare in cats. Causes include small intestinal tumor (e.g., lymphoma, duodenal polyps, adenocarcinoma, mast cell tumor) and vitamin K deficiency (intoxication or a result of malabsorption).

### Diagnostic approach

Ultrasonography is useful when looking for bleeding lesions (e.g., intestinal tumor), but gastroduodenoscopy is the most sensitive test for GUE. If endoscopy is nondiagnostic, contrast radiography may permit detection of small intestinal lesions beyond the reach of the endoscope. Exploratory laparotomy is required for such lesions. It is easy to miss bleeding mucosal lesions when viewing the serosa or palpating the bowel, so intraoperative endoscopy is recommended.

Iron deficiency anemia can result from chronic gastrointestinal blood loss. CBC may reveal microcytosis and hypochromasia, but measurement of total serum iron and total iron binding capacity and staining of bone marrow for iron are more definitive tests.

## TENESMUS (TEXT PP 356-357)

Tenesmus (ineffectual and/or painful straining at urination or defecation) and dyschezia (painful or difficult elimination of feces) are primarily caused by inflammatory or obstructive lesions of the distal colon, urinary bladder, or urethra. Most rectal masses and strictures cause hematochezia; however, some do not disrupt the colonic mucosa and only cause tenesmus.

### Causes

In dogs the major causes of tenesmus and dyschezia include perineal or rectal inflammation and pain (e.g., anal sacculitis, perianal fistulas), tumors, proctitis (either primary disease or secondary to diarrhea or prolapse), histoplasmosis, pythiosis, and colonic or rectal obstruction (e.g., rectal neoplasia or granuloma, perineal hernia, constipation, prostatomegaly, pelvic fracture, pelvic canal masses, rectal foreign object).

In cats the primary causes of tenesmus and dyschezia include urethral obstruction, rectal obstruction (pelvic fracture, perineal hernia), constipation, and abscess near the rectum.

### Diagnostic approach

The first goal, especially in cats, is to distinguish lower urinary tract disease from alimentary tract disease. In cats, tenesmus secondary to urethral obstruction is often misinterpreted as constipation. On abdominal palpation, a distended urinary bladder suggests obstruction; a small, painful bladder suggests inflammation. Urinalysis should be performed, and if necessary the urethra should be catheterized to determine patency.

*Behavior.* Observing the animal defecate may help define the underlying process. Animals with colonic or rectal inflammation often continue to strain after defecating, whereas constipation causes the patient to strain only before feces are produced. Animals with colitis often exhibit tenesmus in a squatting position, whereas tenesmus caused by obstruction usually occurs in a partially walking or partially squatting position.

*Rectal examination.* If alimentary tract disease is suspected, the abdomen and rectum should be palpated and the anus and perineal areas examined. Most strictures, perineal hernias, masses, enlarged prostate glands, pelvic fractures, and rectal tumors can be detected during digital rectal examination. Perianal fistulas are usually visible but may manifest only as perirectal thickenings. The anal sacs should be expressed and their contents examined. Finally, the feces are examined for excessive hardness and abnormal contents (e.g., hair, trash). Do not assume that constipation, if present, is causing the tenesmus. Severe pain (e.g., from proctitis) may make the patient refuse to defecate and may cause secondary constipation.

*Biopsy.* Masses, strictures, and infiltrative lesions should be biopsied. Rectal scraping is sometimes sufficient (e.g., for histoplasmosis), but biopsies that include the submucosa are preferred. Fine-needle aspiration should be performed if an extracolonic mass is found, because abscesses occasionally occur in extracolonic locations.

## CONSTIPATION (TEXT PP 357-358)

Constipation or obstipation (intractable constipation) has many possible causes (Box 28-5). Symptomatic therapy is often successful, but it is better to identify the cause before treatment.

### Diagnostic approach

The history should be evaluated for iatrogenic, dietary, environmental, and behavioral causes. Physical and rectal examinations are used to search for rectal obstruction or infiltration. Feces should be examined for items such as plastic, bones, hair, and popcorn. Evaluation of CBC, serum biochemistry panel, and urinalysis may reveal causes of colonic inertia (e.g., hypercalcemia, hypokalemia, hypothyroidism).

*Diagnostic imaging.* Plain pelvic radiographs help eliminate anatomic abnormalities and undetected colonic obstruction (e.g., prostatomegaly, enlarged sublumbar lymph node). Ultrasonography is preferred when looking for infiltrative disease. Colonoscopy is indicated when obstruction is suspected that is too cranial to detect with digital examination. Ultrasound-guided fine-needle aspiration of infiltrative colonic lesions is sometimes diagnostic, but rigid colonoscopy allows a more reliable biopsy. When a thorough workup fails to identify a cause in a patient with a grossly dilated colon, then idiopathic megacolon may be present.

## FECAL INCONTINENCE (TEXT P 358)

Fecal incontinence is caused by neuromuscular disease (e.g., cauda equina syndrome, lumbosacral stenosis) or partial rectal obstruction. Severe, irritative proctitis may cause urge incontinence. Patients with rectal obstructions continually try to defecate because the anal canal is filled. Proctitis is suspected based on rectal examination and confirmed by proctoscopy and biopsy. Neuromuscular disease is suspected when an abnormal

---

**Box 28-5**

## Causes of Constipation

### IATROGENIC CAUSES
Drugs
Opiates
Anticholinergics
Sucralfate (Carafate)
Barium

### BEHAVIORAL OR ENVIRONMENTAL CAUSES
Change in household or routine
Soiled litter box or no litter box
House training
Inactivity

### REFUSAL TO DEFECATE
Behavioral cause
Pain in rectal or perineal area
Inability to assume position to
    defecate
    Orthopedic problem
    Neurologic problem

### DIETARY CAUSES
Excessive fiber in dehydrated animal
Abnormal diet
Hair
Bones
Indigestible material (e.g., plants,
    plastic)

### COLONIC OBSTRUCTION
Pseudocoprostasis
Deviation of rectal canal
    Perineal hernia

### INTRALUMINAL AND INTRAMURAL DISORDERS
Tumor
Granuloma
Cicatrix (Stricture of oesophagus)
Rectal foreign body
Congenital stricture

### EXTRALUMINAL DISORDERS
Tumor
Granuloma
Abscess
Healed pelvic fracture
Prostatomegaly
Prostatic or paraprostatic cyst
Sublumbar lymphadenopathy

### COLONIC WEAKNESS
Systemic disease
Hypercalcemia
Hypokalemia
Hypothyroidism
Chagas' disease

### LOCALIZED NEUROMUSCULAR DISEASE
Spinal cord trauma
Pelvic nerve damage
Dysautonomia
Chronic, massive dilatation of the
    colon causing irreversible stretching
    of the colonic musculature

### MISCELLANEOUS CAUSES
Severe dehydration
Idiopathic megacolon (especially cats)

---

anal reflex is found, usually with other neurologic defects in the anal, perineal, hind limb, and/or coccygeal region (see Chapter 72).

## WEIGHT LOSS (TEXT PP 358-360)

Weight loss can be caused by many different problems (Box 28-6). If other abnormalities with more defined lists of differential diagnoses (e.g., ascites, vomiting, diarrhea, polyuria and polydipsia) are present, they should be pursued first. If there are no concurrent problems that allow localization of the disease, the first step is to determine how the appetite was when weight loss began. Weight loss despite a good appetite usually indicates maldigestion, malabsorption, excessive use of calories (e.g., hyperthyroidism, lactation), or inappropriate loss of calories (e.g., diabetes mellitus).

---

**Box 28-6**

## Causes of Weight Loss

Food
    Not enough (especially possible if
        multiple animals are present)
    Poor quality or low caloric density
    Inedible
Anorexia (see Box 28-7)
Dysphagia (see Box 28-1)
Regurgitation and vomiting (i.e., losing
    enough calories to account for weight
    loss)
Maldigestive disease
    Exocrine pancreatic insufficiency
        (usually but not always associated
        with diarrhea)
Malabsorptive disease
    Small intestinal disease (may be
        associated with normal stools)
Malassimilation
    Organ failure
        Cardiac failure
        Hepatic failure
        Renal failure
        Adrenal failure
Cancer cachexia

Excessive use of calories
    Lactation
    Increased work
    Extremely cold environment
    Pregnancy
    Increased catabolism resulting
        from fever or inflammation
    Hyperthyroidism
Increased loss of nutrients
    Diabetes mellitus
    Protein-losing nephropathy
    Protein-losing enteropathy
Neuromuscular disease
    Lower motor neuron disease

---

### Diagnostic approach

The history should be reviewed for dietary problems, dysphagia, regurgitation, vomiting, and increased use of calories. The signalment may suggest particular diseases such as hyperthyroidism in older cats or portosystemic shunts in young dogs.

*Physical examination.* Abnormalities that help localize the problem to a particular body system include nasal disease that prevents normal olfaction, dysphagia, arrhythmia, weakness (which suggests neuromuscular disease), abnormally sized or shaped organs, pain, and abnormal fluid accumulations. Retinal examination may identify inflammatory or infiltrative diseases, especially in cats.

*Laboratory tests.* CBC, serum biochemistry profile, and urinalysis should be evaluated for evidence of inflammation, organ failure, or paraneoplastic syndrome. Cats should be tested for FeLV and FIV. Serum $T_4$ and free $T_4$ ($fT_4$) should be measured in older cats.

*Diagnostic imaging.* If laboratory data are unhelpful, thoracic radiographs are obtained; significant thoracic disease cannot be eliminated by physical findings alone. Most cats and some dogs can be palpated well enough that abdominal radiographs are not necessary early in the workup. However, abdominal ultrasonography may reveal lesions that are not evident on abdominal palpation and plain radiographs.

*Further evaluation.* If the cause of weight loss remains undetermined, daily physical examination may be the best means of localizing the problem. Fever of unknown origin is discussed in Chapter 95. Organ function testing (e.g., serum bile acids, ACTH-stimulation tests, serum TLI) may be worthwhile. If serum $T_4$ and $fT_4$ concentrations are normal in a cat with suspected hyperthyroidism, these values should be rechecked or a $T_3$-suppression test performed (see Chapter 51).

*Biopsy.* If the cause remains undiagnosed, gastric and intestinal biopsy (preferably via endoscopy) should be considered. If laparotomy is performed, the entire abdomen should be examined and biopsy samples taken of the alimentary tract (multiple sites), liver, and mesenteric lymph nodes. Biopsy of the pancreas should also be performed in cats.

*Investigating obscure causes.* Difficult-to-diagnose causes of weight loss include feline hyperthyroidism with normal serum $T_4$ and $fT_4$, gastric disease that is not causing vomiting, intestinal disease that is not causing vomiting or diarrhea, hepatic disease with normal serum ALT or SAP, occult inflammatory disease, hypoadrenocorticism with normal serum electrolyte concentrations, occult cancer, "dry" feline infectious peritonitis, and CNS disease without cranial nerve deficits.

Tests to evaluate the CNS (e.g., cerebrospinal fluid analysis, electroencephalography, computed tomography, magnetic resonance imaging) and peripheral nerves and muscles (e.g., electromyography, biopsies of muscle and nerve) may be warranted (see Chapter 66). If the cause remains undiagnosed and the history and physical examination are noncontributory, occult cancer becomes a major differential diagnosis.

## ANOREXIA (TEXT P 360)

The approach to anorexia of uncertain cause is similar to that to weight loss, as are the differential diagnoses (Box 28-7). Inflammatory disease is often detected by means of CBC and/or the presence of fever. Gastric disease may produce anorexia without vomiting. Rarely, cancer cachexia with anorexia as the predominant sign is caused by relatively small tumors that are not grossly detectable. CNS disease must be considered whenever mentation is altered, although altered mentation may resemble the depression and lethargy commonly seen with other diseases.

---

**Box 28-7**

### Major Causes of Anorexia

Inflammatory disease
  Bacterial infections
  Viral infections
  Fungal infections
  Rickettsial infections
  Protozoal infections
  Sterile inflammation
    Immune-mediated disease
    Neoplastic disease
    Pancreatitis
Alimentary tract disease
  Gastric or intestinal disease
  Dysphagia (especially resulting
    from pain)
Nausea
  Stimulation of the medullary
    vomiting center for any reason,
    even if it is not sufficient to
    cause vomiting, especially
    gastric or intestinal disease

Metabolic disease
  Organ failure (e.g., kidney, adrenal,
    liver, heart)
  Hypercalcemia
  Diabetic ketoacidosis
  Hyperthyroidism (usually causes
    polyphagia, but some cats have
    apathetic hyperthyroidism)
Other causes
  Cancer cachexia
  Anosmia
  Central nervous system disease
  Psychologic causes
  Fever

## ABDOMINAL EFFUSION (TEXT PP 360-361)

Abdominal effusion is usually caused by hypoalbuminemia, portal hypertension, and/or peritoneal inflammation. Effusion resulting from alimentary tract disorders is primarily caused by PLE or alimentary tract rupture (septic peritonitis). In some patients with PLE the stools are normal and ascites is the presenting complaint. Malignancies may obstruct lymphatic flow or increase vascular permeability, producing modified transudates or nonseptic peritonitis. Modified transudates also result from hepatic or cardiac disease.

## ACUTE ABDOMEN (TEXT PP 361-362)

The term *acute abdomen* refers to various abdominal disorders that produce hypovolemic or septic shock, sepsis, and/or severe pain (Box 28-8). Treatment is determined by the severity of the clinical signs. The first step is to identify and treat shock and/or gastric dilatation and volvulus. Once these conditions are eliminated or managed, the next major decision is whether exploratory surgery or medical therapy is indicated. Typically, abdominal imaging (plain radiographs and/or ultrasonography) and clinical pathologic studies (CBC, chemistry panel) should be performed before a decision is made to do a laparotomy. A barium study is seldom useful.

Animals with abdominal masses, foreign objects, bunched-up loops of painful small intestine (e.g., linear foreign body), or spontaneous septic peritonitis should undergo surgery as soon as supportive therapy has made the anesthetic risk acceptable. Surgery is not necessarily beneficial and may even be detrimental to patients with pancreatitis, parvoviral enteritis, pyelonephritis, prostatitis, or cholecystitis. But if optimal medical therapy is being given and the patient is (1) clearly deteriorating, (2) not improving after 2 to 5 days, or (3) continuing in excruciating pain, it may be appropriate to recommend exploratory surgery.

---

**Box 28-8**

### Major Causes of Acute Abdomen

Septic inflammation
Septic peritonitis resulting from any
  cause, but especially a perforated or
  devitalized hollow viscus
  Perforating linear foreign body
  Ruptured gallbladder resulting from
    cholecystitis
  Abscess
    Pancreatic
    Splenic
    Hepatic
    Prostatic
    Renal
  Pyometra
Nonseptic inflammation
  Pancreatitis
  Iatrogenic inflammation
    Surgical sponge

Organ distension or obstruction
  Gastric dilatation or volvulus
  Mesenteric volvulus
  Intussusception
  Incarcerated obstruction
  Intestinal obstruction resulting
    from any cause
Ischemia
  Torsion of spleen, testicle, or other
    organ
Other causes of abdominal pain (see
  Box 28-9)
Abdominal hemorrhage
  Abdominal neoplasia
  Trauma
  Coagulopathy
Abdominal neoplasia

---

**Box 28-9**

## Causes of Abdominal Pain

Poor palpation technique
Musculoskeletal system
  Fractures
  Intervertebral disk disease (common)
  Diskospondylitis (common)
  Abscesses
Gastrointestinal tract
  Gastrointestinal ulcer
  Foreign object
  Neoplasm
  Adhesions
  Intestinal ischemia
  Intestinal spasm
  Organ distention or obstruction (see
    Box 28-8)
Hepatobiliary tract
  Hepatitis
  Cholelithiasis or cholecystitis
Pancreas
  Pancreatitis (common)
Spleen
  Torsion (uncommon)
  Rupture
  Neoplasm
  Infection
Peritoneum
  Peritonitis (common)
    Septic
    Nonseptic (e.g., uroabdomen)
  Adhesions

Urogenital system
  Pyelonephritis
  Lower urinary tract infection
  Nonseptic cystitis (common in cats)
  Cystic or ureteral obstruction or
    rupture (common, especially after
    trauma)
  Urethritis or obstruction (common)
  Metritis
  Uterine torsion (rare)
  Neoplasm
  Testicular torsion (rare)
  Prostatitis (common)
  Mastitis (does not cause true
    abdominal pain, but mimics
    abdominal pain)
Miscellaneous causes
  Adrenalitis (associated with
    hypoadrenocorticism)
  Heavy metal intoxication
  Vasculopathy
    Rocky Mountain spotted fever
  Vasculitis
  Infarct
  Autonomic (abdominal) epilepsy
Iatrogenic causes
  Misoprostol
  Bethanechol
  Postoperative causes (especially if
    animal has a tight suture line)

---

## ABDOMINAL PAIN (TEXT PP 362-363)

Abdominal pain must first be localized as true abdominal or extraabdominal (e.g., lumbosacral origin). Animals with true abdominal pain may have obvious discomfort and may whine, growl, or snap if the abdomen is touched. Some dogs stretch out and assume a "praying" position. Other animals have less conspicuous signs (e.g., grunt or try to walk away when palpated; tensed abdomen) that are easily missed. Poor or rough abdominal palpation technique in normal animals may produce a guarding response, mimicking abdominal pain. The major causes of abdominal pain are listed in Box 28-9.

The diagnostic approach depends on severity and progression and whether any causes are obvious. The steps are similar to those used for acute abdomen. Some causes can be difficult to diagnose (e.g., acute pancreatitis, localized peritonitis).

## ABDOMINAL DISTENTION OR ENLARGEMENT (TEXT PP 363-364)

Abdominal distention or enlargement can be associated with an acute abdomen, but it is usually a separate problem. Abdominal distention has five basic causes: tissue, fluid, gas, fat, and weak abdominal muscles (Box 28-10).

---

**Box 28-10**

## Causes of Abdominal Enlargement

**TISSUE**
Pregnancy
Hepatomegaly (infiltrative or inflammatory disease, lipidosis, neoplasia)
Splenomegaly (infiltrative or inflammatory disease, neoplasia, hematoma)
Renomegaly (neoplasia, infiltrative disease, compensatory hypertrophy)
Miscellaneous neoplasia
Granuloma (e.g., pythiosis)

**FLUID**
Contained in organ(s)
Congestion resulting from torsion, volvulus, or right-sided heart failure
Spleen
Liver
Cysts
Paraprostatic cyst
Perinephric cyst
Hepatic cyst
Hydronephrosis
Intestines or stomach (resulting from obstruction or ileus)
Pyometra
Free in abdomen
Transudate, modified transudate, exudate, blood, chyle

**GAS**
Contained in organ(s)
Stomach (gastric dilation or volvulus)
Intestines (resulting from obstruction)
In parenchymatous organs (e.g., liver) resulting from infection with gas-producing bacteria
Free in abdomen
Iatrogenic (after laparoscopy or laparotomy)
Alimentary tract or female reproductive tract rupture
Bacterial metabolism (peritonitis)

**FAT**
Obesity
Lipoma

**WEAK ABDOMINAL MUSCLES**
Hyperadrenocorticism

**FECES**

---

**Diagnostic approach**

The first concern is whether acute abdomen is present. After acute abdomen is eliminated, physical examination and abdominal radiographs and/or ultrasound are used to classify the enlargement. Free abdominal fluid is sampled and analyzed. Biopsy of abdominal masses and enlarged organs should be performed unless there exists a reason not to (e.g., hepatomegaly caused by severe right-sided heart failure). Fine-needle aspiration is usually safe, although leakage of septic contents or implantation of neoplastic cells may occur. Ultrasound helps determine the potential for hemorrhage or leakage (e.g., cyst or mass with characteristics of hemangiosarcoma).

***Other tests.*** CBC, serum biochemistry panel, and urinalysis are used to determine if specific organ involvement (e.g., hyperadrenocorticism) is likely. Contrast alimentary or urinary tract radiographs may be useful in selected cases.

***Interpretation.*** Spontaneous pneumoperitoneum suggests alimentary tract rupture or septic peritonitis and is an indication for immediate surgical exploration. A hollow viscus dilated with gas may indicate obstruction (e.g., gastric dilation, intestinal obstruction) or physiologic ileus. If obstruction seems likely, surgery is indicated. If abdominal muscle weakness is suspected, hyperadrenocorticism should be investigated.

# 29

# Diagnostic Tests for the Alimentary Tract

## *(Text pp 365-386)*

## ROUTINE LABORATORY EVALUATION (TEXT PP 365-366)

### Complete Blood Count

Complete blood count (CBC) is especially important in patients that may have neutropenia (e.g., suspected parvoviral enteritis, sepsis), infection (e.g., aspiration pneumonia), or anemia (e.g., melena, hematemesis) and those that have fever, weight loss, or anorexia of occult cause. If the patient is anemic, CBC should be evaluated for evidence of iron deficiency (e.g., hypochromasia, microcytosis, thrombocytosis, increased red blood cell distribution width). Iron deficiency anemia resulting from gastrointestinal (GI) disease is less common in cats than in dogs.

#### Coagulation profile

Platelet count is recommended if blood loss is suspected. Platelet numbers can be estimated from blood smears. Dogs should have 8 to 30 platelets per oil immersion field; 1 platelet per field suggests a platelet count of approximately 15,000 to 20,000/µl. Coagulation panels may reveal unsuspected coagulopathies (e.g., disseminated intravascular coagulation). Activated clotting times are crude estimates of the intrinsic clotting pathway; partial thromboplastin times are more sensitive.

### Serum Biochemistry Profile

Evaluation of blood urea nitrogen, creatinine, total protein, albumin, alanine aminotransferase, serum alkaline phosphatase, sodium, potassium, calcium, phosphorus, magnesium, bilirubin, and glucose are important in patients with severe vomiting, diarrhea, ascites, unexplained weight loss, or anorexia. Total carbon dioxide is not as definitive as blood gas analysis but helps define the acid-base status.

#### Albumin

Serum albumin is typically a more useful index than total protein, as hyperglobulinemia in a hypoalbuminemic dog can produce a normal serum protein concentration. Severe hypoalbuminemia (<2 g/dl) is important diagnostically; it is more commonly found in animals with infiltrative alimentary disease, parvoviral diarrhea, intestinal lymphangiectasia, GI blood loss, or ascites.

### Urinalysis

Urinalysis is required to accurately evaluate renal function and, in conjunction with urine protein/creatinine ratio, to help identify the cause of hypoalbuminemia. Urine should always be obtained before fluid therapy.

## FECAL EVALUATION (TEXT PP 366-368)

### Fecal Parasites

Fecal flotation is indicated in almost every animal with alimentary tract disease or weight loss, especially in puppies and kittens. Even if it is not the primary problem, parasitism may cause additional debilitation.

#### Flotation techniques

Concentrated salt or sugar solutions are typically used. Zinc sulfate solution is preferred for detecting most nematode ova and *Giardia* cysts (see text). Some parasites intermittently shed small numbers of ova or cysts, necessitating repeated fecal analyses for diagnosis. Whipworm and *Giardia* infections can be especially difficult to diagnose.

Common tapeworm ova are contained in segments and are not found by flotation techniques. *Nanophyetus salmincola* (the fluke responsible for salmon poisoning) is detected by many flotation solutions, but sedimentation techniques are required to detect most other fluke ova. *Cryptosporidia* can be detected by flotation techniques, but higher magnification (×1000) must be used; enzyme-linked immunosorbent assay (ELISA) is more sensitive.

#### Direct examination

Direct fecal examination is not sensitive and should not replace flotation techniques. However, it occasionally allows for a diagnosis of amebiasis, strongyloidiasis, and whipworm infestations missed by flotation procedures. Motile *Giardia* and *Tritrichomonas* trophozoites may be found if the feces are very fresh and the smear is adequately diluted with saline.

### Fecal Digestion Tests

Examining feces for undigested food particles by staining thin fecal smears with Sudan (for fat) and/or iodine (for starch and muscle fibers) is of dubious value. Finding excessive undigested fat suggests exocrine pancreatic insufficiency (EPI); however, false-positive and false-negative results are common. Serum trypsinlike immunoreactivity (TLI) is a better test for EPI (see later).

#### Occult blood

Tests for fecal occult blood are seldom indicated. If this analysis is desired, the animal should be fed a meat-free diet for 3 to 4 days before the test. Repeated testing may be needed to demonstrate intermittent bleeding.

### Miscellaneous Fecal Analyses

The ELISA for canine parvovirus is very specific; however, the virus may not be shed for the first 24 to 48 hours. An ELISA for detecting a *Giardia*-specific antigen in human feces (see text) appears useful but may not be any more accurate than multiple zinc sulfate flotation examinations. An ELISA for detecting cryptosporidial antigens in feces appears to be more sensitive than fecal examinations. Rotavirus can also be diagnosed in feces by ELISA. However, rotavirus infection is of uncertain significance in dogs.

Assays for *Clostridium perfringens* enterotoxin and *Clostridium difficile* toxins have been used in dogs with diarrhea. A single negative test result does not rule out the presence of either organism; the test may need to be performed two or three times before the toxin is found. Not all animals that test positive for clostridial toxins have clinical signs of disease.

### Bacterial Culture of Feces

Fecal culture is seldom indicated unless an infectious disease is suspected or other tests (e.g., endoscopy, biopsy) are nondiagnostic. Fecal culture cannot be used to diagnose antibiotic-responsive enteropathy (ARE; formerly small intestinal bacterial overgrowth).

#### Common pathogens

The pathogens most likely to be cultured from small animal feces are *C. perfringens, C. difficile, Salmonella* spp., *Campylobacter jejuni, Yersinia enterocolitica,* and verotoxin-producing strains of *Escherichia coli.* (Note: Confirmation of verotoxin production requires polymerase chain reaction [PCR] or bioassay.) *Aeromonas* spp. and *Plesiomonas* spp. may also cause diarrhea. However, the mere presence of any of these bacteria in feces does not confirm that they are causing disease.

*Salmonella* spp. can sometimes be cultured from colonic mucosa in dogs with feces that test negative; the PCR technique used to detect *Salmonella* spp. in equine feces may be useful in canine and feline feces. *Candida* is occasionally cultured from feces. It is often of uncertain significance but may cause problems in some animals (e.g., chemotherapy patients).

## Cytologic Evaluation of Feces

Fecal cytology may identify etiologic agents and/or inflammatory cells. A thin, air-dried smear is stained with Gram's or a Romanowsky-type stain (e.g., Diff-Quick). The latter identifies cells better than Gram's stain. Fecal leukocytes indicate transmural colonic inflammation rather than superficial mucosal inflammation. However, their presence does not allow definitive diagnosis.

Excessive numbers of spore-forming bacteria (>3 per ×1000 field) were thought to suggest clostridial colitis. However, this finding is neither specific nor sensitive for clostridial colitis. Short, curved, gram-negative rods suggest campylobacteriosis. The larger spirochetes, which are often plentiful in diarrheic feces, are of questionable pathogenicity. Fungal organisms (e.g., *Histoplasma capsulatum, Candida* spp.) are rarely found by fecal examination; cytologic examination of mucosal scrapings or histologic examination of biopsy specimens is usually needed.

## DIAGNOSTIC IMAGING (TEXT PP 368-377)

### Radiography

Radiographs generally are useful in animals with dysphagia, regurgitation, vomiting, abdominal mass and distention, abdominal pain, or acute abdomen. They are occasionally helpful in animals with constipation, weight loss, or anorexia of unknown cause, but other tests are usually indicated first and often render imaging unnecessary. Plain radiographs are rarely diagnostic in dogs or cats with chronic diarrhea or marked abdominal effusion, and they may not be cost effective when the abdomen can be palpated thoroughly (e.g., in many cats). Although contrast-enhanced radiographs may delineate structures that plain radiographs cannot (e.g., gastric outflow tract obstruction), plain radiography should always precede contrast radiography. Radiographs in at least two views should always be taken, usually the right lateral and ventrodorsal (VD) views.

### Ultrasonography

Ultrasonography is often useful in animals with acute abdomen, abdominal effusion, vomiting, weight loss or anorexia of unknown cause, abdominal mass and distention, or abdominal pain. It aids in the diagnosis of pancreatitis, infiltration in various organs, and intussusceptions that radiographs miss. Ultrasonography can be more informative than radiography in determining whether a patient with acute abdomen needs surgery. It can also provide guidance for percutaneous aspiration and biopsy.

### Imaging of the Oral Cavity and Pharynx

Animals with dysphagia, oral pain, halitosis of unknown cause, or a swelling or mass involving the oral cavity or pharynx should undergo diagnostic imaging. If dysphagia of neuromuscular origin is suspected, fluoroscopy is recommended. Ultrasonography is particularly informative in the evaluation of infiltrates or masses. Lateral, dorsoventral (DV), and oblique radiographic views of the skull are used when looking for foreign objects or fractures. Open-mouth VD views and end-on views of the nose may also help. Foreign objects, fractures, bone lysis, and soft-tissue masses or densities, and emphysema are common findings. The bone surrounding the tooth roots should be examined for lysis, and the temporomandibular joints for arthritis.

## Imaging of the Esophagus

Indications for radiographic evaluation of the esophagus include regurgitation (including pharyngeal dysphagia), pain on swallowing, unexplained recurrent pneumonia, and thoracic masses of undetermined origin. A barium contrast esophagogram is needed unless plain films reveal an esophageal foreign object, evidence of perforation (e.g., pneumothorax, emphysematous mediastinitis, pleural or mediastinal effusion), or an obvious hiatal hernia. Even if megaesophagus is present, a barium contrast study can be used to determine the presence of obstruction at the lower esophageal sphincter (rare) or cricopharyngeal incompetence (worsens prognosis). Ultrasonography is seldom useful unless a thoracic mass is present.

### Radiographic findings

Esophageal dilation, foreign objects, soft-tissue densities, spondylosis suggestive of spirocercosis, and hiatal hernia may often be .dentified on plain films. An air-filled esophagus is not always diagnostic for megaesophagus. Accumulation of food in the classic location for a vascular ring anomaly may also be caused by localized esophageal weakness or a thymic cyst.

*Contrast radiography.* Obstruction is suggested by abrupt termination of the barium column as it travels caudally; weakness usually causes retention of contrast throughout the esophagus. Partial obstruction is suggested by retention of barium-impregnated food but not of liquid or paste. Contrast esophagograms should be considered in patients with unidentified thoracic masses, because many esophageal tumors radiographically resemble pulmonary parenchymal masses.

*Reflux esophagitis.* Gastroesophageal reflux and esophagitis can be difficult to diagnose radiographically. Barium may adhere to severely diseased mucosa, but less severe esophagitis may not be detected. Norma. dogs may have an episode of gastroesophageal reflux during a contrast study, whereas dogs with pathologic gastroesophageal reflux may not have reflux during the examination.

## Imaging of the Stomach and Small Intestine

### Plain radiographs

Plain radiographs may be used to detect masses, foreign objects, gas- or fluid-distended hollow viscus, misshapen or emphysematous parenchymal organs, pneumoperitoneum, abdominal effusion, and displacement of organs suggestive of a mass or adhesion.

*Gastric abnormalities.* Gastric outflow obstruction can be difficult to diagnose with plain radiographs unless gastric distention is marked or foreign objects or masses are seen. However, gastric dilation, especially with volvulus, is easily recognized. Radiolucent gastric foreign objects may be seen if outlined by swallowed air.

*Intestinal distention.* Obstructed intestines typically become distended with air, fluid, and/or ingesta. However, intestinal distention may be caused by inflammation (adynamic or physiologic ileus) as well as obstruction (mechanical, occlusive, or anatomic ileus). Therefore diseases that produce severe inflammation (e.g., parvoviral enteritis) may clinically and radiographically mimic intestinal obstruction.

Anatomic ileus typically produces a greater degree of distention than physiologic ileus, and the distention is nonuniform, with "stacking" of distended loops or sharp bends and turns. If the entire intestinal tract is uniformly distended with gas and the clinical signs fit, mesenteric volvulus may be diagnosed. If marked intestinal distention is found but is very localized and seems out of place, a strangulated or incarcerated intestinal obstruction should be considered.

*Linear foreign bodies.* Linear foreign bodies rarely produce gas-distended bowel loops but tend to cause the intestines to bunch together, sometimes with small gas bubbles. In some cases "pleating" (i.e., accordion-like folding) of the intestines is seen. Pleating is often more obvious on contrast-enhanced films.

*Other intestinal abnormalities.* It is difficult to determine the thickness of intestines on plain radiographs; patients with diarrhea and increased intestinal fluid are often misdiagnosed as having thickened intestinal walls. Decreased serosal contrast (e.g., because of lack of fat or excessive abdominal fluid), displacement of stomach or intestines (suggesting a mass), and abnormal gas accumulations are other important findings. Pneumoperitoneum is diagnosed if both the thoracic and abdominal surfaces of the diaphragm or the serosal surfaces of the liver, stomach, or kidneys are easily seen.

### Ultrasonography
Ultrasonography is useful for (1) detecting intussusceptions, pancreatitis, abdominal infiltrative disease, lymphadenopathy, masses, some radiolucent foreign bodies, and small amounts of effusion not seen radiographically; (2) evaluating the hepatic parenchyma; and (3) identifying abdominal neoplasia in animals with substantial effusion. It may also be used to guide fine-needle aspiration or biopsy.

### Contrast-enhanced gastrogram
Contrast gastrograms are performed in vomiting patients when plain radiographs and ultrasound are unrevealing. Delayed gastric emptying, luminal filling defects (e.g., growths, radiolucent foreign objects), ulcers, pyloric lesions that prevent gastric emptying, and infiltrative lesions may be seen. Some vomiting patients have constrictions and infiltrative lesions (e.g., inflammatory bowel disease, tumors) in the duodenum. Normal structures can resemble an abnormality, so any abnormality must be seen on at least two films before disease can be diagnosed.

*Gastric ulcers.* Ulcers are documented when barium is seen entering the gastric or duodenal wall or when a persistent spot of barium is identified long after the stomach has emptied the contrast agent. Contrast gastrograms are not as sensitive as endoscopy for detection of gastric ulceration, and they cannot be used to detect erosions.

### Contrast-enhanced small intestinal studies
Vomiting is the principal reason for performing contrast studies of the upper small intestines. Contrast radiographs are particularly useful for distinguishing anatomic from physiologic ileus. Cranial obstructions are easier to demonstrate than caudal ones. If a very caudal obstruction is suspected (e.g., ileocolic intussusception), a barium enema (or ultrasonography) is better than an upper GI contrast series. Patients with diarrhea seldom benefit from contrast studies of the intestines.

Normal radiographic findings do not exclude severe intestinal disease, and even when radiographs suggest infiltrative disease, biopsy is still needed to determine the cause. It is usually more cost effective to perform endoscopy (or even surgery). It is easy to overinterpret contrast radiographs of the intestines; abnormalities must be seen on at least two films taken at different times before disease is diagnosed.

*Obstruction.* Complete intestinal obstruction is represented by inability of the barium column to advance beyond a certain point. (There may or may not be intestinal dilation orad to this point.) Partial obstruction may be indicated by delayed passage past a point and/or constriction of the lumen. Focal dilations not caused by obstruction (e.g., diverticula) are rare and usually represent a localized neoplastic infiltrate. In rare instances intestinal blind loops and/or short-bowel syndromes are detected. Motility problems may cause slowed passage of the contrast material through the alimentary tract.

*Enteritis and infiltration.* Enteritis is often diagnosed when a fine "brush border" is seen in the lumen, but this finding is caused by barium that is normally distributing itself among villi, not by enteritis. Infiltration is denoted by scalloped margins ("thumbprinting"); such a pattern may result from neoplasia (e.g., lymphoma), inflammatory bowel disease (e.g., lymphocytic, plasmacytic, or eosinophilic enteritis), fungal infection (e.g., histoplasmosis), or parvoviral enteritis. However, its absence does not eliminate a diagnosis of infiltrative disease.

### Imaging of the Colon and Rectum
If flexible colonoscopy is available, there seldom exists any need for barium enemas. If only rigid colonoscopy is available, barium enemas are needed to evaluate the ascending and transverse colon. When colonoscopy is unavailable, barium enema may also be useful when one is looking for infiltrative lesions (e.g., rectal or colonic neoplasia

causing hematochezia), partial or complete obstruction, and ileocolic or cecocolic intussusception. It can also be used to evaluate the colon orad to a near-complete rectal obstruction to determine if more infiltrative lesions or obstructions are present in addition to the one palpated near the rectum.

Barium enemas unreliably detect mucosal disease (ulcers, inflammation) but can reveal intraluminal filling defects representing ileocolic or cecocolic intussusception, proliferative colonic neoplasia (e.g., polyps, adenocarcinoma), extraluminal compression (smooth-surfaced displacement of barium from the colonic lumen), and infiltrative disease (roughened, partial obstruction, or "apple core" lesion). An abnormality must be found on at least two films to ensure that it is not an artifact.

## PERITONEAL FLUID ANALYSIS (TEXT P 377)

Abdominocentesis is performed with a syringe and needle or, if this fails, a multi-fenestrated catheter. If peritoneal inflammation is suspected but abdominal fluid cannot be retrieved, peritoneal lavage may be performed. Fluid analysis is discussed in Chapter 36.

## DIGESTION AND ABSORPTION TESTS (TEXT P 378)

### Serum Trypsinlike Immunoreactivity

The recommended test for exocrine pancreatic function is serum TLI. Other tests, such as measurement of fecal proteolytic activity and fat absorption with and without pancreatic enzymes, are no longer recommended. TLI is the most sensitive and specific test for EPI. The assay is even valid in animals receiving pancreatic enzyme supplements. It is primarily indicated in dogs with chronic small intestinal diarrhea or chronic weight loss of unknown origin. Feline EPI is rare, so this test is seldom needed in cats.

Normal dogs have serum TLI values of 5.2 to 35 µg/L; values <2.5 µg/L confirm EPI. Cats have higher normal values (28 to 115 µg/L). Pancreatitis, renal failure, and severe malnutrition may increase serum TLI, but this rarely causes misinterpretation of results. If EPI is caused by obstruction of the pancreatic ducts (rare) as opposed to acinar cell atrophy (common), the serum TLI test may not detect maldigestion. In such cases quantitative fecal proteolytic assay is required (see text).

### Intestinal permeability testing

Intestinal permeability can be tested by administering a sugar solution after a fast, then measuring the amounts and ratios of the sugars in blood or urine collected several hours later. Increased permeability seems to be a reliable marker of small intestinal disease, although it is not specific for any particular disease. Currently the major value to such testing is in (1) determining that a patient with clinical signs of uncertain cause has small intestinal disease, and (2) evaluating response to therapy in difficult cases.

## SERUM VITAMIN CONCENTRATIONS (TEXT PP 378-379)

Serum concentrations of cobalamin and folate are sometimes measured in animals with chronic small intestinal diarrhea or chronic weight loss of uncertain cause. Low serum cobalamin is supportive of a diagnosis of ARE or severe small intestinal mucosal disease (especially involving the ileum). Low serum folate may also be found in animals with severe intestinal mucosal disease.

The combination of decreased serum cobalamin and increased serum folate is highly specific for ARE; however, the sensitivity is questionable, because concentrations of these vitamins are normal in some animals with ARE. Serum cobalamin concentrations are usually decreased in dogs with EPI, possibly because the incidence of ARE in these patients is high. B-complex vitamin supplementation can increase serum cobalamin and folate levels.

## OTHER SPECIAL TESTS (TEXT P 379)

### Serum gastrin

Serum gastrin is measured in animals with signs suggestive of gastrinoma: chronic vomiting, weight loss, and diarrhea in older animals, especially if concurrent esophagitis or duodenal ulceration is present. Serum is collected after an overnight fast and rapidly frozen. Serum gastrin may also be increased in patients with gastric outflow obstruction, renal failure, short bowel syndrome, or atrophic gastritis or in those receiving antacid therapy such as a histamine-2 receptor antagonist or proton pump inhibitor. Resting serum gastrin levels vary, with occasional values in the normal range in gastrinoma patients. Stimulating gastrin secretion with ingestion of food or intravenous injection of secretin or calcium is more sensitive in establishing the diagnosis than is baseline serum gastrin.

### Urease activity in gastric mucosa

Testing for urease activity in gastric mucosa is sometimes performed when one is looking for *Helicobacter* spp. However, no evidence suggests that this test is more advantageous than special staining (e.g., Warthin-Starry) of multiple gastric biopsy specimens.

### Acetylcholine receptor antibodies

Antibodies to acetylcholine receptors should be measured when one is looking for causes of dysphagia or esophageal weakness that could be of neuromuscular origin (see Chapter 73). Increased titers strongly suggest a myasthenic-like disease, even if no systemic signs are present.

### 2M antibodies

Antibodies to 2M muscle fibers can help diagnose canine masticatory muscle myositis. Dogs with polymyositis are typically negative for these antibodies, whereas most dogs with masticatory muscle myositis are positive.

## ENDOSCOPY (TEXT PP 379-384)

Endoscopy is often useful when radiographs and ultrasonography are nondiagnostic in patients with chronic vomiting, diarrhea, or weight loss. Although excellent for detection of morphologic changes (e.g., masses, ulcers, obstruction), it is insensitive for revealing abnormal function (e.g., esophageal weakness).

### Esophagoscopy

Esophagoscopy is indicated in patients with suspected or confirmed esophageal masses, obstruction, esophagitis, or regurgitation. Esophageal tumors, foreign objects, inflammation, and obstructions caused by cicatrix are readily diagnosed; foreign objects and cicatrix can sometimes be treated endoscopically. Esophagoscopy may also aid in identification of partial obstructions not detected with contrast esophagograms.

It is important that the stomach be entered and the tip of the scope retroflexed to examine the lower esophageal sphincter area for leiomyomas and other easily missed lesions. Care must be taken to avoid creating potentially fatal tension pneumothorax in patients with esophageal perforation.

### Gastroduodenoscopy

Gastroduodenoscopy and biopsy are indicated in animals with vomiting, apparent gastroduodenal reflux, or small intestinal disease. It is more sensitive and specific for detection of mucosal ulcers, erosions, tumors, and inflammatory lesions than diagnostic imaging techniques. Biopsies of the gastric and duodenal mucosae should always be obtained, because normal visual findings do not rule out severe mucosal disease. As with esophagoscopy, gastroscopy is not sensitive when one is looking for functional problems (e.g., gastric hypomotility).

### Colonoscopy

Proctoscopy or colonoscopy is indicated in animals with chronic large bowel disease that is unresponsive to appropriate dietary, antibacterial, or anthelmintic therapies. Proctoscopy is performed in patients with obvious rectal abnormalities (e.g., stricture felt on digital rectal examination). Colonoscopy allows a more thorough evaluation of the colon. If a flexible scope is used, the ileocolic valve and cecum should be inspected.

Biopsy of the mucosae should always be performed; normal appearance does not eliminate significant disease. Strictured areas with relatively normal-appearing mucosa are usually caused by a submucosal lesion, in which case biopsy must be aggressive enough to include the submucosa. Cytology is sensitive for histoplasmosis and prototothecosis, and it may be useful for some neoplasms and eosinophilic colitis.

*Ileoscopy.* Ileoscopy is indicated in dogs and cats with diarrhea and in cats with vomiting. It is usually performed during flexible colonoscopy and requires thorough colonic cleansing so that the ileocolic valve can be visualized. It is difficult or impossible for the ileum in most cats to be entered, but biopsy forceps can often be passed through the ileocolic valve to perform blind biopsy of the ileal mucosa.

## BIOPSY TECHNIQUES (TEXT PP 384-385)

### Fine-needle aspiration

Fine-needle aspiration or core biopsy of enlarged lymph nodes, abdominal masses, and infiltrated abdominal organs may be done via abdominal palpation or ultrasonography if the structure can be held stationary. A 23- to 25-gauge needle is typically used so that inadvertent intestinal or vascular perforation is insignificant.

### Endoscopic biopsy

Rigid endoscopy usually provides excellent biopsy samples of the descending colon. Flexible endoscopes allow access to most areas of the alimentary tract, but the tissue samples obtained may not always be deep enough to allow diagnosis of submucosal lesions. Ideally, the tissue to undergo biopsy is visualized; however, the biopsy forceps can be passed through the pylorus or ileocolic valve to perform blind biopsy of the duodenum or ileum if necessary. Handling of samples is discussed in the text.

Two common problems with endoscopically obtained tissue samples are insufficient sample size and excessive artifact. Lymphoma is sometimes relatively deep in the mucosa (or submucosal), and a superficial biopsy reveals tissue reaction only above the tumor, resulting in a misdiagnosis of inflammatory bowel disease. Multiple biopsy samples should be taken until at least five samples of excellent size and depth (full mucosal thickness) have been obtained.

*Interpretation.* A squash preparation of one tissue specimen can be evaluated cytologically; the remaining samples are fixed in formalin and evaluated histologically. Cytology of the gastric mucosa may reveal adenocarcinoma, lymphoma, inflammatory cells, or large numbers of spirochetes. Cytology of intestinal mucosa may reveal eosinophilic enteritis, lymphoma, histoplasmosis, prototothecosis, and occasionally giardiasis, bacteria, or *Heterobilharzia.* The absence of cytologic findings suggestive of these disorders does not eliminate them, but finding them cytologically is diagnostic.

### Full-thickness surgical biopsy

Full-thickness biopsies obtained at surgery usually have less artifact and allow evaluation of submucosal tissue. If surgery is performed, the entire abdomen should be examined from the beginning of the stomach to the end of the colon, and all parenchymal organs evaluated. Biopsies should be obtained from all obviously abnormal tissues. Biopsy specimens of the stomach, duodenum, jejunum, ileum, mesenteric lymph nodes, liver, and pancreas (cats) should also be obtained, regardless of their appearance. Even if an obvious lesion (e.g., a large tumor) is found, it is wise to perform biopsies of these other tissues. In emaciated animals, gastrostomy or enterostomy feeding tubes can be placed before the abdomen is exited.

# 30

# General Therapeutic Principles

## (Text pp 387-404)

## FLUID THERAPY (TEXT PP 387-389)

### Electrolyte Needs

Fluid therapy is used primarily to treat shock, dehydration, and electrolyte and acid-base disturbances. Vomiting animals are often assumed to be hypokalemic; however, patients with hypoadrenocorticism or anuric renal failure may be hyperkalemic. Serum electrolytes should be measured, but if fluid therapy must begin before they are available, physiologic saline solution plus 20 mEq of potassium chloride (KCl) per liter is a reasonable choice. A lead II electrocardiographic tracing may be used to identify moderate to severe hyperkalemia (see Chapter 55). Bicarbonate administration is rarely needed. Bicarbonate or lactated Ringer's solution should not be used if alkalosis is likely (e.g., with vomiting of gastric origin).

### Routes of Administration

#### Parenteral

Parenteral administration is indicated when the patient is significantly hypovolemic or if absorption of enteral fluids is uncertain (e.g., with intestinal obstruction, vomiting, ileus). Shock necessitates intravenous (IV) fluid administration. The intramedullary (IMed) route may be used if an IV catheter cannot be placed; the intraperitoneal route is acceptable, but it repletes the intravascular compartment more slowly than the IV and IMed routes.

Subcutaneous (SC) administration is acceptable if the patient is not in shock, can absorb the fluid, and allows repeated SC administration. Multiple SC depots of 10 to 50 ml are given, depending on the patient's size. Severely dehydrated animals may not absorb SC fluids as rapidly as desired, making initial IV or oral (PO) administration more desirable.

#### Oral

Oral rehydration makes use of intestinal sodium absorption. Coadministration of dextrose or an amino acid speeds up sodium and water absorption. This approach works only if the patient can ingest PO fluids without vomiting and has functional intestinal mucosa. Many dogs and cats with acute enteritis not caused by severe parvovirus infection can be rehydrated orally.

### Fluid Rate and Type

Dogs in shock may be given up to 88 ml of isotonic crystalloids per kilogram intravenously during the first hour. (Sometimes this rate must be exceeded to reestablish adequate peripheral perfusion.) In general the initial fluid rate for cats in shock should not exceed 55 ml/kg. Lactated Ringer's or physiologic saline solution is commonly used; fluids given rapidly to treat shock should not contain much supplemental potassium.

### Hypertonic saline

Hypertonic (e.g., 7%) saline solution may be used to treat severe hypovolemic or endotoxic shock at a rate of 4 to 5 ml/kg over 10 minutes. The solution can be readministered in 2 ml/kg aliquots until a total of 10 ml/kg has been given or serum sodium is >160 mEq/L. Isotonic fluids are then continued at a reduced rate (e.g., 10 to 20 ml/kg/hr) until shock is controlled. A mixture of 7% saline plus Dextran 70, given at 3 to 5 ml/kg over 5 minutes, has a longer duration of effect than hypertonic saline alone.

Hypertonic solutions should not be used in patients with hypernatremic dehydration, cardiogenic shock, or renal failure; uncontrolled hemorrhage may also be a contraindication. Dextran is rarely associated with allergic reactions or renal failure but should be used carefully or not at all in patients with coagulopathies.

### Colloids

Colloids (e.g., hetastarch) are also useful for treating shock. Their effects last longer than hypertonic saline, and they do not increase total body sodium. Small volumes (5 to 10 ml/kg, maximum of 20 ml/kg/day) are administered quickly; the subsequent IV fluid rate is reduced to avoid hypertension. Colloids should be used cautiously in patients with bleeding tendencies.

### Hypoproteinemia

Excessive fluids can dilute and further decrease serum albumin and plasma oncotic pressure, causing ascites, edema, and diminished peripheral perfusion. In patients with severe hypoalbuminemia (serum albumin <1.5 g/dl) a plasma transfusion (6 to 10 ml/kg) should be considered. Serum albumin should be measured 8 to 12 hours after the transfusion. Animals with severe protein-losing enteropathies and nephropathies rapidly excrete the supplemented protein, making repeated transfusion necessary.

Hetastarch (5 to 20 ml/kg/day) and Dextran 70 may be used in place of plasma or albumin. Hetastarch may persist in the intravascular space longer than albumin and help maintain plasma oncotic pressure in animals with severe protein-losing enteropathies. When hetastarch is used, the maintenance fluid rate must be reduced to avoid hypertension. Human albumin has been used instead of canine plasma, but glomerulonephritis is a potential complication.

## Estimating Requirements

### Initial fluid needs

Dehydrated animals are treated by replacing the estimated fluid deficit. First, the degree of dehydration must be estimated. Prolonged skin tenting is usually first noticed at 5% to 6% dehydration. Dry, tacky oral mucous membranes usually indicate 6% to 7% dehydration.

Next, multiplication of the estimated percentage of dehydration by the patient's weight (in kilograms) yields the number of liters needed to replace the deficit. This amount is replaced over 2 to 8 hours, depending on the patient's condition. The fluid rate generally should not exceed 88 ml/kg/hr. It is better to overestimate rather than underestimate the fluid deficit, unless the patient has congestive heart failure, anuric or oliguric renal failure, severe hypoproteinemia, severe anemia, or pulmonary edema.

### Maintenance requirements

Maintenance fluids are administered once fluid deficits have been replaced. Maintenance requirements are approximately 60 ml/kg/day. In general, potassium should be supplemented if the patient is anorexic or vomiting, has diarrhea, or is receiving prolonged or intensive fluid therapy (Table 30-1). Cats receiving IV fluids often have an initial drop in serum potassium, even when the fluids contain 40 mEq KCl/L. Oral potassium is often more effective than parenteral supplementation if the animal is not vomiting.

***Continued losses.*** Adequacy of fluid therapy can be gauged by regularly weighing the patient. Progressive weight loss implies inadequate fluid therapy in the face of ongoing fluid loss. A change of 1 pound represents approximately 500 ml of water. Ongoing losses can be estimated from observation of vomiting, diarrhea, and urination; however, underestimation is common.

Table 30-1

## General Guidelines for Potassium Supplementation of IV Fluids

| Plasma potassium concentration (mEq/L) | Amount of KCl to add to fluids given at maintenance rates* (mEq/L) |
|:---:|:---:|
| 3.7-5 | 10-20 |
| 3-3.7 | 20-30 |
| 2.5-3 | 30-40 |
| 2-2.5 | 40-60 |
| <2 | 60-70 |

*Do not exceed 0.5 mEq $K^+$/kg/hr, except in animals in hypokalemic emergencies, and then only with constant, close electrocardiographic monitoring. Be sure to routinely monitor plasma potassium concentrations whenever administering fluids with >30 mEq $K^+$/L.

*KCl,* Potassium chloride.

### Monitoring Fluid Therapy

Development of inspiratory pulmonary crackles, a systolic heart murmur, a gallop rhythm, or edema (especially cervical) suggests overhydration. Central venous pressure (CVP) is an excellent indicator of excessive fluid administration; however, it is rarely needed except in patients with severe cardiac or renal failure and those receiving aggressive fluid therapy. CVP is normally <4 cm $H_2O$ and generally should not exceed 10 cm $H_2O$, even with aggressive fluid therapy.

## DIETARY MANAGEMENT (TEXT PP 389-396)

Symptomatic or specific dietary therapy is often important in animals with gastrointestinal (GI) tract problems. Symptomatic therapy usually involves feeding a bland, easily digested diet. Specific therapy typically involves feeding elimination or hypoallergenic diets, diets with a highly restricted fat content, fiber-supplemented diets, or a combination of these.

### Bland Diets

Bland, easily digestible diets are indicated in animals with acute gastritis or enteritis. Such diets are available commercially but can be homemade (e.g., combinations of boiled poultry, lean hamburger, fish, low-fat cottage cheese, boiled rice, and/or boiled potatoes). Frequent, small amounts are fed until the diarrhea resolves. The diet is then gradually returned to normal. The bland diet may be continued long-term, although it must be nutritionally balanced if it is homemade (especially in puppies and kittens).

### Elimination or Hypoallergenic Diets

Elimination or hypoallergenic diets are indicated if dietary allergy or intolerance is suspected. The diet may be composed of the same ingredients found in bland diets, but it must be formulated to contain food that the patient has not eaten before or that is very unlikely to provoke allergy or intolerance (e.g., potatoes). Commercial elimination diets are available, although it may be best to try a homemade one first (see text).

Elimination diets must be fed for at least 6 weeks (preferably >8 weeks) before their efficacy can be accurately determined. No other foods or treats should be offered, including pills, toys, or medications with flavorings. If signs resolve during this time, the diet should be continued for at least another 4 weeks. If the diet seems effective, a more convenient commercial diet may be substituted. If the homemade diet will be continued, appropriate vitamins, minerals, and fatty acids should be added (see text).

### Partially Hydrolyzed Diets

Partially hydrolyzed diets are formulated to eliminate proteins large enough to cause immunologic reactions. These diets are not hypoallergenic for all animals, but many dogs and cats do not have allergic reactions to them. Another advantage of these diets is that the partially hydrolyzed proteins may be easier for the diseased alimentary tract to digest and absorb.

### Elemental Diets

The nutrients in these diets are supplied as amino acids and simple sugars. Elemental diets are hypoallergenic; they are also extremely easy to digest and absorb in animals with major small intestinal disease, and they do not contribute to further intestinal inflammation in animals with "leaky gut." The elemental diets prepared for people typically contain less protein than desired for dogs and cats, but they can be supplemented with amino acids (see text).

### Low-Fat Diets

Ultra–low-fat diets are indicated in animals with intestinal lymphangiectasia. Medium-chain triglycerides (MCTs) have been recommended as supplements to such diets; however, they have an unpleasant taste, so only small amounts (e.g., 1 tsp/lb of food) should be added to the diet. Using a highly digestible, ultra–low-fat diet usually eliminates the need for supplementing MCTs.

### High-Fiber Diets

Fiber supplementation may help dogs and cats with large intestinal diseases. Insoluble fiber is poorly digested or metabolized by bacteria, so it produces more bulky stool. Some insoluble fibers also help to normalize colonic myoelectrical activity (i.e., help prevent spasms). Soluble fiber is metabolized by bacteria into short-chain volatile fatty acids, which are trophic to colonic mucosa; however, soluble fiber may slow small intestinal absorption of nutrients.

Fiber-enriched diets help correct diarrhea in many animals with large bowel disease, especially those with minimal inflammation; they also lessen constipation not caused by obstruction or pain. Such a diet should be fed for at least 2 weeks, although most patients that respond do so within the first week. A commercial high-fiber diet may be used, or fiber can be added to the current diet. Psyllium hydrocolloid (Metamucil) or coarse, unprocessed wheat bran is added at the rate of 1 to 2 tsp/can or 1 to 4 tbsp/can of food, respectively. Adequate water intake is important to prevent obstipation.

### Special Nutritional Supplementation

Refusal to ingest adequate calories necessitates special supplementation. Daily maintenance requirements should be calculated to avoid underfeeding; 60 kcal/kg/day is a reasonable estimate for mature dogs and cats that are not lactating or experiencing significant energy or protein losses. More precise calculations are recommended if the patient has severe disease or ongoing fluid and nutritional losses (Box 30-1).

#### Appetite stimulants

Simply sending the animal home, warming the food, and offering very palatable foods (e.g., chicken baby food) sometimes ensure adequate intake. Cyproheptadine (2 to 4 mg/cat) stimulates some mildly anorectic cats to eat, but it seldom causes severely anorectic cats (e.g., those with severe hepatic lipidosis) to eat enough. Megestrol acetate is an excellent appetite stimulant but occasionally causes diabetes mellitus, reproductive problems, and tumors. Appetite stimulants are usually less effective in dogs than in cats.

#### Tube feeding

Tube feeding is more reliable for ensuring adequate caloric intake. Intermittent orogastric tube feeding is useful in patients that need nutritional support for only a short time, although it may be used longer in orphaned puppies and kittens.

***Nasoesophageal tube.*** Nasoesophageal tubes are indicated in animals that need nutritional support and have a functional esophagus, stomach, and intestines. They are easy to place but difficult to maintain in vomiting animals. Small-diameter tubes (e.g., 5 French) are needed in small dogs and cats, which limits feeding options to a commercial liquid diet and limits the rate of administration. Some dogs and cats do not tolerate

---

**Box 30-1**

## Calculation of Nutritional Needs and Formulations of Parenteral Solutions

Actual body weight = _____ kg

### BASAL ENERGY REQUIREMENT

30 (weight in kg) + 70 = _____ kcal/day
However, if <2 kg or >25 kg, use 70 (weight in kg)$^{0.75}$

### MAINTENANCE ENERGY REQUIREMENT

Basal requirement × Adjustment factor = _____ kcal/day

| Adjustment factors | Dogs | Cats |
|---|---|---|
| Cage rest | (1.25) | (1.1) |
| After surgery | (1.3) | (1.12) |
| Trauma | (1.5) | (1.2) |
| Sepsis | (1.7) | (1.28) |
| Severe burn | (2) | (1.4) |

### PROTEIN REQUIREMENT

4 g/kg in adult dogs
6 g/kg in cats and hypoproteinemic dogs
If animal has renal failure, use 1.5 g/kg in dogs OR 3 g/kg in cats
Protein requirement = _____ g/day

### SOLUTION FORMATION

- _____ g of protein necessitates _____ ml of an 8.5% or 10% amino acid solution (85 or 100 mg of protein/ml, respectively).
- Determine the calories derived from the protein (4 kcal of protein per gram), and subtract this from the daily caloric needs. Supply the remaining calories with glucose and lipid. _____ kcal needed.
- Provide at least 10%, and preferably 40%, of caloric needs with lipid emulsion. A 20% lipid emulsion has 2 kcal/ml. Do not use in lipemic animals; use with caution in animals with pancreatitis. _____ ml needed. Provide remainder of calories with 50% dextrose, which has 1.7 kcal/ml. _____ ml needed.
- Use half the calculated amount of solution on the first day, and increase it to the calculated amount on the second day, if hyperglycemia, lipemia, azotemia, or hyperammonemia does not occur.
- Either use amino acid solution with electrolytes or add electrolytes so that the solution has sodium at 35 mEq/L, chloride at 35 mEq/L, potassium at 42 mEq/L, magnesium at 5 mEq/L, and phosphate at 15 mmol/L. These concentrations may be adjusted as needed, depending on the animal's serum electrolyte concentrations. Add multiple vitamins and trace elements (especially zinc and copper) that are formulated for use in parenteral nutrition solutions.

---

nasoesophageal tubes and continually pull them out. However, these tubes are usually effective for short-term therapy (1 to 10 days), and some animals tolerate them for weeks. Rhinitis occurs in some patients.

*Pharyngostomy and esophagostomy tube.* Pharyngostomy and esophagostomy tubes are indicated in animals with a functional esophagus, stomach, and intestines that do not tolerate nasoesophageal or intermittent tube feeding. Both types of tube effectively bypass oral lesions. Other advantages include easy placement and removal and minimal complications if the tube is properly inserted. However, it is easy to malposition pharyngostomy tubes such that they cause gagging and regurgitation, especially in cats and small dogs. Vomiting can make it difficult to maintain these tubes, but they may be used for weeks or months. Because the tubes used are larger than nasoesophageal tubes, homemade gruels can be fed.

**Gastrostomy tube.** Gastrostomy tubes can be used in animals with functional stomach and intestines when nasoesophageal, pharyngoesophagostomy, or intermittent gastric tubing are unacceptable. Gastrostomy tubes allow administration of thick gruels and are often tolerated for months. Vomiting is not a contraindication. Surgery, endoscopy, or a special device designed for gastrostomy tube placement is necessary. The major risks are leakage and peritonitis, which is rare but catastrophic. Low-profile gastrostomy tubes can be used if a stoma has been established by a routine gastrostomy tube (see text).

**Enterostomy tube.** Enterostomy tubes are indicated in animals with functional intestines when the stomach must be bypassed (e.g., recent gastric surgery). Laparotomy or laparoscopy is needed to place these tubes (see text). The small diameter of enterostomy tubes typically necessitates administration of commercial liquid diets, which are best infused at a constant rate. If diarrhea develops, the rate is decreased or fiber (e.g., psyllium) is added to the liquid diet.

### Diets for Special Enteral Support
Commercial diets may be used for enteral support. Diets containing glutamine, which is critical for small intestinal mucosal nutrition, may be beneficial. If the feeding tube diameter is sufficient, blended commercial diets can be used. For example, a gruel made by blending one can of Hill's feline p/d with 1.5 cups (350 ml) of water provides approximately 0.9 kcal/ml and is useful in dogs and cats. Elemental diets may be better than blended gruels in animals with intestinal disease. Note: When feeding cats, ensure that the diet contains sufficient taurine.

#### Administration rates
Bolus feeding is usually used with nasoesophageal, pharyngoesophagostomy, or gastrostomy tubes. Animals that have been anorectic for days or weeks should initially receive small amounts (e.g., 3 to 5 ml/kg) every 2 to 4 hours. The amount is gradually increased and the frequency decreased until the patient is receiving its caloric needs in three or four daily feedings. Typically, 22 to 30 ml/kg/feeding is administered to most dogs and cats. Larger volumes may be given if vomiting or distress does not result. Constant-rate infusion is generally used with enterostomy tubes (see text). Constant infusion may also be done through gastrostomy or esophagostomy tubes in animals that readily vomit when fed in boluses (e.g., some cats with severe hepatic lipidosis).

### Parenteral Nutrition
Parenteral nutrition is indicated if the intestines cannot reliably absorb nutrients. It is the most certain method of providing nutrition; however, it is expensive and has potential metabolic and infectious complications.

#### Total parenteral nutrition
When total parenteral nutrition (TPN) is used, daily caloric and protein requirements are determined (see Box 30-1) and the customized solution is administered by constant IV infusion. Body weight, rectal temperature, urine glucose, and serum sodium, chloride, potassium, phosphorus, and glucose must be regularly monitored, and the feeding solution adjusted to prevent or correct serum imbalances. If possible, the patient should also receive some PO feedings to help prevent intestinal villous atrophy.

A central IV line must be dedicated to TPN solution administration only. Aseptic placement and management of the catheter are the best protection against catheter-related sepsis. Prophylactic antibiotics do not replace proper management and are ineffective in preventing infections.

#### Partial parenteral nutrition
Partial parenteral nutrition is similar to TPN, but it (1) aims to supply approximately 50% of the caloric needs; (2) has a lower osmolality, so it can be administered via a

peripheral vein; and (3) is intended to be used for approximately 1 week, with the goal of getting a severely ill or emaciated patient "over the hump" before starting enteral nutrition.

## ANTIEMETICS (TEXT PP 396-397)

Antiemetics are indicated in many patients with acute vomiting or when vomiting is causing discomfort or excessive fluid and electrolyte losses. Peripheral-acting drugs (Table 30-2) are less effective than centrally acting ones but may suffice in patients with mild disease. Also, PO administration is an untrustworthy route in nauseated animals. If it is important to halt the vomiting, a centrally acting drug should be administered parenterally. Suppositories are convenient, but absorption is erratic.

### Centrally Acting Antiemetics
#### Phenothiazine derivatives
Prochlorperazine (Compazine) is an especially effective antiemetic. Emesis is usually prevented at doses that do not cause marked sedation. Chlorpromazine causes vasodilation and can decrease peripheral perfusion in dehydrated patients. Phenothiazines also lower the seizure threshold in animals with epilepsy.
#### Metoclopramide
Metoclopramide (Reglan) inhibits emesis by suppressing the chemoreceptor trigger zone and increasing gastric tone and peristalsis. Therefore it is contraindicated in patients with gastric or duodenal obstruction. Rarely, it worsens vomiting by causing

**Table 30-2**

### Selected Antiemetic Drugs

| Drug | Dosage* |
|---|---|
| **PERIPHERALLY ACTING DRUGS** | |
| Kaopectate | 1-2 ml/kg PO q8-12h |
| Bismuth subsalicylate (Pepto-Bismol) | 1 ml/kg PO q8-24 (dogs only) |
| Anticholinergic drugs | |
| Propantheline (Pro-Banthine) | 0.25-0.5 mg/kg PO q8h |
| Aminopentamide (Centrine) | 0.01-0.03 mg/kg SC or IM q8-12h (dogs only) |
| | 0.02 mg/kg SC or IM q8-12h (cats only) |
| **CENTRALLY ACTING DRUGS** | |
| Phenothiazine derivatives | |
| Chlorpromazine (Thorazine) | 0.3-0.5 mg/kg IM q8h |
| Prochlorperazine (Compazine) | 0.1-0.5 mg/kg IM q6-8h |
| Metoclopramide (Reglan) | 0.25-0.5 mg/kg PO, IM, or IV q8h |
| | 1-2 mg/kg/day, constant IV infusion |
| Ondansetron (Zofran) | 0.1-0.2 mg/kg SC q8h |
| Trimethobenzamide (Tigan) | 3 mg/kg PO or IM q8h (dogs only) |
| Antihistamine | |
| Diphenhydramine (Benadryl) | 2-4 mg/kg PO q8h |
| | 1-2 mg/kg IM q8-12h |
| Narcotics | |
| Not usually recommended as antiemetics, although some are quite effective after producing an initial episode of vomiting | |

*Dosages are for both dogs and cats unless otherwise specified.
*IM,* Intramuscularly; *IV,* intravenously; *PO,* orally; *SC,* subcutaneously

excessive gastric contractions. In patients with severe vomiting, metoclopramide may be more effective if given by constant IV infusion (see Table 30-2). In rare cases, patients exhibit unusual behaviors. Severe renal failure makes these adverse effects more likely.

### Other Drugs

Ondansetron (Zofran) is effective in some animals in which vomiting is not controlled with phenothiazines or metoclopramide (e.g., severe canine parvoviral enteritis). It is not effective in all vomiting animals, especially those with alimentary tract obstructions. Narcotics such as fentanyl, oxymorphone, and butorphanol may cause vomiting initially, but once the drug penetrates to the medullary vomiting center, vomiting is usually inhibited. Trimethobenzamide (Tigan) and antihistamines are effective in some animals, but generally they are untrustworthy antiemetics in dogs and cats.

## ANTACID DRUGS (TEXT P 397)

Antacid drugs (Table 30-3) are indicated when it is appropriate to lessen gastric acidity (e.g., gastric ulcer disease, acid hypersecretion resulting from renal failure, mast cell tumor, gastrinoma). They may also diminish vomiting caused by gastric hyperacidity.

### Antacids

Antacids are typically of limited efficacy. Compounds that contain aluminum or magnesium tend to be more effective and do not cause the gastric acid rebound that sometimes occurs with calcium-containing antacids. Antacids should be administered orally every 4 to 6 hours; however, this may cause diarrhea, especially with magnesium-containing compounds. These antacids may also interfere with absorption of other drugs (e.g., tetracycline, cimetidine). Hypophosphatemia is possible with extensive use of aluminum hydroxide, and hypermagnesemia can occur if magnesium-containing compounds are used in animals with renal failure.

### $H_2$-receptor antagonists

The main indication for histamine-2 ($H_2$) antagonists is treatment of gastric and duodenal ulcers and erosions. They can be used prophylactically to help prevent ulceration associated with stress and use of nonsteroidal antiinflammatory drugs (NSAIDs), but they are most effective in treatment of existing ulcers.

**Table 30-3**

### Selected Antacid Drugs

| Drug | Dosage* |
|---|---|
| **ACID TITRATING DRUGS** | |
| Aluminum hydroxide (many names) | 5-10 ml PO q4-6h |
| Magnesium hydroxide (many names) | 5-10 ml PO q4-6h (dogs) or q8-12h (cats) |
| **GASTRIC ACID SECRETION INHIBITORS** | |
| **$H_2$-receptor antagonists** | |
| Cimetidine (Tagamet) | 5-10 mg/kg PO, IM, or IV q6-8h |
| Ranitidine (Zantac) | 2 mg/kg PO or IV q8-12h (dogs only) |
| | 2.5 mg/kg IV or 3.5 mg/kg PO q12h (cats only) |
| Famotidine (Pepcid, Pepcid AC) | 0.5 mg/kg PO or IM q12-24h |
| **Proton pump inhibitor** | |
| Omeprazole (Prilosec) | 0.7-1.5 mg/kg PO q12-24h (dogs only) |

*Dosages are for both dogs and cats unless otherwise specified.

*IM,* Intramuscularly; *IV,* intravenously; *PO,* orally.

Cimetidine (Tagamet) is effective in controlling gastric acidity but needs to be given three or four times per day. It inhibits hepatic cytochrome P-450 enzymes, slowing metabolism of some drugs. Ranitidine (Zantac), famotidine (Pepcid), and nizatidine (Axid) are equally or more effective when administered one or two times per day and do not affect hepatic enzymes as much as cimetidine does. Nizatidine and ranitidine also have prokinetic effects on the stomach. Parenteral administration, especially rapid IV injection of ranitidine, may cause nausea, vomiting, and/or bradycardia.

### Proton pump inhibitors

Proton pump inhibitors include omeprazole (Prilosec) and lansoprazole (Prevacid). They are the most effective drugs for decreasing gastric acid secretion. Omeprazole is primarily used in patients with severe gastroesophageal reflux or gastrinoma, diseases in which $H_2$ antagonists are often inadequate. It is uncertain whether most patients with gastric ulcers benefit from the enhanced gastric acid secretion blockade, compared with $H_2$-receptor antagonist therapy.

## INTESTINAL PROTECTANTS (TEXT P 398)

Intestinal protectants (Table 30-4) include drugs and inert adsorbents such as Kaopectate and barium sulfate contrast media. Inert adsorbents may provide clinical relief in patients with minor inflammation, but they have no proved efficacy in the treatment of gastritis or enteritis. It is inappropriate to rely on these drugs alone in very sick patients.

### Sucralfate

Sucralfate (Carafate) is indicated for patients with gastroduodenal ulceration and erosion (GUE) but may also be useful for treatment of esophagitis. It does not prevent NSAID-induced ulceration but may help prevent stress ulceration. In patients with severe bleeding, a large initial dose (e.g., 2 to 4 g) may be used.

Sucralfate can be used with $H_2$ antagonists for severe GUE. However, sucralfate may adsorb other drugs, so any other orally administered drugs should be given 1 to 2 hours before or after sucralfate. No absolute contraindications for sucralfate exist. The biggest disadvantage is that it must be given orally, and many patients that need it are vomiting. The major adverse effect is constipation.

### Misoprostol

Misoprostol (Cytotec) is a prostaglandin $E_1$ analog that is used to help prevent NSAID-induced gastroduodenal ulceration. It is primarily used in dogs that require NSAIDs but develop associated anorexia or vomiting. Use of NSAIDs that are associated with a higher risk of GI problems (e.g., naproxen) is another indication. The

### Table 30-4

#### Selected Gastrointestinal Protectants and Cytoprotective Agents

| Drug | Dosage* | Comment |
|---|---|---|
| Sucralfate (Carafate) | 0.5-1 g (dogs) or 0.25 g (cats) PO three or four times daily, depending on animal's size; may administer 2-4 g as a "loading" dose in dogs with severe alimentary tract hemorrhage | Potentially constipating; adsorbs some other orally administered drugs; primarily used to treat existing ulcers |
| Misoprostol (Cytotec) | 2-5 µg/kg PO three times daily (dogs only) | May cause diarrhea or abdominal cramps; primarily used to prevent ulcers; not for use in pregnant animals |
| Kaopectate | 1-2 mg/kg PO four to eight times daily | Questionable efficacy |

*Dosages are for both dogs and cats unless otherwise specified.
*PO,* Orally.

major adverse effects are abdominal cramping and diarrhea (which usually disappears after 2 or 3 days). Pregnancy may be a contraindication. Misoprostol may have immunosuppressant properties, especially when it is combined with other drugs.

## DIGESTIVE ENZYME SUPPLEMENTATION (TEXT P 398)

Pancreatic enzyme supplementation is indicated to treat exocrine pancreatic insufficiency. Products vary greatly in potency. Powdered preparations tend to be more effective than enteric-coated pills. Efficacious products in dogs include Viokase-V and Pancreazyme. The powder should be mixed with the animal's food (1 to 2 tsp/meal). In addition, the feeding of a low-fat diet may help reduce diarrhea. Antacid and/or antibiotic therapy is occasionally needed to prevent gastric acidity or small intestinal bacteria from rendering the enzyme supplement ineffective. Some dogs develop stomatitis, diarrhea, or both if large amounts of enzyme are fed.

## MOTILITY MODIFIERS (TEXT PP 398-399)

### Drugs That Prolong Intestinal Transit Time

Drugs that prolong intestinal transit time (Table 30-5) are primarily used to symptomatically treat diarrhea, particularly when diarrhea causes excessive fluid or electrolyte losses or owners require diarrhea control at home. Opiates tend to be more effective than parasympatholytics (which create ileus). Both classes of drugs also have antisecretory effects. Cats do not tolerate narcotics as well as dogs, so these drugs should be avoided in this species (although loperamide may be used with caution).

Loperamide (Imodium) is so effective at decreasing intestinal flow that it could increase the risk for bacterial proliferation, thereby initiating or perpetuating disease (clinically rare). Overdose can cause collapse, vomiting, ataxia, and hypersalivation, which requires treatment with a narcotic antagonist. Diphenoxylate (Lomotil) is similar to loperamide but is less effective and has greater potential for toxicity. However, some dogs respond to it but not to loperamide. *Do not use diphenoxylate in cats.*

### Drugs That Shorten Transit Time

Prokinetic drugs empty the stomach, increase intestinal peristalsis, or both. Outflow obstruction is a contraindication, because vigorous contractions against such a lesion may cause pain and/or perforation.

**Table 30-5**

### Selected Drugs Used to Treat Diarrhea Symptomatically

| Drug | Dosage* |
|------|---------|
| **INTESTINAL MOTILITY MODIFIERS** | |
| **Anticholinergic drugs** | |
| Methscopolamine (Pamine) | 0.3-1 mg/kg PO q8h (dogs only) |
| Propantheline (Pro-Banthine) | 0.25-0.5 mg/kg PO q8-12h |
| **Opiates** | |
| Diphenoxylate (Lomotil) | 0.05-0.2 mg/kg PO q8-12h (dogs only) |
| Loperamide (Imodium) | 0.1-0.2 mg/kg PO q8-12h (dogs only) |
| | 0.08-0.16 mg/kg PO q12h (cats only) |
| Paregoric | 0.05-0.06 mg/kg PO q12h (dogs only) |
| **ANTIINFLAMMATORY AND ANTISECRETORY DRUG** | |
| Bismuth subsalicylate (Pepto-Bismol) | 1 ml/kg PO q8-12h (dogs only) for 1-2 days |

*Dosages are for both dogs and cats unless otherwise specified.
*PO,* Orally.

### Metoclopramide
Metoclopramide is effective only on the stomach and proximal duodenum. However, it can be administered parenterally.

### Cisapride
Cisapride stimulates normal motility from the lower esophageal sphincter to the anus. It is usually effective unless the tissue has suffered irreparable damage (e.g., megacolon in cats). Primarily used for constipation, it may also be used for gastroparesis or gastroesophageal reflux (usually more effective than metoclopramide) and small intestinal ileus. Rarely, it may benefit dogs with megaesophagus. Cisapride is available only as an oral preparation. It has few adverse effects, although large doses may cause diarrhea, muscle tremors, ataxia, fever, aggression, and other central nervous system (CNS) signs.

### Erythromycin and $H_2$ antagonists
Erythromycin enhances gastric motility at doses lower than required for antibacterial activity (i.e., 2 mg/kg). It may also increase intestinal motility. Nizatidine and ranitidine also have gastric prokinetic effects at routinely used doses.

### Bethanechol
Bethanechol (Urecholine) is an acetylcholine analog that stimulates intestinal motility and secretion. It produces strong contractions that can cause pain or injury; it is therefore infrequently used except to increase urinary bladder contractions. Urinary outflow tract obstruction is a contraindication.

### Pyridostigmine
Pyridostigmine (Mestinon) inhibits acetylcholinesterase and is used to treat myasthenia gravis. This drug is used for acquired megaesophagus associated with antibodies to acetylcholine receptors. It must be used cautiously; overdose can cause signs of parasympathetic overload (e.g., vomiting, miosis, diarrhea). Azathioprine (with or without steroids) is better for long-term treatment of myasthenia gravis.

## ANTIINFLAMMATORY AND ANTISECRETORY DRUGS (TEXT PP 399-401)
Intestinal antiinflammatory or antisecretory drugs (see Table 30-5) are indicated for lessening fluid losses from diarrhea and for controlling intestinal inflammation that is unresponsive to dietary or antibacterial therapy.

### Bismuth subsalicylate
Pepto-Bismol is effective in many dogs with acute enteritis. The main disadvantages are that the salicylate is absorbed (warranting caution in cats and in dogs receiving other nephrotoxic drugs), it turns stools black (which mimics melena), and it must be administered orally (unpalatable). Bismuth is bactericidal for certain organisms including *Helicobacter* spp.

### Salicylazosulfapyridine
Sulfasalazine (Azulfidine) is indicated in animals with significant colonic inflammation, not for empirical therapy of undefined diarrhea. This drug is generally not beneficial for small intestinal problems.

*Dosage.* The dosage in dogs generally is 50 to 60 mg/kg, divided q8h (not to exceed 3 g/day). It may be effective at lower doses when used with glucocorticoids. Many dogs with colitis respond in 3 to 5 days. However, the drug should be given for 2 weeks before deciding that it is ineffective. If signs of colitis resolve, the dose should be gradually reduced.

A dosage of 15 to 20 mg/kg/day, divided q12h, is often tolerated in cats. But cats must be closely observed for salicylate intoxication (lethargy, anorexia, vomiting, hyperthermia, and/or tachypnea). Some cats that vomit or become anorexic may tolerate the medication if enteric-coated tablets are used.

*Precautions.* If the patient cannot be weaned off the drug entirely, the lowest effective dose should be used and the patient monitored regularly for drug-induced adverse effects. Sulfasalazine may cause transient or permanent keratoconjunctivitis sicca. Other complications may include cutaneous vasculitis, arthritis, bone marrow suppression, diarrhea, and any other problem associated with sulfa drugs or NSAIDs.

*Related drugs.* Olsalazine and mesalamine do not contain sulfa, which is responsible for most of the adverse effects of sulfasalazine. They may be as effective as sulfasalazine, but safer. Olsalazine and mesalamine have been used effectively in dogs. Their dose is in general approximately half that of sulfasalazine. Keratoconjunctivitis sicca has been reported in dogs receiving mesalamine.

### Corticosteroids

Corticosteroids are used for chronic alimentary tract inflammation (e.g., moderate to marked lymphocytic, plasmacytic, or eosinophilic inflammatory bowel disease) that is unresponsive to elimination diets. Myasthenia and perianal fistulas may also respond. Relatively high doses (e.g., prednisolone, 2.2 mg/kg/day) are often used initially. Response may be rapid or may take weeks. If PO administration is a problem in a cat, long-acting steroid injections may be used. Sometimes dexamethasone is effective when prednisolone is not, but dexamethasone seems to have more adverse effects.

*Precautions.* Corticosteroids often benefit cats with inflammatory bowel disease, but they may worsen ulcerative or lymphocytic-plasmacytic colitis in some dogs. Iatrogenic Cushing's syndrome is a problem in dogs. It is important to have a definitive diagnosis before high-dose prednisolone therapy is used, because some diseases that mimic steroid-responsive lymphocytic colitis (e.g., histoplasmosis) are absolute contraindications to corticosteroid therapy.

### Retention enemas

Enemas containing corticosteroids or 5-aminosalicylic acid are sometimes indicated in patients with severe distal colitis. These enemas place large doses of antiinflammatory agent directly on the affected area while minimizing systemic effects.

### Budesonide

Budesonide is an orally administered steroid designed to have minimal systemic effects because it is eliminated by first-pass hepatic metabolism. This drug has been used for inflammatory bowel disease and hepatic disease. Iatrogenic hyperadrenocorticism has been reported with its use.

### Immunosuppressive therapy

Treatment with azathioprine or chlorambucil is indicated in animals with severe inflammatory bowel disease that is unresponsive to corticosteroid and dietary therapy. Immunosuppressive therapy allows corticosteroids to be used at lower doses and for shorter periods of time. However, the possibility of adverse effects from these drugs usually limits their use to patients with severe disease. They should be used only if the diagnosis has been confirmed histopathologically.

*Azathioprine (Imuran).* Azathioprine is commonly used for severe lymphocytic-plasmacytic infiltrates. It may also be useful for myasthenia. The dose in dogs is 50 mg/m² daily or every other day. A lower dose (0.3 mg/kg every other day) has been used in cats, but it is not recommended because of the risk of myelotoxicity. In both species it may take 2 to 5 weeks before beneficial effects are seen. In cats the major side effect is neutropenia caused by myelosuppression. If the neutrophil count drops below 2000/μl, the drug should be stopped or the dose decreased. Side effects in dogs include hepatic disease, pancreatitis, and bone marrow suppression.

*Chlorambucil (Leukeran).* Chlorambucil is used for the same intestinal conditions as azathioprine but has fewer adverse effects. A reasonable starting dose in cats is 1 mg twice a week for cats <3.5 kg and 2 mg twice a week for cats >3.5 kg; it may take 4 to 5 weeks before any benefit is seen. If a response is noted, the dose is very slowly decreased over the next 2 to 3 months while the patient is monitored for myelosuppression.

## ANTIBACTERIAL DRUGS (TEXT P 401)

In dogs and cats with GI problems, antibiotics are primarily indicated when aspiration pneumonia, fever, a leukogram suggesting sepsis, severe neutropenia, antibiotic-responsive enteropathy, clostridial colitis, symptomatic *Helicobacter* gastritis, and perhaps hematemesis or melena are suspected. Animals with acute abdomen may be treated with antibiotics while the disease is being defined. In general, however, routine use of anti-microbials is not recommended unless the patient is at significantly increased risk for infection or a specific disorder is being treated.

Occasionally, pets have enteritis caused by specific bacteria, but even that is not necessarily an indication for antibiotics. Clinical signs caused by some bacterial enteri-tidies (e.g., salmonellosis, enterohemorrhagic *Escherichia coli*) generally do not resolve more quickly when the patient is treated with antibiotics, even those to which the organism is sensitive.

### Broad-spectrum coverage

If systemic or abdominal sepsis is suspected to have originated from the alimentary tract (e.g., parvoviral enteritis, perforated intestine), broad-spectrum antimicrobial therapy is indicated. Antibiotics with a good aerobic gram-positive and anaerobic spec-trum (e.g., ampicillin, 20 mg/kg IV q6h or clindamycin, 10 mg/kg IV q8h) combined with antibiotics with excellent activity against most aerobic bacteria (e.g., amikacin, 25 mg/kg IV q24h or enrofloxacin, 15 mg/kg IV q24h) are often effective.

To improve the anaerobic spectrum, especially if a cephalosporin is used instead of ampicillin, metronidazole (10 mg/kg IV q8 to 12h) may be included. Alternatively, a second-generation cephalosporin (e.g., cefoxitin, 22 mg/kg IV q6 to 8h) may be used. In general, it takes 48 to 72 hours before it is clear whether the therapy is effective.

### Helicobacter gastritis

Gastritis associated with *Helicobacter* may be treated with various combinations of drugs. A combination of an antacid (e.g., famotidine or omeprazole) and a macrolide antibiotic (e.g., erythromycin or azithromycin) or amoxicillin is very effective. Adding metronidazole may enhance efficacy. Some patients respond to erythromycin or amoxi-cillin alone. If high doses of erythromycin (e.g., 22 mg/kg q12h) cause vomiting, the dose may be lowered to 10 to 15 mg/kg q12h. A 10- to 14-day course of combination therapy is adequate in most patients, although recurrence is common.

### Metronidazole

Metronidazole (10 to 15 mg/kg q12h) is commonly used in animals with inflam-matory bowel disease (IBD). It has activity against anaerobic bacteria and protozoa (e.g., *Giardia),* as well as having immunomodulatory effects. Adverse effects are uncommon but include salivation, vomiting, CNS abnormalities (e.g., seizures), and neutropenia. These adverse effects usually resolve after drug withdrawal. Some cats and a few dogs with IBD respond to metronidazole better than they do to corticosteroids.

## ANTHELMINTIC DRUGS (TEXT PP 401-402)

Anthelmintics are frequently prescribed for dogs and cats with alimentary disease, even if parasitism is not the primary problem. It is reasonable to use these drugs empirically for suspected parasitic infections in patients with acute or chronic diarrhea. Table 30-6 lists selected anthelmintics.

## ENEMAS, LAXATIVES, AND CATHARTICS (TEXT PP 402-403)

### Enemas

#### Retention enemas

Retention enemas are given so that the administered material stays in the colon until it has its desired effect. Overdistention of the colon and use of drugs that may be absorbed with undesirable effects should be avoided. Suspected or pending colonic rupture is a contraindication (although difficult to predict). Neurosurgical patients receiving corticosteroids (e.g., dexamethasone) may be at increased risk for colonic perforation. Animals with colonic tumors or recent colonic surgery or biopsy also should not receive enemas.

#### Cleansing enemas

Cleansing enemas are used to remove fecal material. Large volumes of warm water are repeatedly infused into the rectum. Volumes of 50 to 100 ml are tolerated by most small dogs, 200 to 500 ml by medium dogs, and 1 to 2 L by large dogs. Care should

**Table 30-6**

## Selected Anthelmintics

| Drug | Dosage* (PO) | Use | Comments |
|---|---|---|---|
| Albendazole (Valbazen) | 25 mg/kg q12h for 3 days (dogs only)<br>25 mg/kg q12h for 5 days (cats only) | G | May cause leukopenia in some animals. Do not use in early pregnancy. Not approved for use in dogs. |
| Fenbendazole (Panacur) | 50 mg/kg for 3 days | H, R, W, G | Not approved for use in cats but can be used for 3-5 days in cats to eliminate *Giardia*. Give with food. |
| Furazolidone | 4.4 mg/kg q12h for 5 days | G | |
| Metronidazole (Flagyl) | 50 mg/kg for 5-10 days (dogs only)<br>25-50 mg/kg for 5 days (cats only) | G | Rarely causes neurologic signs. |
| Pyrantel (Nemex) | 5 mg/kg, repeat in 7-10 days (dogs only)<br>20 mg/kg, once only (cats only) | H, R, P | Give after meal. |
| Ivermectin | 200 µg/kg (dogs only) | H, R, P | Do not use in Collies, Shelties, Border Collies, or Australian Shepherds. Use with caution in Old English Sheepdogs. Approved for use only as heartworm preventive. |
| Milbemycin (Interceptor) | 0.5 mg/kg, monthly | H, R, W | Not approved for use in cats. |
| Praziquantel (Droncit) | 5 mg/kg for dogs >6.8 kg<br>7.5 mg/kg for dogs <6.8 kg<br>6.3 mg/kg for cats <1.8 kg<br>5 mg/kg for cats >1.8 kg | T | 10 mg/kg for juvenile *Echinococcus* spp. |
| Epsiprantel (Cestex) | 5.5 mg/kg for dogs<br>2.75 mg/kg for cats | T | |
| Selamectin (Revolution) | 6 mg/kg topical for cats | H, R | Not approved for use in dogs. |
| Sulfadimethoxine (Albon) | 50 mg/kg on day 1, then<br>27.5 mg/kg q12h for 9 days | C | |
| Trimethoprim-sulfadiazine (Tribrissen) | 30 mg/kg for 10 days | C | May cause dry eyes, arthritis, cytopenia, hepatic disease. |

*Dosages are for both dogs and cats unless otherwise specified.

*C, Coccidia; G, Giardia; H, hookworms; P, Physaloptera; PO, orally; R, roundworms; T, tapeworms; W, whipworms.*

be taken to avoid overdistending or perforating the colon. Rapid infusion often causes vomiting in cats. Suspected or pending colonic perforation is a contraindication for cleansing enemas.

### Hypertonic enemas

Hypertonic enemas are potentially dangerous and should be used cautiously, if at all. They can cause massive, fatal fluid and electrolyte shifts (hyperphosphatemia, hypocalcemia, hypokalemia, or hyperkalemia), especially in cats, small dogs, and any animal that cannot quickly evacuate the enema because of obstipation.

## Cathartics and Laxatives

Cathartics and laxatives (Table 30-7) should be used only to promote defecation in patients that are not obstructed. They are not routinely indicated in small animals, except as part of lower bowel cleansing before contrast abdominal radiographs or endoscopy.

## Irritative laxatives

Bisacodyl stimulates defecation rather than softening feces. It is often used before colonoscopy and in patients that are reluctant to defecate because of altered environment. It is not appropriate for long-term use. A glycerin suppository or a lubricated matchstick is often an effective substitute.

### Bulk and osmotic laxatives

Bulk and osmotic laxatives include various fibers (especially soluble), magnesium sulfate, lactulose, and, in milk-intolerant patients, ice cream or milk. They promote fecal retention of water and are indicated in patients that have overly hard stools not caused by ingestion of foreign objects. These laxatives are more appropriate for long-term use than irritative cathartics. Larger doses may be needed in cats, as they retain fluids better than dogs.

*Fiber.* Fiber, a bulking agent, can be used indefinitely. Commercial high-fiber diets may be used, or existing diets may be supplemented. It is important to supply adequate amounts of water, or the fiber can cause constipation. Too much fiber may cause excessive stool; it can also cause inappetence (decreased palatability), which is a danger in overweight cats at risk for hepatic lipidosis. Fiber should not be given to patients with partial or complete obstruction, as impaction may occur.

### Table 30-7

### Selected Laxatives, Cathartics, Stool-Softening Agents, and Bulking Agents

| Drug | Dosage (PO) | Comments |
|---|---|---|
| Bisacodyl (Dulcolax) | 5 mg (small dogs and cats) 10-15 mg (larger dogs) | Do not break tablets |
| Coarse wheat bran | 1-3 tbsp/454 g of food | |
| Canned pumpkin pie filling | 1-3 tbsp/day (cats only) | Principally for cats |
| Dioctyl sodium sulfosuccinate (Colace) | 10-200 mg q8-12h (dogs only) 50 mg q12-24h (cats only) | Be sure animal is not dehydrated when treating |
| Laculose (Cephulac) | 1 ml/5 kg q8-12h, then adjust dose as needed (dogs only) 5 ml q8h, then adjust dose as needed (cats only) | Can cause severe osmotic diarrhea |
| Psyllium (Metamucil) | 1-2 tsp/454 g of food | Be sure animal has enough water, or constipation may develop |

*PO,* Oral.

*Lactulose (Cephulac).* Lactulose is a very effective osmotic laxative. It is particularly useful in patients that refuse high-fiber diets. The dose necessary to soften feces must be determined in each patient, but 0.5 to 5 ml may be given two or three times per day. Cats often need higher doses (e.g., 5 ml q8h). If gross overdose occurs, so much water can be lost that hypernatremic dehydration ensues.

# 31

# Disorders of the Oral Cavity, Pharynx, and Esophagus

## (Text pp 405-417)

### OROPHARYNX: MASSES, PROLIFERATIONS, AND INFLAMMATION (TEXT PP 405-409)

#### Sialocele

Sialoceles are caused by salivary duct obstruction and rupture with leakage into subcutaneous tissues. Most cases are traumatic, but some are idiopathic. A large, usually painless swelling is found under the jaw or tongue or occasionally in the pharynx. Oral cavity sialoceles may cause dysphagia, whereas pharyngeal sialoceles often produce gagging or dyspnea. If traumatized, they may bleed or cause anorexia because of discomfort.

##### Diagnosis and treatment

Aspiration with a large-bore needle yields thick fluid that resembles mucus and contains some neutrophils. Contrast radiography (contrast sialogram) sometimes defines which gland is involved. Treatment involves opening and draining the mass and excising the associated salivary gland. The prognosis is excellent.

#### Sialoadenitis, Sialoadenosis, or Salivary Gland Necrosis

Sialoadenitis may be idiopathic or may occur secondary to vomiting or regurgitation. It may cause painless enlargement of one or more salivary glands (usually the submandibular glands). The animal may be dysphagic if the gland is substantially inflamed. A syndrome of noninflammatory swelling associated with vomiting and responsive to phenobarbital therapy has been described.

##### Diagnosis and treatment

Biopsy with cytology or histopathology confirms that the mass consists of salivary tissue and determines whether inflammation or necrosis is present. If substantial inflammation and pain are present, surgical removal is most efficacious. If the patient is vomiting, a search should be made for an underlying cause, which, if found, should be treated and the size of the salivary glands monitored. If no other cause for vomiting can be found, phenobarbital may be administered at anticonvulsant doses (see Chapter 69). The prognosis is usually excellent.

## Oral Neoplasms in Dogs

Most soft-tissue masses of the oral cavity are neoplasms; most are malignant (e.g., melanoma, squamous cell carcinoma [SCC], fibrosarcoma). Acanthomatous epulides, oral papillomatosis, fibromatous epulides (Boxers), and eosinophilic granulomas (Siberian Huskies, Cavalier King Charles Spaniels) also occur.

### Clinical features

The most common signs are halitosis, dysphagia, bleeding, or a growth protruding from the mouth. Papillomatosis and fibromatous periodontal hyperplasia may cause discomfort when eating and occasionally cause bleeding, mild halitosis, or tissue protrusion from the mouth.

### Diagnosis

Thorough examination of the oral cavity usually reveals a mass involving the gingiva, although the tonsillar area, hard palate, or tongue can also be affected. Diagnosis requires cytology or histopathology, although papillomatosis and epulis may be strongly suspected from the gross appearance. If malignancy is a consideration, thoracic radiographs should be obtained; metastases are rare but are a very poor prognostic sign if present. Maxillary and mandibular radiographs should also be taken to check for bony involvement. Fine-needle aspiration of regional lymph nodes (even if grossly normal) is indicated to look for metastases, although biopsy may be required for definitive diagnosis.

### Treatment

The preferred approach in patients with confirmed malignant oral neoplasia but with no clinically detectable metastases is aggressive surgical excision of the mass and surrounding tissues (e.g., mandibulectomy, maxillectomy). Enlarged regional lymph nodes should be excised and evaluated histopathologically. Papillomatosis usually resolves spontaneously, although some masses have to be resected if they interfere with eating. Fibromatous epulides may also be resected if they cause problems. Anecdotal reports suggest that piroxicam is beneficial for patients with SCC.

*Radiation and chemotherapy.* Acanthomatous epulis and ameloblastomas may respond to radiation therapy alone, although complete surgical excision is preferred. SCC or fibrosarcomas with residual postoperative disease may benefit from adjunctive radiation therapy. Radiotherapy plus hyperthermia has been successful in some dogs with oral fibrosarcoma, whereas combination chemotherapy may help others. Chemotherapy is usually not beneficial in dogs with SCC, acanthomatous epulis, or melanoma.

### Prognosis

Early, complete excision of gingival or hard palate SCC, fibrosarcomas, acanthomatous epulides, and (rarely) melanomas may be curative. SCC affecting the base of the tongue and tonsillar carcinomas carry a very poor prognosis; complete excision or irradiation usually causes severe morbidity. Melanomas metastasize early and carry a very guarded prognosis.

## Oral Neoplasms in Cats

Oral tumors are less common in cats than in dogs; most are SCC. Eosinophilic granulomas (see later) are relatively common in cats and can closely mimic carcinoma. A large, deep biopsy is needed, because it is crucial to differentiate malignant tumors from eosinophilic granulomas. The surface of many oral masses is ulcerated and necrotic, making it difficult to interpret this part of the mass. Surgical excision is desirable for SCC. Radiation therapy and/or chemotherapy may benefit cats with incompletely excised SCC not involving the tongue or tonsils. In general, however, the prognosis for cats with oral SCC is guarded to poor.

## Feline Eosinophilic Granuloma

Feline eosinophilic granuloma complex includes indolent ulcer, eosinophilic plaque, and linear granuloma. The cause is unknown. Indolent ulcers are classically found on the lip or oral mucosa of middle-aged cats. Eosinophilic plaque usually occurs on the skin of the medial thighs and abdomen. Linear granuloma is typically found on the posterior aspect of the rear legs of young cats but may also occur on the tongue, palate, or other oral mucosae.

### Clinical features and diagnosis

Severe oral involvement typically produces dysphagia, halitosis, and/or anorexia. An ulcerated mass may be found at the base of the tongue or on the hard palate, glossopalatine arches, or anywhere else in the mouth. Deep biopsy is necessary for accurate diagnosis. Affected cats may also have cutaneous lesions; peripheral eosinophilia is inconsistently found.

### Treatment and prognosis

High-dose corticosteroid therapy (e.g., prednisolone, 2.2 to 4.4 mg/kg/day orally [PO]) usually controls the lesions. Sometimes cats are best treated with methyl-prednisolone acetate injections (20 mg every 2 weeks, as needed). Megestrol acetate is also effective, but it may cause diabetes mellitus, mammary tumors, and uterine problems, so it probably should not be used. Chlorambucil might be useful in resistant cases. The prognosis is good, but lesions can recur.

## Gingivitis and Periodontitis

Bacterial proliferation and toxin production, usually associated with tartar buildup, destroy normal gingival structures and cause inflammation in dogs and cats. Immunosuppression resulting from feline leukemia virus or feline immunodeficiency virus infection predisposes some cats to this disease. Many affected animals are asymptomatic, but halitosis, oral discomfort, anorexia, dysphagia, drooling, and tooth loss may occur.

### Diagnosis and treatment

Examination of the gums reveals hyperemia around the tooth margins. Gingival recession may reveal tooth roots. Supragingival and subgingival tartar should be removed and the crowns polished. Antimicrobial drugs effective against anaerobic bacteria (e.g., amoxicillin, clindamycin, metronidazole) may be used before and after teeth cleaning. Regular tooth-brushing and/or oral rinses with specially formulated chlorhexidine solution helps prevent recurrence. The prognosis is good with proper therapy.

## Stomatitis

Causes of stomatitis in dogs and cats include the following:

- Renal failure
- Trauma (e.g., foreign objects, caustic substances, chewed electrical cords)
- Immune-mediated disease (e.g., pemphigus, lupus)
- Upper respiratory viruses (e.g., feline viral rhinotracheitis, feline calicivirus)
- Infection secondary to immunosuppression
- Tooth root abscesses
- Severe periodontitis
- Osteomyelitis
- Thallium intoxication (rare)

### Clinical features and diagnosis

Most dogs and cats with stomatitis have thick, ropy saliva, severe halitosis, and/or anorexia caused by pain. Some animals are febrile and lose weight. Stomatitis is diagnosed by gross examination of the lesions, but an underlying cause should be sought. Biopsies are indicated, as are routine laboratory tests and radiographs of the mandible and maxilla, including the tooth roots.

### Treatment and prognosis

Therapy is both symptomatic and specific, directed at the underlying cause. Thorough cleaning of teeth and aggressive antibacterial therapy (systemic antibiotics effective against aerobes and anaerobes, oral rinses with antibacterial solutions) often help. In some patients, extracting teeth in the most severely affected areas may help. Bovine lactoferrin may ameliorate otherwise resistant lesions in cats. The prognosis depends on the underlying cause.

## Feline Lymphocytic-Plasmacytic Gingivitis and Pharyngitis

Feline lymphocytic-plasmacytic gingivitis, an idiopathic disorder, may be caused by feline calicivirus or any stimulus that produces sustained gingival inflammation. Anorexia and halitosis are the most common signs. Affected cats have reddened gingiva and/or posterior pillars of the pharynx. In severe cases the gingiva may be obviously proliferative and bleeds easily. Dental neck lesions often accompany gingivitis. Teeth chattering is occasionally seen.

### Diagnosis and treatment

Biopsy is needed for diagnosis; histology reveals lymphocytic-plasmacytic infiltration. Serum globulins may be increased. Currently no reliable therapy exists. Proper cleaning and polishing of teeth and antibiotic therapy effective against anaerobic bacteria may help. High-dose corticosteroid therapy (prednisolone, 2.2 mg/kg/day) is often useful. In severe cases multiple tooth extractions may alleviate the source of inflammation. Immunosuppressive drugs such as chlorambucil may be tried in obstinate cases. The prognosis is guarded; severely affected patients often do not respond well to therapy.

## DYSPHAGIA (TEXT PP 409-410)

### Masticatory Muscle Myositis or Atrophic Myositis

Masticatory muscle myositis is an idiopathic, immune-mediated disorder that affects the masticatory muscles in dogs. It has not been reported in cats.

### Clinical features and diagnosis

In the acute stages the temporalis and masseter muscles may be swollen and painful. However, most dogs are not presented until the muscles are severely atrophied and the mouth cannot be opened, even under anesthesia. These signs allow presumptive diagnosis. Biopsy of the temporalis and masseter muscles provides confirmation. Antibodies to type 2M fibers strongly support the diagnosis.

### Treatment and prognosis

High-dose prednisolone therapy (2.2 mg/kg/day) ± azathioprine (50 mg/m$^2$ q24h) is usually curative. Once control is achieved, administration is reduced to every 48 hours, and the dose of prednisolone is slowly tapered. If needed, a gastrostomy tube may be used until the dog can eat. The prognosis is usually good, but continued medication may be needed.

### Cricopharyngeal Achalasia or Dysfunction

Incoordination between the cricopharyngeal muscle and the rest of the swallowing reflex produces obstruction at the cricopharyngeal sphincter during swallowing. The cause is uncertain, but the condition is usually congenital and primarily seen in young dogs. The major sign is regurgitation immediately after or concurrent with swallowing. Some patients become anorectic, which leads to severe weight loss. Clinically this condition may be indistinguishable from pharyngeal dysfunction (see later).

### Diagnosis and treatment

In a young patient the regurgitation of food immediately after swallowing is suggestive, but pharyngeal dysphagia (with normal cricopharyngeal sphincter function) occasionally occurs as a congenital defect. Definitive diagnosis requires fluoroscopy or cinefluoroscopy while the patient is swallowing barium. Cricopharyngeal myotomy is curative, but function in the cranial esophagus must be evaluated before this surgery is considered. The prognosis is good if cicatrix does not occur postoperatively.

### Pharyngeal Dysphagia

Pharyngeal dysphagia is primarily an acquired disorder. Neuropathies, myopathies, and junctionopathies (e.g., localized myasthenia gravis) are the main causes. Inability to form a normal food bolus at the base of the tongue and/or propel the bolus into the esophagus is often associated with lesions of cranial nerves IX or X. Simultaneous dysfunction of the cranial esophagus may cause food retention just caudal to the cricopharyngeal sphincter.

### Clinical features

Although pharyngeal dysphagia primarily is found in older animals, young animals occasionally have transient signs. Pharyngeal dysphagia often mimics cricopharyngeal achalasia, i.e., regurgitation associated with swallowing. Patients with pharyngeal dysphagia sometimes have more difficulty swallowing fluids than solids. Aspiration (especially of liquids) is common.

### Diagnosis

Fluoroscopy or cinefluoroscopy performed while the patient is swallowing barium is required to distinguish pharyngeal from cricopharyngeal dysphagia. In the former the animal does not have adequate strength to push food boluses into the esophagus; in the latter the animal has adequate strength, but the cricopharyngeal sphincter stays shut or opens at the wrong time during swallowing.

### Treatment and prognosis

Either the pharynx must be bypassed (e.g., gastrostomy tube) or the underlying cause resolved (e.g., treat or control myasthenia gravis). Cricopharyngeal myotomy can be disastrous, because it allows food retained in the proximal esophagus to easily reenter the pharynx and be aspirated. The prognosis is guarded. It is often difficult to find and treat the underlying cause, and the animal is prone to progressive weight loss and recurring aspiration pneumonia.

## ESOPHAGEAL WEAKNESS OR MEGAESOPHAGUS (TEXT PP 410-413)

### Congenital Esophageal Weakness

The cause of congenital esophageal weakness (megaesophagus) is unknown. Miniature Schnauzers, Great Danes, and Dalmatians may be at increased risk. In Collies esophageal weakness may be caused by dermatomyositis.

### Clinical features

Affected patients are usually presented because of "vomiting" (actually regurgitation) with or without weight loss. Coughing and other signs of aspiration tracheitis and/or pneumonia are common and may be seen without regurgitation.

### Diagnosis

The history is used to help differentiate regurgitation from vomiting (see Chapter 28). Congenital disease is suspected if regurgitation and/or aspiration began when the pet was very young. However, if signs are relatively mild or intermittent, the diagnosis might not be made until the patient is older. Finding generalized esophageal dilation that is not associated with obstruction allows presumptive diagnosis. Diverticula in the cranial thorax occasionally occur and can easily be confused with vascular ring obstruction. Endoscopy is not as useful as contrast radiography for diagnosing this disorder.

### Treatment

No cure exists; cisapride (0.25 mg/kg) ameliorates signs in rare cases. Dietary management is used to prevent further dilation and aspiration. The animal is fed gruel from a platform that requires the pet to stand nearly vertically. This position is best maintained for 5 to 10 minutes after eating and drinking. Feeding several small meals per day is recommended. Some dogs do better when fed dry food on a free-choice basis throughout the day from a platform. Gastrostomy tubes can provide some relief from regurgitation and/or aspiration. However, animals may still regurgitate saliva, and, if gastroesophageal reflux is present, food.

### Prognosis

In some dogs the dilated esophagus partially returns to normal size and function. Even if the esophagus remains dilated, well-managed dogs may lead a good-quality life. Nevertheless, the prognosis is guarded; some patients respond well, but some continue to have severe regurgitation and/or aspiration despite all treatment efforts. Aspiration pneumonia is the major cause of death.

## Acquired Esophageal Weakness

Acquired esophageal weakness in dogs is usually caused by neuropathy, myopathy, or junctionopathy (e.g., myasthenia gravis). German Shepherds, Golden Retrievers, and Irish Setters may be at increased risk. In cats, gastroesophageal reflux and hiatal hernia seem to be more common causes.

### Clinical features

Patients usually are presented because of "vomiting" (actually regurgitation), but some have a cough and little or no regurgitation. Severe weight loss may occur if the dog regurgitates most of its food.

### Diagnosis

The first step is to establish that regurgitation, not vomiting, is occurring (see Chapter 28). The diagnosis is usually made by finding generalized esophageal dilation without evidence of obstruction on plain and contrast radiographs. Severity of clinical signs does not always correlate with the magnitude of radiographic changes. Some symptomatic patients have only mild retention just behind the cricopharyngeal muscle. It is important to rule out lower esophageal spasm and stricture, which, although rare, radiographically mimic esophageal weakness but require surgical treatment. Radiographs should also be evaluated for evidence of gastroesophageal reflux.

*Investigating the cause.* It is important to search for an underlying cause (see Chapter 28). Antibodies to acetylcholine receptors (indicative of myasthenia gravis) should be sought in dogs. An adrenocorticotropic hormone–stimulation test is indicated to look for occult hypoadrenocorticism. Serum $T_4$, free $T_4$, and thyroid-stimulating hormone concentrations may reveal hypothyroidism. Electromyogram may reveal generalized neuropathies or myopathies. Dysautonomia is suspected based on clinical signs (see later). If an underlying cause cannot be found, the disease is termed *idiopathic acquired megaesophagus.*

### Treatment

Dogs with acquired megaesophagus caused by localized myasthenia gravis, hypoadrenocorticism, or hypothyroid myopathy often respond to appropriate therapy for those conditions. Gastroesophageal reflux may respond to prokinetic and antacid therapy (cisapride, 0.25 mg/kg, and omeprazole, 0.7 to 1.5 mg/kg). Severe esophagitis may cause secondary esophageal weakness, which resolves after appropriate therapy.

*Symptomatic therapy.* If the disease is idiopathic, dietary therapy as described for congenital esophageal weakness is the only recourse. Cisapride may help when there exists concurrent gastroesophageal reflux. Gastrostomy tubes diminish the potential for aspiration, ensure positive nitrogen balance, and help treat esophagitis if present. Some dogs benefit from long-term gastrostomy tube use, but others continue to regurgitate and aspirate because of severe gastroesophageal reflux.

### Prognosis

If the underlying cause can be treated and the esophageal dilation and weakness resolve, the prognosis is good. However, the prognosis for animals with idiopathic megaesophagus that respond to dietary management is guarded, and in unresponsive animals, very poor. All patients with esophageal weakness are at risk for aspiration pneumonia and sudden death.

## Esophagitis

Esophagitis is generally caused by gastroesophageal reflux, persistent vomiting, esophageal foreign objects, or caustic agents. Pills (e.g., tetracycline) may stick in the esophagus and cause severe esophagitis in cats.

### Clinical features and diagnosis

Regurgitation is expected, although anorexia and drooling may predominate if swallowing is painful. If a caustic agent is ingested, the mouth and tongue are often hyperemic and/or ulcerated. A history of vomiting suggests esophagitis secondary to excessive exposure to gastric acid. This may occur with parvoviral enteritis. Plain and contrast radiographs may reveal hiatal hernias, gastroesophageal reflux, or esophageal foreign bodies. Contrast esophagograms do not reliably detect esophagitis; esophagoscopy with or without biopsy is needed for diagnosis.

### Treatment

The goals of treatment are to decrease gastric acidity, prevent reflux of gastric contents, and protect the denuded esophagus. Histamine-2 antagonists (see Table 30-3) may be used, but omeprazole is superior for decreasing gastric acidity. Metoclopramide stimulates gastric emptying, reducing the gastric volume available to reflux into the esophagus, but cisapride (0.25 to 0.5 mg/kg) is more effective.

Sucralfate may help protect the esophageal mucosa (see Table 30-4). Antibiotics effective against anaerobes (e.g., amoxicillin, clindamycin) are used. A gastrostomy feeding tube helps protect the esophagus while the mucosa is healing and ensures a positive nitrogen balance. Corticosteroids (e.g., prednisolone, 1.1 mg/kg/day) can be administered to prevent cicatrix formation, but their efficacy is dubious. Hiatal hernias may need surgical repair.

### Prognosis

The prognosis depends on the severity of the esophagitis and whether an underlying cause can be identified and controlled. Early, aggressive therapy helps prevent cicatrix formation and allows a better prognosis.

## Hiatal Hernia

Hiatal hernia is a diaphragmatic abnormality that allows part of the stomach to prolapse into the thoracic cavity. It may also allow gastroesophageal reflux. The condition may be congenital or acquired; Shar Pei dogs seem to be predisposed.

### Clinical features and diagnosis

Regurgitation is the primary sign in symptomatic animals. Plain or contrast esophagograms may reveal gastric herniation into the thorax; however, herniation may be intermittent and difficult to detect. It is sometimes necessary to put pressure on the abdomen during radiography to cause displacement of the stomach. Hiatal hernias are occasionally found endoscopically.

### Treatment and prognosis

If the hiatal hernia is symptomatic when the animal is at an early age, surgery is more likely to be required to correct it. If signs of hiatal hernia first appear later in life, aggressive medical management of gastroesophageal reflux (e.g., cisapride, omeprazole) is often sufficient. If medical management is not successful, surgery can be considered. The prognosis is good in both cases.

## Dysautonomia

Dysautonomia is an idiopathic condition that causes loss of autonomic nervous system function. Currently in the United States there appears to be an increased incidence in Missouri and surrounding states.

### Clinical features

Clinical signs vary considerably. Megaesophagus and subsequent regurgitation are common (but not invariable). Dysuria with urinary bladder distention, mydriasis and lack of pupillary light response, dry mucous membranes, weight loss, constipation, vomiting, poor anal tone, and anorexia are also reported.

### Diagnosis

Dysautonomia is usually first suspected clinically. Radiographs revealing distention of multiple areas of the alimentary tract (e.g., esophagus, stomach, small intestine) are suggestive. A presumptive antemortem diagnosis is usually made by observing the effects of pilocarpine on pupil size after 1 or 2 drops of 0.05% pilocarpine are placed in one eye only. If the treated eye rapidly constricts but the untreated eye does not, dysautonomia is likely. Finding that a dysuric dog with a large bladder can urinate after administration of bethanechol (0.04 mg/kg subcutaneously [SC]) is also suggestive. Definitive diagnosis requires histopathology of autonomic ganglia, which can be obtained only at necropsy.

**Treatment**

Treatment is palliative. Bethanechol (1.25 to 5 mg q24h) can be given to aid urination. The bladder should be expressed as needed. Gastric prokinetics (e.g., cisapride) may help lessen vomiting.

## ESOPHAGEAL OBSTRUCTION (TEXT PP 413-415)

### Vascular Ring Anomalies

Vascular ring anomalies are congenital defects. Persistent right fourth aortic arch (PRAA) is the most common. These anomalies occur in dogs and cats. Regurgitation is the most common presenting complaint, although signs of aspiration may be found. Signs often begin shortly after solid food is fed for the first time. Some animals have relatively mild signs and are not diagnosed until they are several years old.

**Diagnosis**

Definitive diagnosis is usually made by contrast esophagogram. Typically the esophagus is dilated cranial to the heart and is normal caudal to the heart. Rarely, the entire esophagus is dilated (because of concurrent megaesophagus), except for narrowing at the base of the heart. Endoscopically the esophagus has extramural narrowing near the base of the heart.

**Treatment and prognosis**

Surgical resection of the anomalous vessel is necessary. Dietary management alone is insufficient, because the dilation persists and may progress. Also, the patient is at risk for foreign body occlusion at the site of the PRAA. However, dietary therapy benefits some patients postoperatively. In general, the more severe the preoperative dilation, the more likely regurgitation will continue postoperatively. Although most pets benefit from surgery, a guarded prognosis is appropriate. If postsurgical stricture occurs, esophageal ballooning or a second surgical procedure may be considered.

### Esophageal Foreign Objects

Almost anything can lodge in the esophagus, but objects with sharp points (e.g., bones, fish hooks) are common. Most obstructions occur at the thoracic inlet, at the base of the heart, or immediately cranial to the diaphragm. Dogs are more commonly affected.

**Clinical features**

Regurgitation or anorexia secondary to esophageal pain is common. Acute onset of regurgitation is suggestive of esophageal foreign body. Other signs depend on the site of obstruction, whether it is complete or partial, and whether esophageal perforation has occurred. Complete obstructions cause regurgitation of solids and liquids, whereas partial obstructions may allow passage of liquids. If the object is impinging on an airway, acute dyspnea may occur. Esophageal perforation usually causes fever and anorexia; dyspnea may occur because of pleural effusion or pneumothorax. Subcutaneous emphysema rarely occurs.

**Diagnosis**

Plain thoracic radiographs reveal most esophageal foreign bodies, although poultry bones may be difficult to see. It is also important to look for evidence of esophageal perforation: pneumothorax, pleural effusion, and/or mediastinal fluid. Esophagoscopy is diagnostic and frequently therapeutic; esophagograms are rarely appropriate.

**Treatment**

Foreign objects are best removed endoscopically unless they are too firmly lodged or radiographs suggest perforation; thoracotomy is indicated in these situations. During endoscopy the esophagus should be carefully insufflated to avoid rupturing weakened areas or causing tension pneumothorax. The object should be pushed into the stomach only if the clinician is confident that it is unlikely to cause additional esophageal damage. After the object is removed, the esophageal mucosa should be examined. Thoracic radiographs can be repeated to check for pneumothorax.

Treatment after foreign body removal may include antibiotics, antacids, prokinetic agents, gastrostomy feeding tube, and/or corticosteroids (prednisolone, 1.1 mg/kg/day), depending on residual damage. Perforation usually requires thoracotomy to remove septic debris and close the esophageal defect.

### Prognosis

The prognosis for patients without perforation is usually good. Perforation warrants a guarded prognosis, depending on the severity of thoracic contamination. Cicatrix formation is possible if mucosal and submucosal damage occurs.

## Esophageal Cicatrix

Esophagitis from any cause can produce a stricture in dogs and cats, although severe, deep inflammation of the esophagus (e.g., foreign body obstruction or severe gastro-esophageal reflux) is usually involved.

### Clinical features and diagnosis

The main sign is regurgitation, especially of solids. Some animals are anorectic because of pain when food becomes lodged in the stricture by forceful esophageal peristalsis. Partial obstructions can be difficult to diagnose. Contrast esophagograms (often using barium mixed with food) are needed. Esophagoscopy is definitive, but a partial stricture may not be obvious in large dogs unless a large-diameter endoscope is used and the esophagus is carefully inspected after being dilated.

### Treatment

Treatment consists of correcting the suspected cause (e.g., esophagitis) and/or widening the stricture by ballooning or bougienage. Ballooning may be performed via esophagoscopy. Surgical resection should be avoided, because iatrogenic stricture at the anastomosis site is common. After the esophagus has been dilated, antibiotics with or without corticosteroids (prednisolone, 1.1 mg/kg/day) are often administered to help prevent infection and restricture; however, their efficacy is unknown. If esophagitis is present, it should be treated aggressively. Some animals are cured after one ballooning; others require multiple procedures. Long-term gastrostomy tubes may be needed in some patients.

### Prognosis

The shorter the length of esophagus involved and the sooner the corrective procedure is performed, the better the prognosis. Patients with extensive, mature strictures and/or continuing esophagitis often need repeated dilatory procedures and have a more guarded prognosis. Most patients with benign esophageal strictures can be helped.

### Prevention

Early identification and appropriate treatment of high-risk patients (e.g., those with severe esophagitis, after foreign object removal) help decrease the likelihood of stricture formation. The efficacy of corticosteroids is uncertain, but they are worth trying in selected cases.

## ESOPHAGEAL NEOPLASMS (TEXT PP 415-416)

Primary esophageal sarcomas in dogs are often a result of *Spirocerca lupi*. Primary esophageal carcinomas are of unknown cause. Leiomyomas and leiomyosarcomas are found at the lower esophageal sphincter in older dogs. Thyroid carcinomas and pulmonary alveolar carcinomas may invade the esophagus in dogs. SCC is the most common esophageal neoplasm in cats.

### Clinical features

Animals with primary esophageal tumors may be asymptomatic until the tumor is well advanced. Regurgitation, anorexia, and/or halitosis may occur if the tumor is large or causes esophageal dysfunction. If the esophagus is secondarily involved, signs may result from esophageal dysfunction or tumor effects on other tissues.

### Diagnosis

Plain radiographs may reveal a soft-tissue density in the caudal lung fields. These tumors may be difficult to distinguish from pulmonary lesions without contrast esophagograms. Esophagoscopy reveals intraluminal and intramural masses or strictures and usually finds extraluminal masses that are causing esophageal stricture. Retroflexing the tip of the endoscope in the stomach is the best method of identifying lower esophageal sphincter leiomyomas and leiomyosarcomas.

**Treatment and Prognosis**

Surgical resection is rarely curative (except for leiomyomas at the lower esophageal sphincter), owing to the advanced nature of most esophageal neoplasms when they are diagnosed. Resection may be palliative. Photodynamic therapy may be beneficial in dogs and cats with small, superficial esophageal neoplasms. The prognosis is usually poor.

# 32

# Disorders of the Stomach

## *(Text pp 418-430)*

### GASTRITIS (TEXT PP 418-421)

#### Acute Gastritis

Ingestion of spoiled or contaminated foods, foreign objects, toxic plants, chemicals, or irritating drugs (e.g., nonsteroidal antiinflammatory drugs [NSAIDs]) is a common cause of acute gastritis. Dogs are more often affected than cats. Signs are acute in onset and primarily involve vomiting food or bile (with or without small amounts of blood). Affected animals are uninterested in food and may or may not appear ill. Fever and abdominal pain are uncommon.

##### Diagnosis

Unless the animal was seen eating some irritant, acute gastritis is usually a diagnosis of exclusion based on history and physical findings. Abdominal imaging and routine laboratory tests are indicated if the patient is severely ill or if other disease is suspected. Once alimentary foreign body, obstruction, parvoviral enteritis, uremia, diabetic ketoacidosis, hypoadrenocorticism, hepatic disease, hypercalcemia, and pancreatitis are ruled out, acute gastritis is the tentative diagnosis. The diagnosis is more likely if vomiting resolves after 1 to 2 days of therapy (although pancreatitis should still be considered). Gastroscopy may reveal bile or gastric erosions or hyperemia.

##### Treatment and prognosis

Treatment consists primarily of parenteral fluid therapy; withholding food and water for 24 hours often controls vomiting. If vomiting persists or is excessive or if the patient becomes depressed, centrally acting antiemetics (e.g., prochlorperazine, metoclopramide, ondansetron) may be administered (see Table 30-2). When feeding resumes, small amounts of cool water are offered frequently. If the animal drinks without vomiting, small amounts of a bland diet (e.g., one part cottage cheese or boiled chicken and two parts potato) are offered. The prognosis is excellent as long as fluid and electrolyte balance is maintained.

#### Hemorrhagic Gastroenteritis

Hemorrhagic gastroenteritis classically occurs in small-breed dogs that have not had access to garbage. It may be immune mediated.

### Clinical features and diagnosis
Hemorrhagic gastroenteritis typically causes profuse hematemesis with or without hematochezia. The course of disease is acute and rapidly produces illness. In severe cases the animal may be moribund by the time of presentation. Patients typically are hemoconcentrated (packed cell volume >55%) with normal plasma total protein. This finding plus the acute onset of typical clinical signs allows presumptive diagnosis. Thrombocytopenia and renal or prerenal azotemia may be seen in severely affected patients.

### Treatment and prognosis
Aggressive fluid therapy is necessary to treat or prevent shock, disseminated intravascular coagulation (DIC), and renal failure secondary to hypovolemia. Parenteral antibiotics (e.g., ampicillin, chloramphenicol) are often used but are of uncertain value. The prognosis is good for most patients that are presented early. Inadequately treated patients may die from circulatory collapse, DIC, and/or renal failure.

## Chronic Gastritis
Several types of chronic gastritis exist. Lymphocytic-plasmacytic gastritis may be an immune or inflammatory reaction to a variety of antigens. *Helicobacter* spp. could be responsible in some animals (especially cats). *Physaloptera rara* causes a similar reaction in some dogs. Eosinophilic gastritis may result from an allergic reaction, probably to food antigens. Atrophic gastritis may be the result of chronic gastric inflammatory disease and/or immune mechanisms. *Ollulanus tricuspis* may cause granulomatous gastritis in cats.

### Clinical features and diagnosis
Anorexia and vomiting are the most common signs. Frequency of vomiting varies from once a week to many times a day. Some animals have only anorexia. Clinical pathology is nondiagnostic, although eosinophilic gastritis sometimes causes peripheral eosinophilia. Imaging may reveal mucosal thickening, but this is inconsistent and nondiagnostic. Diagnosis requires gastric mucosal biopsy, preferably via endoscopy. Gastric lymphoma can be surrounded by lymphocytic inflammation, so shallow biopsies may result in an incorrect diagnosis. If *Ollulanus tricuspis* is suspected, vomitus or gastric washings should be examined for the parasites; they might also be found in gastric biopsies. *Physaloptera* organisms are visible endoscopically.

### Treatment
Lymphocytic-plasmacytic gastritis sometimes responds to dietary therapy (low-fat, low-fiber elimination diets) alone. If such therapy is inadequate, corticosteroids (e.g., prednisolone, 2.2 mg/kg/day) can be used concurrently, with the dose gradually decreased to the lowest effective level. Signs may return and be more difficult to control if reduction in dosage occurs too quickly. Sometimes concurrent use of histamine-2 ($H_2$) receptor antagonists (see Table 30-3) is beneficial. Rarely, azathioprine or a similar drug is necessary.

Canine eosinophilic gastritis usually responds to a strict elimination diet. If dietary therapy alone fails, the addition of corticosteroids (e.g., prednisolone, 1.1 to 2.2 mg/kg/day) is usually effective. Atrophic or granulomatous gastritis is more difficult to treat. Bland, low-fat diets may help control signs. Atrophic gastritis may also respond to anti-inflammatory, antacid, and prokinetic therapy. Granulomatous gastritis does not respond well to diet or corticosteroid therapy.

### Prognosis
The prognosis for animals with lymphocytic-plasmacytic gastritis is good with appropriate therapy. The prognosis for canine eosinophilic gastritis is also good. Feline eosinophilic gastritis can be a component of hypereosinophilic syndrome, which often responds poorly to treatment and carries a guarded prognosis.

## *Helicobacter*-Associated Disease
*Helicobacter felis* and *Helicobacter heilmannii (Gastrospirillium hominis)* may be the principal gastric spirochetes in dogs and cats. *Helicobacter pylori* has also been found in cats. A cause-and-effect relationship has not been clearly established between *Helicobacter*

infection and canine or feline gastric disease, but signs resolve in some ill animals with gastric *Helicobacter* infections when the organism is eliminated.

### Clinical features

Affected animals may have nausea, anorexia, and/or vomiting associated with lymphocytic and occasionally neutrophilic infiltrates. However, most infected animals are asymptomatic.

### Diagnosis

Gastric biopsy is required for diagnosis. The organisms are easy to identify with special stains (e.g., Giemsa, Warthin-Starry). The bacteria are not uniformly distributed throughout the stomach, so it is best to perform biopsy of the body, fundus, and antrum. Diagnosis can also be made by cytology of the gastric mucosa or by evaluation of gastric mucosal urease activity (see Chapter 29). It is important to eliminate other conditions that better explain the animal's clinical signs before diagnosing *Helicobacter*-associated disease.

### Treatment and prognosis

A combination of metronidazole, omeprazole (or an $H_2$-receptor antagonist), and either amoxicillin or a macrolide antibiotic is often used. Some animals respond to either erythromycin or amoxicillin alone. Azithromycin has fewer side effects than erythromycin and is very effective. Therapy should continue for at least 10 days. Animals with *Helicobacter*-associated disease respond well to treatment and have a good prognosis, although recurrence of infection is common. Any patient that does not respond should be reexamined for other diseases.

## *Physaloptera rara*

*P. rara* is a nematode that has an indirect life cycle involving cockroaches and beetles. It primarily infests dogs. One parasite is enough to cause intractable vomiting that often is unresponsive to antiemetics. Vomitus may contain bile. The dog is otherwise healthy.

### Diagnosis and treatment

Sodium dichromate or magnesium sulfate solution is needed to identify the eggs in feces, although ova are seldom found because few are passed. Diagnosis is generally made when the parasites are found during gastroduodenoscopy. Only one worm may be present, and it can be difficult to find, especially when attached within the pylorus. Empirical treatment with pyrantel pamoate or ivermectin is a reasonable alternative. If the parasite is found during endoscopy, it can be removed with forceps. Vomiting usually stops as soon as all worms are eliminated.

## *Olluanus tricuspis*

*O. tricuspis* is a nematode that is transmitted directly via vomited material. Cats are most commonly affected, although dogs and foxes are occasionally infected. Infection is more common in catteries; infrequently, pets in single-cat households are infected. Vomiting is the principal sign, although clinically normal cats can harbor the parasite. A few infected animals have severe gastritis and become debilitated.

### Diagnosis and treatment

Looking for parasites in gastric washings or vomitus with a dissecting microscope is the best means of diagnosis. Parasites are occasionally seen in gastric mucosal biopsies. Oxfendazole (10 mg/kg orally [PO] q12h for 5 days) or fenbendazole may be effective.

# GASTRIC OUTFLOW OBSTRUCTION OR STASIS (TEXT PP 421-427)

## Benign Muscular Pyloric Hypertrophy (Pyloric Stenosis)

Pyloric stenosis typically is seen in younger animals, especially brachycephalic dogs and Siamese cats, but it can occur in any animal. The cause is uncertain.

### Clinical features

Patients usually vomit food shortly after eating; the vomiting is sometimes described as projectile. The animal is otherwise clinically normal, although weight loss is occasionally found. Some cats vomit so much that secondary esophagitis and regurgitation develop.

### Diagnosis

Diagnosis requires identification of gastric outflow obstruction with barium radiographs, gastroduodenoscopy, and/or exploratory surgery. Endoscopically, increased folds of normal mucosa may be seen at the pylorus. At surgery the serosa appears normal, but the pylorus is palpably thickened. Thickened pyloric musculature can also be identified with ultrasonography.

Infiltrative disease of the pyloric mucosa must be ruled out via biopsy. Extra-alimentary tract diseases that cause vomiting (see Box 28-2) should also be ruled out. Hypochloremic, hypokalemic alkalosis sometimes occurs but is insensitive and nonspecific for gastric outflow obstruction.

### Treatment and prognosis

Surgical correction is indicated. Pyloroplasty is more consistently effective than pyloromyotomy. However, improperly performed pyloroplasty can cause perforation. Surgery should be curative, and the prognosis is good.

## Gastric Antral Mucosal Hypertrophy

Antral mucosal hypertrophy is idiopathic and is primarily found in older, small-breed dogs. Gastric outflow obstruction is caused by excessive mucosa. Antral hypertrophy clinically resembles pyloric stenosis: patients usually vomit food, especially after meals.

### Diagnosis

Gastric outlet obstruction is diagnosed radiographically, ultrasonographically, or endoscopically, but definitive diagnosis of antral mucosal hypertrophy requires biopsy. Endoscopically, the convoluted mucosal folds may suggest a submucosal neoplasia, although the mucosa is not as firm as expected with an infiltrative tumor. In some cases the mucosa is reddened and inflamed. At surgery one should find no evidence of submucosal infiltration or muscular thickening suggestive of pyloric stenosis or neoplasia. It is important to differentiate mucosal hypertrophy from these other diseases; gastric carcinomas typically have a worse prognosis, and surgery is not always indicated.

### Treatment and prognosis

Antral mucosal hypertrophy is treated by mucosal resection, usually combined with pyloroplasty. The prognosis is excellent.

## Gastric Foreign Objects

Anything that can pass through the esophagus can become a gastric foreign object. Dogs are affected more commonly than cats. Vomiting is a common sign and may result from gastric outlet obstruction, distention, or irritation. Some animals show only anorexia, and others are asymptomatic.

### Diagnosis

Acute onset of vomiting in an otherwise normal animal, especially a puppy, suggests foreign body ingestion. The object may be palpable or may be seen on plain radiographs. Contrast radiographs and endoscopy are the most reliable means of diagnosis. Canine parvoviral infection can mimic foreign object obstruction; it initially causes intense vomiting, and the virus may not be detectable in the feces. Hypokalemic, hypochloremic metabolic alkalosis is consistent with gastric outflow obstruction; however, these changes may be absent in obstructed animals and present in nonobstructed animals.

### Treatment

Small objects that are unlikely to cause damage may be allowed to pass through the gastrointestinal (GI) tract, but most should be removed. Vomiting may induce elimination of the object. In dogs, apomorphine (0.02 mg/kg intravenously [IV] or 0.1 mg/kg subcutaneously [SC]) or hydrogen peroxide (1 to 5 ml/kg of 3% solution PO) may be used as an emetic. In cats, xylazine (0.4 to 0.5 mg/kg IV) is used. If doubt exists regarding the safety of this approach, the object should be removed endoscopically or surgically.

Before the patient is anesthetized for surgery or endoscopy, the electrolyte and acid-base status should be evaluated. Electrolyte changes, especially hypokalemia, are common but unpredictable. Hypokalemia predisposes to cardiac arrhythmias and should be corrected before anesthesia.

### Prognosis

The prognosis is good unless the patient is debilitated or septic peritonitis develops secondary to gastric perforation.

## Gastric Dilation and Volvulus

Gastric dilatation and volvulus (GDV) occurs when the stomach dilates excessively with gas. The stomach may maintain its normal position (dilation) or it may twist (volvulus), in which case the pylorus typically rotates from the right side of the abdomen, below the body of the stomach, to arrive dorsal to the cardia on the left side. Splenic torsion may occur concurrently. The cause is unknown but may involve abnormal gastric motility.

### Risk factors

GDV primarily occurs in large- and giant-breed dogs with deep chests; it is rare in small dogs and cats. Irish Setters with a deeper thorax relative to width are more likely to experience GDV. Dogs with parents that had GDV may also be at increased risk. Eating once a day and eating from an elevated platform seem to increase risk.

### Clinical features

Affected dogs typically retch nonproductively and may show signs of abdominal pain. Marked cranial abdominal distention may be seen later, although it is not always obvious in large, heavily muscled dogs. Eventually depression and a moribund state occur.

### Diagnosis

Signalment and physical findings allow presumptive diagnosis but do not permit differentiation of dilation from volvulus. On plain radiographs (right lateral view), volvulus is identified by displacement of the pylorus and/or a "shelf" of tissue in the gastric shadow. It is impossible to distinguish dilation alone from dilation and volvulus based on ability to pass an orogastric tube into the stomach.

### Treatment

Treatment consists of aggressive therapy for shock (e.g., hetastarch or hypertonic saline) and gastric decompression. If the patient is asphyxiating, the stomach is decompressed first. Serum electrolyte concentrations and acid-base status should be evaluated. Mesenteric congestion predisposes to infection and endotoxemia, so it is reasonable to administer systemic antibiotics (e.g., cefazolin, 20 mg/kg IV).

*Decompression.* Gastric decompression is usually accomplished with an orogastric tube. The stomach is then lavaged with warm water. Most dogs with dilation or volvulus can be decompressed in this manner. The tube should not be forced into the stomach. If it cannot be passed, the stomach can be decompressed by insertion of a large needle (e.g., 12 to 14 gauge, 3 inches long) into the stomach, just behind the rib cage in the left flank. Temporary gastrostomy may instead be performed in the left paralumbar area.

*Surgery.* Once the patient is stabilized, surgery can be performed to reposition the stomach, remove the spleen (if grossly infarcted), remove or invaginate devitalized gastric wall, and perform a gastropexy. If a temporary gastrostomy was performed, it must be closed. Deciding whether to first stabilize the patient or to immediately perform a laparotomy is based on the condition of the dog at initial presentation and on whether the patient would be a much better anesthetic risk after stabilization.

In dogs with gastric dilation without torsion, gastropexy is optional and may even be performed after the dog has completely recovered from the current episode. Gastropexy prevents torsion, but it does not prevent dilation. Prophylactic gastropexy may be performed during other elective procedures (e.g., spay) in animals believed to be at increased risk for GDV.

*Postoperative care.* After surgery the patient should be monitored by electrocardiogram for 48 to 72 hours. Lidocaine, procainamide, or sotolol may be needed if cardiac arrhythmias diminish cardiac output (see Chapter 4). Hypokalemia is common and should be resolved, as it makes arrhythmias refractory to medical control.

### Prognosis

The prognosis depends on how quickly the condition is recognized and treated. Mortality rates of 18% to 28% are reported. Early therapy improves the prognosis. Preoperative arrhythmias, increased blood lactate concentrations, gastric wall necrosis, severe DIC, partial gastrectomy, and splenectomy worsen the prognosis. Although rare, gastric dilation may recur after gastropexy.

## Partial or Intermittent Gastric Volvulus

Dogs with partial or intermittent volvulus do not have the life-threatening, progressive syndrome that characterizes classic GDV. Although it occurs in the same breeds as GDV, partial volvulus usually causes a chronic, intermittent problem. It can occur repeatedly and resolve spontaneously, with the dog appearing normal between bouts.

### Diagnosis and treatment

Occasionally the stomach maintains itself in a twisted position but does not fill with gas. Signs of gastric disease may persist in such patients, and plain radiographs are usually diagnostic. Intermittent torsion may necessitate repeated radiographs and/or contrast studies. Endoscopic diagnosis is difficult because it is possible to cause temporary gastric volvulus by manipulating the gastroscope in an air-distended stomach. Surgical repositioning with gastropexy is usually curative and carries a good prognosis.

## Idiopathic Gastric Hypomotility

The idiopathic gastric hypomotility syndrome is characterized by poor gastric emptying and motility despite lack of anatomic obstruction or inflammation. It primarily occurs in dogs.

### Clinical features and diagnosis

Affected dogs vomit food several hours after eating but otherwise appear to feel well. Some develop weight loss. Fluoroscopy documents decreased gastric motility, but diagnosis requires ruling out gastric outlet obstruction, infiltrative and inflammatory bowel disease, and extraalimentary tract diseases (e.g., renal, adrenal, or hepatic failure; hypercalcemia or severe hypokalemia).

### Treatment and prognosis

Metoclopramide increases gastric peristalsis in some dogs; cisapride or erythromycin may be effective if metoclopramide fails (see Chapter 30). Diets low in fat and fiber also promote gastric emptying. Dogs that respond to medical management have a good prognosis. Those that do not respond may still be acceptable pets.

## Bilious Vomiting Syndrome

Bilious vomiting syndrome may be the result of gastroduodenal reflux when the dog's stomach is empty for long periods (e.g., during an overnight fast). It affects otherwise normal dogs that are fed once daily in the morning. Classically the dog vomits bile-stained fluid late at night or in the morning, just before eating. This history and absence of obstructive or inflammatory GI disorders and extraalimentary tract diseases strongly suggest bilious vomiting syndrome. Feeding the dog an extra meal late at night is often curative. If vomiting continues, a gastric prokinetic (see Chapter 30) may be administered late at night to prevent reflux. The prognosis is excellent. Most animals respond to therapy, and those that do not remain otherwise healthy.

## GI ULCERATION AND EROSION (TEXT PP 427-428)

### Etiology

GI ulceration and erosion (GUE) has several causes, including NSAID use, stress, and neoplasia. Ulceration may be a consequence of severe hypovolemic, septic, or neurogenic shock, such as occurs after trauma, surgery, or endotoxemia. It can also be caused by a variety of other illnesses. Renal and hepatic failure may cause GUE; the latter is important in dogs. Foreign objects rarely cause GUE, but they prevent healing and increase blood loss from existing ulcers. Inflammatory bowel disease occasionally is associated with GUE in dogs.

**NSAIDs.** Use of aspirin, phenylbutazone, ibuprofen, naproxen, piroxicam, flunixin, and other NSAIDs is a major cause of GUE in dogs. Naproxen, ibuprofen, and indomethacin are particularly dangerous. Carprofen and etodolac have less potential to cause GUE, but it can still occur in animals taking these drugs. Concurrent use of more than one NSAID or use of an NSAID plus a corticosteroid (especially dexamethasone) increases the risk of GUE. Steroids alone are seldom a problem, unless dexamethasone is used in high doses or the patient is at increased risk for GUE (e.g., severe anemia). Use of NSAIDs in patients with poor visceral perfusion (e.g., cardiac failure or shock) increases the risk of GUE.

**Neoplasia.** Mast cell tumors may release histamine (especially during radiation or chemotherapy), which induces gastric acid secretion. Gastrinomas are usually found in older dogs (and rarely cats). They secrete gastrin, which causes severe gastric hyperacidity, duodenal ulceration, esophagitis, and diarrhea. Gastric neoplasms and other infiltrative diseases (e.g., pythiosis) may also result in GUE.

### Clinical features
GUE is more common in dogs than in cats. Anorexia can be the primary sign. Vomiting may occur; vomitus may containing fresh or digested blood. Anemia and/or hypoproteinemia occasionally occurs and causes edema, pallor, weakness, and dyspnea. Most affected dogs do not show pain during abdominal palpation. Some ulcers perforate and seal over before generalized peritonitis occurs. In such cases a small abscess may develop at the site and cause abdominal pain, anorexia, and/or vomiting.

### Diagnosis
Presumptive diagnosis is usually based on evidence of GI blood loss (e.g., hematemesis, melena, iron-deficiency anemia) in an animal without a coagulopathy. History and physical examination may identify an obvious cause (e.g., NSAID administration, mast cell tumor). Mast cell tumors can resemble almost any cutaneous lesion, so all cutaneous masses or nodules should be evaluated cytologically. Hepatic and renal failure are usually diagnosed from complete blood count, serum biochemistry profile, and urinalysis.

Contrast radiographs are diagnostic for foreign objects and sometimes for GUE. Ultrasonography may reveal gastric thickening (e.g., infiltrative lesions) and mucosal defects. Gastroduodenoscopy is the most sensitive and specific test and, in conjunction with biopsy, can identify tumors, foreign bodies, and inflammation. Multifocal duodenal erosion suggests gastrinoma. Serum gastrin concentrations should be measured if a gastrinoma is suspected or if no other causes are likely.

### Treatment
Treatment depends on the severity of GUE and whether an underlying cause is detected. Therapy directed at the underlying cause is important, but patients with GUE that is not obviously life threatening may be treated symptomatically.

**Symptomatic therapy.** Depending on the severity, antacids (either $H_2$-receptor antagonists or proton pump inhibitors), sucralfate, parenteral fluids, and withholding of food and/or provision of parenteral nutrition (see Chapter 30) are often effective. If medical therapy is unsuccessful after 5 to 8 days or if the patient has life-threatening bleeding despite therapy, the ulcer(s) should be resected in most cases. The stomach should be examined endoscopically before surgery to determine the number and location of the ulcers.

**Gastrinoma.** In patients with gastrinoma, $H_2$-receptor antagonist therapy is often palliative for months. Animals with high serum gastrin concentrations may require more potent and/or higher doses of $H_2$ blockers (e.g., famotidine) or a proton pump inhibitor such as omeprazole (see Table 30-3).

### Prognosis
The prognosis is favorable if the underlying cause can be controlled and therapy prevents ulcer perforation.

### Prevention
Carafate or an $H_2$-receptor antagonist sometimes helps prevent GUE. Misoprostol is designed to prevent NSAID-induced ulceration and is more effective than $H_2$ antagonists or sucralfate; however, it is not universally successful. These drugs are discussed in Chapter 30.

## INFILTRATIVE GASTRIC DISEASES (TEXT PP 428-429)

### Neoplasia

Neoplastic infiltrations (e.g., adenocarcinoma, lymphoma, leiomyomas, and leiomyosarcomas in dogs; lymphoma in cats) may produce GUE through direct mucosal disruption. Adenocarcinomas are typically infiltrative and decrease gastric emptying by impairing motility and/or obstructing outflow. Gastric lymphoma is typically a diffuse lesion but can produce masses. Benign gastric polyps are of uncertain cause and significance.

#### Clinical features

Dogs and cats with gastric tumors are usually asymptomatic until the disease is advanced. Anorexia is the most common sign. Vomiting because of gastric neoplasia usually signifies advanced disease or gastric outflow obstruction. Weight loss is commonly caused by nutrient loss or cancer cachexia. Hematemesis occasionally occurs; leiomyomas often cause upper GI bleeding. Gastric tumors can cause iron deficiency anemia even if GI blood loss is not obvious. Polyps rarely cause signs unless they obstruct the pylorus.

#### Diagnosis

Iron deficiency anemia in a dog or cat without obvious blood loss suggests GI bleeding, often because of a tumor. Plain and contrast radiographs may reveal gastric wall thickening, decreased motility, and/or mucosal irregularities. The only sign of submucosal adenocarcinoma may be failure of one area to dilate (usually the antrum). Ultrasound-guided aspiration of thickened areas in the gastric wall may be diagnostic for adenocarcinoma or lymphoma. Endoscopically, such areas may appear as multiple mucosal folds extending into the lumen without ulceration or erosion. Some tumors are obvious endoscopically.

When lesions undergo biopsy endoscopically, the sample must be deep enough to include submucosal tissue. Scirrhous adenocarcinomas may be so dense that diagnostic biopsy samples cannot be obtained with flexible endoscopic forceps. Mucosal lymphomas and adenocarcinomas often produce GUE, and tissue samples taken from the edge of the ulcer are usually diagnostic. Polyps usually are obvious endoscopically but should always undergo biopsy to ensure that adenocarcinoma is not present.

#### Treatment

Most adenocarcinomas are advanced before clinical signs are obvious, making complete surgical excision difficult or impossible. Leiomyomas and leiomyosarcomas are more likely to be resectable. Gastroduodenostomy may palliate gastric outflow obstruction resulting from an unresectable tumor. Chemotherapy is rarely helpful except in dogs and cats with lymphoma. Gastric polyps do not need to be resected unless they cause outflow obstruction.

#### Prognosis

The prognosis for patients with adenocarcinoma or lymphoma is poor unless it is detected very early. Leiomyomas and leiomyosarcomas, if diagnosed early, are often cured surgically.

### Pythiosis

Pythiosis is a fungal infection caused by *Pythium insidiosum*. It is most common in the Gulf coast area of the southeastern United States. Any area of the alimentary tract or skin may be affected; the stomach, duodenum, and colon are common sites. Pythiosis primarily affects dogs. Typical signs include vomiting, anorexia, diarrhea, and/or weight loss. Colonic involvement is suggested by tenesmus and hematochezia.

#### Diagnosis

Diagnosis requires biopsy that includes the submucosa. Rigid endoscopy is best; flexible endoscopy rarely allows deep enough samples. Cytology may be diagnostic if an excised piece of submucosa is scraped with a scalpel blade. The fungal hyphae do not stain and appear as "ghosts" with typical Romanowsky-type stains. The organisms can be sparse and difficult to find histologically, even in large tissue samples.

**Treatment and prognosis**

Complete surgical excision provides the best chance for cure. Itraconazole (5 mg/kg PO q12h) or liposomal amphotericin B (2.2 mg/kg) may be beneficial in some patients. Pythiosis often spreads to involve structures that cannot be surgically removed (e.g., root of the mesentery, pancreas surrounding the bile duct), resulting in a grim prognosis.

# 33

# Disorders
# of the Intestinal Tract

## *(Text pp 431-465)*

## ACUTE DIARRHEA (TEXT PP 432-433)

### Acute Enteritis

Acute enteritis can be caused by infectious agents, poor diet, abrupt dietary changes, inappropriate foods, additives, and/or parasites. Except in the case of parvovirus the cause is rarely diagnosed, and most patients spontaneously improve (although supportive therapy may be needed). Diarrhea of unknown cause is common, especially in puppies and kittens.

#### Clinical features

Signs consist of diarrhea with or without vomiting, dehydration, fever, anorexia, depression, crying, and/or abdominal pain. Very young animals may become hypoglycemic and stuporous.

#### Diagnosis

History and findings of physical and fecal examinations are used to identify possible causes. Fecal flotation and direct fecal examination are always indicated, because parasites may worsen the problem even when they are not the main cause. The need for other diagnostic procedures depends on the severity of the illness and whether risk of contagion exists; mild enteritis is usually treated symptomatically without performing additional diagnostics.

*Diagnostic tests.* If the patient is febrile, has hemorrhagic stools, is involved in an outbreak of serious enteritis, or is particularly ill, additional tests are indicated. Tests may include complete blood count (CBC) to identify neutropenia, fecal enzyme-linked immunosorbent assay (ELISA) for parvovirus (dogs), serology for feline leukemia virus (FeLV) and feline immunodeficiency virus (FIV) (cats), blood glucose to identify hypoglycemia, and serum electrolytes to detect hypokalemia. Abdominal imaging should be used to investigate abdominal pain and when masses, obstruction, or foreign body is suspected.

#### Treatment

The goal is to reestablish fluid, electrolyte, and acid-base homeostasis. Patients with severe dehydration (>8%) should receive fluids intravenously (IV); fluids administered subcutaneously (SC) or orally (PO) usually suffice in less severely dehydrated animals. Potassium supplementation is usually indicated; bicarbonate is rarely needed.

   ***Antidiarrheals.*** Antidiarrheals are seldom necessary, except when excessive fecal losses make maintenance of fluid and electrolyte balance difficult. Opiates are usually most effective. Bismuth subsalicylate (see Table 30-5) is useful in dogs with mild to moderate enteritis. However, it is unpalatable, and absorption of the salicylate could cause nephrotoxicity in some patients. Cats rarely need these medications. If antidiarrheals are needed for more than 2 days, the patient should be reassessed.

   ***Antiemetics.*** Severe intestinal inflammation often causes vomiting that is difficult to control. Centrally acting antiemetics (e.g., prochlorperazine, metoclopramide; see Table 30-2) are more effective than peripherally acting drugs. The patient must be well hydrated before receiving phenothiazine derivatives (which can cause hypotension). If these antiemetics fail, ondansetron can be used.

   ***Feeding.*** Withholding food may be necessary if eating causes severe vomiting or explosive diarrhea with substantial fluid loss. However, if feeding does not make the vomiting and diarrhea much worse, offering frequent, small amounts of easily digested, nonirritating foods (e.g., cottage cheese, boiled chicken, potato) is preferable to withholding food. Bowel starvation is to be avoided, if possible. If food was withheld, it should be reoffered as soon as possible. After the enteropathy is clinically resolved, the patient is gradually switched back to its normal diet over 5 to 10 days. If diarrhea returns, the switch is postponed for another 5 days. Some patients with severe enteritis need parenteral nutrition to establish a positive nitrogen balance.

   ***Other recommendations.*** If the patient is febrile, neutropenic, or in septic shock, broad-spectrum systemic antibiotics (e.g., β-lactam plus aminoglycoside) are indicated. Hypoglycemia can develop during septic shock, especially in young animals. Adding dextrose (2.5% to 5%) to the intravenous fluids or administering an intravenous bolus of 50% dextrose (2 to 5 ml/kg) may be needed to counter hypoglycemia. Flunixin meglumine (0.5 to 1 mg/kg IV) seems to help in treatment of septic shock; however, it may cause severe gastric ulceration and impair renal blood flow. If the cause of diarrhea is unknown, the clinician should assume it to be infectious and disinfect the premises accordingly.

### Prognosis
   The prognosis depends on the patient's condition and can be influenced by age and concurrent gastrointestinal (GI) problems. Very young or emaciated animals and those with septic shock or substantial intestinal parasite burdens have a more guarded prognosis. Intussusception may occur secondary to acute enteritis, worsening the prognosis.

## Dietary-Induced Diarrhea
Dietary causes of diarrhea are common, especially in young animals. Poor-quality ingredients (e.g., rancid fat), bacterial enterotoxins or mycotoxins, allergy or intolerance to ingredients, and inability to digest normal foods are common causes.

### Clinical features
   Mild to moderate diarrhea usually begins 1 to 3 days after a new diet is started. The diarrhea typically reflects small intestinal dysfunction (no fecal blood or mucus). Other signs are less common, unless parasites or complicating factors are present.

### Diagnosis
   History and findings of physical and fecal examinations are used to eliminate other common causes. If diarrhea occurs shortly after a suspected or known dietary change, tentative diagnosis of diet-induced disease is reasonable. Intestinal parasitism should be investigated, because it can contribute to the problem.

### Treatment and prognosis
   A bland diet (e.g., potato plus boiled, skinless chicken) fed in multiple small feedings usually resolves the diarrhea in 1 to 3 days. Once the diarrhea resolves, the pet's regular diet can be gradually reintroduced. The prognosis is usually excellent, unless a very young animal with minimal nutritional reserves becomes emaciated, dehydrated, or hypoglycemic.

## INFECTIOUS DIARRHEA (TEXT PP 433-440)

### Canine Parvoviral Enteritis

Classic parvoviral enteritis is caused by canine parvovirus type 2 (CPV-2), which usually causes signs 5 to 12 days after the dog is infected. The most recently recognized strain (CPV-2b) can also infect cats.

#### Clinical features

The clinical syndrome depends on the virulence of the virus, the size of the inoculum, and the host's defenses. Doberman Pinschers, Rottweilers, Pit Bulls, and Labrador Retrievers may be more susceptible than other breeds. Viral destruction of intestinal crypts may produce diarrhea, vomiting, intestinal bleeding, and subsequent bacterial invasion. Some patients have only mild or even subclinical disease.

*"Classic" signs.* Many dogs are initially presented because of depression, anorexia, and/or vomiting (which can resemble foreign object ingestion). Diarrhea is often absent for the first 24 to 48 hours and may not be bloody when it does occur. Intestinal protein loss can develop secondary to inflammation and cause hypoalbuminemia. Vomiting is usually a prominent finding and may be so severe as to cause esophagitis. Damage to bone marrow progenitors may produce transient or prolonged neutropenia, making the patient susceptible to serious bacterial infection. Fever and/or septic shock are common in severely ill dogs. Puppies that are infected in utero or before 8 weeks of age may develop myocarditis.

#### Diagnosis

Tentative diagnosis is often based on history and physical findings. Neutropenia is suggestive of but neither sensitive nor specific for canine parvoviral enteritis.

*Enzyme-linked immunosorbent assay.* Regardless of whether diarrhea occurs, infected dogs shed large numbers of viral particles in the feces ($>10^9$/g), so fecal ELISA for CPV-2 is the best diagnostic test. (Note: Vaccination with a modified-live CPV vaccine may cause a weak positive result for 5 to 15 days after vaccination.)

The ELISA may be negative if performed too early in the clinical course of the disease. It should be repeated in dogs that most likely have parvoviral enteritis but are initially negative. However, shedding decreases rapidly and may be undetectable by 10 to 14 days after infection.

*Other tests.* If the dog dies, typical histologic lesions (e.g., crypt necrosis) and fluorescent antibody techniques can establish a definitive diagnosis.

#### Treatment

Treatment is basically the same for any severe, acute, infectious enteritis (Box 33-1). Fluid and electrolyte therapy is used in combination with antibiotics. Mistakes include inadequate fluid therapy (common), overzealous fluid administration (especially in dogs with severe hypoproteinemia), and failure to recognize and treat sepsis and concurrent GI disease (e.g., parasites, intussusception).

---

**Box 33-1**

### General Guidelines for Treatment of Canine Parvoviral Enteritis*

#### FLUIDS†

- A history of decreased water intake plus increased loss such as vomiting and/or diarrhea confirms dehydration, regardless of whether or not the dog appears to be dehydrated.
- Administer balanced electrolyte solution with 20-40 mEq/L of KCl.
- Dogs with very mild cases may receive SC fluids (IV fluids still preferred), but watch for sudden worsening of the disease.
- Dogs with moderate to severe cases should receive fluids via IV or intramedullary route.

---

*Continued.*

---

Box 33-1—cont'd

## General Guidelines for Treatment of Canine Parvoviral Enteritis*

### FLUIDS†

- Add 2.5% to 5% dextrose to IV fluids if dog has been hypoglycemic or is at risk (e.g., septic shock).
- Administer plasma or hetastarch if serum albumin ≤2 g/dl.

### ANTIBIOTICS†

- Administer antibiotics to febrile or severely neutropenic dogs.
- Administer prophylactic antibiotics for nonfebrile, neutropenic patients (e.g., cefazolin).
- Administer antibiotics to febrile, neutropenic patients (e.g., ampicillin + amikacin).

### ANTIEMETICS

- Prescribe the following as needed:
  - Prochlorperazine (first choice)
  - Metoclopramide
  - Ondansetron or butorphanol (for intractable vomiting when dog does not respond to other medications)

### FLUNIXIN MEGLUMINE (CONTROVERSIAL)

- Sometimes used for patients with severe systemic inflammatory response syndrome (septic shock).
- Use once but not concurrently with corticosteroids; repeated doses or excessive doses can cause life-threatening gastroduodenal ulceration and bleeding; sometimes severe ulceration and bleeding occur even with modest doses.
- Do not use in severely dehydrated dogs.

### ANTHELMINTICS

- Use pyrantel if dog does not vomit it; ivermectin is also acceptable.

### DOGS WITH SECONDARY ESOPHAGITIS

- If regurgitation occurs in addition to vomiting, administer metoclopramide and $H_2$-receptor antagonists (injectable preferred).

### SPECIAL NUTRITIONAL THERAPY

- Administer total parenteral nutrition (TPN) if prolonged anorexia occurs; if TPN cannot be used, recommend partial parenteral nutrition.
- Try to feed dog small amounts as soon as feeding does not cause major exacerbation in vomiting.

### MONITOR PHYSICAL STATUS

Physical examination (1-3 times per day depending on severity of signs)
Body weight (1 or 2 times per day to assess changes in hydration status)
Serum potassium (every 1 or 2 days depending on severity of vomiting and diarrhea)
Serum protein (every 1 or 2 days depending on severity of signs)
Glucose (every 4-12 hr in dogs that have septic shock or were initially hypoglycemic)
Packed cell volume (every 1 or 2 days)
White blood cell count: either actual count or estimated from a slide (every 1 or 2 days in febrile animals)

---

*The same guidelines generally apply to dogs with other causes of acute enteritis or gastritis.
†Usually the first considerations when an animal is presented.
*H*, Histamine; *IV*, intravenous; *KCl*, potassium chloride; *SC*, subcutaneous.

*Antibiotic therapy.* If the patient is in septic shock, an antibiotic combination with a broad aerobic and anaerobic spectrum is recommended (e.g., ampicillin plus amikacin). Renal perfusion must be maintained with fluid therapy when aminoglycosides are administered. Caution should be used when administering enrofloxacin to young, large-breed dogs, as cartilage damage can occur.

*Other medications.* Severe, intractable vomiting complicates therapy and may require administration of prochlorperazine, metoclopramide, or ondansetron (see Table 30-2). If esophagitis occurs, histamine-2 ($H_2$)–receptor antagonists and sucralfate may be useful (see Tables 30-3 and 30-4). Human granulocyte colony-stimulating factor at 5 µg/kg q24h has been used to increase neutrophil numbers in severely neutropenic patients (see text).

*Feeding.* A bland diet can be offered once vomiting has ceased for 18 to 24 hours (see discussion of acute enteritis, earlier). Total or partial parenteral nutrition can be life saving in patients with intractable vomiting.

*Control of infection.* The dog should be kept from other susceptible animals for 2 to 4 weeks after discharge, and the owner should be conscientious about disposal of feces. Vaccination of other dogs in the household should be considered (see later).

When trying to prevent the spread of parvoviral enteritis, it is important to remember that (1) parvovirus persists for months in the environment; (2) asymptomatic dogs may shed virulent CPV-2 in their feces; (3) maternal immunity sufficient to inactivate vaccine virus may persist up to 18 weeks of age; and (4) dilute bleach (1:32) kills the virus.

### Prognosis

Typically, dogs treated promptly and appropriately survive, especially if they live past the first 4 days of clinical disease. Intussusception is a possible sequela and can cause persistent diarrhea in puppies recovering from the viral infection. Dogs that recover develop long-lasting immunity that may be lifelong.

### Prevention

Vaccination of puppies should commence at 5 to 8 weeks of age, preferably with a high-antigen-density vaccine. High-density vaccines are effective in some puppies given a single injection after 12 weeks of age; however, if an inactivated vaccine is administered, it may be best to give a second injection. In general the last vaccination should be administered per manufacturer's recommendations (usually between 12 and 20 weeks of age).

Annual revaccination is generally recommended, although vaccination every 3 years may be sufficient after the initial series. Adults previously unvaccinated usually receive two doses 2 to 4 weeks apart. If one dog in a multiple-dog household develops parvoviral enteritis, booster vaccinations should be given to the other dogs, preferably using an inactivated vaccine.

## Feline Parvoviral Enteritis

Feline parvoviral enteritis (feline distemper, feline panleukopenia) is caused by a parvovirus distinct from CPV-2, although CPV-2b can infect cats and cause clinical disease. Clinical findings, diagnostic techniques, treatment, prognosis, and prevention are similar to those described for canine parvoviral enteritis. Most cats survive with supportive care, as long as overwhelming sepsis is prevented.

## Canine Coronaviral Enteritis

Canine coronaviral enteritis is typically much less severe than "classic" parvoviral enteritis. It rarely causes hemorrhagic diarrhea, septicemia, or death, although small or very young dogs may die from dehydration or electrolyte abnormalities if not properly treated. Clinical signs may last 3 to 20 days. Concurrent parvovirus infection increases morbidity and mortality. Coronaviral enteritis can occur in mature dogs.

### Diagnosis

Canine coronaviral enteritis is seldom definitively diagnosed. Most dogs are treated symptomatically for acute enteritis until they improve. Electron microscopy of feces obtained early in the disease can be diagnostic. However, the virus is fragile and easily disrupted by inappropriate handling of feces.

### Treatment and prognosis

Symptomatic therapy for acute enteritis is usually successful, except perhaps for very young animals. The prognosis for recovery is good. A vaccine is available but of uncertain value, except in high-risk situations (e.g., infected kennels, dog shows).

## Feline Coronaviral Enteritis

The severity of feline coronaviral enteritis is age related. Adults are often asymptomatic, whereas kittens may have mild, transient diarrhea and fever. Death is rare, and the prognosis for recovery is excellent. No vaccine is available. This disease is important because (1) affected animals seroconvert and may be positive on feline infectious peritonitis (FIP) serology, and (2) mutation by the feline coronavirus may be the cause of FIP.

## FeLV-Associated Panleukopenia

FeLV-associated panleukopenia is a nonneoplastic disease caused by FeLV. Intestinal lesions histologically resemble those produced by feline parvovirus. Bone marrow and lymph nodes are inconsistently affected. These patients might also have parvoviral infections that cannot easily be detected.

### Clinical features and diagnosis

Chronic weight loss, vomiting, and diarrhea are common. The diarrhea often has characteristics of large bowel disease (see Chapter 28). Some patients are also neutropenic. Finding FeLV infection in a cat with chronic diarrhea is suggestive of this disorder. The chronic course helps differentiate it from parvoviral enteritis. Intestinal biopsy helps eliminate other causes.

### Treatment and prognosis

Symptomatic therapy for acute enteritis plus elimination of other problems that compromise the intestines (e.g., parasites, poor diet) may be beneficial. This disease is associated with a very poor prognosis because of other FeLV-related complications.

## FIV-Associated Diarrhea

FIV can cause severe, purulent colitis that occasionally results in colonic rupture. Affected patients appear ill, whereas many cats with chronic large bowel disease resulting from inflammatory bowel disease (IBD) or dietary intolerance seemingly feel fine. Detecting antibodies to FIV and finding severe, purulent colitis allow presumptive diagnosis. Therapy is supportive. The long-term prognosis is very poor, although some cats can be maintained for months.

## Salmon Poisoning

Salmon poisoning is caused by *Neorickettsia helminthoeca*. Dogs are infected when they eat fish (primarily salmon) infected with a fluke (*Nanophyetus salmincola*) that carries the rickettsia. This disease is principally found in the Pacific Northwest of the United States.

### Clinical features and diagnosis

Severity of signs varies, and they may include fever, anorexia, vomiting, generalized lymphadenopathy, and/or diarrhea. The diarrhea is typically of small bowel origin but may become bloody. Presumptive diagnosis is usually based on the patient's habitat plus a history of recent consumption of raw fish or exposure to streams or lakes. Finding *Nanophyetus* spp. ova in the stool or rickettsia in fine-needle aspirates of enlarged lymph nodes is confirmatory.

### Treatment and prognosis

Treatment consists of symptomatic control of dehydration, vomiting, and diarrhea, plus elimination of the rickettsia and flukes. Tetracycline, oxytetracycline, doxycycline, or chloramphenicol eliminate the rickettsia. The fluke is killed with praziquantel (see Table 30-6). The prognosis depends on disease severity at the time of diagnosis. Most dogs respond favorably to tetracyclines and supportive therapy. The key to success, however, is awareness of the disease; untreated salmon poisoning carries a poor prognosis.

## Campylobacteriosis

Campylobacteriosis is caused by *Campylobacter jejuni*. Poultry is probably a reservoir. This organism is also found in the intestinal tract of some healthy dogs and cats. Campylobacteriosis is primarily diagnosed in young animals in crowded conditions (e.g., kennels, humane shelters) or as a nosocomial infection. *C. jejuni* may also cause enteritis during recovery from canine parvoviral enteritis.

### Clinical features and diagnosis

Mucoid diarrhea (with or without blood), anorexia, fever, or any or all of these are the primary signs. The disease tends to be self-limiting, but it occasionally causes chronic diarrhea. *C. jejuni* has special culture requirements. The fecal sample must be submitted promptly or appropriate transport media used. Occasionally, classic *Campylobacter* forms ("commas," "seagull wings") are found during cytologic examination of a fecal smear. However, because it may be cultured from normal dogs and cats, appropriate signs, history, or response to therapy is needed to confirm that *C. jejuni* is causing disease.

### Treatment and prognosis

Erythromycin (10 to 15 mg/kg PO q8h) or neomycin (10 to 20 mg/kg PO q12h) is usually effective. Tetracycline may also be a good choice; β-lactam antibiotics (e.g., penicillins, cephalosporins) are often ineffective. The patient should be treated for at least 1 to 3 days beyond resolution of signs. However, antibiotic therapy may not eradicate the bacteria, and reinfection is likely in kennel conditions. Chronic infections may require prolonged therapy (weeks). With appropriate antibiotic therapy, the prognosis for recovery is good.

### *Precautions.*

Infected dogs and cats should be isolated, and people working with a patient or its environment or wastes should wear protective clothing and wash with disinfectants.

## Salmonellosis

Numerous *Salmonella* spp. serotypes can cause disease in dogs and cats. The bacteria may originate from animals shedding the organism or from contaminated foods (especially poultry and eggs). Salmonellosis is seldom confirmed as a cause of canine or feline GI disease, even though the bacteria are often present in the colon and/or mesenteric lymph nodes.

### Clinical features

Salmonellosis can cause acute or chronic diarrhea, septicemia, and/or sudden death, especially in very young or geriatric animals. Salmonellosis in young animals can mimic parvoviral enteritis; occasionally it develops during or after parvoviral enteritis.

### Diagnosis

*Salmonella* spp. may be cultured from normal animals, so definitive diagnosis can be difficult. Culture of *Salmonella* spp. from the blood confirms septicemia. Diagnosis of GI salmonellosis requires (1) appropriate signs, (2) culture of the organism from feces or GI mucosa, (3) elimination of other causes (e.g., parvovirus), and (4) response to therapy. Fecal culture often necessitates use of enrichment and/or selective media. Identification by polymerase chain reaction can be a sensitive method of diagnosis.

### Treatment and prognosis

Treatment depends on disease severity. Septicemic patients should receive supportive therapy and parenteral antibiotics as determined by susceptibility testing. Quinolones, potentiated sulfa drugs, and chloramphenicol are often good initial choices. Patients with diarrhea may need only supportive therapy; antibiotics are of questionable value and might promote a carrier state. The prognosis is usually good in animals with just diarrhea but guarded in septicemic patients.

*Precautions.* Infected patients should be isolated from other animals at least until they are asymptomatic. Even when signs resolve, reculturing of feces is reasonable to ensure that shedding has stopped. People in contact with the patient and its environment and wastes should wear protective clothing and wash with disinfectants (e.g., hexachlorophene).

## Clostridial Diseases

*Clostridium perfringens* and *Clostridium difficile* can be found in clinically normal dogs but appear to cause diarrhea in some. *C. perfringens* may produce an acute, bloody, self-limiting diarrhea or chronic large bowel diarrhea (with or without blood or mucus); this condition is primarily recognized in dogs. Disease associated with *C. difficile* is poorly characterized in small animals.

### Diagnosis

For *C. perfringens,* fecal ELISA to detect enterotoxin appears to hold promise. This infection cannot be reliably diagnosed by finding spore-forming bacteria on fecal smears nor by detecting enterotoxin using reversed passive latex agglutination. Response to treatment with tylosin or amoxicillin allows tentative diagnosis.

*C. difficile* is hard to culture from feces. Infection has been diagnosed with commercial laboratory kits for *C. difficile* toxin in feces; however, false-positive and false-negative results can occur. Response to treatment with metronidazole allows presumptive diagnosis.

### Treatment

If *C. perfringens* colitis is suspected, antimicrobials active against the organism are recommended. Tylosin (20 to 80 mg/kg/day, divided q12h) or amoxicillin (22 mg/kg q12h) is effective and has minimal adverse effects. However, antibiotic treatment does not necessarily eliminate the bacteria, and many dogs need indefinite therapy. Some animals can eventually be maintained with once daily or every other day antibiotic therapy. Some patients with chronic large bowel diarrhea seemingly caused by *C. perfringens* respond to fiber-supplemented diets. If disease caused by *C. difficile* is suspected, supportive fluid and electrolyte therapy may be necessary, depending on the severity of signs.

### Prognosis

The prognosis is excellent in dogs with diarrhea resulting from *C. perfringens* but uncertain in those with diarrhea resulting from *C. difficile.*

## Miscellaneous Bacteria

*Yersinia enterocolitica, Aeromonas hydrophila,* and *Plesiomonas shigelloides* may cause acute or chronic enterocolitis in dogs and cats. *Y. enterocolitica* is primarily found in colder environments; pigs may serve as reservoirs. It is also a cause of food poisoning. Enterohemorrhagic *Escherichia coli* (EHEC) occasionally causes diarrhea in dogs and cats.

### Clinical features

Small bowel diarrhea may be caused by any of these bacteria. Yersiniosis usually affects the colon and produces chronic large bowel diarrhea.

### Diagnosis

Fecal culture is warranted for persistent diarrhea that cannot be diagnosed by routine means (e.g., fecal examination, mucosal biopsy) and for apparently infectious diarrhea (multiple animals and/or people affected). Patients with persistent colitis, especially those that are in contact with pigs, should be cultured for *Y. enterocolitica.* Specific enrichment and selection procedures are recommended. If EHEC is suspected, it is helpful to screen *E. coli* isolates for the ability to ferment sorbitol and then serotype the strains and/or analyze for production of verotoxins. These toxins may also be detected in feces.

### Treatment and prognosis

Therapy is supportive. Appropriate antibiotics as determined by culture and sensitivity are often used, although they do not shorten clinical disease resulting from EHEC. *Y. enterocolitica* is often sensitive to tetracyclines. Treatment should be continued for 1 to 3 days beyond clinical remission. The patient should be isolated from other animals. People in contact with the animal and/or its environment and wastes should wear protective clothing and wash with disinfectants. The prognosis seems to be good if the bacteria can be identified by culture and the infection is treated appropriately.

## Histoplasmosis

*Histoplasma capsulatum* can cause disease that involves the GI, respiratory, and/or reticuloendothelial systems, as well as the bones and eyes. It is mainly found in animals from the Mississippi and Ohio River valleys.

### Clinical features

Alimentary tract involvement is primarily found in dogs; diarrhea (can be bloody and contain mucus) and weight loss are common signs. The lungs, liver, spleen, lymph nodes, bone marrow, bones, and/or eyes may also be affected. Symptomatic GI involvement is much less common in cats; respiratory dysfunction (e.g., dyspnea, cough), fever, and/or weight loss are more common in this species.

*GI disease.* In GI histoplasmosis the colon is usually the most severely affected segment. Diffuse, severe, granulomatous, ulcerative mucosal disease often produces bloody stool, intestinal protein loss, intermittent fever, and/or weight loss. The disease may "smolder" for long periods, causing mild to moderate nonprogressive signs. Occasionally, histoplasmosis causes focal colonic granulomas or is present in grossly normal-appearing colonic mucosa.

### Diagnosis

Dogs that are from endemic areas and that have chronic large bowel diarrhea are suspect. Protein-losing enteropathy is common in dogs with severe histoplasmosis, so hypoalbuminemia in a dog with large bowel disease is suggestive of the disease, regardless of where the animal lives. Diagnosis requires cytologic or histologic identification of the yeast. Serologic tests and fecal culture are unreliable, especially in cats.

*Techniques.* Rectal examination sometimes reveals thickened rectal folds, which can be scraped to obtain material for cytologic preparations. Colonic biopsies are usually diagnostic, but special stains may be necessary. Rarely, mesenteric lymph node samples or repeated colonic biopsy are required.

*Other organs.* Fundic examination occasionally reveals active chorioretinitis. Abdominal radiographs may show hepatosplenomegaly, and thoracic radiographs sometimes demonstrate pulmonary involvement (e.g., miliary interstitial infiltrates, hilar lymphadenopathy). Cytologic evaluation of hepatic or splenic aspirates, bone marrow, or buffy coat smears may reveal the organism. Rarely, CBC reveals yeast in circulating white blood cells. Thrombocytopenia may also be found.

### Treatment

It is crucial to look for histoplasmosis before beginning empiric corticosteroid therapy for canine colonic IBD. Corticosteroids may allow a previously treatable case to rapidly progress and kill the patient. Itraconazole alone or preceded by amphotericin B is often effective. Treatment for 4 to 6 months may be necessary to lessen the chance of relapse.

### Prognosis

Many dogs can be cured if treated early. Multiple organ system involvement worsens the prognosis. Central nervous system (CNS) involvement is a poor prognostic indicator.

## Protothecosis

*Prototheca zopfi* is an invasive algae. Immunodeficiency may be needed for the organism to cause disease, which affects dogs and occasionally cats. Collies may be over-represented. The disease primarily involves the skin, colon, and eyes, but it may disseminate throughout the body.

### Clinical features and diagnosis

Colonic involvement causes bloody stools and other signs of colitis, similar to histoplasmosis (although protothecosis is much less common). Diagnosis requires demonstration of the organism via cytology or histopathology of colonic biopsies.

### Treatment and prognosis

Most drugs work inconsistently. High doses of liposomal amphotericin B might be useful. The prognosis for disseminated disease is poor.

## ALIMENTARY TRACT PARASITES (TEXT PP 440-446)
### Whipworms
*Trichuris vulpis* is primarily found in the eastern United States and mostly affects dogs. Animals acquire the infection by ingesting ova.
#### Clinical features
Whipworms produce a wide spectrum of mild to severe colonic disease, including hematochezia and protein-losing enteropathy. Severe trichuriasis may cause severe hyponatremia and hyperkalemia, mimicking hypoadrenocorticism. Marked hyponatremia may cause CNS signs (e.g., seizures). Whipworms do not affect cats as often or as severely.
#### Diagnosis
*T. vulpis* should always be sought in dogs with bloody stools or large bowel diarrhea. Diagnosis is made by finding ova in the feces or seeing the adults during endoscopy. However, the ova are dense and float only in properly prepared solutions. Also, they are shed intermittently and sometimes can be found only after multiple fecal examinations.
#### Treatment and prognosis
It is reasonable to empirically treat dogs with chronic large bowel disease with fenbendazole or other appropriate drugs (see Table 30-6) before proceeding to endoscopy. If whipworm infection is suspected or confirmed, the dog should be treated again in 3 months. The prognosis for recovery is good, but ova persist in the environment for long periods.

### Roundworms
Roundworms are common in dogs (*Toxocara canis* and *Toxascaris leonina)* and cats (*Toxocara cati* and *T. leonina).* *T. canis* is often contracted transplacentally; both *T. canis* and *T. cati* may use transmammary passage.
#### Clinical features
Roundworms may cause or contribute to diarrhea, stunted growth, poor hair coat, and poor weight gain, especially in young patients. Runts with "pot bellies" often have severe roundworm infection. Sometimes roundworms gain access to the stomach, in which case they may be vomited. If parasites are numerous, they may obstruct the intestines or bile duct.
#### Diagnosis
Diagnosis is easy because ova are readily found by fecal flotation. Occasionally, neonates develop signs of roundworm infestation before the parasites mature and produce ova.
#### Treatment
Various anthelmintics are effective (see Table 30-6); pyrantel is particularly safe for puppies and kittens, especially those with diarrhea. Patients should be retreated at 2- to 3-week intervals.
#### *Prevention.*
High-dose fenbendazole therapy (50 mg/kg/day from day 40 of gestation until 2 weeks postpartum) lessens transplacental and transmammary transmission to puppies. Newborn puppies can be treated with fenbendazole (100 mg/kg for 3 days). Unweaned puppies should be treated at 2, 4, 6, and 8 weeks of age. Unweaned kittens should be treated at 6, 8, and 10 weeks of age.
#### Prognosis
The prognosis for recovery is good unless the animal is already severely stunted.

### Hookworms
*Ancylostoma* spp. and *Uncinaria* spp. are more common in dogs than in cats. Infestation is usually via ingestion of the ova or through transcolostral transmission; freshly hatched larvae may also penetrate the skin. Adults live in the small intestine; in severe infestations, hookworms may also be found in the colon.
#### Clinical features
Dogs are more severely affected than cats. Puppies may have life-threatening blood loss or iron-deficiency anemia, melena, frank fecal blood, diarrhea, and/or failure to

thrive. Hookworms alone rarely cause disease in mature dogs unless infestation is massive. However, they may contribute to disease caused by other intestinal problems.

### Diagnosis
Hookworm infection is suggested by the signalment and clinical signs. Iron-deficiency anemia in a puppy or kitten without fleas is highly suggestive. Finding ova in the feces is diagnostic. However, 5- to 10-day-old puppies may be exsanguinated by transcolostrally obtained hookworms before ova appear in the feces. (Such prepatent infections rarely occur in older animals that have received a sudden, massive exposure.)

### Treatment and prevention
Various anthelmintics are effective (see Table 30-6). Treatment should be repeated in 3 weeks. In anemic puppies and kittens blood transfusions may be life saving. Use of heartworm preventatives containing pyrantel or milbemycin limits hookworm infestation. Treating pregnant bitches with high-dose fenbendazole (see discussion of roundworms, earlier) reduces transcolostral transmission to puppies.

### Prognosis
The prognosis is good in mature dogs and cats but guarded in severely anemic puppies and kittens. Severely stunted puppies and kittens may never attain their anticipated body size.

## Tapeworms
Several species of tapeworm infect dogs and cats, the most common being *Dipylidium caninum*. Fleas and lice are intermediate hosts for *D. caninum;* wild animals (e.g., rabbits) are intermediate hosts for some *Taenia* spp.

### Clinical features
Tapeworms are rarely pathogenic in small animals. The most common sign is anal irritation associated with shed segments. Occasionally a segment enters an anal sac and causes inflammation. Very rarely, large numbers of tapeworms cause intestinal obstruction.

### Diagnosis
*Taenia* spp. and *D. caninum* eggs are confined in segments and therefore are undetected by routine fecal flotation. *Echinococcus* spp. (and some *Taenia* spp.) ova may be found in the feces. Diagnosis is usually made when the owner reports tapeworm segments on the feces or perineum.

### Treatment and prevention
Praziquantel and epsiprantel are effective against all species of tapeworms (see Table 30-6). Prevention involves controlling the intermediate hosts (fleas and lice for *D. caninum*).

## Strongyloidiasis
*Strongyloides stercoralis* principally affects puppies in crowded conditions. Motile larvae can penetrate unbroken skin or mucosa; therefore puppies may be reinfested from their own feces even before larvae are evacuated from the colon. Infested animals can quickly acquire large parasitic burdens.

### Clinical features and diagnosis
Affected animals usually have mucoid or hemorrhagic diarrhea and are systemically ill (e.g., lethargic). Respiratory signs occur if parasites invade the lungs (verminous pneumonia). The diagnosis is made when larvae are found in fresh feces, either by direct examination or with Baermann sedimentation. *Strongyloides* spp. larvae must be differentiated from *Osleri* spp. larvae. The feces must be fresh; if they are old, hookworm ova (which resemble *Strongyloides* spp.) may hatch.

### Treatment and prognosis
Fenbendazole (used for 5 days), thiabendazole, and ivermectin are effective anthelmintics (see Table 30-6). The prognosis is guarded in young animals with severe diarrhea and/or pneumonia.

## Coccidia
*Isospora* spp. are principally found in young cats and dogs. The coccidia invade and destroy villous epithelial cells. Coccidia may be clinically insignificant (especially in

an older animal) or they may cause mild to severe diarrhea, sometimes with blood. Rarely, a kitten or puppy loses enough blood to require a blood transfusion.

### Diagnosis

Coccidiosis is diagnosed by finding oocysts on fecal flotation. However, repeated fecal examinations may be needed, and small numbers of oocysts do not necessarily equate with insignificant infestation. These oocysts must not be confused with giardial cysts. Occasionally, *Eimeria* oocysts are seen in the feces of dogs that eat deer or rabbit excrement.

### Treatment and prognosis

Sulfadimethoxine or trimethoprim-sulfa should be administered for 10 to 20 days (see Table 30-6). Amprolium (50 mg PO q24h for 3 to 5 days) has been used in puppies, but it is potentially toxic in cats. Toltrazuril (15 mg/kg PO q24h for 3 days) decreases oocyst shedding. The prognosis for recovery is good, unless underlying problems allowed the coccidia to become pathogenic in the first place.

## Cryptosporidiosis

*Cryptosporidium parvum* is a coccidian that infests the brush border of small intestinal epithelial cells. Diarrhea is the most common sign in dogs and cats, although many infected cats are asymptomatic. Dogs with diarrhea are usually less than 6 months of age.

### Diagnosis

Diagnosis requires identification of the tiny oocysts (which are easy to miss on fecal examination) or a positive ELISA (more sensitive than fecal examination). Microscopic examination should be at 1000×. Use of acid-fast stains on fecal smears or fluorescent antibody techniques improves sensitivity.

### Treatment and prognosis

No reliable treatment exists. Most young dogs with diarrhea associated with cryptosporidiosis die or are euthanized. Many cats have asymptomatic infections; those with diarrhea have an unknown prognosis.

## Giardiasis

Giardiasis is caused by a protozoan, *Giardia* sp., and is primarily a problem in dogs; cats are occasionally infected. Clinical signs vary from mild to severe diarrhea, which may be persistent, intermittent, or self-limiting. Typically the diarrhea is like a "cow patty," without blood or mucus; however, much variation exists. Some patients lose weight.

### Diagnosis

Giardiasis is diagnosed by finding motile trophozoites in fresh feces or duodenal washes, by finding cysts with fecal flotation techniques, or by finding giardial proteins in feces using ELISA. Zinc sulfate solution is best for demonstrating cysts, especially when centrifugal flotation is performed. At least three fecal examinations should be performed over a 7- to 10-day period before giardiasis is discounted. Washes of the duodenal lumen (performed endoscopically or surgically) or cytologic examination of the duodenal mucosa occasionally reveal *Giardia* organisms when other techniques do not.

### Treatment and prognosis

Metronidazole is approximately 85% effective after 7 days of therapy and has few adverse effects. Furazolidone for 5 days may be as effective and is available as a suspension, making it easy to treat kittens. Albendazole (3 days in dogs, 5 days in cats) and fenbendazole (5 days in dogs and cats) are fairly effective; neomycin given PO may also be useful. However, no drug is 100% effective, so failure to respond to therapy does not rule out giardiasis. The prognosis for recovery is usually good, although the organisms are sometimes difficult to eradicate.

## Trichomoniasis

Trichomoniasis in cats is caused by *Tritrichomonas foetus/suis*. Infection probably occurs via the fecal-oral route. Trichomoniasis typically causes large bowel diarrhea that rarely contains blood or mucus. Most affected cats are otherwise normal, although they may have anal irritation. The diarrhea may spontaneously resolve or it may persist for months.

### Diagnosis

Diagnosis requires identification of motile trophozoites, which requires timely examination of fresh feces diluted with warm saline solution. *Tritrichomonas* trophozoites are often mistakenly identified as *Giardia* trophozoites. If trichomoniasis is diagnosed, it is still important to look for other causes of diarrhea (e.g., *C. perfringens,* diet, *Cryptosporidium* spp.), because treatment for the concurrent problem often results in resolution of the diarrhea.

### Treatment and prognosis

Currently no effective treatment for feline trichomoniasis exists. Many cats improve somewhat while receiving antibiotic therapy. In most cats the diarrhea eventually resolves, although it may recur if the cat undergoes a stressful event (e.g., surgery).

## MALDIGESTIVE DISEASE (TEXT PP 446-447)

### Exocrine Pancreatic Insufficiency

See Chapter 40.

## MALABSORPTIVE DISEASES (TEXT PP 447-450)

IBD is a syndrome of idiopathic intestinal inflammation; it is a diagnosis of exclusion. IBD occurs in both dogs and cats, and can affect any portion of the intestine. Although the cause is unknown, it may be a generic intestinal response to bacterial and/or dietary antigens. Clinical and histologic features can closely resemble those of alimentary lymphoma.

### Canine Lymphocytic-Plasmacytic Enteritis

Lymphocytic-plasmacytic enteritis (LPE) is the most commonly diagnosed canine IBD. Chronic small intestinal diarrhea is common, but some dogs have weight loss with normal stools. If the duodenum is severely affected, vomiting may be the major sign; diarrhea can be either mild or absent. Protein-losing enteropathy occurs in dogs with the more severe forms.

#### Diagnosis

No historic, physical, or laboratory findings are diagnostic for canine LPE, although severe disease may cause hypoalbuminemia with or without hypoglobulinemia. Endoscopy may be suggestive of infiltrative disease. Elimination of known causes plus histologic examination of intestinal mucosa is required for diagnosis. However, histologic diagnosis of LPE is subjective, and biopsy samples are frequently overinterpreted. In addition, it can be difficult to distinguish a well-differentiated lymphocytic lymphoma from severe LPE, even with full-thickness samples (see text).

#### Treatment

Elimination diets and antibiotics should be included in the treatment regimen in case the problem is actually dietary intolerance or antibiotic-responsive enteropathy (ARE), especially in dogs with "mild" IBD. Home-made hypoallergenic diets are optimal. Elemental diets can be invaluable in severely emaciated or hypoproteinemic patients with severe inflammation. Other therapy depends on the severity of LPE.

*Moderate to severe LPE.* Moderate to severe disease (marked inflammatory infiltrates, especially if associated with hypoalbuminemia) usually requires dietary change, antibiotics (e.g., tetracycline), high-dose corticosteroid therapy (e.g., prednisolone, 2.2 mg/kg/day), metronidazole, and sometimes azathioprine, cyclophosphamide, or cyclosporine. Severely affected animals may initially benefit from enteral or parenteral nutritional supplementation.

When severe LPE is treated, azathioprine is started with the other drugs, and the decision whether to continue it is based on the patient's response over the first 2 to 3 weeks of treatment (i.e., before a clinical effect of the drug can be expected). Failure to respond to therapy may be the result of inadequate therapy, owner noncompliance, or misdiagnosis (i.e., diagnosing LPE when the problem is lymphoma).

If the patient responds to therapy, treatment should be continued without change for another 2 to 4 weeks. Once the clinician is convinced that the therapy is effective, the animal should be slowly weaned from the drugs, starting with those that have the greatest potential for adverse effects. Attempts should be made to maintain the dog on every-other-day corticosteroid and azathioprine therapy at the lowest effective dose. Only one change is made at a time, and decreases in dose should not be made more frequently than once every 2 to 3 weeks. Dietary and antibiotic therapy are usually the last to be altered.

### Prognosis

The prognosis depends on the severity of the infiltrate, the presence or absence of hypoalbuminemia, the patient's body condition, and the need for immunosuppressive drugs. Most patients need a special diet for the rest of their lives. Many with moderate to severe disease also need prolonged medical therapy. Iatrogenic Cushing's syndrome should be avoided when corticosteroids are used. LPE has been suggested to be a prelymphomatous lesion in some dogs (see the discussion of immunoproliferative enteropathy in Basenjis); however, the association between LPE and alimentary lymphoma is very uncertain (see text).

## Canine Lymphocytic-Plasmacytic Colitis

Lymphocytic-plasmacytic colitis (LPC) typically causes large bowel diarrhea (soft stools with blood or mucus; no appreciable weight loss). In general these dogs are healthy except for soft stools. Biopsy is required for diagnosis. It is easy to overinterpret tissues and diagnose LPC when other causes (e.g., clostridial colitis, dietary intolerance, fiber-responsive diarrhea) are responsible.

### Treatment and prognosis

Many dogs initially diagnosed with LPC respond to hypoallergenic diets, fiber-supplemented diets, and/or tylosin. Sulfasalazine (Azulfidine), mesalamine, or olsalazine may be used in dogs with moderate to severe LPC. Corticosteroids and/or metronidazole may be effective by themselves or may allow lower doses of sulfasalazine to be effective. The prognosis is better than for dogs with LPE.

## Feline Lymphocytic-Plasmacytic Enteritis

Feline LPE principally causes vomiting, but weight loss, diarrhea, and/or anorexia may also occur. Diarrhea and protein-losing enteropathy are less common than in dogs with LPE. Biopsy and elimination of other causes of the clinical signs are required for diagnosis.

### Treatment

Highly digestible elimination diets may be curative and should always be used if the cat will eat them. High doses of corticosteroids are also used. Low-dose metronidazole (10 to 15 mg/kg PO q12h) may be effective, either alone or in combination with corticosteroids and diet. Chlorambucil is reserved for cats with biopsy-proved, severe LPE that does not respond to other therapy or for cats with well-differentiated lymphoma.

Enteral or parenteral nutritional support may be useful in emaciated cats (see Chapter 30). Parenteral administration of cobalamin to cats with very low serum cobalamin may aid in control of diarrhea. Budesonide (a locally acting steroid) has been used in some patients with difficult-to-control IBD. If the cat responds to therapy, the elimination diet should be continued while attempts are made to gradually taper off the medications, one at a time.

### Prognosis

The prognosis is usually good, but if the cat is emaciated, the prognosis is guarded. As in dogs, it is unclear whether feline LPE is a premalignant lesion.

## Feline Lymphocytic-Plasmacytic Colitis

LPC is much more common in cats than in dogs. It may occur alone or with LPE. Hematochezia is the most common sign; diarrhea is the second most common.

High-fiber and hypoallergenic diets are often beneficial. Most cats also respond to prednisolone and/or metronidazole; sulfasalazine is rarely needed. The prognosis is usually good.

## Canine Eosinophilic Gastroenterocolitis

Canine eosinophilic gastroenterocolitis (EGE) is usually an allergic reaction to dietary substances (e.g., beef, milk). Signs do not always respond to dietary change, so this may represent true IBD in some dogs. It is less common than canine LPE or LPC. German Shepherd Dogs are overrepresented.

### Clinical features and diagnosis

Small and/or large intestinal diarrhea and weight loss are common. Vomiting may occur in dogs with gastric or duodenal involvement. Some patients have concurrent eosinophilic respiratory tract disease; cutaneous allergic reactions may also be seen. Although peripheral eosinophilia is consistent with EGE, it is not always present. Cytologic evaluation of mucosal impression smears from intestinal biopsies may reveal numerous eosinophils (1 to 3/hpf). Biopsy is required for diagnosis.

### Treatment

A strict hypoallergenic diet (e.g., fish or turkey and potato) often resolves the signs. Partially hydrolyzed diets may be helpful, but they are not a panacea. If signs do not resolve with dietary therapy, addition of corticosteroids is usually curative. Corticosteroids should be slowly withdrawn after signs resolve to determine if they are still needed.

Sometimes a patient initially responds to dietary management but relapses because it becomes allergic to one of the ingredients. This necessitates a different elimination diet. In patients prone to developing such intolerances, switching back and forth from one elimination diet to another at 2-week intervals helps prevent the patient from becoming allergic to the new diet.

### Prognosis

The prognosis is usually good, although some dogs are sensitive to many foods.

## Feline Eosinophilic Enteritis or Hypereosinophilic Syndrome

Some cats have eosinophilic enteritis as part of a hypereosinophilic syndrome (HES). The cause of this syndrome is unknown, but immune-mediated and neoplastic mechanisms may be responsible. Less severely affected cats without HES may have a condition similar to canine EGE.

### Clinical features and diagnosis

Small intestinal diarrhea, vomiting, weight loss, or any of these are the principal signs. Mucosal cytology sometimes allows presumptive diagnosis, and peripheral eosinophilia, although inconsistent, is suggestive of this disorder. Intestinal biopsy is necessary for definitive diagnosis. Intestinal eosinophilic infiltrates are the most common finding in HES, although splenic, hepatic, lymph node, and bone marrow infiltrates and peripheral eosinophilia are common.

### Treatment and prognosis

Cats with eosinophilic enteritis not resulting from HES often respond favorably to elimination diets plus corticosteroid therapy. High-dose corticosteroid therapy (e.g., prednisolone, 4.4 to 6.6 mg/kg/day) has been used with little success in cats with HES. The prognosis is guarded to poor for cats with HES. Those with the less severe syndrome may have a fair prognosis.

## Granulomatous Enteritis or Gastritis

### Dogs

Granulomatous enteritis or gastritis is uncommon in dogs and requires biopsy for diagnosis. Signs are similar to those of other forms of IBD. If the disease is localized, surgical resection can be considered. If it is diffuse, corticosteroids, metronidazole, antibiotics, azathioprine, and dietary therapy should be considered. The prognosis is poor.

### Cats

Granulomatous enteritis is a rare IBD in cats that causes weight loss, protein-losing enteropathy, and possibly diarrhea. Diagnosis requires histopathologic confirmation. Affected cats usually respond to high-dose corticosteroid therapy, but attempts to reduce the dose may cause recurrence of clinical signs. The prognosis is guarded.

## Immunoproliferative Enteropathy in Basenjis

Immunoproliferative enteropathy in Basenjis, a breed-specific syndrome, primarily involves the small intestine. It causes an intense lymphocytic-plasmacytic infiltrate, often with villous clubbing, mild lacteal dilation, gastric rugal and/or mucosal hypertrophy, and lymphocytic gastritis. It may have a genetic basis or predisposition; intestinal bacteria may also play an important role. Most affected Basenjis start showing signs by 3 to 4 years of age.

### Clinical features

The disease tends to be a severe form of LPE that waxes and wanes, often worsening when the patient is stressed (e.g., traveling, other disease). Common signs include weight loss, small intestinal diarrhea, vomiting, and/or anorexia.

### Diagnosis

Marked hypoalbuminemia and hyperglobulinemia are common, especially in advanced cases. The early stages resemble many other intestinal disorders. In advanced cases signs are so suggestive that a presumptive diagnosis is often made without biopsy. However, other diseases (e.g., lymphoma, histoplasmosis) may mimic immunoproliferative enteropathy, so biopsy is recommended before aggressive immunosuppressive therapy is begun.

*Asymptomatic dogs.* Performing biopsies of asymptomatic dogs to identify those that will develop the disease is of dubious value. Clinically normal Basenjis may have lesions similar to dogs with diarrhea and weight loss, although the changes tend to be milder.

### Treatment

Therapy includes feeding a highly digestible, elimination, or elemental diet, antibiotics for ARE (see later), high-dose corticosteroids, metronidazole, and azathioprine. Response to therapy is variable, and affected dogs that respond are at risk for relapse, especially if stressed.

### Prognosis

The prognosis for recovery is poor, but some patients can be maintained for prolonged periods with careful monitoring. Many affected dogs die within 2 to 3 years of diagnosis. A few dogs develop lymphoma.

## Enteropathy in Shar Peis

Chinese Shar Peis have a poorly characterized enteropathy that may be unique to them or may be a severe form of IBD. The main clinical signs include diarrhea and/or weight loss. Small intestinal biopsy is necessary for diagnosis. Eosinophilic and lymphocytic-plasmacytic infiltrates are typically found. Serum cobalamin and folate concentrations may help identify concurrent ARE (see later). The patient is treated for IBD (elimination diets and immunosuppressive drugs) and ARE. Affected dogs have a guarded prognosis.

## Antibiotic-Responsive Enteropathy

In ARE the duodenum, the jejunum, or both are contaminated with excessive numbers of bacteria (usually $>10^5$ colony forming units per milliliter), and the host has an abnormal response to these bacteria. Any species of bacteria may be present, but *E. coli,* enterococci, and anaerobes such as *Clostridium* spp. are especially common. Anaerobic bacteria might cause worse problems than aerobic bacteria.

The bacteria may be present because of (1) an anatomic defect that allows retention of food (e.g., partial stricture or area of hypomotility), (2) other diseases (e.g., intestinal mucosal disease), (3) impaired host defenses (e.g., hypochlorhydria, immunoglobulin A deficiency, $H_2$-receptor antagonist therapy decreasing gastric acidity), or (4) no identifiable reason.

### Clinical features and diagnosis

ARE can occur in any dog. The major signs include diarrhea, weight loss, or both, although vomiting may also occur. Multiple, quantitative duodenal fluid cultures are the "gold standard" for diagnosis, but these cultures are difficult to obtain in most private practices. Serum cobalamin and folate concentrations are reasonable screening tools (see Chapter 29). Duodenal mucosal cytology occasionally allows detection of bacteria, although it has poor sensitivity. Because of the difficulty in diagnosing ARE, many clinicians use response to therapy for diagnostic purposes.

### Treatment

Treatment for ARE is reasonable whenever the disorder is suspected. Therapy consists of antibiotics plus correction of potential causes (e.g., blind or stagnant loops of intestine). Broad-spectrum antibiotics effective against aerobes and anaerobes are recommended. Tetracycline (22 mg/kg q12h), tylosin (10 to 80 mg/kg q12h in food), or amoxicillin (22 mg/kg q12h) is usually effective. Occasionally a pure culture of a specific bacterium is found in the duodenum, allowing specific antibiotic therapy. Antibiotics should be continued for 2 to 4 weeks. Because there may exist an underlying cause that cannot be corrected, some patients need long-term or indefinite antibiotic therapy.

### Prognosis

The prognosis is good for control of ARE, but the clinician must be concerned with possible underlying causes.

## PROTEIN-LOSING ENTEROPATHY (TEXT P 451)

Any disease that produces alimentary inflammation, infiltration, congestion, or bleeding can produce protein-losing enteropathy (PLE). IBD and alimentary lymphoma are common causes in adult dogs; hookworms and chronic intussusception are common in very young dogs. When IBD is responsible, it is usually a severe form of LPE, although EGE or granulomatous disease may be responsible. Immunoproliferative enteritis of Basenjis, GI ulceration and erosion, and bleeding tumors can also produce PLE. Cats infrequently have PLE, which is usually a result of LPE or lymphoma.

### Intestinal Lymphangiectasis

Intestinal lymphangiectasia (IL) is a disorder of the canine intestinal lymphatic system. It is unreported in cats. Leakage of lymphatic fat into the intestinal wall may cause granuloma formation, which exacerbates lymphatic obstruction. The disorder has many potential causes, including lymphatic obstruction, pericarditis, infiltrative mesenteric lymph node or intestinal mucosal disease, and congenital malformations. However, most cases are idiopathic. Yorkshire Terriers, Soft-Coated Wheaten Terriers, and Lundehunds appear to be at higher risk.

#### Clinical features

The first sign may be small intestinal diarrhea or transudative ascites. Diarrhea is inconsistent and may occur late in the disease, if at all. Intestinal lipogranulomas (white nodules in the intestinal serosa) are sometimes found during surgery.

#### Diagnosis

Clinical pathology is nondiagnostic, but hypoalbuminemia and hypocholesterolemia are expected. Lymphopenia is common but inconsistent. Diagnosis requires histologic evaluation of intestinal mucosa; cytology is rarely helpful. Feeding fat the night before the biopsy seems to make the lesions more obvious, and classic endoscopic lesions may be seen in the duodenal mucosa. Endoscopic biopsies are often diagnostic, but surgical biopsies are sometimes required. IL may be localized to one area of the intestines (e.g., the ileum) and can be missed during surgery or endoscopy.

**Treatment**

The underlying cause is rarely determined, necessitating reliance on symptomatic therapy. An ultra–low-fat diet restricted in long-chain fatty acids helps prevent further intestinal lacteal engorgement and subsequent protein loss. Prednisolone (1.1 mg/kg/day) sometimes lessens inflammation around the lipogranulomas and improves lymphatic flow. Monitoring serum albumin may be the best way of assessing response to therapy. If the patient improves on dietary therapy, it should probably be fed that diet indefinitely. If prednisolone is also needed, it is reasonable to gradually decrease the dose after clinical control is attained.

**Prognosis**

The prognosis is variable, but most dogs respond well to ultra–low-fat diets, although some require prednisolone as well. Relatively few dogs die despite dietary and prednisolone therapy.

## PLE in Soft-Coated Wheaten Terriers

Soft-Coated Wheaten Terriers have a predisposition to PLE and protein-losing nephropathy. The cause is uncertain, although food hypersensitivity is present in some affected dogs. Individual dogs may have PLE, protein-losing nephropathy, or both. Typical clinical signs may include vomiting, diarrhea, weight loss, and ascites. Affected dogs usually are middle-aged when diagnosed. Panhypoproteinemia and hypocholesterolemia are common. Histopathology of intestinal mucosa may reveal lymphangiectasia, lymphangitis, or IBD. Treatment is as described for IL or IBD. The prognosis is guarded to poor in clinically ill animals; most die within a year of diagnosis.

# FUNCTIONAL INTESTINAL DISEASE (TEXT P 452)

## Irritable Bowel Syndrome

Irritable bowel syndrome (IBS) is an idiopathic large bowel disease in people, characterized by diarrhea or constipation and cramping. An organic lesion cannot be identified, so a "functional" disorder is presumed. Some dogs with chronic large bowel diarrhea have a comparable syndrome.

Some dogs with IBS are of small breeds and are heavily imprinted on a single family member. Clinical signs may develop after separation of the dog from the person. Other dogs with IBS are nervous and high-strung (e.g., police or guard dogs, especially German Shepherd Dogs). Some patients have no apparent initiating cause.

**Clinical features and diagnosis**

Chronic, large bowel diarrhea is the principal sign. Fecal mucus is common, blood infrequent, and weight loss rare. Diagnosis consists of eliminating known causes by physical examination, clinical pathology, fecal analysis, colonoscopy and biopsy, and therapeutic trials.

**Treatment and prognosis**

Treatment with fiber-supplemented diets (7% to 9% fiber on a dry-matter basis) is often helpful. Many patients must receive fiber chronically to prevent relapse. Anticholinergics (e.g., propantheline, 0.25 mg/kg or dicyclomine 0.15 mg/kg up to q8h, as needed) occasionally are useful. The prognosis is good; in most patients the signs are controlled by diet or medical management.

# INTESTINAL OBSTRUCTION (TEXT PP 452-455)

## Simple Intestinal Obstruction

Simple intestinal obstruction (luminal obstruction without peritoneal leakage, venous occlusion, or bowel devitalization) is usually caused by foreign objects. Infiltrative disease and intussusception may also be responsible.

**Clinical features**

Simple obstructions usually cause vomiting along with anorexia, depression, or diarrhea. Abdominal pain is uncommon. The more proximal the obstruction, the more frequent and severe the vomiting tends to be. If the intestine becomes devitalized and septic peritonitis results, the patient may be moribund or in septic shock on presentation.

### Diagnosis

Abdominal palpation, plain radiography, or ultrasonography can be diagnostic if it reveals a foreign object, mass, or dilated intestinal loops. Abdominal ultrasound can reveal dilated or thickened intestinal loops that are not obvious on radiographs or palpation. If it is difficult to distinguish obstruction from physiologic ileus, contrast radiography may be helpful. If an abdominal mass or obstructive ileus is found, ultrasound or exploratory surgery should be performed. Aspirate cytology of masses may be used to diagnose other diseases (e.g., lymphoma).

### Treatment

Laboratory tests (especially serum electrolyte and blood gas analysis) should be performed before exploratory surgery. Vomiting of gastric origin classically produces a hypokalemic, hypochloremic metabolic alkalosis and paradoxic aciduria, whereas vomiting resulting from intestinal obstruction may produce metabolic acidosis and varying degrees of hypokalemia. However, such changes cannot be accurately predicted even when the cause of vomiting is known.

### Prognosis

The prognosis is usually good unless septic peritonitis is present or massive intestinal resection is necessary.

## "Incarcerated" Intestinal Obstructions

Incarcerated or "strangulated" intestinal obstruction is a true surgical emergency; patients deteriorate quickly if the entrapped loop is not removed.

### Clinical features

Acute vomiting, abdominal pain, and progressive depression are typical findings. Palpating the entrapped loop often causes severe pain and occasionally causes vomiting. Physical examination may indicate endotoxic shock (e.g., "muddy" mucous membranes, tachycardia).

### Diagnosis

Presumptive diagnosis is made by finding a distended, painful intestinal loop, especially if the loop is contained within a hernia. Radiographically a markedly dilated segment of intestine is found, possibly outside of the peritoneal cavity. Otherwise, an obviously strangulated loop of intestine is found during exploratory surgery.

### Treatment and prognosis

Immediate surgery and aggressive therapy for endotoxic shock (fluids, antibiotics, and possibly nonsteroidal antiinflammatory drugs) are indicated. Devitalized bowel should be resected, taking care to avoid spillage of septic contents into the abdomen. The prognosis is guarded; prompt recognition and immediate surgery are needed to minimize mortality.

## Mesenteric Torsion and Volvulus

In mesenteric torsion and volvulus the intestines twist around the root of the mesentery, causing severe vascular compromise. Typically, much of the intestine is devitalized by the time surgery is performed. This uncommon cause of intestinal obstruction principally occurs in larger dogs (especially German Shepherd Dogs).

### Clinical features and diagnosis

Mesenteric torsion causes acute onset of severe vomiting, abdominal pain, and depression. Bloody diarrhea may occur; abdominal distention is not as evident as in patients with gastric dilation or volvulus. Abdominal radiographs are often diagnostic and typically show widespread, uniform ileus.

### Treatment and prognosis

Immediate surgery is necessary. The intestines must be repositioned, and devitalized bowel resected. The prognosis is extremely poor; most patients die despite heroic efforts. Patients that live may develop short bowel syndrome if massive intestinal resection was necessary.

## Linear Foreign Objects

Linear foreign objects (e.g., string, thread, nylon stocking, cloth) lodge or "fix" at one point, such as the base of the tongue or the pylorus, while the rest trails off into the intestines. Peristaltic waves cause the small intestine to gather around it. As the intestines continue trying to propel it distally, they become pleated, and the linear object cuts or "saws" into the intestines, often perforating them at multiple sites on the antimesenteric border. Fatal peritonitis can result. Linear foreign objects are more common in cats than in dogs.

### Clinical features

Vomiting of food, bile, or phlegm is common, but some patients are simply anorectic or depressed. A few (especially dogs with chronic linear foreign bodies) are relatively asymptomatic for days or weeks while the foreign body continues to embed itself in the intestines.

### Diagnosis

The history may be suggestive of a linear foreign body, and bunched, painful intestines are occasionally detected by abdominal palpation. The object is sometimes seen lodged at the base of the tongue in cats. If necessary, chemical restraint (e.g., ketamine, 2.2 mg/kg IV) is used to allow adequate oral examination.

*Radiography.* Foreign objects lodged at the pylorus must be diagnosed by imaging or endoscopy. The objects are infrequently seen radiographically and only rarely produce dilated intestinal loops. Plain radiographs may reveal small gas bubbles in the intestines, especially in the region of the duodenum; obvious intestinal pleating is occasionally seen. If contrast radiographs are performed, they typically reveal a pleated or bunched intestinal pattern, which is diagnostic for linear foreign body.

### Treatment

If the patient is otherwise healthy, the object has been present only for 1 or 2 days, and the object is fixed under the tongue, it may be cut loose to see if it will pass through the intestines without further problem. Surgery is indicated if the patient does not clearly improve within 12 to 24 hours.

*Surgery.* If doubt exists regarding how long the object has been present or if it is lodged at the pylorus, surgery is recommended. Endoscopic removal occasionally succeeds, but it is easy to rupture devitalized intestine and cause peritonitis. Surgery is often needed to remove linear objects. If the object has been present for a long time, it may embed itself in the intestinal mucosa, making intestinal resection necessary.

### Prognosis

The prognosis is usually good unless severe septic peritonitis is present or massive intestinal resection is necessary. Extensive resection causing short bowel syndrome has a guarded to poor prognosis.

## INTUSSUSCEPTION (TEXT PP 455-456)

Intussusception may occur anywhere in the alimentary tract, but ileocolic intussusceptions seem more common than other types.

## Ileocolic Intussusception

Ileocolic intussusceptions are often associated with active enteritis, especially in young animals. They may also occur in animals with acute renal failure, leptospirosis, prior intestinal surgery, and other problems.

### Clinical features

Clinical signs can include scant bloody diarrhea, vomiting, abdominal pain, and/or a palpable abdominal mass. Chronic ileocolic intussusceptions typically produce less vomiting, abdominal pain, and hematochezia. These patients often have intractable diarrhea and are typically hypoalbuminemic because of protein loss from the congested mucosa.

### Diagnosis

PLE in a young dog without hookworms or in a puppy that is having an un-expectedly difficult recovery from parvoviral enteritis should prompt suspicion of chronic intussusception. Palpating an elongated, obviously thickened intestinal loop is suggestive; however, some infiltrative diseases produce similar findings. Ileocolic intussusceptions that are short and do not extend far into the descending colon may be difficult to palpate. Occasional intussusceptions "slide" in and out of the colon and can be missed during abdominal palpation. If the intussusception protrudes as far as the rectum, it may resemble a rectal prolapse.

*Diagnostic imaging.* Plain radiographs infrequently allow diagnosis of ileocolic intussusception because intestinal gas accumulation is minimal. A barium contrast enema may reveal a characteristic colonic filling defect caused by the intussuscepted ileum. Abdominal ultrasonography is a quick and sensitive way of detecting intussusceptions. Flexible colonoscopic examination is also definitive.

*Investigating the cause.* A reason for the intussusception (e.g., parasites, mass, enteritis) should always be sought. Feces should be examined for parasites, and full-thickness intestinal biopsies should be performed at the time of surgical correction. In particular the tip of the intussuscepted bowel should be examined for a mass lesion. Additional diagnostic tests may be warranted, depending on the history, physical findings, and results of clinical pathology studies.

### Treatment and prognosis

Intussusceptions must be treated surgically. Some acute ones can be reduced, but chronic ones usually must be resected. Recurrence (in the same or a different place) is common unless the intestines are surgically plicated. The prognosis is good if septic peritonitis has not occurred and the intussusception does not recur.

## Jejunojejunal Intussusception

The principal findings with acute jejunal intussusception include vomiting and/or abdominal pain; hematochezia is uncommon. Mucosal congestion can be severe; intestinal devitalization eventually occurs, and bacteria and their toxins gain access to the peritoneal cavity. In severe cases the intestine may rupture because of ischemia.

### Diagnosis and treatment

Diagnosis is the same as for ileocolic intussusception; jejunal intussusceptions may be easier to palpate because of their location. Plain radiographs may be more likely to demonstrate obstructive ileus (gas-distended bowel loops). Abdominal ultrasonography is the preferred method of diagnosis. Treatment and prognosis are the same as for ileocolic intussusception.

## MISCELLANEOUS INTESTINAL DISEASES (TEXT PP 456-457)

### Short Bowel Syndrome

Short bowel syndrome is an iatrogenic disorder caused by resection of >75% of the small intestine. The remaining intestine is unable to adequately digest and absorb nutrients. Large numbers of bacteria may reach the upper small intestine, especially if the ileocolic valve was removed. However, not all animals with substantial small intestinal resections develop this syndrome. Rarely, short bowel syndrome is caused by congenital defects.

### Clinical features and diagnosis

Affected animals usually have severe weight loss and intractable diarrhea (typically without mucus or blood). Undigested food particles are often seen in the feces. A history of substantial resection and appropriate clinical signs are sufficient for diagnosis. It is wise to determine how much intestine is left by performing barium contrast radiographs; retrospective estimates based on surgery can be surprisingly inaccurate.

### Treatment

If the patient cannot maintain its body weight with oral feeding alone, total parenteral nutrition is needed until intestinal adaptation occurs. It is important to continue feeding the animal to stimulate intestinal mucosal hypertrophy. The diet should be highly digestible (e.g., low-fat cottage cheese and potato) and should be fed in small amounts at least three times per day. Opiate antidiarrheals (e.g., loperamide) and $H_2$-receptor antagonists may be useful in lessening diarrhea and decreasing gastric hypersecretion. Antibiotics might be needed to control the large bacterial populations now present in the small intestine.

### Prognosis

If intestinal adaptation occurs, the animal may eventually be fed a near-normal diet. However, some animals will never be able to resume a regular diet, and others die despite all efforts. Patients that are initially malnourished have a worse prognosis. Some dogs and cats do better than expected.

## SMALL INTESTINAL NEOPLASMS (TEXT PP 457-458)

### Alimentary Lymphoma

Lymphoma often affects the intestines, although extraintestinal forms (e.g., lymph nodes, liver, spleen) are more common in dogs. Alimentary lymphoma is more common in cats. Malabsorption, diverticula, and/or intestinal obstruction may occur in association with the intestinal forms. Lymphoma may be caused by FeLV in cats, but the cause in dogs is unknown. LPE has been suggested to be prelymphomatous in some animals, but malignant transformation of LPE to lymphoma seems rare.

### Clinical features

Chronic, progressive weight loss, anorexia, small intestinal diarrhea, and/or vomiting may be seen. Alimentary lymphoma may cause nodules, masses, diffuse intestinal thickening, dilated sections of intestine, and/or focal constrictions, but lymphoma may be present in normal-appearing intestine. Mesenteric lymphadenopathy is typical but not invariable. Extraintestinal abnormalities (e.g., peripheral lymphadenopathy) are inconsistently found. PLE may occur.

### Diagnosis

Diagnosis requires demonstration of neoplastic lymphocytes. This may be accomplished by fine-needle aspiration, imprint, or squash cytology preparations. However, histopathology of intestinal biopsies is the most reliable diagnostic method. Paraneoplastic hypercalcemia occasionally occurs but is neither sensitive not specific for lymphoma.

*Biopsy interpretation.* If endoscopic biopsies are obtained, a poor quality or shallow sample may be erroneously interpreted as LPE. Occasionally, neoplastic lymphocytes are found only in the serosal layer, and full-thickness surgical biopsies are necessary. Extremely well-differentiated lymphocytic lymphomas may be impossible to distinguish from LPE, even with multiple full-thickness biopsies. In such cases diagnosis depends on finding lymphocytes in organs in which they should not be found (e.g., liver) or by performing immunohistochemical stains to determine if the lymphoid population is monoclonal.

### Treatment and prognosis

Chemotherapy can prolong survival in cats. An appropriate treatment protocol is outlined in Chapter 82. The long-term prognosis is very poor, but some cats with well-differentiated intestinal lymphoma live for years with therapy.

### Intestinal Adenocarcinoma

Intestinal adenocarcinoma is more common in dogs than in cats. It typically causes diffuse intestinal thickening or focal circumferential mass lesions. Primary clinical signs are vomiting (caused by intestinal obstruction) and weight loss.

### Diagnosis

Diagnosis requires demonstration of neoplastic epithelial cells either by cytology or histopathology. Endoscopy, surgery, and ultrasound-guided fine-needle aspiration may each yield diagnostic samples. Scirrhous carcinomas have very dense fibrous connective tissue that often cannot be obtained for biopsy with a flexible endoscope, so surgery is sometimes required in order to obtain diagnostic biopsy specimens.

### Treatment and prognosis

The prognosis is good if complete surgical excision is possible, but metastasis to regional lymph nodes is common by the time of diagnosis. Postoperative adjuvant chemotherapy does not appear beneficial.

## Intestinal Leiomyoma or Leiomyosarcoma

Leiomyomas and leiomyosarcomas are connective tissue tumors primarily found in the small intestine (and stomach) of older dogs; they usually form distinct masses. Primary clinical signs are of intestinal hemorrhage, iron-deficiency anemia, and obstruction. These tumors can also cause hypoglycemia as a paraneoplastic effect.

### Diagnosis and treatment

Diagnosis requires demonstration of neoplastic cells. Ultrasound-guided fine-needle aspirate may be diagnostic, but biopsy is often necessary. Surgical excision may be curative if no metastases are present. Metastasis carries a poor prognosis, although symptoms in some animals are palliated by chemotherapy.

# LARGE INTESTINAL INFLAMMATION (TEXT P 458)

## Acute Colitis or Proctitis

Acute colitis has many causes (e.g., bacteria, diet, parasites). The underlying cause is seldom diagnosed, because this problem tends to be self-limiting. Acute proctitis probably has similar causes but may also be secondary to passage of a rough foreign object. These conditions are more common in dogs than in cats.

### Clinical features

Patients with acute colitis often seem to feel well despite having large bowel diarrhea (e.g., hematochezia, fecal mucus, tenesmus). Vomiting is uncommon. Constipation, tenesmus, dyschezia, hematochezia, and/or depression may be present.

### Diagnosis

Rectal examination is important. Patients with acute colitis may have rectal discomfort and/or hematochezia. Those with acute proctitis may have roughened, thick, and/or ulcerated mucosa. Eliminating obvious causes (e.g., diet, parasites) and resolving the problem with symptomatic therapy allows presumptive diagnosis. Colonoscopy and biopsy are definitive but seldom needed.

### Treatment and prognosis

Withholding food for 24 to 36 hours lessens the severity of clinical signs. Small amounts of a bland diet (e.g., cottage cheese and rice) with or without fiber should then be fed. After resolution the patient may be maintained on this diet or gradually returned to its original diet. Areas of anal excoriation should be cleaned, and an antibiotic-corticosteroid ointment applied. For proctitis, broad-spectrum antimicrobial therapy effective against anaerobes may be used, as well as stool softeners. The prognosis for idiopathic disease is good. Most animals recover within 1 to 3 days.

# LARGE INTESTINAL INTUSSUSCEPTION/PROLAPSE (TEXT PP 458-459)

## Cecocolic Intussusception

Cecocolic intussusception (i.e., inversion of the cecum into the colon) is rare. It primarily occurs in dogs. The cause is unknown, but whipworm-induced typhlitis may be responsible. Hematochezia is the major sign; it may be so severe that the dog becomes anemic. Intestinal obstruction does not develop, and diarrhea is rare. Cecocolic intussusception is rarely palpable. Diagnosis usually requires flexible endoscopy, ultrasonography, and/or barium enema. Typhlectomy is curative, and the prognosis is good.

## Rectal Prolapse

Rectal prolapse is usually secondary to enteritis or colitis in young dogs and cats. They begin to strain because of rectal irritation and eventually prolapse some or all of the rectal mucosa. Mucosal exposure increases irritation and perpetuates straining, which promotes further prolapse. Manx cats may be predisposed to rectal prolapse.

### Clinical features and diagnosis

Colonic or rectal mucosa extending from the anus is obvious during physical examination. Rectal examination is needed to differentiate rectal prolapse from an intussusception protruding from the rectum.

### Treatment and prognosis

Treatment consists of resolving the original cause of straining (if possible), re-positioning the rectal mucosa, and preventing additional straining. A well-lubricated finger is used to reposition the mucosa. If it readily prolapses after being replaced, a purse-string anal suture (with an opening large enough to allow defecation) is used for 1 to 3 days. Occasionally, epidural anesthetic is needed to prevent repeated prolapse.

If the everted mucosa is so irritated that straining continues, kaolin (Kaopectate) retention enemas may provide relief. If a massive prolapse is present or if the rectal mucosa is irreversibly damaged, resection may be necessary. The prognosis is usually good, but in some patients the condition tends to recur.

## LARGE INTESTINAL NEOPLASMS (TEXT P 459)

### Adenocarcinoma

Principally found in dogs, colonic and rectal adenocarcinomas are more common in older patients. These tumors can extend into the lumen or be infiltrative and produce circumferential narrowing. Some of these tumors arise from polyps.

#### Clinical features and diagnosis

Hematochezia is common. Infiltrative tumors are likely to cause tenesmus and/or constipation. Because most colonic neoplasms arise in or near the rectum, digital examination is the best screening test. Colonoscopy is required for more orad masses. Finding carcinoma cells is necessary for diagnosis; histopathology is often more reliable than cytology. Relatively deep biopsy samples obtained with rigid biopsy forceps are required to diagnose submucosal carcinomas. Imaging is used to detect sublumbar lymph node or pulmonary metastases.

#### Treatment and prognosis

Complete surgical excision is curative. However, most tumors cannot be completely excised because of their location, extent of local invasion, and/or tendency to me-tastasize to regional lymph nodes. The prognosis for unresectable adenocarcinomas is poor. Preoperative and intraoperative radiotherapy may be palliative in some dogs with nonresectable colorectal adenocarcinomas.

### Rectal Polyps

Rectal polyps primarily occur in dogs. They cause hematochezia (sometimes considerable) and tenesmus. Obstruction is rare. Rectal palpation often reveals a mass with a narrow attachment to the underlying mucosa, although some large adenomatous polyps resemble sessile adenocarcinomas. Occasionally, multiple small polyps are palpated throughout one segment of the colon, usually within a few centimeters of the rectum. Histopathology is required to distinguish benign polyps from malignancies.

#### Treatment and prognosis

Complete surgical excision is curative. If possible, thorough endoscopic evaluation of the colon should be done before surgery to be certain additional polyps are not present. If incompletely excised, polyps return. Multiple polyps within a defined area may necessitate segmental colonic mucosal resection. The prognosis is good. Most rectal and colonic polyps do not undergo malignant transformation.

## MISCELLANEOUS LARGE INTESTINAL DISEASES (TEXT P 460)

### Pythiosis

Pythiosis is caused by *Pythium insidiosum*. Pythiosis of the large bowel usually occurs in or near the rectum, although it can involve any area of the intestinal tract. It is more common in dogs; cats are rarely affected.

#### Clinical features

Rectal lesions often cause partial obstruction. The dog may be presented because of constipation and/or hematochezia. Fistulas may also develop, resembling perianal fistulas. Patients with advanced disease often lose weight. Rarely, infarction of mucosa or vessels is present, with subsequent ischemia.

### Diagnosis

Because the lesion is submucosal and very fibrotic, rigid biopsy forceps are necessary to obtain deep samples that include submucosa. Special stains (e.g., Warthin-Starry) are needed. Sometimes the organism cannot be found, but pyogranulomatous, eosinophilic inflammation is suggestive. A serologic test developed at Louisiana State University shows promise.

### Treatment and prognosis

Complete surgical excision is recommended. No medication is consistently effective, although itraconazole or liposomal amphotericin B benefits some patients. The prognosis is poor unless the lesion can be completely excised.

## PERINEAL AND PERIANAL DISEASES (TEXT PP 460-461)

### Perineal Hernia

Perineal hernia occurs when the pelvic diaphragm (coccygeus and levator ani muscles) weakens, allowing the rectal canal to deviate laterally. These hernias are principally found in older, intact male dogs (especially Boston Terriers, Boxers, Corgis, and Pekingese); cats are rarely affected.

### Clinical features and diagnosis

Most patients are presented because of dyschezia, constipation, or perineal swelling. Urinary bladder herniation into the defect may cause severe postrenal uremia with depression and vomiting. Digital rectal examination should allow detection of rectal deviation, lack of muscular support, and/or a rectal diverticulum. The clinician should check for retroflexion of the urinary bladder into the hernia. Such herniation can be confirmed using ultrasonography, radiography, bladder catheterization, or aspiration of the swelling to see if urine is present.

### Treatment and prognosis

Postrenal uremia constitutes an emergency; the bladder should be emptied and repositioned, and intravenous fluids administered. The preferred treatment is surgical reconstruction of the muscular support; however, surgery may fail, and clients should be prepared for additional reconstructive procedures. The prognosis is fair to guarded.

### Perianal Fistulas

The cause of perianal fistulation is unknown. Fistulas may develop when impacted anal crypts and/or anal sacs become infected and rupture into deep tissues. However, an immune-mediated mechanism is likely to be involved, as the condition generally responds to immunosuppressive drugs. Perianal fistulas are more common in dog breeds with sloping conformation and/or a broad tail base (e.g., German Shepherd Dogs).

### Clinical features and diagnosis

Typically, one or more painful draining tracts are present around the anus. Animals are usually presented because of constipation, odor, rectal pain, and/or rectal discharge. Diagnosis is made by physical and rectal examination. Draining tracts are sometimes absent, but granulomas and abscesses can be palpated per rectum. Rarely, rectal pythiosis mimics perianal fistula.

### Treatment

Many affected dogs are cured with immunosuppressive therapy (e.g., cyclosporine, 5 mg/kg q12h; azathioprine, 50 mg/m$^2$ q48h; or topical 0.1% tacrolimus) with or without antibiotic therapy (e.g., metronidazole or erythromycin). Generally only one immunosuppressive drug is used at a time. If cyclosporine is used, blood levels of the drug should be monitored to ensure that the dose is appropriate for that patient. Concurrent use of ketoconazole (5 mg/kg PO q12h) may allow a lower dose of cyclosporine to be effective. Hypoallergenic diets may also be beneficial in management of dogs with perianal fistulas. Rarely, patients do not respond to medical therapy and require surgery.

### Prognosis

Medical management is successful in most patients. However, the prognosis is guarded, as repeated medical care or surgery may be needed. Surgery may result in fecal incontinence.

## Anal Sacculitis

Anal sacculitis is relatively common in dogs and occasionally occurs in cats. Small dogs (e.g., Poodles, Chihuahuas) have a higher incidence. The anal sac becomes infected, resulting in an abscess or cellulitis.

### Clinical features

Mild cases cause irritation ("scooting," licking or biting the area); the inflamed anal sacs may bleed onto the feces. In severe cases the animal can have obvious pain, swelling, and/or draining tracts. Dyschezia or constipation may develop because the patient refuses to defecate. Fever may occur with severe sacculitis.

### Diagnosis

Physical and rectal examinations are usually diagnostic. The anal sacs are painful, and their contents, which may appear purulent, bloody, or normal, are increased in volume. In severe cases it may be impossible to express the affected sac. If the sac has ruptured, a fistulous tract is usually found at a 4 o'clock or 7 o'clock position to the anus. Occasionally, an abscess is obvious.

### Treatment

Mild cases require only that the sac be expressed and an aqueous antibiotic-corticosteroid preparation infused (usually only once). Infusion with saline may aid in expressing impacted sacs. Expression of the sacs at home by clients can often prevent impaction and reduce the likelihood of severe complications.

*Severe sacculitis.* Abscesses should be lanced, drained, flushed, and hot packed; systemic antibiotics should also be administered. Hot packs also help soft spots form in early abscesses. If the problem recurs, is severe, or is unresponsive to medical therapy, affected sacs can be resected.

### Prognosis

The prognosis is usually good.

## PERIANAL NEOPLASIA (TEXT PP 461-462)

### Anal Sac (Apocrine Gland) Adenocarcinoma

Anal sac adenocarcinomas are derived from the apocrine glands and are usually found in older female dogs. An anal sac or pararectal mass can often be palpated, but some are not obvious. Paraneoplastic hypercalcemia that causes anorexia, weight loss, vomiting, and polyuria and polydipsia is common. Occasionally, constipation occurs because of the perineal mass or hypercalcemia. Metastatic sublumbar lymphadenopathy occurs early in the disease, but metastasis to other organs is rare.

### Diagnosis

Diagnosis requires cytology and/or histopathology. Hypercalcemia in an older female dog should lead to careful examination of both anal sacs and pararectal structures. Abdominal ultrasonography may reveal sublumbar lymphadenopathy.

### Treatment and prognosis

Hypercalcemia, if present, must be treated. The tumor should be removed, but these tumors have often metastasized to regional lymph nodes by the time of diagnosis. The prognosis is guarded. Palliative chemotherapy is beneficial in some dogs.

## Perianal Gland Tumors

Perianal gland tumors (adenomas and adenocarcinomas) arise from modified sebaceous glands. Male hormones appear to stimulate the growth of perianal adenomas, which are more often found in older male dogs, especially Cocker Spaniels, Beagles, and German Shepherd Dogs.

### Clinical features

Perianal adenomas are often sharply demarcated, raised, and red, and may be pruritic. Commonly found around the anus and base of the tail, they may be solitary or multiple and can spread over the entire caudal half of the dog. Pruritus may lead to licking and ulceration of the tumor. Perianal adenocarcinomas are rare; they are usually large, infiltrative, ulcerated masses with a high metastatic potential.

### Diagnosis

Diagnosis requires cytology and/or histopathology, but neither reliably distinguishes malignant from benign masses. Finding metastases (e.g., regional lymph nodes, lungs) is the most certain method of diagnosing malignancy.

### Treatment and prognosis

Surgical excision is preferred for benign or solitary tumors that have not metastasized. Neutering is recommended for dogs with adenomas. Radiation is recommended for multicentric and some malignant tumors. Chemotherapy (vincristine-adriamycin-cyclophosphamide; see Chapter 79) is effective in dogs with adenocarcinomas. The prognosis is good for benign lesions but guarded for malignant ones.

## CONSTIPATION (TEXT PP 462-463)

Constipation can be caused by any disease that causes rectal pain, colonic obstruction, or colonic weakness. It can also be caused by other disorders (see Box 28-5).

## Old Pelvic Fractures

Prior pelvic trauma is a common cause of pelvic canal narrowing and constipation in cats. Cats appear clinically normal once the pelvic fractures heal, but narrowing of the canal partially obstructs the colon. Digital rectal examination is diagnostic. Radiographs further define the extent of the problem.

### Treatment and prognosis

Minimal pelvic narrowing may be controlled with stool softeners, but orthopedic surgery is needed to widen very narrow canals. The prognosis depends on how severely the colon is distended and on the success of surgery to widen the canal. Unless it is massively stretched, the colon can often resume function if kept empty and allowed to regain its normal diameter. Prokinetic drugs such as cisapride (0.25 mg/kg PO q8 to 12h) may stimulate peristalsis; however, these drugs must not be used if obstruction persists.

## Benign Rectal Stricture

The cause of benign rectal stricture is uncertain, but it may be congenital. Constipation and tenesmus are the primary clinical signs. Digital rectal examination reveals a stricture, although it can be missed in large dogs or if the stricture is beyond the reach of one's digit. Proctoscopy and deep biopsy (including submucosa) of the stricture are needed to differentiate between a benign fibrous lesion and a neoplastic or fungal lesion.

### Treatment and prognosis

In some patients dilation via balloon or retractor tears the stricture and allows normal defecation; other patients require surgery. Owners should be warned that strictures may re-form during healing and that surgery carries a slight risk of causing fecal incontinence. Corticosteroids (e.g., prednisolone, 1.1 mg/kg/day) might impede stricture re-formation. The prognosis is guarded to good.

## Dietary Indiscretion

Eating inappropriate foods or other materials (e.g., paper, popcorn, hair, bones) is common in dogs, especially those that eat trash. It is best diagnosed by examining fecal matter retrieved from the colon. Excessive dietary fiber supplements can cause constipation if the patient becomes dehydrated.

### Treatment

Controlling the pet's eating habits, adding appropriate amounts of fiber to the diet, and feeding a moist diet (especially in cats) help prevent constipation. Repeated retention and cleansing (not hypertonic) enemas may be needed. Manually disrupting hard feces should be avoided; but if necessary, the animal should be anesthetized and instruments or rigid colonoscope and warm-water lavage used to break up the fecal mass.

### Prognosis

The prognosis is usually good. The colon should function normally after cleansing unless the distention has been prolonged and severe.

### Idiopathic Megacolon

Idiopathic megacolon is primarily a feline disease, although dogs are occasionally affected. The cause is unknown but may include behavior (e.g., refusal to defecate) or altered colonic neurotransmitters. Patients may be depressed or anorectic and are often presented because of infrequent defecation. Diagnosis requires palpating a massively dilated colon plus eliminating dietary, behavioral, metabolic, and anatomic causes. Abdominal radiographs should be evaluated if proper abdominal palpation cannot be done.

#### Treatment and prognosis

Impacted feces must be removed. Multiple warm-water retention and cleansing enemas over 2 to 4 days usually are effective. Future fecal impaction is prevented by (1) adding fiber to a moist diet (e.g., Metamucil, pumpkin pie filling), (2) making sure clean litter is always available, and (3) using osmotic laxatives (e.g., lactulose) and/or prokinetic drugs (e.g., cisapride). Bisacodyl is seldom as useful as lactulose. Lubricants are not helpful because they do not change fecal consistency.

If conservative therapy fails or is refused by the client, subtotal colectomy is indicated. Cats typically have soft stools for a few weeks postoperatively and in some cases for the rest of their lives. The prognosis is fair to guarded. Many cats respond well to conservative therapy if they are treated early.

# 34

---

# Disorders of the Peritoneum

## *(Text pp 466-469)*

## INFLAMMATORY DISEASES (TEXT PP 466-468)

### Septic Peritonitis

Spontaneous septic peritonitis is usually caused by alimentary tract perforation or devitalization resulting from neoplasia, ulceration, intussusception, foreign objects, or suture dehiscence. Septic peritonitis can also develop after gunshot wounds, surgery, or hematogenous spread from elsewhere. It occurs more frequently in dogs than in cats.

#### Clinical features

Affected animals are usually depressed, febrile, and vomiting and may have abdominal pain. Abdominal effusion is usually mild to moderate. Typically, signs rapidly progress to septic shock, but some animals have only mild vomiting, slight fever, and copious abdominal fluid and seem relatively well. If it is secondary to suture line dehiscence, septic peritonitis classically develops 3 to 6 days postoperatively.

#### Diagnosis

Most patients have small amounts of abdominal fluid that cannot be detected by physical examination but that decreases serosal detail on plain radiographs. Ultrasonography is sensitive for detecting such small fluid volumes; it may also reveal infiltrations responsible for perforation. Free peritoneal gas strongly suggests alimentary tract leakage or infection with gas-forming bacteria (or recent abdominal surgery). Neutrophilia is common but nonspecific.

*Abdominocentesis.* Centesis (plus diagnostic peritoneal lavage) is indicated if free abdominal fluid is seen or if septic peritonitis is suspected. Retrieved fluid is examined cytologically and cultured. Severely degenerate neutrophils, bacteria (especially if phagocytized by white blood cells), or fecal contents are diagnostic for septic peritonitis. However, fecal contents and bacteria are often not seen despite severe infection. Prior antibiotic use can greatly suppress bacterial numbers and percentages of degenerative neutrophils. Mild neutrophil degeneration in abdominal fluid is expected after recent abdominal surgery.

### Treatment

Patients with spontaneous septic peritonitis usually have an alimentary tract leak and should undergo surgical exploration as soon as they are stable. Preanesthetic complete blood count, serum biochemistry profile, and urinalysis are desirable; however, surgery should not be unnecessarily delayed for laboratory results.

*Surgery.* A careful search should be made for intestinal or gastric defects. Biopsy of tissue surrounding a perforation should be performed to search for underlying neoplasia or inflammatory bowel disease. After the defect is corrected, the abdomen should be repeatedly lavaged with large volumes of warm crystalloid solutions. The abdomen cannot be adequately lavaged via a drain tube or even a peritoneal dialysis catheter except in the mildest of cases. Adhesions re-form quickly; they should not be broken down unless it is necessary in order to examine the intestines. Bowel should be resected only if it is truly devitalized or obviously infiltrated.

*Drainage.* Substantial abdominal contamination may require protracted drainage. Open abdominal drainage is preferred and is accomplished by using a nonabsorbable suture to close the abdomen, except for a 6- to 8-cm opening at its most dependent aspect. This opening is covered with sterile absorbent dressings that are changed as needed, usually 2 to 4 times/day initially and eventually once/day. When the dressing is changed, the opening should be explored with a sterile, gloved hand to ensure that omentum and intestines have not blocked the site. This is repeated until abdominal drainage decreases and most or all of the peritoneal contamination is gone.

A second surgery closes the abdomen, although sometimes the opening closes spontaneously. The abdomen should be recultured at the time of the second surgery. Note: Hypoalbuminemia can occur, especially if abdominal drainage is prolonged and copious.

*Antibiotics.* Systemic antimicrobial therapy should be broad spectrum and parenteral. Combinations of a β-lactam (e.g., ampicillin), an aminoglycoside (e.g., amikacin), and metronidazole are reasonable. Enrofloxacin may be substituted for the aminoglycoside. Cefoxitin (22 mg/kg q6 to 8h) is almost as effective as a β-lactam plus an aminoglycoside. Fluid and electrolyte therapy help prevent aminoglycoside-induced nephrotoxicity.

### Prognosis

The prognosis depends on the cause of the leak and the patient's condition when it is diagnosed. Septic shock and disseminated intravascular coagulation worsen the prognosis.

## Sclerosing, Encapsulating Peritonitis

Sclerosing, encapsulating peritonitis is a chronic condition in which abdominal organs are covered and "encased" in heavy layers of connective tissue. Reported causes include bacterial infection, steatitis, and fiberglass ingestion. This form of peritonitis is rare.

### Clinical features and diagnosis

Typical signs include vomiting, abdominal pain, and ascites. Analysis of abdominal fluid usually reveals red blood cells, mixed inflammatory cells, and macrophages. During exploratory surgery the lesions may mimic those of mesothelioma. The diagnosis is confirmed by biopsy.

### Treatment and prognosis

Antibiotics plus corticosteroids may be tried. Removal of any underlying cause (e.g., steatitis in cats) is desirable, but the cause is rarely found. Most affected animals die despite therapeutic attempts.

## HEMOABDOMEN (TEXT P 468)

Blood in the abdominal cavity is either iatrogenic (e.g., abdominocentesis) or represents spontaneous disease. Clots or platelets in the sample usually mean that the bleeding was iatrogenic or is currently occurring near the site of abdominocentesis. Hemoabdomen is usually the result of a bleeding neoplasm (e.g., hemangiosarcoma, hepatoma), coagulopathy (e.g., rodenticide intoxication), or trauma (e.g., automobile associated). Thrombocytopenia may cause or be caused by abdominal bleeding.

However, most red effusions are blood-tinged transudates, not hemoabdomen. Hemoabdomen is present when the fluid has a hematocrit of >10%. History, physical examination, coagulation studies, and/or abdominal ultrasonography usually establish the diagnosis.

### Abdominal Hemangiosarcoma
#### Etiology

Abdominal hemangiosarcoma often originates in the spleen (see Chapter 84). It can spread throughout the abdomen by implantation, causing widespread peritoneal seepage of blood, or it can metastasize to distant sites (e.g., liver, lungs).

#### Clinical features

Abdominal hemangiosarcoma is principally found in older dogs, especially German Shepherd dogs and Golden Retrievers. Anemia, abdominal effusion, and periodic weakness or collapse from poor peripheral perfusion are common presenting complaints.

#### Diagnosis

Ultrasonography is the most sensitive test for splenic and hepatic masses, especially when copious abdominal effusion exists. Radiographs may reveal a mass if minimal free peritoneal fluid is present. Abdominocentesis typically reveals hemoabdomen but not neoplastic cells. Definitive diagnosis requires biopsy (via laparotomy) Two or more large tissue samples should always be submitted. Fine-needle biopsy (especially fine-needle core biopsy) is sometimes diagnostic.

#### Treatment

Solitary masses should be excised. Chemotherapy may be palliative for some animals with multiple masses; chemotherapy is also indicated as an adjuvant postoperative treatment modality.

#### Prognosis

The prognosis is poor because the tumor metastasizes early.

## MISCELLANEOUS PERITONEAL DISORDERS (TEXT P 469)

### Abdominal Carcinomatosis

The term *abdominal carcinomatosis* refers to widespread, miliary peritoneal carcinomas that may have originated from various sites (e.g., the intestine or pancreas). Weight loss may be the predominant complaint, although some animals are presented because of obvious abdominal effusion.

#### Diagnosis

Physical examination and radiography rarely help establish the diagnosis. Ultrasonography may reveal masses or infiltrates if they are large enough; however, small, miliary lesions can be missed by ultrasound. Fluid analysis reveals a nonseptic exudate or a modified transudate; epithelial neoplastic cells are rarely found. Laparotomy or exploratory abdominal surgery with histologic examination of biopsy specimens is usually needed for diagnosis.

#### Treatment and prognosis

Intracavitary chemotherapy helps some animals, although generally no effective treatment exists. Cisplatin (50 to 70 mg/m$^2$ q3 weeks) and 5-fluorouracil (150 mg/m$^2$ q2 to 3 weeks) are frequently effective in decreasing fluid accumulation in dogs with carcinomatosis; carboplatin (150 to 200 mg/m$^2$ q3 weeks) may be effective in cats. However, the prognosis is guarded to poor.

### Feline Infectious Peritonitis

See Chapter 102.

## Drugs Used in Gastrointestinal Disorders

| Generic name | Trade name | Dogs | Cats |
|---|---|---|---|
| Albendazole | Valbazen | 25 mg/kg PO q12h for 3-4 days | Same for 5 days |
| Aluminum hydroxide | Amphojel | 10-30 mg/kg PO q6-8h | Unknown |
| Amikacin | Amiglyde | 20-25 mg/kg IV q24h | Same |
| Aminopentamide | Centrine | 0.01-0.03 mg/kg PO, IV, SC q8-12h | 0.02 mg/kg PO, SC q8-12h |
| Amoxicillin | — | 22 mg/kg PO, IM, SC, q12h | Same |
| Amphotericin-B | Fungizone | 0.1-0.5 mg/kg IV q2-3days; watch for toxicity | 0.1-0.3 mg/kg IV q2-3days; watch for toxicity |
| Amphotericin B (lipid complex or liposomal) | Abelcet; AmBisome | 1.1-3.3 mg/kg/treatment IV; watch for toxicity | 0.5-2.2 mg/kg/treatment IV; not approved, watch for toxicity |
| Ampicillin | — | 22 mg/kg IV, q6-8h | Same |
| Amprolium | — | 50 mg/kg (puppies) for 3-5 days (not approved) | Do not use |
| Apomorphine | — | 0.02-0.04 mg/kg IV; 0.04-0.1 mg/kg SC | Do not use |
| Atropine | — | 0.02-0.04 mg/kg IV, SC q6-8h; 0.2-0.5 mg/kg IV, IM for organophosphate toxicity | Same |
| Azathioprine | Imuran | 50 mg/m² PO q24h (not approved) | 0.3 mg/kg PO q2days (not approved and not recommended) |
| Azithromycin | Zithromax | 10 mg/kg PO q12-24h (not approved) | 5 mg/kg PO q24h (not approved) |
| Bethanechol | Urecholine | 5-15 mg total dose PO q8h | 1.2-5 mg total dose PO |
| Bisacodyl | Dulcolax | 5-15 mg total dose PO as needed | 5 mg total dose PO q24h |
| Bismuth subsalicylate | Pepto-Bismol | 1 ml/kg PO q8-12h for 1-2 days | Do not use |
| Cefazolin | Ancef | 20-25 mg/kg IV, IM, SC q6-8h | Unknown, probably the same |
| Cefoxitin | Mefoxin | 22-30 mg/kg IV, IM, SC q6-8h (not approved) | 1 mg twice weekly for cats <3.5 kg; 2 mg |
| Chlorambucil | Leukeran | Not used for IBD | twice weekly for cats >3.5 kg (not approved) |
| Chloramphenicol | — | 50 mg/kg PO, IV, SC q8h | Same, but q12h |
| Chlorpromazine | Thorazine | 0.3-0.5 mg/kg IV, IM, SC q8-12h for vomiting | Same |
| Cimetidine | Tagamet | 5-10 mg/kg PO, IV, SC q6-8h | Same |

*Continued.*

## Drugs Used in Gastrointestinal Disorders—cont'd

| Generic name | Trade name | Dogs | Cats |
|---|---|---|---|
| Cisapride | Propulsid | 0.25-0.5 mg PO q8-12h | 2.5-5 mg total dose PO q8-12h (1 mg/kg maximum dose) |
| Clindamycin | Antirobe | 11 mg/kg PO q8h | Same |
| Cyproheptadine | Periactin | Not used for anorexia | 2-4 mg total dose |
| Dexamethasone | Azium | 0.05-0.1 mg/kg IV, SC, PO q24h for inflammation | Same |
| Diazepam | Valium | Not used for anorexia | 0.2 mg IV |
| Dicyclomine | Bentyl | 0.15 mg/kg PO q8h | Unknown |
| Dioctyl sodium sulfosuccinate | Colace | 10-100 mg total dose PO, depending on weight, q8-12h | 10-25 mg total dose PO q12-24h |
| Diphenhydramine | Benadryl | 2-4 mg/kg PO; 1-2 mg/kg IV, IM q8h | Same |
| Diphenoxylate | Lomotil | 0.05-0.2 mg/kg PO q8-12h | Do not use |
| Doxycycline | Vibramycin | 10 mg/kg PO q24h | 2.5-5 mg/kg PO q12h |
| Enrofloxacin | Baytril | 2.5-20 mg/kg PO q12h | Same |
| Epsiprantel | Cestex | 5.5 mg/kg PO once | 2.75 mg/kg PO once |
| Erythromycin | — | 11-22 mg/kg PO q8h (for antimicrobial action); 1 mg/kg PO q8h (for prokinetic activity) | Same |
| Famotidine | Pepcid | 0.5-1 mg/kg PO, IV q12-24h | Same (not approved) |
| Fenbendazole | Panacur | 50 mg/kg PO q24h for 3-5 days | Not approved, but probably the same as for dogs |
| Flunixin meglumine | Banamine | 1 mg/kg IV for septic shock | Not recommended |
| Furazolidone | Furoxone | 4.4 mg/kg PO q12h for 5 days for giardiasis | Same |
| Itraconazole | Sporanox | 5 mg/kg PO q12h | Same |
| Ivermectin | — | 200 µg/kg SC (not in Collies or other sensitive breeds) for intestinal parasites | 250 µg/kg SC |
| Kaopectate | — | 1-2 ml/kg PO q8-12h | Same |
| Ketamine | — | Not used | 1-2 mg/kg IV for 5-10 min of restraint |
| Ketoconazole | Nizoral | 10-20 mg/kg PO q24h | Same (usually divided dose) |
| Lactulose | Cephulac | 0.2 ml/kg PO q8-12h, then adjust (not approved) | 5 ml total dose PO q8h (not approved) |

| | | | |
|---|---|---|---|
| Loperamide | Imodium | 0.1-0.2 mg/kg PO q8-12h (not approved) | 0.08-0.16 mg/kg PO q12h (not approved) |
| Magnesium hydroxide | Milk of Magnesia | 5-10 ml total dose PO q6-8h (antacid) | 5-10 ml total dose PO q8-12h (antacid) |
| Megestrol acetate | Ovaban | Not recommended | Not recommended |
| Mesalamine | Pentasa | 10-20 mg/kg PO q12h (not approved) | Not recommended |
| Methscopolamine | Pamine | 0.3-1 mg/kg PO q8h | Unknown |
| Methylprednisolone acetate | Depo-Medrol | 1 mg/kg IM q1-3wk | 10-40 mg total dose IM q1-3wk |
| Metoclopramide | Reglan | 0.25-0.5 mg/kg IV, PO, IM q8-24h; 1-2 mg/kg/day CRI | Same (not approved) |
| Metronidazole | Flagyl | 25-50 mg/kg PO q24h for 5-7 days for giardiasis; 10-15 mg/kg PO q12h for IBD | 25-50 mg/kg PO q24h for 5 days for giardiasis |
| Milbemycin | Interceptor | 0.5 mg/kg PO monthly | Not approved |
| Misoprostol | Cytotec | 2-5 µg/kg PO q8h (not approved) | Unknown |
| Neomycin | Biosol | 10-20 mg/kg PO q6-12h | Same |
| Nizatidine | Axid | 5 mg/kg PO q24h (not approved) | Unknown |
| Olsalazine | Dipentum | 10 mg/kg PO q12h (not approved) | Unknown |
| Omeprazole | Prilosec | 0.7-1.5 mg/kg PO q12-24h (not approved) | Same (not approved) |
| Ondansetron | Zofran | 0.5-1 mg/kg PO; 0.1-0.2 mg/kg IV q8-24h (not approved) | Unknown |
| Oxazepam | Serax | Not used for anorexia | 2.5 mg total dose PO |
| Oxytetracycline | | 22 mg/kg PO q12h | Same |
| Pancreatic enzymes | Viokase-V; Pancreazyme | 1-3 tsp/454 g of food | Same |
| Paregoric | Corrective mixture | 0.05 mg/kg PO q12h (not approved) | Not recommended |
| Piperazine | — | 44-66 mg/kg PO once | Same |
| Praziquantel | Droncit | See manufacturer's recommendations | See manufacturer's recommendations |
| Prednisolone | — | 1-2 mg/kg PO, IV, SC, q24h or divided, for antiinflammatory effects | Same |
| Prochlorperazine | Compazine | 0.1-0.5 mg/kg IM q8-12h | 0.13 mg/kg IM q12h (not approved) |
| Propantheline | Pro-Banthine | 0.25-0.5 mg/kg PO q8-12h (not approved) | Same (not approved) |
| Psyllium hydrocolloid | Metamucil | 1-2 tsp/454 g of food | Same |
| Pyrantel pamoate | Nemex | 5 mg/kg PO | 20 mg/kg PO |
| Pyridostigmine | Mestinon | 0.5-2 mg/kg PO q8-12h | Not used |
| Ranitidine | Zantac | 2 mg/kg PO, IV, IM, q8-12h (not approved) | 2.5 mg/kg IV; 3.5 mg/kg PO q12h |

*Continued.*

## Drugs Used in Gastrointestinal Disorders—cont'd

| Generic name | Trade name | Dogs | Cats |
|---|---|---|---|
| Selamectin | Revolution | 6 mg/kg topically (not approved) | 6 mg/kg topically |
| Sucralfate | Carafate | 0.5-1 g PO q6-8h, depending on size | 0.25 g q6-12h |
| Sulfadimethoxine | Albon | 50 mg/kg PO first day, then 27.5 mg/kg PO q12h for 9 days | Same |
| Sulfasalazine | Azulfidine | 10-15 mg/kg PO q6-8h | Not recommended, but 7.5 mg/kg PO q12h is used |
| Tetracycline | — | 20 mg/kg PO q8-12h | Same |
| Thiabendazole | Omnizole | 50 mg/kg PO q24h for 3 days (not approved) | Unknown |
| Toltrazuril | Baycox | 5-20 mg/kg PO q24h | Unknown |
| Trimethobenzamide | Tigan | 3 mg/kg IM q8h (not approved) | Unknown |
| Trimethoprim-sulfadiazine | Tribrissen | 30 mg/kg PO q24h for 10 days | Unknown |
| Tylosin | Tylan | 20-40 mg/kg PO q12-24h in food | Same |
| Vitamin $B_{12}$ | — | 100-200 mg PO q24h or 0.25-1 mg IM, SC q7days | 50-100 mg PO q24h |
| Xylazine | Rompun | 1.1 mg/kg IV; 2.2 mg/kg SC, IM | 0.44 mg/kg IM or IV for emesis |

*CRI*, Constant-rate infusion; *IBD*, inflammatory bowel disease; *IM*, intramuscularly; *IV*, intravenously; *PO*, orally; *SC*, subcutaneously.

# PART IV

# Hepatobiliary and Exocrine Pancreatic Disorders

Susan E. Bunch

# 35

# Clinical Manifestations of Hepatobiliary Disease

## (Text pp 472-482)

Clinical signs of hepatobiliary disease in cats and dogs can be extremely variable (Box 35-1), and none of these signs is pathognomonic for hepatobiliary disease. Severity does not necessarily correlate with the degree of liver injury or with the prognosis, although several of these signs are often seen together in animals with end-stage hepatic disease (e.g., ascites, metabolic encephalopathy, bleeding).

---

**Box 35-1**

### Clinical Signs and Physical Examination Findings in Dogs and Cats with Hepatobiliary Disease

**GENERAL, NONSPECIFIC**

Anorexia
Depression
Lethargy
Weight loss
Small body stature
Poor or unkempt haircoat
Nausea, vomiting
Diarrhea
Dehydration

**MORE SPECIFIC, BUT NOT PATHOGNOMONIC**

Abdominal enlargement (organomegaly, effusion, or muscular hypotonia)
Jaundice, bilirubinuria, acholic feces
Metabolic encephalopathy
Behavioral changes (aggression, dementia, hysteria)
Circling, ataxia, staggering, aimless pacing, head pressing, cortical blindness
Intermittent hypersalivation
Tremors
Generalized seizures
Coma
Coagulopathies
Polydipsia, polyuria

---

## ABDOMINAL ENLARGEMENT (TEXT PP 472-476)

Abdominal enlargement may be the presenting complaint or it may be noted during physical examination. Common causes are organomegaly, abdominal effusion, and poor abdominal muscle tone. Abdominal enlargement should be refined to the level of organomegaly, abdominal effusion, or poor muscular tone by physical examination. Additional tests are required to obtain a definitive diagnosis.

### Organomegaly

The organs that most often contribute to increased abdominal size are the liver and spleen. In cats or dogs with pleural effusion or other diseases that expand thoracic volume, the liver may be displaced caudally and appear to be enlarged.

*Hepatomegaly.* Liver enlargement may be generalized or focal. Infiltrative and congestive processes and those that stimulate hepatocellular hypertrophy or mononuclear-phagocytic cell hyperplasia tend to result in smooth or slightly irregular, firm, diffuse hepatomegaly. Focal or asymmetric hepatic enlargement is often seen with proliferative or expansive diseases that form solid or cystic mass lesions. Specific causes are listed in Table 35-1.

*Hepatosplenomegaly.* Smooth, generalized hepatosplenomegaly may have a non-hepatic cause, such as passive congestion secondary to right-sided congestive heart failure or pericardial disease. Hepatosplenomegaly in icteric dogs or cats may be attributable to benign mononuclear-phagocytic cell hyperplasia secondary to immune-mediated hemolytic anemia or to infiltrative processes such as lymphoma, systemic mast cell disease, or myeloid leukemia. Another cause of hepatosplenomegaly is primary hepatic parenchymal disease with sustained intrahepatic portal hypertension, in which case the liver is usually firm and irregular.

### Abdominal Effusion

The origin of abdominal effusion is determined by analysis of a fluid specimen. Ascites is fluid of low protein content and low cell count and is usually related to hepatic or cardiovascular disorders.

#### Intrahepatic causes

Intrahepatic portal venous hypertension is the most common mechanism that leads to ascites in animals with hepatobiliary disease. Inflammatory or neoplastic cellular infiltrates and fibrosis are the most common causes. Sinusoidal obstruction by regenerative nodules, collagen deposition, or cellular infiltrates cause effusion with variable protein content and generally low cell count. Rarely, chylous effusion is present.

#### Prehepatic causes

Prehepatic portal venous occlusion, a large arteriovenous fistula, and mesenteric lymphatic obstruction associated with lymphoma can each lead to ascites. Portal venous occlusion can be caused by intraluminal obstruction (e.g., thrombus), extraluminal compression (e.g., mesenteric lymph node, neoplasm), or portal vein hypoplasia or atresia.

#### Posthepatic causes

Venous congestion from disease of the major hepatic veins and/or distally (thoracic caudal vena cava, heart) increases formation of hepatic lymph, a protein-rich fluid that exudes from superficial hepatic lymphatics. Dogs are more likely to develop abdominal effusion from posthepatic venous congestion than are cats. Concurrent factors in dogs (and rarely cats) with hepatic parenchymal failure, such as hypoalbuminemia (serum albumin of 1.5 g/dl), altered rate of peritoneal resorption, or sodium and water retention, may further enhance movement of fluid into the peritoneal space.

*Feline infectious peritonitis.* Perivenular pyogranulomatous infiltrates in the visceral and parietal peritoneum of cats with the effusive form of feline infectious peritonitis also promote exudation of straw-colored, protein-rich fluid into the peritoneal space. Typically, the fluid is of low to moderate cellularity with a heterogeneous cell population of neutrophils and macrophages.

Table 35-1

## Differential Diagnoses for Changes in Hepatic Size

| Diagnosis | Species |
|---|---|
| **HEPATOMEGALY** | |
| **Generalized** | |
| Infiltration | |
|   Primary or metastatic neoplasia | C, D |
|   Chronic hepatitis complex | D |
|   Cholangitis | C |
|   Extramedullary hematopoiesis* | C, D |
|   Mononuclear-phagocytic cell hyperplasia* | C, D |
|   Amyloidosis (rare) | C, D |
| Passive congestion* | |
|   Right-sided heart failure | C, D |
|   Pericardial disease | D |
|   Caudal vena cava obstruction | D |
|   Caval syndrome | D |
|   Budd-Chiari syndrome (rare) | C, D |
| Hepatocellular hypertrophy | |
|   Lipidosis | C (moderate to marked), D (mild) |
|   Hypercortisolism (steroid hepatopathy) | D |
|   Anticonvulsant drug therapy | D |
|   Acute extrahepatic bile duct obstruction | C, D |
|   Acute hepatotoxicity | C, D |
| | |
| **Focal or asymmetric** | |
| Primary or metastatic neoplasia | C, D |
| Nodular hyperplasia | D |
| Chronic hepatic disease with fibrosis and<br>  nodular regeneration | D |
| Abscess(es) (rare) | C, D |
| Cysts (rare) | C, D |
| | |
| **MICROHEPATIA (GENERALIZED ONLY)** | |
| Reduced hepatic mass[†] | |
|   Chronic hepatic disease with progressive loss of<br>    hepatocytes | D |
|   Decreased portal blood flow with hepatocellular<br>    atrophy | C, D? |
|   Congenital portosystemic shunt | C, D |
|   Intrahepatic portal vein hypoplasia | D |
|   Chronic portal vein thrombosis | D |
| Hypovolemia | |
|   Shock? | ? |
|   Addison's disease | D |

*Concurrent splenomegaly likely.

[†]Loss of portal blood flow to one lobe can cause the lobe to atrophy.

*C,* Primarily cats; *C, D,* cats and dogs; *D,* primarily dogs.

*Hepatic tumors.* Hepatobiliary malignancies or other intraabdominal carcinomas that have disseminated to the peritoneum can elicit an inflammatory reaction with subsequent exudation of lymph and fibrin. The fluid may be serosanguineous, hemorrhagic, or chylous. The protein content is variable, and the fluid is likely to contain exfoliated malignant cells if the primary neoplasm is a carcinoma, mesothelioma, or lymphoma.

*Bile peritonitis.* Extravasation of bile from a ruptured biliary tract elicits a strong inflammatory response and stimulates transudation of lymph by serosal surfaces. Cats and dogs with bile peritonitis may have diffuse or cranial abdominal pain on palpation. The fluid appears dark orange, yellow, or green, and the predominant cell type is the healthy neutrophil, except when the biliary tract is infected.

## Abdominal Muscular Hypotonia

Abdominal distention in the absence of organomegaly and effusion suggests abdominal muscular hypotonia. Reduced muscular strength may result from severe malnutrition or excess endogenous or exogenous corticosteroids. In cats and dogs with hyperadrenocorticism the combination of hepatomegaly, redistribution of fat stores to the abdomen, and muscular weakness causes abdominal distention.

## JAUNDICE, BILIRUBINURIA, AND CHANGE IN FECAL COLOR (TEXT PP 476-479)

### Jaundice

For hyperbilirubinemia to be detectable as yellow-stained tissues (serum bilirubin of 2 mg/dl) or serum (bilirubin of 1.5 mg/dl), either a large and persistent increase in production of bile pigment or major impairment in bile excretion (cholestasis with hyperbilirubinemia) must be present. In the absence of hemolysis, jaundice is attributable to diffuse hepatocellular or biliary disease or to interrupted delivery of bile to the duodenum.

If only one of the bile ducts is obstructed, there may be biochemical clues for localized cholestasis, such as high serum alkaline phosphatase activity, but the liver's overall ability to excrete bilirubin is preserved, and jaundice does not develop. Traumatic or pathologic biliary tract rupture allows leakage of bile into the peritoneal space and some absorption of bile components. Depending on the underlying cause and the time elapsed, jaundice may be mild or moderate. If biliary rupture has occurred, the total bilirubin content of the abdominal effusion is greater than that of the serum.

Nonhepatic diseases such as sepsis occasionally cause jaundice. Mild hyperbilirubinemia (2.5 mg/dl) is detected in approximately 20% of hyperthyroid cats; it resolves with return to euthyroidism.

### Bilirubinemia and bilirubinuria

Reference values for serum total bilirubin concentration are generally <0.3 mg/dl in cats and <0.6 mg/dl in dogs. Bilirubinuria (2+ to 3+ on dipstick) may be normal in canine urine of specific gravity >1.025. Bilirubinuria in cats is always abnormal. Lipemia is a common cause of pseudohyperbilirubinemia in dogs.

### Acholic feces

Acholic (pale) feces result from total absence of bile pigment in the intestine. Mechanical diseases of the extrahepatic biliary tract, such as complete extrahepatic bile duct obstruction (EBDO) or traumatic bile duct avulsion from the duodenum, are the most common causes.

## HEPATIC ENCEPHALOPATHY (TEXT PP 479-481)

Signs of abnormal mentation and neurologic dysfunction can develop in animals with serious hepatobiliary disease. Either the functional hepatic mass is markedly reduced or portal blood flow has been diverted by the development of portosystemic venous anastomoses. Portosystemic shunting can occur via a macroscopic vascular pattern that results from a congenital vascular miscommunication or by a complex of acquired "relief valves" that open in response to sustained portal hypertension secondary to severe primary hepatobiliary disease.

Intrahepatic, microscopic portosystemic shunting or widespread hepatocellular dysfunction accounts for hepatic encephalopathy (HE) in other cases. Rarely, congenital urea enzyme cycle deficiencies and organic acidemias may cause HE. Urinary tract infection with urea-splitting organisms (e.g., *Staphylococcus, Proteus)* could cause transient hyperammonemia and signs of HE if marked urine stasis is present. Animals with systemic diseases that have hepatic manifestations do not undergo sufficient loss of hepatic mass or change in hepatic blood flow to develop signs of HE.

### Clinical features

Subtle, nonspecific signs that could represent chronic or subclinical HE include anorexia, depression, weight loss, lethargy, nausea, fever, hypersalivation (ptyalism), intermittent vomiting, and diarrhea. Certain events might precipitate an acute episode of HE in these patients. Feeding, major gastrointestinal hemorrhage, and drugs that require hepatic biotransformation are possible causes. Other conditions, such as azotemia, metabolic alkalosis, hypokalemia, dehydration, infection, and constipation, could also precipitate HE. Nearly any central nervous system sign may be observed with acute HE, including trembling, ataxia, hysteria, dementia, marked personality change (usually toward aggressiveness), circling, head pressing, cortical blindness, and seizures. In most cases the signs are symmetric.

## COAGULOPATHIES (TEXT PP 481-482)

Subclinical and clinical coagulopathies occur in animals with severe diseases of the hepatic parenchyma and in some patients with complete EBDO or traumatic bile duct transection. Hemorrhagic tendencies may even be a presenting sign in cats and dogs with severe hepatobiliary disease. However, despite the fact that most coagulation proteins and inhibitors are synthesized in the liver, the overall frequency of clinically apparent disturbances in hemostasis is low.

In addition to clotting factor abnormalities, severe hepatic disease can cause bleeding because of portal hypertension–induced vascular congestion and fragility; and some dogs with acute hepatic necrosis are thrombocytopenic. Bleeding most often occurs in the upper gastrointestinal tract (stomach, duodenum), and results in hematemesis and melena. Severe diseases of the hepatic parenchyma predispose the animal to disseminated intravascular coagulation (see Chapter 89).

## POLYURIA AND POLYDIPSIA (TEXT P 482)

Increased thirst and volume of urination can be clinical signs of serious hepatocellular dysfunction in dogs (and rarely in cats). Several factors may be involved, including alterations in serum concentrations of cortisol, urea, sodium, and potassium (see text).

# 36

# Diagnostic Tests for the Hepatobiliary System

## (Text pp 483-505)

No single test adequately identifies liver disease or its underlying cause; a battery of tests must be used to assess the hepatobiliary system. A reasonable package of screening tests for hepatobiliary disease includes a complete blood count, serum biochemical profile, urinalysis, fecal analysis, and survey abdominal radiographs or ultrasonography. Table 36-1 lists the clinically relevant hepatobiliary diseases of cats and dogs.

## COMPLETE BLOOD COUNT (TEXT PP 485-486)

### Red blood cells

Few red blood cell (RBC) changes suggest hepatobiliary disease. Microcytosis (mean corpuscular volume [MCV] <60 fl in dogs other than Japanese Akita and Shiba Inu) with normochromia or slight hypochromia is common in dogs with congenital portosystemic shunting (PSS) and less common in those with chronic hepatic failure and acquired PSS. Most affected animals are not anemic. If anemia is present, it must be distinguished from anemia of inflammatory disease and from iron deficiency anemia associated with chronic gastrointestinal (GI) blood loss.

*Anemia.* Strongly regenerative anemia, with macrocytosis, high reticulocyte count, and normal to slightly increased serum protein concentration in a jaundiced dog, especially if spherocytes are present, suggests hemolytic anemia. Animals with hemolytic anemia typically also have high serum liver enzyme activities and bile acid concentrations. Mild-to-moderate, nonregenerative anemia is common in cats with many different illnesses, including those of the hepatobiliary tract.

*Morphologic abnormalities.* Acanthocytes, leptocytes, and codocytes (target cells) are often seen with serious hepatobiliary disease. Poikilocytosis is a consistent finding in cats with congenital PSS and is occasionally seen with other feline hepatobiliary diseases. Schistocytes (fragmented RBCs) are expected with disseminated intravascular coagulation (DIC); hemangiosarcoma should be considered when an inappropriate number of nucleated RBCs is also found.

### White blood cells

Few white blood cell changes are expected in cats or dogs with hepatobiliary disease, except when an infectious agent is present as the initiating event (e.g., histoplasmosis, bacterial cholangitis, leptospirosis) or when infection complicates a primary hepatobiliary disorder (e.g., gram-negative sepsis in a dog with cirrhosis; septic bile peritonitis). Neutrophilic leukocytosis is likely with bacterial infection. Pancytopenia is typical of disseminated histoplasmosis or severe toxoplasmosis in cats and early infectious canine hepatitis in dogs.

Table 36-1

## Clinically Relevant Hepatobiliary Diseases in Dogs and Cats

| | Primary | Secondary |
|---|---|---|
| **COMMON** | | |
| Cat | Idiopathic lipidosis | Secondary lipidosis |
| | | Lymphoproliferative or metastatic neoplasia (including FeLV-related) |
| | | Hyperthyroidism |
| | | Feline infectious peritonitis |
| Dog | Chronic hepatitis complex | Acute pancreatitis |
| | Congenital portosystemic venous anomaly | Extrahepatobiliary sepsis |
| | Drug- or toxin-induced hepatopathy | Vacuolar hepatopathy (hypercortisolism, diabetes mellitus, hypothyroidism, hyperlipidemia-associated vacuolar hepatopathy in Miniature Schnauzers, other adrenal steroid?) |
| | Cholangitis complex | Right-sided congestive heart failure |
| | | Metastatic neoplasia |
| **LESS COMMON** | | |
| Cat | Extrahepatic bile duct obstruction | Toxoplasmosis |
| | Congenital portosystemic venous anomaly | Histoplasmosis |
| Dog | Biliary tract disease, all kinds | Leptospirosis |
| | Primary neoplasia | Canine distemper |
| | Intrahepatic portal vein hypoplasia | Histoplasmosis |
| | | Rocky Mountain spotted fever |
| | | Ehrlichiosis |
| | | Babesiosis |

**RARE**

| | | |
|---|---|---|
| Cat | Drug- or toxin-induced hepatopathy | Leptospirosis |
| | Hepatic or biliary cysts | Extrahepatobiliary sepsis (?) |
| | Liver flukes (except in predatory Florida cats) | Abscess(es) |
| | Primary neoplasia | |
| | Venoocclusive disease | |
| | Peliosis hepatis | |
| | Biliary cirrhosis | |
| | Intrahepatic arteriovenous fistula | |
| | Intrahepatic portal vein hypoplasia | |
| | Massive necrosis, all causes | |
| Dog | Infectious canine hepatitis | Amyloidosis |
| | Hepatic or biliary cysts | Hepatocutaneous syndrome (superficial necrolytic dermatitis) |
| | Inherited glycogen storage disease | Abscess(es) |
| | Amyloidosis | |
| | Peliosis hepatis | |
| | Destructive cholangiolitis | |
| | Venoocclusive disease | |
| | Intrahepatic arteriovenous fistula | |
| | Massive necrosis, all causes | |

*FeLV,* Feline leukemia virus.

## TESTS OF HEPATOBILIARY STATUS (TEXT PP 486-487)

### Alanine aminotransferase and aspartate aminotransferase

The two enzymes of most diagnostic use are alanine aminotransferase (ALT) and aspartate aminotransferase (AST). ALT most accurately reflects hepatocellular injury, although AST may be a more reliable indicator of liver injury in cats. Generally the magnitude of the elevation approximates the extent of hepatocellular injury: twofold to threefold elevations in serum ALT are associated with mild hepatocellular lesions, fivefold to tenfold elevations are seen with moderately severe lesions, and increases greater than tenfold suggest marked hepatocellular injury.

Other enzyme activities that indicate hepatocellular injury include arginase, succinate dehydrogenase, glutamate dehydrogenase, and lactate dehydrogenase, but they offer little diagnostic advantage over ALT. Arginase activity may be a more precise index of severity of a hepatic lesion.

### Alkaline phosphatase and γ-glutamyltransferase

Increases in serum alkaline phosphatase (AP) and γ-glutamyltransferase (GGT) activities reflect cholestasis. Measurable AP activity is also detectable in nonhepatobiliary tissues, including osteoblasts, intestinal mucosa, renal cortex, and placenta. However, serum activity in healthy adult cats and dogs arises only from the liver.

*Effects of drugs.* Anticonvulsants (phenytoin, phenobarbital, primidone) and corticosteroids can cause striking elevations (up to 100-fold) in serum AP in dogs. Usually no other clinicopathologic or microscopic evidence of cholestasis (e.g., hyperbilirubinemia) is present. Corticosteroids induce a unique AP isoenzyme that is identifiable by electrophoretic and immunoassay techniques. This characteristic is useful in the interpretation of high total serum AP in a dog with subtle clinical signs suggestive of iatrogenic or naturally occurring hypercortisolism (see Chapter 53). Serum GGT also rises in response to corticosteroids, but less spectacularly.

*Relative changes.* The behaviors of serum AP and GGT tend to be parallel in cholestatic hepatopathies of cats and dogs, although elevations are much less dramatic in cats. Therefore measurement of both enzymes can help differentiate drug-induced elevations from cholestatic disease. Relatively small increases in serum activity, especially of GGT, are important signals of hepatic disease in cats. A pattern of high serum AP with a more modest rise in GGT is most consistent with hepatic lipidosis in cats, although extrahepatic bile duct obstruction (EBDO) must also be considered.

## TESTS OF HEPATOBILIARY FUNCTION (TEXT PP 487-490)

A summary of laboratory tests and their interpretation is given in Table 36-2.

### Serum albumin

Hypoalbuminemia may be a manifestation of hepatic inability to synthesize albumin. However, causes other than lack of hepatic synthesis (e.g., massive glomerular or GI loss; bleeding) must be considered before hypoalbuminemia is ascribed to hepatic insufficiency. Renal protein loss can be detected by routine urinalysis. Diseases that cause GI protein loss usually result in an equivalent loss of globulins (panhypoproteinemia), which is not typical of hypoproteinemia of hepatic origin. In fact, globulin concentrations frequently are normal or increased in animals with chronic inflammatory hepatic disease. Loss must approximate 80% of functional hepatocytes before hypoalbuminemia develops; therefore it indicates severe, chronic hepatic insufficiency.

### Blood urea nitrogen

Serum urea concentration is commonly affected by several nonhepatic factors. Most common causes of low blood urea nitrogen (BUN) concentration are complete anorexia and therapeutic reduction in protein intake. BUN concentration can also be decreased by medullary washout associated with sustained polydipsia (PD) and polyuria (PU). If low BUN is noted in a cat or dog with normal water intake, a good appetite, and a diet with an appropriate protein content, the possibility of hepatic inability to produce urea should be investigated.

**Table 36-2**

## Summary of First- and Second-Line Clinicopathologic Tests Useful in the Diagnosis of Hepatobiliary Disease

| Screening test | Principle examined | Comments |
|---|---|---|
| Serum ALT, AST activities | Integrity of hepatocyte membranes; escape from cells | Degree of increase roughly correlates with number of hepatocytes involved |
| Serum AP, GGT activities | Reactivity of liver cells and biliary epithelium to various stimuli; increased synthesis and release | Increase associated with intrahepatic or extrahepatic cholestasis or drug effect (dogs only): corticosteroids, anticonvulsants (AP only, not GGT) |
| Serum albumin concentration | Protein synthesis | Rule out other causes of low concentration (glomerular or intestinal loss); low value indicates ≥80% overall hepatic function loss |
| Serum urea concentration | Protein degradation and detoxification | With low values, rule out prolonged anorexia; dietary protein restriction; severe PU and PD; urea cycle enzyme deficiency (rare); congenital PSS; severe, acquired chronic hepatobiliary disease |
| Serum bilirubin concentration | Uptake and excretion of bilirubin | Rule out marked hemolysis first; if PCV is normal, intrahepatic or extrahepatic cholestasis is present |
| Serum cholesterol concentration | Biliary excretion, intestinal absorption, integrity of the enterohepatic circulation | High values compatible with severe cholestasis of any kind; low values suggest congenital PSS, anticonvulsant drug–induced change, severe, acquired chronic hepatobiliary disease, or severe intestinal malassimilation |
| Serum glucose concentration | Hepatocellular gluconeogenic or glycolytic ability | Low values indicate severe hepatocellular dysfunction or presence of a primary liver tumor |
| Plasma ammonia concentration | Integrity of the enterohepatic circulation, hepatic function and mass | High fasting or postchallenge values suggest congenital or acquired PSS or acute hepatocellular inability to detoxify ammonia to urea (massive necrosis) |
| Serum bile acid concentrations | Integrity of the enterohepatic circulation, hepatic function and mass | High fasting or postprandial values compatible with hepatocellular dysfunction, congenital PSS, or loss of hepatic mass |
| Coagulation profile | Hepatocellular function, adequacy of vitamin K stores | Abnormal values may indicate marked hepatocellular dysfunction, acute or chronic DIC, complete EBDO |

*ALT,* Alanine aminotransferase; *AP,* alkaline phosphatase; *AST,* aspartate aminotransferase; *DIC,* disseminated intravascular coagulation; *EBDO,* extrahepatic bile duct obstruction; *GGT,* γ-glutamyltransferase; *PCV,* packed cell volume; *PSS,* portosystemic shunting; *PU* and *PD,* polyuria and polydipsia.

### Serum bilirubin

Hyperbilirubinemia occurs from greatly increased production or decreased excretion of bile pigment. Increased production of bilirubin from RBC destruction arises from intravascular or extravascular hemolysis and, rarely, resorption of a large hematoma. Under these circumstances, serum bilirubin is usually <10 mg/dl in dogs. Values typically do not increase above 10 mg/dl unless there exists a concurrent flaw in bilirubin excretion. Because increased production *and* decreased excretion of bilirubin occur in dogs with severe hemolysis, serum bilirubin can be as high as 35 mg/dl in these cases.

*Conjugated versus unconjugated bilirubin.* Nearly all diseases associated with hyperbilirubinemia in cats and dogs are characterized by a mixture of conjugated and unconjugated bilirubinemia, so quantifying the two fractions achieves little in discriminating primary hepatic or biliary disease from nonhepatobiliary disease. One exception is acute massive hemolysis, in which total bilirubin may initially consist primarily of the unconjugated form.

*Hemolysis versus cholestasis.* Hyperbilirubinemia is attributed to hemolysis when there exist moderate to marked anemia with strong evidence of regeneration and minimal changes in serum markers of cholestasis (AP, GGT). Because RBC membrane changes are often a component of many primary hepatobiliary disorders, accelerated RBC destruction often contributes to high serum bilirubin content. In such cases clinicopathologic evidence of cholestasis (high serum AP and GGT activities with moderate to high ALT activity) is strong, and, if anemia is present, it is mild and poorly regenerative.

### Serum cholesterol

Hypercholesterolemia is found in cats and dogs with severe intrahepatic cholestasis or EBDO. An abnormal lipoprotein, lipoprotein X, appears in the blood of dogs with EBDO. Hypocholesterolemia is frequently noted in cats and dogs with congenital PSS and in dogs with chronic, severe hepatocellular disease. In other hepatobiliary diseases the total cholesterol values vary considerably within the reference range. Normal values in young kittens (4 weeks old) are higher than those in adults.

### Serum glucose

Hypoglycemia is uncommon in dogs and cats with hepatobiliary disease. It occurs in animals with acquired chronic, progressive hepatobiliary disease when ≤20% functional hepatic mass remains. Hypoglycemia is often a near-terminal event in these patients. Hypoglycemia is also found in dogs with congenital PSS. In each case if hypoglycemia is identified and confirmed by repeated testing, and nonhepatic causes (e.g., sepsis, insulinoma, Addison's disease) are excluded, either a primary hepatic tumor (e.g., hepatocellular carcinoma) or a severe, generalized hepatopathy should be considered.

### Serum electrolytes

Serum electrolyte measurements facilitate supportive care of cats and dogs with hepatobiliary disease but give no particular hints as to the character of the disorder. The most common abnormality is hypokalemia. Metabolic alkalosis may also be found and is usually caused by overzealous diuretic therapy in dogs with chronic hepatic failure and ascites. Hypokalemia and metabolic alkalosis may worsen signs of hepatic encephalopathy.

### Serum bile acids

Serum bile acid (SBA) analysis is a sensitive, relatively specific test of hepatocellular function and integrity of the enterohepatic circulation. Small concentrations of bile acids are found in the peripheral blood of healthy, fasted cats and dogs (total <5 μmol/L by enzymatic method and 5 to 10 μmol/L by radioimmunoassay [RIA]). Two-hour postprandial values in normal animals may increase threefold to fourfold (15 μmol/L enzymatic method for cats and dogs; 25μmol/L RIA method for dogs).

*Abnormal values.* Abnormally high fasting and/or postprandial SBA concentrations reflect a disturbance in hepatic secretion into the bile or at any point along the path of portal venous return to the liver and hepatocellular uptake. Low SBA values may be attributable to ileal malabsorption of bile acids; however, both fasting and postprandial SBA concentrations may be undetectable in healthy animals.

If only one sample can be obtained, the postprandial value is more useful. Biopsy is recommended when enzymatic postprandial SBA exceeds 20 µmol/L in cats and 25 µmol/L in dogs. No pattern of preprandial and postprandial values is pathognomonic for any particular hepatic disorder, although the magnitude of elevation above 20 µmol/L in cats and 25 µmol/L in dogs roughly correlates with the severity of the disorder. In animals with congenital PSS it is relatively common for fasting values to be within normal limits and for postprandial values to be as high as tenfold to twentyfold higher. Generally, secondary hepatic diseases cause more modest hepatobiliary dysfunction (SBA values <100 µmol/L).

**Plasma ammonia**

Fasting plasma ammonia should be measured in any cat or dog with historic or physical examination findings suggestive of HE (see Box 35-1). High plasma ammonia usually indicates reduced hepatic mass and/or the presence of PSS. Fasting plasma ammonia values are 100 µg/dl for normal dogs and 90 µg/dl for normal cats. At least 6 hours of fasting should precede sample collection. Samples must be collected into iced heparinized tubes, spun immediately in a refrigerated centrifuge, and the plasma removed within 30 minutes. Feline plasma can be frozen at –20° C and assayed within 48 hours; canine plasma must be assayed within 30 minutes.

If no signs of HE are present and the results of other tests are equivocal, an ammonium chloride challenge test can be done (Table 36-3). Plasma values after $NH_4Cl$ administration in normal animals do not exceed a twofold increase over baseline values. An exaggerated response most commonly indicates congenital or acquired PSS. It could also result from massive loss of functional hepatocytes.

## URINALYSIS (TEXT PP 490-491)

Common urinalysis findings consistent with hepatobiliary disease include excessive bilirubinuria in a nonanemic dog (2+ in urine of SG <1.025), presence of bilirubinuria in cats, and ammonium biurate crystalluria. (Small numbers of bilirubin crystals may be found in concentrated urine specimens from normal dogs, but ammonium biurate crystals are not found in freshly voided urine.) In dogs excessive bilirubinuria may precede the onset of hyperbilirubinemia and jaundice.

If urine samples are processed properly, repeated absence of urobilinogen suggests (but is not diagnostic for) complete EBDO. Consistently dilute urine (SG as low as 1.005) may be a feature of congenital PSS or severe hepatocellular diseases.

## FECAL EVALUATION (TEXT P 491)

Fecal analysis rarely provides useful information, except for a change in appearance with two specific conditions: absence of fecal pigment (acholic feces) and steatorrhea are consequences of chronic complete EBDO, and dark orange–colored feces reflect increased bilirubin production or excretion after marked hemolysis.

**Table 36-3**

## Summary of Techniques for Ammonium Chloride Challenge Testing* in the Diagnosis of Hyperammonemia

| Route | Dose of ammonium chloride |
|---|---|
| Oral | |
| Via stomach tube | 0.1 g/kg as a 10% solution (1 m/kg, maximum 3 g total dosage) |
| Via gelatin capsule | 0.1 g/kg |
| Rectal | Give cleansing enema first, 0.1 g/kg as a 5% solution (2 ml/kg) |

*Test should be preceded by at least a 6-hr fast; blood samples should be collected for plasma ammonia concentration before and at 30 min after administration of ammonium chloride.

## ABDOMINOCENTESIS (TEXT P 491)

If abdominal fluid is detected during physical examination, radiography, or ultrasonography, a sample should be obtained for analysis. Characteristics and possible causes of the various types of transudate and exudate are given in Table 36-4.

## COAGULATION TESTS (TEXT P 492)

Clinically relevant coagulopathies are unusual in cats and dogs with hepatobiliary disease, except for those with acute hepatic failure, complete EBDO, or active DIC. It is more common to have subtle prolongation of activated partial thromboplastin time (APTT; 1.5 times normal), positive fibrin degradation products, and variable fibrinogen concentration (<100 to 200 mg/dl). Mild thrombocytopenia (130,000-150,000 cells/μl) is usually associated with splenic sequestration or chronic DIC. More severe thrombocytopenia (<100,000 cells/μl) is expected in acute DIC or decompensated chronic DIC.

Some animals with severe hepatic disease and relatively unremarkable routine coagulation profiles have high serum activity of proteins induced by vitamin K antagonism (PIVKA), which could lead to bleeding tendencies.

## DIAGNOSTIC IMAGING (TEXT PP 492-499)

### Survey Radiography

Survey radiography is of little benefit if moderate to marked abdominal effusion is present. Poor detail in emaciated or very young animals that lack abdominal fat stores also makes the detection of subtle hepatic changes difficult.

#### Generalized changes

With generalized hepatomegaly, the liver extends beyond the costal arch; it displaces the gastric axis and pylorus caudally and dorsally on lateral view and shifts the gastric shadow caudally and to the left on ventrodorsal (VD) view. The edges of the liver may appear rounded on lateral view. Occasionally the spleen and liver cannot be differentiated when they are in direct contact (right lateral view). Increased intrathoracic volume associated with deep inspiration, severe pleural effusion, or overinflation of the lungs may result in caudal displacement of the liver, giving the impression of hepatomegaly.

Microhepatia is more difficult to recognize. Changes in the angle of the gastric fundus on right lateral view could indicate a small hepatic shadow if the angle is more upright, especially if the stomach seems closer to the diaphragm. The liver may also seem small in animals with traumatic herniation of liver lobes into the thorax or in those with congenital peritoneopericardial hernia.

#### Focal changes

Focal hepatic enlargement is indicated by displacement of organs adjacent to the affected lobe. The right lateral lobe is most commonly enlarged, shifting the body and pyloric regions of the stomach dorsally (lateral view) and to the animal's left (VD view); the gastric fundus remains in its normal position. Left displacement of the stomach is normal in cats. If the left lateral lobe is enlarged, the gastric fundus moves to the left and caudally, and the lesser curvature may appear indented. Neoplasia, hyperplastic or regenerative nodules, and cysts most commonly account for focal hepatic enlargement or irregular liver margins without enlargement. If the gallbladder is massively enlarged because of EBDO, it may mimic a right cranial abdominal mass or an enlarged liver lobe. Changes in opacity are rare and are usually associated with hepatic or biliary tract infection caused by gas-forming bacteria (patchy and/or linear areas of decreased opacity) or mineralization (focal or diffuse spots of mineralization or mineralized biliary calculi).

#### Contrast studies

Ultrasonography is preferred over contrast radiography to confirm the presence of hepatic masses, cholelithiasis, EBDO, congenital PSS, and other structural diseases. However, portal venography is still necessary to localize some types of congenital PSS. Techniques are described in the text.

**Table 36-4**

**Characteristics of Abdominal Effusion in Hepatobiliary Disease**

| | Appearance | Nucleated cell count | Protein content | Specific gravity | Example(s) |
|---|---|---|---|---|---|
| **TRANSUDATES** | | | | | |
| Pure | Clear, colorless | <2500/μl | <2.5 g/dl | <1.016 | Chronic hepatic failure with marked hypoalbuminemia, intrahepatic portal vein hypoplasia, chronic portal vein thrombosis |
| Modified | Serosanguineous, amber | >2500/μl <7000/μl | ≥2.5 g/dl | 1.010-1.031 | Chronic hepatic failure, right-sided heart failure, pericardial disease, caval syndrome, Budd-Chiari–like syndrome, feline infectious peritonitis |
| **EXUDATES** | | | | | |
| Septic | Cloudy; red, dark yellow, green | >20,000/μl | ≥2.5 g/dl | 1.020-1.031 | Perforated duodenal ulcer, bile peritonitis (fluid bilirubin concentration exceeds that in serum) |
| Nonseptic | Clear; red, dark yellow, green | >7000/μl <20,000/μl | ≥2.5 g/dl | 1.017-1.031 | Feline infectious peritonitis, neoplasia with serosal involvement, ruptured hemangiosarcoma, early bile peritonitis |

## Ultrasonography

The hepatic parenchyma, gallbladder, large hepatic and portal veins, and adjacent caudal vena cava are all visible in the liver of the normal cat and dog. Dilated, anechoic (black) vascular channels and echoic bile ducts can be identified, as well as localized accumulations of anechoic material that represent neoplastic masses, cysts, or abscesses. Hyperechoic (bright) areas indicate increased fibrous tissue, fat, mineralization, or gas pockets. Mixed patterns can be seen in association with parenchymal neoplastic disease, as well as with chronic hepatic disease with nodular regeneration. Whether the lesion is focal or diffuse, ultrasonography can also be used to guide biopsy for cytologic or histopathologic analysis.

### Specific findings

A dilated gallbladder may indicate prolonged anorexia unless dilated bile ducts, particularly the common bile duct, are also seen (which supports a diagnosis of EBDO or chronic cholangitis or cholangiohepatitis in cats). Intrahepatic or extrahepatic anomalous vessels may be identified in animals with PSS. Doppler color-flow imaging confirms the location of the suspicious vessel(s) and the direction of blood flow. Doppler imaging can also provide evidence of intrahepatic portal hypertension by assessing the speed and direction of portal flow. Portal blood flow toward the liver (hepatopetal) is normal; flow away from the liver (hepatofugal) is abnormal. Ultrasonographic findings and interpretation are summarized in Table 36-5.

## Scintigraphy

### Portosystemic shunts

Scintigraphy is used primarily for the diagnosis of PSS. The radiopharmaceutical is placed into the descending colon or spleen and its vascular path is plotted to determine whether the isotope arrives in the liver first (normal) or in the heart and lungs (typical of any kind of portal venous bypass).

This approach evaluates the portal blood supply rather than the hepatic mass, which may or may not be reduced in animals with congenital PSS or primary hepatobiliary disease and acquired PSS. Furthermore, this test does not provide anatomic detail but merely evidence of the presence or absence of congenital or acquired PSS. Transcolonic or splenic portal scintigraphy is most helpful in confirming the presence of congenital PSS in a cat or dog with atypical clinicopathologic findings, equivocal abdominal ultrasonographic findings, and no evidence of portal hypertension (e.g., ascites).

# LIVER BIOPSY (TEXT PP 499-504)

In many primary hepatobiliary diseases, biopsy is needed to establish a diagnosis and prognosis. In some cases bile culture is also needed. Biopsy is indicated to (1) explain abnormal hepatic status and/or function tests, especially if they persist for >1 month; (2) explain hepatomegaly of unknown cause; (3) determine hepatic involvement in systemic illness; (4) stage neoplastic disease; (5) objectively assess response to therapy; and (6) evaluate the progress of previously diagnosed but untreatable disease.

### Percutaneous biopsy or aspiration

Several approaches are available (see text). In general, percutaneous needle core biopsy or aspiration of a single cavitary or solid lesion highly likely to be nonlymphoid cancer should be avoided unless the owner is unwilling to permit surgery for complete resection. Fine-needle aspiration for cytologic analysis is advisable if multiple nodules are noted, as metastatic cancer may have an ultrasonographic appearance similar to that of benign hyperplastic or regenerative nodules. In a small and/or firm, fibrotic liver it is difficult to obtain diagnostic biopsy specimens by percutaneous needle methods.

Correlation between 18-gauge needle biopsy and wedge biopsy is relatively poor (<40%) for certain hepatobiliary diseases (e.g., chronic hepatitis or cirrhosis, cholangitis, portovascular anomaly, fibrosis). If a needle technique is selected, the largest available instrument should be used (at least 16 gauge, preferably 14 gauge). Percutaneous biopsy should *not* be used if chances are good that the disease can be corrected surgically, such

**Table 36-5**

## Ultrasonographic Findings in Dogs and Cats with Hepatobiliary Diseases

| Finding | Possible interpretations |
|---|---|
| **PARENCHYMA** | |
| **Anechogenicity** | |
| Focal | Cyst(s)—may be singular or multiple with septa; thin walled |
| | Abscess(es)—may be poorly demarcated and may have a heterogeneous echotexture |
| | Hematoma(s)—appearance depends on maturity |
| | Lymphoma—may look like cyst if solitary |
| **Hypoechogenicity** | |
| Focal | Focal or multifocal neoplasia |
| | Regenerative nodule |
| | Extramedullary hematopoiesis |
| | Normal liver surrounded by hyperechoic liver |
| | Hematoma(s) |
| Diffuse | Abscess(es) or granuloma(s) |
| | Neoplastic or inflammatory cell infiltrates |
| | Passive congestion |
| | Hepatocellular necrosis |
| **Hyperechogenicity** | |
| Focal | Focal or multifocal neoplasia |
| | Mineralization (creates shadowing artifact) |
| | Fibrosis |
| | Gas (creates reverberation artifact) |
| | Hematoma or abscess |
| | Fatty infiltration (attenuates the sound beam) |
| Diffuse | Fibrosis |
| | Neoplastic or inflammatory cell infiltrates |
| | Steroid hepatopathy (dogs only) |

*Continued.*

**Table 36-5**

## Ultrasonographic Findings in Dogs and Cats with Hepatobiliary Diseases—cont'd

| Finding | Possible interpretations |
| --- | --- |
| **TUBULAR STRUCTURES—BILIARY TRACT** | |
| Dilated intrahepatic and extrahepatic bile ducts | Extra hepatic bile duct obstruction (see Box 37-1); persistent or recently relieved |
| | Severe cholangitis complex (cats) |
| | Choledochal cyst (rare) |
| Distended gallbladder | Normal (prolonged fasting) |
| Distended gallbladder and cystic duct | Cystic duct obstruction |
| Distended gallbladder and common bile duct | Extrahepatic bile duct obstruction (see Box 37-1); persistent or recently relieved |
| Focal areas of gravity-dependent hyperechogenicity within biliary tract or gallbladder that cause acoustic shadowing | Cholelithiasis |
| Focal areas of hyperechogenicity within gallbladder that settle to dependent portion of gallbladder when animal's position changes | "Sludged" or inspissated bile from severe cholestasis, prolonged anorexia, and dehydration |
| Stellate or "kiwi fruit" appearance to gallbladder | Gallbladder mucocele |
| Intraluminal echoic masses in gallbladder | Neoplasia (polyp, malignant neoplasm) |
| | Adherent inspissated bile |
| Apparent thickened gallbladder wall | Cystic hyperplasia (focal) |
| | Cholecystitis, cholangitis |
| | Infectious canine hepatitis |
| | Hypoalbuminemia with edema formation |
| | Abdominal effusion |
| | Neoplasia |

## TUBULAR STRUCTURES—BLOOD VESSELS

| | |
|---|---|
| Dilated hepatic veins and portal veins | Right-sided congestive heart failure |
| | Right atrial mass or thrombus |
| | Pericardial disease |
| | Intrathoracic caudal vena cava occlusion |
| | Hepatic vein occlusion (Budd-Chiari syndrome) |
| Prominent hepatic arteries | Reduced portal blood flow |
| Distended portal vein with reduced velocity and flow | Portal hypertension of any cause (by Doppler imaging) |
| Inapparent hepatic vessels | Cirrhosis |
| | Severe fatty infiltration |
| Inapparent portal veins | Congenital portosystemic shunt |
| | Portal vein thrombus |
| | Intrahepatic portal vein hypoplasia |
| Aberrant vessel that communicates with systemic circulation | Intrahepatic or extrahepatic congenital portosystemic shunt |
| Connection between a portal vein and an artery within one or more liver lobes | Arterioportal venous fistula |
| Many tortuous veins clustered around left kidney and along colon | Acquired portosystemic shunts associated with portal hypertension |

as in EBDO or congenital PSS. Instead a specimen is obtained at the time of surgery to complete the diagnostic evaluation.

**Precautions**

Universal precautions before liver biopsy include fasting the animal for at least 12 hours, measurement of serum albumin, and assessment of coagulation status. Ideally a complete coagulation profile is performed, including one-stage prothrombin time (OSPT), APTT, fibrin degradation products, fibrinogen content, and platelet count; activated clotting time is also worthwhile. Bleeding after ultrasound-guided biopsy is more likely if the platelet count is <80,000 cells/$\mu$l or if the OSPT (dogs) or APTT (cats) is prolonged. If possible, von Willebrand's factor is measured in susceptible breeds. In dogs with type 1 von Willebrand's disease, desmopressin acetate (DDAVP, 1 $\mu$g/kg subcutaneously [SC]) is given before surgery (see Chapter 89).

Mild abnormalities in the coagulation profile do not preclude liver biopsy, although the procedure should be delayed in the presence of clinical evidence of bleeding or marked abnormalities on coagulation tests. Because animals with complete EBDO may be vitamin K deficient (prolonged OSPT and APTT), pretreatment with vitamin $K_1$ (5 mg/kg SC, q12-24h) is indicated for 1 or 2 days before surgery. Repeating the measurement of OSPT and APTT within 24 hours should demonstrate normal or near-normal values; if not, the dose is adjusted and the procedure delayed. If coagulation indexes show minimal improvement, plasma is administered before biopsy. If bleeding is excessive during or after biopsy and cannot be controlled with direct pressure or application of clot-promoting substances, fresh whole blood or plasma is given. (See Chapter 85 for transfusion guidelines.)

# 37

# Hepatobiliary Diseases in the Cat

## (Text pp 506-524)

The clinical signs of most hepatobiliary diseases in adult cats are similar. Other than nonspecific signs such as lethargy, anorexia, and weight loss, the most consistent findings are jaundice and various degrees of hepatomegaly. Other, less common signs include chronic intermittent vomiting, diarrhea, fever, abdominal effusion, and central nervous system (CNS) signs. Hepatic encephalopathy (HE) in cats is most often manifested as depression and ptyalism.

Results of laboratory tests also are often similar among hepatobiliary diseases in cats. For this reason, subtle details of the history and liver biopsy assume an even greater role in cats than in dogs with hepatobiliary disease. Excluding hepatic lipidosis, clinically important acquired hepatic disease in cats tends to be more biliary in distribution than in dogs.

## HEPATIC LIPIDOSIS (TEXT PP 506-513)

Primary or idiopathic hepatic lipidosis is the most common hepatic disease of cats. Proposed factors include protein catabolism in anorectic cats, inadequate protein or carbohydrate intake, arginine or methionine deficiency, and possibly peripheral insulin resistance.

Cats may also develop hepatic lipidosis when they are anorectic as a result of another illness, such as diabetes mellitus, cardiomyopathy, neoplasia, neurologic disease, inflammatory hepatobiliary or intestinal disease, pancreatitis, feline infectious peritonitis (FIP), or chronic renal disease. This condition is termed *secondary hepatic lipidosis*. Hepatic lipid accumulation should resolve once the inciting illness is controlled and the cat's appetite returns to normal.

Whether lipid deposition in hepatocytes occurs with or without a detectable cause, prolonged anorexia seems to be important in the genesis of this syndrome. Clinical illness develops once >50% of hepatocytes are affected.

### Clinical features

Most affected cats are >2 years of age; no breed or gender predilection is apparent. Affected cats commonly are obese, are housed indoors, and have experienced a stressful event or an illness that has caused them to become anorectic and lose weight rapidly. The initiating event is not always known. Anorexia of approximately 2 weeks' duration precedes the development of jaundice, intermittent vomiting, and dehydration. Previously obese cats have extensive loss of muscle mass but maintain certain fat stores (falciform ligament, inguinal region). Cats with concurrent pancreatitis are often underweight.

### Diagnosis

Typical clinicopathologic findings are those of cholestasis. Total bilirubin concentration ranges from normal (<0.3 mg/dl) to 20 mg/dl, with mild to moderate nonregenerative anemia and normal to moderately high (threefold to fivefold increase) alanine aminotransferase (ALT) and high (tenfold to fifteenfold increase) alkaline phosphatase (AP) activities. Serum $\gamma$-glutamyltransferase (GGT) activity is usually normal or only slightly elevated, unlike in other cholestatic diseases. Fasting serum bile acid concentrations are above normal limits in most affected cats. Blood cholesterol and glucose concentrations may also be high, but this is usually attributable to diabetes. Coagulation abnormalities may be noted in cats with concurrent acute pancreatitis.

*Diagnostic imaging.* Hepatomegaly may be confirmed using abdominal radiography. The primary ultrasonographic feature is generalized hyperechogenicity; evidence of localized structural disease (e.g., mass lesions) or of dilated gallbladder and bile ducts suggestive of extrahepatic bile duct obstruction (EBDO) or cholangitis is absent. Abdominal effusion and an irregular pancreas with low or mixed echogenicity suggest coexisting pancreatitis.

*Percutaneous fine-needle aspiration.* Definitive diagnosis requires cytologic or histologic evaluation of a liver specimen. Percutaneous fine-needle aspiration for cytology is usually safe, quick, and easy to perform. It should be performed at the time of ultrasonographic examination and before needle or surgical biopsy is considered. Smears are stained with Wright's or quick hematology stains; Sudan III can be applied to unstained smears to confirm lipid vacuolation in hepatocytes. With primary hepatic lipidosis, inflammatory or other cells are conspicuously absent.

*Liver biopsy.* Cytologic findings correlate inconsistently with histopathologic findings, so if the results of diagnostic evaluation do not fit perfectly with the diagnosis of primary hepatic lipidosis, liver biopsy is needed. With laparoscopy or surgical biopsy, the liver appears pale, friable, and yellow, with a prominent reticular pattern. When placed in buffered 10% formalin, specimens usually float.

*Other tests.* Additional diagnostic tests are performed to determine the presence of concurrent illnesses that could be causing protracted anorexia and secondary hepatic lipidosis. Tests are selected based on the history, physical examination, and clinicopathologic and ultrasonographic evaluations. If there exists no evidence of illness in other body systems or of a single stressful event suspected of having initiated anorexia, then hepatic lipidosis is considered to be primary or idiopathic.

**Treatment**
The most important aspect of treatment is complete nutritional support, along with treatment of known concurrent illnesses. A high-protein diet may hasten recovery.

*Appetite stimulants.* Appetite stimulants such as diazepam (0.2 mg/kg intravenously [IV] q12-24h), oxazepam ($^1/_4$ of a 15-mg tablet orally [PO] q12-24h), or cyproheptadine (1 to 2 mg PO q8-12h) can be given to cats that are minimally affected and are still interested in eating at least one third of their daily maintenance requirements. However, if the total daily nutritional needs are not being met within 2 or 3 days, prompt use of aggressive nutritional support (i.e., tube feeding) is recommended.

*Nutritional support.* Severely affected cats are stabilized with fluid and electrolyte therapy before anesthesia is considered for biopsy and/or feeding tube placement. During this time nutritional support can be provided via nasoesophageal tube with a liquid enteral diet (e.g., Clinicare Feline Liquid Diet). Cats with signs of HE are given a protein-restricted liquid enteral diet (e.g., Clinicare Feline Liquid Diet NF), with other medications as needed to control signs (see Chapter 39).
The total number of calories per day is calculated as follows:

Maintenance energy requirement (MER) in calories = 1.4 (30 [body weight in kg] + 70)

One third of the daily requirement is administered over three or four meals on day 1. On day 2 the size of each meal is increased so that two thirds of the daily requirement is fed. The total MER is fed on day 3 (split into three or four feedings) and is continued for 5 to 7 days. When the cat's condition is stable, a more permanent feeding system can be installed with the patient under general anesthesia (see text).

*Other supportive measures.* Cats that cannot tolerate full feeding because of gastroparesis benefit from potassium supplementation if hypokalemic or from administration of a promotility agent such as metoclopramide (0.2 to 0.5 mg/kg subcutaneously [SC] or via tube, q6-8h, 15 to 20 minutes before feeding). Hypophosphatemia may develop during refeeding and, if severe, can cause hemolytic anemia. If the serum phosphate is <2 mg/dl, supplementation is provided with potassium phosphate (0.015 mmol of phosphate per kilogram per hour, added to 0.9% saline, given IV over 6 to 12 hours or until serum phosphate is near the reference range). For cats with prolonged OSPT and APTT, vitamin $K_1$ (0.5 mg/kg SC q12h) is recommended.

*Pancreatitis.* Cats with concurrent pancreatitis present a nutritional challenge, as the preferred feeding methods for hepatic lipidosis and pancreatitis are diametrically opposed. Enteral tube feeding distal to the pancreas (duodenostomy or jejunostomy) has been successfully used in a small number of cats.

**Prognosis**
When appropriate nutritional support is given, recovery rates are >60%. No known permanent sequelae occur in cats that recover, and no reason exists to believe that the condition will recur. Nevertheless, obesity should be avoided. The prognosis for cats with concurrent pancreatitis is guarded to grave.

# INFLAMMATORY HEPATOBILIARY DISEASE (TEXT PP 513-517)

*Cholangitis* is the term used to define a group of diseases characterized by inflammation of bile ducts, with bile duct proliferation and hyperplasia also observed as a nonspecific response to cholestasis. Ascension of bacteria from the duodenum or digestive enzymes from a subclinically inflamed pancreas are proposed causes. More than 80% of cats with cholangitis have histologic evidence of inflammatory bowel disease, and approximately 50% have changes consistent with mild pancreatitis.

Several types of cholangitis occur in cats, based on histopathologic findings (predominant inflammatory cell type). Despite speculation, there remains insufficient evidence to conclude that these conditions represent phases of a progressive biliary tract disorder that begins with acute inflammation and culminates with biliary cirrhosis. Until this situation is clarified, these conditions are considered as separate entities.

### Clinical features

Cats with cholangitis have no unique historic or physical examination features, although many are males over 4 years old with a history of chronic, waxing-and-waning illness. Common presenting signs include anorexia, depression, weight loss, vomiting, diarrhea, dehydration, hepatomegaly, and jaundice. Approximately 50% of affected cats have hyperglobulinemia; a few have an immunoglobulin G monoclonal gammopathy. The clinical entities described in the following sections are recognized.

*Cholangiohepatitis.*

*Acute cholangiohepatitis.* Acute cholangiohepatitis (CH) tends to be a disease of young to middle-aged cats (median age 3.3 years). Clinical signs are typical of any feline chronic hepatobiliary disease, except that the period of illness is relatively short (<1 month) and findings include fever and an inflammatory leukogram. Most affected cats have an underlying disorder that could favor ascending bacterial invasion of the biliary tract by enteric bacteria, such as biliary anomaly (e.g., bilobed gallbladder), liver flukes, cholelithiasis, cholecystitis, pancreatitis, pancreatic periductal fibrosis, or duodenitis.

*Chronic CH.* Chronic CH may be a later stage of acute CH. It may result from inappropriate treatment of acute CH, or it may represent an immune-mediated response to antigens from the intestine. Affected cats generally are older (median age 9 years).

*Lymphocytic cholangitis.* Cats with lymphocytic cholangitis generally are young to middle aged; Persians appear to be overrepresented. Abdominal effusion of high protein content (>5 g/dl) is present in approximately one third of cases.

*Sclerosing cholangitis.* Sclerosing cholangitis is a rare condition of older cats (>10 years). Signs and clinicopathologic features are typical of severe, chronic cholestasis.

*Lymphocytic portal hepatitis.* Lymphocytic portal hepatitis (LPH), an inflammatory hepatopathy, is seen in asymptomatic cats >10 years of age. It appears to progress and cause illness in some cats, but it is not related to intercurrent intestinal or pancreatic inflammation. Further information is needed to determine the clinical relevance of this condition and whether specific treatment is indicated.

### Diagnosis

The major forms of inflammatory hepatic disease in cats have clinical and clinico-pathologic features typical of intrahepatic cholestasis: mild, nonregenerative anemia; variable leukocytosis; high serum liver-specific enzyme activities; hyperbilirubinemia; and high serum bile acid concentrations. Radiographic findings are nonspecific. Ultrasonographic examination may reveal dilated intrahepatic and extrahepatic bile ducts and gallbladder, with shadowing that often represents "sludged" or inspissated bile. The walls of portal veins appear less clearly identifiable in cats with LPH compared with those in cats with CH. Definitive diagnosis can be established only by liver biopsy.

*Liver biopsy and bile aspiration.* Preliminary impressions of the cytologic nature of the infiltrate can be achieved by fine-needle aspiration, but percutaneous needle biopsy or surgical biopsy is required for definitive diagnosis. Bile for bacterial culture and sensitivity is best obtained from the gallbladder with ultrasound guidance or during exploratory laparotomy. Finding "white bile" (bile completely devoid of bilirubin pigment) indicates severe cholestasis and lack of hepatocellular ability to excrete bilirubin. This observation is most often made in chronic forms of CH, but it has been reported in acute CH. Acholic feces are expected in these cases.

### Features of specific conditions

*Acute CH.* In addition to an inflammatory leukogram, serum liver enzyme activities are typical of a mixed pattern of parenchymal and biliary injury, with normal to twofold elevations in serum AP and as high as tenfold elevations in ALT. Further diagnostic evaluation to identify an underlying disorder is guided by clinical suspicions.

Bacterial culture of bile in these cases most often yields enteric organisms, such as *Escherichia coli, Pseudomonas* spp., and *Enterococcus* spp. However, results may be negative if antimicrobial therapy has already been initiated. Consistent histologic features in liver biopsy specimens include dilated intrahepatic bile ducts that contain an exudate of degenerate neutrophils and neutrophilic invasion of bile duct walls and adjacent periportal hepatocytes.

*Chronic CH.* Histopathologically there is a mixed cellular infiltrate of neutrophils, lymphocytes, and plasma cells in portal tracts around bile ducts. Bile duct hyperplasia and portal fibrosis are prominent features.

*Lymphocytic cholangitis.* Serum biochemical findings are similar to those in cats with acute CH. Because affected cats often have hyperglobulinemia and abdominal effusion, they can be mistaken for having the effusive form of FIP. Liver biopsy is essential for differentiating between these two conditions.

The hepatic lesion of lymphocytic cholangitis is characterized by aggregates of inflammatory cells, predominantly lymphocytes but also smaller numbers of neutrophils, plasma cells, and eosinophils, in portal tracts and around bile ducts. There is also a variable degree of periductal fibrosis. The lesion may progress to biliary cirrhosis. Occasionally the lumina of the bile ducts are obliterated. Some affected cats have lymphocytic aggregates in the pancreas.

*Sclerosing cholangitis.* Thickened extrahepatic and/or intrahepatic bile ducts, with diffuse proliferative fibrosis of their walls, is typical of sclerosing cholangitis. The ducts are distended and their lumina nearly obliterated. The gallbladder may also be involved. Diseases that cause mechanical bile duct obstruction must be excluded before this diagnosis is considered (Box 37-1).

*Lymphocytic portal hepatitis. LPH* is characterized by infiltration of portal areas with lymphocytes and, to a lesser extent, plasma cells. Bile duct proliferation and portal and bridging fibrosis also occur.

**Treatment**

Specific treatment is dictated by the results of hepatic biopsy and bile culture. Until results are known, treatment decisions are guided by clinical features such as signalment and clinicopathologic findings.

*Acute and chronic CH.* Until bile culture results are available, a good empiric antibiotic choice for acute CH is amoxicillin or cefazolin (22 mg/kg PO or IV q8h). Addition of an aminoglycoside (amikacin) or a fluoroquinolone (marbofloxacin) is advised for cats suspected of having systemic involvement. In confirmed cases specific

---

**Box 37-1**

**Causes of Extrahepatic Bile Duct Obstruction**

**EXTRALUMINAL COMPRESSIVE**

Neoplasia
  Biliary
  Pancreatic
  Duodenal
Stricture
  After trauma, pancreatitis, or duodenitis
Diaphragmatic hernia
Congenital anomalies of the extrahepatic biliary tract (e.g., choledochal cyst)*

**INTRALUMINAL OBSTRUCTIVE**

Cholelithiasis
  Mixed composition
  Pigment
  Cholesterol (rare)
Inspissated bile
Liver flukes
  (*Platynosomum concinnum, others*)*

---

*Cats only.

antibiotic treatment should continue for at least 6 weeks. In cats with chronic CH, long-term antibiotic treatment is given first, followed by corticosteroids (see discussion of lymphocytic cholangitis, later) if no improvement is seen.

*Choleretic agents.* Ursodeoxycholic acid (ursodiol) is a valuable adjunct in cats with chronic cholestatic hepatopathies. However, this and other choleretic agents *should not be used in cats with EBDO* (see text p 517). A dosage of 10 mg/kg PO q24h is safe for at least 3 months in normal cats; however, controlled studies of safety and efficacy in cats with cholestatic hepatopathy have not been performed. Preparations are available only in 300-mg capsules, so individual doses must be compounded.

*Diet.* Nutritional support is an important component of medical therapy in cats with CH. A balanced, high-protein maintenance diet (30% to 40% protein on a dry-matter basis) is fed to cats that do not have signs of HE. In cats with HE a combination of boiled rice and cottage cheese can be given over the short term, or a protein-restricted prescription diet (e.g., Feline k/d [Hill's Pet Products] or Veterinary Diet NF [Ralston Purina]) can be used. The preferred route of enteral feeding (e.g., appetite stimulation, nasoesophageal tube, esophagostomy or gastrostomy tube) depends on the degree and duration of anorexia.

*Lymphocytic cholangitis.* Treatment for lymphocytic cholangitis currently centers on modulating the histologic lesion with corticosteroids (e.g., prednisone, 2.2 mg/kg PO q24h initially). The decision as to when to decrease the dose depends on the individual patient; clinical, clinicopathologic, or histopathologic evidence of improvement usually indicates control of the disease. Some cats benefit from a higher dose of prednisone (4 mg/kg PO q24h) or the addition of metronidazole (7.5 mg/kg PO q12h); some cats fail to respond completely.

### Prognosis

The prognosis for cats with acute CH seems to be variable. Most cats that survive the first 1 to 2 months of treatment have a good chance for cure and long-term survival. Some cats with chronic CH, lymphocytic cholangitis, or LPH appear to live comfortably for months to years, with or without corticosteroid therapy.

## NEOPLASIA (TEXT PP 517-518)

Primary hepatobiliary neoplasms are rare in cats. Cholangiocellular carcinoma (CC) and hepatocellular carcinoma (HC) are reported most often. Hepatic metastases with neoplasia arising from other tissues is more common. Most frequently diagnosed are hemolymphatic neoplasms such as lymphoma, myeloproliferative malignancy, systemic mast cell disease, and hemangiosarcoma. Hepatic metastases from carcinomas of the mammary gland, pancreas, kidney, and gastrointestinal tract have also been reported.

### Clinical features

Most affected cats are >10 years old, except for cats with feline leukemia virus–related disease, which are younger. No particular breed predilection for hepatobiliary neoplasia exists. Male cats are predisposed to HC; females are predisposed to CC.

Clinical signs are nonspecific and include lethargy, anorexia, weight loss, and abdominal distention from either hepatomegaly or effusion (ascites or hemoperitoneum). Simultaneous pleural and peritoneal effusion suggests the presence of cancer in both cavities. Whether or not jaundice is present depends on the distribution of neoplasia in the liver; those involving biliary structures or portal tracts cause cholestasis. Neoplasia affecting the liver commonly causes organ enlargement, either in a firm diffuse or nodular pattern that is detectable by physical, radiographic, or ultrasonographic examination.

### Diagnosis

A suspicion that hepatic neoplasia is present may be gained from findings of physical examination, radiography, and ultrasonography. Definitive diagnosis requires cytologic or histopathologic evaluation of a liver specimen. Abnormal liver enzyme activities are common, but unless there exists >75% involvement with neoplasm, functional disturbances do not occur.

Because the liver is often secondarily involved in neoplastic processes, a careful search for a primary site is essential. Certain relatively benign conditions, such as hepatic cysts and bile duct adenomas, must not be mistaken for malignant processes such as CC, which can be cystic.

### Treatment

Surgical resection of a primary hepatobiliary neoplasm that is confined to one liver lobe and has not metastasized may result in prolonged (>1 year) disease-free survival. Treatment of cats with hemolymphatic or metastatic hepatobiliary neoplasia is usually selected according to the cell type of the primary neoplasm (see Chapter 84). Investigational treatments, such as hepatic dearterialization or chemotherapy combined with hyperthermia, may be available through referral institutions.

### Prognosis

The size of the neoplasm is less important in determining the prognosis than the degree of invasiveness and the presence of regional or distant metastases. The prognosis for cats with benign hepatocellular or biliary tumors after resection is good; most cats are free of disease at least 1 year later. The prognosis for malignant neoplasia generally is grave because of the extent of involvement at the time of diagnosis.

## EXTRAHEPATIC BILE DUCT OBSTRUCTION (TEXT PP 518-520)

EBDO is a syndrome with several different underlying causes, categorized as either extraluminal compressive or intraluminal obstructive lesions (see Box 37-1). Choleliths can be a cause of EBDO or an incidental finding. They can form as a result of dehydration, bacterial infection, and infrequent gallbladder evacuation during periods of anorexia. Inspissated bile ("pigment" stones) may be a complication of severe intrahepatic cholestasis from CH or hepatic lipidosis. Liver fluke infections, reported most commonly in cats from Louisiana, Florida, and Hawaii, are most often subclinical but may cause EBDO in severely affected cats.

### Clinical features

Clinical findings may be indistinguishable from those of other severe cholestatic hepatopathies (e.g., anorexia, depression, vomiting, jaundice, hepatomegaly), especially if obstruction is incomplete. A greatly distended gallbladder may be found on abdominal palpation.

### Diagnosis

EBDO is diagnosed by physical examination, clinical pathology, radiography, ultrasonography, and exploratory laparotomy. Complete EBDO causes marked increases in serum AP (up to fivefold), ALT (tenfold to thirtyfold), fasting bile acids (up to 100-fold), and bilirubin (up to 25 mg/dl). High serum GGT activity is also characteristic, with a similar or greater magnitude of elevation to that seen in the serum AP. Acholic feces, vitamin K–responsive coagulopathy, and persistent absence of urobilinogen in correctly processed urine specimens are persuasive evidence of complete bile duct obstruction.

*Ultrasonography.* The most common location of obstruction is the common bile duct (CBD) at or near the duodenum. The gallbladder and bile ducts proximal to the obstruction become distended and tortuous; these, along with generalized hepatomegaly, are discernible ultrasonographically. Mild gallbladder distention associated with anorexia and infrequent evacuation should not be overinterpreted as indicative of EBDO.

*Choleliths.* Choleliths that formed as a result of altered local factors (e.g., dehydration, bacterial infection, infrequent gallbladder evacuation) are greenish-brown or black. They may or may not be radiographically opaque, depending on how much mineral they contain. They can be located in the gallbladder, CBD, or rarely in the cystic, hepatic, or interlobar ducts and are visible with ultrasonography. Because choleliths and inspissated bile can form secondary to primary hepatobiliary disease, liver and/or gallbladder biopsy, bile culture and cytology, and stone analysis are important.

*Liver biopsy.* Hepatic consequences of unrelieved EBDO observed on histologic examination of liver tissue are bile canalicular plugs, biliary epithelial hyperplasia, bile ductule multiplication, periportal fibrosis, and variable degrees of neutrophilic inflammation and necrosis.

**Liver flukes.** Histologic changes associated with fluke infection are not unique, although pleomorphic portal infiltrates consisting of eosinophils, lymphocytes, plasma cells, neutrophils, and macrophages are occasionally seen. The diagnosis is made by finding fluke ova in the feces of cats with compatible clinicopathologic findings, or at surgery.

### Treatment

A combined surgical and medical approach is usually needed. After the patient is stabilized (fluid and electrolyte therapy, vitamin K therapy), the immediate goals are to surgically relieve the obstruction and correct the underlying cause. If the cause cannot be corrected and bile flow reestablished easily, reconstructive procedures (cholecystojejunostomy or cholecystoduodenostomy) may be needed.

**Supportive care.** Supportive care is extremely important postoperatively. Attending to fluid, electrolyte, and nutritional needs is critical to a successful outcome. Biochemical abnormalities associated with EBDO should begin to subside immediately after surgery. Whether the trend continues toward normality will depend on whether the initiating cause has been addressed.

**Liver flukes.** Praziquantel may be effective in treating liver fluke infection; a dosage of 20 mg/kg PO or SC q24h for 3 days is currently recommended. Because use of praziquantel in this situation is an extralabel application, owner consent is recommended.

## CONGENITAL PORTOSYSTEMIC SHUNT (TEXT PP 520-521)

With regard to congenital portosystemic shunts (PSS), the most common anomaly in cats is a single extrahepatic shunt arising from the gastric, splenic, or portal vein and joining with the caudal vena cava. Complete portocaval shunt with intrahepatic portal vein hypoplasia, as well as patent ductus venosus, is occasionally found.

### Clinical features

Male cats <3 years of age seem to be predisposed; mixed-breed, Persian, and Himalayan cats are at increased risk. Typical signs are primarily referable to HE (see Chapter 35). Intermittent ptyalism is a consistent finding and may be a subtle manifestation of HE. Onset of signs often correlates with eating. Severity of additional signs, such as stunted growth, may be related to size and location of the aberrant vessel. Less common features are recurrent urate urolithiasis, prolonged recovery from anesthesia or tranquilization, and improvement of behavioral and neurologic signs with antibiotic therapy.

Most affected cats are underweight, and some have renomegaly, but physical examination findings are otherwise nonspecific. Evidence of additional congenital defects, such as heart murmur or cryptorchidism, may be found. Some clinicians describe a unique copper coloration to the irises in cats of non-Asian breed with congenital PSS.

### Diagnosis

Suspicion arises from routine and liver-specific laboratory test results. The most common abnormalities are postchallenge (food or ammonium chloride) hyperammonemia, and high fasting and/or postprandial serum bile acids. Low blood urea nitrogen, mild changes in liver enzyme activities, microcytosis, poikilocytosis, and decreased urine concentration are seen less often. Evidence of striking hepatocellular injury is not seen unless a superimposing hepatic insult is present. Mild increases in serum AP activity might be attributable to accelerated bone turnover in cats ≤6 months of age.

Diagnosis is confirmed by ultrasonography, transcolonic portal scintigraphy or contrast portal venography, measurement of portal pressures, or hepatic biopsy. Liver size in affected cats is normal or decreased. Hepatic biopsy should be obtained to ensure that the changes characteristic of congenital PSS are present: lobular hepatocellular atrophy, inconspicuous portal vein tributaries, arteriolar duplication, and, occasionally, mild lipidosis and vacuolar change. There should be minimal, if any, necrosis or inflammation.

### Treatment

Definitive treatment is complete surgical ligation of the anomalous vessel, assuming there exists adequate intrahepatic portal venous vasculature to accept redirected blood flow. Cats that have had complete shunt ligation become clinically normal; partial improvement is expected after incomplete shunt ligation.

For cats with congenital PSS that cannot be completely occluded, applying a device that causes progressive narrowing of the shunt vessel over approximately 30 days (ameroid constrictor) may be an option (see text). Older cats (>5 years) or cats with preexisting neurologic signs may be at greater risk for a poor outcome after surgical treatment of congenital PSS.

*Hepatic encephalopathy.* Symptomatic management to control signs of chronic HE preoperatively is wise and should continue for 1 month after corrective surgery (see Chapter 39). The same regimen is used for cats with inoperable PSS. Note: Symptomatic management is not a suitable long-term alternative to surgical correction. Signs of HE are less severe, but without restoration of portal blood flow, hepatic health continues to deteriorate, and CNS changes associated with poorly controlled HE may become permanent.

## ACUTE TOXIC HEPATOPATHY (TEXT PP 521-523)

Toxic hepatopathy is hepatic injury directly attributable to environmental toxins or certain therapeutic agents. A partial list of hepatotoxins is given in Table 37-1. In the case of hepatotoxicity from therapeutic agents (e.g., tetracycline or diazepam) idiosyncratic reactions can occur, but drug overdose is usually the reason for liver injury.

### Clinical Features

In general, drug- or toxin-induced hepatic injury in cats is uncommon, and most reactions are acute (within 5 days of exposure). Adverse hepatic reactions may go unnoticed because the first signs of illness are vomiting and diarrhea, after which the medication is stopped. If the signs resolve, usually no further evaluation is performed.

### Diagnosis

Clinical evidence suggestive of drug- or toxin-induced hepatic damage includes history (e.g., known exposure); normal liver size or mild, generalized, tender hepatomegaly; high serum ALT and/or AST activities; and hyperbilirubinemia. If the exposure was nonlethal, evidence also includes recovery with discontinuation of the agent and specific or supportive care.

No pathognomonic changes occur in the liver, although necrosis with minimal inflammation and lipid accumulation are "classic" findings. Many times all clinicopathologic markers of toxic liver insult are present, but the inciting chemical cannot be identified.

### Treatment

Basic principles for treating toxicoses are applied: prevent further exposure and absorption, manage life-threatening cardiopulmonary and renal complications, hasten elimination of the substance, implement specific therapy if possible, and provide supportive care. Few hepatotoxins have specific antidotes (Table 37-2); therefore successful recovery often requires time and aggressive supportive care.

## SECONDARY HEPATOBILIARY DISEASE (TEXT PP 523-524)

Several systemic illnesses have hepatic manifestations that may be identified by physical, clinicopathologic, or radiographic examination (see Table 36-1). In such cases the hepatic lesion should recede with satisfactory treatment of the primary illness.

Table 37-1

## Therapeutic Agents or Environmental Toxins Observed to Cause Clinically Relevant Hepatic Injury

| | Dosage | |
|---|---|---|
| | Cats | Dogs |
| **THERAPEUTIC AGENTS** | | |
| Acetaminophen | 120 mg/kg | 200 mg/kg |
| Griseofulvin | X | — |
| Megestrol acetate | X | — |
| Ketoconazole | X | X |
| Phenazopyridine | X | — |
| Aspirin | >33 mg/kg/day | X |
| Primidone, phenytoin, phenobarbital | — | X |
| Glucccorticoids | — | X |
| Thiacetarsemide | — | X |
| Phenylbutazone | — | X |
| Mebendazole | — | X |
| Diethylcarbamazine-oxibendazole | — | X |
| Halothane, methoxyflurane | — | X |
| Trimethoprim-sulfa | — | X |
| Mibolerone | — | X |
| Naproxen | — | X |
| Carprofen | — | X |
| Tetracycline | X | — |
| Diazepam | X | — |
| Stanozolol | X | — |
| Nitrofurantoin | X | — |
| Amiodarone | X | — |
| Lomustine (CCNU) | — | X |
| | | |
| **ENVIRONMENTAL TOXINS** | | |
| Pine oil + isopropanol | X | ? |
| Inorganic arsenicals (lead arsenate, sodium arsenate, sodium arsenite) | X | X |
| Thallium | X | X |
| Zinc phosphide | X | X |
| White phosphorus | X | X |
| *Amanita phalloides* (mushroom) | X | X |
| *Zamia floridana* (Cycad) | ? | X |
| Aflatoxin | X | X |
| Dry-cleaning fluid (trichloroethane) | X | X |
| Toluene | X | X |
| Phenols | X | X |
| Zinc | — | X |

*X*, Hepatotoxic; —, not known to be hepatotoxic; ?, possibly hepatotoxic.

**Table 37-2**

### Suggested Specific Treatment for Dogs and Cats Exposed to Hepatotoxins

| Substance | Treatment |
|---|---|
| **THERAPEUTIC AGENT** | |
| Acetaminophen | 140 mg/kg N-acetylcysteine PO or IV as a 20% solution for a loading dose; continue at 70 mg/kg 6 hr later and q6h thereafter for a total of seven treatments; ascorbic acid, 30 mg/kg PO q6h, should also be given |
| **ENVIRONMENTAL TOXINS** | |
| Inorganic arsenicals | 2.5-5 mg/kg BAL IM q4h for 2 days, then q12h until recovery; should be initiated within 36 hr of exposure |
| Thallium | 70 mg/kg diphenylthiocarbazine PO q8h; must be started within 24 hr of exposure; controversial |

*BAL,* British antilewisite; *IM,* intramuscularly; *IV,* intravenously; *PO,* orally.

# 38

# Hepatobiliary Diseases in the Dog

## *(Text pp 525-545)*

Acquired liver disorders in dogs are diverse and are not predictably characterized by jaundice and hepatomegaly. Extensive and sometimes serial testing is often required to reach a diagnosis. Hepatocytes are the target of injury in dogs; the clinical syndrome of hepatic failure with abdominal effusion, acquired portosystemic shunts (PSS), and other complications of portal hypertension is common. Chronic hepatopathies are much more common than acute hepatic diseases in dogs.

## CHRONIC HEPATITIS (TEXT PP 525-531)
### General Features
Chronic hepatitis in dogs is composed of a spectrum of hepatic diseases that share similar historical, clinical, and, possibly, histopathologic features (Table 38-1). Affected dogs are ill for weeks or months, with combinations of anorexia, weight loss, lethargy,

**Table 38-1**

## Acquired Canine Hepatic Diseases Known Collectively as Chronic Hepatitis

| Familial | Drug-associated | Infectious | Idiopathic |
|---|---|---|---|
| Copper hepatotoxicosis<br>Bedlington Terrier | Diethylcarbamazine-oxibendazole<br>Anticonvulsants (phenytoin, primidone, phenobarbital) | Infectious canine hepatitis<br>Acidophil cell hepatitis (Great Britain) | Chronic hepatitis<br>Lobular dissecting hepatitis |
| Doberman Pinscher?<br>West Highland White Terrier | Trimethoprim-sulfa? | Leptospirosis?<br>Subsequent to *Corynebacterium parvum* immunotherapy? | |
| Dalmatian<br>Other copper accumulation associated with cholestasis?<br>Skye Terrier<br>Doberman Pinscher?<br>Labrador Retriever?<br>Cocker Spaniel? | | | |

polyuria (PU) and polydipsia (PD), jaundice, abdominal effusion, signs of hepatic encephalopathy (HE), and hemorrhagic tendencies.

Typical clinicopathologic findings are persistently high serum alanine amino-transferase (ALT) activity with less strikingly elevated alkaline phosphatase (AP) and γ-glutamyltransferase (GGT) activities early in the course of the disease, followed by hypoalbuminemia, low blood urea nitrogen (BUN), and high serum bile acid (SBA) concentrations late in the course. Liver biopsy is crucial for accurate diagnosis and prognosis, although much overlap exists among these diseases. Variable changes include portal and periportal hepatocellular necrosis, mixed inflammatory cell infiltrates, fibrosis, biliary hyperplasia, and nodular regeneration.

Depending on the extent and cause, it may be possible to reverse or control the process with specific therapy, or at least to modulate its course with symptomatic treatment. The specific diseases or syndromes of chronic hepatitis currently recognized in dogs are discussed separately in the following sections. Treatment of chronic liver disease is discussed later.

### Familial Chronic Hepatitis

Chronic hepatopathy characterized by hepatic copper (Cu) accumulation occurs in several breeds, most notably the Bedlington Terrier, Doberman Pinscher, West Highland White Terrier, Skye Terrier, and Dalmatian. The disease in Bedlingtons is inherited as an autosomal recessive trait; in other breeds a familial basis is strongly suspected. Some individuals have hepatic Cu accumulation but no clinical signs or histopathologic abnormalities. (The normal range for hepatic Cu concentration in mixed-breed dogs is 200 to 400 μg/g dry weight [DW].) Treatment for Cu hepatopathy is discussed on page 526 of the text.

#### Bedlington Terriers

In affected Bedlingtons signs of illness generally become evident in middle age. Severity of clinical signs and of clinicopathologic and histopathologic findings are directly related to the degree of hepatic Cu accumulation. Clinical signs usually do not develop until hepatic Cu accumulation is marked (approximately 2000 μg/g DW). Hemolytic anemia can occur if a large number of hepatocytes die suddenly and release Cu into the circulation, but this is rare.

*Diagnosis.* Histopathologic changes are not unique and range from multifocal necrosis with inflammation to more severe changes, including nodular regeneration, bile duct hyperplasia and fibrosis, and macronodular or micronodular cirrhosis. Special stains must be used to confirm that the dark, brownish granules within lysosomes contain Cu.

The normal range for liver Cu in Bedlingtons is 91 to 358 μg/g DW. Most affected (homozygous) dogs have liver Cu >800 μg/g DW, regardless of age, at the time of biopsy.

*Identifying carriers.* Currently the only practical, widely available means of identifying affected homozygous dogs and asymptomatic carriers (purebred heterozygotes and Bedlington crosses) before the onset of signs is by hepatic Cu quantification at 6 months of age, and if necessary, 10 to 12 months later. Carriers have hepatic Cu concentrations in both specimens that are normal or slightly elevated (400 to 700 μg/g DW) but are similar to one another. In affected dogs the hepatic Cu concentration of the second specimen is much greater than that of the first.

Genetic testing has recently been evaluated for identification of affected dogs. As long as several related dogs are available for testing, this method will identify affected, heterozygous, and normal dogs. Carrier and affected dogs should be neutered.

#### Doberman Pinschers

Doberman hepatopathy appears to be a progressive condition that occurs pre-dominantly in middle-aged females. Signs and clinicopathologic abnormalities usually are present for months. This condition is similar to autoimmune chronic-active hepatitis (CAH) in humans, although an immune basis has not been confirmed in dogs. Classic lesions are portal mononuclear cell inflammation with extension into adjacent parenchyma ("piecemeal" necrosis) and other lobules ("bridging" necrosis), and periportal fibrosis. Advanced CAH is characterized by cirrhosis with evidence of ongoing hepatocyte injury.

Serum biochemistry and histopathology reveal more evidence of cholestasis in Dobermans than in Bedlingtons. The role of Cu in Doberman hepatopathy is not fully understood. Typically, hepatic Cu concentration in affected Dobermans is 450 to 3600 µg/g DW.

### West Highland White Terriers

Hepatic disease associated with Cu retention in Westies appears to differ from other familial hepatopathies. The range of hepatic Cu in affected dogs is 450 to 3500 µg/g DW, which is lower than that of many affected Bedlingtons, and liver Cu concentration does not increase with age.

### Skye Terriers

Familial hepatopathy in Skye Terriers is described as mild to moderate periportal and pericentral inflammation, with intracanalicular cholestasis and Cu accumulation. Regenerative parenchymal nodules surrounded by fibrous connective tissue bands are seen in chronic cases. The degree of Cu retention seems to correlate with the degree and duration of cholestasis.

### Dalmatians

Cu-associated liver injury has been reported in a small number of Dalmatians. Clinical signs were nonspecific (anorexia, lethargy, vomiting, diarrhea). Affected dogs ranged in age from 1.5 years to 10 years (median, 5 years). The predominant serum biochemical change was high ALT activity (up to elevenfold increase), with mild increases in AP (normal to fivefold elevation). Liver Cu concentration was >2000 µg/g DW in most affected dogs. Despite treatment with a Cu chelator or zinc (Zn), most dogs died within 3 months of diagnosis.

## Drug Administration

Heartworm prevention and treatment for osteoarthritis, central nervous system disorders, allergic or immune-mediated diseases, and cancer are the most common situations in which drugs given long term might cause chronic adverse hepatic reactions in dogs. The overall frequency is low, and most are probably associated with unique susceptibility. Except for glucocorticoid hepatopathy, hepatic lesions in dogs with drug-induced hepatotoxicity are not unique. Presumptive diagnosis is usually based on careful examination of the history, and improvement on discontinuation of drug therapy.

### Heartworm preventatives

The combination of diethylcarbamazine and oxibendazole (Filaribits Plus) occasionally causes depression, anorexia, weight loss, vomiting, PU and PD, and icterus. Signs are observed within weeks of starting drug administration and resolve shortly after discontinuation of the drug. In some dogs clinicopathologic evidence of persistent hepatobiliary disease is seen.

### Anticonvulsants

Primidone, alone or in combination with other anticonvulsants, can cause clinical hepatic disease. High serum activities of AP (fivefold to eightfold increase) and ALT (twofold to threefold increase) are common; serum GGT activity is usually normal. Dogs that require higher than recommended dosages may develop serious hepatic injury that progresses to cirrhosis. Chronic phenobarbital administration can cause similar changes. In dogs that develop hepatotoxicity associated with primidone or phenobarbital, potassium bromide may be safely substituted for seizure control (see Chapter 69).

### Glucocorticoids

Chronic glucocorticoid administration in dogs causes a unique hepatopathy, characterized by hepatocyte vacuolization (glycogen accumulation). Hepatomegaly and high serum activities of AP (up to 100-fold increase), GGT (sixfold to tenfold increase), and ALT (twofold to fourfold increase) are common, especially in dogs receiving prednisone. The AP is a specific glucocorticoid-induced isoenzyme (see Chapter 36). Mild hepatic dysfunction, demonstrated by high fasting SBA concentrations (up to 50 µmol/L;

can be as high as 100 μmol/L), is gradually reversible on termination of glucocorticoid therapy. Hyperbilirubinemia and histopathologic evidence of cholestasis are absent. Glucocorticoid hepatopathy is rarely severe enough to cause hepatic failure.

### Chemotherapeutic drugs

Most chemotherapeutic agents in current use cause little, if any, clinically relevant chronic hepatic injury. Azathioprine causes hepatic damage more often than other agents; usually this represents an idiosyncratic reaction or inappropriate dosage. Lomustine (CCNU) is hepatotoxic in dogs.

## Infectious Agents

Primary chronic hepatitis caused by infectious organisms appears to be unusual in dogs. The liver is often secondarily involved in many acute systemic illnesses (see Table 36-1), but chronic sequelae are rare. Canine adenovirus type I is responsible for infectious canine chronic hepatitis.

## Idiopathic Chronic Hepatitis

The most common form of chronic hepatitis in mixed-breed and purebred dogs other than those addressed previously is an idiopathic condition described as lobular dissecting hepatitis. Characterized clinically by ascites and clinicopathologic findings consistent with hepatic failure, it occurs in relatively young dogs (7 months to 5 years of age).

Multifocal inflammatory infiltrates, disturbance of lobular architecture by fine collagen and reticulin fibers, and scant inflammation and connective tissue deposition in portal tracts are typical features. Acquired PSS may develop secondary to intrahepatic portal hypertension. The prognosis appears to be extremely poor, although it is possible for individual dogs to survive comfortably for years with supportive care. Corticosteroids appear to improve the hepatic lesions and clinical signs in some dogs.

## Idiopathic Hepatic Fibrosis

Idiopathic hepatic fibrosis was described in 19 dogs, most of which were German Shepherd Dogs (GSD) or GSD crosses. Most dogs were anorectic and lethargic and had microhepatia, ascites, and signs of HE. Clinicopathologic findings included microcytosis and high serum AP activity; several dogs also had mild hyperbilirubinemia.

Three subtypes of fibrosis were noted: central perivenous, diffuse pericellular, and periportal. No evidence of inflammation was present. All dogs received medical treatment for HE and ascites; some also received prednisolone, and others colchicine. Response to treatment was variable.

## CONGENITAL PORTOVASCULAR DISORDERS WITH NORMAL PORTAL PRESSURE (TEXT PP 531-533)

### Congenital PSS

Many different patterns of portovascular anomaly have been described in dogs. The most common are single extrahepatic communications between the portal vein or one of the mesenteric veins and the caudal vena cava or azygous vein in small-breed dogs and patent ductus venosus in large-breed dogs. Hypoplasia or aplasia of intrahepatic portal vasculature could complicate any of these anomalies, but it is unusual. A familial predisposition for single extrahepatic PSS is suspected in the Yorkshire Terrier, Miniature Schnauzer, Lhasa Apso, and Shih Tzu. Retrievers, Irish Setters, Irish Wolfhounds, and other large-breed dogs are predisposed to intrahepatic PSS.

### Clinical features

Common signs in dogs with single intrahepatic or extrahepatic PSS are those of HE and/or gastrointestinal (GI) disturbance, such as vomiting, diarrhea, and pica. Additional historic and physical examination findings are listed in Table 38-2. Age range of affected dogs is 2 months to 10 years, but most cases are seen when the dog is <1 year old. No gender predilection exists.

Table 38-2

## Clinical Features of Congenital Portosystemic Shunt in Dogs and Cats

| | |
|---|---|
| Signalment | Less than 1 yr of age, either gender, purebred |
| History | Neurologic signs, often after a meal (dementia, circling, wall-hugging, personality change, seizures [rare]) |
| | Intermittent vomiting; sometimes diarrhea |
| | Preference for fruits and vegetables (especially dogs) |
| | Hypersalivation (especially cats) |
| | Apparent improvement in neurologic signs with antibiotic treatment |
| | Anesthetic or sedative intolerance |
| | Polydipsia and polyuria (less common) |
| | Recurrent urate urolithiasis in breeds other than the Dalmatian or English Bulldog |
| Physical examination | Small stature |
| | Bilateral renomegaly |
| | Poor or unkempt haircoat |
| | Other congenital anomalies |
| | Cystic calculi (especially in cats and older dogs) |
| | Cryptorchidism |
| | Copper-colored irises in non-Asian cat breeds |

### Diagnosis

Definitive diagnosis is based on demonstration of an abnormal connection between portal vein and systemic vein and characteristic histopathologic findings in dogs with clinical and clinicopathologic evidence of hepatic insufficiency. Regardless of the type of anomaly, findings in >50% of affected dogs include microcytosis, hypoalbuminemia, mild increases in serum AP and ALT activities, hypocholesterolemia, low BUN, post-challenge hyperammonemia, and normal or high fasting SBA with high postprandial SBA.

In many cases the liver is small. Combinations of ultrasonography, transcolonic or splenic scintigraphy, and contrast portal venography may be needed to confirm the location of the anomalous vessel before surgical correction is attempted.

### Treatment and prognosis

Occlusion of the anomalous vessel is the treatment of choice, but surgical correction of both extrahepatic and intrahepatic PSS is challenging. Portal pressure, which is normal in dogs with congenital PSS, should be measured and liver biopsy obtained in all dogs undergoing surgery.

Dogs with a single extrahepatic PSS that can be ligated completely without causing the portal pressure to exceed 18 cm $H_2O$ have the best prognosis for a normal life span and quality of life. Partial recovery is expected in dogs that have extrahepatic PSS that cannot be totally occluded without causing fatal portal hypertension. Ligation of intra-hepatic PSS is technically more difficult; a nonsurgical technique has been developed for gradual closure of intrahepatic PSS (see text).

*Complications.* Generalized motor seizures occasionally develop postoperatively in older dogs (>18 months of age) after ligation of single congenital extrahepatic PSS. These seizures may be intractable and either necessitate euthanasia or result in residual neurologic abnormalities.

*Managing HE.* Signs of HE are managed medically before surgery (see Chapter 39), and these measures are continued for 1 month after surgical correction. For dogs with partially occluded or inoperable PSS, symptomatic management is recommended for life. However, diet is no substitute for surgical correction. Hepatic deterioration associated with poor portal blood flow progresses as long as the abnormal vascular pattern persists.

### Microvascular Dysplasia

Microvascular dysplasia (MVD) is a disorder in which clinical features of congenital PSS are present, but a macroscopic vascular anomaly cannot be identified and there exists microscopic evidence of disordered hepatic vasculature. MVD can occur as a single anomaly or jointly with congenital PSS. In Cairn Terriers it involves the terminal portal veins and apparently is an autosomal inherited trait.

#### Clinical features

MVD occurs in the same breeds that are predisposed to extrahepatic congenital PSS. Typical presenting complaints include vomiting, diarrhea, and signs of HE, especially in dogs with both defects. Dogs with only MVD are somewhat older and many have mild or no signs of illness. Affected Cairn Terriers, and perhaps other breeds such as the Maltese, usually are asymptomatic, although they have clinicopathologic evidence of hepatic dysfunction.

#### Diagnosis

The most important aspects of identifying MVD are ruling out a surgically correctable PSS and obtaining a liver biopsy specimen for confirmation or exclusion of other hepatopathies. Dogs with MVD alone may have some of the same clinicopathologic features of those with congenital PSS; some appear normal except for modest increases in SBA concentrations. In young, purebred dogs that have been screened for congenital PSS before sale or that are ill for nonhepatic reasons, high SBA concentrations may be the only clinicopathologic finding.

*Imaging studies.* Unlike in dogs with congenital PSS, the liver is usually normal in size. Contrast portography using repeated injections and multiple exposures might indicate altered perfusion of the smaller branches of the portal vasculature in one or more liver lobes but no evidence of a macroscopic shunt vessel. Results of transcolonic or splenic scintigraphy are normal.

*Liver biopsy.* Histopathologic changes are identical to those in dogs with congenital PSS. Random juvenile intralobular blood vessels can be seen in dogs with MVD or congenital PSS and may represent a compensatory response to decreased portal blood flow.

#### Treatment and prognosis

No surgical remedy for MVD exists; symptomatic management for HE (if present) is the only treatment. Affected dogs seem to live comfortably in good to excellent condition for at least 5 years without serious consequences.

## CONGENITAL PORTOVASCULAR DISORDERS WITH HIGH PORTAL PRESSURE (TEXT PP 533-535)

### Noncirrhotic Portal Hypertension

Noncirrhotic portal hypertension describes a category of hepatopathies in humans characterized by portal hypertension, a patent portal vein, and relatively unremarkable liver biopsy findings. Two diseases primarily of young dogs (<2.5 years) might fit this description: hepatoportal fibrosis and primary portal vein hypoplasia. Another recently described syndrome in young (<4 years of age), purebred dogs of various breeds (weighing >10 kg) also resembles idiopathic noncirrhotic portal hypertension.

It is possible that all three conditions are variations of the same disorder—intrahepatic portal vein hypoplasia—and that the severity of signs and clinicopathologic changes relates to the degree of portal vasculature affected.

#### Clinical features and diagnosis

Affected dogs do not consistently have signs of HE, commonly have microhepatia, and usually have ascites, GI abnormalities, polydipsia, weight loss, and clinicopathologic features compatible with hepatic failure (including hypoalbuminemia). The presence of multiple extrahepatic PSS is characteristic. Hepatic histopathologic changes are nearly indistinguishable from those in dogs with PSS or MVD.

#### Treatment and prognosis

Symptomatic treatment for ascites and HE is usually indicated. Treatment with colchicine may improve the outcome in dogs with hepatoportal fibrosis. Specific treatment for primary portal vein hypoplasia is not known, but affected dogs can remain in good health for a number of years with medical treatment for HE and ascites. However, duodenal ulceration, urate urolithiasis, and other sequelae to persistent portal hypertension may compromise long-term health.

### Arterioportal Fistula

Intrahepatic arterioportal fistula, causing marked volume overload of the portal circulation and portal hypertension, acquired PSS, and ascites, is seen occasionally in dogs. Abdominal ultrasound with Doppler imaging can usually detect the tortuous tubular structures; sometimes the turbulent blood flow through the fistula can be ausculted through the body wall.

#### Treatment

If only one liver lobe is affected, that lobe can be removed surgically. Assuming intrahepatic portal vasculature is adequate, the acquired PSS regresses once portal overcirculation subsides. More commonly, however, multiple liver lobes are involved, making surgical cure impossible.

## TREATMENT FOR CHRONIC LIVER DISORDERS (TEXT PP 535-537)

Treatment for drug-induced chronic hepatitis is straightforward. Signs and clinicopathologic abnormalities should improve soon after drug administration is suspended. If complete resolution does not occur, liver biopsy is indicated to determine if other hepatic disease is present or if medication is needed to modify persistent pathologic processes. Treatment for other chronic hepatic disease consists of supportive care, dietary modification, and specific medications when indicated. Overall, the prognosis is guarded to poor because the underlying cause often cannot be eliminated.

### Prevention and Treatment of Copper Excess

#### Reducing dietary copper

In Bedlington Terriers and other breeds with familial Cu hepatotoxicosis, decreasing dietary Cu does not remove excess hepatic Cu, but it helps to slow further accumulation. The following are purported to be low-copper diets: (1) Cornucopia Senior or Life (Cornucopia Natural Pet Foods); (2) Canine l/d (Hill's Prescription Diets); and (3) homemade diets that do not contain organ meats, shellfish, or cereals. High-copper snacks such as organ meats, shellfish, cereal, chocolate, nuts, dried fruit, legumes, and mushrooms should be avoided.

#### Reducing intestinal absorption of copper

Administration of Zn salts benefits at-risk West Highland and Bedlington Terriers early in life, before massive accumulation of hepatic Cu has occurred. The recommended dose is 100 mg of elemental Zn, preferably as acetate or sulfate, given orally (PO) q12h without food or with a small amount of tuna. The goal is to maintain serum Zn concentrations (measured every 2 to 3 months) at 200 to 300 $\mu$g/dl and <600 $\mu$g/dl. The dose may be reduced to 50 mg q12h after 3 months, assuming the plasma Zn concentration remains in the target range. If serum Zn is <150 $\mu$g/dl, the dose must remain in the range of 50 to 100 mg PO q12h.

#### Copper chelators

Older dogs with marked Cu accumulation require drugs that chelate Cu and promote its extraction from the liver. The drug most often recommended is D-penicillamine (10 to 15 mg/kg PO q12h 30 min before meals). Vomiting and anorexia are common adverse effects that can be minimized by starting at the lower end of the dose range and increasing the dose after 1 week or dividing the dose and giving it more frequently.

Use of D-penicillamine is recommended in West Highland White Terriers only when the liver Cu is >2000 $\mu$g/g DW. However, decreases in hepatic Cu occur only after several months of therapy, so rapid improvement cannot be expected in severely ill dogs. A decrease in liver Cu of approximately 900 $\mu$g/g DW per year can be anticipated in dogs treated with D-penicillamine.

Trientine (10 to 15 mg/kg PO q12h, 30 minutes before meals) is an equally effective Cu chelator that may be used in dogs that cannot tolerate D-penicillamine. Glucocorticoids may be of greater benefit than Cu chelators in some Doberman Pinschers and perhaps other breeds with Cu-associated hepatopathy of unknown mechanism.

To avoid Cu deficiency, chelation therapy is continued until normal liver Cu concentrations are reached, as determined by liver biopsy. The regimen can then be changed to a preventive protocol consisting of a Cu-restricted diet and Zn administration.

### Glucocorticoids

Use of glucocorticoids for treatment of chronic hepatitis remains controversial. In one study, dogs with chronic hepatitis that were given prednisone (1.1 mg/kg PO q12h for 7 to 10 days, then 1.1 mg/kg/day for 10 days, then 0.6 mg/kg/day) lived three times longer than those that were not given glucocorticoids. Histopathologic lesions progressed in dogs not given glucocorticoids. The authors also recommended ascorbic acid (25 mg/kg/day PO) and Zn supplementation. Whether to give antiinflammatory or immunosuppressive doses of glucocorticoids needs to be clarified.

### Azathioprine

Azathioprine (50 mg/m$^2$ PO q24h) can initially be given with prednisone, then later on alternate days with prednisone (1 mg/kg/day PO). Because of the potential for bone marrow toxicity, complete blood counts (CBCs) should be performed weekly or every other week during azathioprine therapy. Treatment should be suspended for 5 to 7 days if the total neutrophil count is <2000 cells/$\mu$l or if the platelet count is <100,000 cells/$\mu$l. Once hematologic abnormalities have resolved, azathioprine can be reinstituted at 75% of the original dose.

### Antifibrotic agents

Antifibrotic agents can be used as the sole agent for primarily fibrotic hepatopathies (e.g., idiopathic hepatic fibrosis). An antifibrotic agent can also be added to the treatment regimen when chronic hepatitis has a fibrotic component and the dog does not tolerate or is unresponsive to glucocorticoids, especially if clinical manifestations of portal hypertension (ascites and HE) are present. The drug used most often is colchicine (0.03 mg/kg/day PO), but it must be given for months or years to be of benefit.

## Dietary Modification

Dietary modifications are aimed at providing sufficient nutrients and calories to support repair of hepatic tissue while minimizing aberrations in protein metabolism that induce or perpetuate HE. These diets are highly digestible, contain high-quality protein in moderate quantities, and rely on nonprotein sources for most of their calories (see Chapter 39).

## Adjunctive Treatments

### Antioxidants

Several medications have been recommended for their free-radical–scavenging capabilities. Vitamin E (400 to 500 IU/day PO) can protect liver cells from Cu toxic injury and cholestatic concentrations of bile acids, and it appears safe clinically. S-adenosylmethionine (Denosyl SD4; 20 mg/kg PO q24h after an overnight fast) may be of benefit in animals with acute toxic hepatopathy.

### Ursodiol

Ursodiol may be of benefit in patients with chronic hepatitis. It displaces injurious bile acids from the bile acid pool, protects liver cells from oxidant injury, increases bile flow, and modulates cytokine responses. It appears to be safe at a dose of 10 to 15 mg/kg PO q24h.

## ACUTE TOXIC HEPATOPATHY (TEXT PP 537-538)

Drugs or environmental toxins with inherent ability to cause hepatic injury include pesticides, herbicides, cleaning agents, and plant toxins. Most adverse hepatic reactions observed in dogs involve chronic administration of therapeutic agents. A partial list of drugs and environmental toxins reported to be hepatotoxic in dogs is given in Table 37-1.

### Clinical features
Clinical signs are indistinct from those of other hepatopathies, except in onset and perhaps severity. Vomiting is common. Nutritional status and gender are important; females may be more susceptible. Dose, duration of exposure, and chemical composition contribute to how toxicity is expressed.

### Diagnosis
Clinicopathologic findings are typical of hepatocellular damage: high serum ALT and variable increases in serum AP activities. Jaundice is usually of hepatocellular rather than biliary origin. A liver biopsy is performed only if recovery is incomplete and other hepatobiliary diseases are suspected. Histopathologic lesions include centrolobular necrosis or periportal inflammation, either of which can be a feature of other hepatopathies. Therefore a detailed history is the most valuable diagnostic test.

### Treatment and prognosis
Most drug-related hepatotoxicities in dogs are idiosyncratic, so prompt recognition is the best defense. If a drug is suspected of causing hepatic disease, its administration should be suspended. Except for a few hepatotoxic agents for which specific antidotes exist (see Table 37-2), additional treatment is supportive. As soon as exposure is terminated, improvement in clinical signs and clinicopathologic data should be evident. In cases of brief toxic exposure, complete recovery is likely. If a large amount of hepatic mass has been seriously injured, residual hepatic insufficiency may persist.

## BILIARY TRACT DISORDERS (TEXT PP 538-540)

Disorders of the biliary tract generally are classified as primary diseases originating in the biliary tract itself (uncommon in dogs) or diseases of other organ systems that secondarily affect the biliary tract. Primary conditions that involve the bile ducts (cholangitis) and/or gallbladder (cholecystitis) in dogs include extrahepatic bile duct obstruction (EBDO), bile peritonitis, and gallbladder mucocele. Specific causes of EBDO are listed in Box 37-1. Bile peritonitis most often results from abdominal trauma that damages the common bile duct (CBD) or pathologic rupture of a severely diseased gallbladder.

The most common causes of secondary biliary tract disease in dogs are pancreatitis and sepsis arising from nonhepatobiliary sources (see Table 36-1). Rarely, certain drugs (e.g., sulfonamides) cause bile ductule injury or destructive cholangiolitis.

### Clinical features
Clinical signs and physical examination findings for each of these disorders may not differ greatly unless the underlying condition has caused EBDO or bile peritonitis. Regardless of the underlying disorder, typical signs are jaundice, vomiting (acute or chronic), anorexia, depression, weight loss, and in some cases vague cranial abdominal pain. It is sometimes possible to palpate the gallbladder when it is greatly distended.

Early signs of bile peritonitis are nonspecific; jaundice, fever, and abdominal effusion are seen as the condition progresses. Hypovolemia and sepsis may occur in dogs with undetected bile peritonitis. Gallbladder mucocele is reported most often in older, small-breed dogs. Common presenting complaints are anorexia, lethargy, and vomiting. Gallbladder rupture occurs in approximately 50% of cases.

### Diagnosis
After collection of a minimum database, mechanical obstruction is ruled out first, usually by ultrasonography. Then liver, bile, and possibly gallbladder mucosa specimens are obtained for histopathology and microbial culture and sensitivity, preferably before antibiotic treatment is initiated.

*Clinical pathology.* Typical findings with biliary tract disease include hyperbilirubinemia, high serum AP and GGT activities, high fasting and postprandial SBA concentrations, and less severe elevations in serum ALT. Generally, more severe cholestatic lesions cause more severe changes. Inflammatory abdominal effusion is expected in dogs with bile peritonitis, but not with most causes of EBDO (except for malignant effusion associated with pancreatic cancer).

Acholic feces, vitamin K–responsive coagulopathy, and repeated absence of urobilinogen in properly processed urine specimens are found only in cases in which bile flow has been completely interrupted for several weeks. If obstruction is incomplete, these features are not present, and the clinical and clinicopathologic findings resemble those of other, nonobstructive biliary tract disorders.

Note: Monitoring serum bilirubin concentration to determine when to intervene surgically is not worthwhile, because in dogs with EBDO it declines over days or weeks, without relief of obstruction.

*Radiography.* Radiographic findings may include hepatomegaly and a mass effect in the area of the gallbladder. Gas shadows associated with the gallbladder and other biliary structures may indicate ascending infection with gas-forming organisms. Findings consistent with concurrent acute pancreatitis are loss of serosal detail in the area of the pancreas, trapped pockets of gas in the duodenum, and duodenal displacement. Choleliths, which in dogs usually form as a sequela of cholestasis and infection, are radiolucent unless they contain calcium (which occurs in approximately 50% of cases).

*Ultrasonography.* It is often possible to differentiate between medical and surgical causes of jaundice using ultrasonography. Dilated and tortuous hepatic bile ducts and CBD, as well as gallbladder distention, are convincing evidence of EBDO at the CBD or sphincter of Oddi. When dilated biliary structures are seen, it might be difficult to distinguish EBDO that requires surgical intervention from transient, resolving EBDO associated with severe acute pancreatitis or from nonobstructive biliary disease (e.g., bacterial cholecystitis or cholangitis) unless a source of obstruction is identified (e.g., pancreatic mass, cholelith in the CBC).

With gallbladder mucoceles the contents of the gallbladder have a characteristic stellate appearance (like a cross section of a kiwi fruit). Cystic hyperplasia and epithelial polyp formation are common lesions in older dogs, not to be confused with choleliths in the gallbladder. Prolonged fasting causes mild gallbladder enlargement that should not be misinterpreted.

*Tissue and bile specimens.* A liver biopsy and bile specimen should be obtained in all cases. If surgery is not an option, liver and bile samples are obtained via ultrasonographic guidance. To minimize bile leakage, a 22-gauge needle with a 12-ml syringe attached is used for bile retrieval, and an attempt is made to evacuate the gallbladder. Risk of iatrogenic bile or septic peritonitis is greatest with a severely diseased gallbladder wall; surgery is necessary in such cases.

The bile specimen is submitted for cytology and aerobic and anaerobic bacterial cultures if choleliths are found or the biliary structures appear thickened. Enteric organisms similar to those found in cats are usually isolated (see Chapter 37). Some bacteria have a predilection for the gallbladder mucosa, so a specimen of that tissue should also be submitted for culture.

Typical hepatic histopathologic findings in early EBDO are canalicular bile plugs and bile ductular proliferation, with degrees of periportal inflammation and fibrosis found in chronic cases. Confounding biliary infection incites a stronger inflammatory reaction in the periportal region. Mucosal hyperplasia and variable mural necrosis of the gallbladder are common findings in dogs with mucoceles.

### Treatment

Surgery is required in dogs with persistent EBDO, bile peritonitis, or gallbladder mucocele. Surgical goals are to relieve biliary obstruction or leakage and restore bile flow. Reconstructive procedures to divert bile flow can be performed if the cause of EBDO cannot be corrected.

If the distinction between medical and surgical causes of jaundice is not clear, it is safer to proceed surgically. Should a site of obstruction or biliary injury not be identified, at least tissue (liver, gallbladder mucosa) and bile specimens can be obtained for cytology, histopathology, and bacterial culture and sensitivity. It is possible to obtain liver and bile specimens in dogs with suspected nonobstructive biliary disease with ultrasonographic guidance or by laparoscopy, but risk of delayed bile leakage is higher with these techniques.

### Special considerations

Coagulation status and fluid and electrolyte needs should be addressed preoperatively. If clinical or subclinical coagulopathy is present, vitamin $K_1$ is administered (1 mg/kg subcutaneously [SC] q24h) for 24 to 48 hours before and after surgery. Any abdominal fluid is analyzed and cultured for aerobic and anaerobic bacteria. If surgery for bile peritonitis is to be delayed, peritoneal drainage should be established. Administration of bile acids to stimulate bile flow is contraindicated in dogs with EBDO.

*Antibiotic therapy.* Antibiotic therapy is started immediately after bile samples are obtained; ampicillin or amoxicillin (22 mg/kg intravenously [IV], SC, or PO q8h), first-generation cephalosporins (22 mg/kg IV or PO q8h), and metronidazole (7.5 to 15 mg/kg PO q8-12h; use lower dose with severe hepatobiliary dysfunction) are all good initial choices in animals without a long history of antibiotic administration.

### Prognosis

Cholecystectomy is curative in dogs with gallbladder mucocele. The prognosis for dogs with EBDO or bile peritonitis depends on the underlying cause. If the cause can be addressed without surgical reconstruction, the prognosis is fair to good. If extensive biliary reconstruction is needed, the prognosis is guarded because of the potential for recurrent ascending bacterial infections and other complications.

## FOCAL HEPATIC LESIONS (TEXT PP 541-524)

### Abscesses

Hepatic abscesses are usually the result of septic embolization from an abdominal site of bacterial infection. In puppies they are a consequence of omphalophlebitis; in adults they occur most often from inflammatory conditions of the pancreas or hepatobiliary system. Adult dogs with endocrine diseases, such as diabetes mellitus or hypercortisolism, are also at risk. Occasionally infection in a location other than the abdominal cavity (e.g., endocardium, lung) may disseminate to the liver. Aerobic bacteria are isolated most often; gram-negative organisms are common isolates. *Clostridium* spp. may be isolated anaerobically.

### Clinical features

Signalment and physical examination findings depend on the underlying cause. Most affected dogs are >8 years of age. Regardless of the cause, anorexia, lethargy, and vomiting are consistent presenting complaints. Expected findings include fever, dehydration, and abdominal pain. Hepatomegaly may be detected in dogs with diabetes mellitus or hypercortisolism and in some dogs with primary hepatobiliary disease.

### Diagnosis

Neutrophilic leukocytosis with a left shift, and high serum AP and ALT activities are typical but nonspecific findings. Radiographs may reveal irregular hepatomegaly, a mass, or gas opacity within the hepatic parenchyma, but ultrasonography is the imaging modality of choice. One or more hypoechoic or anechoic masses, perhaps with a hyperechoic rim, are characteristic findings. Cytology of a fine-needle aspirate or surgical biopsy specimen distinguishes an abscess from nodular hyperplasia, neoplasm, or granuloma. Ideally, material is obtained for cytology and aerobic and anaerobic bacterial culture from a lesion deep in the liver parenchyma.

### Treatment and prognosis

Treatment consists of surgical removal of infected tissue (if possible), administration of appropriate antibiotics, supportive care, and resolution of any underlying condition. With aggressive medical and surgical management, the prognosis is fair. Surgery is not indicated in animals with multiple abscesses. In these cases, ultrasound-guided centesis and abscess evacuation may be a reasonable adjunct to antimicrobial treatment.

*Antimicrobial therapy.* Antibiotics with a gram-negative and anaerobic spectrum are initiated until culture and sensitivity results are available. Amikacin (10 mg/kg IV or intramuscularly [IM] q8h) or enrofloxacin (2.5 to 5 mg/kg IV or PO q12h) combined with metronidazole (10 mg/kg PO q8-12h, or 7.5 mg/kg PO q8-12h in dogs with hepatic dysfunction) or clindamycin (10 mg/kg IV or PO q12h) is a good empiric choice. Treatment is continued for 6 to 8 weeks or until indicators of septic abscessation are resolved.

## Nodular Hyperplasia

Nodular hyperplasia of the liver is a benign condition of older dogs. It does not cause clinical illness, but it may be misinterpreted on ultrasonography or at surgery as a more serious condition, such as primary or metastatic malignancy or regenerative nodules associated with cirrhosis. Most dogs have multiple, macroscopic nodules; some have a single nodule.

No evidence of hepatic dysfunction is found on serum biochemical analysis, although affected dogs have high serum AP activity (usually 2.5-fold but may be as high as fourteenfold elevation), which prompts investigation for hypercortisolism.

Because the prognosis for the other nodular hepatic conditions differs, and it is important to include the margin of the lesion with adjacent hepatic tissue, wedge biopsy is recommended. Needle specimens are likely to be too small to confidently differentiate nodular hyperplasia from primary hepatocellular carcinoma (HC) or hepatocellular adenoma (HA).

## Neoplasia

Primary hepatic neoplasms are rare in dogs. The most common types are HC and intrahepatic cholangiocellular (bile duct) carcinoma (CC); HA is found less often. Primary sarcomas, such as hemangiosarcoma, are uncommon.

Metastases from distant sites (e.g., GI, pancreatic, and mammary adenocarcinomas; splenic hemangiosarcoma) are much more common. Liver involvement is also common in dogs with hemolymphatic disorders, such as lymphoma, myeloproliferative disorders, and mast cell neoplasia.

Both HC and CC usually metastasize early; the most common sites are regional lymph nodes, lung, and peritoneal surfaces. HA is a benign tumor; its histologic features are very similar to those of nodular hyperplasia (see text).

### Clinical features

Most primary hepatic neoplasms occur in older dogs. Signs and physical examination findings are nonspecific, except for diffuse or nodular hepatomegaly. The left liver lobes are often affected by HC, which can occur in three different patterns: massive (single, large nodule; most common), nodular (multiple, smaller nodules), and diffuse (indistinct nodules throughout). HA most often occurs as a single mass that typically is smaller than the massive form of HC; however, HA can be multifocal.

### Diagnosis

Clinicopathologic findings are nonspecific and may be normal, even in dogs with extensive involvement. Hypoglycemia has been described in association with HC in dogs. When a single, large hepatic mass is identified, distinguishing well-differentiated HC from nodular hyperplasia and HA can be very difficult. Biopsy is required for definitive diagnosis.

### Treatment and prognosis

Surgical resection is the treatment of choice for primary hepatic neoplasms. Other treatments are investigational at this time. The prognosis for HA reportedly is good, but the prognosis for dogs with HC is more variable.

## SECONDARY HEPATIC DISEASE (TEXT PP 542-543)

Hepatic involvement is a component of many systemic illnesses in dogs (see Table 36-1). For most of these diseases, clinical and clinicopathologic evidence of serious hepatic insufficiency is not present, and the hepatic manifestations regress after the primary illness resolves. Liver biopsy is not necessary. Because serious hepatic sequelae are rare with these diseases, no liver-specific treatment is indicated.

### Pancreatitis

Acute pancreatitis typically involves the liver by causing direct extension of inflammation to the liver, and/or transient or persistent EBDO. Liver enzyme activities are typical of a mixed hepatocellular and biliary tract insult: high serum AP and GGT activities with less striking ALT elevation and variable serum bilirubin concentration.

### Sepsis

Cholestasis associated with sepsis can occur in dogs. Gram-negative organisms are cultured most often, but gram-positive and mixed infections have also been reported. Elevations of serum bilirubin (may exceed 30 mg/dl), fasting SBA concentrations, and liver-specific enzyme activities (mild to moderate; serum AP usually greater than ALT) are typically seen.

### Miscellaneous disorders

Hepatomegaly associated with lipid or glycogen accumulation is a common finding in dogs with hypercortisolism, hypothyroidism, or diabetes mellitus. Chronic passive congestion from congestive heart failure or heartworm disease causes generalized hepatomegaly and ascites with normal or minimally abnormal serum liver enzyme activities. Acute hepatic necrosis may be a consequence of heat stroke or other types of thermal injury.

# 39

# Treatment of Complications of Hepatic Failure

## *(Text pp 546-551)*

The clinical syndrome of hepatic failure with abdominal effusion, acquired portosystemic shunt, and other complications of portal hypertension is observed frequently in dogs but rarely in cats. Aggressive management is vital to enable hepatic recovery while specific therapy is taking effect and to permit a reasonable quality of life.

## HEPATIC ENCEPHALOPATHY (TEXT PP 546-548)

### Chronic Hepatic Encephalopathy

The goal in patients with hepatic encephalopathy (HE) is to restore normal neurologic function by decreasing formation of gut-derived encephalotoxins, eliminating precipitating factors, and correcting acid-base and electrolyte abnormalities. The standard approach uses a combination of dietary protein restriction and agents that discourage ammonia formation and absorption (Box 39-1). Generally, patients with chronic HE undergo diet modification first; medications are added if control of signs is inadequate.

### Diet

The ideal diet for long-term management of HE does the following: (1) it uses carbohydrates as the primary energy source; (2) it uses highly digestible protein of high

---

**Box 39-1**

## Medical Management of Hepatic Encephalopathy

### ACUTE

Nothing by mouth

Fluids given intravenously

1. 0.45% saline solution in 2.5% dextrose with added potassium at a maintenance or 1.5 × maintenance rate
2. Add potassium according to serum electrolyte concentration, or use a safe concentration (20 mEq of potassium chloride per liter of administered fluids) until serum electrolyte results are available

Enemas every 6 hr

1. Warm-water cleansing enemas
2. Retention enemas containing povidone-iodine (10%), neomycin sulfate (22 mg/kg), or lactulose (three parts lactulose to seven parts water at 20 ml/kg); instill into colon with aid of Foley catheter; leave in place for 15-20 min

Other

1. Flumazenil (0.02 mg/kg IV; efficacy unproved)
2. Branched-chain amino acid solutions
3. L-Dopa
4. Ion exchange resins

### CHRONIC

Protein-restricted diet (commercial or homemade)

Lactulose (cats: 2.5-5 ml PO q8h; dogs: 2.5-15 ml PO q8h)

Antibiotics

1. Metronidazole (7.5 mg/kg PO q12h)
2. Amoxicillin (22 mg/kg PO q12h)
3. Neomycin sulfate (20 mg/kg PO q8h)

---

*IV,* Intravenously; *PO,* orally.

---

biologic value; (3) it contains low levels of aromatic amino acids and methionine and high levels of branched-chain amino acids and arginine; (4) it has a normal fat content; (5) it has adequate levels of vitamins; and (6) it is supplemented with potassium, calcium, and zinc.

Modified diets based on nonmeat protein are commercially available in feline and canine formulations (e.g., Hill's Prescription Diets l/d and Ralston Purina's Veterinary Diet NF) or can be prepared by owners (see text). Although protein restriction ameliorates the signs of HE, sufficient protein (on a dry-matter basis, approximately 20% for dogs and 30% to 35% for cats) must be provided to curb endogenous protein catabolism and maintain muscle mass and body weight.

***Special needs.*** Some cats and dogs with chronic HE refuse protein-restricted diets. Feeding smaller meals more frequently, adding seasoning, warming the food, providing positive reinforcement, and gradually introducing the new diet can encourage eating. If these measures fail, and no evidence exists of another complication of hepatic failure (e.g., gastrointestinal [GI] ulceration) or unrelated health problem, two choices remain: (1) continue to give the previous diet and rely on other medical measures to control HE, or (2) provide forced nutrition.

Placement of a feeding tube or initiation of total parenteral nutrition is reserved for patients that are likely to achieve short-term survival and improve and that just need additional time. Tube esophagostomy is preferred. Tube gastrostomy placed percutaneously is contraindicated in cats and dogs with ascites but would be acceptable if placed surgically.

### Lactulose
Lactulose (see Box 39-1) helps control signs of HE. The dose is adjusted until two or three soft stools per day are achieved; overdose results in watery diarrhea. No complications of chronic lactulose use in animals are known. Lactulose can also be given by enema to patients with acute HE.

### Antibiotics
If dietary therapy alone or in combination with lactulose is insufficient, antibiotics may be added. Antibiotics that are effective against anaerobes (metronidazole, amoxicillin) and gram-negative urea-splitting organisms (neomycin sulfate) are preferable (see Box 39-1). The lower dose of metronidazole is given to avoid neurotoxicity, a potential adverse effect of delayed hepatic excretion. Rarely nephrotoxicity and malabsorption are seen with long-term neomycin use.

### Controlling precipitating factors
Conditions known to accentuate or precipitate HE should be avoided or treated aggressively when detected. They include a high-protein diet (especially one containing red meat), GI hemorrhage, azotemia, constipation, infection, metabolic alkalosis, hypokalemia, excessive tranquilization, use of methionine-containing compounds (e.g., urinary acidifiers), and transfusion of stored blood or packed red blood cells.

## Acute HE
Acute HE is a true medical emergency. The principles of management for chronic HE apply, but the steps are more aggressive. Giving nothing by mouth, administering enemas, and administering fluids intravenously (IV) constitute the basic therapeutic approach (see Box 39-1). Dehydration can occur if lactulose enemas are used too aggressively without attention to fluid intake.

Intravenous fluids should not contain lactate, as alkalinizing solutions may precipitate or worsen HE. Half-strength (0.45%) saline in 2.5% dextrose is a good choice, with potassium added as necessary (see Table 55-1). Benzodiazepine receptor antagonists, such as flumazenil (0.02 mg/kg IV once), rapidly and dramatically improve the neurologic status in some patients.

## MASSIVE HEPATIC NECROSIS (TEXT P 548)
Massive hepatic necrosis is a syndrome of rapidly progressive, massive liver cell injury, with necrosis and loss of confluent hepatic parenchyma. The most likely cause is ingestion of a toxic substance, such as a massive dose of acetaminophen in a cat, cycad palm seeds or *Amanita phalloides* mushrooms in dogs, and carprofen or trimethoprim-sulfa in susceptible dogs or diazepam in susceptible cats. Clinical signs are attributable to HE, cerebral edema, coagulopathy, and sepsis.

### Treatment
Failure to respond to treatment for HE or rapid central nervous system deterioration is suggestive of brain edema, for which mannitol (1 g/kg of 20% solution IV over 30 minutes; PRN q4h) and furosemide (1 to 2 mg/kg IV q8h for three doses) are given. Glucocorticoids are not indicated. Other complications that can compound the patient's condition (e.g., hypoglycemia, hypokalemia, GI hemorrhage) should be treated aggressively. Mechanical hyperventilation to create hypocapnia may also assist in decreasing intracranial pressure.

### Prognosis
More often, similar clinical signs are observed in animals with acute decompensation of long-term, stable, chronic hepatobiliary disease, with severe HE precipitated by one of the factors discussed previously. The prognosis in either case (true acute hepatic failure or decompensated chronic hepatic failure) is guarded. If hepatic mass is sufficient to regenerate, animals may recover and survive.

## ASCITES (TEXT PP 549-550)

Accumulation of peritoneal fluid as a result of sustained intrahepatic portal hypertension is common in dogs with chronic hepatic failure but is rarely seen in cats (except for some with lymphocytic cholangitis). Occasionally fluid collects in the subcutaneous tissues or the pleural space.

### Treatment

Treatment is indicated if ascites causes respiratory embarrassment or anorexia. A combination of dietary sodium restriction and diuretic therapy is usually needed.

*Diet.* Diets used to manage congestive heart failure (e.g., Canine h/d) are sufficiently sodium restricted; however, the protein composition of severely sodium-restricted diets is not optimal for control of HE. Some protein-restricted commercial diets (e.g., Canine l/d and Veterinary Diet NF) and home-cooked equivalents have moderately reduced sodium content.

*Diuretics.* If sodium restriction alone does not control ascites after 5 to 7 days, diuretic therapy is added. The aim is gradual diuresis to avoid volume depletion. Aldosterone antagonists such as spironolactone (beginning at 0.5 to 1 mg/kg orally [PO] q12h) are the initial agents of choice. The dose may be doubled in dogs that do not respond. Potassium supplementation should not be given when higher doses of spironolactone are used. If improvement is still not seen after 1 to 2 weeks at the higher dose, a loop diuretic such as furosemide (1 mg/kg PO q12h initially) is added or substituted.

Measuring body weight (aim for approximately 2% loss per day), combined with gradually decreasing abdominal girth, is an objective means of assessing efficacy. Once ascites is under control, the diuretic dose is reduced to the minimum necessary, given daily or on alternate days. Complications associated with overzealous furosemide therapy include dehydration, azotemia, hypokalemia, and hyponatremia.

*Abdominocentesis.* When ascites is refractory to dietary manipulation and diuretics, the fluid may be removed by abdominocentesis or with a shunt device containing a one-way valve (see text). It is wise to avoid removal of large volumes of abdominal fluid in patients with a serum albumin <2 g/dl. If fluid removal is necessary (e.g., to provide symptomatic relief or in association with abdominal surgery), re-formation can be slowed by temporarily improving the plasma oncotic pressure with colloids such as hetastarch (20 ml/kg/day IV) or human albumin (12.5 g/20 kg of lean body weight, IV over 24 hours).

## COAGULOPATHY OR GASTROINTESTINAL HEMORRHAGE (TEXT PP 550-551)

Aside from having a subclinical coagulopathy or disseminated intravascular coagulation (DIC), dogs with chronic hepatic failure often have GI bleeding from ulceration. The most common location is the duodenum. GI hemorrhage can cause acute decompensation of a previously stable patient with chronic hepatic failure.

Ulceration and hemorrhage should be suspected in any dog with chronic hepatic failure presented with signs of acute HE. Rectal examination may reveal melena in a dog that is anorectic and not defecating. Subclinical intestinal blood loss can be detected with a commercially available test for fecal hemoglobin (HemoQuant; normal fecal blood loss in dogs is ≤0.043 ml/kg/day). Vague cranial abdominal discomfort during palpation may indicate the presence of a GI ulcer. However, upper GI contrast studies, endoscopy, and/or ultrasonography may be needed for confirmation.

### Treatment

Treatment for GI hemorrhage not caused by DIC centers on antiulcer medications. If blood transfusion is needed, *fresh* whole blood or *fresh* packed red blood cells (RBCs) are used; stored blood or RBCs could precipitate or worsen HE. Nonsteroidal anti-inflammatory drugs, corticosteroids, and other ulcerogenic drugs should be avoided.

*Antiulcer medications.* One of the $H_2$ receptor antagonists, ranitidine (2 mg/kg PO or IV q8h) or famotidine (0.5 mg/kg PO q12-24h), is usually combined with sucralfate

(1 g/25 kg PO q6-8h). Omeprazole (0.7 mg/kg PO q24h) is a more potent gastric acid inhibitor and may be of benefit in nonresponsive dogs.

*Coagulopathy.* DIC in dogs with chronic hepatic failure is managed with heparin therapy if sufficient plasma antithrombin activity is present (>40%; see Chapter 89). Fresh whole blood or plasma transfusion with one dose of heparin (50 to 200 IU/kg) added is recommended. The maintenance heparin dose may need to be lowered in some dogs (see Chapter 89). Impaired heparin degradation is suspected if the activated partial thromboplastin time (APTT) is excessively prolonged (>1.5 times normal) 2 hours after injection. Each subsequent dose is reduced by 20% until the target 2-hour postinjection APTT (1.5 times normal) is reached.

## SEPSIS (TEXT P 551)

Dogs with chronic hepatocellular disease may be more susceptible to infection. If signs or clinicopathologic findings are compatible with sepsis (e.g., fever, leukocytosis with a left shift and toxic neutrophils), specimens for anaerobic and aerobic bacterial culture should be collected. Blood is obtained for culture and sensitivity testing unless a source of infection is obvious. Broad-spectrum bactericidal antibiotics are instituted until results are available. Amikacin (10 mg/kg IV, intramuscularly, or subcutaneously q8h) combined with ampicillin or cephazolin (22 mg/kg IV q8h) is a good initial choice.

# 40

# Exocrine Pancreas

## *(Text pp 552-567)*

Clinical signs of pancreatic disease relate to either tissue injury by digestive enzymes or insufficient secretion of enzymes for normal digestion. Diseases that affect the exocrine pancreas in cats and dogs are listed in Table 40-1.

## ACUTE PANCREATITIS (TEXT PP 552-560)

Acute pancreatitis is much more common in dogs than in cats. Several factors have been implicated in its development (Box 40-1); more than one factor is likely involved. Pancreatic inflammation can extend locally to the stomach, duodenum, and colon. In addition, substances released into the circulation cause the many systemic effects commonly associated with severe pancreatitis: hepatocellular necrosis, pulmonary edema, renal tubular degeneration, cardiomyopathy, hypotension, and disseminated intravascular coagulopathy (DIC).

Pancreatic inflammation ranges from mild (edematous or interstitial) to severe (hemorrhagic, necrotizing, or suppurative). The clinical features coincide roughly with the severity of inflammation.

**Table 40-1**

## Diseases of the Exocrine Pancreas

|  |  | Primary | Secondary |
|---|---|---|---|
| Common | Cat | Nodular hyperplasia (incidental finding in old cats) | Chronic pancreatitis (cholangitis, inflammatory bowel disease) |
|  | Dog | Acute pancreatitis | Acute pancreatitis (trauma: automobile accident, surgical; ischemia; hypercortisolism?; hyperlipoproteinemia; drugs) |
|  |  | Nodular hyperplasia (incidental finding in old dogs) |  |
| Less common | Cat | Acute pancreatitis | Acute pancreatitis (trauma; acute toxoplasmosis) |
|  |  | Subclinical chronic pancreatitis |  |
|  | Dog | Exocrine pancreatic insufficiency | Exocrine pancreatic insufficiency (protein or calorie malnutrition; duodenal hyperacidity; acute, severe, or chronic, relapsing pancreatitis) |
|  |  | Relapsing or chronic pancreatitis | Chronic pancreatitis (diabetes mellitus; idiopathic hyperlipoproteinemia; hyperadrenocorticism?) |
| Rare | Cat | Exocrine pancreatic insufficiency | Chronic pancreatitis (feline infectious peritonitis; toxoplasmosis) |
|  |  | Pancreatic flukes (*Eurytrema procyonis*) |  |
|  |  | Pancreatic adenocarcinoma |  |
|  | Dog | Pancreatic adenocarcinoma | Exocrine pancreatic insufficiency (pancreatic adenocarcinoma) |

---

**Box 40-1**

### Factors Believed to Be Involved in the Development of Acute Pancreatitis*

**NUTRITION**
  Obesity
  High-fat diet

**ISCHEMIA**
  Hypovolemia
  Vasoactive amine–induced vasoconstriction
  Associated with DIC

**HYPERLIPOPROTEINEMIA**
  After ingestion of a large fatty meal
  Idiopathic form in Miniature Schnauzers

**DRUGS**
  L-Asparaginase
  Azathioprine?
  Other chemotherapeutic agents
  Organophosphates
  Corticosteroids (controversial)

**DUODENAL REFLUX**
  Increased intraluminal pressure during severe vomiting

**OTHER**
  Abdominal trauma
  Hypercalcemia
  Cholangitis (cats)
  Infection (toxoplasmosis, feline infectious peritonitis)
  Hyperadrenocorticism?

---

*Uncommon in cats.
*DIC*, Disseminated intravascular coagulation.

### Clinical features

Middle-aged or older dogs of terrier or nonsporting breeds and Domestic Shorthair cats are most often affected. There exists no gender predilection, but neutered cats and dogs are predisposed. Most dogs with idiopathic acute pancreatitis are overweight. The history in dogs often includes recent ingestion of a large, fatty meal.

*Clinical signs.* Findings vary with the stage of illness. They can range from anorexia and depression with vague abdominal pain in mildly affected dogs to severe vomiting, hemorrhagic diarrhea, and shock or even death in more severely affected animals (Table 40-2). Some patients, particularly cats, are icteric at presentation. Complications (Table 40-3) are more likely in patients with severe acute pancreatitis.

### Diagnosis

A broad-based evaluation is necessary, because the clinical features of acute pancreatitis are indistinguishable from those of other disorders that cause an acute condition in the abdomen (e.g., acute enteritis or gastroenteritis, intestinal foreign body, acute toxic enteropathy or hepatopathy, sepsis, peritonitis, pyometra), and because no single test is pathognomonic for pancreatitis.

**Table 40-2**

## Presenting Clinical Signs and Physical Examination Findings in Dogs with Acute Pancreatitis

| Mild | Moderate to severe |
|---|---|
| **COMMON CLINICAL SIGNS** | |
| Depression, anorexia, nausea (ptyalism, licking lips) | Depression, anorexia |
| Vomiting | Vomiting (possibly hematemesis) |
| Behavior indicating abdominal pain (position of relief) | Behavior indicating abdominal pain (position of relief) |
| **OTHER CLINICAL SIGNS** | |
| Diarrhea (can be of large- or small-bowel origin) | Hematochezia or melena |
| | Jaundice |
| | Respiratory distress |
| | Shock |
| **COMMON PHYSICAL EXAMINATION FINDINGS** | |
| Abdominal pain localized to the right cranial quadrant | Abdominal pain localized to the right cranial quadrant or generalized |
| Fever | Fever or hypothermia |
| Dehydration | Dehydration |
| | Hyperemic mucous membranes |
| | Tachycardia, tachypnea |
| **OTHER PHYSICAL EXAMINATION FINDINGS** | |
| Weakness | Jaundice |
| | Abdominal effusion |
| | Mass effect in the region of the pancreas (inflamed pancreas with adhesions?) |
| | Petechiae or ecchymoses |
| | Cardiac arrhythmia |
| | Glossitis, glossal slough |

The basic approach consists of laboratory analysis (complete blood count [CBC], serum biochemistry, serum amylase and lipase activities [dogs only], urinalysis) and abdominal radiographs or ultrasonography. Drug history and intercurrent disease should also be investigated.

*Complete Blood Count.* Dehydration (evidenced by high packed cell volume [PCV] and plasma protein concentration) and leukocytosis are common in dogs with pancreatitis; leukocytosis is an inconsistent finding in cats. A stress leukogram is seen in mild cases, with greater leukocytosis and a mild to severe left shift observed in more severe cases. Platelet numbers usually are adequate, unless DIC is present. The plasma may be lipemic or icteric. Cats with pancreatitis often have moderate, nonregenerative anemia.

*Serum biochemistry profile.* Prerenal azotemia is found in >50% of cats and dogs with acute pancreatitis; renal azotemia and acute renal failure are uncommon but serious complications of severe pancreatitis. Modest hyperglycemia (200 to 250 mg/dl) is found in up to 65% of cats and dogs with pancreatitis. Hypoalbuminemia and hypocalcemia (after correction for albumin concentration) may also be present. Cats with a plasma ionized calcium of <4 mg/dl have a grave prognosis. Hypokalemia is common in cats with acute pancreatitis.

Table 40-3

## Complications of Severe Acute Pancreatitis in Dogs

| Complication | Diagnostic test(s) |
| --- | --- |
| **MEDICAL** | |
| Cardiac arrhythmia (usually ventricular) | Lead II ECG |
| DIC | Coagulation profile (OSPT, APTT, FDPs, D-dimer, fibrinogen concentration, platelet count), antithrombin activity |
| Dyspnea (pleural effusion; pulmonary edema; pulmonary thromboembolism; pulmonary distress syndrome?) | Arterial blood gases, thoracic radiographs, radionuclide lung perfusion scan |
| Acute renal failure | Measurement of urine production, biochemical profile |
| Permanent diabetes mellitus | Hyperglycemia that persists beyond resolution of acute pancreatitis; measure serum insulin? |
| Nodular panniculitis | Biopsy |
| Sepsis | Blood cultures |
| **SURGICAL** | |
| Extrahepatic bile duct obstruction | Biochemical profile, coagulation profile, ultrasonography |
| Pancreatic abscess or pseudocyst | CBC, ultrasonography, aspiration for cytologic analysis and culture (ultrasound guided or at surgery) |
| Intestinal obstruction (usually duodenal) | Abdominal radiographs and ultrasonography; upper gastrointestinal contrast study (if animal can tolerate barium orally) |

*APTT,* Activated partial thromboplastin time; *CBC,* complete blood count; *DIC,* disseminated intravascular coagulation; *ECG,* electrocardiogram; *FDPs,* fibrin degradation products; *OSPT,* one-stage prothrombin time.

High serum activities of alkaline phosphatase (AP; twofold to fifteenfold increase) and alanine aminotransferase (ALT; normal to tenfold increase) are frequent findings; moderate hyperbilirubinemia (twofold to fivefold increase) is seen in 30% to 40% of affected dogs. Greater serum AP and ALT activities and hyperbilirubinemia occur if the common bile duct is obstructed by adjacent pancreatic inflammation.

Hypercholesterolemia (plus hypertriglyceridemia) is seen in cats and dogs with acute pancreatitis. However, fasting hyperlipidemia (predominantly hypertriglyceridemia) and persistent hyperglycemia in dogs other than Miniature Schnauzers is highly suggestive of diabetes mellitus.

***Serum amylase activity.*** Total serum amylase activity is high in >80% of dogs with pancreatitis. However, renal failure alone may cause high serum amylase activities (2.5- to 3-fold increase). Severe duodenitis or duodenal foreign body could also cause elevations in serum amylase and an identical clinical picture. Serum amylase activity is considered an adequate screening test for pancreatitis in dogs (sensitivity approximately 62%, specificity approximately 57%), but it is not a reliable indicator of pancreatic injury in cats.

***Serum lipase activity.*** Elevated serum lipase activity may be a better indicator of acute pancreatitis. However, lipase may be elevated in situations other than pancreatic injury, including azotemia (2.5- to 3-fold increase), glucocorticoid administration, surgical manipulation of the pancreas, and various cancers and hepatobiliary diseases.

In dogs with pancreatitis, serum activity of lipase often does not parallel that of amylase. Many times one or the other is high, or both can be high or normal. Furthermore, the magnitude of elevation does not correlate with the degree of pancreatic inflammation. Currently, serum lipase activity is considered an adequate screening test for pancreatitis in dogs (sensitivity approximately 73%, specificity approximately 55%), but it is unreliable in cats.

### Diagnostic imaging

*Radiography.* There exist no pathognomonic radiographic signs of pancreatitis, only signs that are consistent with regional peritonitis. They include a ground-glass appearance in the right cranial quadrant; trapped gas pockets in the duodenum; and increased opacity in the area of the pancreas that displaces the duodenum laterally, widens the pyloroduodenal angle, and may delay gastric emptying.

Survey radiographs may be helpful in ruling out intestinal foreign body, which can cause similar signs and clinicopathologic abnormalities. However, other disorders (e.g., severe duodenitis and duodenal ulcer) may have radiographic changes similar to those in patients with pancreatitis.

*Ultrasonography.* Abdominal ultrasonography offers more convincing support for the presence of pancreatitis in dogs, but its sensitivity for diagnosing pancreatitis in cats is low. The most consistent changes are a heterogeneous mass effect and hypoechogenicity in the area of the pancreas (attributable to edema, hemorrhage, and inflammatory exudate). Evidence of hyperechoic peripancreatic fat and dilated bile ducts may also be present. Discrete homogeneous fluid-dense structures are likely to be abscesses or pseudocysts, which are complications of severe pancreatitis.

*Abdominal fluid analysis.* When abdominal effusion is present, abdominocentesis should be performed. Results of cytology are usually compatible with a nonseptic exudate. Amylase and lipase activities in abdominal fluid are often higher than in the serum of dogs with pancreatitis, although severe duodenal inflammation or perforation may yield the same result. Up to 50% of cats with pancreatitis have both peritoneal and pleural effusion (usually serosanguineous).

*Definitive tests.* Serum isoamylase separation and measurement of serum trypsin-like immunoreactivity (TLI) are useful in approximately 50% of cats and dogs with pancreatitis. In such cases serum TLI is $>100$ μg/L in cats (normal, 12 to 82 μg/L) and $>50$ μg/L in dogs (normal, 5 to 35 μg/L). Serum TLI must be assessed in light of renal function, as increases can occur with nonazotemic renal disease in dogs. Nevertheless, serum TLI appears to be a sensitive and clinically useful test in cats.

Pancreatic lipase immunoreactivity (PLI) is another highly sensitive and specific test for pancreatic injury in dogs and presumably in cats. The reference range for canine PLI is 2.2 to 102.1 μg/L.

*Surgery.* If diagnosis is still elusive, exploratory laparotomy and pancreatic biopsy can be performed. Edema, hemorrhage, and plaques of peripancreatic fat necrosis are easily identifiable grossly. Whether pancreatic biopsy *causes* pancreatitis is controversial; more likely, the trauma of performing biopsy of an already inflamed pancreas exacerbates existing inflammation.

### Treatment

Acute pancreatitis is a potentially devastating disease and should be treated aggressively. Goals are to (1) remove the inciting cause, if possible; (2) restore and maintain intravascular volume and pancreatic perfusion; (3) reduce pancreatic secretion; (4) relieve pain; (5) manage complications; and (6) provide nutritional support.

The backbone of treatment for mild or severe pancreatitis is twofold: fluid therapy and nothing by mouth (NPO). Balanced electrolyte solutions are given to address dehydration and continuing losses, and to meet maintenance needs during the NPO period, which may be $>72$ hours. The sight and smell of food should be avoided, and all medications given parenterally.

### Mild pancreatitis

For mildly affected cats and dogs, fluids may be given subcutaneously (SC). At least 24 hours after the last episode of vomiting, small amounts of water and then bland food can be given q8h. If water and food are tolerated without vomiting, the quantity of each may be gradually increased until the total daily requirements are being provided, usually over 5 to 6 days. No other medications are necessary. Recovery should be complete in approximately 7 days. The prognosis for dogs with a single bout of mild pancreatitis is good.

*Dietary management.* A diet low in fat, high in carbohydrates, and containing a moderate level of protein (e.g., Canine i/d or w/d) should be fed indefinitely. Access to table scraps, garbage, and food belonging to other pets should be strictly avoided. Obese dogs should lose weight. Marked dietary fat restriction (e.g., Canine r/d) may be required in dogs that have idiopathic hyperlipoproteinemia or that experience repeated bouts of pancreatitis.

### Severe pancreatitis

The same principles apply to severely affected animals, but treatment is more intensive (Box 40-2). Fluids should be given intravenously (IV), preferably via a large vein so that central venous pressure can be monitored. This, along with measurement of urine production, PCV, plasma protein, and body weight, ensures that fluid requirements are being met. Two of the most common mistakes in managing acute severe pancreatitis are giving too little fluid (i.e., underhydration) and reinstituting oral feeding too soon. Keeping the animal on NPO status may be necessary for at least 5 days.

*Drug therapy.* If vomiting is protracted and unrelated to intestinal obstruction, centrally acting antiemetics, such as chlorpromazine or prochlorperazine at 0.25 to 0.5 mg/kg intramuscularly (IM) or SC q6-8h, may be given, as long as intravascular volume is normal. Suitable analgesics include hydromorphone (0.03 to 0.05 mg/kg IM, as needed [prn]) and butorphanol (0.055 to 0.11 mg/kg SC q6-12h; dogs only). The total daily dose of these analgesics can also be given over 24 hours IV as a continuous infusion.

---

**Box 40-2**

### Summary of Treatment Recommendations for Dogs and Cats with Acute Pancreatitis*

#### MILD PANCREATITIS

NPO for 48 to 72 hours; provide fluids at rate to meet maintenance needs and replace ongoing losses using a balanced electrolyte solution by SC or IV route.

Give small amounts of water, then bland food (low-salt meat baby food or fat-restricted balanced pet food) four times daily beginning at least 24 hours after last episode of vomiting.

If vomiting does not recur with feeding, gradually increase amount of food at each feeding until total daily requirements are being met in one or two feedings per day.

Dogs susceptible to recurrent bouts of pancreatitis should receive a fat-restricted diet indefinitely, with no access to table scraps or garbage.

#### SEVERE PANCREATITIS

NPO for at least 48 to 72 hours (if period of NPO status exceeds 5 days, provide nutritional support by tube duodenostomy or jejunostomy or total parenteral nutrition).

Provide fluids to reverse dehydration, meet maintenance requirements, and replace ongoing losses using IV administration of balanced electrolyte solution.

Give fresh or fresh-frozen plasma to supply antiprotease activity.

Administer broad-spectrum antibiotics parenterally.

Use centrally acting antiemetics if vomiting is profuse.

Give analgesics for abdominal pain.

Treat complications as they are detected (see Table 40-3)

---

*More common in dogs than in cats.

*IV*, Intravenous; *NPO*, nothing by mouth; *SC*, subcutaneous.

*Antibiotics.* The necrotic pancreas is a good medium for bacterial growth; also, in some dogs it is difficult to differentiate severe pancreatitis from pancreatic or systemic gram-negative infection. Cefotaxime (6 to 40 mg/kg IM or IV q6h) or trimethoprim-sulfamethoxazole (15 mg/kg IV q12h, diluted and given slowly in a central vein over 60 to 90 minutes) is a good empiric choice for antibiotic coverage. Enrofloxacin (2.5 to 5 mg/kg IM or IV q12h) may also be used in dogs. Other antibiotics recommended for gram-negative sepsis (e.g., amikacin and ampicillin or cephazolin) may also be effective.

*Other therapies.* Transfusion with plasma (an antiprotease source) may be beneficial in dogs; it can be repeated if steady improvement is not seen. Insulin administration is not required for modest hyperglycemia unless ketosis develops or hyperglycemia persists and steadily increases. If insulin is required, the regular formulation should be used every 6 hours at doses that maintain blood glucose in the range of 150 to 200 mg/dl (see Chapter 52). Corticosteroids are not recommended, except for emergency treatment of shock. Peritoneal lavage may improve survival in dogs.

*Patient monitoring.* PCV, plasma protein, serum electrolytes, and blood urea nitrogen or creatinine should be assessed each day. CBC and complete biochemistry profile (including serum amylase and/or lipase if abnormal initially) should be performed every other day until favorable trends are established.

*Maintenance therapy.* Intravenous fluids should be tapered off, and oral food and water resumed only after vomiting has resolved, which may take at least 5 days. (Elevated serum amylase or lipase and liver enzyme activities may persist for longer.) If vomiting recurs, a 24-hour period of NPO status should be reinstituted. If total NPO time exceeds 5 days, total parenteral nutrition is commenced, or a duodenal or jejunal feeding tube is placed surgically and an elemental diet fed via continuous infusion. The dietary plan outlined for mild pancreatitis should be followed after discharge.

*Complications.* Complications should be treated as they develop. Some (e.g., DIC, acute renal failure, cardiac arrhythmia) are managed medically. Common bile duct obstruction is usually transient, but persistent obstruction after acute pancreatitis has resolved must be addressed surgically. Progressive increases in serum AP and ALT activities, increasing hyperbilirubinemia, and ultrasonographic evidence of a dilated extrahepatic biliary tree are justification for surgery.

*Surgery.* Surgical evaluation and pancreatic débridement are also indicated when (1) apparent recovery is followed by relapse of signs, or (2) persistent fever and leukocytosis with a left shift and toxic neutrophils persist, along with physical, radiographic, or ultrasonographic evidence of a mass in the area of the pancreas.

Although pancreatic mass lesions are usually sterile, specimens should be obtained before surgery via ultrasound guidance, if possible, for bacterial culture and sensitivity testing. Surgery can be delayed or avoided in patients that are steadily improving with medical management. In such cases ultrasound-guided drainage (repeated as needed) is an acceptable alternative to surgery.

## FELINE ACUTE PANCREATITIS—COMPARATIVE ASPECTS (TEXT P 560)

The syndrome of pancreatitis previously described is rare in cats. Pancreatitis in cats generally is subclinical, occurring as a component of multisystemic disease, such as toxoplasmosis, or in association with inflammatory bowel disease.

### Clinical features

The same clinical signs and clinicopathologic features seen in dogs with acute pancreatitis may be noted, but they are more subtle. Two types of severe pancreatitis are recognized in cats: acute necrotizing (more common, similar to canine pancreatitis) and acute suppurative. The acute suppurative form is seen more often in younger cats (mean age 3.5 years). Lethargy, anorexia, vomiting, dehydration, weight loss, jaundice, and hypothermia are typical presenting signs with both forms.

### Diagnosis and treatment

Antemortem diagnosis can be difficult. The diagnostic and treatment approaches discussed in the previous section are recommended for cats, except for the duration of NPO status. Because of the potential for hepatic lipidosis in cats, enteral tube feeding (via duodenostomy or jejunostomy) is recommended as soon as pancreatitis is diagnosed. Both forms of acute pancreatitis in cats are severe and may be difficult to diagnose, so the prognosis is guarded.

## RELAPSING AND CHRONIC PANCREATITIS (TEXT P 560)

Some cats and dogs appear to have repeated bouts of acute pancreatitis with periods of recovery in between. Such cases could be considered to be relapsing pancreatitis. Approximately one third of cats with acute necrotizing pancreatitis also have histopathologic evidence of chronic pancreatitis. Most cats with chronic pancreatitis are older Domestic Shorthair cats. Clinical signs in >50% of cases include anorexia, weight loss, and intermittent vomiting.

### Diagnosis

Chronic pancreatitis is diagnosed primarily by the combined findings of high serum TLI and characteristic microscopic features in pancreatic biopsy specimens (interstitial mononuclear cell inflammation and fibrosis). Chronic pancreatitis can coexist with inflammatory hepatic and/or intestinal disease, all of which can have similar clinical signs.

### Treatment and prognosis

Relapsing and chronic pancreatitis are primarily controlled by strict nutritional management, using a highly digestible diet with high fiber and limited fat content. With strict adherence to a controlled diet the prognosis is good. However, persistent (usually subclinical) inflammation results in progressive loss of functional pancreatic tissue, so exocrine pancreatic insufficiency and diabetes mellitus may develop. Pancreatic enzyme supplements and insulin, respectively, are indicated in such cases.

## EXOCRINE PANCREATIC INSUFFICIENCY (TEXT PP 560-564)

When >85% of pancreatic acinar function is lost, clinical signs of nutrient malassimilation develop. In dogs a single bout of severe acute pancreatitis or repeated bouts of less severe pancreatitis are uncommon causes of exocrine pancreatic insufficiency (EPI). Most cases are caused by inherited (German Shepherd Dog) or adult-onset (idiopathic, in any breed) pancreatic acinar atrophy. The opposite may be true of feline EPI; in many cases the suspected cause is progressive destruction of acinar tissue associated with chronic, subclinical pancreatitis.

### Clinical features

Cats and dogs with EPI typically are presented for chronic weight loss despite a vigorous, even ravenous, appetite. Owners may also report pica and coprophagia. The feces may be normal, soft and voluminous, or watery. Affected German Shepherd Dogs usually are presented by 2 years of age, whereas dogs of other breeds tend to be middle aged when first presented. Rarely, affected animals have prolonged bleeding after venipuncture because of severe malabsorption of vitamin K. Few abnormal physical examination findings are present, except for weight loss, poor-quality haircoat, and possibly oily staining of the perineal region (steatorrhea). Affected animals are bright, alert, and hungry.

### Diagnosis

Results of CBC, serum biochemistry profile, and urinalysis usually are normal. Some dogs have high serum ALT activity (twofold to threefold increase), and many have hypocholesterolemia. Serum cobalamine (vitamin $B_{12}$) concentration is low in almost all cats and many dogs with EPI.

*Screening tests.* History, physical examination, and routine laboratory data cannot differentiate primary small intestinal malabsorption from EPI. Two screening tests, triglyceride challenge and qualitative fecal analysis for trypsin activity and undigested food particles, can be used to arrive at a presumptive diagnosis (Box 40-3). Both tests are subject to differences in technique, interpretation, and daily variation. If triglyceride malabsorption and persistent absence of trypsin activity with evidence of unprocessed

---

**Box 40-3**

## Screening Tests for Diagnosis of Exocrine Pancreatic Insufficiency

### TRIGLYCERIDE CHALLENGE TEST

1. After a 12-hour fast, obtain serum sample, then give corn oil, 3 to 4 ml/kg PO
2. Measure serum triglyceride concentration at 0, 2, and 3 hours after corn oil
   a. Normal: twofold to threefold increase over baseline value in post–corn oil samples
   b. Abnormal: no change from baseline value in post–corn oil samples
3. If abnormal, repeat test the following day but add 2 tsp of pancreatic enzyme powder (Viokase-V) to dose of corn oil
   a. Pancreatic enzyme–responsive: twofold to threefold increase in serum triglyceride concentration over baseline value
   b. Not pancreatic enzyme–responsive: no change in serum triglyceride concentrations in post–corn oil serum samples; consider primary small intestinal disease (see Part 3: Digestive System Disorders)

### QUALITATIVE FECAL ANALYSIS

1. Fecal proteolytic (trypsin) activity
   a. Mix 1 ml of feces with 9 ml of 5% sodium bicarbonate; incubate with tubes of gelatin for 30 to 60 min at 37° C; perform test at least three times on each patient
   b. Normal: gelatin dissolves if trypsin is present and few intact striated muscle fibers are seen on Wright's-stained fresh fecal smears
2. Fecal amylase activity
   a. Stain fresh fecal smears with 2% Lugol's iodine solution
   b. Normal: few starch granules (blue-black in color) are present
3. Fecal lipase activity
   a. Stain fresh fecal smears with Sudan III
   b. Normal: few fat globules (red-orange in color) are present

---

*PO*, Orally.

nutrients in serial fresh fecal specimens are present, a stronger case for EPI can be made and specific treatment instituted pending the results of definitive tests.

*Serum TLI.* The definitive test for EPI in cats and dogs is measurement of serum TLI. The concentration is not affected by feeding in healthy cats, but ideally the serum sample is collected after a 12-hour fast. Normal values in dogs are 5 to 35 µg/L; values <2 µg/L are diagnostic for EPI, and values of 2 to 5 µg/L are equivocal. The normal range in cats is 12 to 82 µg/L; values <8 µg/L are diagnostic for EPI; values of 8 to 12 µg/L are equivocal.

Protein content in the diet may influence serum TLI: the lower the dietary protein, the lower the serum TLI. Nevertheless, dogs with normal pancreatic function fed low-protein diets still have serum TLI values within the reference range. Serum TLI is accurate even when pancreatic enzyme supplementation has been started.

*Pancreatic duct obstruction.* Pancreatic duct obstruction is suspected in animals with clinical findings consistent with EPI but normal triglyceride challenge and serum TLI values and no evidence of primary small intestinal disease. An example is pancreatic fluke *(Eurytrema procyonis)* infestation in cats. If initial testing yields serum TLI values in the equivocal range, treating for EPI and repeating the test 1 to 2 months later is recommended.

### Treatment

The goals are to replace intraluminal pancreatic enzymes and reverse nutritional imbalances. Most cats and dogs can be managed by adding 1 tsp (cat) to 2 tsp (20-kg dog) of a pancreatic enzyme supplement to a balanced ration. The feces should improve in appearance and volume immediately, and the animal should steadily gain weight. Treatment usually is needed lifelong.

*Other recommendations.* Use of $H_2$-receptor antagonists may be of benefit in intractable cases. Adding medium-chain triglycerides (MCT oil; 1 to 2 mg/kg/day orally [PO]) to the diet may improve weight gain. Confirmed vitamin deficiencies should be corrected. Animals with low serum $B_{12}$ concentrations require supplementation (100 to 250 µg for cats, 250 to 500 µg for dogs, SC or IM) weekly until serum concentrations normalize. Injections can then be given every 3 months, and serum $B_{12}$ measured annually.

Persistence of bacterial overgrowth in dogs may cause continued diarrhea despite adequate enzyme supplementation. In such cases antibiotics (metronidazole, 7.5 to 15 mg/kg PO q8-12h; tetracycline, 22 mg/kg PO q8h; or tylosin, 20-30 mg/kg/day with meals) should be given for 6 weeks.

### Prognosis

Most cats and dogs respond to this regimen and have a favorable prognosis for good quality of life. Recently, mesenteric torsion was reported in 10% of German Shepherd Dogs with EPI. All dogs died despite surgical intervention.

## EXOCRINE PANCREATIC NEOPLASIA (TEXT P 564)

Primary neoplasia of the exocrine pancreas (adenocarcinoma) is rare in dogs and cats. It is seen in older animals; Airedales may be overrepresented. Affected animals most commonly have signs of pancreatitis or extrahepatic bile obstruction and, rarely, EPI. Common sign include lethargy, anorexia, and weight loss.

### Diagnosis

A mass in the region of the pancreas may be detectable by palpation or radiography. Results of routine laboratory testing are merely indicative of the consequences of the neoplasm (e.g., extrahepatic bile duct obstruction). Wide fluctuations in serum glucose concentrations are occasionally observed. Ultrasonography usually identifies a pancreatic mass and possibly metastases in the peripancreatic region and liver. Histopathologic examination of a biopsy specimen or cytologic examination of an aspirate from the mass is required for definitive diagnosis. The primary differential diagnosis is chronic pancreatitis.

### Treatment and prognosis

These neoplasms are rapidly metastatic, and currently no effective treatment is available. Surgical excision of the primary tumor may prolong survival, but most affected animals die within 6 months of diagnosis.

## Drugs Used in Dogs and Cats with Hepatobiliary and Exocrine Pancreatic Disorders

| Indication | Drug | Trade Name | Dose |
|---|---|---|---|
| **DIAGNOSTIC USES** | | | |
| Detect hyperammonemia | NH₄Cl | — | 0.1 g/kg<br>In gelatin capsules PO<br>As 10% solution PO<br>As 5% solution (per rectum) |
| Detect fat malabsorption | Corn oil (long-chain triglyceride) | — | 3-4 ml/kg PO |
| Determine portal venous anatomy | Iothalamate sodium | Conray 400 | 0.5-1 ml/kg as a rapid injection |
| Confirm mechanical bile duct obstruction | 99mTc disofenin | Hepatolite | 1 μC IV once |
| Detect presence or absence of portosystemic shunting | 99mTc pertechnetate | — | 1 μC instilled into the descending colon once |
| **THERAPEUTIC USES** | | | |
| Analgesic | Butorphanol | Torbugesic | 0.2-0.8 mg/kg SC, IM, or IV q1-2h (D);<br>0.1-0.4 mg/kg SC, IM, or IV q2-6h (C) |
| | Hydromorphone | — | 0.03-0.05 mg/kg IM prn |
| Antidote for acetaminophen toxicity | N-acetylcysteine | Mucomyst | 140 mg/kg PO or IV as a 20% solution (loading dose), followed 6 hr later by 70 mg/kg PO or IV q6h for seven treatments; also give ascorbic acid, 30 mg/kg PO q6h (C) |
| Antidote for inorganic arsenical toxicity | Dimercaprol | BAL in oil | 2.5-5 mg/kg IM q4h for 2 days; then q12h until recovery |
| Antidote for thallium toxicity | Diphenylthiocarbazone | — | 70 mg/kg PO q8h (controversial) |
| Antiemetic | Chlorpromazine | Thorazine | 0.25-0.5 mg/kg SC or IM q6-8h |
| | Prochlorperazine | Compazine | 0.25-0.5 mg/kg SC or IM q6-8h |
| Antiinflammatory or antifibrotic | Azathioprine | Imuran | 50 mg/m² PO q24h initially, then q48h |
| | Colchicine | — | 0.03 mg/kg/day PO |
| | Prednisone | — | 1 mg/kg PO q12h (D); 1- 2 mg/kg PO q12h (C), then q24h, then q48h |
| | Ursodeoxycholic acid | Ursodiol | 10-15 mg/kg PO q24h |

| Antimicrobial | Amikacin | — | 10 mg/kg IV or SC q8h |
|---|---|---|---|
| | Ampicillin, amoxicillin | — | 22 mg/kg IV or PO q8h |
| | Cephazolin | — | 22 mg/kg IV q8h |
| | Cephalexin | — | 22 mg/kg PO q8h |
| | Cefotaxime | Claforan | 6-40 mg/kg IV or IM q6h |
| | Clindamycin | Antirobe | 10 mg/kg IV or PO q12h |
| | Enrofloxacin | Baytril | 2.5 mg/kg IV or PO q12h |
| | Marbofloxacin | Zeniquin. | 2.75-5.5 mg/kg PO q24h |
| | Metronidazole | Flagyl | 7.5-15 mg/kg PO q12h or q8h (use lower dose if severe hepatic dysfunction present) |
| | Praziquantel | Droncit | 20 mg/kg SC q24h for 3 days |
| | Trimethoprim-sulfamethoxasole | Septra | 15 mg/kg IV q12h |
| | Tylosin | Tylan 40 | 20-30 mg/kg/day PO |
| Antioxidants | Vitamin E | | 400-500 IU/day PO (water-soluble form) |
| | S-adenosylmethionine | Denosyl SD4 | 20 mg/kg PO q24h (after an overnight fast) |
| Appetite stimulant | Cyproheptadine | Periactin | 1-2 mg PO q12h or q8h (C) |
| | Diazepam | Valium | 0.2 mg/kg IV q12-24h (C) |
| | Oxazepam | | 4 mg PO q24h or q12h (C) |
| Caloric supplement | MCT oil | — | 1-2 ml/kg/day PO |
| Cupretic | D-penicillamine | Cuprimine | 10-15 mg/kg PO q12h, 30 min before meal |
| | Trientine | Syprine | 10-15 mg/kg PO q12h, 30 min before meal |
| | Zinc acetate or sulfate | — | 5-10 mg/kg PO q12h |
| Diuresis | | | |
| Acute (massive hepatic necrosis) | Furosemide | Lasix | 1-2 mg/kg IV q8h for 3 doses |
| | Mannitol | — | 1 g/kg of 20% solution IV over 30 min; can repeat q4-6h for three additional doses |
| Chronic | Furosemide | Lasix | 1-2 mg/kg PO q12h or q8h initially, then q24h or q12h |
| | Spironolactone | Aldactone | 0.5-1 mg/kg PO q12h; can be doubled if no effect initially |

*Continued.*

## Drugs Used in Dogs and Cats with Hepatobiliary and Exocrine Pancreatic Disorders—cont'd

| Indication | Drug | Trade Name | Dose |
|---|---|---|---|
| **Hemorrhagic tendency** | | | |
| Intestinal | Cimetidine | Tagamet | 5-10 mg/kg IV, SC, or PO q8h |
| | Famotidine | Pepcid | 0.05 mg/kg PO q12h or q24h |
| | Ranitidine | Zantac | 2 mg/kg IV or PO q12h |
| | Omeprazole | Prilosec | 0.7 mg/kg PO q24h |
| | Sucralfate | Carafate | 1 g/25 kg PO q8h or q6h |
| Generalized | Desmopressin acetate for VWD | — | 1 μg/kg intranasal preparation SC 1 hr preoperatively (See Parts 11 and 12: Oncology; Hematology and Immunology) |
| | Heparin for DIC | — | 1 mg/kg SC q24h |
| Hyperammonemia | Vitamin K₁ | — | 2.5-5 ml (C) or 2.5-15 ml (D) PO q8h, or as retention enema left in place 15-20 min (3 parts lactulose and 7 parts water, 20 ml/kg) |
| | Lactulose | — | |
| | Lactitol | Lacty | 50 mg/kg PO q8h (estimate) |
| | Neomycin sulfate | Biosol | 20 mg/kg PO q8h |
| | Flumazenil | Romazicon | 0.01-0.02 mg/kg IV once; can be repeated once 30 min later (used primarily for diazepam overdose) |
| Nutritional supplement | Elemental diet | CliniCare Liquid Diet | 1 kcal/ml |
| Stimulate gastric motility | Metoclopramide | Reglan | 0.2-0.5 mg/kg PO, SC, or IV 30 min before meal |
| | Cisapride | — | 0.5 mg/kg PO q8-12h |
| Other | Ascorbic acid | — | 25 mg/kg/day PO |
| | Heparin for pancreatitis | — | 50-75 IU/Kg SC q8-12h |
| | Pancreatic enzyme powder or crushed tablets | Viokase V, Pancreazyme, Pancreatic Plus Powder | 1-2 tsp mixed with each meal |
| | Vitamin B₁₂ | — | 100-250 μg SC or IM q7days initially (C); 250-500 μg SC or IM q30days (D) |

*BAL,* British antilewisite; *C,* cat; *D,* dog; *IM,* intramuscularly; *IV,* intravenously; *MCT,* medium-chain triglyceride; *PO,* orally; *SC,* subcutaneously; *prn,* as needed; *VWD,* von Willebrand's disease; ⁹⁹ᵐTc, technetium 99m.

# PART V

# Urinary Disorders

GREGORY F. GRAUER

# 41

# Clinical Manifestations of Urinary Disorders

## (Text pp 568-583)

### POLLAKIURIA, DYSURIA, AND STRANGURIA (TEXT PP 568-572)

Inflammation of the lower urinary tract usually results in increased frequency of urination (pollakiuria) and difficult urination (dysuria) with straining (stranguria). In dogs the inflammation is often caused by bacterial infection; primary bacterial infection of the urinary tract is relatively rare in cats. Sterile inflammation can result from urolithiasis, neoplasia, or cyclophosphamide administration.

#### General diagnostic approach

Abdominal palpation may confirm a distended bladder, thickened bladder wall, bladder mass, or urolithiasis. Digital rectal examination in smaller patients often allows evaluation of the trigone of the bladder and the pelvic urethra for masses or uroliths.

Urinalysis, urine bacterial culture, ultrasonography of the bladder, and/or plain or contrast radiographs of the bladder and urethra usually reveal the cause of pollakiuria, dysuria, and stranguria. If systemic signs (e.g., depression, lethargy, anorexia, vomiting) are present, complete blood count (CBC) and serum biochemistry profile should also be obtained, and the kidneys, prostate gland, and uterus or uterine stump considered as possible sources of inflammation.

### Urethral Obstruction

Urethral obstruction, either functional (e.g., reflex dyssynergia, urethral spasm) or anatomic (e.g., urolithiasis, granulomatous urethritis, neoplasia), usually causes pollakiuria and/or dysuria and stranguria, with an attenuated or absent urine stream. A urethral catheter passes relatively easily in patients with functional obstruction, whereas "grating," difficult passage, or inability to pass the catheter is found with anatomic obstructions. If complete obstruction exists, the degree of postrenal azotemia and hyperkalemia should be assessed immediately, and hyperkalemia treated promptly (see Chapters 46 and 47).

### Urinary Tract Infection

The number of organisms isolated from the urine of a normal dog or cat varies with the collection method. With cystocentesis (ideal), bacterial numbers are clinically relevant when >1000/ml are found; 100 to 1000/ml is of questionable significance, and <100/ml signifies contamination. With catheterization, >10,000/ml is clinically relevant; 1000 to 10,000/ml is questionable, and <1000/ml indicates contamination. When a voided or expressed urine sample is used, >100,000/ml is clinically relevant, <10,000/ml indicates contamination, and intermediate values are of questionable significance.

#### Further evaluation

Patients with recurrent or unresponsive urinary tract infections (UTIs) should be evaluated by ultrasonography or contrast radiography to rule out underlying anatomic disorders. Bladder tumors or polyps, uroliths, pyelonephritis, prostatitis, and urachal remnants are common causes. In some cases systemic disorders (e.g., hyperadreno-corticism, chronic renal insufficiency and failure, diabetes mellitus) are associated with recurrent UTI, as is long-term corticosteroid treatment. UTIs are discussed further in Chapter 45.

## Transitional Cell Carcinoma

Transitional cell carcinoma (TCC) is the most common malignant bladder tumor in dogs and should be suspected in dogs with hematuria, pollakiuria, and dysuria and stranguria. TCCs are rare in cats. These tumors most frequently arise in the bladder trigone region, so they can often be detected by rectal palpation. Ultrasonography or double contrast cystography can confirm that a bladder mass exists. In some cases unilateral or bilateral hydroureter-hydronephrosis is found. Biopsy should be used to confirm the tumor type and stage and to direct specific treatment.

## Urolithiasis

Bladder and urethral uroliths can often be palpated via the abdomen or rectum; however, a thickened, inflamed bladder wall may obscure the presence of small uroliths. In male dogs with dysuria the urethra should be palpated subcutaneously from the ischial arch to the os penis. Ultrasonography or plain and/or contrast radiography is necessary to confirm urolithiasis. Calcium oxalate and struvite uroliths are the most radiodense, whereas urate uroliths are relatively radiolucent and may require contrast radiography for diagnosis (see Chapter 46).

### Urinalysis

Urinalysis often indicates inflammation: hematuria, pyuria, increased numbers of epithelial cells, and proteinuria. Urine pH varies depending on stone type, presence or absence of infection, and diet. In general, struvite uroliths are associated with alkaline urine (especially if urease-producing bacteria are present); cystine uroliths with acidic urine; and oxalate, urate, and silicate uroliths with neutral or acidic urine.

*Crystalluria.* Presence of crystals depends on urine concentration, pH, and temperature. Crystalluria may exist without uroliths, and uroliths may be present without crystalluria; but if the two coexist, the identity of the crystals is usually the same as that of the urolith. (Note: Silicate or calcium oxalate uroliths may be complicated by a urease-producing bacterial infection that could generate struvite crystals.) Specific aspects of crystalluria and urolithiasis are discussed in Chapters 46 (dogs) and 47 (cats).

*Culture.* Urine bacterial culture and sensitivity testing should be performed in all cases of urolithiasis. If cystotomy is performed for stone removal, a small piece of bladder mucosa and/or urolith should be submitted for bacterial culture.

*Qualitative urolith analysis.* Qualitative analysis should be performed if uroliths are passed or removed surgically, as identification of the urolith type facilitates the use of specific measures to dissolve them or prevent their recurrence. Commercial kit analysis is not recommended, however, as these kits do not detect silicic acid salts, frequently fail to detect calcium-containing uroliths, and yield false-positive results for uric acid in >50% of animals with cystine uroliths. Qualitative urolith analysis is available at most teaching hospitals and reference laboratories.

## Feline Lower Urinary Tract Inflammation

Cats with feline lower urinary tract inflammation (FLUTI) usually have pollakiuria, dysuria and stranguria, microscopic or gross hematuria, and inappropriate voiding. Other signs and physical examination findings depend on whether urethral obstruction is present (see Chapter 47).

### Diagnostic approach

Acute onset of pollakiuria, dysuria and stranguria, and hematuria in an otherwise healthy cat suggests FLUTI. Physical examination should include digital rectal palpation of the caudal bladder and urethra to rule out masses and calculi. Abdominal palpation of the bladder before and after voiding should be performed to determine the residual urine volume and presence of intraluminal masses or uroliths. Complete urinalysis, preferably on urine obtained via cystocentesis, should always be performed in cats with pollakiuria, dysuria, and stranguria.

Further evaluation of cats without obstruction is not warranted if the urine is alkaline and struvite crystals are found in the sediment. In most cases the urine is sterile and signs respond to dietary therapy (see Chapter 47). However, if signs persist beyond 5 to 7 days of dietary therapy, a second urinalysis with culture and sensitivity testing, abdominal radiographs, ultrasound, and/or contrast cystogram-urethrogram should be performed. These procedures should also be performed in cats with signs of FLUTI when the urine is acidic and no struvite crystals are present, in an attempt to find an underlying disease process.

## HEMATURIA (TEXT PP 572-575)

Hematuria with pollakiuria, dysuria, and stranguria is usually associated with lower urinary tract inflammation, whereas hematuria alone often indicates an upper urinary tract problem. Hematuria may be gross (macroscopic) or occult (microscopic; >5 red blood cells [RBCs]/hpf). Occult hematuria is common in dogs and cats with pollakiuria, dysuria, and stranguria. Myoglobin, hemoglobin, drugs, and food colorants can also discolor the urine (pseudohematuria); in such cases the urine supernatant remains discolored after centrifugation.

### Etiology

In most cases hematuria is caused by inflammation, trauma, or neoplasia of the urogenital tract. Exceptions include hematuria caused by bleeding disorders, strenuous exercise, heat stroke, renal infarcts, renal telangiectasia in Welsh Corgies, and renal hematuria in Weimaraners.

#### Timing relative to voiding.

Hematuria that occurs at the beginning of voiding suggests hemorrhage originating from the bladder neck, urethra, vagina, vulva, penis, or prepuce. Proestrus, metritis, pyometra, prostatic disease, and genital tract neoplasia are possible extraurinary causes. Hematuria that occurs either at the end of voiding or throughout urination usually indicates hemorrhage originating from the bladder, ureters, or kidneys (Table 41-1).

### Clinical signs

In patients with inflammation, trauma, or neoplasia of the lower urinary tract, hematuria may be accompanied by pollakiuria, dysuria, and stranguria. Hematuria associated with upper urinary tract disease may be associated with systemic signs (e.g., depression, lethargy, anorexia, vomiting, diarrhea, weight loss, abdominal pain), but some patients are asymptomatic. Occasionally, upper urinary tract hemorrhage results in the formation of blood clots in the bladder with subsequent dysuria and stranguria.

When hematuria is caused by genital tract hemorrhage, spontaneous bleeding unassociated with urination may be observed. Additional signs can include purulent vaginal or urethral discharge, behavioral changes (e.g., proestrus), and, with prostatic disease, straining to defecate and a stilted gait.

### Diagnostic approach

When possible the kidneys should be palpated and assessed for size, shape, consistency, symmetry, and presence of pain. The bladder should be palpated before and after the patient voids. Voiding should be observed to confirm the timing of hematuria, the character of the urine stream, and the presence or absence of dysuria; this also allows collection of a voided urine sample.

#### Digital palpation.

Rectal palpation allows evaluation of the pelvic urethra and, in male dogs, the prostate gland; the trigone of the bladder can also be palpated in small dogs and cats. In larger female dogs, vaginal palpation and use of a speculum allow evaluation of the urethral orifice for masses, strictures, and lacerations. In male dogs the urethra should be palpated subcutaneously from the ischial arch to the os penis, and the penis should be extruded and examined for masses, signs of trauma, and urethral prolapse. Catheterization of the urethra in dysuric animals allows assessment of urethral patency.

Table 41-1

## Potential Causes of Hematuria

| Urinary causes | Extraurinary causes |
|---|---|
| **INITIAL HEMATURIA** | |
| Urethral cause | Spontaneous bleeding unassociated with voiding; |
|   Trauma |   may also occur with the following: |
|   Infection |   Prostatic: infection, cyst, abscess, tumor |
|   Urolithiasis |   Uterine: infection, tumor, proestrus, subinvolution |
|   Neoplasia |   Vaginal: tumor, trauma |
| Granulomatous urethritis |   Preputial or penile: tumor, trauma |
| Bladder trigone region | |
|   Neoplasia | |
| | |
| **TOTAL OR TERMINAL HEMATURIA** | |
| Pseudohematuria | Prostatic (see above) |
| Kidney, ureter, bladder | Bleeding disorders |
| Trauma | Heat stroke |
| Infection | Exercise induced |
| Urolithiasis | |
| Tumor | |
| Parasitism | |
| Drug induced (cyclophosphamide) | |
| Feline lower urinary tract | |
|   inflammation syndrome | |
| Renal infarct | |
| Renal telangiectasia | |
| Idiopathic renal hematuria | |

*Urinalysis.* Comparison between urine obtained by cystocentesis and voided urine helps differentiate lower urinary or genital tract disease from upper urinary tract disease. Abnormal findings in urine collected by cystocentesis indicate involvement of the bladder, ureters, kidneys, or prostate (reflux into the bladder). Note: Cystocentesis, catheterization, and bladder expression may each result in traumatic hematuria.

Urinalysis should be performed within 30 minutes after urine collection. The sediment should be examined for RBCs, white blood cells (WBCs), epithelial cells, tumor cells, casts, crystals, parasite ova, and bacteria. Reagent strips used for the detection of blood in urine reveal hemoglobin from lysed cells, but myoglobinuria also causes a positive result.

*Clinicopathologic.* CBC and serum biochemistry profile should be evaluated in animals with hematuria and systemic signs. An inflammatory leukogram is compatible with metritis and pyometra, acute bacterial pyelonephritis, or prostatitis. Azotemia with hematuria usually indicates renal parenchymal disease or a rent in the urinary excretory pathway, although prerenal causes of azotemia should be ruled out. If blood loss caused by hematuria is severe or if signs of generalized bleeding exist, a hemostasis profile, platelet count, and bleeding time should be evaluated.

### Further evaluation

Plain and contrast radiography, ultrasonography, and/or cystoscopy often help in determining the location and cause of hematuria. In some cases, exploratory surgery and biopsy may be necessary for diagnosis. Biopsies may be obtained from the kidneys, bladder, and prostate gland. If indicated, ureteral catheterization via cystotomy or visualization via cystoscopy may be performed to determine if renal hematuria is unilateral or bilateral.

## DISORDERS OF MICTURITION (TEXT PP 575-577)

Disorders of micturition include urine retention and urine leakage (incontinence). Incontinence may be caused by congenital abnormalities or acquired disorders. It is helpful to determine if the bladder is distended, small, or normal in size. Causes of incontinence that are usually associated with a distended bladder include neurogenic disorders (lower and upper motor neuron lesions and reflex dyssynergia) and obstruction to urinary outflow. Incontinence associated with a small or normal-sized bladder is usually caused by either bladder hypercontractility or decreased urethral resistance. Specific causes of urinary incontinence are listed in Table 41-2.

### Geriatric Incontinence

Incontinence may also be caused by senility, decreased bladder capacity, or decreased mobility in senior animals. Polyuric-polydipsic disorders such as chronic renal insufficiency and failure and diabetes mellitus in senior animals often exacerbate incontinence, as do diuretic and corticosteroid therapy. Urinary incontinence is discussed further in Chapter 48.

## POLYDIPSIA AND POLYURIA (TEXT PP 577-579)

### Etiology

Polydipsia (PD) and polyuria (PU) are defined as water consumption >100 ml/kg/day and urine production >50 ml/kg/day, respectively. It is possible, however, for individuals to have abnormal thirst and urine production within these normal values. PD and PU usually coexist, and determination of the primary component is one of the initial diagnostic considerations.

### Primary polydipsia

In animals with primary PD, thirst is abnormally stimulated, resulting in water consumption in excess of physiologic need. Renal function is usually normal, and secondary PU occurs to rid the body of excess water. Usually the cause is either psychogenic or hepatic (insufficiency or portosystemic shunt).

Table 41-2

## Causes of Urinary Incontinence and Associated Clinical Signs

| Disorders | Clinical signs |
|---|---|
| **LARGE BLADDER** | |
| Lower motor neuron lesions | Dribbling of urine, distended bladder that is easily expressed, history of trauma or surgery in pelvic region |
| Upper motor neuron lesions | Distended bladder that is difficult to express; paresis or paralysis may be present |
| Reflex dyssynergia | Often large-breed, male dog; distended bladder that is difficult to express but easy to catheterize; urine stream initiated and then interrupted |
| Outflow tract obstruction | Usually male animals; dysuria-stranguria, dribbling of urine; distended bladder that is difficult to express and catheterize |
| **SMALL BLADDER** | |
| Urethral sphincter mechanism incompetence | Middle-aged or older neutered or spayed dogs; dribbling of urine usually occurs when animal is relaxed or asleep; normal voiding otherwise |
| Detrusor hyperreflexia or instability | Pollakiuria, dysuria-stranguria, hematuria, bacteriuria |
| Congenital abnormalities | Young animal; constant dribbling of urine may occur; voiding may be normal otherwise |

### Primary polyuria

Primary PU associated with a relative or absolute lack of antidiuretic hormone (ADH) is termed *central* or *pituitary diabetes insipidus*, whereas PU caused by non-responsiveness to ADH is termed *nephrogenic diabetes insipidus* (see Chapter 49). Nephrogenic diabetes insipidus has many possible causes, including the following:

- renal—insufficiency or failure, postobstructive diuresis, renal medullary solute washout, normoglycemic glucosuria
- metabolic—hyperadrenocorticism or hypoadrenocorticism, hyperthyroidism, diabetes mellitus
- electrolyte imbalances—hypercalcemia, hypokalemia
- hepatic insufficiency
- pyometra
- iatrogenic disease
- drugs

### Diagnostic approach

History and physical examination may suggest the underlying cause. A minimum database consisting of CBC, serum biochemistry profile, urinalysis, thoracic radiographs, and abdominal radiographs or ultrasonographs may confirm or suggest a diagnosis in many cases of primary PU. However, further specific tests are often necessary to confirm a diagnosis (Table 41-3).

**Table 41-3**

### Ancillary Diagnostic Tests That May Be Used to Evaluate Dogs and Cats with Polydipsia and Polyuria

| Suspected disorder | Further diagnostic tests |
|---|---|
| Primary polydipsia | Plasma osmolality, modified water deprivation, rule out hepatic insufficiency or PSS |
| Pituitary diabetes insipidus | Plasma osmolality, modified water deprivation test, response to exogenous antidiuretic hormone |
| Nephrogenic diabetes insipidus | |
| Renal insufficiency or failure | Serum urea nitrogen and creatinine concentrations, creatinine clearance, electrolyte fractional clearance, biopsy |
| Hyperadrenocorticism | ACTH-stimulation test, dexamethasone-suppression test, urine cortisol/creatinine ratio |
| Hypoadrenocorticism | Serum sodium/potassium ratio, ACTH-stimulation test |
| Hepatic insufficiency or PSS | Serum bile acids preprandially and postprandially, abdominal ultrasonography ± Doppler, $^{99}$Tc scan, portal angiography, biopsy |
| Pyometra | Abdominal radiography or ultrasonography, vaginal cytology |
| Hypercalcemia | Serum calcium concentrations (total and ionized), radiography, lymph node cytology or biopsy, bone marrow cytology, PTH and PTHrp assays |
| Hypokalemia | Serum potassium concentration, potassium fractional clearance |
| Glucosuria | Concurrent serum glucose concentration |
| Hyperthyroidism | Serum total and free thyroxine concentrations, triiodothyronine-suppression test, cardiac evaluation, $^{99}$Tc scanning |
| Renal medullary solute washout | Repeat water deprivation and exogenous ADH testing after gradual water restriction and dietary salt and protein supplementation for 10 to 14 days |

*ACTH,* Adrenocorticotropic hormone; *ADH,* antidiuretic hormone; *PSS,* portosystemic shunt; *PTH,* parathyroid hormone; *PTHrp,* parathyroid hormone–related peptide; $^{99}$Tc, technetium 99.

***Urine specific gravity.*** Urine specific gravity (SG) can be helpful in determination of the underlying cause and confirmation of whether the animal is truly polyuric. Interpretation of random urine SG requires knowledge of the patient's hydration status, blood urea nitrogen (BUN) and serum creatinine concentrations, and current medications. Normal dogs and cats should produce hypersthenuric urine (SG >1.030 in dogs and >1.035 in cats) in response to dehydration.

It is unusual for dogs and cats with PD and PU to have consistently hypersthenuric urine; this finding should warrant confirmation of PD and PU by measurement of water consumption. Patients with primary PD or central diabetes insipidus usually have hyposthenuric urine (SG 1.001 to 1.007), whereas urine in patients with nephrogenic diabetes insipidus is most likely isosthenuric (SG 1.008 to 1.012) or minimally concentrated (SG 1.013 to 1.030 or 1.035).

### Further evaluation

If the history, physical examination, and minimum data base are unrewarding, specialized diagnostic tests, including plasma osmolality, water deprivation testing, and response to exogenous ADH, may be necessary (see Chapter 42).

## PROTEINURIA (TEXT PP 579-581)

### Etiology

Proteinuria may be caused by physiologic or pathologic conditions (Table 41-4). Physiologic or benign proteinuria is often transient and abates when the underlying cause is corrected. Pathologic proteinuria may arise from renal or nonrenal sources. Nonrenal proteinuria is most frequently associated with lower urinary tract inflammation or hemorrhage. Changes in the urine sediment usually reflect the underlying cause (e.g., urolithiasis, neoplasia, trauma, bacterial cystitis).

Renal proteinuria is most often caused by glomerular lesions (e.g., glomerulonephritis, amyloidosis; see Chapter 43). Persistent proteinuria with normal urine sediment or hyaline casts is strongly suggestive of glomerular disease. Renal proteinuria may also be caused by inflammatory or infiltrative disorders of the kidney (e.g., neoplasia,

Table 41-4

## Classification of Proteinuria

| Type | Causes |
|---|---|
| Physiologic | Strenuous exercise |
| | Seizures |
| | Fever |
| | Exposure to heat or cold |
| | Decreased activity level (strict cage rest) |
| Pathologic | |
| Nonurinary | Bence Jones proteinuria |
| | Hemoglobinuria or myoglobinuria |
| | Congestive heart failure |
| | Genital tract inflammation |
| Urinary | |
| Nonrenal | Cystourolithiasis |
| | Bacterial cystitis |
| | Trauma or hemorrhage |
| | Neoplasia |
| | Drug-induced cystitis (e.g., cyclophosphamide) |
| Renal | Glomerular lesions |
| | Abnormal tubular resorption |
| | Renal parenchymal inflammation or hemorrhage |

pyelonephritis) or by tubular abnormalities that result in decreased resorption of filtered protein (e.g., Fanconi syndrome).

### Identifying proteinuria

The dipstick test is most sensitive for albumin. False-positive results may occur with alkaline urine or urine contaminated with quaternary ammonium compounds or if the dipstick is left in contact with the urine too long. False-negative results may be found with Bence Jones proteinuria or with dilute or acidic urine. Ideally the supernatant from centrifuged urine samples should be used for all physicochemical analysis. Quantifying proteinuria is discussed in Chapter 42.

### Diagnostic approach

Proteinuria should always be interpreted in light of urine SG. Clinically relevant proteinuria may be missed if the urine is dilute. Conversely, "trace" or 1+ protein may be normal in concentrated urine. Urine protein is frequently increased in patients with lower urinary tract inflammation or hemorrhage, so proteinuria should also be interpreted in relation to sediment changes that are compatible with inflammation or hemorrhage (e.g., bacteria and increased numbers of WBCs, RBCs, and epithelial cells).

Prerenal (physiologic and pathologic nonurinary), postrenal (pathologic urinary [nonrenal]), and inflammatory renal proteinuria can usually be differentiated on the basis of history, physical examination, and urine sediment changes. Renal proteinuria caused by abnormal tubular resorption is frequently accompanied by normoglycemic glucosuria and abnormal urinary loss of electrolytes, which helps differentiate tubular from glomerular proteinuria.

## AZOTEMIA (TEXT PP 581-583)

When a patient is presented with azotemia, decreased renal excretory function should be the main diagnostic consideration. Decreased excretion of urea nitrogen and creatinine may result from both extrarenal (prerenal and postrenal) and primary renal causes.

### Prerenal Azotemia

Any condition that decreases renal blood flow can result in prerenal azotemia, including hypovolemia (e.g., dehydration, hypoadrenocorticism), hypotension (e.g., anesthesia, cardiomyopathy), and aortic or renal arterial thrombosis. Hypersthenuric urine with relatively low sodium and high creatinine concentrations is usually produced (Table 41-5). Correction of the underlying disorder (e.g., fluid therapy to correct hypovolemia) results in rapid resolution of the azotemia unless the underlying disorder persisted long enough or was severe enough to cause renal parenchymal damage.

### Disproportionate changes in BUN and creatinine

Disproportionate increases in BUN relative to creatinine can be caused by high-protein diets, upper gastrointestinal hemorrhage, and increased tubular resorption of urea nitrogen associated with prerenal azotemia. Conversely, a disproportionately low BUN can be observed with decreased liver function, portosystemic shunts, low-protein diets, and prolonged diuresis.

**Table 41-5**

### Differentiation of Prerenal Azotemia from Acute Renal Failure

| Indexes | Prerenal azotemia | Acute renal failure |
|---|---|---|
| Urine specific gravity | Hypersthenuric | Isosthenuric or minimally concentrated |
| Fractional clearance of sodium* | <1% | >2% |
| Urine creatinine-to-serum creatinine ratio | >20:1 | <10:1 |

*(Urine$_{Na}$ × Serum $_{Cr}$)/(Urine$_{Cr}$ × Serum$_{Na}$)

## Postrenal Azotemia

Postrenal azotemia is usually caused by obstruction to urine outflow or rupture of the urine outflow tract. Urine SG varies depending on the patient's hydration status. In cases of urethral obstruction, dysuria and stranguria are common and catheterization is difficult.

Rupture of the urinary tract usually involves the bladder or urethra, is more common in males, and frequently results in abdominal effusion or SC fluid accumulation. Fluid obtained by abdominocentesis is usually sterile and contains a higher concentration of creatinine than the serum. Positive contrast urethrography and/or cystography confirms urethral obstruction or rupture of the urethra or bladder.

## Renal Azotemia

Renal azotemia occurs as a result of nephron loss or damage and is usually associated with renal failure. The diagnosis is confirmed when azotemia is persistently associated with isosthenuria or minimally concentrated urine (see Table 41-5).

### Prerenal versus renal azotemia

Differentiating prerenal from renal azotemia is difficult in some patients. Azotemia caused by dehydration, accompanied by decreased urine-concentrating ability, can be confused with renal azotemia. Examples include furosemide treatment that creates dehydration and hypercalcemia that compromises urine-concentrating ability and causes dehydration secondary to vomiting. Frequently response to fluid therapy is the best way to differentiate prerenal from renal azotemia: renal azotemia does not completely resolve with fluid therapy alone.

## Renal Failure

Renal failure is a state of decreased renal function in which azotemia and inability to concentrate urine persist concurrently. Treatment and prognosis vary for patients with acute versus chronic renal failure. Acute renal failure occurs within hours or days; associated signs and laboratory data are listed in Table 41-6. Chronic renal failure occurs over a period of weeks, months, or years; clinical signs are often relatively mild for the magnitude of azotemia. Renal failure is discussed further in Chapter 44.

## RENOMEGALY (TEXT P 583)

Renal enlargement is usually detected on physical examination or abdominal radiography or ultrasonography. Normal kidney length on abdominal radiographs should be approximately 2.5 to 3 times the length of L2 in cats and 2.5 to 3.5 times the length of L2 in dogs.

### Table 41-6

**Differentiation of Acute from Chronic Renal Failure on the Basis of History, Clinical Signs, and Clinical Pathology Data**

| Acute renal failure | Chronic renal failure |
| --- | --- |
| History of ischemia or toxicant exposure | History of renal disease or polydipsia and polyuria |
| Normal or high hematocrit | Nonregenerative anemia |
| Swollen kidneys | Small, irregular kidneys |
| Hyperkalemia (with oliguria) | Normal or hypokalemia |
| More severe metabolic acidosis | Normal or mild metabolic acidosis |
| Active urine sediment | Inactive urine sediment |
| Good body condition | Weight loss |
| Relatively severe clinical signs for level of dysfunction | Relatively mild clinical signs for level of dysfunction |

### Etiology

Enlarged kidneys with a normal shape can be caused by edema, acute inflammation, diffusely infiltrating neoplastic disease, unilateral compensatory hypertrophy, trauma (intracapsular hemorrhage), or hydronephrosis. Enlarged, abnormally shaped kidneys may be caused by renal neoplasia, cysts, abscesses, hydronephrosis, or hematomas.

### Diagnostic approach

Ultrasonography and intravenous urography can be used to further define kidney shape and reveal internal details. Ultrasonography is particularly useful for evaluating enlarged kidneys associated with fluid accumulation (e.g., hydronephrosis, abscesses, and perirenal and parenchymal cysts) and can also be used to guide fine-needle aspiration or needle biopsy of the affected kidney. Kidney biopsy is often necessary to confirm the cause of the renomegaly; however, biopsy is contraindicated if only one kidney is present or if a bleeding disorder, hydronephrosis, a cyst, or an abscess is suspected.

# 42

# Diagnostic Tests for the Urinary System

## (Text pp 584-599)

## RENAL EXCRETORY FUNCTION (TEXT PP 584-586)

### Glomerular Filtration Rate

Serum urea nitrogen (BUN) and creatinine (Cr) concentrations provide a crude index of glomerular filtration rate (GFR). However, renal azotemia does not develop until approximately 75% of the nephrons in both kidneys have been destroyed. This percentage may even be higher in animals with chronic, progressive renal disease. Measurement of renal clearance can provide more accurate information about renal excretory function, especially in early renal disease.

#### Creatinine clearance

Renal clearance of insulin is the gold standard for determining GFR. However, creatinine (Cr) clearance is easier to measure and therefore more practical. GFR can be calculated as follows:

$$\text{GFR (ml/min)} = \text{Urine}_{Cr}\ [\text{mg/dl}] \times \text{Urine volume [ml/min]}/\text{Serum}_{Cr}\ [\text{mg/dl}]$$

This value is divided by the patient's body weight (in kilograms) and expressed in milliliters per minute per kilogram. (Note: Prerenal and postrenal factors, as well as renal parenchymal lesions, influence plasma clearance.)

*Endogenous Cr clearance.* Measurement of endogenous Cr clearance requires urine collection for 24 hours, thereby necessitating indwelling or repeated urinary catheterization, or a metabolism cage. It is used clinically to evaluate renal excretory function when dysfunction is suspected but BUN and Cr are within normal ranges. Less commonly, endogenous Cr clearance can be used to better quantify renal excretory function when azotemia is present. Sample collection is discussed in the text. Normal endogenous Cr clearance is 2.8 to 3.7 ml/min/kg in dogs and 2 to 3 ml/min/kg in cats.

*Exogenous Cr clearance.* Measurement of exogenous Cr clearance is most appropriate in nonazotemic patients. Cr (100 mg/kg) is injected subcutaneously (SC); 40 minutes later, urine is collected for 20 minutes, and serum samples are obtained at the start and end of the collection period. The average of the two serum Cr concentrations is used. Normal exogenous Cr clearance is 3.5 to 4.5 ml/min/kg in dogs and 2.4 to 3.3 ml/min/kg in cats.

### Plasma clearance of iohexol

Measurement of plasma clearance of iohexol allows reliable estimation of GFR in dogs and cats without urine collection. Plasma iohexol can be measured at university teaching hospitals and some reference laboratories.

### Scintigraphy

Renal scintigraphy using technetium 99m ($^{99m}$Tc)–diethylenetriaminepentaacetic acid also allows evaluation of GFR and is available at several universities and major referral centers.

### Fractional Clearance

Expressing the renal clearance of a solute as a percentage of Cr clearance indicates the body's attempt to conserve or excrete the solute. Fractional clearance (FC) of a solute (S) is calculated as follows:

$$FC_S = (Urine_S / Serum_S)/(Urine_{Cr}/Serum_{Cr})$$

In normal dogs and cats, FC of sodium, chloride, and calcium is <1%; values for potassium and phosphorus are more variable and may be as high as 20% and 39%, respectively.

### Indications

Determining the FC of electrolytes may be helpful with (1) primary hyperparathyroidism, in which FC of phosphorus is increased; (2) tubular dysfunction such as Fanconi syndrome, in which FC is increased for all electrolytes; and (3) differentiation of prerenal azotemia from acute renal failure (ARF; see Table 41-5). FC of electrolytes can also be monitored daily in dogs and cats receiving potentially nephrotoxic drugs (e.g., gentamicin); twofold to threefold increases can indicate tubular damage before overt azotemia occurs.

### Preparation

Timed urine collection is not necessary, although FC of electrolytes should be performed only after a 12- to 15-hour fast. The alternative is to feed the patient a standard diet for several days before FC determination.

## QUANTIFICATION OF PROTEINURIA (TEXT P 586)

If the dipstick method or sulfosalicylic acid test for proteinuria suggests clinically relevant proteinuria, and the urine sediment is normal, urine protein excretion should be quantified at a reference laboratory.

### Urine protein/Cr ratio

By dividing urine protein ($U_{pr}$; mg/dl) by urine Cr ($U_{cr}$; mg/dl), the effect of urine volume on protein concentration is negated. Multiplying the value by 20 allows conversion to mg/kg/24 hr. Normal urine protein excretion in dogs and cats is <20 mg/kg/24 hr; therefore a $U_{pr}/U_{cr}$ of <1 is normal.

*Interpretation.* The $U_{pr}/U_{cr}$ ratio cannot differentiate glomerular proteinuria from proteinuria associated with lower urinary tract inflammation or hemorrhage. Therefore complete urinalysis should always be performed before or along with assessment of $U_{pr}/U_{cr}$. If evidence of inflammation is present, protein determination should be repeated after successful treatment of the inflammatory disorder.

The magnitude of glomerular proteinuria is roughly correlated with the nature of the glomerular lesion. In general, urine protein excretion is greater in dogs with glomerulonephritis than in dogs with glomerular atrophy or interstitial nephritis but less than in dogs with amyloidosis.

### Microalbuminuria

An antigen-capture enzyme-linked immunosorbent assay for dogs is commercially available for the detection of concentrations of albumin in urine that are too low to be detected by standard dipstick tests (urine albumin of 1 to 30 mg/dl). In certain instances microalbuminuria is an accurate predictor of overt proteinuria and renal disease (see text).

### Electrophoresis

Urine and serum protein electrophoresis may help identify the source of proteinuria and establish a prognosis. Proteinuria associated with hemorrhage into the urinary tract has an electrophoretic pattern similar to that of the serum. Early glomerular damage usually results primarily in albuminuria; with progression, increasing amounts of globulin may also be lost. Marked hypoalbuminemia and decreased serum concentrations of larger molecular weight proteins suggest severe glomerular proteinuria and nephrotic syndrome.

## OSMOLALITY, WATER DEPRIVATION, AND ANTIDIURETIC HORMONE (TEXT PP 587-588)

### Plasma and Urine Osmolality

Measurement of plasma osmolality may aid in identifying the primary component of PD and PU syndromes. Normal plasma osmolality is 280 to 310 mOsm/kg. In patients with primary PD, plasma osmolality is usually low (275 to 285 mOsm/kg). Patients with primary PU often have high plasma osmolality (305 to 315 mOsm/kg). However, considerable overlap can exist in plasma osmolalities between primary PD (polydipsia) and primary PU (polyuria) disorders.

#### Urine:plasma osmolality

The ratio of urine to plasma osmolality allows a more precise determination of urine concentration than does urine SG alone. In response to dehydration, normal dogs and cats should be able to form urine that is five to six times more concentrated than plasma.

### Water Deprivation Tests

Water deprivation tests allow evaluation of the neurohypophyseal-renal axis. They are used to differentiate diabetes insipidus from primary PD and should be performed only after other causes of PU and PD have been ruled out with physical examination and minimum data base.

#### Precautions

These tests are potentially dangerous; they should be performed only with the patient under close observation and after gradual reduction in its water intake. Failure to produce concentrated urine (i.e., diabetes insipidus) can result in severe dehydration and possibly ischemic renal injury.

#### Guidelines

The test is ended when the patient (1) loses 5% of its body weight as a result of dehydration, (2) becomes azotemic, (3) becomes hyperosmolemic (plasma osmolality >320 mOsm/kg), or (4) produces hypersthenuric urine (SG >1.030 in dogs and >1.035 in cats).

The time necessary to reach the end-point is variable; small dogs and cats may dehydrate within several hours, whereas in large dogs marked dehydration may not occur for 36 to 48 hours. Patients that fail to produce hypersthenuric urine have a form of diabetes insipidus, either pituitary or nephrogenic (see subsequent discussion of response to exogenous antidiuretic hormone [ADH]).

Plasma osmolality is a good indicator of hydration status during water deprivation, and in fact it may obviate the need for a water deprivation test. A baseline plasma osmolality of 320 mOsm/kg in a nondehydrated patient with hyposthenuria or isosthenuria suggests failure of the neurohypophyseal-renal axis. Similarly, a water deprivation test should not be performed on a patient that is clinically dehydrated or azotemic and that has hyposthenuria, isosthenuria, or minimally concentrated urine.

## Response to Exogenous ADH

Administration of ADH may be used to differentiate pituitary diabetes insipidus (lack of ADH) from nephrogenic diabetes insipidus (lack of response to ADH). Aqueous ADH (3 to 5 U, intramuscularly [IM]) is usually given, although synthetic DDAVP nasal spray (given as drops into the conjunctival sac) or injectable DDAVP (3 to 5 U, SC) may also be used.

### Guidelines

In patients that fail to respond to water deprivation, ADH should be administered at the end-point of the water deprivation test, before water is offered. It is important that the patient's bladder be emptied immediately before administration of ADH so that urine produced in response to ADH is not diluted by previously formed urine. Patients with pituitary diabetes insipidus usually respond by producing urine with a greatly increased SG within 2 hours. Lack of an increase in urine SG in response to both water deprivation and exogenous ADH administration indicates the presence of nephrogenic diabetes insipidus.

### Renal medullary washout

Patients with primary PD or pituitary diabetes insipidus may develop medullary washout, which makes them appear to have nephrogenic diabetes insipidus. Gradual reduction in water intake over 10 to 14 days (10% reduction every other day until the patient is drinking 80 to 90 ml/kg/day) may correct medullary washout before the water deprivation test is performed. A lightly salted, high-protein diet should be fed during this time. Water restriction should be discontinued if the patient becomes overly aggressive for water or becomes lethargic or weak. Lack of response to water deprivation and exogenous ADH after gradual water reduction indicates a type of nephrogenic diabetes insipidus other than medullary washout.

## BLADDER AND URETHRAL FUNCTION (TEXT P 588)

### Urethral Pressure Profile

The urethral pressure profile (UPP) assesses the perfusion pressure or minimal distention pressure within the neck of the bladder and urethra during the storage phase of micturition. Functional urethral length (length of urethra with pressure greater than intravesical pressure) and maximal urethral closure pressure (greatest urethral pressure minus intravesical pressure) can be determined from the UPP. Electromyogram may be combined with UPP to define the portion of urethral resistance contributed to by periurethral-striated muscle (external sphincter).

*Indications.* UPP can be used to assess urethral sphincter tone in cases of suspected sphincter incompetence or functional urethral obstruction or spasm. UPP can also be used to evaluate sphincter response to treatment with α-adrenergic drugs or estrogens and for preoperative assessment in patients with ectopic ureters and vaginal strictures (because the incidence of urethral sphincter incompetence is increased in animals with these anomalies).

### Cystometrography

Cystometrography records changes in intravesicular pressure during bladder filling and detrusor contraction. It allows evaluation of the detrusor reflex, maximal detrusor contraction pressure, and bladder capacity and compliance in cases of suspected detrusor atony, instability, and decreased capacity or compliance.

### Uroflowmetry

Uroflowmetry measures urine flow during voiding and defines the relationship between urine flow and detrusor contraction. Normal, increased, or decreased urethral resistance can therefore be established.

## BACTERIAL ANTIBIOTIC SENSITIVITY TESTING (TEXT PP 588-589)

Concentration of antibiotic by the kidneys frequently results in organism sensitivity, even when disk-diffusion indicates resistance. However, if an organism infecting the urinary tract is highly resistant on disk sensitivity (e.g., susceptible only to amino-glycosides), minimum inhibitory concentration (MIC) can be helpful in determining if alternative antibiotics will be effective. As a rule, if the MIC is 25% of the expected mean urine concentration (Table 42-1), the organism should be susceptible. Note: In cases of pyelonephritis or bladder infections with a thickened bladder wall, drug concentrations within these tissues will be closer to serum concentrations, and MIC sensitivity should not be used.

## DIAGNOSTIC IMAGING (TEXT PP 589-596)

### Plain Radiography

It is relatively difficult to visualize the kidneys (especially the right kidney) on plain abdominal radiographs. Nevertheless, plain radiographs should be used to determine kidney number, location, size, shape, and density. Kidney size is best estimated by comparing kidney length to the adjacent lumbar vertebra (see Chapter 41). Any mineral-type radiopacity within the kidney is abnormal.

### Ultrasonography

Ultrasonography is used to evaluate renal tissue architecture. Relatively hypoechoic renal cortices may be observed in patients with acute tubular necrosis, polycystic kidney disease, abscesses, or renal edema associated with ARF. Relatively hyperechoic renal cortices are associated with end-stage renal failure, nephrocalcinosis, amyloidosis, feline infectious peritonitis, or calcium oxalate nephrosis secondary to ethylene glycol ingestion. With glomerular and tubulointerstitial disease, the echotexture may be normal or hyperechoic, depending on chronicity. Renal lymphoma may make the renal cortices appear hypoechoic or hyperechoic. Hydronephrosis and hydroureter are easily diagnosed by ultrasonography.

#### Resistive index

Resistance to renal blood flow (resistive index) can be calculated with color flow Doppler imaging. It is increased in several renal diseases (see text).

**Table 42-1**

### Urine Concentration of Selected Antimicrobial Agents Determined in Healthy Dogs with Normal Renal Function

| Antibiotic | Dose* | Route | Urine concentration (µg/ml; mean ± standard deviation) |
|---|---|---|---|
| Penicillin G | 40,000 U/kg q8h | PO | 294 ± 211 |
| Ampicillin | 25 mg/kg q8h | PO | 309 ± 55 |
| Amoxicillin | 11 mg/kg q8h | PO | 202 ± 93 |
| Tetracycline | 20 mg/kg q8h | PO | 138 ± 65 |
| Chloramphenicol | 33 mg/kg q8h | PO | 124 ± 40 |
| Sulfisoxazole | 22 mg/kg q8h | PO | 1466 ± 832 |
| Cephalexin | 30 mg/kg q12h | PO | 805 ± 421 |
| Trimethoprim-sulfa | 15 mg/kg q12h | PO | 55 ± 19 |
| Enrofloxacin | 2.5 mg/kg q12h | PO | 43 ± 12 |

*Doses are the same for cats, except that the dosage of chloramphenicol in cats is 20 mg/kg q8h for 1 wk.
*PO*, Orally.

### Evaluating the bladder

Ultrasonography is particularly useful for differentiating intraluminal masses (e.g., calculi, blood clots, tumors, polyps). The prostate gland and sublumbar lymph nodes are also readily evaluated. Ultrasonography may be less effective for detection of mucosal irregularities, small uroliths, and bladder rupture than contrast cystography (see next section).

## Contrast Studies

Intravenous urography can aid in evaluation of the renal vessels, parenchyma, pelvis, and ureters. Potential indications include kidney abnormalities noted on plain radiographs or ultrasonography, inability to visualize one or both kidneys, and hematuria of suspected renal origin. Urography also provides a qualitative assessment of individual kidney excretory function, so it should be performed before nephrectomy or nephrotomy. Its utility diminishes with azotemia; good renal opacification becomes more difficult as azotemia increases. This test should be avoided in dehydrated patients and in those receiving potentially nephrotoxic drugs. The technique is described in the text.

### Evaluating the ureters

Normal ureteral diameter is 1 to 2 mm, and apparent filling defects are frequently caused by normal peristaltic contractions. Indications for urographic evaluation of the ureters include suspected obstructive uropathy, trauma (rupture or laceration), calculi, ectopic ureters, neoplasia, and ureterocele.

### Evaluating the bladder

Retrograde contrast radiographic studies are used to visualize the bladder and its relationship to other structures in the caudal abdomen. Negative (air or carbon dioxide [$CO_2$]) or positive (iodinated) contrast may be used; however, double-contrast studies provide the best information about the bladder mucosal surface. Potential abnormalities include mucosal and mural lesions, luminal filling defects, urachal remnants, diverticuli, vesicoureteral reflux, extraluminal mass lesions, and bladder tears.

### Evaluating the urethra

Contrast urethrography is most often performed in males to rule out urethral obstruction and/or rupture. It may be used to identify the presence and location of mucosal and mural lesions, luminal filling defects, strictures, extramural compression, and urethral rupture or laceration.

## Computed Tomography

Plain and contrast-enhanced computed tomography is increasingly being used for evaluation of renal pathology in university hospitals and other referral centers.

## CYSTOSCOPY (TEXT PP 596-598)

Cystoscopy allows visualization and biopsy of the urethral and bladder mucosae. In some cases bladder mucosal lesions can be resected and uroliths removed or crushed via cystoscopy. This procedure can also be used to catheterize the ureters for urine samples and retrograde pyelography. Indications for cystoscopy include lower urinary tract inflammation; evaluation of potential anatomic abnormalities (e.g., urolithiasis, polyps, ectopic ureters, urachal remnants) in patients with recurrent urinary tract infections, urine retention, or leakage; evaluation and biopsy of bladder or urethral masses; and differentiation of unilateral and bilateral renal hematuria.

## RENAL BIOPSY (TEXT P 598)

Renal biopsy should be considered if the diagnosis is in question or if treatment or prognosis may be altered on the basis of the histopathology results. In most cases of renal disease a specific diagnosis is required for appropriate treatment, and specific diagnosis frequently requires biopsy. Prognosis for renal disease is best based on the severity of dysfunction, response to treatment, and renal histopathology.

Renal biopsy should be considered only after less invasive tests have been completed and blood clotting ability has been assessed. Contraindications include a solitary kidney, a bleeding abnormality, severe systemic hypertension, and renal lesions associated with fluid accumulation (e.g., hydronephrosis, renal cysts or abscesses). The technique and precautions are discussed in the text.

# 43

# Glomerulonephropathies

## (Text pp 600-607)

Glomerulonephritis (GN) is the most common type of glomerulonephropathy and one of the major causes of chronic renal insufficiency (CRI) and chronic renal failure (CRF). Deposition of amyloid within the glomerulus is another important, although less common, glomerulonephropathy. Loss of plasma proteins, principally albumin, in the urine is the hallmark of glomerulonephropathy.

### Etiology
Most glomerulonephropathies in dogs and cats are immune mediated; immune complexes in the glomerular capillary wall initiate glomerular damage. Cellular proliferation (proliferative GN), thickening of the glomerular basement membrane (membranous GN), and, eventually, hyalinization and sclerosis occur in the glomerulus as a result. The initial pathophysiologic consequence of proliferative and/or membranous GN is proteinuria. Azotemia is not an early finding; it occurs when >75% of the nephrons are damaged and become nonfunctional.

Several infectious and inflammatory diseases have been associated with GN (Table 43-1). In many cases, however, the antigen source or underlying disease process is not identified, and the glomerular disease is referred to as *idiopathic*.

*Amyloidosis.* Glomerular amyloidosis is a progressive disease that frequently leads to CRF. The reactive systemic form, in which amyloid is deposited in several organs including the kidneys, occurs in dogs and cats. It is usually associated with an underlying inflammatory or neoplastic process; however, in many patients no predisposing factors can be identified.

*Familial amyloidosis.* Renal amyloidosis is a familial disease in Abyssinian cats and results in medullary amyloid deposition as a part of systemic amyloidosis. Suspected familial medullary amyloidosis has also been reported in young Chinese Shar Pei dogs. Intermittent fever and tibiotarsal joint swelling that resolve regardless of treatment are often observed in these dogs.

Note: The medullary deposition of amyloid in Abyssinian cats and Shar Pei dogs makes proteinuria uncommon. Renal failure, however, is a common sequela.

### Clinical features
The clinical signs associated with mild to moderate urinary protein loss are usually nonspecific (e.g., weight loss, lethargy), but many patients with low-grade proteinuria appear normal. When protein loss is severe, edema and/or ascites often develops (Table 43-2). If glomerular disease is extensive, renal failure with azotemia, polydipsia and polyuria, anorexia, nausea, and vomiting may occur. Occasionally, signs associated

Table 43-1

## Diseases Associated with Glomerulonephritis in Dogs and Cats

**INFECTIOUS**

**Dogs**

Canine adenovirus I
Bacterial endocarditis
Brucellosis
Dirofilariasis
Ehrlichiosis
Leishmaniasis
Pyometra
Borelliosis
Chronic bacterial infections (gingivitis, pyoderma)
Rocky Mountain spotted fever
Trypanosomiasis
Septicemia
Helicobacter?

**Cats**

Feline leukemia virus
Feline immunodeficiency virus
Feline infectious peritonitis
Mycoplasma polyarthritis
Chronic bacterial infections

**NEOPLASIA**

**INFLAMMATORY**

Pancreatitis
Systemic lupus erythematosus
Other immune-mediated diseases
Prostatitis (dogs)
Hepatitis (dogs)
Chronic skin disease (cats)
Inflammatory bowel disease (dogs)

**OTHER**

Idiopathic
Familial
Nonimmunologic—hyperfiltration?
Diabetes mellitus
Hyperadrenocorticism and long-term high
    dose corticosteroids? (dogs)

Table 43-2

## Signs Associated with Different Manifestations of Glomerular Disease

| Manifestation | Clinical signs | Clinicopathologic findings |
|---|---|---|
| Mild to moderate proteinuria* | Lethargy, mild weight loss, decreased muscle mass | Serum albumin 1.5-3 g/dl |
| Marked proteinuria (>3.5g/day) | Severe muscle wasting; weight gain may occur, however, as a result of edema or ascites | Serum albumin <1.5 g/dl; hypercholesterolemia |
| Renal failure | Depression, anorexia, nausea, vomiting, weight loss, polyuria and polydipsia | Azotemia, isosthenuria or minimally concentrated urine, hyperphosphatemia; nonregenerative anemia |
| Pulmonary thromboembolism | Acute dyspnea or severe panting | Hypoxemia; normal or low $Pco_2$; fibrinogen >300 mg/dl; antithrombin <70% of normal |
| Retinal hemorrhage and/or detachment | Acute blindness | Systolic blood pressure >180 mm Hg |

*Microalbuminuria (see Chapter 42) may precede proteinuria and therefore may be an early diagnostic tool.
$Pco_2$, Partial pressure of carbon dioxide.

with an underlying infectious, inflammatory, or neoplastic disease are the reason for presentation.

In rare instances a dog may be presented because of acute dyspnea or severe panting caused by pulmonary thromboembolism, or because of acute blindness caused by retinal hemorrhage or detachment secondary to systemic hypertension (see later).

**Nephrotic syndrome.** Persistent proteinuria can lead to signs of nephrotic syndrome: marked proteinuria, hypoalbuminemia, ascites or edema, and hypercholesterolemia. This syndrome is more common in dogs than in cats. Systemic hypertension and hypercoagulability are common complications in dogs.

**Hypertension.** Hypertension has been associated with immune-mediated GN, glomerulosclerosis, and amyloidosis. In one study 84% of dogs with glomerular disease were found to be hypertensive. Retinal changes (hemorrhage, detachment, papilledema) are suggestive of hypertension.

**Thromboembolism.** Hypercoagulability and thromboembolism associated with nephrotic syndrome occur secondary to several clotting abnormalities (e.g., mild thrombocytosis; platelet hypersensitivity; loss of antithrombin in urine; and increases in fibrinogen and clotting factors V, VII, VIII, and X). The pulmonary arterial system is the most common casualty. Dogs with pulmonary thromboembolism are usually dyspneic, hypoxic, and hypocapneic with minimal pulmonary radiographic abnormalities.

### Diagnosis

Persistent, severe proteinuria with normal urine sediment (plus hyaline casts) is the hallmark of glomerulonephropathy. The urine protein/creatinine ratio ($U_{pr}/U_{cr}$) is used to quantify the magnitude of protein loss. Microalbuminuria may precede overt proteinuria (see Chapter 42). Definitive diagnosis of protein-losing nephropathy is made by evaluation of renal cortical histopathology.

Blood pressure measurement can help in the evaluation and management of animals with glomerular disease. With identification and control of hypertension, the progression of the glomerular disease, as well as damage in other target organs, may be attenuated.

### Treatment

The most important therapeutic approach for glomerular disease is identification and correction of underlying disease processes. However, because an antigen source or underlying disease frequently is not identified or is impossible to eliminate, immunosuppressive drugs and supportive therapies have been recommended for animals with GN (Box 43-1).

**Immunosuppressive drugs.** In many instances immunosuppressive treatment is of no benefit, and in some cases it exacerbates the glomerular lesions and proteinuria. If immunosuppressive drugs are used, proteinuria should be quantified ($U_{pr}/U_{cr}$) frequently to assess treatment efficacy.

Corticosteroid treatment of GN may be more efficacious in cats than in dogs. Corticosteroids probably should not be used in dogs with GN because iatrogenic hyperadrenocorticism has been associated with GN and thromboembolism. The exception would be a corticosteroid-responsive underlying disease such as systemic lupus erythematosus.

**Antiplatelet therapy.** Antiplatelet therapy (e.g., aspirin, indomethacin, dipyridamole, platelet-activating factor antagonists) has proved beneficial in several studies. Low-dose aspirin therapy is most often recommended (see Box 43-1). Concurrent treatment with prostaglandin analogs or dietary supplementation with marine (n-3) polyunsaturated fatty acids may also attenuate glomerular disease.

**Dimethyl sulfoxide.** Experimentally, dimethyl sulfoxide (DMSO) can dissolve amyloid fibrils, and its antiinflammatory effects may decrease production of acute phase reactant SAA (see text). Decreased urinary protein excretion was observed in one dog with amyloidosis treated with DMSO (80 mg/kg subcutaneously three times per week). However, in other studies DMSO was ineffective in dogs with amyloidosis.

**Colchicine.** Although colchicine has been recommended to prevent medullary amyloidosis in Shar Peis with fever and tibiotarsal joint swelling, no controlled studies

---

**Box 43-1**

## Treatment Guidelines for Dogs and Cats with Glomerulonephritis

1. Identify and eliminate any underlying diseases
2. Immunosuppressive treatment (usually not recommended for dogs)
   a. Cyclophosphamide, 50 mg/m$^2$ PO q48h (dogs) or 200-300 mg/m$^2$ PO q3wk (cats), or
   b. Azathioprine, 50 mg/m$^2$ PO q24h for 7 days, then q48h (dogs only), or
   c. Cyclosporin, 15 mg/kg PO q24h (dogs only)
   d. Prednisone, 1 to 2 mg/kg PO q12-24h (cats only)
3. Antiinflammatory-hypercoagulability treatment: aspirin, 0.5 to 5 mg/kg PO q12h (dogs); 0.5 to 5 mg/kg PO q48h (cats)
4. Supportive care
   a. Dietary: sodium restriction, high-quality–low-quantity protein
   b. Hypertension: dietary sodium restriction; ACEIs (e.g., enalapril, 0.5 mg/kg PO q12-24h, and benazepril, 0.25-0.5 mg/kg PO q24h; ACEIs often have anti-proteinuric effects as well) and/or calcium channel blockers
   c. Edema and ascites: dietary sodium restriction; furosemide, 2.2 mg/kg PO q8-24h, if necessary

---

*ACEIs,* Angiotensin-converting enzyme inhibitors; *PO,* orally.

have been performed. The recommended dose is 0.025 mg/kg orally q24h. Increasing the frequency to q12h may be considered if the patient tolerates the initial dose for 2 weeks. However, adverse effects of colchicine include bone marrow toxicity.

*Angiotensin-converting enzyme inhibitors.* Angiotensin-converting enzyme inhibitors (ACEIs) such as enalapril decrease proteinuria, intrarenal hypertension, and systolic blood pressure in many nephrotic patients. Doses are given in Box 43-1. Note: ACEIs decrease renal excretory function in some patients.

Treatment with enalapril improved renal function and prolonged survival in male Samoyeds with hereditary nephritis, a primary glomerular disease that results in proteinuria and CRF in affected dogs before they are 1 year of age.

*Anticoagulant therapy.* Measurement of plasma antithrombin and fibrinogen concentrations helps determine which patients should be treated with anticoagulants. Dogs with antithrombin <70% of normal and fibrinogen >300 mg/dl are candidates for therapy. Antiplatelet drugs, heparin, and coumarins have been used. Low-dose aspirin (see Box 43-1) is easily administered at home and does not require extensive monitoring. Because fibrin accumulation within the glomerulus is a frequent consequence of GN, anticoagulant therapy may serve a dual purpose.

*Supportive care.* Supportive therapy is important in cats and dogs with GN or amyloidosis. High-quality, reduced-quantity protein diets are recommended; replacing urine protein loss with supplemental dietary protein is not recommended, because it tends to exacerbate proteinuria. Sodium-reduced diets (approximately 0.3% dry matter) are often recommended, but they are without proved benefit. Vasodilators and diuretics may be used as necessary to control systemic hypertension (see Box 43-1).

*Monitoring.* Monitoring $U_{pr}/U_{cr}$ and serum urea nitrogen and creatinine concentrations is important in patients undergoing immunosuppressive or antihypertensive treatment. If immunosuppressive therapy exacerbates the glomerular lesions and proteinuria, treatment should be altered or discontinued. Although proteinuria generally occurs before the onset of azotemia, GN can lead to CRI and failure, in which both GFR and proteinuria decrease. Management guidelines for CRF are given in Chapter 44.

### Prognosis

The prognosis for dogs and cats with immune-complex GN is fair to guarded unless the underlying disease process can be identified and corrected. Monitoring $U_{pr}/U_{cr}$ and serum urea nitrogen and creatinine concentrations during treatment helps determine the prognosis. Renal amyloidosis carries a guarded to poor prognosis. No specific treatment has proved to be effective, and the disease is progressive, ultimately resulting in CRF.

# 44

# Renal Failure

## *(Text pp 608-623)*

Renal failure occurs when approximately 75% of the nephrons of both kidneys cease to function. Acute renal failure (ARF) results from abrupt reduction in renal function and is usually caused by ischemic or toxic insult to the kidneys, although leptospirosis is reemerging as an important cause of ARF. Resulting tubular lesions and dysfunction may be reversible. In contrast, nephron damage associated with chronic renal failure (CRF) is usually irreversible. It occurs over weeks, months, or years and is a leading cause of death in dogs and cats. A specific cause is rarely determined once end-stage kidney damage is present.

## ACUTE RENAL FAILURE (TEXT PP 608-615)

ARF has the following three distinct phases:

1. Initiation. During this phase, therapies that reduce the renal insult can prevent development of established ARF.
2. Maintenance. This phase is characterized by tubular lesions and established nephron dysfunction. Therapeutic intervention during this phase is often lifesaving but usually does little to diminish existing renal lesions, improve function, or hasten recovery.
3. Recovery. This is the period during which renal lesions are repaired and function improves. Although new nephrons cannot be produced and irreversibly damaged nephrons cannot be repaired, hypertrophy of surviving nephrons may adequately compensate for the decrease in nephron numbers.

### Etiology

Boxes 44-1 and 44-2 present partial lists of potential nephrotoxicants and ischemic causes of ARF, respectively.

### Clinical features

Clinical signs of ARF are often nonspecific and include lethargy, depression, anorexia, vomiting, diarrhea, and dehydration; occasionally, uremic breath and/or oral ulcers are present. Signs tend to be severe when compared with those of CRF with the same magnitude of azotemia (see Table 41-6).

---

**Box 44-1**

## Partial List of Potential Nephrotoxicants in Dogs and Cats

**THERAPEUTIC AGENTS**
Antimicrobials
Aminoglycosides
Cephalosporins
Nafcillin
Polymyxins
Sulfonamides
Tetracyclines
Antifungals
Amphotericin B
Anthelmintics
Thiacetarsamide
Analgesics
Piroxicam
Ibuprofen
Phenylbutazone
Naproxen

**HEAVY METALS**
Lead
Mercury
Cadmium
Chromium

**ORGANIC COMPOUNDS**
Ethylene glycol
Carbon tetrachloride
Chloroform
Pesticides
Herbicides
Solvents

**PIGMENTS**
Hemoglobin
Myoglobin

**INTRAVENOUS AGENTS**
Radiographic contrast agents

**CHEMOTHERAPEUTIC AGENTS**
Cisplatin
Methotrexate
Doxorubicin

**ANESTHETICS**
Methoxyflurane

**MISCELLANEOUS AGENTS**
Hypercalcemia
Snake venom

---

**Box 44-2**

## Partial List of Potential Causes of Decreased Renal Perfusion and Ischemia in Dogs and Cats

Dehydration
Hemorrhage
Hypovolemia
Decreased oncotic pressure
Deep anesthesia
Increased blood viscosity
Sepsis
Shock and vasodilation
Administration of nonsteroidal antiinflammatory drugs
Hyperthermia
Hypothermia
Burns
Trauma
Renal vessel thrombosis or microthrombus formation

### Diagnosis

ARF occurs within hours or days of exposure to the insult. Unique signs and clinico-pathologic findings include enlarged or swollen kidneys, normal to high hematocrit, good body condition, active urine sediment (e.g., granular casts and renal epithelial cells), and relatively severe hyperkalemia and metabolic acidosis (especially in the face of oliguria). The diagnosis is confirmed when azotemia with concurrent isosthenuria or minimally concentrated urine persists.

*Prenal versus renal azotemia.* Prerenal dehydration and azotemia superimposed on an inability to concentrate urine (e.g., Addison's disease, hypercalcemia, or over-zealous use of furosemide) initially mimics renal failure, but volume replacement results in resolution of prerenal azotemia.

*Ultrasonography.* Ultrasonographic findings are usually nonspecific (normal or diffuse, slightly hyperechoic renal cortical echotexture). In patients with calcium oxalate nephrosis from ethylene glycol ingestion, the renal cortices can be very hyperechoic. Doppler estimation of resistive index in renal arcuate arteries is increased in many dogs with ARF.

*Biopsy.* Histopathologic examination of renal cortical biopsies reveals varying degrees of tubular necrosis. Evidence of tubular epithelial regeneration can be observed as early as 3 days after the acute insult. Histopathology does not allow differentiation between toxicant- and ischemia-induced ARF, but it is often helpful in establishing a prognosis. Evidence of tubular regeneration and generally intact basement membranes are good prognostic findings. Conversely, large numbers of granular casts, extensive tubular necrosis, and interstitial mineralization and fibrosis with disrupted tubular basement membranes are poor prognostic signs.

### Preventing ARF

#### Assessing risk

In many cases ARF inadvertently is caused in conjunction with diagnostic or thera-peutic procedures (e.g., use of potentially nephrotoxic drugs; hypotension and decreased renal perfusion during anesthesia and surgery). An important aspect of prevention of hospital-acquired ARF is identification of patients at increased risk. In some situations, predisposing factors can be eliminated or corrected before any potential renal insult occurs.

The following factors predispose dogs to ARF:

- preexisting renal disease or renal insufficiency
- dehydration
- decreased cardiac output
- sepsis, pyometra
- disseminated intravascular coagulation
- fever
- liver disease
- electrolyte abnormalities—e.g., hypokalemia, hypercalcemia
- concurrent use of potentially nephrotoxic drugs (see Box 44-1)
- concurrent use of diuretics and potentially nephrotoxic drugs (e.g., amino-glycosides)
- decreased dietary protein
- diabetes mellitus

These risk factors are additive, and any complication occurring in high-risk patients increases the potential for ARF. Patients with shock, acidosis, sepsis, vasculitis, fever, or major organ system failure and those undergoing prolonged anesthesia are at increased risk for ARF. These patients are also likely to require anesthesia or drugs that are potentially damaging to the kidneys. In otherwise healthy patients a combination of factors may also increase the potential for ARF (e.g., concurrent administration of furosemide and gentamicin).

*Potassium and gentamicin.* Reduced dietary potassium intake exacerbates gentamicin-induced nephrotoxicity, as potassium-depleted cells may be more susceptible to necrosis. Furthermore, high-dose gentamicin treatment increases urinary excretion of potassium, which could result in potassium depletion (especially if it occurs in combination with prolonged anorexia, vomiting, or diarrhea), and therefore increases the risk for gentamicin-induced nephrotoxicity.

***Nonsteroidal antiinflammatory drugs.*** Use of nonsteroidal antiinflammatory drugs (NSAIDs) increases the risk of ARF. Anesthesia, sodium and/or volume depletion, sepsis, congestive heart failure, nephrotic syndrome, and hepatic disease are conditions in which NSAIDs should be avoided. If NSAIDs are used preoperatively to reduce postoperative pain, the patient's hydration status and blood pressure should be carefully monitored during surgery.

### Monitoring at-risk patients

High-risk patients undergoing anesthesia and animals receiving potentially nephrotoxic drugs should be monitored closely. Urine production is an excellent parameter to monitor during anesthesia. Ideally, urine production is >2 ml/kg/hr. For patients receiving potentially nephrotoxic drugs, increased urinary excretion of protein, glucose (normoglycemic glucosuria), or casts may be an early indication of renal tubular damage.

***Enzymuria.*** Detection and quantification of urine enzymes can be used to identify early nephrotoxicity in dogs, as enzymuria usually precedes other manifestations of nephrotoxic proximal tubular injury by several days. Ratios of urine γ-glutamyltransferase (GGT) and *N*-acetyl glucosaminidase (NAG) to creatinine (Cr) accurately reflect 24-hour urine GGT and NAG excretion if measured before the onset of azotemia. Baseline urine GGT/Cr and NAG/Cr should be obtained in all dogs receiving potentially nephrotoxic drugs; twofold to threefold increases above baseline suggest clinically relevant tubular damage. Drug therapy should be discontinued at that point.

### Intervention

If renal damage is suspected, all potentially nephrotoxic drugs should be discontinued. Induction of emesis or gastric lavage should be considered in order to decrease the absorption of recently ingested toxicants. Gastrointestinal (GI) adsorbents and cathartics (e.g., activated charcoal and sodium sulfate) may also be beneficial. Peritoneal dialysis can be used to decrease blood concentrations of dialyzable toxicants (e.g., ethylene glycol, gentamicin). Diuresis should be initiated with isotonic saline intravenously (IV).

### Treatment guidelines

Treatment of ARF is outlined in Box 44-3. The goals are to correct renal hemodynamic disorders and alleviate water and solute imbalances in order to "buy time" for nephron repair and hypertrophy. A positive response is indicated by a decrease in serum Cr concentration and an increase in urine production. Identification and elimination of any prerenal or postrenal abnormalities also are essential.

### Fluid therapy

Fluid deficits should be replaced IV within 6 hours. Maintenance needs and replacement of continuing losses should be provided over a 24-hour period using 0.45% saline in 2.5% dextrose to prevent worsening of the potential hypernatremia and hyperkalemia.

***Monitoring urine output.*** Oliguria is common in patients with ARF; however, nonoliguric ARF can occur, so urine production should be quantified to properly assess fluid needs. Measurement of urine volume also allows assessment of endogenous Cr clearance (see Chapter 42), which provides a more accurate estimation of glomerular filtration rate (GFR) than does serum Cr alone. (Note: Uremic patients have depressed cellular immunity, and infection is a leading cause of death. Intermittent catheterization is usually preferable to indwelling catheters for timed urine collections.)

Diuresis decreases serum urea nitrogen and potassium concentrations and lessens the tendency for overhydration to occur. However, GFR and renal blood flow frequently are unchanged, and any increase in urine production is actually a result of decreased tubular resorption of filtrate. It is important to remember that increased urine production alone does not indicate an improvement in GFR.

***Acid-base status.*** During rehydration, acid-base and electrolyte status should be addressed. Metabolic acidosis and hyperkalemia are common in patients with oliguric

**Box 44-3**

## Treatment Guidelines for Dogs and Cats with Acute Renal Failure

Discontinue all potentially nephrotoxic drugs; consider measures to decrease absorption (e.g., induction of emesis and administration of activated charcoal and sodium sulfate).

Start specific antidotal therapy if applicable (e.g., alcohol dehydrogenase inhibitors for ethylene glycol).

Identify and treat any prerenal or postrenal abnormalities.

Start intravenous fluid therapy with normal saline solution or 0.45% saline solution in 2.5% dextrose:
  a. Rehydrate animal within 6 hours.
  b. Provide maintenance fluid and replace continuing fluid losses.

Assess volume of urine production.

Correct acid-base and electrolyte abnormalities; rule out hypercalcemic nephropathy.

If necessary to increase urine production, provide mild volume expansion while monitoring urine volume, body weight, plasma total solids, hematocrit, and central venous pressure.

Administer vasodilators, diuretics, or both, if necessary, to increase urine production:
  a. Mannitol or
  b. Furosemide and dopamine

Base subsequent fluid volumes on urine production plus 20 ml/kg/24 hr.

Consider peritoneal dialysis if no response to above treatment occurs; perform biopsy of kidney at time of dialysis catheter placement.

Control hyperphosphatemia:
  a. Phosphate-restricted diet and, if necessary,
  b. Enteric phosphate binders

Treat vomiting and gastroenteritis with the following:
  a. Metoclopramide or
  b. Trimethobenzamide or
  c. Chlorpromazine

Treat gastric hyperacidity with histamine-2 blockers.

Provide caloric requirements (70 to 100 kcal/kg/day).

ARF, but bicarbonate therapy should be reserved for patients whose blood pH is ≤7.15. Overzealous sodium bicarbonate therapy can create ionized calcium (Ca) deficits and sodium excesses.

***Treating hyperkalemia.*** Hyperkalemia is a life-threatening condition that occurs in dogs and cats with ARF. It is best diagnosed on the basis of serum potassium concentration; however, bradycardia and electrocardiographic changes (see Box 46-1) are other indicators. Hyperkalemia should be promptly treated with a slow intravenous bolus of 1 to 2 mEq/kg of sodium bicarbonate, or regular insulin (0.25 to 0.5 U/kg IV) followed by dextrose (4 ml of 50% dextrose per unit of insulin). Alternatively, calcium gluconate (0.5 to 1 ml/kg of 10% solution slowly IV while the electrocardiogram is monitored) may be used.

***Diuretics.*** If oliguria persists after rehydration, and no signs of overhydration are present, mild volume expansion with 3% to 5% of the patient's body weight in fluid may be initiated. If fluid therapy alone fails to induce diuresis, either mannitol or a combination of dopamine and furosemide can be administered. Doses are given in Table 44-7.

The combination of dopamine and furosemide is more effective for ischemic ARF than for toxicant-induced ARF, and it is a better choice than mannitol in overhydrated

## Potassium Supplementation Guidelines

| Measured serum potassium concentration (mEq/L) | Amount of KCl (mEq) to be added to each liter of fluid* |
|:---:|:---:|
| 3-3.5 | 28 |
| 2.5-3 | 40 |
| 2-2.5 | 60 |
| <2 | 80 |

*Do not administer at a rate of more than 0.5 mEq/kg/hr.

*KCl,* Potassium chloride.

patients. However, furosemide may potentiate gentamicin-induced nephrotoxicosis. Once diuresis occurs, polyionic solutions (e.g., Normosol or lactated Ringer's) should be used for maintenance. Potassium supplementation is often necessary and should be determined by measuring the serum potassium concentration (Table 44-1).

*Other measures.* Peritoneal dialysis should be considered in patients with severe, persistent azotemia, acidosis, or hyperkalemia. Dialysis may also be used to treat over-hydration and in some cases may hasten the elimination of toxicants. Renal biopsy should be performed if the diagnosis is in doubt, if the patient does not respond to therapy within 3 to 5 days, or if peritoneal dialysis is considered.

### Diet

Provision of daily caloric requirements is important; endogenous protein catabolism not only causes weight loss and muscle wasting but also increases blood urea nitrogen (BUN) concentrations. Reduced-protein diets and enteric phosphate binders (e.g., aluminum hydroxide or carbonate) should be used to reduce BUN concentrations and combat hyperphosphatemia in uremic dogs and cats (see the dietary guidelines for CRF given later). In some instances, adequate renal function can be regained, but reduced-protein diets should probably be continued if BUN concentrations are $>60$ mg/dl.

*Encouraging eating.* Inappetence resulting from gastric hyperacidity and vomiting can usually be controlled with histamine-2 ($H_2$)–receptor blockers (e.g., ranitidine) and central antiemetics (e.g., trimethobenzamide, metoclopramide; see Table 44-2). Administration of food mixed with water via stomach tube may be tolerated by animals that are anorexic but not vomiting.

### Prognosis

The long-term prognosis for animals with ARF is usually fair to good if the patient survives the period of renal regeneration and compensation (which may take several weeks or months). Severity of azotemia, histopathologic lesions, and response to therapy are the most important prognostic indicators. Recognition and appropriate treatment of renal injury in the initiation phase improve the prognosis.

## CHRONIC RENAL FAILURE (TEXT PP 615-622)

### Etiology

The cause of CRF is usually difficult to determine because the histologic end-point of irreversible glomerular or tubular damage is usually the same. Box 44-4 lists potential causes of CRF.

### Clinical features

CRF occurs over a period of weeks, months, or years, and signs are often relatively mild for the magnitude of azotemia (see Table 41-6). Unique features include a history of weight loss, polydipsia and polyuria, poor body condition, nonregenerative anemia, and small, irregular kidneys.

*Uremic syndrome.* Uremic syndrome occurs as a result of increasing plasma concentrations of substances normally excreted by the kidneys. Components include

---

**Box 44-4**

## Potential Causes of Chronic Renal Failure in Dogs and Cats

Immunologic disorders
  Systemic lupus erythematosus
  Glomerulonephritis
  Vasculitis (feline infectious peritonitis)
Amyloidosis
Neoplasia
  Primary
  Secondary
Nephrotoxicants
Renal ischemia
Inflammatory or infectious causes
  Pyelonephritis
  Leptospirosis
  Renal calculi
Hereditary and congenital disorders
  Renal hypoplasia or dysplasia
  Polycystic kidneys
  Familial nephropathies (Lhasa Apsos, Shih Tzus, Norwegian Elkhounds, Rottweilers, Bernese Mountain Dogs, Chow Chows, Newfoundlands, Bull Terriers, Pembroke Welsh Corgis, Chinese Shar Peis, Doberman Pinschers, Samoyeds, Golden Retrievers, Standard Poodles, Soft-Coated Wheaten Terriers, Cocker Spaniels, Beagles, Keeshonds, Bedlington Terriers, Cairn Terriers, Basenjis, Abyssinian cats)
Urinary outflow obstruction
Idiopathic

---

sodium and water imbalance, anemia, carbohydrate intolerance, neurologic disturbances, pneumonitis, GI disturbances, osteodystrophy, immunologic incompetence, and metabolic acidosis.

### Diagnosis
The diagnosis of CRF is usually based on a combination of historical, physical examination, and clinicopathologic findings. Small kidneys may be evident on plain radiographs. Ultrasonography usually reveals diffusely hyperechoic renal cortices (fibrosis) with loss of the normal corticomedullary boundary. Radiology and ultrasonography can also help rule out potentially treatable causes of CRF such as pyelonephritis and renal urolithiasis. Renal biopsy is not routinely performed on patients with CRF unless the diagnosis is in question.

### Treatment guidelines
Box 44-5 outlines the treatment approach for patients with CRF. Even though CRF is usually irreversible, the severity of the signs can generally be reduced. Treatment is directed at disorders that may contribute to the progression of renal failure (e.g., systemic hypertension, soft-tissue mineralization).

*Hydration.* It is important that animals with CRF always have water available. Dehydration can occur as a consequence of gastroenteritis and may cause a rapid and severe decline in renal function. If anorexia, vomiting, or diarrhea results in dehydration, deficits should be aggressively replaced parenterally. The volume of fluids needed depends on the degree of dehydration and on maintenance needs and continuing fluid losses.

Maintenance fluid needs in animals with CRF are higher than those of normal animals because of polyuria. Polyuria also results in increased loss of vitamins B and C,

---

**Box 44-5**

### Treatment Guidelines for Dogs and Cats with Chronic Renal Failure

Discontinue all potentially nephrotoxic drugs.

Identify and treat any prerenal or postrenal abnormalities.

Rule out or identify any treatable conditions such as pyelonephritis and renal urolithiasis by means of radiography or ultrasonography.

Measure blood pressure; consider treatment with ACEIs or calcium channel blockers if animal has systemic hypertension.

Initiate dietary protein reduction if moderate to severe azotemia (blood urea nitrogen 60 mg/dl) is present.

If animal has hyperphosphatemia, start a phosphorus-restricted diet and add enteric phosphate binders; consider use of calcitriol.

Treat vomiting and gastroenteritis, if present, with the following:
  a. Metoclopramide or
  b. Trimethobenzamide or
  c. Chlorpromazine
  d. $H_2$ blockers

Treat anemia, if present, with the following:
  a. Anabolic steroids
  b. Human recombinant erythropoietin

Provide caloric requirements (70-100 kcal/kg/day); consider the placement of a gastrostomy or esophagostomy tube if the animal is not vomiting.

---

*ACEIs,* Angiotensin-converting enzyme inhibitors; $H_2$, histamine 2.

---

which should be compensated for by dietary supplementation. If the patient is not able to drink enough to keep up with its urine output, daily subcutaneous fluids may be indicated; many owners are able to do this for their pets at home.

*Hypertension.* Hypertension is common in dogs and cats with CRF (approximately 60% of cases). Reduction of dietary salt intake is often recommended first, but in many cases angiotensin-converting enzyme inhibitors (ACEIs) or Ca channel blockers also are necessary (see Table 44-2 for doses). ACEIs may even slow the rate of progression of CRF.

*Acidosis.* Sodium bicarbonate or potassium citrate should be supplemented at a dose of 8 to 12 mEq/kg orally (PO) q12h to minimize metabolic acidosis. However, care must be taken, as overzealous bicarbonate treatment may aggravate hypertension and create ionized Ca deficits. When urine pH increases above 7 or plasma bicarbonate increases above 18 to 20 mEq/L, bicarbonate supplementation should be reduced or discontinued. Many protein-reduced prescription diets are already supplemented with potassium citrate, so further supplementation may be unnecessary.

*Hyperphosphatemia.* Management of hyperphosphatemia is closely related to dietary protein reduction (see below), in that restricting protein intake also reduces phosphorus (P) intake. Enteric phosphate binders (see Table 44-2) may also be necessary; however, they generally are ineffective if dietary P is not reduced.

#### Lowering serum parathyroid hormone concentration

Parathyroid hormone (PTH) production is indirectly stimulated by hyperphosphatemia. The consequences of hyperparathyroidism can be severe and include osteodystrophy, neuropathy, bone marrow suppression, and soft-tissue mineralization (which, if it occurs in the kidney, causes irreversible nephron damage and progressive decline in renal function).

*Calcitriol.* Reducing dietary P intake and using enteric phosphate binders usually lowers but does not normalize serum PTH concentration. Addition of ultra–low-dose calcitriol is effective when started early. Daily oral doses of 1.5 to 3.5 ng/kg in dogs and 1.5 ng/kg in cats are recommended. The proper calcitriol dose for that animal should be formulated by a compounding pharmacy.

Note: Calcitriol should be used only after hyperparathyroidism has been documented and the animal is well hydrated and is eating a P-reduced diet in conjunction with enteric phosphate binders (avoiding Ca-containing enteric phosphate binders). Ideally, serum PTH concentration should be measured before and 1, 3, and 6 months after starting calcitriol treatment to ensure that it has decreased and remains within the normal range (see text).

**Monitoring serum P and Ca.** Serum P should be <6 mg/dl before and during calcitriol treatment, and the product of Ca × P should be <70 mg/dl. Calcitriol can be given to CRF patients that are hypercalcemic, but serum Ca and Ca × P values must be evaluated frequently to ensure that they are improving.

A serum biochemistry profile should be obtained at 1 week and 1 month and then monthly. Hypercalcemia caused by ultra–low-dose calcitriol is rare and should resolve within 4 days of discontinuing the treatment; if it does not resolve, other potential causes (e.g., hypercalcemia of malignancy) should be investigated. If hyperphosphatemia develops during calcitriol treatment, further dietary P reduction and/or increased administration of enteric phosphate binders may be necessary.

### Diet

A reduction in dietary protein intake is the cornerstone of CRF management; it is usually recommended when the patient's BUN is 60 to 80 mg/dl. However, if dietary protein is too restricted, reduced renal hemodynamics, signs of protein depletion (decreased body weight, muscle mass, and serum albumin concentration), anemia, and acidosis can develop or worsen. Regardless, the patient's dietary carbohydrate and fat requirements must be met. Inadequate caloric intake stimulates the catabolism of endogenous proteins for energy, which exacerbates the signs of renal failure.

**Suitable diets.** Ideally, all essential amino acid requirements are met without excesses by feeding reduced quantities of high-biologic-value protein. Most commercial pet foods have a relatively high protein content. Suitable commercial diets include Hill's Prescription Diet k/d, Purina NF-formula diets, Iams Early and Advanced Stage renal failure diets, and Waltham Veterinarium medium- and low-protein diets. Homemade reduced-protein recipes are also available (see text).

Minimum protein requirements for patients with CRF are higher than those of normal animals. Dogs and cats with CRF should receive a minimum of 2 g and 3.3 g of protein/kg/day, respectively. A favorable response is indicated by stable body weight and serum Cr and albumin concentrations, with decreasing serum urea nitrogen and P concentrations.

### Managing GI signs

Vomiting may be treated with trimethobenzamide, metoclopramide, or chlorpromazine (see Table 44-2). Metoclopramide is the drug of choice. Chlorpromazine may cause hypotension and decreased renal blood flow, so it should be used only if other antiemetics are ineffective.

$H_2$-receptor blockers (e.g., ranitidine) effectively decrease gastric acid secretion, which may attenuate vomiting in dogs and cats with CRF (see Table 44-2). In dogs, xylocaine viscous (0.5 to 1 ml PO) before feeding often decreases pain associated with oral ulcers and encourages the patient to eat.

**Feeding tubes.** If vomiting can be controlled but the animal still will not eat enough to meet its daily caloric requirements, a feeding tube may be indicated. Gastrostomy tubes are tolerated very well by most cats, and they can remain in place for months. Esophagostomy and gastrostomy tubes also provide a relatively stress-free route for fluid therapy.

### Managing anemia

Anabolic steroids may be of benefit by promoting red cell production and a positive nitrogen balance. However, treatment extending over several months is usually required before a response is observed, and benefits are generally minimal.

***Erythropoietin.*** Recombinant human erythropoietin (r-HuEPO; Epogen, 100 U/kg subcutaneously three times per week) can be effective in dogs and cats with anemia of CRF. It often improves appetite, weight gain, strength, and the sense of well-being. The dose is decreased or the dose interval lengthened once the target packed cell volume (35% to 40% in dogs and 30% to 35% in cats) is reached. Oral iron supplementation may be necessary during treatment because rapid erythropoiesis can deplete iron stores.

Note: Potential for antibody formation against r-HuEPO exists. These antibodies may also react with endogenous erythropoietin, making the dog or cat transfusion dependent.

### Other recommendations

Uremic animals are more susceptible to life-threatening infections. Indwelling urinary catheters should be used only if necessary and only with aseptic technique and closed collection systems. Prophylactic antibiotic therapy is not recommended, however; instead, treatment of urinary tract infections should be based on bacterial culture and sensitivity results. Potentially nephrotoxic antibiotics such as gentamicin should be avoided.

***Drugs.*** Patients with CRF are good candidates for adverse drug reactions. Package inserts should be studied to determine the route of drug excretion, potential for toxicity, and dosage adjustment (increased interval or decreased dosage) for patients in renal failure. Usually, dosage adjustment is not necessary if serum Cr is <2.5 mg/dl.

***Stress.*** Stressful situations should be avoided. Many patients with CRF are geriatric animals that respond better to outpatient treatment than to hospitalization.

***Reassessment.*** Follow-up examinations should be performed every 2 to 4 months. Body weight, complete blood count, serum biochemistry, and urinalysis should be assessed at each recheck.

### Prognosis

Renal lesions associated with CRF are usually irreversible and often progressive; treatment rarely improves renal function.

**Table 44-2**

## Drugs Used in Dogs and Cats with Acute and Chronic Renal Failure

| Drug | Action | Dosage |
|---|---|---|
| Aluminum hydroxide (Dialume, Amphojel) | Enteric phosphate binder | 10-30 mg/kg q8h PO, with or immediately after meals |
| Amlodipine besylate (Norvasc) | Calcium antagonist | 2.5 mg/dog or 0.1 mg/kg PO q24h (dog); 0.625 mg/cat/day PO (cats) |
| Benazepril (Lotensin) | ACEI | 0.25-0.5 mg/kg q24h |
| Chlorpromazine (Thorazine) | Antiemetic | 0.25-0.5 mg/kg q6-8h IM, SC, PO, after rehydration only |
| Cimetidine (Tagamet) | $H_2$ blocker | 2.5-5 mg/kg q6-8h PO, IV, IM |
| Dopamine (Intropin) | Renal vasodilator | 2-10 µg/kg/min IV |
| Enalapril (Enacard) | ACEI | 0.25-0.5 mg/kg q12-24h PO (dogs); 6.25 mg/cat q12h PO (cats) |
| Erythropoietin (r-HuEPO) (Epogen) | Erythropoieses | Doses range from 35-50 U/kg three times per week to 400 U/kg/week IV, SC (adjust dose to PCV of 30%-35%) |
| Famotidine (Pepcid) | $H_2$ blocker | 0.5 mg/kg q12-24h IM, SC, PO |
| Furosemide (Lasix) | Loop diuretic | 2-4 mg/kg q8-12h IV, PO |
| Hydralazine (Apresoline) | Arterial vasodilator | 0.5-2 mg/kg q8-12h PO (dogs); 2.5-5 mg/cat q12-24h PO (cats) |
| Lisinopril (Prinivil, Zestril) | ACEI | 0.5 mg/kg PO q24h (dogs) |
| Mannitol | Osmotic diuretic | 0.5-1 g/kg as 20%-25% solution, slow IV bolus over 5-10 min |
| Metoclopramide (Reglan) | Antiemetic | 0.2-0.5 mg/kg q8-24h PO, SC |
| Nandrolone decanoate (Deca-Durabolin) | Anabolic steroid | 1-1.5 mg/kg every week IM (dogs); 1 mg/cat every week IM (cats) |
| Ranitidine (Zantac) | $H_2$ blocker | 2 mg/kg q24h PO, IV (dogs); 2.5 mg/kg q12h IV, 3.5 mg/kg q12h PO (cats) |
| Sodium bicarbonate or potassium citrate | Alkalinization | 8-12 mEq/kg q12h PO |
| Trimethobenzamide (Tigan) | Antiemetic | 3 mg/kg q8h IM (dogs) |

*ACEI*, Angiotensin-converting enzyme inhibitor; $H_2$, histamine 2; *IM*, intramuscularly; *IV*, intravenously; *r-HuEPO*, recombinant human erythropoietin; *PCV*, packed cell volume; *PO*, orally; *SC*, subcutaneously.

# 45

# Urinary Tract Infections

## *(Text pp 624-630)*

Urinary tract infections (UTIs) are more common in dogs than in cats. Most UTIs in dogs involve bacterial inflammation of the lower urinary tract, although ascension of bacteria to the ureters and kidneys is a potential sequela. Mycoplasmal, chlamydial, viral, and fungal UTIs are rare.

### Etiology

The most common pathogens are *Escherichia coli* (45%), *Staphylococcus* (13%), and *Proteus* (10%). Pathogens isolated in <10% of cases include *Enterococcus, Klebsiella, Streptococcus, Enterobacter,* and *Pseudomonas.* Although UTIs usually involve a single organism, mixed infections are found in 20% to 30% of cases. Anaerobes rarely cause UTI.

***Contributing factors.*** Bacterial virulence, the number of invading organisms, and host defense mechanisms are important factors that influence the establishment of UTIs. Disorders that decrease the frequency and/or volume of voided urine or that result in increased urine residual volume predispose animals to UTI; and conditions that result in dilute urine (e.g., polydipsia and polyuria disorders) reduce the antibacterial properties of normal, concentrated urine. Urethral length and bactericidal prostatic secretions in male dogs contribute to the lower incidence of UTI compared with that in female dogs.

***Catheterization.*** Catheterization of the bladder is a considerable risk factor for UTI. Any time the bladder is catheterized, bacteria are carried up the urethra to the bladder. If the catheter damages the bladder mucosa, the chance of infection increases greatly.

***Uncomplicated versus complicated UTIs.*** Uncomplicated UTIs are infections without underlying structural or functional abnormalities. The infection is usually cleared soon after appropriate antibiotic treatment is initiated.

Defective host defense mechanisms, such as anatomic defects, mucosal damage (e.g., urolithiasis, neoplasia), and conditions that alter urine volume or composition (e.g., renal failure, hyperadrenocorticism, prolonged corticosteroid administration, neoplasia, diabetes mellitus), can complicate UTIs. Elimination of infection with antibiotic treatment alone usually does not occur; signs either persist during treatment or recur shortly after antibiotic withdrawal. Any UTI in a male dog should be considered a complicated infection.

### Clinical features

Lower urinary tract inflammation often results in pollakiuria, stranguria or dysuria, and gross or microscopic hematuria. Patients with acute bacterial pyelonephritis or prostatitis may manifest nonspecific systemic signs (e.g., lethargy, depression, anorexia, fever, leukocytosis), which rarely occur with lower UTIs. However, systemic signs are often absent in patients with chronic pyelonephritis and prostatitis.

### Diagnosis

Cystocentesis is the best method of urine collection for analysis and bacterial culture. When catheterization, voiding, or bladder expression is used, the number of organisms per milliliter must be determined to differentiate infection from contamination (see Chapter 41). Urine bacterial culture and antibiotic sensitivity testing should be used to confirm the presence and type of bacteria, to guide antibiotic choices, and, in cases of recurrent UTI, to help differentiate relapse from reinfection (see text p 626).

*Urinalysis.* Findings compatible with lower UTI include bacteriuria, hematuria, pyuria, and increased numbers of transitional epithelial cells in the urine sediment. Increased protein concentration and alkaline pH may also be observed. However, bacteria and sediment abnormalities are not always found, especially with hyposthenuric or isosthenuric urine. (Note: Some urine dipsticks have a nitrate pad to detect nitrate-reducing bacteria. This test is inaccurate in dogs and cats.)

*Lower versus upper UTI.* Differentiating lower urinary infection from upper tract involvement or prostatitis is difficult, but it should be attempted to prevent renal damage in patients with pyelonephritis. Cylindruria, especially white blood cell (WBC) casts, indicates the presence of renal disease and, if coupled with a significant bacteriuria, is highly suggestive of bacterial pyelonephritis. Abnormalities that can be associated with bacterial pyelonephritis are summarized in Box 45-1.

*Further investigation.* It is important to identify patients with immune system disorders that predispose to UTI. Examples include diabetes mellitus, hyperadrenocorticism, chronic renal failure, urolithiasis, urachal remnants, excessive perivulvar skin folds or pyoderma, and incontinence. Complete physical examination should be performed on all animals with signs of UTI. Also, urinalysis and culture should be performed on all animals with suspected immune system defects.

## Management

Treatment guidelines are summarized in Box 45-2. Verification of appropriate antibiotic selection can be made after 3 to 5 days of therapy by ensuring that the urine is sterile. (Note: Urine sediment may still be abnormal at this time.) Therapy can be discontinued once signs have resolved, urine sediment is normal, and urine culture is negative. In general, uncomplicated lower UTI should be treated for 2 to 3 weeks, and complicated UTI should be treated for a minimum of 4 weeks.

### Acute, uncomplicated UTI

If bacterial sensitivity results are unavailable, antibiotic choice should be based on bacterial identification. Table 45-1 lists antibiotic sensitivities for the common urinary pathogens. If bacterial identity is unknown, treatment should be based on the gram-staining characteristics: ampicillin, amoxicillin, or amoxicillin-clavulanic acid for gram-positive (G+) bacteria, and trimethoprim-sulfa or enrofloxacin for gram-negative (G–) bacteria.

---

**Box 45-1**

### Clinicopathologic Findings That Can Be Associated with Bacterial Pyelonephritis in Dogs and Cats

Fever, leukocytosis, renal pain

Cellular casts in urine sediment

Renal failure (e.g., azotemia, inability to concentrate urine, polydipsia-polyuria)

Excretory urogram and ultrasonographic abnormalities (i.e., renal pelvis dilatation or asymmetric filling of diverticula, dilatec ureters)

Bacteria in inflammatory lesions identified by renal histologic studies

Positive result from bacterial culture of ureteral urine obtained at cystoscopy (Stamey test)

Positive result from bacterial culture of urine obtained after rinsing bladder with sterile saline solution (Fairley test)

Positive result from bacterial culture of fluid aspirated from the renal pelvis (pyelocentesis) under ultrasound guidance

---

**Box 45-2**

### Ideal Steps to Follow in the Management of Urinary Tract Infections in Dogs and Cats

Determine diagnosis on the basis of history, urine sediment, and, ideally, urine culture and sensitivity findings.

Select an antimicrobial agent.

Reculture urine in 3-5 days to ascertain effectiveness of selected antimicrobial agent.

Examine urine sediment 3 or 4 days before discontinuing antibiotic treatment.

Repeat urinalysis and culture 10-14 days after cessation of antibiotic therapy.

Patients with recurrent urinary tract infections should undergo contrast-enhanced radiography or ultrasonography, complete blood count, and serum biochemistry profile to determine whether they have underlying predisposing factors.

Frequent reinfections may need to be treated with prophylactic doses of antibiotics after the initial inflammation has been cleared up in response to standard-dose antibiotic treatment.

---

**Table 45-1**

### Antimicrobial Agents to Which >90% of Urinary Isolates Are Susceptible in Vitro at Concentrations <25% of the Expected Urine Concentration

| Organism | Antimicrobial agents |
| --- | --- |
| Escherichia coli* | Trimethoprim-sulfa |
| | Fluoroquinolone |
| | Amoxicillin–clavulanic acid |
| Coagulase-positive *Staphylococcus* spp. | Amoxicillin |
| | Chloramphenicol |
| | Trimethoprim-sulfa |
| | Cephalosporin (first generation) |
| *Proteus mirabilis* | Amoxicillin |
| | Fluoroquinolone |
| | Cephalosporin (first, second, or third generation) |
| | Amoxicillin–clavulanic acid |
| *Klebsiella pneumoniae** | Cephalosporin (first, second, or third generation) |
| | Fluoroquinolone |
| | Amoxicillin–clavulanic acid |
| | Trimethoprim-sulfa |
| *Streptococcus* spp. | Amoxicillin |
| | Amoxicillin–clavulanic acid |
| | Chloramphenicol |
| | Cephalosporin (first, second, or third generation) |
| *Pseudomonas aeruginosa* | Tetracycline |
| | Fluoroquinolone |
| | Carbenicillin |
| *Enterobacter* spp.* | Trimethoprim-sulfa |
| | Fluoroquinolone |
| *Enterococcus* spp. | Fluoroquinolone |
| | Trimethoprim-sulfa |
| | Chloramphenicol |
| | Tetracycline |

*These bacteria are capable of undergoing major changes in their susceptibility to antibiotics and are therefore less predictable.

### Complicated UTI

Long-term (4- to 6-week) antibiotic treatment is required for complicated UTI, and careful follow-up examinations should be performed. When antibiotic treatment is used for this period of time, adverse effects should be considered. Keratoconjunctivitis sicca may occur with long-term use of trimethoprim-sulfa (rare), and nephrotoxicity is always a concern with aminoglycosides, even with short-term treatment.

### Unresponsive cases

Several possible reasons exist for a poor response to therapy:

- use of ineffective drugs or ineffective duration of therapy
- failure of owner to administer prescribed dose at proper intervals
- decreased drug absorption—e.g., gastrointestinal disease, concurrent intake of certain foods or drugs
- impaired drug action—e.g., bacteria are not multiplying or are sequestered in an inaccessible site (prostate gland, urolith)
- failure to recognize and eliminate predisposing causes
- presence of a mixed bacterial infection in which one or more pathogens is not susceptible to the antimicrobial agent being used
- iatrogenic reinfection caused by catheterization
- development of drug resistance in the bacteria involved

### Recurrent infection

Recurrence of UTI can be classified as relapse or reinfection. Relapses are caused by the same bacteria and occur within days or weeks of the end of treatment. They can result from use of improper antibiotic or dosage, emergence of drug-resistant pathogens, or failure to eliminate predisposing causes. Relapses in male dogs can be caused by chronic prostatic infections.

With reinfection, antibacterial treatment cleared the first infection, but the urinary tract subsequently became infected with another bacterium. The interval between re-infections (>2 weeks) generally is longer than the interval between relapses. Reinfection often indicates failure to eliminate predisposing causes; alternatively the infection may be iatrogenic (e.g., catheterization). Reinfection with less invasive bacteria (e.g., *Pseudomonas aeruginosa*, *Klebsiella pneumoniae*, *Enterobacter cloacae*) suggests that the host's immune system is compromised.

*Evaluation.* Recurrent UTI should always be evaluated by urine culture and sensitivity, and intensified attempts should be made to identify contributing factors. Double-contrast cystography and ultrasonography may rule out anatomic abnormalities, mucosal bladder lesions, and urolithiasis. In intact male dogs, semen and prostatic wash cytology and culture and ultrasonography should be used to rule out bacterial prostatitis. Excretory urography, ultrasonography, and renal biopsy may confirm the presence of pyelonephritis, although results may be normal in animals with chronic pyelonephritis. Finally, asymptomatic hyperadrenocorticism should be considered, especially when low numbers of WBCs and red blood cells are present in the urine sediment.

*Antibiotic therapy.* For animals with frequent reinfection associated with host defense mechanism problems that cannot be cured, low-dose (one third to one half dose) antimicrobial therapy, given at bedtime, may be useful. The drug remains in the bladder overnight, supplementing the animal's defense mechanisms. For recurrences caused by G+ bacteria, penicillins are recommended; for recurrences caused by G–bacteria, trimethoprim-sulfa or enrofloxacin is recommended. However, it is important to bear in mind that low-dose, long-term antibiotic treatment can predispose to resistant UTIs.

*Urinary acidifiers.* Ammonium chloride has been advocated as adjunctive therapy. Acidic urine is mildly antibacterial, and it may also optimize the effect of certain antibiotics (e.g., penicillin, ampicillin, carbenicillin, tetracycline, nitrofurantoin). Ammonium chloride (60 to 100 mg/kg orally [PO] q12h) is given to maintain urine pH at 6.5. This strategy is not without risk, however, especially in male dogs. Oxalate, silicate, urate, and cystine are less soluble in acidic urine, and urolithiasis can result from excessive acidification.

***Urinary antiseptics.*** Urinary antiseptics have also been advocated as adjunctive therapy. Antiseptics are less effective than specific antimicrobial therapy but are probably more effective than urinary acidifiers. Methenamine mandelate (10 mg/kg PO q6h in dogs) is the most commonly used drug. It should be used with ammonium chloride to enhance its effectiveness. Methylene blue is a weak urinary antiseptic agent that used to be common in combination products designed to treat lower urinary tract inflammation. However, methylene blue should not be used in cats because of its potential to cause Heinz bodies and anemia. Phenazopyridine, a urinary tract analgesic, also should not be used in cats.

# 46

# Canine Urolithiasis

## *(Text pp 631-641)*

Most uroliths in dogs are found in the bladder or urethra; only approximately 5% are located in the kidneys or ureters. Uroliths are usually named according to their mineral content. Approximately 50% of canine uroliths are composed of struvite (magnesium ammonium phosphate). Other types include calcium oxalate (33%), urate (8%), cystine (1%), and silicate (1%). Mixed uroliths (containing <70% of any one mineral type) constitute approximately 7% of all uroliths.

### Etiology
Conditions that contribute to crystallization of salts and urolith formation include (1) high urinary concentration of salts, (2) urine retention, (3) favorable urine pH for crystallization, (4) a nidus on which crystallization can occur, and (5) inadequate concentrations of crystallization inhibitors in the urine. The greater the urine concentration of salts and the less often voiding occurs (e.g., decreased water intake), the greater the chance of urolith formation. High dietary intake of minerals and protein and the ability of dogs to produce highly concentrated urine contribute to urine supersaturation.

Certain breed and gender predispositions are recognized for specific types of urolithiasis in dogs. These and other features are summarized in Table 46-1.

***Struvite uroliths.*** Most canine diets are rich in minerals and protein, which frequently results in urine supersaturation with magnesium, ammonium, and phosphate. Consistently high urine pH, potentially caused by drugs, diet, or renal tubular disorders, also facilitates struvite urolith formation. Urinary tract infection (UTI) is another important predisposing factor, as bacterial infection may increase the production of ammonium and phosphate ions.

***Calcium oxalate uroliths.*** Factors involved in formation of calcium oxalate stones are not completely understood but likely include increased urine calcium concentrations. Hypercalciuria can occur with defective tubular resorption of calcium, overt hypercalcemia (e.g., primary hyperparathyroidism, neoplasia, vitamin D intoxication), certain drugs (e.g., glucocorticoids, furosemide), and dietary supplementation with calcium or salt. An association between hyperadrenocorticism and calcium-containing uroliths has been identified in dogs.

**Table 46-1**

## Factors That Help Predict Urolith Composition

| Urolith type | Clinicopathologic abnormalities | Common affected ages (yr) | Commonly affected breeds | Gender predisposition | Urinary tract infection | Usual urine pH | Radiographic density (1-3 scale) |
|---|---|---|---|---|---|---|---|
| Magnesium ammonium phosphate (struvite) | Usually none | 1-8 | Miniature Schnauzer, Bichon Frise, Cocker Spaniel, Miniature Poodle | Female (>80%) | Very common, especially urease-producing bacteria (e.g., *Staphylococcus, Proteus*) | Neutral to alkaline | 2.5 |
| Calcium oxalate | Occasional hypercalcemia | 5-12 | Miniature Schnauzer, Miniature Poodle, Yorkshire Terrier, Lhasa Apso, Bichon Frise, Shih Tzu, Cairn Terrier | Male (>70%) | Rare | Acidic to neutral | 3 |
| Urate | Decreased BUN and serum albumin and abnormal preprandial and postprandial SBA in dogs with PSS | 1-4 | Dalmatian, English Bulldog, Miniature Schnauzer (PSS), Yorkshire Terrier (PSS) | Male (>90%) | Uncommon | Acidic to neutral | 1 |
| Cystine | Usually none | 1-7 | Dachshund, Basset Hound, English Bulldog, Yorkshire Terrier, Irish Terrier, Rottweiler, Chihuahua, Mastiff, Tibetan Spaniel | Male (>95%) | Rare | Acidic | 1.5 |
| Silicate | Usually none | 4-9 | German Shepherd, Golden Retriever, Labrador Retriever, Old English Sheepdog | Male (>95%) | Uncommon | Acidic to neutral | 2.5 |

*BUN,* Serum urea nitrogen; *PSS,* portosystemic shunt; *SBA,* serum bile acids.

Decreased urine concentrations of calcium oxalate crystallization inhibitors (glycosaminoglycans, Tamm-Horsfall protein, osteopontine, citrate), defective urinary nephrocalcin, or increased dietary intake of oxalate (e.g., vegetables, grass, vitamin C) may also play a role in dogs.

Calcium oxalate solubility is increased in urine with a pH >6.5, whereas a urine pH of <6.5 favors calcium oxalate crystal formation. The overall prevalence of these uroliths in dogs has increased significantly in recent years, perhaps because of the increased use of urine-acidifying diets. Obesity also appears to increase the risk for calcium oxalate urolithiasis.

**Urate uroliths.** Most urate uroliths are composed of ammonium acid urate. These stones are more common in Dalmatians and English Bulldogs, but they can occur in any dog with hepatic insufficiency resulting from portosystemic shunt (PSS) or cirrhosis. UTIs, especially those caused by urease-producing bacteria, facilitate ammonium acid urate crystallization.

Approximately 60% of urate uroliths occur in Dalmatians, and approximately 75% of uroliths in Dalmatians are urate. Urinary uric acid excretion in Dalmatians is approximately 10 times that of other dogs; however, only a small percentage of Dalmatians form urate stones. Males are at greater risk than females (approximately 16:1).

**Cystine uroliths.** Cystinuria is an inherited disorder of renal tubular transport and a primary factor in cystine urolith formation, although not all dogs with cystinuria develop cystine uroliths. These stones are most often found in male Dachshunds.

**Silicate uroliths.** Silicate uroliths frequently have a jack-shaped appearance, although not all jackstones are silicates (ammonium urate and struvite uroliths may also be jack-shaped). The cause is unknown but is probably related to dietary intake of silicates (e.g., consumption of corn gluten and/or soybean hulls).

### Clinical features

Clinical signs depend on the number, type, and location of the uroliths. Most stones are located in the bladder, so signs of cystitis (hematuria, pollakiuria, dysuria, and stranguria) are common; mucosal irritation is more severe with jack-shaped uroliths.

In males small uroliths may pass into the urethra, causing partial or complete obstruction and signs of bladder distention, dysuria and stranguria, and postrenal azotemia (depression, anorexia, vomiting). Uroliths frequently lodge at the caudal aspect of the os penis. Occasionally, the bladder or urethra ruptures, resulting in abdominal effusion or subcutaneous perineal fluid accumulation and postrenal azotemia.

**Renal and ureteral uroliths.** Patients with unilateral renal uroliths may be asymptomatic, or they may have hematuria and chronic pyelonephritis. Bilateral renal uroliths, especially if associated with pyelonephritis, frequently lead to chronic renal failure. Dogs with ureteral uroliths may also be asymptomatic, or they may have hematuria and abdominal pain. Unilateral obstruction of a ureter often results in unilateral hydronephrosis without evidence of decreased renal function.

### Diagnosis

Diagnosis is usually based on history, physical examination, and radiography or ultrasonography. In male dogs with dysuria and stranguria, attempted passage of a urinary catheter is often met with "gritty-feeling" resistance if urethral stones are present. Uroliths >10 mm in any dimension are likely to be struvite. Struvite uroliths in the bladder are most likely to be smooth, blunt-edged or faceted, or pyramidal.

The diagnosis can usually be confirmed with plain or retrograde positive contrast urethrography. Some cystouroliths can be detected by abdominal palpation. Plain radiographs and ultrasonography usually confirm their presence unless the stones are radiolucent (see Table 46-1) or very small. Double-contrast cystography is the most sensitive diagnostic tool. Ultrasonography works well for confirming the presence of renoliths and hydronephrosis or hydroureter.

### Treatment

Treatment must include relief of urethral obstruction and decompression of the bladder, if necessary. Options include passage of a small-bore urethral catheter, cystocentesis, dislodgment of urethral calculi by hydropulsion, or emergency urethrotomy.

---

**Box 46-1**

### Electrocardiographic Findings and Treatment Recommendations for Dogs and Cats with Hyperkalemia

**ELECTROCARDIOGRAPHIC FINDINGS**
Bradycardia
Flattened waves
Prolonged PR interval
Widened QRS complexes
Tall or spiked T waves
Arrhythmias

**TREATMENT RECOMMENDATIONS**
Fluid therapy with 0.9% saline solution
Slow IV bolus of regular insulin (0.25-0.5 U/kg), followed by 50% dextrose (4 ml/U of administered insulin), or
Slow IV bolus of sodium bicarbonate (1-2 mEq/kg), or
Slow IV bolus of 10% calcium gluconate (0.5-1 ml/kg while monitoring the ECG)

---

*ECG,* Electrocardiogram; *IV,* intravenous.

Fluid therapy should be initiated to restore water and electrolyte balance if postrenal azotemia or uremia exists.

*Hyperkalemia.* Potentially life-threatening hyperkalemia can occur in dogs with urethral obstruction or rupture of the bladder or urethra. Serum potassium, BUN, and creatinine concentrations should be measured in patients with suspected obstruction. Alternatively, bradycardia and electrocardiographic findings suggestive of hyperkalemia (Box 46-1) support the need for aggressive treatment to lower the serum potassium concentration.

*Medical versus surgical management.* Although medical dissolution of struvite, urate, and cystine uroliths can be effective (Table 46-2), the choice between surgical removal and medical dissolution is not always clear. Surgery allows definitive diagnosis of urolith type, correction of predisposing anatomic abnormalities (e.g., urachal remnants, bladder polyps), and bladder mucosal sampling for bacterial culture if urine yields no growth; however, it usually does not decrease the rate of urolith recurrence.

Medical treatment decreases the concentration of calculogenic salts in the urine and increases urine salt solubility and urine volume, but a high level of owner commitment is required over several weeks or months. Also, some uroliths (calcium oxalate, calcium phosphate, silicate, and mixed uroliths) are not responsive to medical dissolution. Patients with obstructive uropathy cannot be treated with medical management alone, although voiding urohydropulsion (see text) or catheter urolith retrieval can be used to nonsurgically remove some cystouroliths. Lithotripsy (available at some referral centers) has been used successfully to treat nephroliths and ureteroliths in dogs.

*Reevaluation.* Whenever medical dissolution is attempted, the patient should be reexamined at least monthly. Complete urinalysis should be done, and abdominal radiography or ultrasonography performed to assess urolith size. If urinalysis findings are suggestive of UTI, bacterial culture and sensitivity should be performed and antibiotic treatment initiated or adjusted accordingly. If urolith size is not decreased after 2 months of treatment, then owner compliance, control of infection, and urolith type should be reassessed, and surgical removal considered.

*Recurrence rates.* Recurrence occurs in up to 25% of cases; it is relatively common for individual dogs to have three or more episodes of urolithiasis. Recurrence is greatest in dogs with metabolic uroliths (calcium oxalate, urate, cystine) or familial predispositions

Table 46-2

## Treatment and Prevention of Urolithiasis in Dogs

| Urolith type | Treatment options | Prevention |
|---|---|---|
| Struvite | Surgical removal or dissolution:<br>Hill's s/d diet<br>Control infection<br>Urease inhibitor?<br>Keep urine pH <6.5, BUN <10 mg/dl, and uSG <1.020 | Hill's c/d diet<br>Monitor urine pH and sediment, and treat any infections quickly and appropriately |
| Calcium oxalate | Surgical removal | Hill's u/d diet?<br>Potassium citrate? |
| Urate | Surgical removal or dissolution:<br>Hill's u/d diet<br>Allopurinol (7-10 mg/kg q8-24h PO)<br>Control infection | Hill's u/d diet<br>Allopurincl if necessary |
| Silicate | Surgical removal | Hill's u/d diet<br>Prevent consumption of dirt and grass |
| Cystine | Surgical removal or dissolution:<br>Hill's u/d diet<br>N-(2-mercaptopropionyl)-glycine (15-20 mg/kg q12h PO) | Hill's u/d diet<br>Thiol-containing drugs, if necessary |

*BUN,* Blood urea nitrogen; *PO,* orally; *uSG,* urine specific gravity.

(e.g., Miniature Schnauzers with struvite uroliths). Appropriate preventive measures and frequent reevaluation are important.

### Prevention

General preventive measures include induction of diuresis and eradication of UTI. Addition of 0.5 to 1 g of salt/day (1 tsp = 3.5 g of sodium chloride) to the diet is often recommended, with certain important exceptions. Some commercial diets formulated for the management of canine urolithiasis are high in salt and should not be further supplemented. Prevention or dissolution of calcium oxalate and cystine uroliths should not include increased dietary salt. Salt should not be used in hypertensive patients.

Maintenance of urine specific gravity <1.020 is ideal, and dogs should be given frequent opportunities to void. Urine sediment and pH should be monitored regularly, and UTIs treated promptly on the basis of bacterial culture and sensitivity (see Chapter 45).

### Struvite uroliths

Struvite uroliths can usually be dissolved by feeding Hill's Canine Prescription Diet s/d. The average time for dissolution is 8 to 10 weeks (range, 2 weeks to 7 months, depending on urolith size). Sterile uroliths usually dissolve more rapidly than those associated with UTIs (range, 1 to 3 months). Hill's s/d should be fed for at least 1 month after the calculi have disappeared radiographically.

*Precautions.* Hill's s/d cannot be fed as a maintenance diet and should not be used during pregnancy, lactation or growth or after surgery. It should not be fed to dogs with congestive heart failure, hypertension, or nephrotic syndrome. This diet will not dissolve nonstruvite uroliths, and it is not effective if UTI persists or if anything in addition to s/d is fed. In Miniature Schnauzers the high fat content of s/d may exacerbate any lipid abnormalities and increase the risk for pancreatitis.

*Controlling UTI.* Elimination of any bacterial UTI is essential. Antibiotics should be given throughout the course of medical dissolution; selection is based on urine culture and sensitivity. When severe or persistent UTIs are caused by urease-producing bacteria, acetohydroxamic acid may be added at a dose of 12.5 mg/kg PO q12h. Treatment with urinary acidifiers in conjunction with the s/d diet usually is not recommended.

*Long-term management.* Measures to prevent recurrence include prevention and control of UTI, maintenance of acidic urine, and decrease in dietary intake of calculogenic salts. Hill's Canine Prescription Diet c/d is a good maintenance diet; 0.5 g of salt (approximately 1/8 tsp) should be added daily to increase water consumption and urine production.

In dogs with recurrent UTIs, predisposing abnormalities and hyperadrenocorticism should be ruled out (see Chapter 45). Occasionally, long-term, lower-dose antibiotic treatment is necessary. Routine urinalysis should be performed every 2 to 4 months in asymptomatic patients, and follow-up urine cultures in patients with signs of lower urinary tract inflammation.

### Calcium oxalate uroliths

Medical dissolution of oxalate uroliths currently is not possible. Moderate restriction of dietary protein, calcium, oxalate, and sodium is recommended to prevent recurrence after surgical removal. Hill's Canine u/d is preferred, without added salt. Potassium citrate (40 to 75 mg/kg PO q12h) may also be beneficial; however, overzealous urine alkalization may result in the formation of calcium phosphate stones. Thiazide diuretics such as hydrochlorothiazide (2 mg/kg PO q12h) decrease urine calcium excretion in dogs, an effect that can be enhanced by combining treatment with the u/d diet.

### Urate uroliths

For urate uroliths that are not associated with hepatic insufficiency, medical dissolution consists of a low-protein diet, urine alkalization, allopurinol, and elimination of UTI. Hill's Canine u/d is recommended for dissolution and prevention; 0.5 to 1 g of salt/day (1/8 to 1/4 tsp) may be added to increase water consumption and urine production in nonhypertensive patients.

*Allopurinol.* Allopurinol is given at a dose of 10 to 15 mg/kg PO q12-24h, and if necessary sodium bicarbonate or potassium citrate (Urocrit-K, starting with 1/4 tablet PO q8h) is added to maintain a urine pH of 7. Long-term use of allopurinol may increase the risk for xanthine urolithiasis, but in patients with multiple episodes of urate urolithiasis, the benefits may outweigh the risks.

*Hepatic insufficiency.* In dogs with urate stones secondary to hepatic insufficiency, the underlying disorder should be corrected if possible. If hepatic function can be improved, urolith dissolution may occur spontaneously. Even so, it is usually recommended that cystotomy be performed for urolith removal at the time of PSS correction. In dogs with inoperable PSS the u/d diet may decrease urine saturation with ammonium urate and reduce signs of hepatic encephalopathy.

### Silicate uroliths

Medical dissolution of these stones is not yet feasible. Recommendations to decrease recurrence after surgical removal include dietary change, increasing urine volume, and urine alkalization (see recommendations for other uroliths). Hill's canine u/d may be beneficial, with 0.5 to 1 g of salt per day added. Consumption of dirt and grass, which may contain silicates, should be discouraged.

### Cystine uroliths

Recommendations for medical dissolution and prevention include dietary protein and methionine restriction, urine alkalization, and thiol-containing drugs. Hill's Canine u/d is most appropriate. Urine pH should be maintained at approximately 7.5 with potassium citrate (as recommended for calcium oxalate uroliths); sodium bicarbonate should be avoided.

*Thiol-containing drugs.* D-Penicillamine decreases urine cystine concentrations. However, it may interfere with surgical wound healing, so it should not be started earlier than 2 weeks after surgery. Other adverse effects include immune-complex glomerulonephritis, fever, lymphadenopathy, and skin hypersensitivity. *N*-(2-mercaptopropionyl)-glycine (see Table 46-2) may have fewer adverse effects.

# 47

# Feline Lower Urinary Tract Inflammation

## (Text pp 642-649)

Feline lower urinary tract inflammation (FLUTI) is characterized by one or more of the following signs: pollakiuria, hematuria, dysuria and stranguria, inappropriate urination, and partial or complete urethral obstruction. These signs have historically been termed *feline urologic syndrome*.

### Epidemiologic features

In general the prevalence of FLUTI is equally divided between males and females, and most cases occur in cats 2 to 6 years of age. When struvite uroliths are the cause (see later), female cats 1 to 2 years old are most often affected. Overweight cats and indoor cats are predisposed to FLUTI. The prevalence often increases in winter and spring. Recurrence occurs in 30% to 70% of cats. Mortality rates range from 6% to 36%. Hyperkalemia and uremia are major causes of death in males with urethral obstruction. Chronic renal failure secondary to ascending pyelonephritis is a possible long-term sequela, especially after repeated urethral catheterization.

### Etiology

FLUTI can be divided into two categories based on the presence or absence of struvite (magnesium ammonium phosphate) crystalluria or uroliths. Cats with struvite-related FLUTI may have overt urolithiasis, crystalluria without obstruction, or urethral obstruction with struvite-containing mucous plugs. (However, apparently normal cats can have struvite crystalluria, and mucous plugs without struvite crystals can cause urethral obstruction). As with canine urolithiasis, formation of crystals or uroliths requires a high concentration of urolith-forming constituents in the urine, favorable pH for crystallization, and adequate time in the urinary tract (see Chapter 46).

Cats in the non–struvite-related group usually have urinary tract inflammation without detectable struvite crystals or urolith formation. A small percentage (<5%) of young cats in both groups have primary bacterial urinary tract infection (UTI), although bacterial UTI is more common in older cats with compromised host defense mechanisms (e.g., chronic renal failure). In most cats with FLUTI the cause of the inflammation is unknown.

**Diet.** Dietary factors, especially high dietary magnesium (Mg), play a role in the development of struvite crystals and uroliths. Obesity is linked to struvite-associated FLUTI, probably because of excessive food and therefore Mg consumption. In general, dry cat foods contain more Mg per kilocalorie than do canned or semimoist foods and require greater total intake to meet caloric needs. Consumption of dry food also results in greater fecal volume and fecal water loss, which may decrease urine volume, increasing the concentration of Mg and other calculogenic substances in the urine and increasing the time these substances are present in the urinary tract.

**Urine pH.** More important than urine Mg is urine pH. Struvite is approximately 100 times more soluble at a urine pH of 6.4 than at 7.7. Many standard cat foods produce a postprandial increase in urine pH of approximately 1 unit that lasts 3 to 5 hours. Cats fed standard foods on an ad libitum basis may have a higher daily average urine pH than meal-fed cats.

*Infection.* Most feline struvite uroliths form in sterile urine. (However, struvite-associated FLUTI may alter normal host defense mechanisms and allow bacterial colonization of the bladder or urethra.) When bacterial infection is present, the most common organism is a urease-producing *Staphylococcus* sp. Feline calicivirus, bovine herpesvirus 4, and feline syncytia-forming virus have been implicated in FLUTI, although the role of these viruses is undetermined.

*Catheterization.* Perhaps the biggest predisposition for bacterial cystitis is urethral catheterization (especially placement of indwelling urinary catheters) combined with fluid therapy and formation of dilute urine. Trauma created by urethral catheterization may also cause urethritis or periurethral inflammation, leading to urethral compression and subsequent obstruction.

*Anatomic factors.* Obstruction is more common in male cats because of the length and diameter of the urethra; many cases are caused by mucus and struvite plugs that lodge in the penile urethra. Anatomic abnormalities or partial obstructions may interfere with normal voiding and increase urine residual volume. Chronic inflammation with fibrosis and thickening of the bladder wall may result in decreased detrusor tone and incomplete voiding.

*Other stones.* Approximately 30% of feline uroliths are struvite, but other uroliths can cause signs of FLUTI. Calcium (Ca)-oxalate stones account for approximately 50% of feline uroliths, and urates constitute approximately 7%. Burmese, Persian, and Himalayan cats are at higher risk for Ca-oxalate uroliths. These stones are more common in neutered males than in females, have a higher prevalence in older animals, and involve the kidneys more often than do struvite stones.

The prevalence of Ca-oxalate uroliths is increasing, possibly because of the widespread use of acidifying diets to prevent struvite-related FLUTI. Cats fed diets low in sodium or potassium or formulated to maximize urine acidity have a decreased risk of developing struvite stones but an increased risk of developing Ca-oxalate stones. Feeding a single brand of cat food and maintaining cats in an indoor-only environment are other risk factors for Ca-oxalate urolithiasis.

*Environmental factors.* Decreased urine volume and frequency of urination may facilitate development of both types of FLUTI. Possible causes include a dirty or poorly available litter box, decreased physical activity (e.g., cold weather, castration, obesity, illness, confinement), and decreased water consumption caused by water taste, availability, or temperature. Stress (e.g., boarding, cat shows, a new pet in the home) may also contribute.

### Clinical features

Clinical signs depend on which component of the disease complex is present (Box 47-1). In unobstructed cats the signs may be missed in cats that live primarily outdoors. On physical examination unobstructed cats are apparently healthy, except for a small, easily expressed bladder; the bladder wall may be thickened, and abdominal palpation may cause pain.

*Urethral obstruction.* In male cats with urinary obstruction, presenting signs depend on how long the obstruction has been present. Within 6 to 24 hours most obstructed cats make frequent attempts to urinate, and they pace, vocalize, hide, lick their genitalia, and display anxiety. If the obstruction is not relieved within 36 to 48 hours, signs of postrenal azotemia may develop (see Box 47-1).

The most relevant physical examination findings in obstructed cats are a turgid, distended bladder that is difficult or impossible to express and pain on abdominal palpation. Care should be taken, because manipulation of a distended bladder can lead to rupture. In males with urethral obstruction the penis may be congested and protrude from the prepuce; the cat may lick his penis until it becomes excoriated and bleeds. Occasionally a urethral plug is observed extending from the urethral orifice.

---

**Box 47-1**

**Clinical Signs Associated with Feline Lower Urinary Tract Inflammation**

---

**CYSTITIS AND URETHRITIS**
Hematuria
Pollakiuria
Dysuria and stranguria
Vocalizing during voiding
Licking at genitalia
Urination in inappropriate places

**PARTIAL OR COMPLETE URETHRAL OBSTRUCTION**
Inability to urinate, straining in the litter box
Hiding behavior
Vocalizing during voiding
Painful abdomen
Licking at genitalia
Congested penis extended from prepuce
Signs of postrenal azotemia
Depression
Weakness
Anorexia
Emesis
Dehydration
Hypothermia
Acidosis and hyperventilation
Electrolyte disturbance (hyperkalemia)
Bradycardia

---

**Diagnosis**

Diagnosis of urethral obstruction is usually straightforward, based on history and physical examination findings. In unobstructed cats with FLUTI, urinalysis usually reveals hematuria; if not, behavioral causes of abnormal urination should be considered.

*Struvite-related FLUTI.* When urine pH is alkaline and struvite crystals are found in the sediment, struvite-associated disease is likely. Radiography or ultrasonography and urine culture should be used to rule out overt urolithiasis and UTI, especially if the patient has no response to an Mg-restricted, acidifying diet (Box 47-2).

*Non–struvite-related FLUTI.* When the urine is acidic, radiography or ultrasonography helps rule out anatomic abnormalities (e.g., thickened bladder wall, polyps, tumors, nonstruvite urolithiasis). Cystoscopy is also a valuable tool in cats with FLUTI. Nonspecific findings include prominent mucosal vascularity and submucosal petechial hemorrhages. Radiography (plain and double-contrast cystography), ultrasonography, or cystoscopy and urine culture should be performed in all cats with recurrent FLUTI.

*Differential diagnoses.* Bacterial cystitis and urethritis, viral cystitis, and mycoplasmal or ureaplasmal cystitis can each cause or mimic signs of FLUTI, as can neoplasia, trauma, irritant cystitis and urethritis, urolithiasis, vesicourachal diverticuli, urethral strictures, extraluminal inflammation and masses, and neurologic disorders.

*Vesicourachal diverticuli.* Vesicourachal diverticuli are found in approximately 25% of cats with FLUTI. Although these diverticuli may be congenital or acquired, most are thought to develop secondary to FLUTI, and therefore are not a major initiating factor. Acquired diverticuli are primarily found in cats >1 year old (mean, 3.7 years)

---

**Box 47-2**

## Diagnostic and Therapeutic Plan for Cats with FLUTI

1. Rule out urethral obstruction; relieve obstruction, if present.
2. Assess degree of hyperkalemia with an electrocardiogram; measure serum urea nitrogen, creatinine, and potassium concentrations; and initiate intravenous fluid therapy if cat is obstructed and depressed.
3. In both obstructed and unobstructed cats obtain a urine sample by cystocentesis, if possible, for the evaluation of urine pH and urine sediment. Culture urine if there is evidence of a UTI (pyuria, bacteriuria).
4. Manage cats with suspected struvite-associated FLUTI using a diet containing less than 20 mEq of magnesium per 100 kcal and acidify urine (between 6.2 and 6.4) with ammonium chloride or methionine, if necessary.
5. Obtain a urine sample in cats with non–struvite-associated FLUTI or in cats with struvite-associated FLUTI with persistent or recurring clinical signs:
   a. If no evidence suggests urinary tract infection, examine the bladder using radiography or ultrasonography or examine the bladder and urethra using contrast-enhanced radiography or cystoscopy.
   b. If no evidence suggests UTI, perform bacterial culture and sensitivity testing and treat with an appropriate antibiotic. If signs persist or recur, examine the bladder using radiography or ultrasonography or examine the bladder and urethra using contrast-enhanced radiography or cystoscopy.
6. In cases of idiopathic FLUTI, try antiinflammatory treatment.

---

*FLUTI,* Feline lower urinary tract inflammation.

---

and are twice as likely to occur in males as in females; increased intravesicular pressure and bladder inflammation during urethral obstruction may play a role. Although a urachal diverticulum may be an incidental finding in an asymptomatic cat, hematuria and dysuria are common.

## Management of FLUTI
### Unobstructed cats

Unobstructed cats with idiopathic dysuria and stranguria and hematuria often become asymptomatic within 5 to 7 days, whether or not therapy is instituted. Treatment and/or initiation of preventive measures is recommended for cats with struvite crystalluria (see Box 47-2).

***Struvite-related FLUTI.*** If alkaline urine with struvite crystalluria is found, the cat should be fed an Mg-restricted, acidifying diet to maintain an average urine pH of <6.4. Urine culture and sensitivity should be performed if pyuria or bacteriuria is observed in the sediment, and appropriate antibiotics administered if culture is positive. Several sources of fresh water should be made available to the cat, and litter boxes should be cleaned frequently and placed in convenient locations.

***Dissolving uroliths.*** Hill's Feline Prescription Diet s/d can be used to dissolve struvite uroliths. Average dissolution time for sterile struvite uroliths is 36 days; 79 days is the average for those associated with bacterial infection. The diet should be fed for 30 days beyond the point at which the uroliths are no longer visible radiographically.

***Preventing recurrence.*** If struvite crystalluria and alkaline urine recur repeatedly, longer-term dietary therapy is warranted. Suitable diets for prevention include Hill's Feline Prescription Diet c/d (canned or dry), Science Diet Feline Maintenance (canned or dry), Iams pH/S, Purina UR-Formula Feline Diet, and Waltham Veterinarium Feline Control pHormula Diet.

The length of treatment with a struvite-prevention diet is controversial, but 2 months is a good initial trial. If struvite-associated FLUTI recurs after initial treatment, a longer therapeutic trial is indicated. However, lifetime feeding of a struvite-prevention diet to a cat that has had only one or two episodes of struvite-related FLUTI usually is not recommended.

*Urine acidifiers.* Ideally, urine pH 4 to 8 hours after feeding is in the range of 6.2 to 6.4. If acidic urine cannot be maintained with these diets (which is rare), urinary acidifiers may be added. Ammonium chloride (800 mg [approximately 1/4 tsp] /day on food) is the most effective urinary acidifier, although diarrhea, vomiting, and anorexia are potential adverse effects. If diarrhea persists after 7 to 10 days, methionine (500 mg q12h) may be substituted.

A urease-producing bacterial infection and dietary indiscretion should be suspected if alkaline urine is found to persist during dietary therapy. Excessive urine acidification may result in chronic metabolic acidosis and increased serum Ca and phosphorus concentrations. Some cats with renal tubular disorders develop hypokalemia and weakness when fed acidifying diets.

*Non–struvite-related FLUTI.* In most cases of FLUTI the urine is acidic and no struvite crystals are found; Mg-restricted, acidifying diets are not recommended in these cats. A urine sample should be obtained by cystocentesis for urine culture; radiography or ultrasonography, contrast-enhanced radiography of the bladder and urethra, or cystoscopy should be performed to rule out anatomic abnormalities if the urine is sterile.

Numerous treatments including antibiotics, tranquilizers, anticholinergics, antispasmodics, and antiinflammatory drugs (e.g., dimethyl sulfoxide, glucocorticoids) have been recommended for idiopathic cystitis in cats. More recently, glycosaminoglycans, amitriptyline, and nonsteroidal antiinflammatory drugs have been recommended. However, no controlled studies have demonstrated efficacy for any of these treatments in the management of idiopathic FLUTI.

### Obstructed cats

Blocked cats that are alert and not azotemic may be sedated for urethral catheterization without further diagnostics or treatment. In a depressed cat with urethral obstruction, serum potassium concentration should be measured or an electrocardiographic rhythm strip evaluated to assess the degree of hyperkalemia (see Table 46-2), and an IV catheter placed for administration of normal (0.9%) saline solution. When hyperkalemia is suspected or confirmed, the cat should be treated aggressively to counter the effects of hyperkalemia on cardiac conduction (see Table 46-2).

*Restraint.* The degree of restraint required for urethral catheterization depends on the patient's temperament and physical status. If necessary, ketamine (1 to 2 mg/kg given intravenously [IV]), thiamylal or thiopental (1 mg/kg IV until effective), or propofol (until effective) may be used. Additional doses of ketamine should be avoided in severely azotemic cats.

*Relieving obstruction.* In some cases the obstruction can be relieved with penile massage and gentle expression of the bladder. If these measures do not result in urine flow, palpation of the urethra per rectum may dislodge a urethral plug or calculus. Sterile isotonic saline can be used to hydropulse urethral plugs into the bladder (see text). If difficulty is encountered catheterizing the bladder, cystocentesis may decrease intravesical pressure and allow the urethral obstruction to be backflushed into the bladder.

*Catheterization.* The following are indications for using an indwelling urethral catheter: (1) inability to restore a normal urine stream, (2) abundance of debris that cannot be extracted via repeated bladder lavage, (3) detrusor atony when the bladder cannot be manually expressed four to six times per day, and (4) intensive care of critically ill patients when urine production is monitored to guide fluid therapy. Catheter placement and maintenance are discussed in the text.

Secondary bacterial UTI is common in cats with indwelling urinary catheters that are on IV fluids to promote diuresis. Nevertheless, prophylactic antibiotics are not recommended; instead, the urine sediment should be examined daily for bacteria and white blood cells, and the urine cultured if necessary.

*Azotemia.* The degree of postrenal azotemia should be assessed by measuring blood urea nitrogen (BUN) and serum creatinine and potassium concentrations. IV fluid therapy is indicated, especially in azotemic cats. Maintenance (60 to 70 ml/kg/day) and replacement therapy (% dehydration/100 × body weight [grams] = amount to administer [milliliters]) should be given IV over 24 hours. Subcutaneous administration of a balanced electrolyte solution may be acceptable once the initial uremic crisis has passed.

*Postobstructive diuresis.* Large-volume, postobstructive diuresis develops in some cats. Measurement of urine volume every 4 to 8 hours aids appropriate replacement therapy; intravenous fluids are essential. BUN and serum creatinine and electrolytes should be reassessed as needed. Occasionally, hypokalemia occurs with prolonged and severe diuresis. If hematuria is severe, the hematocrit should be monitored once or twice a day.

*Managing bladder atony.* Detrusor atony associated with bladder overdistention is common in cats obstructed for >24 hours. If the bladder can be expressed four to six times per day, an indwelling catheter may not be necessary. If the bladder cannot be expressed at least four times per day, an indwelling catheter is indicated.

Bethanechol (2.5 mg orally q8h) can be administered to stimulate detrusor contractility, *but only after urethral patency has been assured* by the presence of a wide urine stream or placement of an indwelling urinary catheter. Acepromazine and phenoxybenzamine can significantly lower intraurethral pressure and may be helpful in the management of functional urethral obstruction in cats with FLUTI.

*Surgery.* If the obstruction cannot be relieved medically, uremic cats must be stabilized before surgery. Repeated cystocentesis should be used to keep the bladder empty until hyperkalemia, acidosis, and uremia are corrected. Elective perineal urethrostomy is occasionally recommended for male cats with recurrent obstruction. However, this procedure does not decrease recurrence of cystitis; in fact, cats with cystitis and perineal urethrostomy are more susceptible to bacterial UTI. Perineal urethrostomy is rarely required for emergency relief of urethral obstruction.

*Diet.* If struvite crystalluria is present, dietary management is similar to that of an unobstructed cat with struvite crystalluria and alkaline urine.

### Follow-up

Urinalysis and urine culture should be repeated in 5 to 7 days in all cats that have been catheterized. All cats receiving corticosteroids should also have follow-up urinalysis and urine culture. Ascending pyelonephritis is a major concern in patients with any UTI, and it is a potential complication of FLUTI, especially if corticosteroids are used.

*Periodic reevaluation.* Periodic assessment of urine pH is beneficial in cats with struvite-associated disease on dietary management. Urine pH 4 to 8 hours after eating should be ≤6.4. Yearly urinalysis and bacterial culture are especially important after perineal urethrostomy.

*Owner education.* Probably the most important aspect of long-term patient monitoring is ensuring that the owner recognizes the signs of urethral obstruction. Any straining in the litter box in male cats with a history of urethral obstruction is cause for alarm.

### Prognosis

The prognosis for male cats with recurrent urethral obstruction is guarded; perineal urethrostomy should be considered, especially if a second obstruction occurred during medical management designed to prevent recurrence. The prognosis for cats with recurrent, nonobstructed FLUTI is fair to good, although pyelonephritis, renal urolithiasis, and chronic renal failure are potential complications or sequelae.

# 48

# Disorders of Micturition

## (Text pp 650-659)

Disorders of micturition encompass problems with urine storage (incontinence) and bladder emptying (urine retention). The most common forms of urinary incontinence are detrusor hyperreflexia or instability and urethral sphincter mechanism incompetence (USMI).

### Etiology

Disorders of micturition can be divided into two broad categories: those associated with a distended bladder and those associated with a small or normal-sized bladder (Table 48-1). In geriatric patients incontinence may also be caused by cognitive disorders, decreased bladder capacity, or decreased mobility. Polyuria (PU) and polydipsia (PD) disorders (e.g., chronic renal insufficiency and failure) and administration of diuretics or corticosteroids can exacerbate incontinence in animals of any age.

### Distended bladder

Disorders associated with a large bladder include neurogenic (upper motor neuron [UMN] or lower motor neuron [LMN] disease, functional urethral obstruction, reflex dyssynergia) and anatomic obstructive disorders. Neurologic disorders can be caused by any condition that creates compression, damage, or degeneration of the spinal cord, pelvic nerve, or pudendal nerve. Conversely, prolonged overdistention of the bladder can lead to neurogenic incontinence by affecting detrusor muscle tone.

### UMN versus LMN lesions

If neurologic lesions or deficits are detected on neurologic examination, the status of the bladder helps localize the lesion and classify the injury as UMN (above L5) or LMN (at or below L5). The most characteristic sign of an LMN lesion affecting the bladder is a distended bladder that is *easily expressed*. If the lesion involves spinal cord segments S1 to S3, both perineal and bulbocavernosus reflexes of the pudendal nerve are absent.

UMN lesions that affect the bladder are characterized by a large, distended bladder that is *difficult to express;* the UMN lesion may also cause paresis or paralysis. Even though it is a primary urine retention disorder, urinary incontinence occurs when intravesical pressure exceeds the outflow resistance and urine leaks through the urethral sphincter (paradoxic incontinence).

### Reflex dyssynergia

Detrusor-urethral (or reflex) dyssynergia is created by active contraction of the detrusor without relaxation of the internal or external urethral sphincters. Reflex dyssynergia is seen primarily in larger-breed male dogs. The cause is usually difficult to determine but may include neurologic lesions of the spinal cord or autonomic ganglia.

Characteristic signs include normal or near-normal initiation of voiding, followed by a narrowed urine stream. Urine may be delivered in spurts, or the stream may be completely disrupted; the patient often strains to urinate and dribbles urine while walking away. It is difficult to express urine from the bladder, although urethral catheterization is usually easy.

### Table 48-1

## Disorders of Micturition

| Disorder | Cause |
|---|---|
| **DISTENDED BLADDER** | |
| Neurogenic | |
| Lower motor neuron disease | Lesion to S1-S3 spinal cord segments (at or below fifth lumbar vertebral body), neoplasia, trauma, cauda equina syndrome |
| | Trauma to pelvic nerve, detrusor atony, canine and feline dysautonomia |
| Upper motor neuron disease | Lesion cranial to S1 spinal cord segment (above fifth lumbar vertebral body), intervertebral disc protrusion, neoplasia, trauma, fibrocartilaginous infarct, meningitis |
| | Cerebral disease, cerebellar disease, brainstem disease |
| Reflex dyssynergia (detrusor-urethral dyssynergia) | Unknown |
| Functional urethral obstruction | Urethral muscular spasm, often associated with urethral inflammation or trauma |
| Anatomic outflow tract obstruction | Urethral stricture, neoplasia, cystic or urethral calculi, granulomatous urethritis, prostatic disease |
| **SMALL OR NORMAL-SIZED BLADDER** | |
| Urethral sphincter mechanism incompetence | Deficient bladder or urethral support, hormone-responsive |
| Detrusor hyperreflexia or instability | Bladder irritation, urethral irritation |
| Congenital incontinence | Ectopic ureters, patent urachus, urethral fistula (rectal or vaginal), pseudohermaphroditism, vaginal strictures |

#### Outflow obstruction

Incontinence in an animal with urinary outflow obstruction occurs when intravesical pressure exceeds urethral pressure, allowing urine to leak past the obstruction. Signs associated with a functional or anatomic urethral obstruction include urine dribbling, unproductive straining to urinate, restlessness, and abdominal pain.

*Anatomic obstruction.* The most common causes of anatomic urethral obstruction are calculi and neoplasia in dogs and struvite-mucus plugs in cats. Urethral strictures and granulomatous urethritis can also obstruct urine flow. Any type of prostatic disease can create outflow obstruction in dogs. Stranguria and tenesmus in older male dogs can be caused by benign prostatic hyperplasia, but bacterial prostatitis, prostatic neoplasia, or abscess is a more likely cause.

*Functional obstruction.* Nonneurogenic functional urethral obstruction, in which resting and voiding urethral pressures are abnormally high, has been associated with prostatic disease, urinary tract infection, urethral muscular spasm, and urethral inflammation, hemorrhage, or edema in dogs and cats. Affected animals have clinical signs and histories similar to those of dogs with reflex dyssynergia. Resting urethral pressure profilometry is usually necessary to differentiate these two syndromes.

#### Small or normal-sized bladder

Disorders associated with a small or normal-sized bladder are caused by increased detrusor contractility or decreased outflow resistance. Causes include USMI, detrusor muscle hyperreflexia and/or instability, and congenital abnormalities.

#### Hormone-responsive incontinence

Hormone-responsive incontinence is a type of USMI that occurs in middle-aged or older, spayed female dogs; it is a consequence of decreased estrogen production (and, in some dogs, defective bladder and urethral support mechanisms). Incontinence is most pronounced when the animal is asleep or relaxed and often responds to estrogen replacement therapy or α-adrenergic drugs. Occasionally, male dogs develop incontinence after castration, especially dogs castrated at an older age; this problem often responds to α-adrenergic therapy or hormone replacement. Diagnosis of hormone-responsive incontinence is based on history, physical examination, urinalysis (absence of lower urinary tract inflammation), and response to therapy.

#### Detrusor hyperreflexia or instability

Detrusor hyperreflexia or instability is characterized by an inability to control voiding, resulting from a strong urge to urinate. Inflammation of the bladder or urethra may create a sensation of bladder fullness that triggers the voiding reflex. Signs include pollakiuria, dysuria and stranguria, and frequently hematuria.

Bacterial UTI is the most common cause in dogs, and sterile inflammation of the lower urinary tract is the most common cause in cats. Detrusor hyperreflexia or instability may also be a primary or idiopathic disorder, not associated with bladder or urethral inflammation.

Evidence of infection or inflammation on urinalysis (e.g., bacteriuria, pyuria, hematuria) supports the tentative diagnosis. If signs persist after appropriate treatment, further diagnostics (ultrasonography, contrast radiography, cystoscopy) are indicated, as infiltrative diseases of the bladder (e.g., neoplasia, chronic cystitis), polyps, uroliths, and urachal remnants can also cause pollakiuria and stranguria.

#### Congenital defects

Urinary incontinence in a young animal can be caused by a variety of congenital defects of the urinary or genital system. The most common defects are ectopic ureters and vaginal strictures; patent urachus, urethrorectal and urethrovaginal fistulas, and female pseudohermaphroditism can also cause urinary incontinence.

***Ectopic ureters.*** Ectopic ureters are most common in female dogs. Breeds at higher risk include Siberian Huskies, Miniature and Toy Poodles, Labrador Retrievers, Fox Terriers, West Highland White Terriers, Collies, and Welsh Corgis. Ectopic ureters are rare in cats; the prevalence is higher in males than in females.

The most common sign is constant urine dribbling, although dogs and cats with a unilateral ectopic ureter may void normally. Because 70% of ectopic ureters in dogs terminate in the vagina, vaginoscopy may reveal the opening of the ectopic ureter, although it can be difficult to find. Intravenous urography and retrograde vaginourethrography are the diagnostic tests of choice.

***Vaginal stricture.*** Incontinence associated with a vaginal stricture is often intermittent, occurring with changes in body position. Diagnosis is made by digital vaginal examination, vaginoscopy, or contrast vaginography.

### Diagnostic Approach to Urinary Incontinence

Clinical features often help determine the underlying problem. Medical problems, especially polyuric disorders and disabilities that impair mobility, should be evaluated and treated. If increased thirst and large urine volume are described by the owner, conditions that cause PD and PU (e.g., diabetes mellitus, pyometra, chronic renal insufficiency and failure, hyperadrenocorticism, hypercalcemia) should be ruled out with appropriate diagnostic tests.

#### Initial evaluation

Age of onset, sexual status, age at neutering, current medications, and history of trauma or previous urinary tract disorders are important aspects of the history.

Physical examination should include evaluation of the perineum for urine scalding or staining. Palpation of the bladder for size and wall thickness and rectal examination for assessment of anal tone and the prostate gland, pelvic urethra, and trigone region of the bladder should be performed in all cases. Digital vaginal examination and vaginoscopy may be used to identify congenital defects in larger female dogs.

**Neurologic examination.** The patient's neurologic status should be thoroughly evaluated. The perineal reflex causes contraction of the anal sphincter and ventroflexion of the tail in response to pinching of the perineal skin. The bulbospongiosus reflex causes contraction of the anal sphincter in response to gentle compression of the bulb of the penis or the vulva. If both reflexes are normal, the pudendal reflex arc (in sacral segments S1 to S3) is intact.

**Observation of voiding.** Dogs should be walked outside so that voiding posture and urine stream can be observed. Immediately after the animal has attempted to void, the bladder should be palpated. Catheterization to quantify residual volume (normally 0.2 to 0.4 ml/kg) is indicated if a large bladder is palpable after voiding.

**Urinalysis.** Urinalysis should be performed in all patients with urinary incontinence. When urine culture is indicated, cystocentesis is the preferred method of collection, except in patients with a distended bladder; ideally these patients are catheterized, without cystocentesis.

### Pharmacologic testing and treatment

Diagnosis often involves assessment of the patient's response to pharmacologic testing or therapy. Detrusor hypocontractility should improve with a parasympathomimetic drug such as bethanechol. Decreased urethral tone should respond to α-adrenergic agents (e.g., phenylpropanolamine) or hormone replacement therapy.

Increased urethral tone is treated with α-sympatholytics (e.g., phenoxybenzamine) and skeletal muscle relaxants (e.g., diazepam). Detrusor hypercontractility often responds to treatment of the underlying inflammatory process; however, smooth muscle antispasmodics (e.g., oxybutinin) and parasympatholytics (e.g., propantheline) may be useful in cases of severe inflammation. Doses for these drugs are given in the table at the end of this section.

### Treatment and prognosis

Treatment guidelines for the specific disorders of micturition are discussed in the following sections. Doses for the drugs mentioned are given in the table at the end of this chapter.

Regardless of the cause, periodic urinalysis to identify or rule out urinary tract infections constitutes an important aspect of follow-up care in an animal with any disorder of micturition. The frequency of urinalysis depends on the nature of the disorder. Owners can be instructed to evaluate the color and odor of the urine and to bring in a urine sample immediately if they suspect an infection; however, routine monitoring is the cornerstone of the prevention of severe urinary tract infections.

## Management of Urinary Incontinence

### LMN disorders

Patients with sacral spinal cord lesions or dysautonomia require expression or strict aseptic catheterization of the bladder at least three times per day; an indwelling urinary catheter can be used if necessary. These procedures may need to be continued for days or weeks if detrusor atony is present.

Urinalysis or examination of the urine sediment should be performed every 3 or 4 days initially, and bacterial culture and antibiotic sensitivity tests performed if any evidence of urinary tract inflammation is present. Urine scalding should be prevented by applying petroleum jelly to the perivulvar or peripreputial and abdominal skin.

**Bethanechol.** Once urethral patency has been ensured by expressing the bladder and increased outflow resistance has been ruled out, bethanechol may be used to increase detrusor contractility. Adverse effects include salivation, vomiting, diarrhea, and intestinal cramping. When they occur, these signs are seen within 1 hour of drug administration; they should prompt reduction in the dose of bethanechol.

### Prognosis

In general the prognosis for animals with neurogenic incontinence is poor. The long-term prognosis for most spinal cord lesions is unfavorable, unless an intervertebral disc protrusion can be successfully decompressed or an extradural mass successfully removed or treated with chemotherapy or radiotherapy. Even if the spinal cord is decompressed, micturition may not completely normalize. Damage to the pudendal nerve, pelvic nerve, or sacral nerve roots carries a more favorable prognosis.

### UMN disorders

Management depends on the presence or absence of a reflex or "autonomic" bladder (spontaneous, incomplete reflex voiding), which often develops 5 to 10 days after spinal cord injury.

*Initial management.* Before autonomic bladder develops, treatment should include aseptic catheterization three times per day. Use of corticosteroids for the neurologic disease may create polyuria, necessitating more frequent catheterization. Corticosteroids also predispose patients to urinary tract infections. Initially, urinalysis or sediment examination should be performed every 3 or 4 days, and bacterial culture and antibiotic sensitivity should be obtained if evidence of urinary tract inflammation is present. Prevention of urine scalding with appropriate bedding and nursing care is important.

*Autonomic bladder.* When autonomic bladder is present, the bladder should be palpated after urination to determine residual urine volume. It may still be necessary to catheterize (express, if possible) the bladder two or three times per day to minimize urine stasis. Urinalysis should be performed monthly (weekly if the animal is receiving corticosteroids), and owners should be instructed to bring in a urine sample if a change in color or odor is noted. Nursing care to prevent urine scalding should be continued.

### Prognosis.

As discussed previously for LMN disorders, the prognosis for recovery of normal micturition in most animals with neurogenic incontinence is poor. Long-term urinary care of paralyzed animals often is necessary. Many owners can be taught to express the bladder, and some can learn to catheterize the urinary bladder; however, some owners are unable to deal with an incontinent animal.

### Reflex dyssynergia

Reflex dyssynergia often responds to pharmacologic management, although the response may take several days. Drugs commonly used include α-blockers (e.g., prazosin, phenoxybenzamine), skeletal muscle relaxants (e.g., diazepam), and occasionally, bethanechol. Intermittent urinary catheterization should be used as necessary to keep the bladder small.

*Phenoxybenzamine.* Phenoxybenzamine has a slow onset of action, so the dose should be increased only at 3- or 4-day intervals and only if a favorable response is not seen. Rapid dose changes should be avoided. Hypotension is the major adverse effect; the dose should be decreased if the animal shows lethargy, weakness, or disorientation. Nausea can be minimized by giving the medication with a small meal.

*Other drugs.* The urine stream is a useful indicator of drug effectiveness. If the stream is weak but continuous and of normal diameter, bethanechol may be used to increase detrusor contractility; however, it must not be used until urethral obstruction has been relieved.

If the urine stream is intermittent or narrowed, increased doses of diazepam, phenoxybenzamine, or both are required. Diazepam has a very short duration of action (1 to 2 hours when given orally [PO]), so giving it 30 minutes before walking the animal sometimes aids in the management of reflex dyssynergia.

It may be several weeks before the appropriate combination of drugs is determined, and drug dosages may need modification over time. Periodic urinalysis is indicated to detect urinary tract inflammation and infection at early stages.

*Prognosis.* In most cases reflex dyssynergia responds to pharmacologic management, but occasionally the underlying disease process worsens, making previously successful therapy ineffective. Drug doses can be reevaluated and increased, but this approach is not always successful. Myelography, epidurography, computed tomography, or magnetic resonance imaging may be indicated in these refractory cases. Catheterization may be necessary for the long-term management of affected animals.

### Functional urethral obstruction

Nonneurogenic functional urethral obstruction has been associated with a range of conditions that affect the urethra itself or urethral patency (e.g., prostatic disease). When treatment of the underlying disorder fails to decrease the outflow resistance, α-blockers (e.g., prazosin, phenoxybenzamine) and skeletal muscle relaxants (e.g., diazepam) should be used.

### Anatomic urethral obstruction

In cases of anatomic obstruction the size and nature of the lesion can usually be determined by retrograde positive-contrast urethrography. Prevention of renal damage and detrusor atony are the main priorities. If the obstruction is caused by a urethral urolith, retropulsion of the stone into the bladder can be successful. If the urolith cannot be moved this way, temporary or permanent perineal urethrostomy may be necessary.

*Prostatic enlargement.* In dogs with benign prostatic hyperplasia, castration usually leads to a rapid decrease in prostate size. Use of estrogens to decrease prostatic size is not recommended. Surgical drainage and marsupialization may be necessary to manage prostatic abscess or cysts. In some cases of prostatic neoplasia, partial or complete prostatectomy may be beneficial; however, this surgery frequently results in neurologic damage and USMI.

*Neoplasia and chronic urethritis.* In most cases trigonal or urethral neoplasia is inoperable, because signs usually are not observed until the tumor is advanced. Therefore the prognosis is poor. In contrast, most female dogs with granulomatous (chronic, active) urethritis respond well to a combination of prednisolone, cyclophosphamide, and antibiotics.

### Urethral sphincter mechanism incompetence

Treatment includes hormone replacement (diethylstilbestrol [DES] for females, testosterone for males) and/or use of α-adrenergic drugs such as phenylpropanolamine (PPA).

*Diethylstilbestrol.* The usual induction therapy for estrogen-responsive incontinence is DES at 0.1 to 1 mg PO q24h for 3 to 5 days. The frequency is then decreased to the lowest effective dose; in some dogs it can be successfully tapered to every 7 to 10 days. Development of estruslike signs and bone marrow toxicity are possible adverse effects of higher-dose DES; endocrine alopecia is another adverse effect. PPA should be tried if the required DES dose is high.

*PPA.* PPA at a dose of 1.5 to 2 mg/kg PO q8h can be used as an alternative or in addition to DES. Owners should watch dogs for hyperexcitability, panting, and anorexia and should decrease the dose if these signs develop. In some animals the dose interval of timed- or precision-release PPA can be decreased to once or twice a day.

*Testosterone.* USMI in neutered male dogs is best treated with α-adrenergic drugs. If testosterone is used, it should be given parenterally. Depository forms injected intramuscularly may be effective for 4 to 6 weeks. Dogs receiving testosterone should have regular rectal examinations to evaluate prostate size. Note: *Testosterone should not be used* in dogs that were neutered because of a testosterone-responsive disease (e.g., benign prostatic hypertrophy, perianal adenomas) or behavioral disorder (e.g., aggression).

*Prognosis.* The prognosis for dogs with hormone-responsive incontinence usually is excellent, although some dogs require multiple drugs for management.

### Detrusor hyperreflexia or instability

Smooth muscle relaxants and anticholinergics (e.g., dicyclomine, oxybutynin, propantheline bromide, imipramine, flavoxate) are used to decrease inappropriate, involuntary detrusor contractions associated with urinary tract inflammation. However, their use should be reserved for patients that do not respond to treatment of the primary disorder. Products containing phenazopyridine dyes (e.g., Azo-Gantrisin) should be avoided because they can cause Heinz body hemolysis and methemoglobinemia, especially in cats.

Dogs treated for inflammatory incontinence secondary to a urinary tract infection should undergo follow-up urinalysis or urine culture to confirm that the infection has been eliminated. Animals with chronic or recurrent cystitis require thorough investigation of the cause. Antispasmodics may provide some relief; however, identification and elimination of the underlying inflammatory disorder should be the priority. In cases in which the detrusor hyperreflexia or instability is primary or idiopathic, anticholinergic agents may be beneficial.

### Congenital disorders

Correction of congenital defects depends on the nature and extent of the defect. Patent urachus and urachal diverticulum are surgically correctable, as are many forms of ectopic ureters. However, USMI may occur in conjunction with ectopic ureter, so surgical reimplantation of the ureter does not guarantee continence. Use of α-adrenergic drugs after surgery increases the likelihood of success. Urethral pressure profiles can be used to detect sphincter incompetence and measure response to α-adrenergic drugs before surgery.

## Drugs Used in Dogs and Cats with Urinary Tract Disorders

| Drug | Trade name | Action | Dose |
|------|-----------|--------|------|
| Allopurinol | Zyloprim | Xanthine oxidase inhibitor | 10 mg/kg PO q8-24h (dogs) |
| Aluminum carbonate, aluminum hydroxide | Basal gel, Amphojel | Enteric phosphate binders | 10-30 mg/kg PO q8h with or immediately after meals |
| Amitriptyline | Elavil | Anticholinergic effects, decreased histamine release from mast cells, increased bladder compliance | 5-10 mg PO q24h (evening) (cats) |
| Amlodipine | Norvasc | Calcium antagonist | 2.5 mg q24h (dogs); 0.625 mg q24h (cats) |
| Ammonium chloride | — | Urinary acidifier | 100 mg/kg PO q12h (dogs); 800 mg daily mixed with food (approximately 1/4 tsp) (cats) |
| Aspirin | — | Antiplatelet, antiinflammatory | 0.5-5 mg/kg q12h (dogs); 0.5-5 mg/kg q24h (cats) |
| Azathioprine | Imuran | Immunosuppressant | 50 mg/m$^2$ PO q24h for 7 days, then q48h (dogs only) |
| Benazepril | Lotensin | Angiotensin-converting enzyme inhibitor | 0.25-0.5 mg/kg PO q24h |
| Bethanechol | Urecholine | Cholinergic (increases detrusor contractility) | 5-15 mg PO q8h (dogs); 1.25-5 mg PO q8h (cats) |
| Chlorpromazine | Thorazine | Antiemetic | 0.25-0.5 mg/kg IM, SC, PO q6-8h (after rehydration only) |
| Cimetidine | Tagamet | H$_2$-blocker | 2.5-5 mg/kg PO, IV, IM q12h |
| Cyclophosphamide | Cytoxan, Neosar | Immunosuppressant | 50 mg/m$^2$ PO q48h (dogs); 200-300 mg/m$^2$ PO q3wk (cats) |
| Cyclosporin | Neoral, Sandimmune | Immunosuppressant | 10 mg/kg q12-24h, adjust dose via monitoring |
| Diazepam | Valium | Skeletal muscle relaxant | 2-5 mg PO q8h |
| Dicyclomine | Bentyl, Bentylol | Antispasmodic, antimuscarinic | 10 mg PO q6-8h (dogs) |

*Continued.*

## Drugs Used in Dogs and Cats with Urinary Tract Disorders—cont'd

| Drug | Trade name | Action | Dose |
|---|---|---|---|
| Diethylstilbestrol (DES) | — | Increased urethral sphincter tone | 0.1-1 mg (dogs), 0.05-0.1 mg (cats) PO q24h for 3-5 days, then same dose q3-7days |
| 1,25-Dihydroxycholecalciferol, calcitriol | Rocaltrol | Active vitamin $D_3$, decreases parathyroid hormone | 1.5-3.5 ng/kg PO q24h |
| Dopamine | Intropin | Renal vasodilator | 2-10 µg/kg/min IV |
| Enalapril | Enacard | Angiotensin-converting enzyme inhibitor | 0.5 mg/kg PO q12-24h (dogs); 0.25-0.5 mg/kg PO q12h (cats) |
| Ephedrine | — | α-Adrenergic, increased urethral sphincter tone | 12.5-50 mg PO q8-12h (dogs); 2-4 mg/kg PO q8-12h (cats) |
| Erythropoietin (r-HuEPO), epoetin alfa | Epogen | Stimulate erythrogenesis | 35-50 U/kg, SC 3 times/wk or 400 U/kg, SC weekly; adjust dose to PCV of 30%-35% |
| Famotidine | Pepcid | $H_2$-blocker | 0.5 mg/kg IM, SC, PO q12-24h |
| Flavoxate | Urispas | Muscle relaxant | 100-200 mg q6-8h |
| Furosemide | Lasix | Loop diuretic | 2-4 mg/kg IV, PO q8-12h |
| Hydralazine | Apresoline | Arterial vasodilator | 0.5-2 mg/kg PO q12h (dogs); 2.5 mg PO q12-24h (cats) |
| Imipramine | Tofranil | Antimuscarinic, adrenergic agonist, muscle relaxant | 5-15 mg PO q12h (dogs); 2.5-5 mg PO q12h (cats) |
| Lisinopril | Prinivil, Zestril | Angiotensin-converting enzyme inhibitor | 0.5 mg/kg PO q24h (dogs) |
| Mannitol | Osmitrol | Osmotic diuretic | 0.5-1 g/kg as 20%-25% solution IV, slow bolus over 5-10 min |
| N-(2-mercaptopropionyl)-glycine | — | Disulfide bond formation with cysteine | 10-15 mg/kg PO q12h (dogs) |
| Metoclopramide | Reglan | Antiemetic | 0.2-0.5 mg/kg PO, SC q8h |
| Nandrolone decanoate | Deca-Durabolin | Anabolic steroid | 1-1.5 mg/kg IM weekly (dogs); 1 mg IM weekly (cats) |

| Generic Name | Trade Name | Mechanism | Dosage |
|---|---|---|---|
| Oxybutynin | Ditropan | Direct antispasmodic effect on smooth muscle | 0.2-0.5 mg/kg PO q8-12h (dogs) |
| D-Penicillamine | Cuprimine | Disulfide bond formation with cysteine | 10-15 mg/kg PO q12h (dogs) |
| Phenoxybenzamine | Dibenzyline | α-Blocker, decreased urethral sphincter tone | 0.2-0.5 mg/kg PO q24h (dogs); 0.5 mg/kg PO q24h (cats) |
| Phenylpropanolamine | Propagest | α-Adrenergic, increased urethral sphincter tone | 1.5-2 mg/kg PO q8-12h |
| Prazosin | Minipress | α-Blocker | 1 mg/15 kg PO q6-8h |
| Propantheline bromide | Pro-Banthine | Anticholinergic, decreases detrusor contractility | 0.25-0.5 mg/kg PO q8-12h |
| Racemethionine | Uroeze, Methio-Form | Urinary acidifier | 150-300 mg/kg/day PO (dogs); 1-1.5 g/day PO (cats) |
| Ranitidine | Zantac | $H_2$-blocker | 2 mg/kg PO, IV q8h (dogs); 2.5 mg/kg IV or 3.5 mg/kg PO q12h (cats) |
| Testosterone cypionate | Andro-Cyp | Increased urethral sphincter tone | 1-2.2 mg/kg IM monthly (dogs) |
| Trimethobenzamide | Tigan | Antiemetic | 3 mg/kg PO, IM q8h (dogs) |

$H_2$, Histamine 2; *IM*, intramuscularly; *IV*, intravenously; *PCV*, packed cell volume; *PO*, orally; *SC*, subcutaneously.

# PART VI

# Endocrine Disorders

RICHARD W. NELSON

# 49

# Disorders of the Hypothalamus and Pituitary Gland

## (Text pp 660-680)

### POLYURIA AND POLYDIPSIA (TEXT PP 660-661)

Polyuria (PU) and polydipsia (PD) in dogs and cats can be defined as urine production >50 ml/kg/day and water consumption >100 ml/kg/day, respectively. (Normal water intake in both species is 20 to 70 ml/kg/day, and normal urine output is 20 to 45 ml/kg/day.) However, it is possible for individual animals to have abnormal thirst and urine production within the normal limits. Polyuria and polydipsia usually coexist, and determination of the primary component is one of the initial diagnostic considerations.

#### Determining the cause

A variety of metabolic disturbances can cause PU and PD (Table 49-1). Primary polyuric disorders can be classified as (1) primary pituitary or nephrogenic diabetes insipidus, (2) secondary nephrogenic diabetes insipidus, (3) osmotic diuresis-induced PU and PD, or (4) hypothalamic or pituitary dysfunction.

Primary polydipsic disorders resulting from a defect in the thirst center have not been reported in dogs and cats. A psychogenic or behavioral basis for compulsive water consumption (psychogenic polydipsia) is described in dogs.

**Table 49-1**

#### Endocrine Disorders That Cause Polyuria and Polydipsia in Dogs and Cats

| Disorder | Tests to establish the diagnosis |
| --- | --- |
| Diabetes mellitus | Fasting blood glucose, urinalysis |
| Hyperadrenocorticism | ACTH stimulation test, low-dose dexamethasone suppression test |
| Hypoadrenocorticism | Blood electrolytes, ACTH stimulation test |
| Primary hyperparathyroidism | Blood calcium and phosphorus, serum PTH concentration, surgical exploration |
| Hyperthyroidism | Serum thyroxine concentration |
| Diabetes insipidus | Modified water deprivation test, response to dDAVP therapy |
| Acromegaly | Baseline growth hormone concentration, CT or MRI |
| Primary hyperaldosteronism | Blood electrolytes; ACTH stimulation test (measure aldosterone) |

*ACTH,* Adrenocorticotropic hormone; *CT,* computed tomography; *dDAVP,* desmopressin acetate; *MRI,* magnetic resonance imaging; *PTH,* parathyroid hormone.

*Initial investigation.* Most endocrinopathies that cause PU and PD are suspected from the history, physical examination findings, and initial database (complete blood count [CBC], serum biochemistry panel, urinalysis). Urinalysis is a particularly useful tool in the initial investigation of an animal with PU and PD (Table 49-2), even though specific tests may be necessary to confirm the diagnosis.

Occasionally the physical examination findings and initial database are normal. Possible causes of PU and PD in these cases include diabetes insipidus, psychogenic polydipsia, unusual hyperadrenocorticism, renal insufficiency without azotemia (uncommon), and possibly mild hepatic insufficiency. The last three should be ruled out before one performs tests for diabetes insipidus or psychogenic polydipsia.

*Urine specific gravity.* Urine specific gravity (SG) varies widely in healthy dogs, in some cases ranging from 1.006 to 1.040 within a 24-hour period. (Wide fluctuations in urine SG have not been reported in healthy cats.) For urine SG in a dog with suspected PU and PD to be accurately assessed, it is wise to have the owner collect several urine samples at different times of the day for 2 to 3 days (storing each sample separately in the refrigerator until analyzed). Evaluation of urine SG in several different samples allows more accurate investigation of the underlying disorder.

*Isosthenuria.* If the urine SG is consistently in the isosthenuric range (1.008 to 1.015), renal insufficiency is the primary differential diagnosis, especially if the blood urea nitrogen (BUN) and serum creatinine are high normal or increased (25 mg/dl and >1.8 mg/dl, respectively) and proteinuria is present (see Table 49-2).

Isosthenuria is also relatively common in dogs with hyperadrenocorticism, psychogenic polydipsia, hepatic insufficiency, pyelonephritis, and partial diabetes insipidus with concurrent water restriction. However, urine SG above the isosthenuric range (e.g., pyelonephritis, psychogenic polydipsia) or below it (e.g., hyperadrenocorticism, partial diabetes insipidus) also occurs with these disorders. If the urine SG is <1.005, renal insufficiency and pyelonephritis are ruled out, and diabetes insipidus, psychogenic polydipsia, and hyperadrenocorticism should be considered.

### Further evaluation

Diagnosis of diabetes insipidus and psychogenic polydipsia should be based on results of a modified water deprivation test, plasma osmolality, and response to synthetic vasopressin (AVP). These tests are described in the following sections.

## DIABETES INSIPIDUS (TEXT PP 661-667)

### Etiology

Defective synthesis or secretion of AVP by the hypothalamus or inability of the renal tubules to respond to AVP causes the syndrome of diabetes insipidus. These abnormalities are termed *central* and *nephrogenic diabetes insipidus,* respectively.

*Central diabetes insipidus.* Central diabetes insipidus (CDI) results from insufficient AVP. It can be caused by any condition that damages the neurohypophyseal system. Idiopathic CDI is the most common form, appearing at any age, in any breed, in either gender. The most common identifiable causes of CDI are head trauma, intracranial tumors (e.g., craniopharyngioma, pituitary chromophore adenoma or adenocarcinoma, metastatic tumors), and hypothalamic or pituitary malformations (e.g., cysts). Head trauma can cause transient or permanent CDI.

*Nephrogenic diabetes insipidus.* Nephrogenic diabetes insipidus (NDI) results from impaired responsiveness of the nephrons to AVP. Plasma AVP concentrations are normal or increased in these animals. NDI is classified as primary (familial) or secondary (acquired). Primary NDI is a rare congenital disorder of unknown etiology; familial NDI has been reported in Huskies. The most common form of diabetes insipidus is secondary NDI, in which the renal tubules lose the ability to respond adequately to AVP. Most of these acquired forms are reversible after correction of the underlying disorder.

### Clinical features

There exists no apparent breed, gender, or age predilection for CDI in dogs. Most cats with CDI are Domestic Shorthair or Longhair, although the disorder also has been

**Table 49-2**

## Results of Urinalysis in Dogs with Selected Disorders That Cause Polyuria and Polydipsia

| Disorder | No. of dogs | Urine Specific Gravity | | Proteinuria (%) | WBC (>5/hpf)(%) | Bacteriuria (%) |
|---|---|---|---|---|---|---|
| | | Mean | Range | | | |
| Central diabetes insipidus | 20 | 1.005 | 1.001-1.012 | 5 | 0 | 0 |
| Psychogenic polydipsia | 18 | 1.011 | 1.003-1.023 | 0 | 0 | 0 |
| Hyperadrenocorticism | 20 | 1.012 | 1.001-1.027 | 48 | 0 | 12 |
| Renal insufficiency | 20 | 1.011 | 1.008-1.016 | 90 | 25 | 15 |
| Pyelonephritis | 20 | 1.019 | 1.007-1.045 | 70 | 75 | 80 |

*hpf,* High-power field; *WBC,* white blood cells.

documented in Persians and Abyssinians. Age at the time of diagnosis in cats ranges from 8 weeks to 6 years (mean, 1.5 years). Primary NDI is identified in puppies, kittens, and young adult dogs and cats (<18 months of age).

*Clinical signs.* PU and PD are the hallmark signs of diabetes insipidus and are typically the only signs seen with congenital and idiopathic CDI and with primary NDI. Affected animals can appear incontinent because of the PU. Additional signs can be found in dogs and cats with secondary CDI or NDI. The most worrisome are neurologic signs, which suggest an expanding hypothalamic or pituitary tumor (in the absence of head trauma).

*Physical examination.* Physical findings are usually unremarkable, although some dogs and cats are thin. As long as access to water is unrestricted, hydration, mucous membrane color, and capillary refill time remain normal. Presence of neurologic abnormalities is variable with trauma-induced CDI or neoplastic destruction of the hypothalamus or pituitary gland. Many animals have no perceptible neurologic alterations; others show mild to severe neurologic signs, including stupor, disorientation, ataxia, circling, pacing, and convulsions. Severe hypernatremia can also cause neurologic signs in traumatized dogs or cats with undiagnosed CDI given inadequate fluid therapy. Persistent hypernatremia and hyposthenuria should raise a suspicion of diabetes insipidus.

### Diagnosis

The diagnostic approach should first rule out causes of secondary NDI. Recommended initial tests include CBC, serum biochemistry panel, urinalysis with bacterial culture, abdominal ultrasonography or radiography, and adrenocorticotropic hormone (ACTH) stimulation test. Results are usually normal with CDI, primary NDI, and psychogenic polydipsia, although low-normal BUN concentration (5 to 10 mg/dl) can be found. Urine SG is usually <1.006, and often 1.001 when access to water is unlimited. Urine osmolality is <300 mOsm/kg.

Urine SG in the isosthenuric range (1.008 to 1.015) does not rule out diabetes insipidus, especially when the urine has been obtained after water is withheld. Erythrocytosis (packed cell volume 50% to 60%), hyperproteinemia, hypernatremia, and azotemia may also be found when access to water is restricted. Diagnostic tests to confirm and differentiate CDI, primary NDI, and psychogenic PD are discussed in the next sections. They can be accurately interpreted only after secondary NDI has been ruled out.

*Differentiating absolute and partial CDI.* Absolute AVP deficiency causes persistent hyposthenuria and severe diuresis. Urine SG usually remains 1.006, even in severely dehydrated patients. Partial deficiency (partial CDI) also causes persistent hyposthenuria and marked diuresis, as long as the animal has unlimited access to water. During periods of water restriction, dogs and cats with partial CDI can increase their urine SG into the isosthenuric range but typically cannot concentrate their urine above 1.020, even when severely dehydrated. The more severe the AVP deficiency, the less concentrated the urine SG during dehydration.

*Modified water deprivation test.* The modified water deprivation test is the best diagnostic test to differentiate between the primary causes of PU and PD. The test consists of two phases.

Phase I evaluates AVP secretory capabilities and renal responsiveness by assessing the effects of dehydration (water restriction until the patient loses 3% to 5% of body weight) on urine SG. Normal dogs and cats and those with psychogenic polydipsia should be able to concentrate urine to >1.030 (1.035 in cats). Dogs and cats with partial and complete CDI and primary NDI have an impaired ability to concentrate urine in the face of dehydration (Table 49-3).

The time required to attain 5% dehydration can also be helpful in establishing the diagnosis. Dogs and cats with complete CDI often reach 5% dehydration in <6 hours, whereas in those with partial CDI and psychogenic polydipsia it often takes >8 hours.

Phase II is indicated for patients that do not concentrate urine to >1.030 during phase I. Phase II determines what effect exogenous AVP has on renal tubular ability to concentrate urine in the face of dehydration (see text).

**Table 49-3**

## Guidelines for Interpretation of the Water Deprivation Test

| Disorder | Initially | Urine Specific Gravity | | Time to 5% Dehydration | |
|---|---|---|---|---|---|
| | | 5% Dehydration | Post ADH | Mean (hr) | Range (hr) |
| Central DI | | | | | |
| Complete | <1.006 | <1.006 | >1.008 | 4 | 3-7 |
| Partial | <1.006 | 1.008-1.020 | >1.015 | 8 | 6-11 |
| Primary nephrogenic DI | <1.006 | <1.006 | <1.006 | 5 | 3-9 |
| Primary polydipsia | 1.002-1.020 | >1.030 | NA | 13 | 8-20 |

*ADH*, Antidiuretic hormone; *DI*, diabetes insipidus; *NA*, not applicable.

*Response to desmopressin.* An alternative approach is evaluation of the response to trial therapy with synthetic AVP, desmopressin acetate (dDAVP). With this method, $1/2$ to 1 of the 0.1-mg or 0.2-mg dDAVP tablets is given orally (PO) q8h, or 1 to 4 drops of dDAVP nasal spray is given via an eyedropper into the conjunctival sac q12h for 5 to 7 days. Owners should notice a decrease in PU and PD by the end of the treatment period if these signs are caused by CDI.

Urine SG should be measured on several urine samples collected by the owner during the last 2 days of trial therapy. An increase in urine SG of >50% compared with pretreatment values supports a diagnosis of CDI, especially if the urine SG is >1.030.

Dogs and cats with primary NDI show minimal improvement with dDAVP therapy, although a response may be observed with very high doses. Those with psychogenic PD can exhibit a mild decrease in urine output and water intake.

*Cautions.* This approach requires that *all other causes* of PU and PD, except CDI, primary NDI, and psychogenic PD, *be ruled out first.* Tests for hyperadrenocorticism should always be evaluated before trial therapy with dDAVP is considered. Dogs with hyperadrenocorticism typically have a positive (albeit moderate) response to dDAVP, which can be misinterpreted as evidence of partial CDI.

*Random plasma osmolality.* Random measurement of plasma osmolality (normally 280 to 310 mOsm/kg) may help diagnose primary or psychogenic PD. As a guide, plasma osmolality of <280 mOsm/kg, obtained while the animal has free access to water, suggests psychogenic PD; plasma osmolality of >280 mOsm/kg is consistent with CDI, NDI, or psychogenic PD.

*Additional diagnostic procedures.* Further diagnostic procedures may be warranted in older dogs and cats with CDI or primary NDI. Pituitary or hypothalamic neoplasia should be considered with CDI. A complete neurologic evaluation (e.g., evaluation of cerebrospinal fluid, computed tomography [CT], magnetic resonance imaging [MRI]) may be warranted before idiopathic CDI is diagnosed. Similarly, a more complete evaluation of the kidney (e.g., abdominal ultrasonography, renal biopsy) may be warranted in an older dog or cat tentatively diagnosed with primary NDI.

### Treatment

Therapeutic options for diabetes insipidus are summarized in Box 49-1.

*dDAVP.* Treatment with dDAVP is the standard therapy for CDI. The intranasal preparation is used most commonly. Intranasal administration is possible but not recommended. Instead, the nasal preparation is transferred to a sterile eyedropper bottle, and drops are placed into the conjunctival sac. A dose of 1 to 4 drops q12-24h is sufficient to control signs of CDI in most animals.

Oral dDAVP tablets can be used in dogs (and presumably in cats), but the response is variable. The initial dose in dogs is 0.1 mg PO q8h. The dose is gradually increased until effective if unacceptable PU and PD persist after 1 week. A decrease in frequency to q12h can be tried once a clinical response is seen. The parenteral formulation of dDAVP can be used in lieu of eye drops or oral tablets. The initial dose is 0.5-2 µg subcutaneously (SC) q12-24h.

Regardless of the route, maximal effect occurs 2 to 8 hours after administration, and duration of action ranges from 8 to 24 hours. Larger doses increase the antidiuretic effects and prolong the duration of action; however, expense becomes a limiting factor. The medication can be administered only in the evenings to prevent nocturia.

*Other measures.* Chlorpropamide, thiazide diuretics, and salt restriction have limited efficacy for the treatment of NDI. dDAVP may control clinical signs if administered in massive amounts (5 to 10 times that recommended for CDI), but the cost may be prohibitive.

Therapy for CDI or NDI is not mandatory as long as the dog or cat has unlimited access to water and is housed in an environment that cannot be damaged by severe PU. *A constant water supply is essential,* however, as relatively short periods of water restriction can have catastrophic results.

### Prognosis

Dogs and cats with idiopathic or congenital CDI usually become relatively asymptomatic with appropriate therapy, and with proper care they have an excellent life

---

**Box 49-1**

**Therapies Available for Polydipsic and Polyuric Dogs with Central Diabetes Insipidus, Nephrogenic Diabetes Insipidus, or Primary (Psychogenic) Polydipsia**

A. Central diabetes insipidus (severe)
  1. dDAVP (desmopressin acetate)
    a. Effective
    b. Expensive
    c. May require drops in conjunctival sac if oral form is ineffective
  2. LVP (lypressin [Diapid])
    a. Short duration of action; less potent than dDAVP
    b. Expensive
    c. Requires drops in nose or conjunctival sac
  3. No treatment—provide continuous source of water
B. Central diabetes insipidus (partial)
  1. dDAVP
  2. LVP
  3. Chlorpropamide
    a. 30%-70% effective
    b. Inexpensive
    c. Pill form
    d. Takes 1-2 weeks to obtain effect of drug
    e. May cause hypoglycemia
  4. Clofibrate—untested in veterinary medicine
  5. Thiazides
    a. Mildly effective
    b. Inexpensive
    c. Pill form
    d. Should be used with low-sodium diet
  6. Low-sodium diet
  7. No treatment—provide continuous source of water
C. Nephrogenic diabetes insipidus
  1. Thiazides—as above
  2. Low-sodium diet
  3. No treatment—provide continuous source of water
D. Primary (psychogenic) polydipsia
  1. Water restriction at times
  2. Water limitation
  3. Behavior modification
    a. Exercise
    b. Another pet
    c. Larger living environment

---

expectancy. Without therapy these animals often lead acceptable lives as long as water is constantly provided.

PU and PD frequently resolve in dogs and cats with trauma-induced CDI, often within 2 weeks. Animals with hypothalamic and pituitary tumors have a guarded to grave prognosis. Neurologic signs typically develop within 6 months after diagnosis of CDI.

The prognosis for animals with primary NDI is guarded to poor because of limited therapeutic options and the generally poor response to therapy. The prognosis for secondary NDI depends on the primary problem.

## PRIMARY (PSYCHOGENIC) PD (TEXT P 667)

Primary PD is defined as a marked increase in water intake that cannot be explained as a compensatory mechanism for excessive fluid loss. Mechanisms are discussed in the text. Psychogenic PD may be induced by concurrent disease (e.g., hepatic insufficiency, hyperthyroidism), or it may represent a learned behavior that follows a change in the pet's environment. PU is compensatory.

### Diagnosis

Psychogenic PD is diagnosed by exclusion of other causes of PU and PD and by demonstration that the dog or cat can concentrate urine to an SG >1.030 during water deprivation. Dogs, and presumably cats, with psychogenic PD have renal medullary solute washout. These dogs can concentrate urine in excess of 1.030, but depending on the severity of solute washout, it may take 12 to 24 hours of water deprivation for concentrated urine to be attained.

### Treatment

Treatment is aimed at *gradually* limiting water intake to amounts in the high-normal range. The volume of water provided is reduced by 10% each week until water volumes of 60 to 80 ml/kg/day are reached. The total 24-hour volume of water is divided into several aliquots, with the last aliquot given at bedtime. Oral salt (1 g/30 kg q12h) and/or sodium bicarbonate (0.6 g/30 kg q12h) may be administered for 3 to 5 days to help reestablish the renal medullary concentration gradient.

For dogs that fail to respond to water restriction, changing the dog's environment or daily routine should be considered; for example, initiate a daily exercise routine, bring a second pet into the home, provide some distraction, or move the dog to an area with an increased amount of contact with humans.

## ENDOCRINE ALOPECIA (TEXT PP 667-670)

Endocrine alopecia is a common problem in dogs and, to a lesser extent, cats. Potential causes are listed in Table 49-4. The alopecia typically is bilaterally symmetric, with a variable distribution pattern. Hairs are easily epilated, and the skin is often thin and hypotonic; hyperpigmentation is common. Other skin lesions such as scales, crusts, and papules are absent, although seborrhea and pyoderma can develop, depending on the underlying cause.

### Diagnostic approach

If the history and physical examination fail to provide insight into the cause, the clinician should sequentially rule out the causes of endocrine alopecia, beginning with the most likely ones. In dogs the most common causes are hypothyroidism and glucocorticoid excess (iatrogenic or spontaneous). Feline endocrine alopecia is perhaps the most common cause in cats.

The diagnostic workup should begin with CBC, serum biochemistry panel, and urinalysis. If initial lab work is not helpful, definitive tests for hypothyroidism and hyperadrenocorticism should be performed concurrently. Diagnosis becomes more difficult once these two endocrinopathies have been ruled out. Growth hormone (GH)–responsive dermatosis and gonadal- or adrenal-dependent sex hormone imbalance are the primary differential diagnoses. Follicular dysplasia can cause a similar clinical picture and should also be considered. GH-responsive dermatosis is discussed separately on p 436.

*Gonadal-dependent sex hormone imbalance.* Endocrine alopecia can result from an excess or deficiency of one of the sex hormones, or it may be responsive to treatment with estrogens or androgens. Dermatologic manifestations are similar for most sex hormone–responsive dermatoses and include endocrine alopecia that initially begins in the perineal, genital, and ventral abdominal regions and spreads cranially; dull, dry, easily epilated hair; failure of the haircoat to regrow after clipping; and variable presence of seborrhea and hyperpigmentation.

Additional signs of hyperestrogenism may include gynecomastia, pendulous prepuce, attraction of other male dogs, squatting to urinate, and unilateral testicular atrophy

**Table 49-4**

## Disorders That Cause Endocrine Alopecia

| Disorder | Common clinicopathologic abnormalities | Diagnostic tests |
|---|---|---|
| Hypothyroidism | Hypercholesterolemia, mild nonregenerative anemia | Baseline $T_4$, free $T_4$, and TSH measurement |
| Hyperadrenocorticism | Stress leukogram, increased SAP, hypercholesterolemia, hyposthenuria, urinary tract infection | ACTH-stimulation test, low-dose dexamethasone-suppression test, urine cortisol/creatinine ratio |
| Growth hormone deficiency—pituitary dwarfism | None | Signalment, physical findings, growth hormone response test |
| Growth hormone-responsive dermatosis—adult dog | None | Growth hormone response test, response to growth hormone supplementation |
| Castration-responsive dermatosis | None | Response to castration |
| Hyperestrogenism | | |
| Functional Sertoli cell tumor—male dog | None (bone marrow depression uncommon) | Physical findings, histopathologic findings, plasma estrogen and inhibin concentration |
| Hyperestrogenism in intact female dog | None (bone marrow depression uncommon) | Abdominal ultrasonography, plasma estrogen concentration, response to ovariohysterectomy |
| Hypoestrogenism (?) | | |
| Estrogen-responsive dermatosis of spayed female dogs | None | Response to estrogen therapy |
| Feline endocrine alopecia | See below | See below |
| Hypoandrogenism(?) | | |
| Testosterone-responsive dermatosis—male dog | None | Response to testosterone therapy |
| Feline endocrine alopecia | None | Response to combined estrogen-testosterone or progestin therapy |
| Telogen defluxion (effluvium) | None | History of recent pregnancy or diestrus |
| Diabetes mellitus | Hyperglycemia, glucosuria | Blood and urine glucose measurement |
| Adrenal sex hormone dermatosis | None | Sex hormones and precursors before and after ACTH stimulation |
| Progestin excess | None | Blood progesterone and 17-OH-progesterone concentration |

*ACTH,* Adrenocorticotropic hormone; *SAP,* serum alkaline phosphatase; *$T_4$,* tetraiodothyronine; *TSH,* thyroid-stimulating hormone.

(contralateral to the testicular tumor) in male dogs; and vulvar enlargement and persistent proestrus, estrus, or anestrus in females.

*Diagnosis.* The dermatologic manifestations can mimic GH-responsive dermatosis, creating a diagnostic challenge, especially when the alopecia occurs in a breed with a known predisposition for GH-responsive dermatosis (e.g., Pomeranians).

Diagnosis is based on the signalment, history, findings on physical examination, results of routine biochemical and hormonal tests used to rule out other causes of endocrine alopecia, and response to treatment. Histologic assessment of a skin biopsy specimen can be used to identify nonspecific endocrine-related alterations and support the diagnosis of endocrine alopecia.

Identification of an increased plasma estrogen concentration would support the presence of a functional Sertoli cell tumor in a male dog and hyperestrogenism in a bitch (assuming that she is not in proestrus or early estrus). Abdominal ultrasonography may identify ovarian cysts or neoplasia in a bitch with hyperestrogenism.

*Treatment.* Treatment for sex hormone–responsive alopecia is summarized in Table 49-5. Because of potentially serious adverse effects of hormone therapy, the more common causes of endocrine alopecia should always be ruled out before one initiates treatment with one of the sex hormones. If the haircoat does not improve within 3 months of the start of therapy, another diagnosis should be considered.

**Adrenal-dependent sex hormone imbalance.** Adrenal-dependent sex hormone imbalance can occur as a primary disorder or in association with hyperadrenocorticism.

**Table 49-5**

## Treatment for Sex Hormone–Induced or Sex Hormone–Responsive Endocrine Alopecia

| Disorder | Primary treatment | Potential adverse reactions to therapy |
|---|---|---|
| Sertoli cell neoplasia | Castration | None |
| Castration-responsive dermatosis | Castration | None |
| Hyperestrogenism in the intact female dog | Ovariohysterectomy | None |
| Estrogen-responsive dermatosis of spayed female dogs | Diethylstilbestrol, 0.1-1 mg PO q24h, 3 weeks per month; once animal responds, 0.1-1 mg q4-7d | Aplastic anemia |
| Feline endocrine alopecia | Megestrol acetate, 2.5-5 mg/cat q48h until hair regrows; then 2.5-5 mg/cat q7-14days | Adrenocortical suppression, benign mammary hypertrophy, mammary neoplasia, pyometra (female cats); infertility (male cats); diabetes mellitus |
| Testosterone-responsive dermatosis | Methyltestosterone, 1 mg/kg (maximum, 30 mg) PO q48h until hair regrows, then q4-7days | Aggression, hepatopathy |
| Telogen defluxion (effluvium) | None | None |
| Adrenal sex hormone dermatosis | Growth hormone, castration, melatonin, mitotane | Diabetes mellitus, hypoadrenocorticism |

*PO,* Orally.

With adrenal-dependent hyperadrenocorticism, increases in sex hormones can affect the dermatologic manifestations of the primary disease. Progesterone-secreting adrenocortical tumors have been described in cats; clinical features mimic hyperadrenocorticism. An increase in baseline and/or post-ACTH plasma 17-hydroxyprogesterone has been documented in dogs with clinical manifestations of hyperadrenocorticism but normal plasma cortisol concentrations after administration of ACTH or dexamethasone.

*Congenital adrenal hyperplasia-like syndrome.* Congenital adrenal hyperplasia-like syndrome, a form of adrenal-dependent sex hormone imbalance, mimics GH-responsive dermatosis. Breeds most commonly affected include the Pomeranian, Chow-Chow, Keeshond, and Samoyed. Both sexes are affected, but males are overrepresented. Elevations in progesterone and its precursors are common in affected dogs. Skin biopsies show the typical changes of endocrine alopecia and may also show features of follicular dysplasia. Diagnosis requires evaluation of sex hormones and their precursors before and after ACTH administration.

Treatment has included castration, methyltestosterone, growth hormone, melatonin (3 to 6 mg q12-24h for 6 weeks), and *o,p'*DDD (mitotane; 15 to 25 mg/kg/day until post-ACTH plasma cortisol is 2 to 5 µg/dl, then maintenance therapy; see p 495). Affected dogs are otherwise healthy, and many owners elect not to treat their dogs because of the expense and/or risk of complications associated with treatment.

## GROWTH HORMONE–RESPONSIVE DERMATOSIS IN ADULT DOGS (TEXT PP 670-673)

GH-responsive dermatosis is a poorly defined disorder that affects adult dogs. The cause is unknown. Baseline plasma GH concentrations in affected dogs are low, and no increase occurs in plasma GH after stimulation of the somatotrophs. Given the strong breed predisposition (see later), genetics must play a role, at least in some breeds. Gender may also play a part, as this condition is more common in males than in females. The lesion does not appear to be progressive or to affect other endocrine functions of the pituitary gland.

Other, as yet poorly characterized, causes of endocrine dermatosis exist that mimic GH-responsive dermatosis. These dogs have the typical signalment and clinical signs of GH-responsive dermatosis, yet they have normal baseline serum insulin-like growth factor I (IGF-I) concentrations. These cases indicate that some dogs that do not have GH deficiency may still respond to GH therapy.

### Clinical features

GH-responsive dermatosis can be found in many different breeds, but Chow-Chows, Pomeranians, Toy and Miniature Poodles, Keeshonds, American Water Spaniels, and Samoyeds are overrepresented. (Congenital adrenal hyperplasia-like syndrome also occurs in these breeds, so GH irregularities in these dogs may be coincidental or a secondary problem.) There seems to be a predilection for males. Clinical signs usually develop in young animals (1 to 4 years of age).

*Clinical signs.* Hyposomatotropism in mature dogs primarily affects hair growth and skin pigmentation. It is characterized by bilaterally symmetric alopecia of the trunk, neck, pinnae, tail, and caudomedial thighs. Alopecia frequently begins in areas of friction or wear (e.g., beneath the collar). Initially a gradual loss of guard (primary) hairs in affected areas occurs, giving the haircoat a puppylike appearance; with time, undercoat (secondary) hairs are lost. Truncal primary hairs are then gradually lost, followed by secondary hairs; however, complete truncal alopecia is uncommon.

The head is not involved, and the legs are involved to a lesser degree than the trunk. Hair in affected areas is easily epilated, and the remaining haircoat is usually dry and dull. Hyperpigmentation develops in alopecic areas. In chronic cases the skin becomes thin and hypotonic. These dogs are otherwise normal.

### Diagnosis

Definitive diagnosis is based on results of a GH stimulation test, in which plasma GH is measured after administration of a secretagogue (see text). However, the means to measure GH in dogs are severely limited. Diagnosis is therefore based on the signalment, history, physical examination findings, absence of alterations on CBC, serum biochemistry panel, urinalysis, supportive dermatohistopathologic findings on skin biopsy (see text), and the ruling out of more common causes of endocrine alopecia. If all findings support a diagnosis of GH-responsive dermatosis, response to GH replacement therapy can be used to help establish the diagnosis.

### Treatment
Treatment of GH-responsive dermatosis involves the administration of GH. However, an effective GH product is not readily available for use in dogs. Porcine GH is immunologically similar to canine GH; if it is available, the recommended dose is 0.1 U (0.05 mg/kg) SC given 3 times per week for 4 to 6 weeks. Hypersensitivity reactions (including angioedema), carbohydrate intolerance, and overt diabetes mellitus (DM) are the primary adverse effects. The animal should be monitored frequently for glucosuria and hyperglycemia, and GH therapy stopped if either develops.

Regrowth of hair and thickening of the skin are used to assess response to therapy. The haircoat should improve within 6 weeks. Clinical remission in dogs that respond to GH treatment is variable in duration but may last up to 3 years. A 1-week course of GH therapy should be given when dermatologic signs begin to recur.

*Other options.* Alternatives to GH therapy that may be effective include castration, melatonin, and *o,p'*DDD (see text, pp 671-673). Response to treatment other than GH casts doubt on the role of GH in the development of this syndrome and emphasizes the difficulty of separating GH-responsive, sex hormone–induced, and sex hormone–responsive endocrine alopecia.

### Prognosis
The long-term prognosis is good, even in untreated dogs. Without treatment, affected dogs eventually lose most of the hair on the thorax and abdomen, and the skin turns black. The dogs are otherwise healthy. Spontaneous regrowth of hair has occurred in some untreated dogs.

## FELINE ACROMEGALY (TEXT PP 673-677)
Feline acromegaly is caused by a functional adenoma of the pituitary pars distalis. Chronic, excessive secretion of GH results in proliferation of bone, cartilage, and soft tissues and in organomegaly, most notably of the kidneys and heart. Excess GH also leads to carbohydrate intolerance, hyperglycemia, and eventually insulin-resistant DM. Most but not all cats with acromegaly have DM at the time acromegaly is diagnosed, and most eventually develop severe insulin resistance.

### Clinical features
Acromegaly typically occurs in older (8 to 14 years), male, Domestic Shorthair or Longhair cats. The earliest signs are usually PU, PD, and polyphagia, which can become quite intense. Weight loss is variable; in most cases acromegaly is considered only when insulin therapy is ineffective in establishing glycemic control of the diabetic state. Insulin doses in cats with acromegaly frequently exceed 2 U/kg q12h, with no apparent decline in blood glucose concentration.

Clinical signs related to the anabolic actions of excess GH (Box 49-2) may be evident at the time DM is diagnosed but more commonly become apparent several months afterward. Because of the insidious onset and slowly progressive nature of these signs, owners are often unaware of the subtle changes in the cat's appearance. *Weight gain in a cat with poorly regulated DM is an important diagnostic clue* for acromegaly. With time, organomegaly, especially of the heart, kidney, liver, and adrenal gland, develop. Diffuse thickening of the soft tissues in the pharyngeal region can lead to upper airway obstruction and respiratory distress.

### Neurologic signs
Neurologic abnormalities can develop as a result of pituitary tumor growth and invasion or compression of the hypothalamus and thalamus. Signs include stupor, somnolence, adipsia, anorexia, temperature deregulation, circling, seizures, and changes

---

**Box 49-2**

## Clinical Signs Associated with Acromegaly in Dogs and Cats

**ANABOLIC, IGF-I–INDUCED**

Respiratory
  Inspiratory stridor
  Transient apnea
  Panting
  Exercise intolerance
  Fatigue
Dermatologic
  Myxedema
  Excessive skin folds
  Hypertrichosis
Conformational
  Increased size
  Increased soft tissue in oropharyngeal
    or laryngeal area
Enlargement of
  Abdomen
  Head
  Feet
  Viscera
Broad face
Prominent jowls
Prognathia inferior
Increased interdental space
Rapid toenail growth
Degenerative polyarthropathy

**CATABOLIC, GH-INDUCED**

Polyuria, polydipsia
Polyphagia

**IATROGENIC**

Progestins
  Mammary nodules
  Pyometra

**NEOPLASIA-INDUCED**

Lethargy, stupor
Adipsia
Anorexia
Temperature deregulation
Papilledema
Circling
Seizures
Pituitary dysfunction
  Hypogonadism
  Hypothyroidism
  Hypoadrenocorticism

*GH*, Growth hormone; *IGF-I*, insulin-like growth factor I.

in behavior. Blindness is uncommon. Papilledema may be found during an ophthalmic examination. Peripheral neuropathy that causes weakness, ataxia, and a plantigrade stance may develop as a result of poorly controlled DM.

### Diagnosis

Poorly controlled DM is responsible for most of the abnormalities identified on serum biochemistry panel and urinalysis, including hyperglycemia, glucosuria, hypercholesterolemia, and mild increases in alanine aminotransferase and alkaline phosphatase activities. Ketonuria is uncommon. Mild erythrocytosis, mild hyperphosphatemia without azotemia, and hyperproteinemia with a normal electrophoretic pattern may also be found. Renal failure is a potential sequela and, when present, causes azotemia, isosthenuria, and proteinuria.

*Diagnostic criteria.* Definitive diagnosis requires documentation of increased baseline serum GH; however, a commercial GH assay is not available for use in cats. The diagnosis is therefore based on (1) conformational alterations (e.g., increased body size, large head, prognathia inferior, organomegaly) in a cat with insulin-resistant DM, (2) persistent increase in body weight in a cat with poorly regulated DM, and (3) documentation of a pituitary mass with CT or MRI. Hyperadrenocorticism must be ruled out before a tentative diagnosis of acromegaly can be made.

*Serum IGF-I.* Further confirmation can be gained by measuring baseline serum IGF-I, which is elevated in cats with acromegaly, although values may be in the upper range of normal in the early stages. Repeating the test 3 to 4 months later usually demonstrates an increase in serum IGF-I if acromegaly is present. The clinical picture and severity of insulin resistance must always be taken into consideration when one interprets serum IGF-I results.

### Treatment

Radiotherapy (cobalt teletherapy) is currently the best treatment option, although response to therapy is unpredictable, ranging from none to dramatic. Typically, tumor size, plasma GH, and serum IGF-I decrease, and insulin responsiveness improves. However, hypersomatotropism usually recurs 6 to 18 months after treatment.

*Managing insulin resistance.* DM is difficult to control, even with large doses of insulin (>20 U q12h). Nevertheless, *administration of large doses of insulin should be avoided.* The severity of insulin resistance fluctuates unpredictably in cats with acromegaly, and severe, life-threatening hypoglycemia may suddenly develop after months of insulin resistance and blood glucose concentrations >400 mg/dl. To prevent severe hypoglycemia, one should not exceed insulin doses of 15 U per injection.

### Prognosis

The short-term prognosis for tumor-induced acromegaly is guarded to good, but the long-term prognosis is poor. Survival times range from 4 to 60 months (typically 1.5 to 3 years). Most cats eventually die or are euthanized because of severe congestive heart failure, renal failure, respiratory disease, neurologic signs of an expanding pituitary tumor, or coma caused by severe hypoglycemia.

## PITUITARY DWARFISM (TEXT PP 677-680)

Pituitary dwarfism results from a congenital deficiency of GH. In dogs, and probably in cats, it is most commonly associated with pituitary hypoplasia or pressure atrophy of the anterior lobe resulting from an anomaly involving the craniopharyngeal duct (Rathke's pouch). Pituitary dwarfism may be due solely to GH deficiency, or it may be part of a combined pituitary hormone deficiency, most often including thyroid-stimulating hormone (TSH) and prolactin.

Pituitary dwarfism is encountered most often as a simple, autosomal-recessive inherited abnormality in German Shepherd Dogs; a similar mode of inheritance has been reported in Carnelian Bear dogs. Other breeds in which pituitary dwarfism has been described include the Weimaraner, Spitz, and Toy Pinscher. It has also been reported in cats.

### Clinical features

The most common manifestations are lack of growth (i.e., short stature), endocrine alopecia, and hyperpigmentation of the skin (Box 49-3). Affected animals are usually normal in size during the first 1 to 2 months of life, after which growth rate is slower than that of their littermates. By 3 to 4 months of age, affected dogs and cats are obviously runts and usually never attain full adult dimensions.

Dwarfs with an isolated GH deficiency typically maintain a normal body contour and proportions as they age (i.e., proportionate dwarfism). Dwarfs with combined deficiencies (most notably TSH) may acquire the square or chunky contour typical of congenital hypothyroidism (i.e., disproportionate dwarfism). Hypogonadism may also develop, although normal reproductive function has been reported in some pituitary dwarfs. In males, testicular atrophy, azoospermia, and a flaccid penile sheath are typical; in females, estrous activity is absent.

*Skin and haircoat.* The most notable dermatologic sign is retention of the lanugo or secondary hairs and absence of the primary or guard hairs. As a result the haircoat is initially soft and wooly. The hairs are easily epilated, and bilateral symmetric alopecia gradually develops. The skin is initially normal but with time becomes progressively hyperpigmented, thin, wrinkled, and scaly. Comedones, papules, and secondary pyoderma frequently develop in adult dwarfs. Secondary bacterial infections of the skin and respiratory tract are common long-term complications.

---

**Box 49-3**

## Clinical Signs Associated with Pituitary Dwarfism

### MUSCULOSKELETAL

Stunted growth
Thin skeleton, immature facial features
Scuare, chunky contour (adult)
Bone deformities
Delayed closure of growth plates
Delayed dental eruption

### REPRODUCTIVE

Testicular atrophy
Flaccid penile sheath
Failure to have estrous cycles

### DERMATOLOGIC

Soft, woolly haircoat
Retention of lanugo hairs
Lack of guard hairs
Alopecia
  Bilaterally symmetric
  Trunk, neck, proximal extremities
Hyperpigmentation of skin
Thin, fragile skin
Wrinkles
Scales
Comedones
Papules
Pyoderma
Seborrhea sicca

### OTHER SIGNS

Mental dullness
Shrill, puppylike bark
Signs of secondary hypothyroidism
Signs of secondary adrenal insufficiency (uncommon)

---

### Diagnosis

The signalment, history, and physical examination usually provide sufficient evidence to include pituitary dwarfism among the tentative diagnoses of short stature. Strong presumptive evidence can be obtained by ruling out other potential causes of small size (Table 49-6).

Results of CBC, serum biochemistry panel, and urinalysis are usually normal in animals with uncomplicated pituitary dwarfism. Hypophosphatemia may result from GH deficiency; and mild hypoalbuminemia, anemia, and azotemia may develop from GH and IGF-I deficiencies. Concurrent hypothyroidism may cause other clinicopathologic alterations (see Chapter 51).

Definitive diagnosis requires evaluation of somatotroph responsiveness to provocative testing. With most pituitary dwarfs no increase occurs in serum GH after administration of a GH secretogogue. However, as discussed earlier, measurement of serum GH is not readily available for use in dogs and cats. Baseline serum IGF-I concentrations

**Table 49-6**

### Some Potential Causes of Small Stature in Dogs and Cats

| Endocrine causes | Nonendocrine causes |
| --- | --- |
| Hyposomatotropism | Malnutrition |
| Hypothyroidism | Gastrointestinal tract disorders |
| Hyperadrenocorticism | Maldigestion |
| Hypoadrenocorticism | Pancreatic exocrine insufficiency |
| Diabetes mellitus | Malabsorption |
| | Heavy intestinal parasitism |
| | Hepatic disorders |
| |    Portosystemic vascular shunt |
| |    Glycogen storage disease |
| | Renal disease |
| | Cardiovascular disease, anomalies |
| | Skeletal dysplasia, chondrodystrophy |
| | Mucopolysaccharidoses |
| | Hydrocephalus |

are low in dogs with pituitary dwarfism, but breed size should be considered when test results are evaluated.

**Treatment**

Therapy involves administration of GH, as discussed on p 437. Subnormal concentrations of thyroid hormone may diminish the effectiveness of GH therapy, so concurrent thyroid hormone supplementation should be given to dogs and cats with suspected panhypopituitarism (see Chapter 51). A beneficial response in the skin and haircoat usually occurs within 8 weeks. An increase in height is dependent on the status of the growth plates at the time treatment is initiated.

Improvement in clinical signs has been reported in two German Shepherd dwarfs treated with medroxyprogesterone acetate at 3- to 6-week intervals. (Progestogens indirectly result in GH secretion from the mammary gland and therefore increased plasma GH and IGF-I.) Adverse effects included pruritic pyoderma in both dogs, mucometra in the female dog, and signs of acromegaly in the male dog.

**Prognosis**

The long-term prognosis is poor. Most animals die by 3 to 5 years of age despite therapy. Death is usually a result of infections, degenerative diseases, or neurologic dysfunction.

# 50

# Disorders
# of the Parathyroid Gland

## (Text pp 681-690)

### HYPERPARATHYROIDISM (TEXT PP 681-686)

Hyperparathyroidism is a sustained increase in parathyroid hormone (PTH) secretion. It can result from (1) a normal physiologic response to decreased serum ionized calcium (Ca) concentrations (renal or nutritional secondary hyperparathyroidism) or (2) a pathologic condition resulting from excessive synthesis and secretion of PTH by abnormal, autonomously functioning parathyroid chief cells (primary hyperparathyroidism, or PHP). With PHP, increased secretion of PTH is maintained regardless of the serum ionized Ca concentration.

#### Secondary hyperparathyroidism

With renal failure, hyperparathyroidism develops as a result of phosphate retention and hyperphosphatemia, which decreases serum ionized Ca and therefore stimulates PTH secretion. The net effect is increased serum phosphorus (P), normal to low serum ionized Ca, increased serum PTH, and diffuse parathyroid gland hyperplasia. The etiogenesis is similar in nutritional secondary hyperparathyroidism, except that the decrease in Ca results from feeding diets with low Ca:P ratios, such as beef heart or liver. Dietary Ca deficiency or P excess decreases serum Ca, inducing increased PTH secretion and parathyroid gland hyperplasia.

#### Primary hyperparathyroidism

PHP is a disorder resulting from excessive, relatively uncontrolled secretion of PTH by one or more abnormal parathyroid glands. It is uncommon in dogs and rare in cats. Parathyroid adenoma is the most common cause; parathyroid carcinoma and adenomatous hyperplasia have also been described. Clinical signs stem from the physiologic actions of excessive PTH secretion, which include hypercalcemia and hypophosphatemia (Table 50-1).

##### Clinical features

PHP occurs in older dogs (mean, 10 years; range, 4 to 16 years). A genetic predisposition is suspected in Keeshonds. In cats with PHP the mean age is 12 years (range, 8 to 15 years). Females and Siamese cats may be overrepresented.

*Clinical signs.* Clinical signs are absent in most dogs and cats with mild PHP, and hypercalcemia is discovered fortuitously. When signs do develop, they tend to be insidious in onset and nonspecific initially. Clinical signs in dogs typically are renal, gastrointestinal, and neuromuscular in origin. The more common signs include polyuria and polydipsia, listlessness, urinary incontinence, weakness, and exercise intolerance. Less common signs include dysuria, pollakiuria, hematuria, inappetence, shivering, muscle wasting, vomiting, constipation, and stiff gait. The most common clinical signs in cats with PHP are anorexia and lethargy.

*Physical examination.* In most cases physical examination is unremarkable, which is important when one is differentiating PHP from hypercalcemia of malignancy.

**Table 50-1**

**Biologic Actions of the Hormones That Affect Calcium and Phosphorus Metabolism**

| Hormone | Bone | Kidney | Intestine | Net Effect | |
|---|---|---|---|---|---|
| | | | | Serum Ca | Serum PO$_4$ |
| Parathyroid hormone | Increased bone resorption | ↑ Ca absorption<br>↑ PO$_4$ excretion | No direct effect | ↑ | ↓ |
| Calcitonin | Decreased bone resorption | ↓ Ca resorption<br>↓ PO$_4$ resorption | No direct effect | ↓ | ↓ |
| Vitamin D | Maintain Ca transport system | ↓ Ca resorption | ↑ Ca absorption<br>↑ PO$_4$ absorption | ↑ | ↑ |

*Ca*, Calcium; *PO$_4$*, phosphorus (phosphate); ↑, increased; ↓, decreased.

Lethargy, generalized muscle atrophy, weakness (variable, but usually subtle), and cystic calculi (Ca-phosphate, Ca-oxalate, or both) are noted in some dogs with PHP. Rarely, parathyroid adenoma is identified by palpation of the ventral neck in dogs. If a mass is palpable, the possibility of a carcinoma should be considered. Cats with PHP can have a palpable mass in the region of the thyroid gland, although hyperthyroidism is a much more likely cause than PHP.

### Diagnosis

PHP should be suspected in a dog or cat with persistent hypercalcemia and normal or low serum P. Serum total Ca typically is 12 to 15 mg/dl but can exceed 16 mg/dl. Serum ionized Ca typically is 1.4 to 1.8 mmol/L but can exceed 2 mmol/L. Serum P typically is <4 mg/dl, unless concurrent renal insufficiency is present.

*Differential diagnoses.* Hypercalcemia in dogs and cats has several possible causes (Table 50-2), but the primary differential diagnoses for hypercalcemia and hypophosphatemia are hypercalcemia of malignancy and PHP. The diagnosis can usually be established based on the history, physical examination findings, results of routine

**Table 50-2**

## Causes of Hypercalcemia in Dogs and Cats

| Disorder | Tests to help establish the diagnosis |
|---|---|
| Primary hyperparathyroidism | Serum PTH concentration, cervical ultrasound, surgery |
| Hypercalcemia of malignancy<br>Humorally mediated: LSA, apocrine gland adenocarcinoma, carcinoma (nasal, mammary gland, gastric, thyroid, pancreatic, pulmonary)<br>Locally osteolytic (multiple myeloma, LSA, squamous cell carcinoma, osteosarcoma, fibrosarcoma) | Physical examination, thoracic and abdominal radiography, abdominal ultrasonography, lymph node and bone marrow aspiration, serum PTHrp |
| Hypervitaminosis D<br>Cholecalciferol rodenticides, plants<br>Excessive supplementation | History, serum biochemistry panel, serum vitamin D concentration |
| Hypoadrenocorticism | Serum $Na^+$, $K^+$, ACTH stimulation test |
| Renal failure | Serum biochemistry panel, urinalysis |
| Granulomatous disease (rare)<br>Systemic mycosis—blastomycosis<br>Schistosomiasis, FIP | Thoracic radiography, fundic examination, cytologic studies of tracheal wash or intestinal biopsy specimens, serum fungal titer |
| Nonmalignant skeletal disorder (rare)<br>Osteomyelitis<br>Hypertrophic osteodystrophy | Radiography of peripheral skeleton |
| Iatrogenic disorder (rare)<br>Excessive calcium supplementation<br>Excessive oral phosphate binders | — |
| Dehydration (mild hypercalcemia) | — |
| Factitious disorder<br>Lipemia<br>Postprandial measurement<br>Young animal (<6 months) | — |
| Laboratory error | — |
| Idiopathic (cats) | — |

*ACTH,* Adrenocorticotropic hormone; *FIP,* feline infectious peritonitis; *$K^+$,* potassium; *LSA,* lymphosarcoma; *$Na^+$,* sodium; *PTH,* parathyroid hormone; *PTHrp,* parathyroid hormone–related protein.

blood and urine tests, thoracic radiography, abdominal and cervical ultrasonography, and measurement of serum PTH and PTH-related protein (PTHrp) concentrations.

With PHP, clinical signs are usually mild or absent, physical examination is normal, and results of routine blood work, thoracic and abdominal radiography, and abdominal ultrasonography are unremarkable, except for hypercalcemia and hypophosphatemia. Additional tests to identify lymphoma (e.g., bone marrow and lymph node aspirates, serum PTHrp) also are normal. Ultrasonography of the thyroparathyroid complex may reveal enlargement of one or more parathyroid glands.

*Renal indexes.* Urine specific gravity of <1.015 is common. Hematuria, pyuria, bacteriuria, and crystalluria may be identified if cystic calculi and secondary bacterial cystitis develop. Prolonged, severe hypercalcemia may cause progressive renal damage with a resultant increase in blood urea nitrogen (BUN), serum creatinine, and serum P. Serum ionized Ca is increased in dogs with PHP-induced renal failure and normal or low when hypercalcemia is induced by primary renal failure.

*Serum PTH.* Measurement of serum PTH helps confirm a diagnosis of PHP. Assays that measure the intact PTH molecule are recommended. Interpretation must be done in conjunction with the serum Ca concentration. If the parathyroid gland is functioning normally, serum PTH is low or undetectable in the face of hypercalcemia. Mid-normal or increased serum PTH is inappropriate in the face of hypercalcemia and is indicative of an autonomously functioning parathyroid gland.

Increased serum PTH can be found in dogs with renal secondary hyperparathyroidism. Because of the influence of the kidney on circulating PTH concentration, *renal function must be normal* in a hypercalcemic dog for evaluation of serum PTH to be meaningful. It may, however, be useful to evaluate serum PTH in conjunction with serum ionized Ca, which typically is normal or low in animals with renal failure and increased in those with PHP. Serum PTH is increased in both disorders.

*Tumor versus hyperplasia.* Parathyroid adenomas typically are small (4 to 8 mm), single, well-encapsulated, light brown to red tumors in close apposition to the thyroid gland. The remaining parathyroid glands are normal or atrophied. Grossly, parathyroid carcinomas appear similar to adenomas, so the diagnosis is based on histologic features (e.g., capsular or vascular invasion). Parathyroid hyperplasia is tentatively diagnosed if more than one parathyroid gland is grossly and microscopically abnormal and renal and nutritional secondary hyperparathyroidism have been ruled out.

Differentiation between hyperplasia and adenoma has important prognostic implications. Surgical removal of a solitary parathyroid adenoma results in cure, assuming that at least one normal parathyroid gland remains. In contrast, persistent hyperparathyroidism is likely in animals with parathyroid hyperplasia, unless all abnormal parathyroid tissue is removed; also, recurrence of hyperparathyroidism weeks or months after surgery is common.

*Surgery.* Ultimately, surgical exploration of the neck is required to establish a diagnosis of PHP. If the signalment, history, and physical examination findings are consistent with PHP, a thorough diagnostic evaluation has failed to identify another cause for the hypercalcemia, and serum PTH is inappropriately increased, the likelihood of PHP is high and surgical exploration of the neck is warranted. Ultrasonographic evaluation of the thyroparathyroid complex provides useful information before surgery regarding the number and location of hyperfunctioning parathyroid glands.

### Treatment

Surgical removal of the abnormal parathyroid tissue is the treatment of choice. Ethanol injection or heat ablation of abnormal parathyroid tissue under ultrasound guidance is also an effective treatment for PHP, although anesthesia is still required, posttreatment hypocalcemia is not avoided, and results are less consistent than with surgical removal.

During surgery, it is important to evaluate all four parathyroid glands before deciding on which gland(s) to remove, and an attempt must be made to ensure that at least one parathyroid gland remains intact to maintain Ca homeostasis and prevent permanent hypocalcemia. Almost all dogs and cats with PHP have a solitary, easily identified parathyroid adenoma. Enlargement of more than one parathyroid gland indicates either multiple adenomas or, more likely, parathyroid hyperplasia.

When more than one enlarged gland is identified, the concern is whether primary or secondary (i.e., renal or nutritional) hyperparathyroidism is present. A thorough presurgical evaluation should rule out secondary causes. A decision to remove three versus four glands should be based on the clinical status and renal function and on the ability of the owner to treat permanent hypoparathyroidism. If none of the glands appears enlarged or if all appear small, the diagnosis of PHP must be questioned, and a diagnosis of occult neoplasia, ectopic parathyroid tumor, or nonparathyroid PTH-producing tumor should be considered.

*Postoperative monitoring.* Surgical removal of the parathyroid tumor results in a rapid decline in circulating PTH and subsequent development of hypocalcemia 1 to 7 days after surgery. The higher the presurgical serum Ca and/or the more chronic the condition, the more likely it is that clinical hypocalcemia will develop. As a guide, if serum total or ionized Ca before surgery is <14 mg/dl or <1.6 mmol/L, respectively, the patient should be kept in the hospital for 5 to 7 days, and serum Ca monitored twice daily.

Treatment for hypocalcemia is not initiated unless clinical signs of hypocalcemia develop or the serum total or ionized Ca drops below 9 mg/dl or 0.9 mmol/L, respectively. In most cases the remaining parathyroid glands are capable of secreting adequate amounts of PTH to prevent severe hypocalcemia, and the hypocalcemia gradually resolves over the ensuing week, so postoperative Ca and vitamin D supplementation is not required.

*Ca and vitamin D therapy.* Serum total or ionized Ca >14 mg/dl or >1.6 mmol/L, respectively, suggests chronic hypercalcemia, marked atrophy of the remaining parathyroid glands, and a high probability that signs of hypocalcemia will develop after surgery. In such animals Ca and vitamin D therapy should be started once a decrease in serum total or ionized Ca is documented (which usually occurs within 6 to 8 hours of surgery). In animals with severe hypercalcemia (total or ionized Ca >18 mg/dl and >2 mmol/L, respectively), vitamin D therapy can begin 24 to 36 hours *before* surgery.

Therapy for hypocalcemia involves intravenous (IV) or subcutaneous (SC) administration of Ca to control existing clinical signs and long-term oral administration of Ca and vitamin D to maintain serum Ca between 9 and 10 mg/dl until the remaining parathyroid glands regain control of Ca homeostasis.

*Withdrawing therapy.* Once serum Ca is stable, the Ca and vitamin D supplements can be gradually withdrawn over 3 to 6 months. Vitamin D therapy should be withdrawn first by gradually increasing the number of days between doses. It can be discontinued once the dog or cat is clinically normal, serum Ca is stable between 9 and 11 mg/dl, and the administration interval is no less than every 7 days. Ca supplementation can then be gradually reduced and discontinued over the subsequent month.

### Prognosis

The prognosis depends on the severity of renal changes induced by hypercalcemia and on the ability to prevent severe postoperative hypocalcemia. If serious renal damage has not occurred and severe postoperative hypocalcemia is avoided, the prognosis is excellent. Hypercalcemia may recur weeks or months after surgery in dogs and cats with PHP caused by parathyroid hyperplasia if one or more parathyroid glands are left in situ.

## PRIMARY HYPOPARATHYROIDISM (TEXT PP 686-689)

### Etiology

Primary hypoparathyroidism results from an absolute or relative deficiency in PTH secretion. Most cases are classified as idiopathic (i.e., no evidence of trauma, malignant or surgical destruction, or other obvious damage to the neck or parathyroid glands). This disorder may have an immune-mediated component. Iatrogenic hypoparathyroidism after bilateral thyroidectomy is common in cats. This form of hypoparathyroidism may be transient or permanent, depending on the viability of the parathyroid gland(s) saved.

Transient hypoparathyroidism may develop secondary to severe magnesium (Mg) depletion (serum Mg <1.2 mg/dl). Mild hypocalcemia and hyperphosphatemia ensue. Mg repletion reverses the hypoparathyroidism. In general, serum Mg in dogs and cats with primary hypoparathyroidism is normal.

### Clinical features

Age at onset of clinical signs in dogs ranges from 6 weeks to 13 years, with a mean of 4.8 years. A gender predisposition for females may exist. No definite breed predisposition exists, although Toy Poodles, Miniature Schnauzers, Labrador Retrievers, German Shepherd Dogs, and Terriers are commonly affected. Few cases of primary hypoparathyroidism have been reported in cats. To date, affected cats have been young to middle aged (6 months to 7 years) and more often male.

*Clinical signs.* The major clinical signs are directly attributable to hypocalcemia, which most notably affects the neuromuscular system. Neuromuscular signs include nervousness, generalized seizures, rear leg cramping or pain, focal muscle fasciculations or twitching, ataxia, and weakness. Additional signs include stiff gait, intense facial rubbing, aggressive behavior, panting, inappetence, listlessness, lethargy, and intense biting or licking at the paws.

Onset of signs tends to be abrupt and severe and occurs more frequently during exercise, excitement, or stress. Signs also tend to be episodic, with bouts of clinical hypocalcemia interspersed with relatively normal periods, lasting minutes to days, even though hypocalcemia persists during these "normal" periods.

*Physical examination.* The most common findings are related to muscular tetany. Fever, panting, and nervousness, often to the point of interfering with the examination, are also common. Potential cardiac abnormalities include paroxysmal tachyarrhythmias, muffled heart sounds, and weak femoral pulses. Cataracts have been reported in a few dogs and in one cat. Occasionally, physical examination is normal despite a history of neuromuscular signs.

### Diagnosis

Primary hypoparathyroidism should be suspected in a dog or cat with persistent hypocalcemia, hyperphosphatemia, and normal renal function. The serum total and ionized Ca usually are <7 mg/dl and <0.8 mmol/L, respectively, and serum P usually is >6 mg/dl.

Hypocalcemia and hyperphosphatemia can also be encountered with nutritional and renal secondary hyperparathyroidism; after administration of a phosphate-containing enema; and with tumor lysis syndrome. The diagnosis of primary hypoparathyroidism is established when serum PTH is undetectable in the face of severe hypocalcemia and other causes of hypocalcemia have been ruled out (Table 50-3). Most causes of hypocalcemia can be identified after evaluation of the history, physical examination findings, and results of routine blood and urine tests and abdominal ultrasonography.

*Serum PTH.* Measurement of serum PTH helps confirm the diagnosis of primary hypoparathyroidism. Blood for this test should be obtained before Ca and vitamin D therapy is started. Assays that measure the intact PTH molecule are recommended, and results must be interpreted in conjunction with serum Ca concentration.

If the parathyroid glands are functioning normally, serum PTH is increased in the face of hypocalcemia. Low or undetectable serum PTH in a hypocalcemic animal is strongly suggestive of primary hypoparathyroidism. Patients with non–parathyroid-induced hypocalcemia have normal or high serum PTH (except those with disorders that cause severe hypomagnesemia).

### Treatment

Therapy involves administration of Ca and vitamin D supplements. Acute therapy to control hypocalcemic tetany involves slow IV administration of Ca-gluconate (*not* Ca-chloride) until effective (Table 50-4). Once signs of hypocalcemia are controlled,

Table 50-3

## Causes of Hypocalcemia in Dogs and Cats

| Disorder | Tests to help establish the diagnosis |
|---|---|
| Primary hypoparathyroidism<br>  Idiopathic<br>  Postthyroidectomy | History, serum PTH concentration, rule out other causes |
| Puerperal tetany | History |
| Renal failure<br>  Acute<br>  Chronic | Serum biochemistry panel, urinalysis |
| Ethylene glycol toxicity | |
| Acute pancreatitis | Physical findings, serum lipase or amylase activities |
| Intestinal malabsorption syndromes | History, digestion or absorption tests, intestinal biopsy |
| Hypoproteinemia or hypoalbuminemia | Serum biochemistry panel |
| Hypomagnesemia | Serum total and ionized Mg |
| Nutritional secondary hyperparathyroidism | Dietary history (what dog or cat eats) |
| Tumor lysis syndrome | History |
| Phosphate-containing enemas | History |
| Anticonvulsant medications | History |
| $NaHCO_3$ administration | History |
| Laboratory error | History |

*Mg,* magnesium; *NaHCO₃* sodium bicarbonate; *PTH,* parathyroid hormone.

Ca-gluconate is continued by continuous IV infusion or SC injection (at the IV dose, but diluted at least 1:1 with saline, and repeated q6-8h), and oral Ca and vitamin D therapy initiated.

Serum Ca should be measured twice daily during this time, and the dose or frequency of SC Ca administration adjusted to control clinical signs and maintain the serum Ca between 8 and 10 mg/dl. (Serum Ca >10 mg/dl is unnecessary to avoid tetany and increases the likelihood of hypercalcemia.) Once serum Ca has remained >8 mg/dl for 48 hours, SC Ca is discontinued by gradually increasing the interval between doses.

*Maintenance therapy.* Maintenance therapy should keep the serum Ca between 9 and 10 mg/dl through daily administration of Ca and vitamin D supplements (Tables 50-4 and 50-5). Ideally, the patient remains hospitalized until the serum Ca stays between 8 and 10 mg/dl without parenteral support. Thereafter, serum Ca should be monitored weekly, and the vitamin D dose adjusted to maintain a serum Ca of 9 to 10 mg/dl.

Once the serum Ca is stabilized in the target range, attempts can be made to slowly taper the oral Ca and then vitamin D to the lowest effective dose. Most dogs and cats with primary hypoparathyroidism require permanent vitamin D therapy, but the Ca supplement can often be gradually tapered over 2 to 4 months and then stopped. Supplementing the diet with Ca-rich foods (e.g., dairy products) helps ensure adequate Ca intake. Reevaluation of serum Ca every 3 to 4 months is advisable.

### Prognosis

With owner compliance, proper therapy, and timely reevaluations, the prognosis is excellent. The more frequent the rechecks, the better the chance of avoiding extremes in serum Ca, and the better the chance of a normal life expectancy.

**Table 50-4**

## Injectable and Oral Calcium Preparations

| Preparation | Dosage form | Approximate calcium content | Dose |
|---|---|---|---|
| **INJECTABLE (IV)** | | | |
| Calcium gluconate | 10% solution | 9.3 mg of Ca per ml | 0.5-1.5 ml/kg (5-15 mg of Ca per kg) |
| Calcium chloride | 10% solution | 27.2 mg of Ca per ml | 0.25-0.75 ml/kg (5-15 mg of Ca per kg) |
| **ORAL** | | | |
| Calcium gluconate | 325-, 500-, 650-, and 1000-mg tablets | 30, 45, 60, and 90 mg of Ca per tablet | 25 mg of Ca per kg q8-12h |
| Calcium lactate | 325- and 650-mg tablets | 42 and 85 mg of Ca per tablet | As above |
| Calcium carbonate | 500-, 650-, and 1250-mg tablets | 200, 260, and 500 mg of Ca per tablet | As above |
| Calcium carbonate and gluconate | 700-mg tablets | 250 mg of Ca per tablet | As above |

**Table 50-5**

## Vitamin D Preparations

| Preparation | Dosage form | Dose | Time for maximal effect | Time for relief of toxicity |
|---|---|---|---|---|
| Vitamin D₂ (ergocalciferol) | Capsules: 25,000 U, 50,000 U<br>Syrup: 8000 U/ml*<br>IM injectable: 50,000 U/ml | Initial: 4000-6000 U/kg/day<br>Maintenance: 1000-2000 U/kg once daily to once every 7-14 days | 5-21 days | 1-18 weeks |
| Dihydrotachysterol | Tablets: 0.125 mg,* 0.2 mg, 0.4 mg<br>Capsules: 0.125 mg*<br>Oral solution: 0.25 mg/ml* | Initial: 0.02-0.03 mg/kg/day<br>Maintenance: 0.01-0.02 mg/kg every 24-48h | 1-7 days | 1-3 weeks |
| 1,25-Dihydroxy vitamin D₃ | Capsules: 0.25 µg | Initial: 0.02-0.03 µg/kg/day<br>Maintenance: 0.005-0.015 µg/kg/day | 1-4 days | 2-14 days |

*Dosage form suitable for administration in cats.

# 51

# Disorders
# of the Thyroid Gland

## *(Text pp 691-728)*

## HYPOTHYROIDISM IN DOGS (TEXT PP 691-709)

### Etiology

Primary hypothyroidism is the most common form of the disorder in dogs; it results from problems within the thyroid gland, most often immune-mediated lymphocytic thyroiditis or idiopathic atrophy. Genetics likely play a role in lymphocytic thyroiditis. Idiopathic atrophy may be a primary degenerative disorder, or it could represent the end stage of lymphocytic thyroiditis. Congenital defects in thyroid hormonogenesis (congenital primary hypothyroidism) are rare in dogs. Secondary hypothyroidism results from pituitary dysfunction. Specific causes of hypothyroidism are listed in Box 51-1.

*Goiter.* Whether or not goiter (thyroid gland enlargement) develops depends on the underlying problem. If the hypothalamic-pituitary-thyroid axis is intact (as occurs with an iodine organification defect), goiter will develop. If the axis is not intact (as occurs with pituitary thyroid-stimulating hormone [TSH] deficiency), goiter will not develop.

### Clinical features

With primary hypothyroidism, signs usually develop during middle age (2 to 6 years). Breeds at increased risk (Box 51-2) tend to develop signs at an earlier age. Clinical signs are quite variable and depend in part on the age of the dog at the time a thyroid hormone deficiency develops. Signs may also differ among breeds.

In adult dogs, the most consistent signs result from the effects of decreased cellular metabolism on the dog's mental status and activity level (Box 51-3). Most dogs with hypothyroidism have some degree of mental dullness, lethargy, exercise intolerance or unwillingness to exercise, and a propensity to gain weight without a corresponding increase in appetite or food intake. These signs are often gradual in onset and subtle.

*Dermatologic signs.* Alterations in the skin and haircoat are common. Classic signs include bilateral symmetric, nonpruritic truncal alopecia; however, alopecia may be local or generalized, may be symmetric or asymmetric, may involve only the tail ("rat tail"), and often starts over points of wear. Nonpruritic endocrine alopecia is not pathognomonic for hypothyroidism, but when present in a dog with lethargy, weight gain, and no polyuria (PU) or polydipsia (PD), hypothyroidism is the most likely diagnosis.

Seborrhea and pyoderma are also common; all forms of seborrhea are possible. Seborrhea and pyoderma may be focal, multifocal, or generalized; both frequently result in pruritus. Therefore hypothyroid dogs with secondary pyoderma or seborrhea may be presented with a pruritic skin disorder.

The haircoat is often dull, dry, and easily epilated, and hair regrowth is slow. Hyperkeratosis leads to scales and dandruff. Variable degrees of hyperpigmentation may also be noted. Chronic otitis externa is seen in some dogs. Myxedema (skin thickening) occurs predominantly in the forehead and face, resulting in rounding of the temporal

---

**Box 51-1**

## Potential Causes of Hypothyroidism in Dogs

### PRIMARY HYPOTHYROIDISM

Lymphocytic thyroiditis
Idiopathic atrophy
Neoplastic destruction
Iatrogenic causes
    Surgical removal
    Antithyroid medications
    Radioactive iodine treatment
    Drugs (e.g., sulfamethoxazole)

### SECONDARY HYPOTHYROIDISM

Pituitary malformation
    Pituitary cyst
    Pituitary hypoplasia
Pituitary destruction
    Neoplasia
Pituitary thyrotropic cell suppression
    Naturally acquired
        hyperadrenocorticism
    Euthyroid sick syndrome
Iatrogenic causes
    Drug therapy, most notably with
        glucocorticoids
    Radiation therapy
    Hypophysectomy

### TERTIARY HYPOTHYROIDISM

Congenital hypothalamic
    malformation (?)
Acquired destruction of
    hypothalamus (?)

### CONGENITAL HYPOTHYROIDISM

Thyroid gland dysgenesis (aplasia,
    hypoplasia, ectasia)
Dyshormonogenesis: iodine
    organification defect
Deficient dietary iodine intake

---

**Box 51-2**

## Dog Breeds Reported to Have an Increased Prevalence of Thyroid Hormone Autoantibodies

Pointer
English Pointer
German Wirehaired Pointer
Boxer
Kuvasz
American Staffordshire Terrier
American Pit Bull Terrier
Giant Schnauzer
Golden Retriever
Chesapeake Bay Retriever
Brittany Spaniel
Australian Shepherd
Malamute

English Setter
Skye Terrier
Old English Sheepdog
Maltese
Petit Basset Griffon Vendeen
Beagle
Dalmatian
Rhodesian Ridgeback
Shetland Sheepdog
Siberian Husky
Borzoi
Doberman Pinscher
Cocker Spaniel

From Nachreiner RF, Refsal KR, Graham PA et al: Prevalence of serum thyroid hormone autoantibodies in dogs with clinical signs of hypothyroidism, *J Am Vet Med Assoc* 220:466, 2002.

---

**Box 51-3**

## Clinical Manifestations of Hypothyroidism in Adult Dogs

**METABOLIC**
Lethargy*
Mental dullness*
Inactivity*
Weight gain*
Cold intolerance

**REPRODUCTIVE**
Persistent anestrus
Weak or silent estrus
Prolonged estrual bleeding
Inappropriate galactorrhea or
    gynecomastia
Testicular atrophy(?)
Loss of libido(?)

**OCULAR**
Corneal lipid deposits
Corneal ulceration
Uveitis

**CARDIOVASCULAR**
Decreased contractility
Bradycardia
Cardiac arrhythmias

**GASTROINTESTINAL**
Esophageal hypomotility(?)
Diarrhea
Constipation

**DERMATOLOGIC**
Endocrine alopecia*
    Symmetric or asymmetric
    "Rat tail"
Dry, brittle haircoat
Hyperpigmentation
Seborrhea sicca or oleosa, or
    dermatitis*
Pyoderma*
Otitis externa
Myxedema

**NEUROMUSCULAR**
Weakness*
Knuckling
Ataxia
Circling
Vestibular signs
Facial nerve paralysis
Seizures
Laryngeal paralysis

**HEMATOLOGIC**
Anemia*
Hyperlipidemia*
Coagulopathy

**MISCELLANEOUS**
Behavioral abnormalities (?)

---

*Common.

region, puffiness and increased thickness of facial skin folds, and, in conjunction with drooping upper eyelids, development of a "tragic facial expression."

*Neuromuscular signs.* Neurologic signs predominate in some dogs. Signs may be referable to the central nervous system (CNS) or peripheral nervous system (see Box 51-3). CNS signs are often present with vestibular signs or facial nerve paralysis. Other peripheral neuropathies include weakness and knuckling or dragging of the feet with excessive toenail wear. Muscle wasting may also be evident. Thyroxine-responsive unilateral forelimb lameness has also been described.

The relationship between hypothyroidism and laryngeal paralysis or esophageal hypomotility remains controversial. It is difficult to prove a cause-and-effect relationship, and treatment of hypothyroidism usually does not improve the clinical signs of these other disorders.

*Reproductive signs.* Hypothyroidism may cause prolonged interestrus intervals and failure to cycle. Maternal hypothyroidism may also result in weak puppies that die shortly after birth. Other abnormalities are listed in Box 51-3.

*Behavioral changes.* Anecdotal reports link hypothyroidism with behavioral problems such as aggression. However, a cause-and-effect relationship has not been established. The benefits, if any, of using thyroid hormone to treat behavioral disorders in dogs remains to be clarified.

*Miscellaneous signs.* Ocular, cardiovascular, digestive, and clotting abnormalities are uncommon clinical manifestations of hypothyroidism. More commonly, biochemical or functional abnormalities of these organ systems are identified in dogs that exhibit the more common signs of hypothyroidism. Echocardiography may identify a decrease in cardiac contractility that is usually mild and asymptomatic, but that may become relevant during a surgical procedure requiring prolonged anesthesia and aggressive fluid therapy.

*Von Willebrand factor deficiency.* A reduction in von Willebrand factor (vWF) activity is sometimes seen, but it is uncommon for hypothyroid dogs to be presented with clinical signs of a bleeding disorder. Evaluation of the coagulation cascade or vWF activity is not indicated unless a bleeding problem is present. (Thyroid hormone supplementation has a variable and sometimes deleterious effect on the blood concentration of vWF in euthyroid dogs with von Willebrand's disease.)

*Cretinism.* Hypothyroidism in puppies is termed *cretinism*. As the age of onset increases, the clinical appearance is similar to that of adult hypothyroidism. Growth retardation and impaired mental development are the hallmarks of cretinism. Dogs with cretinism appear disproportionate, with large, broad heads; shortened mandibles; thick, protruding tongues; wide or square trunks; and short limbs. This picture is in contrast to the proportionate dwarfism caused by growth hormone deficiency (see Chapter 49).

Cretins are mentally dull and lethargic and lack normal playfulness. Other signs can include persistence of the puppy haircoat, dry hair and thickened skin, alopecia, inappetence, delayed dental eruption, goiter, kyphosis, constipation, dyspnea, and gait abnormalities. The presence of goiter is variable and dependent on the underlying cause. Differential diagnoses for failure to grow include endocrine and nonendocrine causes (see Table 49-6).

*Immunoendocrinopathy syndromes.* Lymphocytic thyroiditis can occur in association with other immune-mediated endocrinopathies, although this is uncommon. Hypothyroidism, hypoadrenocorticism, and to a lesser extent diabetes mellitus, hypoparathyroidism, and lymphocytic orchitis are recognized combined syndromes. In most affected dogs each endocrinopathy is manifested separately, with additional disorders following one by one after a variable time (weeks to months). Diagnosis and treatment are directed at each disorder as it becomes recognized. Immunosuppressive drug therapy is not indicated.

### Clinical pathology

The most consistent clinicopathologic abnormalities are elevations in serum cholesterol and triglycerides (e.g., lipemia). Hypercholesterolemia is found in approximately 75% of hypothyroid dogs and can exceed 1000 mg/dl. Fasting hypercholesterolemia and lipemia can be associated with several other disorders, but their presence in a dog with appropriate clinical signs is strongly supportive of hypothyroidism.

A mild normocytic, normochromic, nonregenerative anemia (packed cell volume [PCV] 28% to 35%) is a less consistent finding. Evaluation of red blood cell morphology may reveal increased numbers of leptocytes (target cells). The white blood cell count typically is normal, and platelet counts are normal or increased. A mild to moderate increase in lactate dehydrogenase, aspartate aminotransferase (AST), alanine aminotransferase (ALT), alkaline phosphatase (AP), and, rarely, creatine kinase activities may also be identified. However, these findings are extremely inconsistent and may not be directly related to the hypothyroid state. Mild hypercalcemia is found in some dogs with congenital hypothyroidism. Results of urinalysis usually are normal.

### Dermatohistopathology

Skin biopsies are often performed in dogs with suspected endocrine alopecia. Nonspecific histologic changes are associated with various endocrinopathies, including hypothyroidism. A variable inflammatory cell infiltrate may be present if secondary pyoderma has developed. Presence of "hypothyroid-specific" histopathologic alterations is an indication for further evaluation of thyroid function.

## Tests of thyroid function

Thyroid gland function typically is assessed by measuring baseline serum thyroid hormone concentrations. Tests are available for measurement of thyroxine ($T_4$), free $T_4$ ($fT_4$), 3,5,3'-triiodothyronine ($T_3$), free $T_3$ ($fT_3$), 3,3',5'-triiodothyronine (reverse $T_3$, or $rT_3$), and endogenous TSH. Tests that measure $T_4$ and $fT_4$, in conjunction with TSH, are currently recommended for dogs suspected of having hypothyroidism. Serum $T_3$ concentration is a poor indicator of thyroid function.

***Baseline serum $T_4$.*** Measurement of $T_4$ can be used as the initial test for hypothyroidism or as part of a thyroid panel ($T_4$, $fT_4$, TSH, and antibody test for lymphocytic thyroiditis). Measurement of $T_4$ by radioimmunoassay (RIA) is more accurate than in-clinic enzyme-linked immunosorbent assay methods.

Theoretically interpretation is straightforward, in that dogs with hypothyroidism have low $T_4$ values (generally <1.5 μg/dl). However, the range in hypothyroid dogs overlaps that in healthy dogs, and this overlap becomes more evident in euthyroid dogs with concurrent illness (in which $T_4$ may be <0.5 μg/dl). Therefore $T_4$ must be evaluated in context with the history, physical examination findings, and other clinicopathologic data.

In general, the higher the $T_4$, the more likely it is that the dog is euthyroid, except in hypothyroid dogs with circulating antithyroid hormone antibodies (see p 458). Conversely, the lower the $T_4$, the more likely it is that the dog has hypothyroidism (see Table 51-1), assuming that the history, physical examination findings, and clinicopathologic data are consistent with the disease. If the index of suspicion for hypothyroidism is not high but the $T_4$ is low, then other factors such as euthyroid sick syndrome must be considered (see p 458).

***Baseline $fT_4$.*** The modified equilibrium analysis (MED) technique is the most accurate, and the preferred, method for measuring serum $fT_4$. In general, $fT_4$ values >1.5 ng/dl are consistent with euthyroidism, and values <1 ng/dl (especially those <0.5 ng/dl) are suggestive of hypothyroidism, assuming that the history, physical examination, and clinicopathologic abnormalities are consistent with the disorder. Serum $fT_4$ is not affected by concurrent illness to the same extent as $T_4$, although severe illness can cause $fT_4$ to decrease below 0.5 ng/dl. Circulating antithyroid hormone antibodies do not affect the $fT_4$ results determined by MED, making it a more reliable screening test than total $T_4$.

***Baseline canine TSH.*** Currently there exist two validated tests for measurement of endogenous canine TSH (cTSH). However, the ranges overlap between hypothyroid dogs and euthyroid dogs with concurrent illness, and approximately 20% of hypothyroid dogs have normal cTSH values (<0.6 ng/ml). Endogenous cTSH should always be interpreted in conjunction with $T_4$ or $fT_4$ measured in the same blood sample, and it should never be used as the sole test of thyroid gland function.

Finding a low $T_4$ or $fT_4$ and a high cTSH in a dog with appropriate history and physical examination findings supports the diagnosis of primary hypothyroidism. Finding normal $T_4$, $fT_4$, and cTSH results rules out hypothyroidism. Any other combination of $T_4$, $fT_4$, and cTSH results is difficult to interpret.

Normal $T_4$ or $fT_4$ and increased cTSH may be found in the early stages of primary hypothyroidism. Clinical signs are usually not evident, and treatment with levothyroxine is not indicated. Instead, assessment of thyroid gland function should be repeated in 2 to 4 months, especially if results of antibody tests for lymphocytic thyroiditis are positive. If progressive destruction of the thyroid gland is occurring, $T_4$ and $fT_4$ will gradually decrease and cTSH will increase over time, and clinical signs will eventually develop.

***TSH and thyrotropin-releasing hormone stimulation tests.*** The main advantage of stimulation tests using TSH or thyrotropin-releasing hormone (TRH) is differentiation of hypothyroidism from euthyroid sick syndrome in dogs with low basal $T_4$ or $fT_4$. Although the TSH stimulation test is preferred, TSH for injection is no longer available at a reasonable cost. The TRH stimulation test is still available for use in dogs and cats, although TRH for injection is becoming difficult to obtain. Several different protocols have been published; it is important to follow the protocol recommended by the laboratory performing the measurements. Interpretation of results is discussed in the text.

### Tests for lymphocytic thyroiditis

The finding of circulating autoantibodies against thyroid hormones ($T_4$ and $T_3$) and thyroglobulin (Tg) is believed to be correlated with the presence of lymphocytic thyroiditis. Tg autoantibody measurement is a better screening test for lymphocytic thyroiditis than $T_4$ and $T_3$ autoantibodies.

*Tg autoantibodies.* Presence of Tg autoantibodies implies pathology in the thyroid gland but provides no information about the severity or progressive nature of the condition or the extent of thyroid gland involvement, nor is this test an indicator of thyroid gland function. Tg autoantibodies should not be used alone in the diagnosis of hypothyroidism. Dogs with confirmed hypothyroidism can be negative and euthyroid dogs can be positive for Tg autoantibodies. Identification of Tg autoantibodies would support hypothyroidism caused by lymphocytic thyroiditis if the dog has clinical signs, physical findings, and thyroid hormone test results consistent with the disorder. The value of serum Tg autoantibodies as a marker for eventual development of hypothyroidism remains to be clarified (see text).

*$T_4$ autoantibodies.* Testing for $T_4$ autoantibodies is indicated in dogs with unusual $T_4$ values. $T_4$ autoantibodies may interfere with the RIA used to measure $T_4$, thereby yielding spurious results (see text). Serum $fT_4$ measured by MED is not affected by $T_4$ autoantibodies and should be evaluated in lieu of total $T_4$ in dogs suspected of having $T_4$ autoantibodies.

### Factors that affect thyroid function tests

Many factors can affect both baseline $T_4$ and $fT_4$ and endogenous cTSH concentrations (see Table 51-2). Many of these factors decrease baseline $T_4$ and $fT_4$ and can increase cTSH in euthyroid dogs, potentially causing misdiagnosis of hypothyroidism. Most common are concurrent illness (euthyroid sick syndrome), drugs (especially glucocorticoids), and random fluctuations of thyroid hormone concentrations (which occur in healthy dogs, euthyroid dogs with concurrent illness, and hypothyroid dogs).

*Concurrent illness.* Euthyroid dogs with concurrent illness often have $T_4$ values of 0.5 to 1 µg/dl; with severe illness (e.g., cardiomyopathy, severe anemia), values can be <0.5 µg/dl. Alterations in $fT_4$ and cTSH are more variable and probably depend on the illness involved. In general, $fT_4$ values tend to be decreased, but to a lesser extent than total $T_4$, although $fT_4$ can be <0.5 ng/dl in severe illness.

If pituitary function is suppressed, cTSH is normal or undetectable; if the pituitary response to changes in $fT_4$ is not affected by the concurrent illness, cTSH increases in response to a decrease in $fT_4$. Serum cTSH values can easily exceed 1 ng/ml in dogs with euthyroid sick syndrome.

Treatment of euthyroid sick syndrome should be aimed at the concurrent illness. Thyroid hormone concentrations normalize once the concurrent illness is eliminated. Treatment with levothyroxine is not recommended.

### Diagnosis

Specific tests for thyroid function and lymphocytic thyroiditis are discussed later and further elucidated in Tables 51-1 and 51-2. The recommended approach to diagnosis developed at the 1996 International Symposium on Canine Hypothyroidism is summarized in Box 51-4.

*Response to trial therapy.* Trial therapy should be used only when thyroid hormone supplementation does not pose a risk to the patient. Response to trial therapy with levothyroxine is nonspecific; a dog that has a positive response to therapy has either hypothyroidism or "thyroid-responsive disease."

If a positive response is observed, thyroid supplementation should be gradually discontinued once clinical signs have resolved. If clinical signs recur, hypothyroidism is confirmed and the supplement should be reinitiated. If clinical signs do not recur, a "thyroid-responsive disorder" or a beneficial response to concurrent therapy (e.g., antibiotics, flea control) should be suspected.

*Diagnosis in a previously treated dog.* Exogenous thyroid hormone suppresses pituitary TSH secretion and causes thyroid gland atrophy in healthy euthyroid dogs.

**Table 51-1**

## Interpretation of Baseline Serum Thyroxine and Free Thyroxine Concentrations in Dogs with Suspected Hypothyroidism

| Serum thyroxine concentration (µg/dl) | Serum free thyroxine concentration (ng/dl) | Probability of hypothyroidism |
|---|---|---|
| >2 | >2 | Very unlikely |
| 1.5-2 | 1.5-2 | Unlikely |
| 1-1.5 | 0.8-1.5 | Unknown |
| 0.5-1 | 0.5-0.8 | Possible |
| <0.5 | <0.5 | Very likely* |

*Assuming that a severe systemic illness is not present.

**Table 51-2**

## Variables That May Affect Baseline Serum Thyroid Hormone Function Test Results in Dogs

| Factor | Effect |
|---|---|
| Age | Inversely proportional effect |
| Neonate (<3 mo) | Increased $T_4$ |
| Aged (>6 yr) | Decreased $T_4$ |
| Body size | Inversely proportional effect |
| Small (<10 kg) | Increased $T_4$ |
| Large (>30 kg) | Decreased $T_4$ |
| Breed | |
| Sight hounds (e.g., Greyhound) | $T_4$ and $fT_4$ lower than normal range established for dogs; no difference for TSH |
| Gender | No effect |
| Time of day | No effect |
| Weight gain or obesity | Increased |
| Weight loss or fasting | Decreased $T_4$; no effect on $fT_4$ |
| Strenuous exercise | Increased $T_4$; decreased TSH; no effect on $fT_4$ |
| Estrus (estrogen) | No effect on $T_4$ |
| Pregnancy (progesterone) | Increased $T_4$ |
| Surgery and anesthesia | Decreased $T_4$ |
| Concurrent illness* | Decreased $T_4$ and $fT_4$; depending on illness, TSH may increase, decrease, or not change |
| Drugs | |
| Carprofen | Decreased $T_4$, $fT_4$, and TSH |
| Etodolac | No effect on $T_4$, $fT_4$, or TSH |
| Glucocorticoids | Decreased $T_4$ and $fT_4$; decreased or no effect on TSH |
| Furosemide | Decreased $T_4$ |
| Methimazole | Decreased $T_4$ and $fT_4$; increased TSH |
| Phenobarbital | Decreased $T_4$ and $fT_4$; delayed increase in TSH |
| Phenylbutazone | Decreased $T_4$ |
| Potassium bromide | No effect on $T_4$, $fT_4$, or TSH |
| Progestagens | Decreased $T_4$ |
| Propylthiouracil | Decreased $T_4$ and $fT_4$; increased TSH |
| Sulfonamides | Decreased $T_4$ and $fT_4$; increased TSH |
| Ipodate | Increased $T_4$; decreased $T_3$ |
| Dietary iodine intake | If excessive, decreased $T_4$ and $fT_4$; increased TSH |
| Thyroid hormone autoantibodies | Increased or decreased $T_4$; no effect on $fT_4$ or TSH |

*A direct correlation exists between the severity and systemic nature of the illness and suppression of the serum $T_4$ concentration.

$fT_4$, Free thyroxine; $T_3$, 3,4,3′-triiodothyronine; $T_4$, thyroxine; *TSH*, thyroid-stimulating hormone.

## Diagnostic Recommendations for Evaluating Thyroid Gland Function in Dogs*

1. The decision to assess thyroid gland function should be based on results of the history, physical examination, and routine bloodwork (CBC, serum biochemistry panel, urinalysis).
2. Initial single screening tests include baseline serum $T_4$ and $fT_4$ (measured by MED).
   a. Treatment is indicated if the $T_4$ or $fT_4$ is low and initial evaluation of the dog strongly supports the diagnosis of hypothyroidism.
   b. Treatment is not indicated if the $T_4$ or $fT_4$ is normal and initial evaluation of the dog does not strongly support the diagnosis of hypothyroidism.
   c. Additional diagnostic tests (e.g., endogenous cTSH, Tg, or $T_4$ autoantibodies) are indicated if the $T_4$ is normal but initial evaluation of the dog strongly supports the diagnosis of hypothyroidism or if the veterinarian is uncertain whether hypothyroidism exists after evaluation of the history, physical examination, routine bloodwork, and serum $T_4$ or $fT_4$ levels.
3. Commonly used screening protocols using two diagnostic tests include baseline serum $T_4$ or $fT_4$ (measured by MED) and serum cTSH.
   a. Treatment is indicated if the $T_4$ or $fT_4$ is low and initial evaluation of the dog strongly supports the diagnosis of hypothyroidism, regardless of the serum cTSH concentration.
   b. Treatment is not indicated if all of these tests are normal and initial evaluation of the dog does not strongly support the diagnosis of hypothyroidism.
   c. Treatment is not indicated and the tests should be repeated in 8-12 wk if the $fT_4$ is normal and the cTSH is increased.
   d. Evaluation for serum Tg or $T_4$ autoantibodies is indicated if serum $T_4$ is normal, cTSH is increased, and initial evaluation of the dog strongly supports the diagnosis of hypothyroidism.
4. Common components of a thyroid panel include serum $T_4$, $fT_4$ (measured by MED), cTSH, and an antibody test for lymphocytic thyroiditis.
   a. Treatment is indicated if all results of the tests for thyroid gland function are abnormal and initial evaluation of the dog strongly supports the diagnosis of hypothyroidism, regardless of the thyroid hormone antibody test results.
   b. Treatment is not indicated if all results of the tests for thyroid gland function are normal and initial evaluation of the dog does not strongly support the diagnosis of hypothyroidism, regardless of the thyroid hormone antibody test results. Positive thyroid hormone antibody test results support the presence of lymphocytic thyroiditis and the need to monitor tests of thyroid gland function every 3-6 mo.
   c. When discordant thyroid gland function test results are obtained, the decision to treat should be based on initial evaluation of the dog, the index of suspicion for hypothyroidism, and a critical evaluation of each thyroid gland function test result. Serum $fT_4$ by MED is the most accurate test of thyroid gland function.

*Modified from the International Symposium on Canine Hypothyroidism, *Canine Pract* 22:56, 1997.
*CBC,* complete blood count; *cTSH,* canine thyroid-stimulating hormone; *fT₄,* free thyroxine; *MED,* modified equilibrium dialysis; *Tg,* thyroglobulin; *T₄,* thyroxine.

Serum $T_4$, $fT_4$, and cTSH are decreased or undetectable, depending on the severity of thyroid gland atrophy. Serum $T_4$ and $fT_4$ results are often suggestive of hypothyroidism, even in a previously euthyroid dog, if testing is performed within a month of discontinuation of treatment. Thyroid hormone supplementation must be discontinued and the pituitary-thyroid axis allowed to regain function before meaningful $T_4$ results can be obtained. As a general guide, thyroid hormone supplements should be discontinued for at least 4 weeks, but preferably 6 to 8 weeks, before thyroid gland function is critically assessed.

***Diagnosis of hypothyroidism in puppies.*** A similar approach is used to diagnose congenital hypothyroidism, although cTSH results are dependent on the underlying disorder. Serum cTSH is increased in dogs with primary dysfunction of the thyroid gland and an intact hypothalamic-pituitary-thyroid gland axis, whereas cTSH is normal or undetectable in dogs with pituitary or hypothalamic dysfunction. A TRH stimulation test can help localize the site of the problem.

***Summary.*** Although $T_4$ can be used as an initial screening test, evaluation of a thyroid panel that includes $T_4$, $fT_4$ (measured by MED), cTSH, and Tg autoantibodies provides a more informative analysis of the pituitary-thyroid axis and thyroid gland function. Low $T_4$ and $fT_4$ and increased cTSH in a dog with appropriate clinical signs and clinicopathologic abnormalities strongly supports the diagnosis of hypothyroidism. Concurrent presence of Tg autoantibodies suggests lymphocytic thyroiditis as the underlying cause. Unfortunately, discordant test results are common. When this occurs, the appropriateness of clinical signs, clinicopathologic abnormalities, and index of suspicion become the most important parameters when determining whether to treat the dog.

### Treatment

Synthetic levothyroxine ($T_4$) is the treatment of choice. The initial dose is 0.02 mg/kg (0.1 mg/10 lb; maximum dose, 0.8 mg) q12h. Because of variability in absorption and metabolism, the dose and frequency may require adjustment before a satisfactory response is seen. Thyroid supplementation should be continued for at least 6 weeks before its effectiveness is critically evaluated.

***Response to therapy.*** With appropriate therapy all the clinical signs and clinicopathologic abnormalities associated with hypothyroidism are reversible. An increase in mental alertness and activity usually occurs in the first week of treatment and is an important early indicator that the diagnosis is correct. Although some hair regrowth usually occurs within the first month in dogs with alopecia, it may take several months for complete regrowth and marked reduction in hyperpigmentation of the skin to occur. (Note: The haircoat may worsen initially as large amounts of hair in the telogen stage are shed.) Improvement in neurologic signs is usually evident within 2 weeks, although complete resolution is unpredictable and may take 3 to 6 months of treatment.

***Treatment failure.*** Problems with levothyroxine therapy should be suspected if clinical improvement is not seen within 8 weeks. Poor response to therapy has a number of possible causes. Incorrect diagnosis is the most obvious. Hyperadrenocorticism can sometimes be mistaken for hypothyroidism. Failure to recognize the impact of concurrent illness on thyroid hormone test results is another common cause for misdiagnosing hypothyroidism. Concurrent disease (e.g., allergic skin disease, flea hypersensitivity) is common in hypothyroid dogs and may affect the clinical impression of response to levothyroxine therapy.

Poor response to therapy may also be a result of owner compliance problems, use of an inactivated or outdated product, inappropriate dose or frequency, or poor intestinal absorption. Therapeutic monitoring can be undertaken to identify these possibilities, once owner noncompliance has been ruled out.

***Therapeutic monitoring.*** Serum $T_4$ and cTSH should be measured 4 to 8 weeks after initiation of therapy whenever signs of thyrotoxicosis develop (see later) or when there has been little or no response to therapy. They should also be measured 2 to 4 weeks after an adjustment in levothyroxine therapy in dogs that show poor response to treatment.

Serum $T_4$ and cTSH typically are evaluated 4 to 6 hours after administration of levothyroxine in dogs receiving medication twice daily and just before and 4 to 6 hours after administration in dogs on once-a-day treatment. In dogs with $T_4$ autoantibodies, $fT_4$ should be measured in lieu of $T_4$.

If the dose and schedule are appropriate, $T_4$ should be >2.5 µg/dl 4 to 6 hours after thyroid hormone administration, and cTSH should be <0.6 ng/ml in all samples. A reduction in dose is recommended whenever $T_4$ exceeds 6 µg/dl.

*Thyrotoxicosis.* Development of thyrotoxicosis from excessive administration of levothyroxine is unusual. It is more likely with high doses, twice daily treatment, and in dogs with concurrent renal or hepatic insufficiency. Signs include panting, nervousness, aggressive behavior, PU and PD, polyphagia, and weight loss. Documentation of elevated serum thyroid hormone concentrations supports the diagnosis, although values may be within the normal range, and they are commonly increased in dogs with no signs of thyrotoxicosis. Adjustments in the dose and/or frequency of administration is indicated. Supplementation may need to be discontinued for a few days if signs of toxicosis are severe. Therapeutic monitoring is recommended 2 to 4 weeks after the levothyroxine dose has been adjusted.

### Prognosis

The prognosis depends on the underlying cause. With appropriate therapy the life expectancy of an adult dog with primary hypothyroidism should be normal. Most, if not all, of the clinical manifestations resolve with thyroid hormone supplementation. The prognosis for puppies with hypothyroidism (i.e., cretinism) is guarded and dependent on the severity of skeletal and joint abnormalities. Musculoskeletal problems, especially degenerative osteoarthritis, can result from abnormal bone and joint development. The prognosis for secondary hypothyroidism caused by malformation or destruction of the pituitary gland is guarded to poor.

## HYPOTHYROIDISM IN CATS (TEXT PP 709-712)

### Etiology

Hypothyroidism is most often iatrogenic in cats, resulting from bilateral thyroidectomy, radioactive iodine therapy, or overdose of antithyroid drugs. Naturally acquired, adult-onset primary hypothyroidism is rare. Congenital primary hypothyroidism that causes disproportionate dwarfism is seen more frequently than adult-onset hypothyroidism; causes include a defect in thyroid hormone biosynthesis (most notably an iodine organification defect) and thyroid dysgenesis. Although rare, iodine deficiency has been reported to cause hypothyroidism in kittens fed a strict all-meat diet.

### Clinical features

The most common signs of hypothyroidism in adult cats are lethargy, inappetence, obesity, and seborrhea sicca (Table 51-3). Lethargy and inappetence may become severe. Alopecia, when present, may be asymmetric or bilaterally symmetric, initially involving the lateral neck, thorax, and abdomen.

The clinical signs of congenital hypothyroidism are similar to those in dogs. Affected kittens typically appear normal at birth, but a decrease in growth rate usually becomes evident by 6 to 8 weeks of age. Disproportionate dwarfism develops over the ensuing months.

### Diagnosis

Diagnosis should be based on the history, physical findings, baseline serum $T_4$ or $fT_4$, and, if indicated, response to exogenous TRH (all discussed in the previous section on canine hypothyroidism). Hypercholesterolemia and mild anemia (normocytic, normochromic, nonregenerative) are occasionally identified in cats with iatrogenic or congenital hypothyroidism. Therefore initial screening tests should include complete blood count (CBC), serum cholesterol, and serum $T_4$ or $fT_4$. A normal $T_4$ or $fT_4$ result supports euthyroidism. Low $T_4$ or $fT_4$ in a cat that has undergone thyroidectomy or radioactive iodine therapy or in a kitten with disproportionate dwarfism supports the diagnosis of hypothyroidism.

Low $T_4$ or $fT_4$ in other adult cats is almost always caused by euthyroid sick syndrome or some other nonthyroidal factor. Therefore hypothyroidism should not be diagnosed solely on $T_4$ or $fT_4$ results in an adult cat that has not undergone treatment for hyperthyroidism. A TRH stimulation test should be performed to confirm the diagnosis. Response to trial therapy with levothyroxine is nonspecific and does not, by itself, prove the diagnosis. If trial therapy is attempted and a positive response is observed, thyroid

Table 51-3

## Clinical Manifestations of Feline Hypothyroidism

| Adult-onset hypothyroidism | Congenital hypothyroidism |
|---|---|
| Lethargy | Disproportionate dwarfism |
| Inappetence | Failure to grow |
| Obesity | Large head |
| Dermatologic | Short, broad neck |
|   Seborrhea sicca | Short limbs |
|   Dry, lusterless haircoat | Lethargy |
|   Easily epilated hair | Mental dullness |
|   Poor regrowth of hair | Constipation |
|   Endocrine alopecia | Hypothermia |
|   Alopecia of pinnae | Bradycardia |
|   Thickened skin | Retention of kitten haircoat |
|   Myxedema of the face | Retention of deciduous teeth |
| Reproduction | |
|   Failure to cycle | |
|   Dystocia | |
| Bradycardia | |
| Mild hypothermia | |

supplementation should be gradually discontinued after clinical signs have resolved. Hypothyroidism is likely if clinical signs recur and resolve after treatment is reinstituted.

### Treatment

For cats with iatrogenic hypothyroidism, treatment with levothyroxine is indicated if appropriate clinical signs are present. Asymptomatic cats with low $T_4$ or $fT_4$ should not be treated until clinical signs develop. This approach allows time for atrophied or ectopic thyroid tissue to become functional.

Treatment is similar to that described for dogs. The initial dose of levothyroxine in cats is 0.05 or 0.1 mg once or twice daily. A minimum of 4 weeks should elapse before the response to therapy is assessed. Subsequent reevaluations should include history, physical examination, and measurement of serum $T_4$. The goal is to resolve the signs while avoiding hyperthyroidism; it can usually be accomplished by maintaining serum $T_4$ between 1 and 2.5 μg/dl. The dose and frequency of levothyroxine administration are modified as necessary. If serum thyroid hormone concentrations are normal after 4 to 8 weeks of therapy but no clinical response occurs, the diagnosis should be reviewed.

### Prognosis

The prognosis depends on the underlying cause and on the cat's age when signs develop. With appropriate therapy the life expectancy of an adult cat with primary hypothyroidism is normal. The prognosis for kittens with congenital hypothyroidism is guarded and dependent on the severity of the skeletal changes, as discussed previously for puppies.

## HYPERTHYROIDISM IN CATS (TEXT PP 712-724)

### Etiology

Hyperthyroidism results from excess thyroid hormone secretion from one or both thyroid lobes. Multinodular adenomatous goiter is the most common lesion; thyroid adenoma and carcinoma are far less common. One or both thyroid lobes can be affected. More than 70% of hyperthyroid cats have bilateral involvement; of those, 10%

to 15% have symmetric enlargement, and the remainder have asymmetric enlargement. Approximately 5% of thyrotoxic cats have hyperactive thyroid tissue in the anterior mediastinum, with or without a palpable mass in the neck.

The pathogenesis of adenomatous hyperplasia remains unclear. Epidemiologic studies have identified consumption of commercial canned cat foods as a risk factor, which suggests that a goitrogenic compound (e.g., excess iodine, soy isoflavones) may be involved. Other environmental factors may also play a role.

### Clinical features
Hyperthyroidism is the most common endocrinopathy that affects cats >8 years of age. Average age at initial presentation is 13 years (range, 4 to 20 years). Domestic Shorthair and Longhair are the most frequently affected breeds. Siamese and Himalayans have a decreased risk.

*Clinical signs.* The classic signs are weight loss (which may progress to cachexia), polyphagia, and restlessness or hyperactivity. In some cats, lethargy, weakness, and anorexia are the dominant clinical features, in addition to weight loss. Other signs include haircoat changes (patchy alopecia, matted hair, absent or excessive grooming behavior), PU and PD, vomiting, and diarrhea (Table 51-4). Some cats become aggressive. Because of the multisystemic effects, variable clinical signs, and resemblance to many other diseases, hyperthyroidism should be suspected in any cat >10 years of age that has medical problems.

### Physical examination
Findings are listed in Table 51-4. A discrete thyroid mass is palpable in approximately 90% of cases. However, palpation of a cervical mass is not pathognomonic for hyperthyroidism; some cats with palpable thyroid glands are clinically normal, and not all cervical masses are thyroid glands. A thyroid mass is commonly palpated at the thoracic inlet. Migration of the abnormal thyroid lobe(s) into the anterior mediastinum should be suspected in hyperthyroid cats without a palpable cervical mass. It is often difficult to accurately assess unilateral or bilateral thyroid lobe involvement with palpation alone. A solitary mass is frequently palpated in cats with bilateral thyroid lobe involvement.

### Common concurrent problems
*Thyrotoxic cardiomyopathy.* Hypertrophic and, less commonly, dilitative thyrotoxic cardiomyopathy may develop in cats with hyperthyroidism. Findings include

---

**Table 51-4**

### Clinical Signs and Physical Examination Findings in Cats with Hyperthyroidism

| Clinical signs | Physical examination findings |
|---|---|
| Weight loss* | Palpable thyroid* |
| Polyphagia* | Thin* |
| Unkempt haircoat, patchy alopecia* | Hyperactive, difficult to examine* |
| Polyuria and polydipsia* | Tachycardia* |
| Vomiting* | Hair loss, unkempt haircoat* |
| Nervous, hyperactive | Small kidneys |
| Diarrhea, "bulky" stools | Heart murmur |
| Decreased appetite | Easily stressed |
| Tremor | Dehydrated, cachectic appearance |
| Weakness | Premature beats |
| Dyspnea, panting | Gallop rhythm |
| Decreased activity, lethargy | Aggressive |
| Anorexia | Depressed, weak |
| | Ventral flexion of the neck |

*Common.

tachycardia, a "pounding" heartbeat, and, less frequently, pulse deficits, gallop rhythms, cardiac murmur, and muffled heart sounds (pleural effusion). Electrocardiographic abnormalities include tachycardia, increased R-wave amplitude in lead II, and, less commonly, right bundle branch block, left anterior fascicular block, widened QRS complexes, and atrial and ventricular arrhythmias.

Thoracic radiographs may reveal cardiomegaly, pulmonary edema, or pleural effusion. Echocardiographic abnormalities are discussed in the text. Both forms of cardiomyopathy can result in congestive heart failure. After correction of the hyperthyroid state, hypertrophic thyrotoxic cardiomyopathy is usually reversible, but dilative thyrotoxic cardiomyopathy is not.

*Renal insufficiency.* Hyperthyroidism and renal insufficiency are common diseases of older cats and often occur concurrently. Finding small kidneys on physical examination or increased blood urea nitrogen (BUN), creatinine, and low urine specific gravity (SG; 1.008 to 1.020) should raise suspicion for concurrent renal insufficiency. However, as hyperthyroidism increases the glomerular filtration rate (GFR) and other renal dynamics, the clinical and biochemical manifestations of renal failure may be masked in hyperthyroid cats with renal disease.

Renal perfusion and GFR can acutely decrease, and azotemia or clinical signs of renal insufficiency can become apparent or significantly worsen, after treatment for hyperthyroidism. Because it is not easy to determine what impact hyperthyroidism is having on renal function, cats with hyperthyroidism should initially be given reversible therapy (i.e.. oral antithyroid drugs) until the impact of euthyroidism on renal function can be determined.

*Systemic hypertension.* Systemic hypertension is common in cats with hyperthyroidism, although it usually is clinically silent. Retinal hemorrhages and retinal detachment are the most common complications of systemic hypertension, but ocular lesions are not commonly identified in cats with hyperthyroidism.

*Gastrointestinal disorders.* Gastrointestinal (GI) signs are common in cats with hyperthyroidism. They include polyphagia, weight loss, anorexia, vomiting, diarrhea, increased frequency of defecation, and increased volume of feces. Inflammatory bowel disease is a common concurrent disorder that should be considered in any hyperthyroid cat that has persistence of GI signs after correction of the hyperthyroid state. Intestinal neoplasia, most notably lymphoma, is the most important differential diagnosis in cats with polyphagia and weight loss.

### Diagnosis

Diagnosis is based on appropriate clinical signs, palpation of a thyroid nodule, and documentation of an increase in serum $T_4$ (see later). Occult hyperthyroidism, in which the cat has mild clinical signs, a palpable nodule in the ventral neck, and high-normal $T_4$ (2.5 to 3.5 μg/dl), presents a diagnostic challenge. This nondiagnostic $T_4$ result may be the result of random fluctuations of $T_4$ into the normal range in a cat with mild hyperthyroidism or a decrease in $T_4$ as a result of concurrent nonthyroid illness (e.g., neoplasia, systemic infection, organ system failure) in a hyperthyroid cat. Additional tests (e.g., $fT_4$, radionuclide thyroid scan) are often needed to establish a diagnosis of hyperthyroidism in these cats.

*Clinical pathology.* The CBC is usually normal. The most common abnormalities are a mild increase in PCV and mean corpuscular volume. Neutrophilia, lymphopenia, eosinopenia, or monocytopenia is identified in <20% of cases. Common serum biochemical abnormalities include mild to moderate increases in the activities of ALT, AP, and AST. An increase occurs in one or more of these liver enzymes in approximately 90% of hyperthyroid cats. Additional evaluation of the liver should be considered if these enzyme values are >500 U/L. Increases in BUN and creatinine are found in approximately 30% of cases, and hyperphosphatemia in 20%.

Urine SG ranges from 1.008 to >1.050. In most hyperthyroid cats it is >1.035, which is useful in differentiating primary renal insufficiency from prerenal azotemia in cats with increased BUN. Urinalysis is helpful in ruling out diabetes mellitus in hyperglycemic cats.

***Baseline serum T<sub>4</sub>.*** Random measurement of $T_4$ is reliable in differentiating hyperthyroid cats from those without thyroid disease. An abnormally high $T_4$ strongly supports the diagnosis of hyperthyroidism, especially if appropriate clinical signs are present. A low $T_4$ rules out hyperthyroidism, except in cats with severe, life-threatening, nonthyroid illness.

However, hyperthyroidism should not be excluded on the basis of one normal test result, especially in a cat with appropriate clinical signs and a palpable cervical mass. If the $T_4$ result is not definitive, $T_4$ and $fT_4$ (using the MED technique) should be measured 1 to 2 weeks later. If the diagnosis still is not established, these tests should be repeated in 4 to 8 weeks, or a radionuclide thyroid scan (preferred) or $T_3$ suppression test should be performed (see text). It is important to bear in mind, however, that the thyroid nodule may be nonfunctional and that the clinical signs may be the result of another disease.

***Serum fT<sub>4</sub>.*** Measurement of $fT_4$ by the MED technique is a more reliable test for thyroid gland function than is total $T_4$. Serum $fT_4$ is increased in many cats with occult hyperthyroidism that have normal $T_4$ results. Because of its cost, measurement of $fT_4$ by MED is often reserved for cats with suspected hyperthyroidism when $T_4$ values are borderline.

Occasionally, concurrent illness causes an increase in $fT_4$ above the reference range. For this reason $fT_4$ should always be interpreted in conjunction with total $T_4$ measured from the same sample. An increase in $fT_4$ and high-normal or increased total $T_4$ is supportive of hyperthyroidism. An increase in $fT_4$ in conjunction with a low-normal or low $T_4$ is supportive of euthyroid sick syndrome.

### Treatment

Hyperthyroidism in cats can be managed with thyroidectomy, oral antithyroid medications, or radioactive iodine. Surgery and radioactive iodine can provide a permanent cure; oral antithyroid drugs merely control hyperthyroidism and must be given daily for their effect to be achieved and maintained. Which mode is chosen depends on a number of factors, including general health and age of the cat, renal function, severity of concurrent disease (e.g., thyrotoxic cardiomyopathy), type of thyroid lesion, unilateral versus bilateral lobe involvement, size of the thyroid masses if bilateral, availability of radioactive iodine, surgical expertise, ease of administration of oral medications, and owner's preference (Table 51-5).

*Initial therapy.* The cat should first be treated with oral methimazole to reverse the hyperthyroid-induced metabolic and cardiac derangements, decrease the anesthetic risk associated with thyroidectomy, and assess the impact of treatment on renal function. If renal parameters remain static or improve after resolution of the hyperthyroid state, a more permanent treatment can be recommended.

If significant azotemia or signs of renal insufficiency develop during methimazole therapy, the treatment protocol should be modified to achieve the best possible control of both disorders, and treatment for renal insufficiency instituted. Maintaining a mildly hyperthyroid state may be necessary to improve renal function and avoid the uremia of renal failure.

*Oral antithyroid drugs.* Oral antithyroid drugs (e.g., methimazole, propylthiouracil, carbimazole) are inexpensive, readily available, relatively safe, and effective. Indications include (1) trial therapy to assess the effect of resolving hyperthyroidism on renal function, (2) initial treatment to improve or resolve any associated medical problems before thyroidectomy or radioactive iodine treatment, and (3) long-term treatment of hyperthyroidism. Methimazole (Tapazole) is currently the drug of choice because of the lower incidence of adverse reactions compared with propylthiouracil.

*Oral methimazole.* Adverse reactions are less likely to occur with this drug when the dose is started low (subtherapeutic dose initially) and gradually increased until effective. The recommended initial dosage is 2.5 mg orally (PO) q24h for 2 weeks. If no adverse reactions occur, physical examination reveals no new problems, CBC and platelet count are normal, and serum $T_4$ is $>2$ μg/dl after 2 weeks of therapy, the dose is increased to 2.5 mg PO q12h, and the same indexes are evaluated 2 weeks later.

**Table 51-5**

**Indications, Contraindications, and Disadvantages of the Three Modes of Therapy for Hyperthyroidism in Cats**

| Therapy | Indications | Relative contraindications | Disadvantages |
|---|---|---|---|
| Methimazole, propylthiouracil, carbimazole | Long-term therapy for all forms of hyperthyroidism; initial therapy to stabilize cat's condition and assess renal function before thyroidectomy or radioactive iodine | None | Daily therapy required; no effect on growth of tumor; mild adverse reactions common; severe reactions possible |
| Thyroidectomy | Unilateral lobe involvement; bilateral lobe involvement, asymmetric sizes | Ectopic thyroid lobe; metastatic carcinoma; bilateral, symmetric, large lobes (high risk of hypocalcemia); severe systemic signs; cardiac arrhythmias or failure | Anesthetic risks; relapse of disease; postoperative complications, especially hypocalcemia |
| Radioactive iodine ($^{131}$I) | Therapy for all forms of hyperthyroidism; treatment of choice for ectopic thyroid lobe and thyroid carcinoma | None | Limited availability; prolonged hospitalization; potential for retreatment; hazardous to humans |

The dose is increased in increments of 2.5 mg/day every 2 weeks until the $T_4$ is 1 to 2 µg/dl or adverse reactions develop. Clinical improvement is usually noted within 2 to 4 weeks once good control of $T_4$ is achieved. Methimazole is then continued indefinitely at the effective dose for that cat.

*Transdermal methimazole.* Topical application of methimazole to the pinna of the ear is an alternative to oral administration. Custom veterinary pharmacies offer transdermal methimazole in a pluronic lecithin organogel (PLO), typically at a concentration of 5 mg/0.1 ml of gel. The dosage and frequency are the same as for oral methimazole. Bioavailability after a single dose is poor; nevertheless, transdermal methimazole in a PLO can be efficacious with chronic dosing.

*Adverse effects.* Adverse reactions to methimazole are uncommon and, when they do occur, typically develop within the first 4 to 8 weeks of therapy. CBC, platelet count, and assessment of renal function should be performed every 2 weeks during the first 3 months of therapy. Thereafter, these indexes should be evaluated every 3 to 6 months.

When the administration protocol described previously is used, lethargy, vomiting, and anorexia occur in <10% of cats; these signs are usually mild and transient and often resolve despite continued administration of the drug. Mild methimazole-induced CBC changes occur in <10% of cats and include eosinophilia, lymphocytosis, and transient leukopenia. More worrisome but less common (<5% of cats) alterations include severe thrombocytopenia, neutropenia, and immune-mediated hemolytic anemia. Hepatic toxicity occurs in <2% of cats.

If any of these serious complications develop, methimazole should be discontinued and supportive care (e.g., intravenous fluids, blood transfusions, antibiotics) given. Signs typically resolve within 1 week of discontinuation of methimazole. It is common for these potentially life-threatening reactions to recur, regardless of the antithyroid drug used, so alternative therapy (i.e., surgery, radioactive iodine) is recommended in cats that develop severe adverse reactions to methimazole.

*Carbimazole.* Carbimazole (Neo-Mercazole) is converted to methimazole in vivo; it is an effective alternative if methimazole is not available. An initial dose of 5 mg q8h is recommended. Euthyroidism is typically attained within 2 weeks. Long-term, twice-daily schedules are effective in controlling hyperthyroidism. Adverse reactions are similar to those seen in cats receiving methimazole, but they occur less frequently. Cats being treated with carbimazole should be monitored in the same manner as cats receiving methimazole.

*Surgery.* Thyroidectomy is the treatment of choice unless the cat is an unacceptable anesthetic risk, renal function is questionable, the likelihood of postoperative hypocalcemia is great, ectopic thyroid tissue is present in the thorax, or thyroid carcinoma with metastases is suspected. If possible, an ultrasound examination of the ventral neck or a pertechnetate scan should be performed before surgery to identify the location of the abnormal thyroid tissue, differentiate unilateral from bilateral lobe involvement, and provide some insight into the probability that hypocalcemia will develop postoperatively. Thyroidectomy is discussed further in the text.

*Radioactive iodine.* Irradiation of functional thyroid tumors using iodine 131 ($^{131}$I) is a valuable option in cats with (1) bilateral, markedly enlarged thyroid lobes identified at surgery or via ultrasound or pertechnetate scan; (2) hyperfunctioning, nonaccessible ectopic thyroid masses; and (3) metastatic or nonresectable thyroid carcinoma. Depending on the dose used, >80% of cats become euthyroid within 3 months (most within 1 week), and >95% are still euthyroid at 6 months.

The only recognized adverse reaction is hypothyroidism, which is more likely to develop in cats with bilateral, large, diffusely affected thyroid lobes. Approximately 2% of cats develop clinical signs and laboratory data consistent with hypothyroidism; 2% to 4% require a second $^{131}$I treatment; and 2% have a relapse of hyperthyroidism within 1 to 6 years. Hypothyroidism can be treated with levothyroxine, as discussed earlier in the chapter.

### Prognosis

The prognosis depends on the cat's physical condition at the time of diagnosis, the presence and severity of concurrent disease (especially renal insufficiency), the histologic diagnosis (hyperplasia or adenoma versus carcinoma), choice of therapy, and whether adverse reactions to therapy developed. All three treatment modalities are successful when used under appropriate circumstances. Hyperthyroid cats with hyperplasia or adenoma can be maintained on methimazole for years, assuming adverse reactions to the medication are avoided. Recurrence of hyperthyroidism may occur months or years after thyroidectomy or [131]I therapy, or not at all. Renal-related problems and neoplasia are the most common health problems that limit long-term survival.

## CANINE THYROID NEOPLASIA (TEXT PP 724-728)

### Etiology

Most thyroid adenomas in dogs are small, nonfunctional masses that do not cause clinical signs. Thyroid carcinomas are more common and typically are large, solid masses that cause clinical signs recognizable by owners. They frequently extend into the esophagus, trachea, cervical musculature, nerves, and thyroid vessels. Metastasis to the lungs and the retropharyngeal lymph nodes is common; metastasis to the liver, kidneys, heartbase, bones, and spinal cord can also occur. Because of the high likelihood of malignancy, all thyroid masses should be assumed to be malignant until proved otherwise. Most dogs with thyroid tumors are euthyroid or hypothyroid; approximately 10% of dogs have functional tumors that cause hyperthyroidism.

### Clinical features

Average age at presentation is 10 years (range, 5 to 15 years). Although any breed can be affected, Boxers, Beagles, and Golden Retrievers may be at increased risk. Dogs with nonfunctional thyroid tumors are usually presented because the owner has seen or felt a mass in the neck or because the mass is causing clinical signs related to compression of adjacent structures or metastases. When present, clinical signs of hyperthyroidism are similar to those described in cats.

*Physical examination.* Most thyroid tumors are palpable as firm, asymmetric, lobulated, nonpainful masses in the thyroid region. In most cases the mass is not freely movable. Additional findings may include dyspnea, cough, dysphagia, anorexia, weight loss, lethargy, Horner's syndrome, dehydration, and altered bark. A dry, lusterless coat is common, but alopecia is rare. Regional cervical lymph nodes may be enlarged. Dogs with functional thyroid tumors may be restless, thin, and panting, and auscultation of the heart frequently reveals tachycardia; however, many dogs are remarkably healthy on physical examination.

### Diagnosis

Results of CBC, serum biochemistry panel, and urinalysis usually are unhelpful. Hypercalcemia has been reported in a few cases. Baseline serum $T_4$ and $fT_4$ are increased and cTSH is undetectable in dogs with a functional thyroid tumor that is causing hyperthyroidism. However, most canine thyroid tumors are nonfunctional, and most of these dogs are euthyroid; approximately 25% are hypothyroid.

*Diagnostic imaging.* Ultrasonography of the neck can confirm the presence of a thyroid mass; distinguish among cavitary, cystic, and solid tumors; identify the presence and extent of local tumor invasion; identify metastatic sites in the cervical region; and allow representative tissue for cytologic or histologic evaluation to be obtained by fine-needle aspiration or percutaneous biopsy.

Because pulmonary metastasis is common with thyroid carcinoma, thoracic radiographs should be included in the diagnostic evaluation. Cervical radiographs may also be useful. Abdominal ultrasonography can be used to identify abdominal (most notably hepatic) metastatic lesions.

Where available, computed tomography, magnetic resonance imaging, and nuclear imaging studies can be used to assess the size of the thyroid mass and define the extent of tumor invasion into surrounding structures—information that is valuable if surgery is being considered. Nuclear imaging may also identify sites of ectopic thyroid tissue (neoplastic or normal), provided the cells in ectopic or metastatic sites retain the ability to trap iodine.

*Histopathology.* Definitive diagnosis requires histologic evaluation of a biopsy specimen. Fine-needle aspiration and cytologic examination are recommended initially to confirm that the mass is of thyroid origin. Contamination of the aspirate with blood is very common, however, and differentiation between adenoma and carcinoma is difficult with these small specimens. Large-bore needle biopsy, surgical exploration, or ultrasound-guided biopsy is often required to confirm the diagnosis.

### Treatment

Treatment depends, in part, on the size of the mass, extent of invasion into surrounding tissues, functional status (with regard to thyroid hormone secretion), and histologic diagnosis (adenoma versus carcinoma). All thyroid tumors should be considered malignant until proved otherwise. Therefore surgical removal is the treatment of choice whenever possible, regardless of the functional status of the tumor.

Radiation therapy and chemotherapy are indicated after removal of a thyroid carcinoma, especially if surgical debulking was incomplete or metastasis is suspected (e.g., histologic identification of vascular invasion) and before surgical debulking of a large mass. Radioactive iodine and methimazole can be used to treat functional thyroid tumors causing hyperthyroidism, especially if surgery does not provide a cure. Surgery, chemotherapy, radioactive iodine therapy, cobalt teletherapy, and oral antithyroid drugs are discussed further in the text.

### Prognosis

The prognosis is excellent after surgical resection of thyroid adenomas. Resection of small, well-encapsulated carcinomas also carries a good prognosis. Unfortunately, most dogs have relatively large thyroid masses that have already invaded surrounding tissues or metastasized at the time of diagnosis. In these dogs aggressive therapy using multiple modalities can alleviate the clinical signs and, in some cases, dramatically reduce the tumor burden. However, the long-term prognosis remains guarded to poor, with survival times ranging from 6 to 24 months, depending on the aggressiveness of therapy.

# 52

## Disorders of the Endocrine Pancreas

### (Text pp 729-777)

#### HYPERGLYCEMIA (TEXT P 729)

Hyperglycemia is present when the blood glucose concentration is >130 mg/dl, although clinical signs do not develop until blood glucose exceeds 180 mg/dl in dogs and 200 mg/dl (sometimes up to 280 mg/dl) in cats. The most common cause is diabetes mellitus (DM); severe hyperglycemia can also occur in stressed cats (Box 52-1).

Glycosuria and resulting polyuria (PU) and polydipsia (PD) are the hallmarks of severe hyperglycemia. When a dog or cat with mild hyperglycemia (<180 mg/dl) is presented with PU and PD, a disorder other than DM should be suspected. Disorders that cause insulin resistance should be considered if mild hyperglycemia persists in fasted, unstressed animals, especially if blood glucose increases over time.

---

**Box 52-1**

**Causes of Hyperglycemia in Dogs and Cats**

Diabetes mellitus*
Stress (cats)*
Postprandial effects (diets containing monosaccharides, disaccharides, and propylene glycol)
Hyperadrenocorticism*
Acromegaly (cats)
Diestrus (bitches)
Pheochromocytoma (dogs)
Head trauma
Pancreatitis
Exocrine pancreatic neoplasia
Renal insufficiency
Drug therapy*
Glucocorticoids
Progestagens
Megestrol acetate
Thiazide diuretics
Dextrose-containing fluids*
Parenteral nutrition*

*Common cause.

---

## HYPOGLYCEMIA (TEXT PP 729-731)

### Etiology

Hypoglycemia is present when the blood glucose concentration is <60 mg/dl. Potential causes are listed in Box 52-2. Clinical signs usually develop when blood glucose drops below 45 mg/dl, although this occurrence is quite variable. Signs may be persistent or intermittent and may include seizures (intermittent), weakness, collapse, ataxia and, less commonly, lethargy, blindness, bizarre behavior, and coma. Resulting catecholamine release causes restlessness, nervousness, hunger, and muscle fasciculations.

### Diagnosis

Hypoglycemia should always be confirmed before one attempts to identify the cause. History, physical findings, and routine bloodwork (complete blood count [CBC], serum biochemistry panel, urinalysis) usually provide clues to the cause. Hypoglycemia in puppies and kittens is usually caused by idiopathic hypoglycemia, starvation, liver

---

**Box 52-2**

### Causes of Hypoglycemia in Dogs and Cats

β-Cell tumor (insulinoma)
Extrapancreatic neoplasia
  Hepatocellular carcinoma, hepatoma
  Leiomyosarcoma, leiomyoma
  Hemangiosarcoma
  Carcinoma (mammary, salivary, pulmonary)
  Leukemia
  Plasmacytoma
  Melanoma
Hepatic insufficiency*
  Portocaval shunts
  Chronic fibrosis, cirrhosis
Sepsis*
Hypoadrenocorticism
Hypopituitarism
Idiopathic hypoglycemia*
  Neonatal hypoglycemia
  Juvenile hypoglycemia (especially toy breeds)
  Hunting dog hypoglycemia
Renal failure
Exocrine pancreatic neoplasia
Hepatic enzyme deficiencies
  Von Gierke's disease (type I glycogen storage disease)
  Cori's disease (type III glycogen storage disease)
Severe polycythemia
Prolonged starvation
Prolonged sample storage*
Iatrogenic*
  Insulin therapy
  Sulfonylurea therapy
  Ethanol ingestion
  Ethylene glycol ingestion
Artifact
  Portable blood glucose–monitoring devices
  Laboratory error

---

*Common cause.

insufficiency (e.g., portal shunt), or sepsis. In young adults it is usually caused by liver insufficiency, hypoadrenocorticism, or sepsis. In older animals, liver insufficiency, β-cell neoplasia, extrapancreatic neoplasia, hypoadrenocorticism, and sepsis are the most common causes.

### Treatment

In most cases clinical signs of hypoglycemia can be controlled with glucose administration. Recurrence of hypoglycemia depends on the ability to correct the underlying cause. If clinical signs of hypoglycemia persist, chronic therapy to increase blood glucose may be necessary (see Box 52-9); this is usually necessary for metastatic β-cell or extrapancreatic neoplasia.

If collapse, seizures, or coma develops, blood glucose should be measured before administration of 50% dextrose intravenously (IV; slowly, in aliquots of 2 to 15 ml until signs of hypoglycemia resolve). Caution is necessary in dogs with β-cell neoplasia to minimize rebound hypoglycemia. A continuous intravenous infusion of 2.5% to 5% dextrose in water or of glucagon may be required for several hours or days until other therapy effectively maintains an adequate blood glucose concentration (see Box 52-8).

Occasionally, patients with severe central nervous system (CNS) signs (e.g., blindness, coma) caused by hypoglycemia do not respond to initial glucose therapy. Irreversible cerebral lesions can result from prolonged, severe hypoglycemia. The prognosis in these animals is guarded to poor.

## DIABETES MELLITUS IN DOGS (TEXT PP 731-749)

### Etiology

At initial diagnosis virtually all dogs with DM have insulin-dependent DM (IDDM), which is characterized by hypoinsulinemia, no increase in endogenous serum insulin after administration of glucose or glucagon, failure to establish glycemic control with diet and/or oral hypoglycemic drugs, and an absolute necessity for exogenous insulin.

DM in dogs is multifactorial. Genetic predisposition, infection, insulin-antagonistic diseases and drugs, obesity, immune-mediated insulitis, and pancreatitis are inciting factors. Loss of β-cell function is irreversible in dogs with IDDM, and lifelong insulin therapy is mandatory.

***Transient or reversible DM.*** Transient or reversible DM is uncommon in dogs. The most common scenario is correction of insulin antagonism after spay in a bitch in diestrus that has subclinical DM. A similar situation can occur in dogs with subclinical DM that are treated with insulin-antagonistic drugs (e.g., glucocorticoids) or in the very early stages of an insulin-antagonistic disorder (e.g., hyperadrenocorticism). Failure to quickly correct the insulin antagonism results in IDDM and the need for lifelong insulin therapy.

A "honeymoon" period occurs in some dogs with newly diagnosed IDDM, characterized by excellent glycemic control in response to small doses of insulin (<0.2 U/kg). However, glycemic control becomes more difficult and insulin doses usually increase within 3 to 6 months as residual functioning β cells are destroyed.

***Non–insulin-dependent DM.*** It is very uncommon for non–insulin-dependent DM (NIDDM) to be recognized clinically in dogs, despite documentation of obesity-induced carbohydrate intolerance in dogs and identification of residual β-cell function in some diabetic dogs. A juvenile form of NIDDM has been described in dogs but is rare.

### Clinical features

Most dogs are between 4 and 14 years of age at the time of diagnosis (typically, 7 to 9 years). Juvenile-onset diabetes occurs in dogs <1 year of age but is uncommon. Females are affected approximately twice as often as males. The following breeds are at increased risk: Keeshond, various Terriers (Australian, Fox, Cairn, and Yorkshire), Standard and Miniature Schnauzers, Bichon Frise, Spitz, Miniature and Toy Poodles, Samoyed, and Lhasa Apso. The following breeds are at decreased risk: German Shepherd, Collie, Shetland Sheepdog, Golden Retriever, Cocker Spaniel, Australian Shepherd, Labrador Retriever, Boston Terrier, and Rottweiler.

Table 52-1

## Complications of Diabetes Mellitus in Dogs and Cats

| Common | Uncommon |
|---|---|
| Iatrogenic hypoglycemia | Peripheral neuropathy (dogs) |
| Persistent polyuria, polydipsia, weight loss | Glomerulonephropathy, glomerulosclerosis |
| Cataracts (dogs) | Retinopathy |
| Bacterial infections, especially in the urinary tract | Exocrine pancreatic insufficiency |
| Pancreatitis | Gastric paresis |
| Ketoacidosis | Diabetic diarrhea |
| Hepatic lipidosis | Diabetic dermatopathy (dogs), i.e., superficial necrolytic dermatitis |
| Peripheral neuropathy (cats) | |

*Clinical signs.* The history almost always includes PU and PD, polyphagia, and weight loss. Occasionally, an owner presents a dog because of sudden blindness caused by cataract formation. If the clinical signs associated with uncomplicated DM are not noticed by the owner and impaired vision caused by cataracts does or does not develop, a diabetic dog is at risk for systemic illness as ketoacidosis develops. Signs of diabetic ketoacidosis (DKA) are discussed on p 485. The time from onset of initial signs of DM to the development of DKA is unpredictable, ranging from days to weeks.

*Physical examination.* Findings depend on the presence and severity of DKA, the duration of DM before diagnosis, and the nature of any concurrent disorder. Patients with nonketotic diabetes have no classic physical findings. Many diabetic dogs are obese but otherwise in good physical condition. Dogs with prolonged, untreated diabetes may have lost weight but are rarely emaciated unless concurrent disease (e.g., pancreatic exocrine insufficiency) is present. Diabetes-induced hepatic lipidosis may cause hepatomegaly. Lenticular changes (cataract formation) are common in diabetic dogs. Other complications are listed in Table 52-1. Additional abnormalities may be identified in dogs with DKA.

### Diagnosis
Diagnosis of DM requires the presence of (1) appropriate signs and (2) persistent fasting hyperglycemia *and* glycosuria. Hyperglycemia differentiates DM from primary renal glycosuria; and glycosuria differentiates DM from other causes of hyperglycemia (see Box 52-1), particularly stress-induced hyperglycemia. Presence of ketonuria establishes a diagnosis of DKA.

*Minimum database.* A thorough evaluation of the dog's overall health is recommended in order to identify any disease that may be causing or contributing to carbohydrate intolerance (e.g., hyperadrenocorticism), that may result from carbohydrate intolerance (e.g., bacterial cystitis), or that may mandate a modification of therapy (e.g., pancreatitis). Possible complications of DM are listed in Table 52-1. Minimum laboratory evaluation includes CBC, serum biochemistry panel, serum trypsinlike immunoreactivity, and urinalysis with bacterial culture. Serum progesterone should also be measured if DM is diagnosed in an intact bitch. Potential abnormalities are listed in Box 52-3.

*Further evaluation.* Abdominal ultrasound is indicated to check for pancreatitis, adrenomegaly, pyometritis (intact bitch), and abnormalities affecting the liver and urinary tract (e.g., changes consistent with pyelonephritis or cystitis). Measurement of baseline serum insulin or an insulin response test is not routinely done. Additional tests may be warranted based on the history, physical examination, and minimum database.

### Treatment
The primary goal of therapy is to eliminate the clinical signs. Persistence of signs and development of chronic complications are directly related to the severity and

---

**Box 52-3**

### Clinicopathologic Abnormalities Commonly Found in Dogs and Cats with Uncomplicated Diabetes Mellitus

**COMPLETE BLOOD COUNT**
Typically normal
Neutrophilic leukocytosis, toxic neutrophils if pancreatitis or infection present

**BIOCHEMISTRY PANEL**
Hyperglycemia
Hypercholesterolemia
Hypertriglyceridemia (lipemia)
Increased alanine aminotransferase activity (typically <500 U/L)
Increased alkaline phosphatase activity (typically <500 U/L)

**URINALYSIS**
Urine specific gravity typically >1.025
Glycosuria
Variable ketonuria
Proteinuria
Bacteriuria

**ANCILLARY TESTS**
Hyperlipasemia if pancreatitis present
Hyperamylasemia if pancreatitis present
Serum trypsinlike immunoreactivity usually normal
  Low with pancreatic exocrine insufficiency
  High with acute pancreatitis
  Normal to high with chronic pancreatitis
Variable serum baseline insulin concentration
  IDDM: low, normal
  NIDDM: low, normal, increased
  Insulin resistance induced: low, normal, increased

---

*IDDM*, Insulin-dependent diabetes mellitus; *NIDDM*, non–insulin-dependent diabetes mellitus.

duration of hyperglycemia. Limiting blood glucose fluctuations and maintaining near-normal glycemia helps control the signs and prevent complications. These goals are accomplished through proper insulin therapy, diet, exercise, and prevention and control of concurrent inflammatory, infectious, neoplastic, and hormonal disorders. While attempting to normalize the blood glucose concentration, one must avoid inducing hypoglycemia, a serious and potentially fatal complication of overzealous insulin therapy.

*Initial insulin therapy.* Intermediate-acting insulin (lente or NPH; Table 52-2) is recommended for establishing glycemic control. Recombinant human-source insulin should be used. Therapy is begun with lente or NPH insulin at an approximate dose of 0.25 U/kg twice a day.

Diabetic dogs require several days to equilibrate to changes in insulin dose or preparation. Therefore newly diagnosed diabetic dogs typically are hospitalized for only 24 to 48 hours (until diagnostic evaluation is completed and insulin therapy is initiated). During hospitalization, blood glucose is measured at the time insulin is administered and at 11 AM, 2 PM, and 5 PM. The intent is to identify hypoglycemia (blood glucose <80 mg/dl) in those dogs that are unusually sensitive to insulin. If hypoglycemia occurs, the insulin dose is decreased before the dog is sent home.

**Table 52-2**

**Properties of Recombinant Human Insulin Preparations Used in Dogs and Cats***

| Type of insulin | Route of administration | Onset of effect | Time of Maximum Effect (hr) | | Duration of Effect (hr) | |
|---|---|---|---|---|---|---|
| | | | Dogs | Cats | Dogs | Cats |
| Regular crystalline | IV | Immediate | 1/2-2 | 1/2-2 | 1-4 | 1-4 |
| | IM | 10-30 min | 1-4 | 1-4 | 3-8 | 3-8 |
| | SC | 10-30 min | 1-5 | 1-5 | 4-10 | 4-10 |
| NPH (isophane) | SC | 1/2-2 hr | 2-10 | 2-8 | 6-18 | 4-12 |
| Lente† | SC | 1/2-2 hr | 2-10 | 2-10 | 8-20 | 6-18 |
| Ultralente | SC | 1/2-8 hr | 4-16 | 4-16 | 6-24 | 6-24 |

*Purified pork insulin has similar properties; beef and pork insulin mixtures are less potent and may have a longer duration of action than recombinant human insulins.
†Initial insulin of choice for diabetic dogs and cats. Beef-pork protamine-zinc insulin is also a good initial insulin for diabetic cats.
*IM,* Intramuscular; *IV* intravenous; *SC* subcutaneous.

The insulin dose is not adjusted in dogs that remain hyperglycemic during the first few days of insulin therapy. The objective during the first visit is *not* to establish perfect glycemic control, but rather to begin to reverse the metabolic derangements induced by the disease, allow the patient to equilibrate to the insulin and diet change, and give the owner a few days to become accustomed to treating the diabetic dog at home. Adjustments are made on subsequent evaluations.

**Dietary therapy.** Adjustments in diet and feeding practices are directed at correcting or preventing obesity, maintaining consistency in the timing and caloric content of the meals, and furnishing a diet that helps minimize the postprandial increase in blood glucose. Recommendations are summarized in Box 52-4.

High-fiber diets are beneficial for treating obesity and improving glycemic control (see text). However, these diets should not be fed to thin or emaciated diabetic dogs. Instead, glycemic control is reestablished through insulin therapy and a more calorie-dense, lower-fiber diet designed for maintenance. Once normal body weight is attained, a diet containing more fiber can be gradually substituted.

**Exercise.** Exercise is important in maintaining glycemic control. The daily routine should include exercise, preferably at the same time each day. Strenuous and sporadic exercise can cause severe hypoglycemia and should be avoided. In dogs that sporadically perform strenuous exercise (e.g., hunting dogs), the insulin dose should be decreased on days when the dog performs more than its usual amount of exercise. Reducing the dose by 50% initially is recommended, with further adjustments based on the occurrence of symptomatic hypoglycemia and the severity of PU and PD that develops in the ensuing 24 to 48 hours. The owner must be aware of the signs of hypoglycemia and have a source of glucose (e.g., Karo syrup, candy, food) readily available in case any of these signs develop.

---

**Box 52-4**

## Recommendations for Dietary Treatment of Diabetes Mellitus in Dogs

I. Dietary composition
   Increased fiber content
   Increased digestible carbohydrate content (45%-60% ME)
   Decreased fat content (<25% ME)
   Adequate protein content (15%-30% ME)
II. Feed canned and/or dry kibble foods; avoid diet containing monosaccharides, disaccharides, and propylene glycol
III. Caloric intake and obesity
   Average daily caloric intake in geriatric pet: 40-60 kcal/kg
   Adjust daily caloric intake on individual basis
   Eliminate obesity, if present, by:
      Increasing daily exercise
      Decreasing daily caloric intake
      Feeding low–calorie-dense, low-fat, high-fiber (preferred in diabetics) or low–calorie-dense, low-fat, low-fiber diet designed for weight loss
      Eliminating treats
IV. Feeding schedule
   Maintain consistent caloric content of the meals
   Maintain consistent timing of feeding
   Feed within time frame of insulin action
   Feed one half the total daily caloric intake at time of each insulin injection
   Let "nibbler" dogs continue to nibble throughout day and night

---

*ME,* Metabolizable energy.

***Acarbose.*** Acarbose is a complex oligosaccharide that delays absorption of glucose from the small intestine and decreases postprandial blood glucose concentrations. It improves glycemic control in some dogs with IDDM. However, the high prevalence of adverse effects (e.g., diarrhea, weight loss) and the expense limit its usefulness to dogs with poorly controlled DM in which the cause for poor glycemic control cannot be identified and insulin therapy by itself is ineffective in prevention of clinical signs.

The initial dose should be kept low (12.5 to 25 mg/dog at each meal) and always administered at the time of feeding. A stepwise increase to 50 mg/dog and, in large dogs, a further increase to 100 mg/dog can be considered in those that fail to show improvement in glycemic control after 2 weeks.

***Addressing concurrent problems.*** Any concurrent inflammatory, infectious, hormonal, or neoplastic disorder or administration of insulin-antagonistic drugs can cause insulin resistance and interfere with the effectiveness of insulin therapy. The severity of insulin resistance depends, in part, on the cause. Insulin resistance may be mild and easily overcome by increasing the dose of insulin or it may be severe, causing marked hyperglycemia regardless of the type and dose of insulin administered.

Identification and treatment of concurrent problems plays an integral role in the successful management of the diabetic dog. A thorough history, physical examination, and complete diagnostic evaluation are imperative in the newly diagnosed diabetic dog. Possible causes of insulin resistance are listed in Table 52-3.

***Adjustments to insulin therapy.*** Diabetic dogs typically are evaluated every week until an effective insulin protocol is established, which usually takes approximately 1 month (assuming unidentified insulin-antagonistic disease is not present). During this month, changes in insulin dose, type, and frequency of administration are common and should be anticipated by the owner.

At each evaluation the owner's opinion of water intake, urine output, and overall health of the dog is discussed, a complete physical examination is performed, and any change in body weight is noted; blood glucose is measured serially between 7 and 9 AM and 4 and 6 PM. Adjustments in insulin therapy are based on this information, and the dog is reevaluated in 1 week.

**Table 52-3**

**Recognized Causes of Insulin Ineffectiveness or Insulin Resistance in Diabetic Dogs and Cats**

| Caused by insulin therapy | Caused by concurrent disorder |
|---|---|
| Inactive insulin | Diabetogenic drugs |
| Diluted insulin | Hyperadrenocorticism |
| Improper administration technique | Diestrus (bitch) |
| Inadequate dose | Acromegaly (cats) |
| Somogyi phenomenon | Infection, especially of oral cavity and urinary tract |
| Inadequate frequency of administration | Hypothyroidism (dogs) |
| Impaired insulin absorption, especially ultralente insulin | Hyperthyroidism (cats |
| Antiinsulin antibody excess | Renal insufficiency |
| | Liver insufficiency |
| | Cardiac insufficiency |
| | Glucagonoma (dogs) |
| | Pheochromocytoma |
| | Chronic inflammation, especially pancreatitis |
| | Pancreatic exocrine insufficiency |
| | Severe obesity |
| | Hyperlipidemia |
| | Neoplasia |

Glycemic control is attained when clinical signs of DM have resolved, the dog is healthy and interactive at home, body weight is stable, the owner is satisfied with the progress of therapy, and, ideally, the blood glucose remains between 100 and 250 mg/dl throughout the day.

*Long-term management.* The insulin dose required to maintain glycemic control typically changes (increases or decreases) over time. Once the insulin dose range required to maintain glycemic control becomes apparent, and as confidence is gained in the owner's ability to recognize signs of hypoglycemia and hyperglycemia, the owner is eventually allowed to make *slight* adjustments in the insulin dose (while staying within an agreed-on range) at home, based on observations of the dog's well-being. If the insulin dose is at the upper or lower end of the established range and the dog is still symptomatic, the owner is instructed to call the veterinarian before making further adjustments in the insulin dose.

*Techniques for monitoring glycemic control.* The most important indexes to assess when evaluating glycemic control are the severity of clinical signs and overall health of the dog, as assessed by the owner; physical examination findings; and stability of body weight. Control is adequate if the owner is satisfied with the results of treatment, physical examination is supportive of good glycemic control, and the dog's body weight is stable.

*Morning blood glucose concentration.* The preference is to evaluate the dog at the beginning of the day (7:30 to 9:00 AM), before or within 1 hour of insulin administration, and to obtain blood for measurement of glucose and serum fructosamine (see below) at that time. In most well-regulated diabetic dogs the blood glucose measured between 7:30 and 9:00 AM and before or within 1 hour of insulin administration is 150 to 250 mg/dl.

An early-morning blood glucose <150 mg/dl raises concern for development of hypoglycemia several hours after insulin administration that is either subclinical or not being recognized by the owner. Measurement of serum fructosamine is indicated in this situation; low serum fructosamine (<350 μmol/L) suggests prolonged periods of hypoglycemia and a need to reduce the insulin dose.

Poor glycemic control should be suspected and additional diagnostics (i.e., serial blood glucose curve, serum fructosamine concentration, tests for concurrent disorders) or a change in insulin therapy considered if the owner reports clinical signs (e.g., PU and PD, lethargy, signs of hypoglycemia), if physical examination identifies problems consistent with poor glycemic control (e.g., animal is thin or emaciated, poor haircoat is poor), if the dog is losing weight, or if the morning blood glucose is >300 mg/dl.

*Serum fructosamine.* Documenting an increase in blood glucose does not by itself confirm poor glycemic control, as stress or excitement can cause marked hyperglycemia. If a discrepancy exists among the history, physical examination findings, and blood glucose values, especially if the dog is nervous or excited, serum fructosamine should be measured to further evaluate glycemic control.

The serum fructosamine concentration is directly related to the average blood glucose concentration during the previous 2 to 3 weeks. The higher the average blood glucose, the higher the serum fructosamine; and the lower the average blood glucose, the lower the serum fructosamine. The serum fructosamine concentration is not affected by acute increases in blood glucose (as occur with stress or excitement).

The normal range for serum fructosamine is 225 to 375 μmol/L. Interpretation in a diabetic dog must take into consideration the fact that hyperglycemia is common, even in well-controlled diabetic dogs. Most owners are happy with the dog's response to insulin therapy if serum fructosamine can be kept between 350 and 450 μmol/L. Values >500 μmol/L suggest inadequate diabetic control and a need for insulin adjustments; values >600 μmol/L indicate serious lack of glycemic control.

Concentrations in the lower half of the normal range (<300 μmol/L) or below normal should raise concern for significant periods of hypoglycemia. Glucose counter-regulation (the Somogyi phenomenon) should be suspected if clinical signs (PU and PD, polyphagia, weight loss) are present in a diabetic dog with a serum fructosamine <400 μmol/L.

*Urine glucose monitoring.* Occasional monitoring of urine for glycosuria and ketonuria is helpful in diabetic dogs that have problems with recurring ketosis or hypoglycemia. The owner is instructed not to adjust daily insulin doses based on morning urine glucose measurements, except to decrease the insulin dose in dogs with recurring hypoglycemia and persistent absence of glycosuria. A weekend evaluation of multiple urine samples obtained throughout the day and early evening is recommended. The well-controlled diabetic dog should have urine that is free of glucose for most of each 24-hour period. Persistent glycosuria throughout the day and night suggests a problem that may require evaluation via in-hospital or at-home blood glucose measurements.

*Serial blood glucose curve.* Generation of a serial blood glucose curve allows the clinician to assess the effectiveness of the administered insulin in lowering the blood glucose and to determine the glucose nadir and duration of insulin effect. Evaluation of a serial blood glucose curve is mandatory during initial regulation of the diabetic patient, is periodically of value in assessment of glycemic control, and is necessary for reestablishment of glycemic control in the patient with clinical manifestations of hyperglycemia or hypoglycemia.

The insulin and feeding schedule used by the owner should be followed and blood glucose measured every 1 to 2 hours throughout the day. Ideally, all glucose values will fall within the range of 100 to 250 mg/dl during the period between insulin injections. Typically, but not always, the highest reading occurs at the time of insulin injection. If the blood glucose nadir is >150 mg/dl, the insulin dose may need to be increased, and if the nadir is <80 mg/dl, the insulin dose should be decreased. Protocols and interpretation are discussed further in the text.

**Insulin therapy during surgery.** Generally, surgery should be delayed in a diabetic dog until the patient's clinical condition is stable and the diabetic state is controlled with insulin. The exceptions are situations in which surgery is required to eliminate insulin resistance (e.g., ovariohysterectomy in a diestrus bitch) or to save the animal's life.

Insulin must be administered during the perioperative period to prevent severe hyperglycemia and minimize ketone formation. To compensate for the lack of food intake and prevent hypoglycemia, the insulin dose is decreased and dextrose is administered IV as needed. To correct marked hyperglycemia, regular crystalline insulin is administered intramuscularly (IM) or by continuous intravenous infusion.

The day before surgery the animal is given its normal dose of insulin and fed as usual; food is withheld after 10 PM. On the morning of the procedure, blood glucose is measured before the animal is given insulin. If the blood glucose is <100 mg/dl, insulin is not given and an intravenous infusion of 2.5% to 5% dextrose is initiated. If the blood glucose is 100 to 200 mg/dl, one fourth of the animal's usual morning dose of insulin is given and an intravenous infusion of dextrose is initiated. If the blood glucose is >200 mg/dl, one half of the usual morning dose of insulin is given, but the intravenous dextrose infusion is withheld until the blood glucose drops below 150 mg/dl.

Blood glucose is measured every 30 to 60 minutes during the surgical procedure and perioperative period. The goal is to maintain the blood glucose between 150 and 250 mg/dl. When the blood glucose exceeds 300 mg/dl, the dextrose infusion should be discontinued and the blood glucose evaluated 30 and 60 minutes later. If the blood glucose remains >300 mg/dl, regular crystalline insulin is administered IM at approximately 20% of the dose of long-acting insulin being used at home. Subsequent doses of regular crystalline insulin should be given no more frequently than q4h, and the dose should be adjusted based on the effect of the first insulin injection on blood glucose.

The day after surgery the patient can usually be returned to the routine schedule of insulin administration and feeding. An animal that is not eating can be maintained with intravenous dextrose infusions and regular crystalline insulin injections given subcutaneously (SC) q6-8h until it is eating regularly.

### Complications of insulin therapy

*Hypoglycemia.* Hypoglycemia is a common complication of insulin therapy. It is most likely to occur after sudden, large increases in the insulin dose, with excessive overlap of insulin action in dogs receiving insulin twice a day, and after prolonged inappetence. In many diabetic dogs the signs are not apparent to owners, and hypoglycemia is identified during evaluation of a serial blood glucose curve or serum fructosamine concentration. Clinical signs and treatment of hypoglycemia are discussed on p 470.

Insulin therapy should be stopped until hyperglycemia and glycosuria recur. Adjustment in the subsequent insulin dose is somewhat arbitrary; as a general rule of thumb, the insulin dose should be decreased 25% to 50% and subsequent adjustments based on clinical response and blood glucose values.

*Recurrence of signs of DM.* Recurrence or persistence of clinical signs is perhaps the most common "complication" of insulin therapy in diabetic dogs. It is usually caused by problems with owner technique in administering insulin; problems relating to the insulin type, dose, species, or frequency of administration; or problems with responsiveness to insulin caused by concurrent inflammatory, infectious, neoplastic, or hormonal disorders (e.g., insulin resistance). These problems are summarized in Table 52-3 and discussed further in the text.

*Insulin-binding antibodies.* Antibodies against insulin are detected in the serum in approximately 5% of dogs treated with recombinant human insulin and in approximately 45% of dogs treated with insulin from a beef-pork source. Presence of insulin antibodies causes erratic and often poor glycemic control or inability to maintain glycemic control over time, necessitates frequent adjustments in insulin dose, and occasionally causes development of severe insulin resistance. Recombinant human-source insulin should be used in diabetic dogs to avoid these problems.

*Allergic reactions to insulin.* Allergic reactions to insulin are poorly documented in diabetic dogs. Pain on injection of insulin is usually caused by inappropriate injection technique or site of injection. Chronic injection of insulin in the same area of the body may cause thickening of the skin and subcutaneous tissues, which may impair insulin absorption, resulting in recurrence of clinical signs of DM. Rotation of the injection site helps prevent this problem.

Rarely, diabetic dogs develop focal subcutaneous edema and swelling at the site of insulin injection. Insulin allergy is suspected in these animals. Treatment includes switching to a less antigenic insulin and to a more purified insulin preparation (see text).

### Prognosis

The prognosis depends on the presence and reversibility of concurrent diseases, ease of regulation of the diabetic state with insulin, and owner commitment. Mean survival time for diabetic dogs is approximately 3 years from the time of diagnosis, but diabetic dogs that survive the first 6 months can easily live >5 years with the disease.

## DIABETES MELLITUS IN CATS (TEXT PP 749-762)

In many respects the clinical features, diagnosis, and management of DM in cats are the same as those in dogs. In this section only the features of DM that are unique to cats or that are particularly pertinent to the management of DM in cats are discussed. The reader is referred to the previous section on DM in dogs for a more comprehensive discussion of DM.

### Etiology

The most commonly recognized form of DM in cats is IDDM. Common histologic abnormalities include islet-specific amyloidosis, β-cell vacuolation and degeneration, and chronic pancreatitis. The role of immune destruction and genetic factors remains to be determined.

NIDDM is diagnosed in approximately 30% of diabetic cats. The etiopathogenesis is multifactorial and includes islet-specific amyloid deposition. If amyloid deposition is progressive, it may eventually lead to IDDM. The presence and severity of concurrent insulin resistance strongly influence the clinical impact of partial destruction of the pancreatic islets.

Secondary insulin resistance may be caused by concurrent obesity, drugs, or diseases such as chronic pancreatitis and other chronic inflammatory diseases, infection, hyperthyroidism, hyperadrenocorticism, and acromegaly (see Table 52-3). Even chronic hyperglycemia itself can result in permanent suppression of β-cell function (glucose toxicity). Therefore identification and correction of concurrent problems that affect insulin sensitivity is critical to the successful management of DM in cats.

### Difficulties with classification

Classifying diabetic cats as either IDDM or NIDDM based on their need for insulin treatment can be confusing, because some diabetic cats initially appear to have NIDDM that progresses to IDDM, and some cats alternate between IDDM and NIDDM as the severity of insulin resistance and impairment of β-cell function waxes and wanes.

*"Transient" DM.* Approximately 20% of diabetic cats become 'transiently' diabetic, usually within 4 to 6 weeks of being diagnosed and treated for DM. In these cats, hyperglycemia, glycosuria, and clinical signs of DM resolve, and insulin treatment can be discontinued. Some diabetic cats never require insulin therapy again, but others become permanently insulin dependent weeks or months after resolution of a prior diabetic state.

Cats with transient DM are theoretically in a subclinical diabetic state that becomes clinical when the pancreas is stressed by exposure to a concurrent insulin-antagonistic drug or disease, most notably glucocorticoids, megestrol acetate, or chronic pancreatitis. These cats have some abnormality of the islets that impairs their ability to compensate for concurrent insulin resistance and results in carbohydrate intolerance. Insulin therapy and treatment of the concurrent disorder resolves the apparent IDDM state. The future requirement for insulin therapy depends on status of the islets. If the problem is progressive (e.g., amyloidosis), eventually enough β cells are destroyed and permanent IDDM develops.

### Clinical features

DM can be diagnosed in cats of any age, but most diabetic cats are >9 years of age at the time of diagnosis. DM occurs predominantly in neutered male cats; no apparent breed predisposition exists.

### Clinical signs

The history in virtually all diabetic cats includes PU and PD, polyphagia, and weight loss. A common complaint by owners is the frequent need to change the litter. Additional signs include lethargy; decreased interaction with family members; lack of grooming behavior and development of a dry, lusterless, unkempt or matted haircoat; and decreased jumping ability, rear limb weakness, or development of a plantigrade posture. If signs of uncomplicated diabetes are not observed by the owner, diabetic cats may be at risk for development of systemic illness as progressive DKA develops.

*Physical examination.* Findings depend on the presence and severity of DKA and on the nature of any concurrent disorder. No classic findings occur in nonketotic diabetic cats. Many diabetic cats are obese but are otherwise in good physical condition. Cats with prolonged, untreated diabetes may have lost weight but are rarely emaciated unless concurrent disease (e.g., hyperthyroidism) is present.

Diabetes-induced hepatic lipidosis may cause hepatomegaly. Weakness in the rear limbs, ataxia, knuckling, a plantigrade posture (with the cat's hocks touching the ground when it walks), muscle atrophy, depressed limb reflexes, and deficits in postural reaction testing may be evident if the cat has developed diabetic neuropathy. Distal muscles of the rear limbs may feel hard on digital palpation, and cats may object to palpation or manipulation of the rear limbs. Additional abnormalities may be identified in cats with DKA.

### Diagnosis

As discussed for DM in dogs, the diagnosis is based on identification of appropriate clinical signs, hyperglycemia, and glycosuria. Transient, stress-induced hyperglycemia is a common problem in cats and can cause the blood glucose to exceed 300 mg/dl. Glycosuria usually does not develop in cats with stress hyperglycemia. For this reason, persistent hyperglycemia and glycosuria should always be documented when one is establishing a diagnosis of DM in cats. If the diagnosis is in doubt, the cat can be sent home and the owner instructed to monitor urine glucose at home.

*Serum fructosamine.* Serum fructosamine can be measured if uncertainty exists regarding whether hyperglycemia is stress induced. Documenting an increase in the serum fructosamine supports the presence of sustained hyperglycemia. However, serum fructosamine can be in the upper range of normal in symptomatic cats that have only recently developed DM.

### Concurrent disorders

Simply establishing the diagnosis of DM does not provide the whole picture. A thorough evaluation for concurrent disorders that may affect insulin sensitivity and evaluation of response to treatment are important when one is trying to determine if a diabetic cat has IDDM, NIDDM, or transient DM.

The minimum database in every diabetic cat should include CBC, serum biochemical panel, serum thyroxine concentration, and urinalysis with bacterial culture. If available, abdominal ultrasound should be a routine part of the diagnostic evaluation because of the high prevalence of chronic pancreatitis in diabetic cats. Additional tests may be warranted based on the history and physical examination. Box 52-3 lists potential clinical pathologic abnormalities.

### Serum insulin

The information used to establish a diagnosis of DM does not give any indication of the status of pancreatic islet health and function or the severity and reversibility of concurrent insulin resistance. Serum insulin >15 µU/ml in a newly diagnosed, untreated diabetic cat supports the presence of functional β cells and partial destruction of the islets. However, low or undetectable serum insulin levels do not rule out partial islet cell loss because of the suppressive effects of glucose toxicity. For this reason, measurement of baseline serum insulin or an insulin response test is not routinely performed in cats.

### Treatment

Treatment of DM is discussed at length in the earlier discussion of DM in dogs. Only the aspects of management that are unique or particularly pertinent to cats are discussed here.

The ultimate differentiation between IDDM and NIDDM in cats is often made retrospectively, after the clinician has had several weeks to assess the response to initial therapy (dietary changes, oral hypoglycemic drugs, and control of current diseases). The initial decision between insulin therapy and oral hypoglycemic drugs is based on the severity of clinical signs, the presence of ketoacidosis, the general health of the cat, and the owner's wishes. Glycemic control can be maintained in some diabetic cats simply with dietary changes, oral hypoglycemic drugs, and control of concurrent diseases.

### Insulin therapy

Diabetic cats are notoriously unpredictable in their response to exogenous insulin. No single type of insulin is routinely effective in maintaining glycemic control, even with twice-a-day administration, and it is not possible to predict which type of insulin will work best in individual diabetic cats. Properties of the recombinant human insulin preparations used in cats are summarized in Table 52-2.

*Ultralente insulin.* Ultralente insulin is the longest-acting but least potent of the commonly used commercial insulins. It must be administered twice a day in most diabetic cats, and absorption is inadequate for control of glycemia in approximately 25% of cats.

*Lente and NPH insulin.* Lente and NPH insulin are more potent than ultralente and are more consistently and rapidly absorbed after subcutaneous injection. However, the duration of effect of lente and especially NPH insulin is considerably shorter than 12 hours in some diabetic cats, resulting in inadequate glycemic control despite twice-a-day administration.

Currently, lente insulin of recombinant human origin is initially given at a dose of 1 to 2 U/cat twice daily. The prevalence of insulin antibodies that cause problems with glycemic control is uncommon in cats treated with recombinant human insulin.

*Protamine-zinc insulin.* A protamine-zinc insulin (PZI) of beef-pork origin has recently been shown to be very effective in improving glycemic control in poorly controlled diabetic cats previously treated with ultralente or NPH insulin. PZI is a longer-acting insulin that is more consistently absorbed than ultralente insulin and has a more acceptable duration of effect than NPH insulin. However, the timing of the glucose nadir is quite variable and occurs within 9 hours of PZI administration in >80% of diabetic cats. Therefore PZI is routinely given twice a day.

*Adjustments in insulin therapy.* The approach to adjusting insulin therapy in cats is similar to that in dogs. Most owners of diabetic cats are satisfied with the response to insulin therapy if the blood glucose ranges between 100 and 300 mg/dl throughout the day. Diabetic cats can have problems with insulin-induced hyperglycemia (Somogyi phenomenon) at relatively small doses (2 to 3 U/injection). Therefore it is best to have owners administer a fixed dose of insulin once glycemic control is attained and not adjust the insulin dose without first consulting their veterinarians.

*Surgery.* Management of diabetic cats that require surgery is the same as that described for diabetic dogs.

*Complications of insulin therapy.* Complications are similar to those discussed for dogs. The most common complications of insulin therapy in diabetic cats are recurring hypoglycemia, insulin overdose that causes the Somogyi phenomenon (glucose counter-regulation), incorrect assessment of glycemic control caused by stress-induced hyperglycemia, inadequate absorption of longer-acting insulins, short duration of effect of intermediate-acting insulins, and insulin resistance caused by concurrent inflammatory and hormonal disorders, most notably chronic pancreatitis. These problems are discussed in the text.

Symptomatic hypoglycemia is most likely to occur after sudden large increases in the insulin dose, after sudden improvement in concurrent insulin resistance, with excessive overlap of insulin action in cats receiving insulin twice a day, after prolonged inappetence, and in insulin-treated cats that have reverted to a non–insulin-dependent state. The treatment approach is the same as in dogs.

### Dietary therapy

The principles of dietary therapy for cats are summarized in Box 52-5. Obesity is common in diabetic cats and results from excessive caloric intake typically caused by free-choice feeding of dry cat food. Obesity causes insulin resistance that resolves as obesity is corrected. Control of glycemia often improves, and some diabetic cats revert to a subclinical diabetic state after weight reduction.

The other main goal of dietary therapy is to minimize the impact of a meal on blood glucose concentrations. Half of the cat's total daily caloric intake should be offered at the time of each insulin injection and remain available to the cat to consume when it wishes. Preliminary studies suggest that carbohydrate-restricted diets may be as effective in improving glycemic control as diets moderate in protein, fat, and digestible carbohydrate content and high in fiber (see text).

### Oral hypoglycemic drugs

Oral hypoglycemic drugs are primarily used for the treatment of NIDDM. Sulfonylureas (e.g., glipizide, glyburide) are the most commonly used of the oral hypoglycemic drugs in diabetic cats. Some pancreatic insulin secretory capacity must exist for sulfonylureas to be effective in improving glycemic control. Other hypoglycemic drugs are discussed in the text.

*Glipizide.* Glipizide (Glucotrol) is effective in improving clinical signs and severity of hyperglycemia in approximately 30% of diabetic cats. It has been used successfully as an alternative to insulin therapy in healthy, newly diagnosed diabetic cats. Clinical response is variable, ranging from excellent (blood glucose <200 mg/dl) to partial (clinical improvement but failure to resolve hyperglycemia) to no response. Cats with a partial response to glipizide may have severe NIDDM or the early stages of IDDM.

Glipizide is initially given at a dose of 2.5 mg orally twice a day, with a meal, in diabetic cats that are nonketotic and relatively healthy on physical examination. The cat is examined weekly during the first month of therapy. History, complete physical examination, body weight, urine glucose and ketones, and blood glucose are evaluated

---

**Box 52-5**

## Recommendations for Dietary Treatment of Diabetes Mellitus in Cats

 I. Dietary composition
   Option 1—moderate carbohydrate and fat, high fiber content
   Option 2—high protein, low carbohydrate, low fiber content
   Option 3—high fat, low carbohydrate, low fiber content
   Diet options can be used interchangeably
   Which diet composition improves glycemic control the most is unpredictable
 II. Feed canned and/or dry kibble foods; avoid diets containing monosaccharides, disaccharides, propylene glycol
 III. Caloric intake and obesity
   Average daily caloric intake in geriatric pet: 40-60 kcal/kg
   Adjust daily caloric intake on individual basis
   Eliminate obesity, if present, by:
     Decreasing daily caloric intake
     Feeding diets designed for weight loss
 IV. Feeding schedule
   Maintain consistent caloric content of meals
   Maintain consistent timing of feeding
   Feed within time frame of insulin action
   Feed one half the total daily caloric intake at time of each insulin injection
   Let "nibbler" cats continue to nibble throughout day and night

---

**Table 52-4**

## Adverse Reactions to Glipizide Treatment in Diabetic Cats

| Adverse reaction | Recommendation |
|---|---|
| Vomiting within 1 hour of administration | Vomiting usually subsides after 2-5 days of glipizide therapy; decrease dose or frequency of administration if vomiting is severe; discontinue if vomiting persists >1 wk |
| Increased serum hepatic enzyme activities | Continue treatment and monitor enzymes every 1-2 wk initially; discontinue glipizide if cat becomes ill (lethargy, inappetence, vomiting) or the alanine aminotransferase activity exceeds 500 U/L |
| Icterus | Discontinue glipizide treatment; reinstitute treatment at lower dose and frequency once icterus resolves (usually within 2 wk); discontinue permanently if icterus recurs |
| Hypoglycemia | Discontinue glipizide treatment; recheck blood glucose in 1 wk; reinstitute therapy at lower dose or frequency if hyperglycemia recurs |

at each visit. If adverse reactions (Table 52-4) have not occurred after 2 weeks of treatment, the dose is increased to 5 mg twice a day.

Therapy is continued as long as the cat is stable. If euglycemia or hypoglycemia develops, the glipizide dose may be tapered down or discontinued and blood glucose reevaluated 1 week later to assess the need for continued therapy. If hyperglycemia recurs, the dose is increased or glipizide is reinitiated, with a dose reduction in those cats that previously developed hypoglycemia.

Glipizide is discontinued and insulin therapy initiated if clinical signs continue to worsen, the cat becomes ill or develops ketoacidosis or peripheral neuropathy, the blood glucose remains >300 mg/dl after 1 to 2 months of therapy, or the owner becomes dissatisfied with the treatment.

*Glyburide.* Glyburide (Micronase) has a longer duration of action than glipizide and is usually administered once a day. An initial dose of 0.625 mg/cat (¹/₂ of 1.25-mg tablet) once daily is recommended. Response to therapy and adverse reactions are similar to those described for glipizide.

*Vanadium and chromium.* The trace elements vanadium (V) and chromium (Cr) exert insulin-like effects in vitro. Unpublished studies suggest that V may be effective in improving glycemic control in cats in the early stages of NIDDM. The dose is 0.2 mg of V per kg per day, given once a day in food or water. Adverse effects include anorexia and vomiting. Long-term toxicity is related to accumulation of V in the liver, kidneys, and bone. Acute renal failure has been reported in one cat treated with V for 1 year; renal failure resolved after discontinuation of V supplementation.

The effect of Cr-tripicolinate on glucose tolerance is controversial in cats, ranging from no effect in obese and nonobese healthy cats to a small but significant dose-dependent improvement in glucose tolerance in nonobese healthy cats. The effect of Cr-tripicolinate in diabetic cats has not been reported. Supplementation did not improve glycemic control in a group of dogs with IDDM.

*Acarbose.* Acarbose slows absorption of glucose from the intestine. The feeding of a carbohydrate-restricted diet is recommended instead of acarbose treatment in diabetic cats.

### Techniques for monitoring glycemic control

The techniques for monitoring glycemic control in diabetic cats are similar to those in dogs. One important factor that affects monitoring in diabetic cats is the propensity to develop stress-induced hyperglycemia caused by visits to the veterinary hospital. Once stress-induced hyperglycemia develops, it is a perpetual problem, and blood glucose measurements can no longer be considered accurate. Failure to identify stress hyperglycemia and its impact on interpretation of blood glucose is one of the most important reasons for misinterpretation of the status of glycemic control in diabetic cats.

Micromanaging diabetic cats should be avoided, and serial blood glucose curves should be performed only when the clinician perceives a need to change insulin therapy. The determination of good versus poor glycemic control should be based on the owner's opinion of the presence and severity of clinical signs and the overall health of the cat, ability of the cat to jump, its grooming behavior, findings on physical examination, and stability of body weight. A protocol for generating a blood glucose curve at home and the role of serum fructosamine are discussed in the text.

### Complications of DM

Complications resulting from the diabetes (e.g., peripheral neuropathy) or the therapy (e.g., hypoglycemia) are common in cats (see Table 52-1). The most common complications are hypoglycemia, chronic pancreatitis, weight loss, poor grooming behavior that is causing a dry, lusterless, and unkempt haircoat, and peripheral neuropathy of the hind limbs. Diabetic cats are also at risk for ketoacidosis.

*Diabetic neuropathy.* Diabetic neuropathy occurs in approximately 10% of diabetic cats. Clinical signs and physical examination findings are discussed in the text. Signs can progress to include the thoracic limbs. No specific therapy exists. Aggressive glucoregulation with insulin may improve nerve conduction and reverse the posterior weakness and plantigrade posture; however, response to therapy is variable. Generally, the more severe and long-standing the neuropathy, the less likely that improvement of glycemic control will reverse the clinical signs.

### Prognosis

The prognosis for diabetic cats is similar to that for diabetic dogs. The mean survival time in diabetic cats is approximately 3 years from the time of diagnosis. Diabetic cats that survive the first 6 months can easily live >5 years with the disease.

## DIABETIC KETOACIDOSIS (TEXT PP 762-769)

### Etiology

DKA is a complex condition that is usually affected by concurrent clinical disorders. Virtually all dogs and cats with DKA have a relative or absolute insulin deficiency; some patients develop DKA despite receiving daily insulin injections. It is rare for animals with DKA not to have some coexisting disorder, such as pancreatitis, infection, or renal insufficiency. Recognition and treatment of these disorders are essential for successful management of DKA.

### Clinical features

History and physical findings are variable. DKA occurs most commonly in dogs and cats with previously undiagnosed DM. Less commonly it develops in diabetic patients that are receiving an inadequate dose of insulin and have a concurrent infectious, inflammatory, or insulin-resistant hormonal disorder.

*Clinical signs.* The classic signs of uncomplicated DM (PU and PD, polyphagia, weight loss) develop initially but either go unnoticed or are considered insignificant by the owner. Systemic signs (e.g., lethargy, anorexia, vomiting) ensue as progressive ketonemia and metabolic acidosis develop; the severity of systemic signs is directly related to the degree of acidosis and the nature of concurrent disorders. Time from onset of initial signs of DM to development of systemic signs of DKA ranges from a few days to >6 months. Once ketoacidosis begins to develop, however, severe illness usually becomes evident within 7 days.

*Physical examination.* Common findings include dehydration, depression, weakness, tachypnea, vomiting, and sometimes a strong odor of acetone on the breath. With severe metabolic acidosis, slow, deep breathing (Kussmaul respiration) may be observed. Gastrointestinal (GI) signs such as vomiting, abdominal pain, and abdominal distention are common, because concurrent acute or chronic pancreatitis is common in diabetic dogs and cats. Other intraabdominal disorders should also be considered.

### Diagnosis

Diagnosis of DM requires the presence of appropriate clinical signs and persistent fasting hyperglycemia and glucosuria. Concurrent documentation of ketonuria with reagent test strips that measure acetoacetic acid (e.g., KetoDiastix) establishes the diagnosis of DKA. If ketonuria is not present but DKA is suspected, the serum or urine can be tested for acetone using Acetest tablets.

### Treatment

*"Healthy" patient with diabetic ketosis or DKA.* If signs of systemic illness are absent or mild and metabolic acidosis is mild (total venous carbon dioxide [$CO_2$] or arterial bicarbonate ($HCO_3$) >16 mEq/L), short-acting regular crystalline insulin can be administered SC q8h until ketonuria resolves (usually within 2 to 4 days). The insulin dose should be adjusted based on blood glucose values. To minimize hypoglycemia, the patient should be fed one third of its daily caloric intake with each insulin injection.

Prolonged ketonuria is suggestive of a significant concurrent illness or inadequate blood insulin concentrations to suppress ketogenesis. Once the ketoacidosis has resolved and the patient is eating and drinking, longer-acting insulin preparations may be instituted. Management of DM in dogs and cats is discussed on pp 472 and 481, respectively.

*Sick patient with DKA.* An aggressive therapeutic plan is indicated if the patient has signs of systemic illness; physical examination reveals dehydration, depression, weakness, and/or Kussmaul respiration; blood glucose is >500 mg/dl; or severe metabolic acidosis (total venous $CO_2$ or arterial $HCO_3$ <12 mEq/L) is present. The minimum database includes urinalysis, hematocrit, total plasma protein, blood glucose, venous total $CO_2$ or arterial acid-base evaluation, and serum creatinine and electrolytes (sodium, potassium, calcium, phosphate). Abnormalities frequently associated with DKA are listed in Box 52-6. Other diagnostic tests, such as radiography and abdominal ultrasound, are usually needed to identify concurrent disorders.

The treatment goals are as follows: (1) to provide adequate amounts of insulin to suppress ketogenesis and hepatic gluconeogenesis, (2) to restore water and electrolyte

---

**Box 52-6**

**Common Clinicopathologic Abnormalities Identified in Dogs and Cats with Diabetic Ketoacidosis**

Neutrophilic leukocytosis, signs of toxicity if septic
Hemoconcentration
Hyperglycemia
Hypercholesterolemia, lipemia
Increased alkaline phosphatase activity
Increased alanine aminotransferase activity
Increased blood urea nitrogen and serum creatinine concentrations
Hyponatremia
Hypochloremia
Hypokalemia
Metabolic acidosis (decreased total carbon dioxide concentration)
Hyperlipasemia
Hyperamylasemia
Hyperosmolality
Glycosuria
Ketonuria
Urinary tract infection

---

losses, (3) to correct acidosis, (4) to identify precipitating factors for the present illness, and (5) to provide a carbohydrate substrate (e.g., dextrose) when necessary to allow continued administration of insulin without causing hypoglycemia. Osmotic and biochemical problems can be created by overly aggressive therapy, as well as by the disease process itself, so abnormal parameters should be slowly returned toward normal over 24 to 48 hours.

*Insulin therapy.* Resolution of ketoacidosis can be achieved only through insulin therapy, which should be initiated within 1 to 4 hours of establishment of the diagnosis of DKA. The more severe the hypokalemia, the longer the delay should be before insulin therapy is begun. If hypokalemia or hypophosphatemia is a concern, the initial insulin dose can be reduced to slow the intracellular shift of these electrolytes while lipolysis and generation of free fatty acids are still decreased.

The amount of insulin needed by an individual dog or cat is difficult to predict, so an insulin with a rapid onset of action and short duration of effect should be used. Insulin therapy and other measures for treating severe DKA are outlined in Box 52-7 and discussed in detail in the text.

**Complications of therapy**

Complications induced by therapy for DKA are common and usually result from overly aggressive treatment, inadequate patient monitoring, and failure to frequently reevaluate biochemical parameters. Severe hypokalemia is the most common complication that develops during the first 24 to 36 hours of treatment. Others include hypoglycemia, CNS signs (secondary to cerebral edema), severe hypernatremia and hyperchloremia, and hemolytic anemia (from hypophosphatemia).

Fluid, insulin, and bicarbonate therapy typically require modification three or four times during the initial 24 hours. During this initial period, blood glucose should be measured every 1 to 2 hours and serum electrolytes and blood gases every 6 to 8 hours.

**Prognosis**

Despite all precautions and diligence, a fatal outcome cannot be avoided in some cases; approximately 30% of animals with severe DKA die or are euthanized during initial hospitalization. Death is usually the result of severe underlying illness, severe acidosis (arterial pH <7), or complications of therapy.

---

**Box 52-7**

## Initial Management of Dogs or Cats with Severe Diabetic Ketoacidosis

### FLUID THERAPY

Type: 0.9% saline solution

Rate: 60-100 ml/kg/24 hr initially; adjust based on hydration status, urine output, persistence of fluid losses

Potassium supplement: based on serum $K^+$ concentration; if unknown, initially add 40 mEq of KCl to each liter of fluids

Phosphate supplement: administer if serum P is <1.5 mg/dl; initial IV infusion rate is 0.01-0.03 mmol/kg/hr in calcium-free fluids (e.g., 0.9% saline)

Dextrose supplement: not indicated until blood glucose is <250 mg/dl, then begin 5% dextrose infusion

### BICARBONATE THERAPY

Indication: administer if plasma $HCO_3^-$ is <12 mEq/L or total venous $CO_2$ is <12 mmol/L; if not known, do not administer unless animal is severely ill, and then only once

Amount: mEq $HCO_3^-$ = body weight (kg) × 0.4 × (12 – animal's $HCO_3^-$) × 0.5; if animal's $HCO_3^-$ or total $CO_2$ is unknown, use 10 in place of (12 – animal's $HCO_3^-$)

Administration: add to IV fluids and give over 6 hr; do not give as bolus infusion

Retreatment: only if plasma bicarbonate remains <12 mEq/L after 6 hr of therapy

### INSULIN THERAPY

Type: regular crystalline insulin

Administration technique:

*Intermittent intramuscular method*—initial dose, 0.2 U/kg intramuscularly (IM); then 0.1 U/kg IM hourly until blood glucose is <250 mg/dl, then switch to regular subcutaneous insulin q6-8h

*Low-dose IV infusion method*—initial rate, 0.05 to 0.1 U/kg/hr diluted in 0.9% NaCl and administered via infusion or syringe pump in a line separate from that used for fluid therapy; adjust infusion rate based on hourly blood glucose measurements; switch to subcutaneous regular insulin q6-8h once blood glucose is <250 mg/dl

Goal: gradual decline in blood glucose, preferably approximately 75 mg/dl/hr, until concentration is <250 mg/dl

### ANCILLARY THERAPY

Concurrent pancreatitis is common in DKA; nothing by mouth and aggressive fluid therapy usually indicated

Concurrent infections are common in DKA; use of broad-spectrum, parenteral antibiotics usually indicated

Additional therapy may be needed, depending on the nature of concurrent disorders

### PATIENT MONITORING

Blood glucose measurement every 1-2 hr initially; adjust insulin therapy and begin dextrose infusion when decreases below 250 mg/dl

Hydration status, respiration, pulse every 2-4 hr; adjust fluids according to findings

Serum electrolyte and total venous $CO_2$ concentrations every 6-12 hr; adjust fluid and bicarbonate therapy according to findings

Urine output, glycosuria, ketonuria every 2-4 hr; adjust fluid therapy according to findings

Body weight, packed cell volume, temperature, and blood pressure daily

Additional monitoring, depending on concurrent disease

---

*$CO_2$,* Carbon dioxide; *DKA,* diabetic ketoacidosis; *$HCO_3^-$,* bicarbonate; *IV* intravenous; *$K^+$,* potassium; *KCl,* potassium chloride; *NaCl,* sodium chloride; *P,* phosphorus.

## INSULIN-SECRETING β-CELL NEOPLASIA (TEXT PP 769-775)

### Etiology

Functional tumors arising from the pancreatic islet β cells are malignant tumors that secrete insulin, independent of the suppressive effects of hypoglycemia. β-Cell tumors are uncommon in dogs and rare in cats. Virtually all β-cell tumors in dogs are malignant, and most have microscopic or grossly visible metastases at the time of surgery. Common sites include the lymphatics and lymph nodes (duodenal, mesenteric, hepatic, splenic), liver, and peripancreatic mesentery and omentum.

### Clinical features

Insulin-secreting tumors typically occur in middle-aged or older dogs (mean age, 9.5 years; range, 3-14 years). These tumors are found in a wide variety of breeds but are most common in large-breed dogs such as the German Shepherd, Labrador Retriever, Golden Retriever, and Irish Setter.

*Clinical signs.* Clinical signs are caused by hypoglycemia and a resulting increase in circulating catecholamines; they include seizures, weakness, collapse, ataxia, muscle fasciculations, and bizarre behavior. Other signs that may be observed include polyphagia, weight gain, posterior weakness (neuropathy), and either lethargy or nervousness.

The severity of the signs depends on the duration and severity of hypoglycemia. Dogs with chronic or recurrent hypoglycemia tolerate very low blood glucose (20 to 30 mg/dl) for prolonged periods without showing signs. However, fasting, excitement, exercise, and even eating can trigger clinical signs in these dogs. Clinical signs tend to be episodic and are generally observed for only a few seconds to minutes at a time. Seizures are often self-limiting, lasting from 30 seconds to 5 minutes.

*Physical examination.* Physical examination is surprisingly unremarkable; affected dogs are usually free of visible and palpable abnormalities. Peripheral neuropathy has been reported and can cause rear limb weakness, proprioception deficits, depressed reflexes, and muscle atrophy.

### Diagnosis

Diagnosis of an insulin-secreting tumor requires confirmation of hypoglycemia, inappropriate insulin secretion, and presence of a pancreatic mass (via ultrasonography or celiotomy). Considering the potential causes of hypoglycemia (see Box 52-2), a tentative diagnosis of insulin-secreting tumor can often be made based on the history, physical examination, and absence of abnormalities other than hypoglycemia on routine blood tests.

Abdominal ultrasound can be used to identify a mass in the region of the pancreas and to look for metastases in the liver and surrounding structures. However, because of the small size of most insulin-secreting tumors, negative findings on ultrasound do not rule out such tumors.

*Serum insulin concentration.* The diagnosis is established by measuring serum insulin at a time when hypoglycemia is present (blood glucose <60 mg/dl, preferably <50 mg/dl). Invariably, dogs with insulin-secreting tumors have inappropriate excesses in serum insulin. If the blood glucose is low, then a high-normal or increased serum insulin value is indicative of an insulin-secreting tumor. Serum insulin must be evaluated at the same time as blood glucose. Most dogs with these tumors are persistently hypoglycemic; if the dog is euglycemic, a 4- to 12-hour fast may be necessary to induce hypoglycemia.

Serum insulin in a healthy, fasted dog is usually 5 to 20 μU/ml. Serum insulin >20 μU/ml in a dog with a blood glucose <60 mg/dl, in combination with appropriate clinical signs and clinicopathologic findings, strongly supports the diagnosis of insulin-secreting tumor. However, insulin values in the high-normal range (10 to 20 μU/ml) are possible in dogs with these tumors, and values in the low-normal range (5 to 10 μU/ml) do not rule out an insulin-secreting tumor.

Confidence in identifying inappropriate hyperinsulinemia is dependent on the severity of the hypoglycemia: the lower the blood glucose, the more confident one can be in identifying inappropriate hyperinsulinemia, especially when the serum insulin is within the normal range.

## Treatment

Surgical exploration is the best diagnostic, therapeutic, and prognostic tool. Even in dogs with nonresectable tumors or those with obvious metastases, "debulking" the tumor often results in remission of, or at least reduction in, clinical signs and improved response to medical therapy for weeks or months. Survival time also is longer in dogs that underwent surgical debulking followed by medical therapy than in dogs treated only medically.

*Avoiding severe hypoglycemia.* Until surgery is performed, the dog must be protected from episodes of severe hypoglycemia by frequent feeding of small meals and use of glucocorticoids. A continuous intravenous infusion of balanced electrolyte solution containing 2.5% to 5% dextrose before, during, and immediately after surgery is important. The goal is to maintain the blood glucose >35 mg/dl. If dextrose infusion is ineffective in prevention of severe hypoglycemia perioperatively, a constant rate infusion of glucagon should be considered (dose is given in Box 52-8).

*Complications of surgery.* The most common postoperative complications are pancreatitis and either hyperglycemia or hypoglycemia. Polyionic fluids with 2.5% to 5% dextrose (60 to 100 ml/kg/24 hr IV) and nothing by mouth before, during, and for 24 to 48 hours after surgery, followed by appropriate dietary therapy, help avoid pancreatitis.

Occasionally, dogs develop transient DM after surgery. Until the atrophied normal cells regain their secretory capabilities, the animal may require exogenous insulin. Insulin therapy is indicated only when hyperglycemia and glucosuria persist for >2 days after dextrose-containing intravenous fluids are discontinued.

Initial insulin therapy should be conservative (NPH or lente insulin at 0.25 U/kg once daily); subsequent adjustments should be based on clinical response and on serial blood glucose and serum fructosamine measurements. The need for insulin therapy

---

**Box 52-8**

## Medical Therapy for Hypoglycemic Seizures Caused by an Insulin-Secreting β-Cell Tumor

### SEIZURES AT HOME

Step 1. Rub or pour sugar solution on pet's gums.
Step 2. Once pet is sternal, feed a small meal.
Step 3. Call the veterinarian.

### SEIZURES IN HOSPITAL

Step 1. Administer 1-5 ml of 50% dextrose IV *slowly* over 10 min.
Step 2. Once animal is sternal, feed a small meal.
Step 3. Initiate long-term medical therapy (see Box 52-9).

### INTRACTABLE SEIZURES IN HOSPITAL

Step 1. Administer 2.5% to 5% dextrose in water IV at 1.5-2 times maintenance fluid rate.
Step 2. Add 0.5-1 mg of dexamethasone per kilogram to IV fluids and administer over 6 hr; repeat q12–24h, as necessary.
Step 3. Administer glucagon IV by constant rate infusion at an initial dose of 5-10 ng/kg/min.
Step 4. Administer somatostatin analog (Octreotide), 20-40 μg SC q8-12h.
Step 5. If previous steps fail, anesthetize animal with pentobarbital for 4-8 hr while continuing above therapy; consider surgery to debulk functional tumor.

---

*IV,* Intravenously; *SC,* subcutaneously.

is usually transient (a few days to several months); rarely, a dog will remain diabetic for >1 year.

Dogs that remain hypoglycemic after surgery likely have functional metastases. Medical therapy should be initiated in such dogs. During the initial 48 to 72 hours after surgery, intravenous dextrose should be continued. Additional therapy may be needed if hypoglycemic seizures occur (see Box 52-8).

***Medical treatment for chronic hypoglycemia.*** The goals of long-term therapy are simply to reduce the frequency and severity of clinical signs and avoid an acute hypoglycemic crisis, not to reestablish euglycemia. Medical management is outlined in Box 52-9 and discussed in the text.

### Prognosis

The long-term prognosis is guarded to poor. Survival time is dependent, in part, on the willingness of the owner to treat the disease. A median survival time after diagnosis of only 74 days (range, 8 to 508 days) is reported for dogs treated medically, compared with 381 days (range, 20 to 1758 days) in dogs that initially underwent surgery.

---

**Box 52-9**

### Long-Term Medical Therapy for Dogs with β-Cell Neoplasia

#### STANDARD TREATMENTS

1. Dietary therapy
   a. Feed canned or dry food in three to six small meals daily
   b. Avoid foods that contain monosaccharides, disaccharides, or propylene glycol
   c. Limit exercise
2. Glucocorticoid therapy
   a. Prednisone, 0.5 mg/kg PO divided q12h initially
   b. Gradually increase dose and frequency of administration as needed
   c. Goal is to control signs, not to reestablish euglycemia
   d. Consider alternative treatments if signs of iatrogenic hypercortisolism become severe or glucocorticoids become ineffective

#### ADDITIONAL TREATMENTS

1. Diazoxide therapy
   a. Continue standard treatment; reduce glucocorticoid dose to minimize adverse signs
   b. Diazoxide, 5 mg/kg q12h initially
   c. Gradually increase dose as needed, not to exceed 60 mg/kg/day
   d. Goal is to control clinical signs, not to reestablish euglycemia
2. Somatostatin therapy
   a. Continue standard treatment; reduce glucocorticoid dose to minimize adverse signs
   b. Octreotide, 10-40 g/dog SC q8-12h
3. Streptozotocin therapy
   a. Continue standard treatment; reduce glucocorticoid dose to minimize adverse signs
   b. 0.9% saline diuresis for 3 hr, then streptozotocin, 500 mg/m$^2$, in 0.9% saline and administered IV over 2 hr, then 0.9% saline diuresis for 2 more hours
   c. Administer antiemetics immediately after streptozotocin administration to minimize vomiting
   d. Repeat treatment every 3 wk until hypoglycemia resolves or adverse reactions develop (e.g., pancreatitis, renal failure)

*IV,* Intravenously; *PO,* orally; *SC,* subcutaneously.

The ability of surgery to alter the prognosis depends on the stage of the disease, especially the extent of metastases. Of the dogs that undergo surgery, 10% to 15% die or are euthanized at the time, or within 1 month, of surgery because of severe metastatic disease, uncontrollable postoperative hypoglycemia, or complications related to pancreatitis. Another 20% to 25% of dogs die or are euthanized within 6 months of surgery because of severe metastatic disease and recurrence of clinical hypoglycemia. The remaining 60% to 70% live >6 months postoperatively, many >1 year, before uncontrollable hypoglycemia results in death or euthanasia. Additional surgery to debulk metastatic sites may improve responsiveness to medical therapy and prolong survival time in some dogs.

## GASTRINOMA: ZOLLINGER-ELLISON SYNDROME (TEXT PP 775-776)

Gastrinoma is a malignant, gastrin-secreting pancreatic tumor. Hypergastrinemia induces excessive gastric secretion of hydrochloric acid, which causes esophageal, gastric, and duodenal ulcers and disrupts intestinal digestive and absorptive functions.

### Clinical features

The most consistent clinical signs are vomiting, weight loss, anorexia, lethargy, depression, and diarrhea. Other possible signs include hematemesis, hematochezia, melena, inappetence, PD, and abdominal pain. Physical examination findings can vary from relatively unremarkable to extremely severe. Animals with gastrinoma can be lethargic, thin or emaciated, febrile, dehydrated, and in shock. Mucous membranes can be pale as a result of bleeding ulcers. Compensatory tachycardia and abdominal tenderness also can be found.

### Diagnosis

Gastrinoma should be included among the differential diagnoses for any dog or cat presented for melena or hematemesis or in which severe gastric and duodenal ulceration is identified (by gastroscopy or radiography). The probability of gastrinoma increases if a pancreatic mass is identified on ultrasound, the dog or cat is unresponsive to medical therapy directed at GI inflammation and ulceration, or clinical signs and ulceration recur after discontinuation of antiulcer therapy. Definitive diagnosis requires histologic and immunocytochemical evaluation of the pancreatic mass excised at surgery.

### Treatment

Treatment involves surgical excision of the tumor and control of gastric acid hypersecretion. GI ulceration can usually be managed successfully with histamine-2 receptor antagonists (e.g., ranitidine, famotidine), proton pump inhibitors (e.g., omeprazole), GI protectants (e.g., sucralfate), or prostaglandin E1 analogs (e.g., misoprostol). (See Chapter 30 for more information on these drugs.)

# 53

# Disorders
of the Adrenal Gland

## (Text pp 778-815)

### HYPERADRENOCORTICISM IN DOGS (TEXT PP 778-798)

#### Etiology

Hyperadrenocorticism (Cushing's disease) is classified as pituitary dependent, adrenocortical dependent, or iatrogenic.

*Pituitary-dependent hyperadrenocorticism.* Pituitary-dependent hyperadrenocorticism (PDH) accounts for 80% to 85% of all cases of spontaneous hyperadrenocorticism and is usually caused by a functional adrenocorticotropic hormone (ACTH)–secreting pituitary tumor. Tumor types include adenoma of the pars distalis (most common), adenoma of the pars intermedia (less common), and functional pituitary carcinoma (uncommon). The primary derangement with PDH is excessive ACTH secretion, which causes bilateral adrenocortical hyperplasia and excess cortisol secretion.

*Adrenocortical tumors.* Adrenocortical tumors (ATs) are responsible for 15% to 20% of spontaneous hyperadrenocorticism cases. Adenoma and carcinoma occur with equal frequency; carcinomas tend to be larger and can invade local structures (e.g., kidney, liver, vena cava) or metastasize to the liver and lung. Bilateral tumors are rare. ATs randomly secrete excessive cortisol (independent of pituitary control), which results in cortical atrophy of the uninvolved adrenal and atrophy of normal cells in the involved gland.

*Iatrogenic hyperadrenocorticism.* Excessive administration of glucocorticoids, including topical preparations, can lead to hyperadrenocorticism. Results of ACTH stimulation tests are consistent with spontaneous hypoadrenocorticism, despite clinical signs of hyperadrenocorticism.

#### Clinical features

Hyperadrenocorticism typically develops in dogs 6 years of age (median, 10 years), but it has been documented in dogs as young as 1 year old. PDH and ATs are diagnosed in numerous breeds. All Poodle breeds, Dachshunds, various Terrier breeds, German Shepherd Dogs, Beagles, and Labrador Retrievers are commonly represented; Boxers and Boston Terriers are at increased risk for PDH. Whereas PDH tends to occur more frequently in small dogs (<20 kg), approximately 50% of dogs with functional ATs weigh >20 kg.

*Clinical signs.* Clinical signs are variable. The most common signs are polyuria (PU) and polydipsia (PD), polyphagia, panting, abdominal enlargement, endocrine alopecia, mild muscle weakness, and lethargy (Table 53-1). Some dogs are presented with isolated PU and PD, bilaterally symmetric endocrine alopecia, or, less commonly, panting. The more signs and physical findings present, the greater the index of suspicion for hyperadrenocorticism.

*Concurrent diabetes.* Hyperadrenocorticism causes insulin resistance and can lead to diabetes mellitus; clinical signs (other than PU and PD) and physical findings

**Table 53-1**

## Clinical Signs and Physical Examination Findings in Dogs with Hyperadrenocorticism

| Clinical signs | Physical examination findings |
|---|---|
| Polyuria, polydipsia | Endocrine alopecia |
| Polyphagia | Epidermal atrophy |
| Abdominal enlargement | Comedones |
| Endocrine alopecia | Calcinosis cutis |
| Weakness | Hyperpigmentation |
| Lethargy | Abdominal enlargement |
| Calcinosis cutis | Hepatomegaly |
| Hyperpigmentation | Muscle wasting |
| Neurologic signs (PMA) | Bruising |
|   Stupor | Testicular atrophy |
|   Ataxia | Neurologic signs (PMA) |
|   Circling | Dyspnea (pulmonary thromboemboli) |
|   Aimless wandering | |
|   Pacing | |
|   Behavioral alterations | |
| Respiratory distress-dyspnea (pulmonary thromboemboli) | |

*PMA,* Pituitary macroadenoma.

suggestive of hyperadrenocorticism are often lacking in dogs with concurrent diabetes. Clinical suspicion develops after evaluation of routine blood work or when resistance to insulin therapy is identified (see Chapter 52).

*Pituitary macrotumor syndrome.* In dogs with PDH, neurologic signs can develop as a result of growth and expansion of the pituitary tumor. Signs typically develop >6 months after PDH has been diagnosed and medical therapy initiated. In 10% to 20% of dogs, neurologic signs are present at the time of or shortly after diagnosis and may constitute the primary clinical manifestation of the disease. The most common sign is stupor; other neurologic signs are listed in Table 53-1. Severe compression of the hypothalamus can cause autonomic dysfunction, leading to adipsia, loss of thermoregulation, erratic heart rate, and inability to be roused from a sleeplike state. Definitive diagnosis requires computed tomography (CT) or magnetic resonance imaging (MRI).

### Medical complications

Prolonged steroid excess can cause cardiovascular disease (systemic hypertension, congestive heart failure), renal problems (pyelonephritis, cystic calculi, glomerulopathy), pancreatitis, diabetes mellitus, and pulmonary thromboembolism (PTE). The latter is most common in dogs that have recently undergone medical treatment for PDH or adrenalectomy. Common signs of PTE include acute respiratory distress, orthopnea, and, less commonly, a jugular pulse. Diagnosis and management are discussed in Chapter 22. The prognosis is guarded to grave.

### Diagnosis

Thorough evaluation of any dog suspected of having hyperadrenocorticism should include complete blood count (CBC), serum biochemistry panel, urinalysis with bacterial culture, and, if available, abdominal ultrasonography.

*Clinical pathology.* Stress leukogram and mild erythrocytosis are common. Biochemical derangements can include increased serum activities of alkaline phosphatase (SAP) and alanine aminotransferase (ALT), hypercholesterolemia, lipemia, and hyperglycemia. Serum bilirubin is normal in dogs with hyperadrenocorticism and steroid hepatopathy. Preprandial and postprandial serum bile acids may be mildly increased.

Increases in SAP (>150 U/L, sometimes >1000 U/L) and cholesterol are the most reliable indicators of hyperadrenocorticism. However, no correlation exists between the magnitude of the increase in SAP and the severity of hyperadrenocorticism, magnitude of hepatocellular injury, response to therapy, or prognosis. The SAP activity is normal in some affected dogs. Serum activity of the steroid-induced isoenzyme of SAP (SIAP), while not specific for hyperadrenocorticism, is a sensitive test for the disease, in that absence of SIAP in the serum helps rule out hyperadrenocorticism.

*Urinalysis.* Common abnormalities include hyposthenuria or isosthenuria, proteinuria, and evidence of urinary tract infection. Urine specific gravity (SG) is typically <1.015 when the dog has free access to water. Water-deprived hyperadrenal dogs can concentrate urine, although concentrating ability usually remains less than normal. Glycosuria may be found with concurrent diabetes mellitus. The urine protein/creatinine (Cr) ratio is usually <4, although values >8 may be found.

Hyposthenuria and the antiinflammatory effects of glucocorticoids commonly interfere with the identification of bacteria or inflammatory cells in the urine. When hyperadrenocorticism is suspected, cystocentesis with bacterial culture and antibiotic sensitivity testing is recommended, regardless of the findings on urinalysis.

### Diagnostic imaging

*Radiography.* The most consistent radiographic findings are enhanced abdominal contrast (increased abdominal fat), hepatomegaly, enlarged urinary bladder (PU), and dystrophic calcification of the trachea, bronchi, and occasionally the skin and abdominal blood vessels. The most important, but least common, finding is a soft-tissue mass or calcification in the area of an adrenal gland. The larger the mass, the more likely the tumor is a carcinoma. Approximately 50% of ATs (both adenomas and carcinomas) are calcified. Metastasis of an adrenocortical carcinoma to the pulmonary parenchyma is occasionally evident on thoracic radiographs.

*Ultrasonography.* Abdominal ultrasonography is used to examine the abdomen for abnormalities (e.g., cystic calculi, masses), evaluate the size and shape of the adrenal glands, and screen for metastases. Bilaterally normal-sized or large adrenals (maximum width >0.75 cm) in a dog with hyperadrenocorticism is strong evidence for adrenal hyperplasia caused by PDH. Surrounding blood vessels and organs are not invaded in these patients. Other specific features are described in the text.

ATs are typically identified as adrenal masses that distort the contour of the gland to a greater or lesser degree, depending on the size of the mass (which can range from 1.5 cm to >8 cm in width). With large adrenal masses (>3 cm in width), invasion into surrounding blood vessels and compression of adjacent organs may be seen. These findings suggest adrenocortical carcinoma; generally, the larger the mass, the more likely that it is a carcinoma. With ATs, the contralateral unaffected adrenal is small or undetectable (maximum width typically <0.3 cm).

Bilateral adrenomegaly with the appearance of multiple nodules of varying size is suggestive of macronodular hyperplasia, which may represent an anatomic variant of PDH. Finding normal-sized adrenal glands in a dog with hyperadrenocorticism is most consistent with PDH. Failure to identify either adrenal is inconclusive, and the examination should be repeated.

*CT and MRI.* CT and MRI can be used to assess the size and symmetry of the adrenal glands, but the primary indication is to confirm the presence of a visible pituitary tumor in a dog with clinical signs suggestive of macrotumor, particularly if the owner is willing to consider radiation therapy should a pituitary mass be found. MRI is superior to CT for detection of small pituitary tumors, detection of associated abnormalities (e.g., edema, cysts, hemorrhage, necrosis), and imaging of the adrenal glands.

*Evaluating the pituitary-adrenocortical axis.* Once a diagnosis of hyperadrenocorticism is established, discriminatory testing may be warranted to identify the cause (PDH versus AT), identify the most appropriate therapy, and more accurately determine the prognosis. The need to perform discriminatory testing depends, in part, on the abdominal ultrasound findings and on the owner's willingness to consider adrenalectomy should an AT be found.

Discriminatory tests include low-dose dexamethasone suppression (LDDS), high-dose dexamethasone suppression (HDDS), and baseline plasma endogenous ACTH concentration. These tests are outlined in Table 53-2 and discussed in detail in the text. Baseline morning plasma cortisol level, by itself, is of no diagnostic value. Determination of the urine cortisol/Cr ratio rules out hyperadrenocorticism if the ratio is normal, but an increased ratio does not establish the diagnosis.

The tests I use most commonly to diagnose hyperadrenocorticism and differentiate PDH from AT are the ACTH stimulation test, LDDS test, and abdominal ultrasonography.

### Medical treatment with mitotane

Chemotherapy using mitotane (o,p'DDD; Lysodren) is the most commonly used treatment for PDH. Mitotane is also a viable alternative to adrenalectomy for treatment of AT, especially in aged dogs or dogs with worrisome concurrent disease. Mitotane has two treatment options: (1) the traditional approach, in which the goal is to control the hyperadrenal state without causing clinical signs of hypoadrenocorticism, and (2) medical adrenalectomy, in which the goal is to destroy the adrenal cortex (thereby converting hyperadrenocorticism to hypoadrenocorticism).

The traditional approach is preferred initially; medical adrenalectomy is considered only in dogs that fail to respond to the traditional approach or that become unresponsive to mitotane after months or years of therapy. The traditional approach has two phases: induction (to gain control of the disorder) and maintenance (lifelong therapy to prevent recurrence of clinical signs).

*Induction protocol.* Before induction therapy is begun, the owner should determine the dog's water consumption at home for several 24-hour periods. Once daily water consumption is established, mitotane is begun at 40 to 50 mg/kg/day (25 to 35 mg/kg for dogs without PD or with concurrent diabetes mellitus), divided into two doses. Mitotane is more effective when each dose is ground up, mixed with a small amount of vegetable oil, and given with food.

*Glucocorticoids.* Low doses of glucocorticoids (e.g., prednisone at 0.25 mg/kg orally [PO] q24h) can be administered during induction therapy. However, glucocorticoid therapy can mask the clinical indications that hyperadrenocorticism is being controlled (e.g., resolution of polyphagia and PU and PD) and mask the signs of mitotane overdose (Box 53-1).

Regardless of whether glucocorticoids are used during induction therapy, *they should always be dispensed* before mitotane therapy is begun, so that the owner has them on hand should adverse reactions to mitotane develop.

*Monitoring therapy.* The induction phase is typically performed with the dog at home. Owner awareness of the dog's activity, mental awareness, appetite, water consumption, and overall well-being is essential for avoidance of severe hypoadrenocorticism during induction. The owner is instructed to stop mitotane therapy and contact the veterinarian if lethargy, inappetence, vomiting, weakness, decreased water intake, or any other change in the dog is observed. The owner should be called every day to check on the dog's health and possible development of signs related to hypocortisolism.

The induction phase is complete when reduction in appetite is noted or daily water consumption decreases to 80 ml/kg. Confirmation is based on results of an ACTH stimulation test performed 5 to 7 days after therapy is begun. In dogs that have responded clinically, therapy is withheld until results of the ACTH stimulation test are evaluated. Dogs that have not yet responded clinically should have an ACTH stimulation test but should also remain on daily mitotane therapy pending the results.

The goal is relative hypoadrenocorticism (post-ACTH plasma cortisol of 2 to 5 µg/dl). Daily mitotane therapy and weekly ACTH stimulation tests should be continued until post-ACTH cortisol falls within the desired range or signs of hypocortisolism develop. If the post-ACTH cortisol is <2 µg/dl and the dog appears healthy, maintenance therapy is initiated (but at 25 mg/kg). Mitotane is discontinued and prednisone initiated if the dog is systemically ill.

Table 53-2

**Diagnostic Tests to Assess the Pituitary-Adrenocortical Axis in Dogs**

| Test | Purpose | Protocol | Results and Interpretation | |
|---|---|---|---|---|
| Endogenous ACTH | Differentiate PDH from AT | Plasma sample obtained between 8 and 10 AM; special handling required | <10 pg/ml | Nondiagnostic |
| | | | 10-45 pg/ml | AT |
| | | | >45 pg/ml | PDH |
| ACTH stimulation | Diagnose Cushing's syndrome | 2.2 U of ACTH gel* per kilogram IM; plasma before and 2 hr after ACTH administration | *Post-ACTH cortisol:* | |
| | | | >24 µg/dl | Strongly suggestive† |
| | | or | 19-24 µg/dl | Suggestive‡ |
| | | 0.25 mg of synthetic ACTH* per dog IM; plasma before and 1 hr after ACTH administration | 8-18 µg/dl | Normal |
| | | | <8 µg/dl | Iatrogenic Cushing's syndrome |
| Low-dose dexamethasone suppression test | Diagnose Cushing's syndrome and differentiate PDH from AT | 0.01 mg of dexamethasone per kilogram IV; plasma before and 4 and 8 hr after dexamethasone administration | *Postdexamethasone cortisol:* | |
| | | | *4 hr after:* | *8 hr after:* |
| | | | — | <1.4 µg/dl    Normal |
| | | | <1.4 µg/dl or <50% of "before" value | >1.4 µg/dl    PDH |
| | | | — | >1.4 µg/dl and    PDH <50% of "before" value |
| | | | >1.4 µg/dl | >1.4 µg/dl    PDH or AT |

| Test | Purpose | Protocol | Cortisol concentration: After dexamethasone | After ACTH | Interpretation |
|---|---|---|---|---|---|
| Combination dexamethasone suppression and ACTH stimulation test | Diagnose Cushing's syndrome | 0.1 mg of dexamethasone per kilogram IV; plasma before and 2 hr after dexamethasone; then 2.2 U of ACTH gel per kilogram or 0.25 mg of synthetic ACTH per dog IM; plasma 1 and 2 hr (ACTH gel) or 30 and 60 min (synthetic ACTH) after ACTH | <1.5 µg/dl | 8-18 µg/dl | Normal |
| | | | >1.5 µg/dl | 8-20 µg/dl | Suggestive |
| | | | >1.5 µg/dl | >20 µg/dl | Strongly suggestive |
| | | | <1.5 µg/dl | >20 µg/dl | Suggestive |
| | | | <1.5 µg/dl | <8 µg/dl | Iatrogenic Cushing's syndrome |

| Test | Purpose | Protocol | Postdexamethasone cortisol: | | Interpretation |
|---|---|---|---|---|---|
| High-dose dexamethasone suppression test | Differentiate PDH from AT | 0.1 mg of dexamethasone/kg IV; plasma before and 8 hr after dexamethasone | <50% of "before" value | | PDH |
| | | | <1.4 µg/dl | | PDH |
| | | | >50% of "before" value | | PDH or AT |

*ACTH gel: Cortigel, Savage Laboratories; synthetic ACTH: Cortrosyn, Organon Pharmaceuticals.

†Strongly suggestive of hyperadrenocorticism.

‡Suggestive of hyperadrenocorticism.

AT, Adrenocortical tumor; IM, intramuscularly; IV, intravenously; PDH, pituitary-dependent hyperadrenocorticism.

---

**Box 53-1**

## Adverse Effects of Mitotane in Dogs

**DIRECT EFFECT\***

Lethargy
Inappetence
Vomiting
Neurologic signs
Ataxia
Circling
Stupor
Apparent blindness

**GROWTH OF PMA(?)**

Stupor
Disorientation
Circling
Ataxia
Aimless wandering
Pacing
Behavioral alterations

**SECONDARY TO OVERDOSE\***

Hypocortisolism
    Lethargy
    Anorexia
    Vomiting
    Diarrhea
    Weakness
Hypoaldosteronism (hyperkalemia,
    hyponatremia)
    Lethargy
    Weakness
    Cardiac disturbances
    Hypovolemia
    Hypotension

---

\*Adrenocorticotropic hormone stimulation test, serum electrolyte concentration, response to discontinuation of mitotane, and response to glucocorticoid therapy are used to differentiate these categories of adverse reactions.
*PMA*, Pituitary macroadenoma.

In most dogs clinical signs resolve and a post-ACTH cortisol of <5 μg/dl is achieved within 5 to 10 days of the start of mitotane therapy. A small number of dogs respond in <5 days; an equally small number show minimal improvement after 3 to 4 weeks of therapy.

***Managing concurrent diabetes mellitus.*** Hyperadrenocorticism and diabetes mellitus are common concurrent diseases. For most affected dogs, glycemic control remains poor despite insulin therapy, and good glycemic control generally is not possible until hyperadrenocorticism is controlled. The initial focus should be on treatment of the hyperadrenal state. Insulin therapy is indicated during induction therapy; however, aggressive efforts to maintain the blood glucose below 250 mg/dl should not be attempted. Rather, a conservative dose (0.5 to 1 U/kg) of intermediate-acting insulin (lente or NPH) is administered twice a day to prevent ketoacidosis and severe hyperglycemia (blood glucose >500 mg/dl).

Monitoring induction therapy in these dogs is similar to that described previously, except that water consumption is not reliable in a dog with concurrent diabetes mellitus. Owners are asked to test the dog's urine for glucose, preferably 2 or 3 times each day during induction. Absence of glycosuria is an indication for a 10% to 20% reduction in insulin dose. Mitotane therapy is discontinued and an ACTH stimulation test performed once the urine tests negative for glucose. Critical assessment of glycemic control and adjustments in insulin therapy, if indicated, are initiated once hyperadrenocorticism is controlled and maintenance therapy initiated (see text).

***Maintenance therapy.*** Periodic mitotane administration must be continued to prevent recurrence of clinical signs. The typical weekly maintenance dose is 50 mg/kg PO divided into two or three doses and administered on 2 or 3 days of each week (e.g., Monday and Thursday; Monday, Wednesday, and Friday). Adverse reactions to mitotane are less likely to occur when the weekly dose is divided and given over several days. Subsequent adjustments to the starting dose are based on results of ACTH stimulation tests, performed 3 to 4 weeks after maintenance therapy is initiated and repeated periodically thereafter (see text). The goals are maintenance of post-ACTH cortisol of 2 to 5 μg/dl and an asymptomatic dog.

With time (months to years) the dose and frequency of mitotane usually need to be increased. Periodic ACTH stimulation testing allows the clinician to adjust the mitotane protocol before clinical signs of hyperadrenocorticism recur, thereby avoiding the necessity of another round of induction therapy. Alternative therapies (e.g., medical adrenalectomy using mitotane; ketoconazole; trilostane) should be considered in dogs that become insensitive to mitotane. These therapies are discussed in the text.

***Adverse reactions.*** Adverse reactions to mitotane result from drug sensitivity or excessive administration and subsequent development of glucocorticoid and, if severe, mineralocorticoid deficiency (see Box 53-1). The most common reactions are gastric irritation and vomiting.

If signs of hypocortisolism develop, glucocorticoid therapy is warranted. Clinical improvement is usually seen within hours after administration of prednisone (0.25 to 0.5 mg/kg PO). Glucocorticoid therapy should be continued for 3 to 5 days, then gradually discontinued over the ensuing 1 to 2 weeks. Mitotane therapy should be stopped until the dog is normal without glucocorticoids. The weekly dose of mitotane is reduced when therapy is reinitiated (once the post-ACTH cortisol approaches 2 μg/dl).

Hypoaldosteronism should be considered in any dog with signs of hypocortisolism that does not respond to glucocorticoid therapy. Hyponatremia and hyperkalemia support hypoaldosteronism and are indications for mineralocorticoid therapy.

Neurologic signs caused by mitotane are usually transient (24 to 48 hours) and are more likely to occur in patients that have received the drug for >6 months. The primary differential diagnoses are pituitary macrotumor, hypoadrenocorticism, and thromboembolism. Adjustments in dose or frequency or temporary discontinuation of the drug may alleviate these signs. An alternative mode of therapy should be considered if neurologic signs persist.

### Adrenalectomy

Adrenalectomy is the treatment of choice for AT, unless metastasis or invasion of surrounding organs or blood vessels is identified during the preoperative evaluation, the dog is a poor anesthetic risk, or the probability of PTE is high. Treatment with mitotane or ketoconazole is a viable alternative, especially for aged dogs or those at increased risk for anesthetic, surgical, or postsurgical problems (see text).

Glucocorticoids are not indicated before adrenalectomy and may predispose to worsening hypertension and overhydration and increase the risk for thromboembolism. However, acute hypocortisolism occurs after adrenalectomy, so once the tumor is identified by the surgeon, dexamethasone infusion should be given. Intraoperative and postoperative management are discussed further in the text.

### Radiation therapy

Radiation therapy has successfully reduced tumor size and lessened or eliminated neurologic signs in dogs with pituitary macrotumor syndrome. However, reduction in hormone secretion by the tumor is variable. Mitotane or another form of medical therapy usually is necessary in addition to irradiation.

### Prognosis

The prognosis for dogs with PDH depends on the age and overall health of the dog, and owner commitment to therapy. Mean life span after diagnosis is 30 months. Younger dogs may live considerably longer (4 years). Dogs ultimately die or are euthanized because of complications related to hyperadrenocorticism (e.g., pituitary macrotumor, thromboembolism, infection) or other geriatric disorders.

Average life expectancy for dogs that survive adrenalectomy is 36 months. Dogs with adrenocortical adenoma and nonmetastatic adenocarcinoma (uncommon) have a good prognosis. Dogs with metastatic adenocarcinoma (common) have a poor prognosis, typically succumbing to the disease within 1 year.

Response to radiation can be divided into three equal categories: dogs that fail to respond or that die during radiation treatment (approximately 33%), dogs that show some response and survive for a few months (approximately 33%), and dogs with complete resolution of signs and years of survival (approximately 33%).

## HYPERADRENOCORTICISM IN CATS (TEXT PP 798-804)

Hyperadrenocorticism is uncommon in cats. Many of the clinical features of the disease in cats are the same as those in dogs, described in the preceding section. However, some important differences exist. Most notable are the very strong association with diabetes mellitus; the progressive, relentless weight loss that leads to cachexia; and dermal and epidermal atrophy that leads to extremely fragile, thin, easily torn and ulcerated skin (feline fragile skin syndrome). Establishment of the diagnosis is difficult, and effective medical treatment for hyperadrenocorticism in cats has yet to be identified.

### Etiology

As in dogs, hyperadrenocorticism in cats is classified as PDH, AT, or iatrogenic. Approximately 75% of hyperadrenal cats have PDH, and 25% have AT (equally distributed between adenoma and carcinoma). Iatrogenic hyperadrenocorticism is uncommon in cats; typically it takes months of prednisone administration before clinical signs occur.

### Clinical features

Hyperadrenocorticism is a disease of older (average, 10 years), mixed-breed cats. Carbohydrate intolerance is present in all cats with hyperadrenocorticism, and insulin-resistant diabetes mellitus is also present in many. The most common initial signs of feline hyperadrenocorticism (PU and PD, polyphagia) are more likely caused by diabetes. Other signs and physical findings are not as common and tend to be very subtle in the early stages (Box 53-2).

### Diagnosis

Hyperadrenocorticism is an elusive diagnosis in cats, in part because the clinical signs are often vague and easily attributed to concurrent diabetes mellitus until late in the disease and because none of the diagnostic tests used to establish the diagnosis in dogs are reliable in cats. Ultimately, the diagnosis is based on clinical signs, physical

---

**Box 53-2**

### Clinical Features of Hyperadrenocorticism in Cats

**CLINICAL SIGNS**
Polyuria, polydipsia*
Polyphagia*
Patchy alopecia*
Unkempt haircoat*
Symmetric alopecia
Lethargy
Thin, easily torn skin (feline fragile skin syndrome)*
Weight loss*
Drooping of pinna

**ADDITIONAL PHYSICAL FINDINGS**
"Pot-bellied" appearance*
Hepatomegaly*
Muscle wasting*
Skin infections

---

*Common.

examination findings, abdominal ultrasound, clinicopathologic abnormalities, tests of the pituitary-adrenocortical axis, and the clinician's index of suspicion for the disease.

In the early stages, hyperadrenocorticism may be suspected when causes of insulin ineffectiveness in a cat with diabetes mellitus are ruled out (see Table 52-7). With time, hyperadrenocorticism becomes more apparent as affected cats become progressively more debilitated despite administration of high doses of potent insulin and when cachexia and fragile skin syndrome manifest. (The primary differential diagnosis for insulin resistance, cachexia, and fragile skin syndrome is hyperprogesteronemia, as occurs with progesterone-secreting adrenal tumors.)

*Clinical pathology.* The most common abnormalities are hyperglycemia, glycosuria, hypercholesterolemia, and a mild increase in ALT activity. These alterations indicate concurrent, poorly regulated diabetes mellitus. Abnormalities often found in dogs, such as a stress leukogram, increased SAP activity, isosthenuric or hyposthenuric urine, proteinuria, pyuria, and bacteriuria, are uncommon in cats.

*Evaluating the pituitary-adrenocortical axis.* The tests used to diagnose hyperadrenocorticism in cats and dogs are similar, but some important differences exist in the testing protocol and interpretation of results (Table 53-3). I rely most heavily on the urine cortisol/Cr ratio, dexamethasone suppression test, and abdominal ultrasonography. Normal results of the ACTH stimulation test are common in cats with hyperadrenocorticism.

*Urine cortisol/Cr ratio.* The urine cortisol/Cr ratio may be used as the initial screening test for hyperadrenocorticism in cats. A normal urine cortisol/Cr ratio ($<1.5 \times 10^{-5}$) is a strong finding *against* the diagnosis; an increased ratio does not by itself establish the diagnosis, but it supports performance of the dexamethasone suppression test.

*Diagnostic imaging.* Abdominal ultrasound is used to identify adrenal masses. Generally, the adrenal glands are difficult to identify in cats. Failure to identify the adrenals is an inconclusive finding but is more consistent with normal adrenals than with PDH. Adrenomegaly should be suspected when the maximum width is >0.5 cm; a maximum width >0.8 cm is strongly suggestive of adrenomegaly. Easily visualized, bilaterally large adrenals in a cat with appropriate clinical signs and physical findings and abnormal pituitary-adrenocortical axis tests is strong evidence for adrenal hyperplasia caused by PDH.

CT and MRI can be used to check for pituitary macroadenoma. The primary differential diagnosis is acromegaly (see Chapter 49). Hyperadrenocorticism and acromegaly both cause insulin-resistant diabetes mellitus; however, additional clinical signs differ dramatically between these two disorders.

### Treatment

Treatment of hyperadrenocorticism in cats is problematic. Adrenalectomy is the treatment of choice for cats with an adrenal mass. Unfortunately, a reliable medical treatment for PDH has not been identified in cats. The most viable option is bilateral adrenalectomy. Medical treatment with metyrapone or aminoglutethemide (see later) is usually necessary for 4 to 6 weeks before surgery to reverse the catabolic state, improve skin fragility and wound healing, and decrease the potential for perioperative complications. Adrenalectomy and postoperative management are discussed in the text. Insulin therapy can be discontinued in approximately 50% of cats once hyperadrenocorticism is eliminated, and diabetes is easier to control using less insulin in the remaining cats.

*Medical therapy.* Medical therapy can be tried if the owner is unwilling to consider surgery or if metastatic lesions are identified. However, consistently effective medical therapy remains to be identified. Metyrapone (Metopirone, 65 mg/kg PO q12h) has been successful in controlling clinical signs of hyperadrenocorticism in a few cats, but signs may recur as early as 1 month after the start of therapy. Metyrapone can be useful in stabilizing the cat's condition before adrenalectomy; however, availability can be a problem, and the drug causes gastrointestinal (GI) problems (vomiting, diarrhea) in some cats.

**Table 53-3**

## Diagnostic Tests to Assess the Pituitary-Adrenocortical Axis in Cats

| Test | Purpose | Protocol | Results | Interpretation |
|---|---|---|---|---|
| Endogenous ACTH | Identify PDH | Plasma sample obtained between 8 and 10 AM; special handling required | <45 pg/ml<br>>45 pg/ml | Nondiagnostic<br>PDH |
| ACTH stimulation | Diagnose Cushing's syndrome | 2.2 U of ACTH gel* per kilogram IM; plasma before and 1 and 2 hr after ACTH administration<br>or<br>0.125 mg of synthetic ACTH* per cat IM; plasma before and 30 and 60 min after ACTH administration | *Post-ACTH cortisol concentration:*<br>>15 µg/dl<br>12-15 µg/dl<br>6-12 µg/dl<br><6 µg/dl | Strongly suggestive[†]<br>Suggestive[‡]<br>Normal<br>Iatrogenic Cushing's syndrome |
| Dexamethasone suppression test | Diagnose Cushing's syndrome | 0.1 mg of dexamethasone per kilogram IV; plasma before and 4, 6, and 8 hr after dexamethasone administration | *8 hr postdexamethasone:*<br><1 µg/dl<br>1-1.4 µg/dl<br>>1.4 µg/dl and 4 or 6 hr <1.4 µg/dl<br>>1.4 µg/dl and 4 and 6 hr<br>>1.4 µg/dl | Normal<br>Nondiagnostic<br>Suggestive<br><br>Strongly suggestive |

*ACTH gel: Cortigel, Savage Laboratories; Synthetic ACTH: Cortrosyn, Organon Pharmaceuticals.

[†]Strongly suggestive of hyperadrenocorticism.

[‡]Suggestive of hyperadrenocorticism.

*ACTH,* Adrenocorticotropic hormone; *IM,* intramuscularly; *IV,* intravenously; *PDH,* pituitary-dependent hyperadrenocorticism.

Aminoglutethimide (Cytadren, 30 mg/cat PO q12h) has been successful in controlling clinical signs of hyperadrenocorticism and hyperprogesteronemia in cats with progesterone-secreting tumors. It may also be useful in stabilizing the cat's condition before adrenalectomy and appears to maintain its efficacy for a longer period (months) than metyrapone.

Cobalt irradiation can be tried in cats with pituitary macrotumor, although signs of hypercortisolemia may persist despite shrinkage of the tumor.

### Prognosis

The prognosis in cats is guarded to poor. Unilateral (AT) or bilateral (PDH) adrenalectomy has the potential for excellent success; however, outcome depends on correction of the debilitated state and skin fragility before surgery, expertise of the surgeon, avoidance of perioperative complications, and owner commitment to managing the iatrogenic adrenal insufficiency after bilateral adrenalectomy. Periodic evaluation of serum electrolytes and review of the treatment protocol are important, as an Addisonian crisis can occur months after surgery.

## HYPOADRENOCORTICISM (TEXT PP 804-809)

### Etiology

Adrenocortical insufficiency can be primary or secondary.

*Primary adrenocortical insufficiency.* Primary adrenocortical insufficiency is the more common form of hypoadrenocorticism. It involves a deficiency of both mineralocorticoid and glucocorticoid secretion. Most cases are classified as idiopathic, although immune-mediated adrenocortical destruction is a likely cause. Bilateral destruction of the adrenal cortex by neoplasia (e.g., lymphoma), granulomatous disease, or arterial thrombosis can also cause primary adrenocortical insufficiency. The destruction is progressive, although variable in rate, ultimately leading to complete loss of adrenocortical function. A partial deficiency syndrome may occur initially, with signs manifested only during times of stress (e.g., boarding, travel, surgery).

*Secondary adrenocortical insufficiency.* Secondary adrenocortical insufficiency involves only a deficiency of glucocorticoid secretion. Destructive lesions (e.g., neoplasia, inflammation) in the pituitary gland or hypothalamus and chronic administration of exogenous glucocorticoids or megestrol acetate (cats) are the most common causes.

### Clinical features

Hypoadrenocorticism is typically a disease of young to middle-aged (mean, 4 years; range, 2 months to 12 years) female dogs. No significant breed predilection exists, although genetics probably play a role in Standard Poodles and Portuguese Water Spaniels. The disease is rare in cats. There exists no apparent gender predisposition in cats, but young to middle-aged cats (average, 6 years) are most often affected.

*Clinical signs and physical findings.* The most common clinical manifestations are related to mental status and GI function; they include lethargy, anorexia, vomiting, weight loss, and weakness. Additional findings may include dehydration, bradycardia, weak femoral pulses, and abdominal pain. PU and PD, diarrhea, and shivering are occasionally reported.

*Addisonian crisis.* If hyponatremia and hyperkalemia are severe, the resulting hypovolemia, prerenal azotemia, and cardiac arrhythmias may result in an Addisonian crisis. In severe cases the patient may be presented in shock and moribund. Addisonian crisis must be differentiated from other life-threatening disorders such as diabetic ketoacidosis, necrotizing pancreatitis, and septic peritonitis.

### Diagnosis

Hypoadrenocorticism is often tentatively diagnosed on the basis of history, physical findings, clinical pathology, and, for primary adrenal insufficiency, characteristic electrolyte abnormalities.

*Clinical pathology.* Abnormalities that may be identified on CBC, serum biochemistry panel, and urinalysis are listed in Box 53-3. Hyperkalemia, hyponatremia, and hypochloremia are the classic electrolyte alterations. Serum sodium ranges from normal

---

**Box 53-3**

### Clinicopathologic Abnormalities Associated with Primary Hypoadrenocorticism in Dogs and Cats

**HEMOGRAM**

Nonregenerative anemia
± Neutrophilic leukocytosis
± Mild neutropenia
± Eosinophilia
± Lymphocytosis

**BIOCHEMISTRY PANEL**

Hyperkalemia
Hyponatremia
Hypochloremia
Prerenal azotemia
Hyperphosphatemia
± Hypercalcemia
± Hypoglycemia
Metabolic acidosis (low total $CO_2$, $HCO_3$)

**URINALYSIS**

Isosthenuria to hypersthenuria

---

*$CO_2$,* Carbon dioxide; *$HCO_3$,* bicarbonate.

---

to 105 mEq/L, and serum potassium ranges from normal to >10 mEq/L. The sodium/potassium ratio often is <27 and may be <20 in animals with primary adrenal insufficiency (normal is between 27:1 and 40:1).

However, normal serum electrolyte concentrations do not rule out adrenal insufficiency, as electrolyte abnormalities may not be evident in the early stages of primary insufficiency and do not develop with secondary adrenal insufficiency caused by pituitary failure. Furthermore, various hepatic, GI, and urinary disorders can cause similar alterations in serum electrolytes (see Chapter 55).

*Differentiating from acute renal failure.* Most challenging is differentiation between acute renal failure and primary adrenal insufficiency. Compensatory increases in urine SG (>1.030) aid differentiation. However, many hypoadrenal animals have impaired ability to concentrate urine; some have urine SGs in the isosthenuric range (1.007 to 1.015). Therefore differentiation of these two disorders relies on testing of the pituitary-adrenocortical axis and response to initial fluid and other supportive therapy.

*Electrocardiography.* Hyperkalemia causes characteristic alterations on the electrocardiogram (ECG; see Table 55-3). The severity of the ECG abnormalities correlates with the severity of the hyperkalemia. Therefore the ECG can be used to identify and estimate the severity of hyperkalemia and to monitor changes in serum potassium during therapy.

*Diagnostic imaging.* Abdominal ultrasound may reveal small adrenal glands, suggesting adrenocortical atrophy. However, finding normal-sized adrenal glands does not rule out hypoadrenocorticism. Rarely, megaesophagus is evident on radiographs.

*ACTH stimulation tests.* Confirmation requires evaluation of an ACTH stimulation test (see Tables 53-2 and 53-3). Baseline plasma cortisol and urine cortisol/Cr ratios are unreliable for confirming the diagnosis. One major diagnostic criterion is abnormally decreased post-ACTH plasma cortisol (<2 μg/dl). Normal plasma cortisol (>5 μg/dl) after ACTH stimulation rules out adrenal insufficiency.

Table 53-4

### Differentiation of Primary versus Secondary Hypoadrenocorticism

|  | Primary hypoadrenocorticism | Secondary hypoadrenocorticism |
|---|---|---|
| Serum electrolytes | Hyperkalemia Hyponatremia | Normal |
| ACTH stimulation test |  |  |
| Post-ACTH cortisol | Decreased | Decreased |
| Post-ACTH aldosterone | Decreased | Normal |
| Endogenous ACTH | Increased | Decreased |

*ACTH,* Adrenocorticotropic hormone.

The ACTH stimulation test does not distinguish between primary adrenal insufficiency and secondary insufficiency or adrenocortical destruction caused by mitotane overdose. Differentiation between primary and secondary adrenal insufficiency can be made by periodically measuring serum electrolytes, baseline endogenous ACTH (>100 pg/ml in primary and <45 pg/ml in secondary hypoadrenocorticism), or possibly serum or plasma aldosterone during the ACTH stimulation test (Table 53-4).

**Treatment**

Aggressiveness of therapy depends on the clinical status of the patient and the nature of the insufficiency (glucocorticoid, mineralocorticoid, or both). Many dogs and cats with primary adrenal insufficiency are presented in Addisonian crisis and require immediate, aggressive therapy. In contrast, secondary insufficiency often has a chronic course.

***Addisonian crisis.*** Treatment is directed toward (1) correcting hypotension, hypovolemia, electrolyte imbalances, and metabolic acidosis; (2) improving vascular integrity; and (3) providing an immediate source of glucocorticoids. Recommendations are outlined in Box 53-4 and discussed in the text. Rapid correction of hypovolemia is the first priority.

Most patients show dramatic improvement within 24 to 48 hours of appropriate fluid and glucocorticoid therapy. Over the ensuing 2 to 4 days, a gradual transition from intravenous fluids to oral water and food is undertaken, and maintenance mineralocorticoid and glucocorticoid therapy is initiated. Failure to make this transition smoothly should raise suspicion of insufficient glucocorticoid supplementation, concurrent endocrinopathy (e.g., hypothyroidism), or concurrent illness (especially renal damage).

**Maintenance therapy for primary adrenal insufficiency**

Maintenance therapy is initiated once the patient is stable. Both mineralocorticoids and glucocorticoids are required for maintenance of dogs and cats with primary adrenal insufficiency.

***Desoxycorticosterone pivalate.*** The preferred mineralocorticoid is injectable desoxycorticosterone pivalate (DOCP) at an initial dose of 2.2 mg/kg intramuscularly or subcutaneously every 25 days. Serum electrolytes are measured 12 and 25 days after each injection for the first 2 or 3 treatments, and the dose is adjusted accordingly. If hyponatremia or hyperkalemia is found on day 12, the next dose is increased by approximately 10%. If the day-12 electrolyte profile is normal but the day-25 profile is abnormal, the interval between injections should be decreased by 2 days. Most dogs (and presumably cats) receiving DOCP also require low-dose glucocorticoid therapy (e.g., prednisone, 0.22 mg/kg PO q12h initially).

DOCP is very effective in normalizing serum electrolyte concentrations, and adverse reactions are not observed. However, availability is a problem. The owner can be taught to give the injection subcutaneously at home to avoid the inconvenience and expense of monthly visits to the veterinarian for the injection. However, the

---

**Box 53-4**

### Initial Treatment for Acute Addisonian Crisis

#### FLUID THERAPY
Type: 0.9% saline solution
Rate: 30-80 ml/kg IV initially
Potassium supplementation: contraindicated
Dextrose: 5% dextrose infusion (100 ml, 50% dextrose per liter of intravenous fluids)

#### GLUCOCORTICOID THERAPY
Hydrocortisone hemisuccinate or hydrocortisone phosphate,* 2-4 mg/kg IV, or prednisolone sodium succinate,* 4-20 mg/kg IV, then dexamethasone sodium phosphate, 0.05-0.1 mg/kg in intravenous fluids q12h; alternatively, dexamethasone sodium phosphate, 0.1-2 mg/kg IV, then 0.05-0.1 mg/kg in intravenous fluids q12h[†]

#### MINERALOCORTICOID THERAPY
Desoxycorticosterone pivalate (DOCP; Percoten-V; Novartis), 2.2 mg/kg IM q25d initially

#### BICARBONATE THERAPY
Indicated if $HCO_3^-$ <12 mEq/L or total venous $CO_2^-$ <12 mmol/L or animal is severely ill; mEq $HCO_3^-$ = body weight (kg) × 0.5 × base deficit (mEq/L); if base deficit unknown, use 10 mEq/L; add one quarter of calculated $HCO_3^-$ dose to intravenous fluids and administer over 6 hr; repeat only if plasma $HCO_3^-$ remains <12 mEq/L

---

*Hydrocortisone and prednisolone are assayed by most cortisol radioimmunoassays, interfering with interpretation of the adrenocorticotropic hormone stimulation test result.
[†]Higher doses of glucocorticoids may be required if the dog or cat is in shock.
$HCO_3^-$, Bicarbonate; *IM*, intramuscularly; *IV*, intravenously.

owner should be instructed to bring the patient to the clinic for a complete physical examination and measurement of serum electrolytes every third or fourth treatment. The expense can also be reduced by decreasing the dose and giving DOCP every 21 days.

*Fludrocortisone.* Fludrocortisone acetate (Florinef) is a commonly used mineralocorticoid. The initial dose is 0.02 mg/kg/day PO divided into two doses. Adjustments in dose are based on serum electrolyte concentrations, which are initially assessed every 1 to 2 weeks. Typically, the dose must be increased during the first 6 to 18 months of therapy, which may reflect continuing destruction of the adrenal cortices. After this time the dose usually plateaus and remains relatively stable.

Its use has several major drawbacks: the wide range in dose required to control serum electrolyte concentrations; development of PU and PD and incontinence in some dogs (presumably caused by the potent glucocorticoid activity of the drug); and ineffectiveness (persistent mild hyperkalemia and hyponatremia) in some animals. Addition of hydrocortisone hemisuccinate or salt may help alleviate the electrolyte derangements in animals in which fludrocortisone alone is not completely effective. Alternatively, DOCP could be used.

*Glucocorticoids.* Glucocorticoid supplementation is indicated in all dogs and cats with primary adrenal insufficiency. Prednisone is used at an initial dose of 0.22 mg/kg PO twice a day. Over the ensuing 1 to 2 months it should be gradually reduced to the lowest daily dose that prevents signs of hypocortisolism (e.g., inappetence, vomiting, diarrhea). Approximately 50% of dogs receiving fludrocortisone ultimately do not require glucocorticoid medication, except during times of stress (e.g., boarding). Use of DOCP increases the need for daily glucocorticoid replacement.

The most common reason for persistence of clinical signs despite appropriate treatment is inadequate glucocorticoid supplementation. When healthy and not stressed, dogs and cats with adrenal insufficiency typically require small amounts of prednisone, if any. However, when stressed or ill, these same animals may require large amounts of prednisone (0.5 to 1 mg/kg twice a day). The amount of prednisone required to offset the effects of stress and illness is variable and unpredictable. It is best to err on the high end of the dose range and then gradually decrease the dosage over the ensuing 1 to 2 weeks.

**Secondary adrenal insufficiency.** With one notable exception, therapy for secondary adrenal insufficiency involves administration of glucocorticoids, as described previously. When adrenal insufficiency is caused by overzealous use of glucocorticoids or megestrol acetate, therapy involves gradual reduction in the dose and frequency, and eventual discontinuation of the medication. Periodic measurement of serum electrolytes is advisable, as some dogs and cats believed to have secondary insufficiency ultimately develop primary insufficiency.

### Prognosis
The prognosis for either type of adrenocortical insufficiency usually is excellent with adequate owner education and commitment.

## PHEOCHROMOCYTOMA (TEXT PP 809-812)

### Etiology
Pheochromocytoma is a catecholamine-producing tumor originating in the adrenal medulla. Such tumors are uncommon in dogs and rare in cats. They are usually solitary, slow-growing tumors, ranging in size from <0.5 cm to >10 cm in diameter. Pheochromocytoma is a malignant tumor in dogs. Involvement of the caudal vena cava is common. Mural invasion and/or luminal narrowing of the aorta, renal vessels, adrenal vessels, and hepatic veins can also occur. Sites of metastasis include the liver, lung, regional lymph nodes, spleen, heart, kidney, bone, pancreas, and central nervous system.

### Clinical features
Pheochromocytomas occur most commonly in older dogs and cats (mean age, 11 years). The most common signs are generalized weakness and episodic collapse. Common physical findings involve the respiratory, cardiovascular, and musculoskeletal systems (Table 53-5). Pheochromocytoma may cause periodic clinical signs (e.g., episodes of collapse or tachypnea), and in some cases it results in sudden death. Systemic hypertension and its clinical manifestations tend to be paroxysmal and are not usually evident when the dog is examined.

### Diagnosis
Because clinical signs and physical examination findings are vague, nonspecific, and easily associated with other disorders, pheochromocytoma is often not considered until an adrenal mass is identified with abdominal ultrasound. Diagnosis requires a high index of suspicion on the part of the clinician. A history of acute or episodic collapse, the finding of appropriate respiratory and cardiac abnormalities, and the documentation of systemic hypertension (particularly if paroxysmal) are helpful in establishing a tentative diagnosis. However, failure to document systemic hypertension does not rule out pheochromocytoma.

**Ultrasonography.** Assessment of adrenal size using abdominal ultrasonography is the best screening test. Identification of adrenomegaly (adrenal mass) with a normal-sized contralateral adrenal gland provides further evidence of a pheochromocytoma in a dog or cat with appropriate physical findings. However, a normal-sized adrenal gland does not rule out the diagnosis. Ultrasonography may also provide information regarding metastasis, local invasion, or concurrent problems; pheochromocytoma and adrenocortical tumor can occur simultaneously.

**Other tests.** Many of the clinical signs (e.g., panting, weakness) and blood pressure alterations are similar for hyperadrenocorticism (common) and pheochromocytoma

Table 53-5

## Clinical Signs and Physical Examination Findings Associated with Pheochromocytomas in Dogs

| Clinical signs | Physical examination findings |
|---|---|
| Weakness* | Panting, tachypnea* |
| Collapsing episodes* | Weakness* |
| Lethargy | Tachycardia |
| Inappetence | Cardiac arrhythmias |
| Vomiting | Weak pulses |
| Panting | Pale mucous membranes |
| Polyuria, polydipsia | Muscle wasting |
| Diarrhea | Lethargy |
| Weight loss | Abdominal pain |
| Abdominal distention | Hemorrhage (nasal, surgery site) |
| Rear limb edema | Ascites |
| | Palpable abdominal mass |
| | Rear limb edema |

*Common signs and physical examination findings.

(uncommon), so it is important to rule out hyperadrenocorticism. Measurement of urinary catecholamine concentrations or their metabolites can strengthen the tentative diagnosis of pheochromocytoma. Definitive diagnosis relies on histologic evaluation of the surgically excised adrenal mass.

### Treatment

Medical therapy followed by surgical removal of the tumor is the treatment of choice. Potentially life-threatening complications of surgical excision are common, especially during anesthetic induction and manipulation of the tumor during surgery. Most worrisome are episodes of acute, severe hypertension (systolic pressure >300 mm Hg), severe tachycardia (>250 beats/min), arrhythmias, and hemorrhage. Preoperative α-adrenergic blockade is indicated to minimize the impact of these complications.

*Medical therapy.* Phenoxybenzamine (Dibenzyline) is the drug of choice for α-adrenergic blockade. It is administered for at least 2 weeks before surgery. The initial dose is 0.25 mg/kg PO q12h. Therapy is effective if the clinical signs are reduced and blood pressure is stabilized. An increase in the dose should be considered if clinical signs do not improve after 2 weeks of treatment. (Note: Mitotane is ineffective for treatment of tumors of the adrenal medulla, such as pheochromocytoma.)

### Prognosis

The prognosis depends in part on whether there exists concurrent disease (and the nature of the disease, if present); on the size of the tumor; on whether metastasis or local invasion has occurred; and on whether perioperative complications are avoided. Dogs with surgically excisable tumors have a guarded to good prognosis with appropriate perioperative medical management and care during anesthesia and surgery. Dogs treated medically can live for more than 1 year if the tumor is relatively small (<3 cm), vascular invasion is not present, and medical treatment is effective in minimizing the effects of periodic catecholamine secretion.

## Drugs Used In Endocrine Disorders

| Generic name (trade name) | Purpose | Recommended Dose | |
|---|---|---|---|
| | | Dogs | Cats |
| Acarbose (Precose) | Treat canine diabetes mellitus | 12.5-25 mg/dog PO initially and given with meal | Not applicable |
| Aminoglutethimide (Cytadren) | Treat feline hyperadrenocorticism | Not applicable | 30 mg/cat PO q12h |
| Calcium-injectable and oral preps | Treat hypocalcemia, hypoparathyroidism | See Table 50-4, p 449 | See Table 50-4, p 449 |
| Carbimazole (Neo-Mercazole) | Treat feline hyperthyroidism | Not applicable | 5 mg PO q8h initially |
| Chlorothiazide (Diuril) | Treat central and renal diabetes insipidus | 20-40 mg/kg PO q12h | 20-40 mg/kg PO |
| Chlorpropamide (Diabinese) | Treat partial central diabetes insipidus | 5-20 mg/kg PO q12h | Unknown |
| Desmopressin (DDAVP) | Treat central diabetes insipidus | 1-4 drops of nasal spray in eye q12-48h; 0.1-mg tablets PO q8-12h | 1-4 drops of nasal spray in eye q12-48h; 0.1-mg tablets q8-12h |
| Desoxycorticosterone pivalate (DOCP; Percorten-V) | Treat hypoadrenocorticism | 2.2 mg/kg IM or SC q25d | 2.2 mg/kg IM or SC q25d |
| Dexamethasone sodium phosphate | Treat acute Addisonian crisis | 0.05-0.1 mg/kg in fluids q12h | 0.05-0.1 mg/kg in fluids q12h |
| Diazoxide (Proglycem) | Supportive treatment for β-cell tumor | 5 mg/kg PO q12h initially; increase as needed | Unknown |
| Diethylstilbesterol | Treat estrogen-responsive dermatosis of spayed female dogs | 0.1-1 mg PO q24h 3 wk/mo; once dog responds, 0.1-1 mg q4-7days | Not applicable |
| Doxorubicin (Adriamycin) | Treat canine thyroid neoplasia | 30 mg/m² BSA IV q3-6wk | Not applicable |
| Fludrocortisone acetate (Florinef) | Treat hypoadrenocorticism | 0.01 mg/kg PO q12h initially | 0.05-0.1 mg/cat PO q12h |
| Glipizide (Glucotrol) | Treat feline NIDDM | Not applicable | 2.5-5 mg/cat PO q12h |
| Glucagon USP | Treat hypoglycemia caused by β-cell neoplasia | 5-10 ng/kg/min as continuous intravenous infusion; adjust dose until effective | Unknown |
| Glyburide (Diabeta, Micronase) | Treat feline NIDDM | Not applicable | 0.625-1.25 mg/cat PO q24h |
| Growth hormone—porcine origin | Treat growth hormone–responsive dermatosis; treat pituitary dwarfism | 0.1 U/kg SC three times per week for 4-6 wk | Unknown |

*Continued.*

## Drugs Used In Endocrine Disorders—cont'd

| Generic name (trade name) | Purpose | Recommended Dose Dogs | Recommended Dose Cats |
|---|---|---|---|
| Hydrocortisone sodium succinate (Solu-Cortef) | Treat acute Addisonian crisis | 2-4 mg/kg IV, then administer dexamethasone in intravenous fluids | 2-4 mg/kg IV, then administer dexamethasone in intravenous fluids |
| Insulin | Treat diabetic ketoacidosis; treat diabetes mellitus; supportive treatment for hyperkalemia | See Box 52-7, p 487; See Table 52-2, p 474, and p 473 | See Box 52-7, p 487; See Table 52-2, p 474, and p 481 |
| Ketoconazole (Nizoral) | Treat hyperadrenocorticism | See Table 55-4, p 525 | See Table 55-4, p 525 |
| L-Deprenyl (Eldepryl) | Treat canine hyperadrenocorticism | 10-15 mg/kg PO q12h | 10-15 mg/kg PO q12h |
| Megestrol acetate (Ovaban) | Treat feline endocrine alopecia | 1 mg/kg PO q24h initially | Not applicable |
| Melatonin | Treat congenital adrenal hyperplasia-like syndrome | Not applicable | 2.5-5 mg/cat PO q48h; once cat responds, then q7-14d |
| Metformin (Glucophage) | Treat feline NIDDM | 3-6 mg PO q12-24h | Not applicable |
| Methimazole (Tapazole) | Treat hyperthyroidism | Not applicable | 10-25 mg/cat PO q12-24h |
| | | 2.5 mg/kg PO q12h initially; increase q2-4wk until effective | 2.5 mg/cat PO q24h initially; increase q2-4wk until effective |
| Methyltestosterone | Treat testosterone-responsive dermatosis | 1 mg/kg (max, 30 mg) PO q48h; once dog responds, then q4-7days | Not applicable |
| Metyrapone (Metopirone) | Treat feline hyperadrenocorticism | Not applicable | 65 mg/kg PO q12h |
| Mitotane (o,p'DDD; Lysodren) | Treat canine hyperadrenocorticism | Induction: 12-25 mg/kg PO q12h until effective; Maintenance: 25-50 mg/kg PO once weekly initially | Not applicable |

| Drug | Indication | Dog dose | Cat dose |
|---|---|---|---|
| Phenoxybenzamine (Dibenzyline) | Supportive treatment for pheochromocytoma | 0.25 mg/kg PO q12h initially | Unknown |
| Prednisone | Chronic treatment of hypoadrenocorticism; supportive treatment for β-cell tumor | 0.2-0.5 mg/kg PO q12h initially; 0.25 mg/kg PO q12h initially; increase as needed | 2.5-5 mg/cat PO q12-24h initially; 0.25 mg/kg PO q12h initially; increase as needed |
| Prednisolone sodium succinate (Solu-Delta-Cortef) | Treat acute Addisonian crisis | 4-20 mg/kg IV, then administer dexamethasone in intravenous fluids | 4-20 mg/kg IV, then administer dexamethasone in intravenous fluids |
| Propylthiouracil (PTU) | Treat hyperthyroidism | 50 mg/dog PO q8-12h | 50 mg/cat PO q8-12h |
| Sodium levothyroxine—synthetic $T_4$ | Treat hypothyroidism | 0.02 mg/kg PO q12h initially | 0.05-0.1 mg/cat PO q12-24h |
| Sodium liothyronine—synthetic $T_3$ | Treat hypothyroidism | 4-6 µg/kg PO q8h initially | 25 µg/cat PO q8-12h |
| Somatostatin (Sandostatin, octreotide) | Supportive treatment for β-cell tumor | 10-40 µg/dog SC q8-12h | Unknown |
| Streptozotocin | Treat canine β-cell tumor | 500 mg/m$^2$ BSA IV during saline diuresis q3wk; see Box 52-9 | Not applicable |
| Trilostane (Modrenal) | Treat hyperadrenocorticism | 2-10 mg/kg PO q24h, adjust based on clinical response | 30 mg/cat PO q24h |
| Vitamin D preparations | Treat hypoparathyroidism | See Table 50-5, p 450 | See Table 50-5, p 450 |

BSA, Body surface area; IM, intramuscularly; IV, intravenously; NIDDM, non–insulin-dependent diabetes mellitus; PO, orally; SC, subcutaneously.

# PART VII

# Metabolic and Electrolyte Disorders

RICHARD W. NELSON

DENISE A. ELLIOTT

# 54

# Disorders of Metabolism

## (Text pp 816-827)

### POLYPHAGIA WITH WEIGHT LOSS (TEXT P 816)

The most common cause of polyphagia and weight loss is inadequate caloric intake; other possible causes are listed in Table 54-1. Daily caloric requirements are variable and depend on a number of factors, such as age and amount of physical activity. Average daily requirements for dogs and cats are 60 to 85 kcal of metabolizable energy per kilogram of body weight; requirements for younger animals and smaller breeds of dog are greater. For any size or age, daily caloric requirements may vary by as much as 50% above or below this average.

#### Investigating the cause

Endocrinopathies and gastrointestinal (GI) disorders can also cause polyphagia and weight loss. The history and physical findings usually provide clues to the underlying cause. Complete blood count (CBC), serum biochemistry panel, baseline thyroxine concentration, urinalysis, and fecal examination for parasites should be performed if the history and physical findings are unremarkable. Additional tests may be required to establish a definitive diagnosis (see Table 54-1).

If the initial blood work is unremarkable, inadequate nutrition should be suspected. Changes in the type of diet, daily caloric intake, and feeding routine should be made

Table 54-1

### Differential Diagnosis for Polyphagia and Weight Loss

| Etiology | Definitive diagnostic tests |
| --- | --- |
| Inadequate nutrition | Response to diet change |
| Hyperthyroidism | Baseline $T_4$ and free $T_4$ concentrations |
| Diabetes mellitus | Blood glucose concentration and urinalysis |
| Gastrointestinal disease | |
|   Parasitism | Fecal examination, trial therapy |
|   Infiltrative bowel disease: plasmacytic, lymphocytic, eosinophilic lymphosarcoma | Intestinal biopsy |
|   Histoplasmosis | Intestinal biopsy, serology |
|   Lymphangiectasia | Intestinal biopsy |
|   Pancreatic exocrine insufficiency | Serum trypsinlike immunoreactivity, response to therapy |
| Protein-losing nephropathy | Urinalysis, urine protein/creatine ratio |
| Hypothalamic mass | Computed tomography, magnetic resonance imaging |

$T_4$, Thyroxine.

to ensure that the animal receives adequate amounts of a palatable and nutritionally complete diet. Body weight should be measured 2 and 4 weeks after an appropriate diet is initiated. Failure to gain weight suggests problems with owner compliance or occult disease, most likely involving the GI tract.

## OBESITY (TEXT PP 817-822)

Obesity is a clinical syndrome that involves excess accumulation of body fat. It is the most common form of malnutrition in small animal practice; 25% to 40% of cats and dogs presented to veterinary clinics are obese. Obesity has been associated with an increased incidence of arthritis, diabetes mellitus, hepatic lipidosis, feline lower urinary tract disease (FLUTD), urinary incontinence in spayed bitches, constipation, dermatitis, cardiovascular problems, respiratory problems, and increased anesthetic and surgical risk.

### Contributing factors

Obesity develops when energy intake consistently exceeds daily energy expenditure (which varies with environmental temperature, life stage, and activity level). Several dog breeds are at increased risk for obesity, including the Labrador Retriever, Golden Retriever, Cocker Spaniel, Collie, Dachshund, Cairn Terrier, Shetland Sheepdog, Beagle, Cavalier King Charles Spaniel, and Basset Hound. Obesity is more common in female neutered dogs and male neutered cats.

Obesity results from a disease process or drug administration in <5% of cases. Endocrine abnormalities associated with obesity include hypothyroidism, hyperadrenocorticism, hyperinsulinism, and acromegaly. Drugs such as progestagens and corticosteroids have been associated with the development of obesity.

### Diagnosis

Although numerous methods exist to determine body fat, measurement of body weight, body condition score (BCS), and morphometric measurements remain the most clinically useful techniques.

*Body condition score.* BCS provides a quick and simple subjective assessment of the animal's body condition. The two most commonly used scoring systems in small animal practice are a 5-point system, in which a BCS of 3 is considered ideal (Table 54-2); and a 9-point system, in which a BCS of 5 is considered ideal.

*Morphometric measurements.* Circumferential measurements can be used to estimate the percent body fat in cats. The Feline Body Mass Index (FBMI) is determined by measuring the rib cage circumference at the level of the ninth cranial rib and determining the leg index measurement (LIM), which is the distance from the patella to the calcaneal tuber. The percent body fat can be calculated as 1.5 to 9 (rib cage measurement minus LIM) or determined from a reference chart (see text). Cats with >30% body fat are candidates for a weight loss program. Pelvic circumference in relation to the distance from hock to stifle can be used in a similar way in dogs.

### Treatment

The weight management program is based on determination of the pet's ideal body weight, which can be estimated either by reviewing the medical record for the body weight when the pet was in an ideal body condition or by using breed-specific body weight charts. The optimum body weight for most cats is 3.5 to 5 kg. A thorough

Table 54-2

| Five-Point Body Condition Scoring System for Cats and Dogs | | |
|---|---|---|
| 1 | Thin | Underweight; no obvious body fat |
| 2 | Lean | Skeletal structure visible; little body fat |
| 3 | Optimum | Rib cage easily palpable but not showing; moderate amount of body fat |
| 4 | Overweight | Rib cage barely palpable; body weight more than normal |
| 5 | Obese | Rib cage not palpable; large amount of body fat; physical impairment resulting from excessive body fat |

dietary history should be obtained to calculate the current daily caloric intake of the pet (including snacks and treats).

*Weight loss goals.* It is very important to set realistic and obtainable goals for weight loss in order to maintain client compliance. If the ideal body weight is >15% less than the current body weight, it is crucial to use a stepwise process to gradually achieve the ideal body weight. The initial goal should be a 15% body weight loss. Once this goal has been achieved, a new target body weight can be selected until the pet has reached the ideal body weight. The estimated daily caloric intake to achieve a 15% body weight loss is calculated as follows:

- Cats—intake (kcal/day) = 30 × initial body weight (kg)
- Dogs—intake (kcal/day) = 55 × initial body weight $(kg)^{0.75}$

When animals are fed at this level, 15% body weight loss will be achieved in approximately 18 weeks for cats and approximately 12 weeks for dogs.

*Diet type.* Diets specifically formulated for weight reduction are preferable to feeding lesser amounts of a maintenance diet (a strategy that may supply inadequate amounts of essential nutrients, such as amino acids, vitamins, minerals, and essential fatty acids). High-fiber diets may not be the best approach, particularly in obese cats, as these diets are unpalatable to some animals; refusal to eat the offered food puts the obese cat at risk for developing hepatic lipidosis. High-protein diets may be superior to other types of reduction diets, as they increase the proportion of fat loss while preserving or even increasing lean body mass. Feeding strategies for achieving and maintaining an ideal body weight are discussed further in the text.

*Other management strategies.* In addition to reduction of the daily caloric intake, every effort should be made to increase the daily energy expenditure by encouraging exercise. Providing the client with written instructions for weight loss typically improves both compliance and success. Photographing the pet before beginning the weight reduction program helps clients to see the effects of the weight loss on their pets.

Pets on weight reduction programs should be reevaluated every 2 weeks. The body weight, BCS, and/or FBMI should be recorded and the dietary history reviewed. Ideally, cats should achieve approximately a 1% body weight loss per week. More rapid weight loss in cats increases the risk for hepatic lipidosis. Dogs should achieve a 1% to 2% body weight loss per week. If the rate of weight loss exceeds 2% per week, the number of calories fed to the pet should be increased by 10% to 15%. If no weight loss has occurred, the dietary history should be reevaluated for additional calories. If none are found, then the daily caloric intake should be further reduced by 10% to 15%.

### Prevention

The key to obesity management is prevention. Prevention should begin at the time that the pet is neutered. Owners should be counseled about the risk factors for obesity (male neutered cats; female neutered dogs; inactive, indoor lifestyle; inappropriate feeding practices) and the consequences of obesity (e.g., increased incidence of FLUTD, diabetes mellitus, arthritis). It is important that owners be instructed on both how to feed their pets and how to regularly determine a pet's body condition, so that owners can maintain the ideal body condition of their pets. Weight education should be reinforced at each annual health examination.

## HYPERLIPIDEMIA (TEXT PP 822-827)

### Etiology

Hyperlipidemia is defined as an increased concentration of triglycerides (hyper-triglyceridemia), cholesterol (hypercholesterolemia), or both, in the blood. Postprandial hyperlipidemia is the most common form in dogs and cats. It is a normal physiologic manifestation that results from the production of triglyceride-rich chylomicrons and usually resolves within 2 to 10 hours.

### Fasting hyperlipidemia

In the fasted state hyperlipidemia is an abnormal finding that represents either accelerated production or delayed degradation of lipoproteins. Pathologic abnormalities in plasma lipids and lipoproteins may be of genetic or familial origin (primary) or a consequence of disease or drugs (secondary). Primary causes include idiopathic hyperlipoproteinemia in Miniature Schnauzers and idiopathic hyperchylomicronemia and lipoprotein lipase deficiency in cats. Idiopathic hyperchylomicronemia has also been reported in dogs. Similar to the condition in cats, it is characterized by hypertriglyceridemia, hyperchylomicronemia, and normal serum cholesterol concentrations. Idiopathic hypercholesterolemia has been reported in Doberman Pinschers and Rottweilers.

Secondary causes of hyperlipidemia include hypothyroidism, diabetes mellitus, hyperadrenocorticism, pancreatitis, cholestasis, hepatic insufficiency, nephrotic syndrome, and administration of glucocorticoids or megestrol acetate (cats). Hypothyroidism is the most common cause of hypercholesterolemia in dogs.

### Clinical features

Waxing-and-waning vomiting, diarrhea, and abdominal discomfort are the most common clinical presentations associated with hypertriglyceridemia (Table 54-3). Severe hypertriglyceridemia (>1000 mg/dl) has been associated with pancreatitis, lipemia retinalis, seizures, cutaneous xanthomas, peripheral nerve paralysis, and behavioral changes. Cutaneous xanthomas are the most common manifestation of hypertriglyceridemia in cats. Severe hypercholesterolemia has been associated with arcus lipoides corneae, lipemia retinalis, and atherosclerosis.

### Effects on other biochemical tests

Hypertriglyceridemia may interfere with the results of several routine biochemical tests. The presence of lipemia falsely *increases* the serum concentrations of bilirubin (total and conjugated), phosphorus, total protein (using a refractometer), lipase (dogs), alanine aminotransferase (ALT; dogs), and, in dogs and cats with severe hyperlipemia, serum alkaline phosphatase and glucose. The presence of lipemia falsely *decreases* the serum concentrations of creatinine, total carbon dioxide, cholesterol (dogs), blood urea nitrogen (dogs), and ALT (cats).

The degree of interference depends on the specific assay used, the species (dog versus cat), and the severity of hypertriglyceridemia. Hyperlipidemia may also cause hemolysis, which in turn can interfere with the results of some biochemical assays. Conversely, hyperbilirubinemia can cause the cholesterol concentration to be falsely lower. These potential alterations must be considered when interpreting results in animals with hyperlipidemia. Fortunately, many laboratories attempt to clear hypertriglyceridemia before performing the biochemical assays.

### Table 54-3

### Clinical Signs and Potential Consequences of Hypertriglyceridemia and Hypercholesterolemia

| Clinical signs | Consequences |
|---|---|
| Seizures | Hypertriglyceridemia |
| Blindness | Seizures |
| Abdominal pain | Pancreatitis |
| Anorexia | Lipid-laden aqueous humor: uveitis, blindness |
| Vomiting | Lipemia retinalis |
| Diarrhea | Xanthomas |
| Behavioral changes | |
| Lipemia retinalis | |
| Uveitis | |
| Xanthoma formation | |
| Peripheral neuropathy | Hypercholesterolemia |
|   Horner's syndrome | Corneal arcus lipoides |
|   Tibial nerve paralysis | Lipemia retinalis |
|   Radial nerve paralysis | Atherosclerosis |

### Diagnostic approach

The presence of milklike, opaque serum (lactescence) suggests that the animal is hypertriglyceridemic and that the triglyceride concentration is >1000 mg/dl. Animals that are purely hypercholesterolemic do not exhibit lipemic or lactescent serum. Blood samples to confirm hyperlipidemia should be obtained after a 12- to 18-hour fast. Serum, rather than whole blood or plasma, should be submitted. Reference ranges for serum triglycerides are typically 50 to 150 mg/dl for adult dogs and 20 to 110 mg/dl for adult cats. Reference ranges for serum cholesterol are typically 125 to 300 mg/dl for adult dogs and 95 to 130 mg/dl for adult cats.

*Chylomicron test.* The chylomicron test is a simple test that can help determine whether the lipemia is predominantly a chylomicron or a very–low-density lipoprotein (VLDL) defect. A serum sample is refrigerated for 12 hours. Chylomicrons will float to the top of the sample to form an opaque, cream layer over clear serum. If hypertriglyceridemia is a result of excess VLDL particles, the plasma will remain turbid. Formation of a cream layer over a cloudy serum layer suggests excess of both chylomicrons and VLDL particles.

*Other tests.* Lipoprotein electrophoresis can be used to distinguish the lipoproteins, and ultracentrifugation can provide a quantitative measurement of each of the lipoprotein classes. However, these procedures are time consuming and are not routinely available. The activity of lipoprotein lipase can be assessed by the heparin release test (see text).

*Investigating the cause.* Every effort should be made to determine whether the hyperlipidemia is primary or secondary to an underlying disease process. A full history, physical examination, CBC, serum biochemistry panel, serum lipase and thyroxine concentrations, and urinalysis should be assessed in every hyperlipemic animal. Additional tests, such as abdominal ultrasound and an adrenocorticotropic hormone stimulation test, may be required to establish a diagnosis.

### Treatment of hypertriglyceridemia

In general, severe hypertriglyceridemia (>1000 mg/dl) requires treatment aimed at decreasing the triglyceride concentration in order to prevent possible complications, such as pancreatitis. In other situations, recommendations are influenced by additional variables, including the underlying disease process. A realistic goal is to reduce the triglyceride concentration to <400 mg/dl.

*Dietary therapy.* Restriction of dietary fat is the cornerstone of therapy. The dietary history should be reviewed and the diet altered to one that contains <20% fat (see text). Nutritional management of hypertriglyceridemia in cats is more difficult because of the limited availability of low-fat diets for cats. In addition to a low-fat diet, the absolute caloric intake should be evaluated. If the animal is overweight, caloric restriction is indicated and beneficial.

Plasma triglycerides should be measured after the animal has been fed a low-fat diet for 4 weeks. If the reduction in triglycerides is less than ideal, the dietary history should be reevaluated to ensure that no extra fat calories are being added from treats, that the animal has no access to other pet foods, and that no one is inadvertently providing the animal with dietary fat. If the low-fat commercial products are not able to control the hypertriglyceridemia, then a complete and balanced ultra–low-fat, home-prepared diet can be formulated specifically for the animal by a veterinary clinical nutritionist.

*Dietary supplements.* Some authors recommend menhaden fish oil (200 mg per kilogram of body weight per day) for dogs with hypertriglyceridemia. Niacin (100 mg/ day in dogs) reduces serum triglycerides; however, adverse effects are common and include vomiting, diarrhea, erythema, pruritus, and abnormalities in liver function tests.

*Drug therapy.* Treatment of hypertriglyceridemia with drugs, all of which have the potential for toxicity, should be undertaken with particular care. In general, drugs should not be used in animals in which serum triglyceride level is <500 mg/dl. Until further studies are performed to evaluate the dose, effect, and toxicity, drug therapy is indicated only in animals that have clinical signs associated with severe hypertriglyceridemia that cannot be ameliorated by dietary therapy.

### Treatment of hypercholesterolemia

Hypercholesterolemia is most often associated with the presence of an underlying disease and generally resolves with control of the altered metabolic state. Specific therapy is indicated only for animals with a prolonged, marked increase in serum cholesterol (>800 mg/dl). Nutritional therapy with a low-fat diet is the initial treatment of choice. The addition of soluble fiber to the diet may help reduce serum cholesterol.

***Drug therapy.*** Cholestyramine (1 to 2 g orally [PO] q12h) is effective for lowering serum cholesterol; however, its use has been associated with constipation, it interferes with the absorption of several oral medications, and it may increase hepatic VLDL synthesis, resulting in an increase in serum triglycerides. Lovastatin (10 to 20 mg PO q24h) may be tried in dogs with persistent, severe idiopathic hypercholesterolemia that does not respond to diet alone. Potential adverse effects include lethargy, diarrhea, muscle pain, and hepatotoxicity. Lovastatin should not be administered to dogs with hepatic disease.

# 55

# Electrolyte Imbalances

## *(Text pp 828-846)*

## HYPERNATREMIA (TEXT PP 828-830)

### Etiology

Hypernatremia exists when serum sodium (Na) exceeds 160 mEq/L. It most commonly develops when water is lost in excess of Na. Causes include the following:

- Pure water loss–diabetes insipidus (central or nephrogenic),* hypodipsia-adipsia,* neurologic disease (abnormal thirst mechanism, defective osmoregulation of vasopressin release), inadequate access to water, high environmental temperature, fever
- Hypotonic fluid loss–gastrointestinal (GI) fluid loss (vomiting, diarrhea),* renal failure (chronic or acute polyuric)*
- Osmotic diuresis–diabetes mellitus, mannitol infusion, diuretic administration, postobstructive diuresis
- Cutaneous burns
- Third-space loss–pancreatitis, peritonitis
- Excess Na retention–primary hyperaldosteronism
- Iatrogenic–salt poisoning, hypertonic saline infusion, sodium bicarbonate therapy, parenteral nutrition*

### Clinical features

Signs of hypernatremia originate in the central nervous system (CNS) and include lethargy, weakness, muscle fasciculations, disorientation, behavioral changes, ataxia, seizures, stupor, and coma. Skin turgor often is normal, which falsely implies adequate

---

*Common causes.

hydration, despite significant fluid loss. Signs typically become apparent when plasma osmolality exceeds 350 mOsm/kg (serum Na >170 mEq/L). Severity is related to the absolute increase in serum Na and especially the rapidity with which hypernatremia and hyperosmolality develop. With rapid onset, signs may develop at a serum Na concentration of 170 mEq/L or less.

### Diagnosis

Measurement of serum Na identifies hypernatremia. Careful evaluation of the history, physical findings, and routine clinical pathology (complete blood count [CBC], serum biochemistry panel, urinalysis) usually provides clues to the cause. Evaluation of urine specific gravity (SG) is especially helpful: hypernatremia and hyperosmolality result in hypersthenuric urine. Urine SG <1.008 in a dog or cat with hypernatremia is consistent with central or nephrogenic diabetes insipidus. Urine SG >1.030 in dogs and 1.035 in cats suggests Na retention, primary hypodipsia or adipsia, or GI or insensible water loss. Urine SG between 1.008 and 1.030 (dog) or 1.035 (cat) suggests a primary renal disorder.

### Treatment

The goals of treatment are as follows: (1) to restore extracellular fluid (ECF) volume and correct water deficits at a fluid rate that avoids significant complications, and (2) to identify and correct the underlying cause of the hypernatremia.

*Restore ECF volume.* In animals with modest volume contraction (e.g., tachycardia, dry mucous membranes, slow skin turgor), fluid deficits should be corrected with 0.45% saline supplemented with an appropriate amount of potassium (Table 55-1). With severe dehydration, 0.9% saline or plasma should be used. When one is replacing deficits, rapid fluid administration is contraindicated unless significant hypovolemia is present. Fluid should be administered in a volume only large enough to correct hypovolemia. Worsening neurologic status or sudden onset of seizures during fluid therapy generally is indicative of cerebral edema and the need for hypertonic saline solution or mannitol therapy.

*Correct water deficit.* Once ECF deficits have been replaced, serum Na should be reevaluated and water deficits corrected if hypernatremia persists. An approximation of the water deficit in liters may be calculated using the following formula:

$$\text{Water deficit (L)} = 0.6 \times \text{body weight (kg)} \times (1 - [\text{serum Na}^+_{desired}/\text{serum Na}^+_{present}])$$

Half-strength (0.45%) saline with 2.5% dextrose is used to correct the water deficit in hypernatremic animals with no signs of dehydration; it should also be used in dehydrated animals with persistent hypernatremia after the correction of fluid deficits. A 5% dextrose in water ($D_5W$) solution can be used instead to correct the water deficit in hypernatremic animals; and $D_5W$ can be substituted for 0.45% saline–2.5% dextrose if the hypernatremia does not abate after 12 to 24 hours. When possible, oral fluid administration is preferable for correcting water deficits.

The water deficit should be replaced slowly: approximately 50% in the first 24 hours, and the remainder over the ensuing 24 to 48 hours. Serum Na should decline slowly (preferably at <1 mEq/L/hr). Deterioration in CNS status indicates the presence of

**Table 55-1**

### Guidelines for Potassium Supplementation in Intravenous Fluids

| Serum potassium (mEq/L) | Potassium supplement per liter of fluids* |
|---|---|
| >3.5 | 20 |
| 3-3.5 | 30 |
| 2.5-3 | 40 |
| 2-2.5 | 60 |
| <2 | 80 |

*Total hourly potassium administration should not exceed 0.5 mEq/kg of body weight.

cerebral edema and the immediate need to reduce the fluid rate. Frequent monitoring of serum electrolytes, with appropriate adjustments in the type and rate of fluid administered, is important

**Hypernatremia with increased ECF volume.** On rare occasions a hypernatremic animal is presented with an increase in ECF volume. Such animals are difficult to treat. The goal is to lower the serum Na without exacerbating the increase in ECF volume and causing pulmonary congestion and edema. To slowly correct hypernatremia in these animals, loop diuretics (e.g., furosemide, 1 to 2 mg/kg orally [PO] or intravenously [IV] q8-12h) are administered to promote Na loss in the urine in conjunction with the judicious administration of $D_5W$.

## HYPONATREMIA (TEXT PP 830-832)

### Etiology

Hyponatremia is present when serum Na is <140 mEq/L. It can result from excessive Na loss (primarily via the kidneys), from increased water conservation, or both. In most cases hyponatremia results from abnormalities in water balance (principally a defect in renal water excretion) rather than Na balance. Causes include the following:

- With normal plasma osmolality—hyperlipidemia, hyperproteinemia
- With high plasma osmolality—hyperglycemia,* mannitol infusion
- With low plasma osmolality and hypervolemia—advanced liver failure,* advanced renal failure,* nephrotic syndrome,* congestive heart failure
- With low plasma osmolality and normovolemia—primary polydipsia, inappropriate antidiuretic hormone secretion, myxedema coma of hypothyroidism, iatrogenic (hypotonic fluid administration, antidiuretic drugs such as barbiturates and β-adrenergics)
- With low plasma osmolality and hypovolemia—hypoadrenocorticism,* GI fluid loss,* third-space loss (pleural effusions, peritoneal effusions, pancreatitis), cutaneous burns, diuretic administration

**Pseudohyponatremia.** Hyponatremia must be differentiated from pseudohyponatremia, which is a false decrease in serum Na as a result of laboratory methodology; plasma osmolality is normal. Pseudohyponatremia occurs in the presence of hyperlipidemia or severe hyperproteinemia when flame photometry is used to measure serum Na. Pseudohyponatremia can usually be identified if the method used to measure serum Na is known, a blood sample is examined for the presence of gross lipemia, and a CBC and serum biochemistry panel are performed.

**Effect of osmolality.** Hyponatremia may also occur after an increase in the concentration of osmotically active solutes (e.g., glucose, mannitol) in the ECF. Serum Na decreases 1.3 to 1.6 mEq/L for every 100 mg/dl increase in serum glucose. Estimation of the plasma osmolality is helpful in differentiating the cause of hyponatremia. Hyponatremia is usually associated with hyposmolality (<290 mOsm/kg), whereas pseudohyponatremia is associated with normal plasma osmolality; and hyponatremia caused by an increase in osmotically active solutes in the ECF is associated with hyperosmolality. Plasma osmolality can be estimated using the following formula:

$$\text{Plasma osmolality} = (2 \times \text{Na}) + \left(\frac{\text{Glucose}}{18}\right) + \left(\frac{\text{Urea nitrogen}}{2.8}\right)$$
$$\text{(mOsm/kg)} \qquad \text{[mEq/L]} \quad \text{[mg/dl]} \qquad \text{[mg/dl]}$$

Normal plasma osmolality in dogs and cats is 280 to 310 mOsm/kg.

### Clinical features

Signs of hyponatremia include lethargy, anorexia, vomiting, weakness, muscle fasciculations, disorientation, seizures, and coma. Onset and severity depend on the rapidity with which hyponatremia develops and on its degree. Clinical signs develop when the

---

*Common cause.

decrease in plasma osmolality occurs faster than the brain's defense mechanisms can counter the influx of water into the neurons.

### Diagnosis

Hyponatremia is obvious from measurement of serum electrolytes, although it must be differentiated from pseudohyponatremia. In most dogs and cats the cause is readily apparent after evaluation of the history, physical examination findings, CBC, serum biochemistry panel, and urinalysis findings, but further diagnostic tests may be necessary. Careful assessment of the urine SG, the hydration status of the animal, and, if necessary, the fractional excretion of Na ($FE_{Na}$) help localize the problem. The $FE_{Na}$ can be determined by first measuring urine Na ($U_{Na}$), plasma Na ($P_{Na}$), urine creatinine ($U_{Cr}$), and plasma creatinine ($P_{Cr}$) and then applying the following formula:

$$FE_{Na} = (U_{Na}/P_{Na}) \times (P_{Cr}/U_{Cr}) \times 100$$

In a hypovolemic animal with hyponatremia, $FE_{Na}$ >1% is consistent with hypo-adrenocorticism, Na-losing nephropathy, or use of diuretics. $FE_{Na}$ <1% may be indicative of GI loss, ascites, or edema formation. If a hyponatremic patient is *hyper*volemic, $FE_{Na}$ >1% indicates renal failure; $FE_{Na}$ <1% can signal nephrotic syndrome, congestive heart failure, or hepatopathy.

### Treatment

The goals of therapy are to treat the underlying disease and, if necessary, to increase the serum Na and plasma osmolality. Hyponatremia is corrected by raising the ratio of Na to water in the ECF using intravenous fluid therapy, water restriction, or both. The approach to treatment and the type of fluid used depend on the underlying cause, the severity of the hyponatremia, and the presence or absence of clinical signs.

*Fluid type.* Chronic hyponatremia in an asymptomatic animal is best treated conservatively. Lactated Ringer's or Ringer's solution can be used for mild hyponatremia (serum Na >135 mEq/L) and normal saline solution for more severe hyponatremia (serum Na <135 mEq/L). Normal saline is typically used in symptomatic animals with severe hyponatremia. Hypertonic saline solutions (i.e., 3% sodium chloride [NaCl]) can be considered for the treatment of severe hyponatremia (serum Na <120 mEq/L); however, this fluid should be used with caution and only if severe neurologic signs are present. The Na concentrations of the various parenteral fluid solutions are shown in Table 55-2.

*Rate of replacement.* Fluid and electrolyte balance should be gradually restored over 24 to 48 hours, with periodic measurement of serum electrolytes. The more acute and severe the hyponatremia, the more slowly the serum Na should be corrected. In animals with acute, severe hyponatremia and neurologic signs, a rapid increase in serum Na to >125 mEq/L is dangerous to the CNS and should be avoided. Instead, serum Na should be gradually increased to >125 mEq/L over 6 to 8 hours. Dietary Na restriction and diuretic therapy should be considered in edematous animals.

## HYPERKALEMIA (TEXT PP 832-834)

### Etiology

Hyperkalemia is present when serum potassium exceeds 5.5 mEq/L. Common causes include the following:

- Decreased urinary excretion—e.g., hypoadrenocorticism, acute oliguric-anuric renal failure, urethral obstruction, ruptured bladder (uroabdomen)
- Excessive administration of potassium-containing fluids

Less common causes include metabolic or respiratory acidosis (including diabetic ketoacidosis [DKA]), acute tumor lysis syndrome, reperfusion postthrombus dissolution, end-stage chronic renal failure, certain types of gastroenteritis (e.g., trichuriasis, salmonellosis), chylothorax with repeated pleural fluid drainage, and hyporeninemic hypoaldosteronism. Iatrogenic causes also include administration of potassium-sparing diuretics, angiotensin-converting enzyme inhibitors (e.g., captopril), prostaglandin

**Table 55-2**

## Parenteral Fluid Solutions

| Solution | Electrolyte concentration (mEq/L) | | | Buffer (mEq/L) | Osmolality (mOsm/L) | Calories (kcal/L) |
|---|---|---|---|---|---|---|
| | Sodium | Potassium | Chloride | | | |
| **ELECTROLYTE REPLACEMENT SOLUTIONS** | | | | | | |
| Lactated Ringer's (LRS) | 130 | 4 | 109 | Lactate 25 | 273 | 9 |
| Ringer's | 147 | 4 | 156 | — | 310 | — |
| Normal saline | 154 | — | 154 | — | 308 | — |
| Normosol R | 140 | 5 | 98 | Acetate 27 | 295 | 18 |
| **MAINTENANCE SOLUTIONS** | | | | | | |
| 2½% dextrose/0.45% saline | 77 | — | 77 | — | 280 | 85 |
| 2½% dextrose/half-strength LRS | 65 | 2 | 54 | Lactate 14 | 263 | 89 |
| Normosol M | 40 | 13 | 40 | Acetate 16 | 112 | — |
| Normosol M in 5% dextrose | 40 | 13 | 40 | Acetate 16 | 363 | 175 |
| **COLLOIDAL SOLUTIONS** | | | | | | |
| Dextran 70 (6% w/v in 0.9% saline) | 154 | — | 154 | — | 300-303 | — |
| Hetastarch (6% in 0.9% saline) | 154 | — | 154 | — | — | — |
| Plasma (average values, dog) | 145 | 4 | 108 | 20 | 300 | — |
| **OTHER SOLUTIONS** | | | | | | |
| 5% dextrose in water | — | — | — | — | 252 | 170 |

Modified from Senior DF: Fluid therapy, electrolyte, and acid-base control. In Ettinger SJ, ed: *Textbook of veterinary internal medicine*, ed 3, Philadelphia, 1989, WB Saunders.

inhibitors (e.g., indomethacin), digitalis, β-blockers (e.g., propranolol), or α-adrenergic agonists (e.g., phenylpropanolamine).

*Pseudohyperkalemia.* *Pseudohyperkalemia* refers to an increase in potassium in vitro and can occur in association with severe hypernatremia (dry reagent methods), leukocytosis (white blood cells >100,000/mm$^3$), or thrombocytosis (>1 × 10$^6$/mm$^3$) or when blood is obtained from fluid lines or catheters contaminated with potassium-containing fluids. In Akitas and in English Springer Spaniels with phosphofructokinase deficiency, it can also occur with hemolysis.

### Clinical features

The clinical manifestations reflect changes in cell membrane excitability and the magnitude and rapidity of onset of hyperkalemia. Mild to moderate hyperkalemia (<6.5 mEq/L) typically is asymptomatic. Generalized skeletal muscle weakness develops as hyperkalemia becomes more severe. The most prominent manifestation is cardiac dysfunction: hyperkalemia decreases myocardial excitability, increases the refractory period, and slows conduction (Table 55-3). These effects can cause life-threatening cardiac rhythm disturbances.

### Diagnosis

Measurement of serum potassium or evaluation of an electrocardiogram (ECG) identifies hyperkalemia. Careful review of the history, physical findings, CBC, serum biochemistry panel, and urinalysis usually provides clues as to the cause. Differentiating renal dysfunction from hypoadrenocorticism can pose a diagnostic challenge. An ACTH stimulation test is needed to confirm hypoadrenocorticism (see Chapter 53); measurement of serum aldosterone before and after ACTH administration should be considered, especially if plasma cortisol is normal and no other causes of hyperkalemia are identified. Small rents in the urinary bladder can be difficult to identify and frequently require contrast radiography or surgical exploration to confirm.

### Treatment

Therapy is directed at treating the underlying cause. Symptomatic therapy for hyperkalemia (Table 55-4) should be initiated if serum potassium is >7 mEq/L or if significant cardiac toxicity (e.g., complete heart block, premature ventricular contractions, arrhythmia) is identified on ECG. The goal in such patients is to reverse the cardiotoxic effects and, if possible, reestablish normokalemia. Asymptomatic animals with normal

**Table 55-3**

### Electrocardiographic Alterations Associated with Hypokalemia and Hyperkalemia in Dogs and Cats

| Hypokalemia | Hyperkalemia |
| --- | --- |
| Depressed T-wave amplitude | Serum potassium 5.6-6.5 mEq/L |
| Depressed ST segment | Bradycardia |
| Prolonged QT interval | Tall, narrow T waves |
| Prominent U wave | Serum potassium 6.6-7.5 mEq/L |
| Arrhythmias | Decreased R-wave amplitude |
| Supraventricular | Prolonged QRS interval |
| Ventricular | Serum potassium 7-8.5 mEq/L |
| | Decreased P-wave amplitude |
| | Prolonged PR interval |
| | Serum potassium >8.5 mEq/L |
| | Invisible P wave |
| | Deviation of ST segment |
| | Complete heart block |
| | Ventricular arrhythmias |
| | Cardiac arrest |

Table 55-4

## Potential Therapies for the Management of Hyperkalemia in Dogs and Cats

| Solution | Dose | Route of administration | Duration of effect |
|---|---|---|---|
| Physiologic saline | 60-100 ml/kg/day | IV | Hours |
| Dextrose | 5%-10% in IV fluids, *or* | IV, continuous | Hours |
| | 1-2 ml/kg 50% dextrose | IV, slow bolus | Hours |
| Regular insulin and dextrose | 0.5-1 U/kg in parenteral fluids *plus* | IV | Hours |
| | 2 g of dextrose per unit of insulin administered | IV | |
| | Note: Monitor blood glucose | | |
| Sodium bicarbonate | 1-2 mEq/kg | IV, slow bolus | Hours |
| 10% Calcium gluconate | 2-10 ml | IV, slow infusion | 30-60 min |
| | Note: Monitor cardiac function | | |

*IV,* Intravenous

urine output and chronic hyperkalemia of <7 mEq/L may not require immediate treatment, but a search for the underlying cause should be initiated.

*Fluid therapy.* Intravenous fluids are administered in amounts designed to correct fluid deficits. Normal saline is the fluid of choice. Potassium-containing fluids (e.g., lactated Ringer's solution; see Table 55-2) can be used if normal saline is unavailable. Dextrose may be added to make a 5% to 10% solution, but fluids containing >5% dextrose should be given into a central vein.

Rarely, additional therapy is required to reverse the cardiotoxic effects of hyperkalemia. Sodium bicarbonate and regular insulin with dextrose shift potassium from the extracellular to the intracellular space. Intravenous calcium (Ca) blocks the effects of hyperkalemia on cell membranes but has no effect on blood potassium concentration. Doses are given in Table 55-4.

## HYPOKALEMIA (TEXT PP 834-836)

### Etiology

Hypokalemia is present when serum potassium (K) is <3.5 mEq/L. Common causes include the following:

- GI fluid loss—e.g., vomiting, diarrhea
- Chronic renal failure, especially in cats
- DKA
- Secondary hyperaldosteronism—e.g., liver insufficiency, congestive heart failure, nephrotic syndrome
- Inappropriate fluid therapy—potassium-free fluids (e.g., 0.9% saline), parenteral nutrition solutions, insulin and glucose-containing fluids, sodium bicarbonate therapy
- Diuretic use—loop (e.g., furosemide) or thiazide diuretics
- Low dietary intake

Less common causes include metabolic alkalosis, hypokalemic periodic paralysis (Burmese cats), diet-induced hypokalemic nephropathy in cats, renal tubular acidosis, postobstructive diuresis, primary hyperaldosteronism, hyperthyroidism, and hypomagnesemia.

*Pseudohypokalemia.* Pseudohypokalemia is uncommon and depends on the method used to measure serum K. Hyperlipidemia, hyperproteinemia (>10 g/dl), hyperglycemia (>750 mg/dl), and azotemia (blood urea nitrogen >115 mg/dl) each potentially cause pseudohypokalemia when dry reagent methods are used.

### Clinical features

The clinical consequences of severe hypokalemia primarily involve the neuromuscular and cardiovascular systems. The most common sign is generalized skeletal muscle weakness. In cats, ventroflexion of the neck, forelimb hypermetria, and a broad-based hindlimb stance may also be seen. Onset of weakness is extremely variable, and cats seem more susceptible than dogs. Signs in dogs may not be evident until serum K is <2.5 mEq/L, whereas in cats, signs may be seen when serum potassium is 3 to 3.5 mEq/L. However, most dogs and cats with mild to moderate hypokalemia (3 to 4 mEq/L) are asymptomatic.

*Cardiac and metabolic manifestations.* Cardiac consequences include decreased myocardial contractility, decreased cardiac output, and disturbances in cardiac rhythm. Cardiac disturbances have variable clinical expression and are often evident only on evaluation of the ECG (see Table 55-3). Other metabolic effects include (1) hypokalemic nephropathy, which is characterized by chronic tubulointerstitial nephritis, impaired renal function, and azotemia and manifested clinically as polyuria (PU) and polydipsia (PD) and impaired urine concentrating capability; (2) hypokalemic polymyopathy, characterized by increased serum creatine kinase and electromyographic abnormalities; and (3) paralytic ileus, manifested as abdominal distention, anorexia, vomiting, and constipation. Hypokalemic nephropathy and polymyopathy are more common in cats than in dogs.

### Diagnosis

Measurement of serum K identifies hypokalemia. Careful review of the history, physical findings, CBC, serum biochemistry panel, and urinalysis usually provides clues as to the cause. If a cause is not readily apparent, less likely causes for hypokalemia should be considered, such as renal tubular acidosis or another renal K-wasting disorder, primary hyperaldosteronism, or hypomagnesemia. To help differentiate renal and nonrenal sources of K loss, it may be necessary to determine the fractional excretion of potassium ($FE_K$), as outlined for Na on p 522, or determine 24-hour urine K excretion (see text).

### Treatment

Therapy is indicated when (1) serum K is <3 mEq/L, (2) clinical signs of hypokalemia are present, or (3) reduction in serum K is anticipated and the patient's ability to compensate is impaired (e.g., insulin therapy for DKA). The goal is to reestablish and maintain normokalemia without inducing hyperkalemia.

*Oral supplements.* K supplementation should be given PO whenever possible. Problems with oral preparations include poor palatability and GI irritation (e.g., vomiting, diarrhea, melena). K gluconate as an elixir (Kaon Elixir) or protein base (Tumil-K) is well accepted and has minimal GI side effects. The recommended dose is 2.2 mEq of $K^+$ per 100 calories of required energy intake per day, or 2 mEq of $K^+$ per 4.5 kg of body weight twice a day. Subsequent adjustments are based on clinical response and serum K concentration.

*Parenteral administration.* Parenteral supplementation is indicated when oral therapy is not possible (e.g., vomiting, anorexia). K chloride is most commonly used; in patients with DKA, addition of K phosphate is indicated to avoid hypophosphatemia (see Chapter 52). Intravenous administration is preferred, although K chloride can be given subcutaneously (SC) as long as the solution contains <30 mEq $K^+$/L. The amount of K to be added to intravenous fluids depends on the serum K concentration (see Table 55-1) and the type of fluid used (see Table 55-2). In any case, the rate of intravenous K should not exceed 0.5 mEq/kg/hr.

*Monitoring.* It is difficult to estimate the amount of K required to reestablish normal potassium balance based on the serum K concentration, because K is primarily an intracellular cation. Serial measurement of serum K is important during treatment and should initially be performed every 6 to 8 hours if K is being administered IV. The ECG can also be used as a crude index of serum K concentration (see Table 55-3).

Adjustments are made accordingly, with the goal of establishing a normal serum K concentration and then maintaining the serum K in the normal range as treatment is withdrawn. In patients with normal renal function, the maintenance amount of K is approximately 0.5 mEq/kg/day.

Clinical signs of hypokalemia usually resolve within 1 to 5 days after correction of hypokalemia. Depending on the underlying cause, long-term oral supplementation may be required to prevent the recurrence of hypokalemia.

## HYPERCALCEMIA (TEXT PP 836-839)

Hypercalcemia is present when serum total Ca is >12 mg/dl or serum ionized Ca is >1.45 mmol/L. Mild increases in total Ca (<13 mg/dl), ionized Ca (<1.55 mmol/L), phosphate (<10 mg/dl), and alkaline phosphatase in a healthy puppy are normal. Serum total Ca does not fluctuate with age in cats, but ionized Ca may be a little higher in cats <2 years of age compared with older cats.

In dogs, alternations in plasma protein, particularly albumin, can affect serum total Ca (but not ionized Ca). Therefore serum albumin should be measured when serum total Ca is determined. The following formula can be used to determine the corrected total Ca:

$$\text{Corrected Ca (mg/dl)} = \text{Serum Ca (mg/dl)} - \text{Serum albumin (g/dl)} + 3.5$$

The formula should not be used in dogs <6 months of age, because high values may be obtained. Nor should it be used in cats, because no linear relationship between serum total Ca and serum albumin exists in cats. Note: Even in adult dogs, corrected serum total Ca may not be a reliable indicator of Ca homeostasis.

### Etiology

Hypercalcemia is uncommon in dogs and cats. Humoral hypercalcemia of malignancy (HHM) is the most common cause in both species, with lymphoma being the malignancy most often associated with hypercalcemia; squamous cell carcinoma is another common cause of HHM in cats. Other causes of hypercalcemia include chronic renal failure, primary hyperparathyroidism, hypoadrenocorticism (dogs), hypervitaminosis D (dogs), and idiopathic hypercalcemia (cats). Calcium oxalate urolithiasis and consumption of acidifying diets are commonly identified in cats with hypercalcemia, but their role, if any, in causing the disorder is unknown.

***Renal failure.*** Hypercalcemia can develop in dogs and cats with chronic or, less commonly, acute renal failure. Conversely, prolonged hypercalcemia, especially in conjunction with high-normal or increased serum phosphorus, can cause renal insufficiency and azotemia. Determining whether the renal failure is primary or secondary in a dog with hypercalcemia, hyperphosphatemia, and azotemia poses a diagnostic challenge.

***Idiopathic hypercalcemia.*** Idiopathic hypercalcemia is an increasingly common diagnosis in young and middle-aged cats. The cause is unknown. Hypercalcemia is usually mild (<13 mg/dl) and asymptomatic. Serum phosphorus and renal indexes are normal, and results of a complete diagnostic evaluation are unremarkable. Primary hyperparathyroidism has not been confirmed in any of these cats; serum parathyroid hormone (PTH) is normal or low. Nephrocalcinosis and urolithiasis may develop, presumably secondary to increased urinary Ca excretion. Effective treatment has not been identified. Serum Ca has decreased in some cats after a dietary change to a high-fiber diet or after prednisone treatment was initiated, but the response has been unpredictable.

### Clinical features

Although all tissues can be affected by hypercalcemia, the neuromuscular, GI, renal, and cardiac systems are the most important clinically. Signs include PU and PD, lethargy, anorexia, vomiting, constipation, weakness and, rarely, seizures. Cardiac arrhythmias may develop in animals with severe hypercalcemia (>18 mg/dl), although this is rare. Prolongation of the PR interval and shortening of the QT interval may be found on

ECG with milder hypercalcemia. Clinical signs resulting from the development of Ca uroliths may also occur (see Chapter 46).

Clinical signs are often absent with mild hypercalcemia. When signs do develop, they tend to be insidious in onset. The severity of clinical signs depends on the severity, rate of onset, and duration of hypercalcemia. Clinical signs become more severe as the magnitude of the hypercalcemia increases. Signs are usually mild when serum Ca is <14 mg/dl, are readily apparent with values >14 mg/dl, and become potentially life threatening (i.e., cardiac arrhythmias) when serum Ca exceeds 18 mg/dl.

### Diagnosis

Hypercalcemia should always be reconfirmed, preferably from a nonlipemic blood sample obtained after a 12-hour fast, before one embarks on an extensive diagnostic evaluation. Results of CBC, serum biochemistry panel, and urinalysis, in conjunction with the history and physical examination findings, often provide clues to the diagnosis (see Table 50-2).

*Serum biochemistry panel.* Special attention should be paid to the serum electrolytes and renal indexes. Hypoadrenocorticism-induced hypercalcemia occurs in conjunction with mineralocorticoid deficiency, so hyponatremia, hyperkalemia, and prerenal azotemia also are present. Serum phosphorus is low-normal or low with HHM and primary hyperparathyroidism. If serum phosphorus is increased and renal function is normal, hypervitaminosis D and osteolysis from metastatic or primary bone neoplasia are the primary differential diagnoses.

*Primary versus secondary renal failure.* When hyperphosphatemia and hypercalcemia coexist with azotemia, determining whether renal failure is primary or secondary to hypercalcemia caused by another disorder can be difficult. Measurement of serum ionized Ca may help identify dogs and cats with renal failure–induced hypercalcemia: ionized Ca typically is normal or decreased in renal failure and increased in hypercalcemia caused by other disorders.

*Hypercalcemia alone.* When serum phosphorus is normal or low, HHM and primary hyperparathyroidism are the primary differentials. Systemic signs of illness suggest HHM; dogs and cats with primary hyperparathyroidism are usually healthy, and any clinical signs are mild (see Chapter 50). In either case the appendicular skeleton, peripheral lymph nodes, abdomen, and rectum should be carefully palpated for masses, lymphadenopathy, hepatomegaly, splenomegaly, or pain on digital palpation of the long bones.

*Further evaluation.* Various diagnostic tests may be needed to identify the underlying cause, including thoracic and abdominal radiography; abdominal and cervical ultrasonography; cytologic evaluation of aspirates of the liver, spleen, lymph nodes, and bone marrow; and measurement of serum ionized Ca, PTH, and PTH-related peptide (PTHrP).

*Ionized Ca, PTH, and PTHrP.* Measurement of serum ionized Ca, PTH, and PTHrP from the same blood sample is helpful in differentiating primary hyperparathyroidism from HHM. A profile of increased ionized Ca, nondetectable PTH, and detectable PTHrP is diagnostic for HHM. Lymphoma is the most common cause of detectable PTHrP, but other tumors, including apocrine gland adenocarcinoma and various carcinomas (e.g., mammary gland, squamous cell, bronchogenic), can also cause hypercalcemia by this mechanism.

A profile of increased ionized Ca, normal-to-increased PTH, and nondetectable PTHrP is diagnostic for primary hyperparathyroidism. Ultrasonography of the thyroparathyroid complex may reveal enlargement of one or more parathyroid glands (see Chapter 50); the parathyroid glands are small or undetectable in patients with HHM.

*L-Asparaginase.* Measurement of serum Ca following L-asparaginase administration (20,000 $U/m^2$ IV) should be considered for patients with hypercalcemia of undetermined cause. Serum Ca is measured before and every 12 hours after administration for up to 72 hours. A decline in serum Ca, usually into the normal range, is strongly suggestive of occult lymphoma. Hypersensitivity reactions are the most common adverse effect of L-asparaginase administration; pretreatment with an antihistamine is recommended.

---

**Box 55-1**

## Nonspecific Therapy for Control of Hypercalcemia

### ACUTE THERAPY
1. Correct fluid deficits
2. Physiologic saline diuresis, 60-180 mg/kg/day IV
3. Furosemide, 2-4 mg/kg IV, IM, PO q8-12h
4. Once diagnosis is established: prednisone, 1-2 mg/kg q12h

Additional therapy if above fails:
1. Sodium bicarbonate, 1-4 mEq/kg given in intravenous fluids
2. Salmon calcitonin, 4 U/kg IV, then 4-8 U/kg SC q12-24h
3. Peritoneal dialysis or hemodialysis

### LONG-TERM THERAPY
1. Furosemide (see above)
2. Prednisone (see above)
3. Low-calcium diet: prescription diet k/d, u/d, s/d
4. Intestinal phosphate binders if hyperphosphatemia present
5. Bisphosphonates (etidronate, 10-40 mg/kg PO divided q8-12h)

---

*IM,* Intramuscularly; *IV,* intravenously; *PO,* orally; *SC,* subcutaneously.

### Treatment

Therapy is directed at correcting the underlying cause. Supportive therapy to decrease serum Ca is indicated if (1) signs are severe, (2) serum Ca is >16 mg/dl, (3) the Ca × phosphorus product is >60 (implying metastatic soft-tissue mineralization), or (4) azotemia is present. Supportive therapy must not interfere with attempts to establish a definitive diagnosis, however. As a general rule, saline diuresis followed by diuretic therapy can be initiated without compromising the results of diagnostic tests (Box 55-1).

Because of the high incidence of lymphoma in hypercalcemic patients, glucocorticoids should not be administered unless the cause has been identified. Calcitonin may be useful in animals with severe hypercalcemia and could be used in place of prednisone until a diagnosis is established. However, although calcitonin may rapidly decrease the magnitude of hypercalcemia, its effect may be short-lived (hours), and resistance often develops within a few days, limiting its usefulness in hypercalcemic patients that require prolonged supportive care.

*Prolonged therapy.* If prolonged supportive therapy is required (e.g., cholecalciferol-containing rodenticide toxicity or nontreatable malignancy), furosemide, corticosteroids, and a low-Ca diet can be used to help control the hypercalcemia. Non–Ca-containing intestinal phosphorus binders (e.g., aluminum hydroxide) should be administered if hyperphosphatemia is present, with the dosage based on serial serum phosphorus measurements. Oral bisphosphonates such as etidronate (Didronel) may reduce hypercalcemia caused by lymphoma, myeloma, primary hyperparathyroidism, or hypervitaminosis D in dogs. However, acute renal failure is a possible sequela of therapy.

## HYPOCALCEMIA (TEXT PP 840-841)

### Etiology

Hypocalcemia is present when serum total Ca is <9 mg/dl (<7 mg/dl in dogs and cats <6 months old) or ionized Ca is <1 mmol/L. The most common causes are puerperal tetany in lactating animals, renal failure (acute or chronic), malassimilation syndromes, and primary hypoparathyroidism (e.g., after thyroidectomy in hyperthyroid cats). Other causes include ethylene glycol toxicity, acute pancreatitis, and acute-onset hyperphosphatemia.

Hypocalcemia occurs with hypoalbuminemic states, although ionized Ca is unaffected. Total serum Ca should be adjusted for low serum albumin before making a diagnosis of hypocalcemia. However, the association between the total serum Ca and serum albumin is weak, and serum ionized Ca can be decreased despite a "corrected" serum total Ca that is in the normal range.

### Clinical features

Clinical manifestations vary from none to severe neuromuscular dysfunction. The presence and severity of signs depend on the magnitude, rapidity of onset, and duration of hypocalcemia. Serum total Ca of 7.5 to 9 mg/dl often is clinically silent, whereas values <7.5 mg/dl usually cause clinical signs.

The most common signs are nervousness, behavioral changes, focal muscle twitching (especially ear and face), muscle cramping, stiff gait, tetany, and seizures (usually without loss of consciousness or urinary incontinence). Early indicators, especially in cats, include lethargy, anorexia, intense facial rubbing, and panting. Exercise, excitement, and stress may induce or worsen clinical signs. Additional findings may include fever, "splinted" abdomen, cardiac abnormalities (e.g., weak femoral pulses, muffled heart sounds, tachyarrhythmias), and cataracts.

### Diagnosis

Hypocalcemia should be confirmed before the cause is investigated. History, physical findings, CBC, serum biochemistry panel, serum lipase concentration, and urinalysis usually provide the necessary clues to establish a diagnosis. Primary hypoparathyroidism is the most likely diagnosis in a nonazotemic, nonlactating dog or cat with signs of hypocalcemia. A low or undetectable serum PTH concentration confirms this diagnosis (see Chapter 50).

### Treatment

Therapy is directed at correcting the underlying cause. Vitamin D and/or Ca therapy is indicated if signs of hypocalcemia are present, or if serum total Ca is <7.5 mg/dl or ionized Ca is <0.8 mmol/L. If hypocalcemic tetany is present, calcium gluconate should be administered IV, slowly until effective (see Chapter 50). Auscultation and electrocardiographic monitoring is advisable; if bradycardia or QT shortening occurs, intravenous infusion should be suspended. Ca-rich fluids must be infused with caution in hyperphosphatemic patients because they increase the probability of metastatic soft-tissue calcification, especially in the kidney.

*Maintenance therapy.* Once signs of hypocalcemic tetany have been controlled, oral or subcutaneous Ca and oral vitamin D may be needed to prevent recurrence of clinical signs. Ca-gluconate can be injected SC at the same intravenous dose used to control tetany, but diluted 50:50 with saline. (Note: Calcium chloride should not be administered SC.)

If the cause of hypocalcemia is readily reversible (e.g., weaning puppies from a bitch with puerperal tetany), a single subcutaneous injection of Ca-gluconate may be all that is necessary. In animals with disorders that cause prolonged hypocalcemia (e.g., primary hypoparathyroidism), Ca-gluconate can be injected SC q6-8h until oral vitamin D and Ca supplements become effective in maintaining normocalcemia.

Alternatively, Ca-gluconate can be administered by continuous intravenous infusion at an initial rate of 60 to 90 mg of $Ca^+$ per kilogram per day (10 ml of 10% Ca-gluconate provides 93 mg of $Ca^+$). Note: Ca salts should not be added to fluids that contain lactate, acetate, bicarbonate, or phosphates, as precipitation can result. Serum Ca should be measured daily and subcutaneous or intravenous Ca therapy gradually decreased and then discontinued once serum total Ca is consistently >8 mg/dl or ionized Ca is >0.9 mmol/L.

*Chronic therapy.* Long-term maintenance therapy is most commonly required for the control of idiopathic hypoparathyroidism and hypoparathyroidism that occurs after bilateral thyroidectomy in cats with hyperthyroidism. Oral vitamin D administration is the primary mode of treatment for the management of chronic hypocalcemia; oral Ca supplements are also needed initially (see Chapter 50).

## HYPERPHOSPHATEMIA (TEXT PP 841-842)

### Etiology

Hyperphosphatemia is present when serum phosphate is >6.5 mg/dl (>9 mg/dl in puppies, especially large- and giant-breed dogs, and >8.1 mg/dl in kittens <6 months old). The most common nonphysiologic causes are renal failure (acute or chronic), pre-renal or postrenal azotemia, hypervitaminosis D (e.g., cholecalciferol rodenticides), and primary hypoparathyroidism.

Other causes include excess dietary intake, jasmine toxicity, osteolytic bone lesions (neoplasia), hyperthyroidism, acromegaly, metabolic acidosis, tumor cell lysis syndrome, tissue trauma or rhabdomyolysis, hemolysis, and administration of phosphorus-containing intravenous fluids or enemas, anabolic steroids, diuretics (furosemide, hydrochlorothiazides), or minocycline. Laboratory error, lipemia, and hyperproteinemia can each falsely elevate the serum phosphorus.

### Clinical features

By itself, hyperphosphatemia does not cause clinical signs; it is simply a marker of underlying disease. An acute increase in serum phosphorus can cause hypocalcemia and its associated neuromuscular signs. Sustained hyperphosphatemia can cause secondary hyperparathyroidism, fibrous osteodystrophy, and metastatic calcification in extra-osseous sites. Fortunately, most causes of hyperphosphatemia cause a decrease in serum Ca, so the Ca-phosphorus solubility product ($[Ca] \times [Pi]$) remains <60. The risk of soft-tissue mineralization increases when $Ca \times P > 60$, such as can occur with chronic renal failure.

### Treatment

Hyperphosphatemia usually resolves with correction of the underlying disease. In dogs and cats with renal failure, hyperphosphatemia can initially be lowered with aggressive fluid therapy. Low-phosphorus diets and orally administered phosphate binders are the most effective way to treat sustained hyperphosphatemia caused by renal failure (see Chapter 44).

## HYPOPHOSPHATEMIA (TEXT PP 842-843)

### Etiology

Hypophosphatemia is present when serum phosphorus is <3 mg/dl, but it usually is not clinically worrisome until serum phosphorus is <1.5 mg/dl. Clinically significant hypophosphatemia most often occurs within the first 24 hours of therapy for DKA (see Chapter 52). Other common causes of hypophosphatemia include primary hyper-parathyroidism, hypercalcemia of malignancy, use of phosphate-binding antacids, and parenteral administration of sodium bicarbonate or glucose.

Less common causes include vitamin D deficiency, renal tubular disorders (Fanconi syndrome), eclampsia, respiratory or metabolic alkalosis, hypothermia, administration of proximally acting diuretics or parenteral nutritional solutions, and possibly decreased dietary intake, malabsorption, and steatorrhea.

### Clinical features

Clinical signs may develop when serum phosphorus is <1.5 mg/dl, although signs are quite variable, and severe hypophosphatemia is clinically silent in many animals. Hemolytic anemia is the most common sequela, although hemolysis is usually not iden-tified until serum phosphorus is <1 mg/dl. Hemolytic anemia can be life threatening if not recognized and treated. Other signs associated with hypophosphatemia include weakness, ataxia, and seizures, as well as anorexia and vomiting secondary to intestinal ileus.

### Treatment

Hypophosphatemia usually resolves after correction of the underlying cause. Phosphate therapy probably is not indicated for asymptomatic animals in which serum phosphorus is >1.5 mg/dl and is unlikely to decrease further. Phosphate therapy is indicated if clinical signs or hemolysis are identified or if serum phosphorus is

<1.5 mg/dl, especially if a further decrease is possible. It should also be considered during the initial 24 hours of therapy for DKA, especially if serum phosphorus is low at the time DKA is diagnosed. Phosphate supplementation is not indicated in patients with hypercalcemia, hyperphosphatemia, oliguric renal failure, or suspected tissue necrosis.

*Phosphate supplementation.* The goal is to maintain serum phosphorus >2 mg/dl without causing hyperphosphatemia. Oral supplementation is preferred, using a buffered laxative (e.g., Phospho-Soda), balanced commercial diet, or milk. Intravenous supplementation usually is required to correct severe hypophosphatemia, especially with DKA. Potassium phosphate solutions typically are used; if potassium supplementation is contraindicated, sodium phosphate can be substituted.

The initial dose of phosphate is 0.01 to 0.03 mmol/kg/hr, preferably administered by constant-rate infusion in Ca-free intravenous fluids (e.g., 0.9% saline, $D_5W$). Alternatively, the amount of potassium supplementation required can be determined and then provided with 50:50 potassium chloride and potassium phosphate.

Adverse effects of overzealous phosphate administration include iatrogenic hypocalcemia and its associated neuromuscular signs, hypernatremia, hypotension, and calcification of soft tissues. Because the dose of phosphate necessary for repletion and the animal's response to therapy cannot be predicted, it is important that serum phosphorus be monitored every 6 to 8 hours initially and the phosphate infusion adjusted accordingly.

## HYPERMAGNESEMIA (TEXT P 843)

### Etiology
Hypermagnesemia is present when serum magnesium is >2.5 mg/dl. It is an uncommon clinical problem. Hypermagnesemia occurs with renal insufficiency or failure, or it is iatrogenically induced (e.g., excessive intravenous administration, antacids, laxatives). Excess magnesium is rapidly excreted by the healthy kidney, so iatrogenic hypermagnesemia is more likely in patients with renal insufficiency. Hypermagnesemia has also been reported in cats with thoracic neoplasia and pleural effusion.

### Clinical features
Clinical manifestations include lethargy, weakness, and hypotension. Loss of deep tendon reflexes and ECG changes (prolonged PR intervals, widened QRS complexes, heart block) occur with severe hypermagnesemia.

### Treatment
Therapy begins with discontinuation of all exogenous sources of magnesium. Additional therapy depends on the severity of hypermagnesemia, clinical presentation, and renal function. Most animals with healthy kidneys require only supportive care. Treatment to improve renal function is indicated in patients with renal insufficiency. Dogs and cats with cardiac conduction disturbances or hypotension should be treated with intravenous Ca (see Chapter 50) until cardiac function normalizes. Administration of magnesium-free crystalloid fluids and furosemide can be used to accelerate renal magnesium excretion.

## HYPOMAGNESEMIA (TEXT PP 843-845)

### Etiology
Hypomagnesemia is present when serum magnesium (Mg) is <1.5 mg/dl. The most common causes are chronic diarrhea and vomiting, DKA (especially during the first 24 hours of therapy), prolonged intravenous fluid therapy, and administration of diuretics.

Less common causes include inadequate dietary intake, malabsorption syndromes, acute pancreatitis, cholestatic liver disease, nasogastric suction, renal dysfunction (glomerulonephritis, acute tubular necrosis, drug-induced tubular injury [e.g., aminoglycosides, cisplatin]), postobstructive diuresis, digitalis therapy, hypercalcemia, hypokalemia, hyperthyroidism, primary hyperparathyroidism, primary hyperaldosteronism, sepsis, hypothermia, massive blood transfusion, peritoneal dialysis or hemodialysis, total parenteral nutrition, and acute administration of insulin, glucose, or amino acids.

### Clinical features

Hypomagnesemia is the most common electrolyte disorder found in critically ill dogs and cats, and it may predispose to a variety of cardiovascular, neuromuscular, and metabolic complications. However, clinical signs usually do not occur until serum magnesium is <1 mg/dl; even then, many patients remain asymptomatic. Mg deficiency can result in several nonspecific clinical signs, including lethargy, anorexia, muscle weakness (including dysphagia and dyspnea), muscle fasciculations, ataxia, seizures, and coma. Concurrent hypokalemia, hyponatremia, and hypocalcemia can occur and may influence the clinical manifestations.

***Changes in ECG.*** Changes in the ECG that may be seen with hypomagnesemia include prolonged PR interval, widened QRS complex, depressed ST segment, peaked T waves, and arrhythmias (atrial fibrillation, supraventricular or ventricular tachycardia, ventricular fibrillation). Hypomagnesemia also predisposes patients to digitalis-induced arrhythmias.

### Diagnosis

Assessing Mg status is difficult because there exists no accurate laboratory test to measure total body Mg; only 1% of the body's Mg is present in the serum. Low serum Mg supports a total body Mg deficiency; however, normal serum Mg levels can occur in the presence of total body Mg deficiency. Measurement of serum ionized Mg more accurately assesses total body Mg and is recommended.

### Treatment

Magnesium supplementation is indicated when serum Mg is <1 mg/dl or in the presence of clinical signs or refractory hypokalemia or hypocalcemia. Mild hypomagnesemia may resolve with treatment of the underlying disease, administration of Mg-containing fluids, or correction of hypophosphatemia (if present). Dogs on long-term diuretic and digoxin therapy may benefit from oral Mg supplementation or use of potassium- (and Mg-) sparing diuretics. Renal function must be assessed before supplementation; the Mg dose should be reduced by 50% to 75% in azotemic patients and serum Mg monitored frequently. Use with digitalis cardioglycosides can cause serious conduction disturbances.

***Oral and Intravenous supplements.*** Mg oxide or hydroxide (1 to 2 mEq of $Mg^{++}$ per kilogram per day) is used for oral therapy. The primary adverse effect is diarrhea. Parenteral solutions of Mg sulfate and Mg chloride are available; the intravenous dose is 0.75 to 1 mEq of $Mg^{++}$ per kilogram per day, administered by continuous-rate infusion in $D_5W$. For treatment of life-threatening ventricular arrhythmias, 0.15 to 0.3 mEq of $Mg^{++}$ per kilogram is administered IV over 5 to 15 minutes. The Mg solution should be diluted to 20% in $D_5W$. (Note: Mg is incompatible with sodium bicarbonate, Ca, hydrocortisone, and dobutamine hydrochloride.)

### Monitoring

Serum Mg, Ca, and potassium levels should be monitored daily. The goal is resolution of clinical signs and/or refractory hypokalemia and hypocalcemia. Parenteral administration of magnesium sulfate may cause significant hypocalcemia such that Ca infusion may be necessary. Other adverse effects of magnesium therapy include hypotension, atrioventricular and bundle branch blocks, and, with overdose, respiratory depression and cardiac arrest. Overdose is treated with calcium gluconate, 10 to 50 mg/kg IV.

## Drugs Used in Electrolyte and Metabolic Disorders

| Generic name (trade name) | Purpose | Recommended dose | |
|---|---|---|---|
| | | Dogs | Cats |
| Calcitonin—salmon (Calcimar) | Treat hypercalcemia | 4 U/kg IV, then 4-8 U/kg q12-24h | Unknown |
| Calcium—injectable and oral preparations | Treat hypocalcemia | See Table 50-4 | See Table 50-4 |
| Calcium gluconate—10% | Treat hyperkalemia | 2-10 ml IV, slow infusion; 0.5-1 ml/kg, slow IV infusion | 2-10 ml IV, slow infusion |
| Cholestyramine (Questran) | Treat idiopathic hypercholesterolemia | 1-2 g PO q12h | Unknown |
| Clofibrate (Atromid-S) | Treat idiopathic hypertriglyceridemia | 500 mg PO q12h | Unknown |
| Etidronate disodium (Didronel) | Treat hypercalcemia | 10-40 mg/kg PO divided q8-12h | 10-40 mg/kg PO divided q8-12h |
| Furosemide (Lasix) | Treat hypercalcemia and hypermagnesemia | 2-4 mg/kg PO, IV q8-12h | 2-4 mg/kg PO, IV q8-12h |
| Gemfibrozil (Lopid) | Treat idiopathic hypertriglyceridemia | 200 mg PO q24h | 10 mg/kg PO q12h |
| Insulin—regular crystalline | Treat hyperkalemia | 0.5-1 U/kg plus 2 g dextrose per unit of insulin in parenteral fluids IV | 0.5-1 U/kg plus 2 g dextrose per unit of insulin in parenteral fluids IV |
| Lovostatin (Mevacor) | Treat idiopathic hypercholesterolemia | 10-20 mg PO q24h | Unknown |
| Magnesium—injectable and oral preparations | Treat hypomagnesemia | See p 533 | See p 533 |
| Marine-life oil supplements | Treat idiopathic hypertriglyceridemia | 10-30 mg/kg PO q24h | 10-30 mg/kg PO q24h |
| Niacin | Treat idiopathic hypertriglyceridemia | 100 mg PO q24h | Unknown |
| Potassium gluconate (Kaon Elixir; Tumil-K) | Treat hypokalemia | 2.2 mEq K+/100 kcal food consumed or 2 mEq K+/ 4.5 kg PO q12h | 2.2 mEq K+/100 kcal food consumed or 2 mEq K+/4.5 kg PO q12h |
| Prednisone | Treat hypercalcemia | 1-2 mg/kg PO q12h | 1-2 mg/kg PO q12h |
| Sodium bicarbonate | Treat hyperkalemia | 1-2 mEq/kg IV, slow bolus | 1-2 mEq/kg IV, slow bolus |
| Vitamin D preparations | Treat hypocalcemia | See Table 50-5 | See Table 50-5 |

*IV,* Intravenously; *K+,* potassium; *PO,* orally.

# PART VIII

# Reproductive System Disorders

CHERI A. JOHNSON

# 56

# Disorders
# of the Estrous Cycle

## (Text pp 847-869)

### DIAGNOSTIC TESTS (TEXT PP 853-859)

#### Vaginal Cytology

Vaginal cytology is used to determine the present stage of the estrous cycle, breeding and whelping dates, and the nature of certain abnormal processes within the reproductive tract. Its importance in breeding management and in the evaluation of reproductive disorders cannot be overemphasized. Specimens can be stained with Wright's, Wright-Giemsa, Diff-Quik, trichrome, or new methylene blue.

Vaginal cytology is very useful in the breeding management of bitches, especially when the female does not exhibit strong behavioral estrus or when the breeding pair are geographically separate and either the animals or semen must be transported. The transition from proestrus, through estrus, and into diestrus usually is adequately monitored by cytologic evaluation every other day.

Throughout the estrous cycle, vaginal cytology in queens is similar to that in bitches, except that red blood cells (RBCs) are much less common. Following is a brief description of vaginal cytologic changes during the normal estrous cycle in bitches.

##### Proestrus

Proestrus is characterized by vulvar swelling, serosanguineous vulvar discharge, and attraction of males but unwillingness to allow copulation. During early proestrus, parabasal and intermediate epithelial cells predominate >80%). As proestrus progresses, parabasal cells disappear as superficial cells increase in number. By late proestrus, superficial and anuclear squamous cells account for 70% to 80% of the epithelial cells. RBCs are present throughout proestrus, and white blood cells (WBCs) decrease in number. Extracellular bacteria may be seen. (Note: On the basis of a single cytologic specimen, early to mid proestrus cannot be distinguished from diestrus.)

##### Estrus

Estrus is characterized by acceptance of mating. The vulva is less swollen and the discharge is usually less bloody than during proestrus. However, normal bitches often have a sanguineous discharge throughout proestrus and estrus, so changes in the gross appearance of the discharge are not a reliable indicator of the transition into estrus. Vaginal cytology during estrus is characterized by a predominance (90%) of superficial and anuclear squamous cells and a clear background. WBCs are absent, but RBCs and extracellular bacteria are often present.

##### Diestrus and anestrus

Diestrus begins with the bitch's refusal to mate. No external signs mark the onset of diestrus other than cessation of the signs of estrus. Diestrus is characterized cytologically by a sudden reduction in superficial cells and the reappearance of intermediate cells, neutrophils, and background debris. On the first day of diestrus, parabasal and intermediate cells outnumber superficial and anuclear squamous cells; sheets of intermediate cells are often seen. WBCs return in high numbers during the first 1 or 2 days, and RBCs and bacteria disappear. This initial dramatic change is followed by a gradual change to anestrous cytology, which is quite hypocellular and primarily consists of parabasal cells and small intermediate epithelial cells.

## Vaginoscopy
Vaginoscopy is useful for determining the stage of the estrous cycle, evaluating anatomic abnormalities, determining the source of vulvar discharge (vestibule, vagina, or uterus), and determining the nature and extent of lesions within the vestibule and vagina. Samples for cytology, microbiology, and histopathology can easily be obtained through the endoscope. Equipment and techniques are discussed in the text.

## Vaginal Bacterial Culture
Bacterial infections of the reproductive tract are relatively common. Bacterial culture is indicated in many reproductive disorders, including infertility, purulent vulvar discharge, pyometra, metritis, and abortion or stillbirth. Vaginal culture is often performed in place of uterine culture. The normal bacterial flora of the canine vagina are listed in Box 56-1. The normal flora of the feline vagina are similar, with *Staphylococcus* spp., *Streptococcus canis*, and *Escherichia coli* the most common organisms.

Most of the organisms that constitute the normal flora are potential pathogens, but isolation of such organisms is not necessarily proof of infection. In normal bitches and queens, mixed populations of these organisms are usually recovered in small numbers. *Brucella canis* is always considered a pathogen, however, even in the absence of clinical signs. Heavy growth of a single organism may also be significant.

## Virology
Canine herpesvirus and feline herpesvirus I (feline viral rhinotracheitis) cause respiratory disease, as well as genital lesions, failure to conceive, abortion, and neonatal death.

---

**Box 56-1**

### Normal Bacterial Flora of the Canine Vagina

| AEROBIC BACTERIA | ANAEROBIC BACTERIA |
|---|---|
| Escherichia coli | *Bacteroides melaninogenicus* |
| Coagulase-positive and coagulase-negative staphylococci | *Corynebacterium* |
| α-Hemolytic and β-hemolytic streptococci | *Haemophilus aphrophilus* |
| Nonhemolytic streptococci | *Bacteroides* |
| *Proteus* | *Enterococcus* |
| *Bacillus* | *Peptostreptococcus* (hemolytic and nonhemolytic) |
| *Corynebacterium* | *Mycoplasma** |
| *Pseudomonas* | *Ureaplasma** |
| *Klebsiella* | |
| *Neisseria* | |
| *Micrococcus* | |
| *Haemophilus* | |
| *Moraxella* | |
| *Pasteurella* | |
| *Acinetobacter* | |
| *Flavobacterium* | |
| *Lactobacillus* | |
| *Enterobacter* | |

*See discussion of these infectious agents in Chapter 63.

Respiratory disease and neonatal death are the most common manifestations; rarely, vesicular lesions are found on the mucosa of the vestibule or prepuce. The virus may be isolated from nasal, conjunctival, tracheal, vaginal, or preputial scrapings from symptomatic animals. If clinical signs are compatible, any detectable serum antibody titer for canine herpesvirus is significant. Panleukopenia, feline infectious peritonitis, and feline leukemia virus infection are other potential causes of infertility in queens.

## Measurement of Reproductive Hormones

Reproductive hormones are released in a cyclic, episodic, or pulsatile manner, so the results of hormone testing must be interpreted with this in mind. Serial measurements or provocative testing is often needed. Most hormone assays depend on immunologic reactions; for reliable results the laboratory must have validated the procedures and determined reference ranges for each species and each hormone to be tested.

### Progesterone

Measurement of serum progesterone can be used to identify functional corpora lutea, confirm that ovulation occurred, monitor diestrus and, in bitches, approximate the time of impending ovulation. Point-of-care enzyme-linked immunosorbent assay (ELISA) kits (Status Pro, Progest Assay; Ovucheck; PreMate) provide immediate results and allow in-clinic serial monitoring of serum progesterone. The Canine Ovulation Timing Test (ICG-Status-Pro), which is marketed for use in dogs, is also useful for assessing serum progesterone in cats.

***Normal values.*** In bitches serum progesterone remains at basal levels (<1 ng/ml or <3.2 nmol/L) during proestrus and rises to >2 ng/ml (>6 nmol/L) at or shortly before the preovulatory luteinizing hormone (LH) surge; ovulation follows the LH surge by approximately 2 days. Therefore serial measurement of serum progesterone during proestrus can be used to estimate the time of ovulation. Serum progesterone increases rapidly after ovulation in both bitches and queens and plateaus 2 to 4 weeks later. It then gradually declines, reaching basal levels in nonpregnant bitches 60 to 90 days after the LH surge. In nonpregnant queens that ovulated, progesterone declines to basal levels by 30 to 40 days after ovulation.

***Breeding management.*** Some investigators recommend timing insemination to occur 3 to 6 days after the initial rise in serum progesterone. Others recommend timing insemination with a specific progesterone concentration or range; pregnancy rates are best when insemination is performed while serum progesterone is between 8 and 19 ng/ml (25.4 to 60 nmol/L).

***Other uses.*** High diestrual serum progesterone confirms that ovulation did occur, an important finding in the workup of infertility, recognition of "silent" or unobserved heat, and confirmation of ovarian remnant syndrome. Adequacy of luteal function can be monitored by measuring serum progesterone weekly throughout pregnancy. The date of parturition can also be predicted by monitoring serum progesterone. In bitches (but not necessarily in queens), parturition occurs within 48 hours after serum progesterone falls below 2 ng/ml (6 nmol/L).

### Estradiol

Measurement of serum estradiol can help identify follicular ovarian cysts, estrogen-secreting ovarian or testicular tumors, and estrus in females suspected of having "silent" or unobserved heats or ovarian remnant syndrome. However, serum estradiol is often at or below the limits of detection for the assays used by many commercial endocrine laboratories. It also fluctuates widely and rapidly, and the high concentrations that occur during proestrus may be detectable for only 1 or 2 days. Pathologic increases, such as occur with ovarian follicular cysts or Sertoli cell tumors, may still be less than the detectable limits of many assays. Therefore measurement of estradiol does not often yield diagnostic results.

Because estrogen causes proliferation and cornification of vaginal epithelial cells, vaginal cytology is often preferable to the measurement of serum estradiol in females. The preputial epithelium is also responsive to estrogen, exhibiting changes similar to those of the vaginal epithelium, so preputial cytology may be helpful for demonstrating estrogen-secreting testicular tumors in male dogs.

### LH and follicle-stimulating hormone

Concentrations of LH and follicle-stimulating hormone (FSH) are low during most of proestrus, increase in a preovulatory surge, and then decline, although LH may increase during diestrus. Identification of the preovulatory LH surge can be useful in canine breeding management, but because the LH surge lasts only 24 to 72 hours, frequent (at least once per day) sampling is necessary. Because of the expense and frequent sampling required, serum progesterone is often used in place of LH to estimate the timing of ovulation.

In identification of animals with inadequate gonadotropin secretion, multiple measurements of LH (e.g., three samples every 20 minutes) are more likely than a single measurement to distinguish normal from abnormal animals. The secretory capacity of the pituitary gonadotropins can also be assessed by measuring LH (and/or FSH) before and after administration of gonadotropin-releasing hormone (GnRH).

*Other uses.* Elevated LH has been noted in bitches with ovarian dysplasia and in animals with primary ovarian failure or previous oophorectomy. Evaluation of LH is therefore helpful in distinguishing between ovariectomized and sexually intact bitches: low serum LH in a single blood sample confirms the presence of negative feedback from ovarian tissue. However, high serum LH in a single sample is not necessarily a reliable indicator of ovariectomy because it could also represent the normal pulsatile release of LH during the ovarian cycle. The commercially available ELISA test (ICG Status-LH Canine Ovulation Timing Test) is suitable for this purpose.

### GnRH stimulation test

Exogenous GnRH can be used to evaluate the pituitary-gonadal axis and to determine whether functional gonads are present. After administration of GnRH to normal dogs and cats, a prompt (<30 min) increase occurs in serum LH. GnRH causes ovulation and a subsequent increase in serum progesterone only if administered during estrus to females with mature ovarian follicles; serum progesterone should not change substantially in response to GnRH administration at other times. Serum testosterone increases after GnRH in normal males. Absence of an increase in serum LH after GnRH administration suggests a pituitary problem. Protocols are discussed in the text.

### Relaxin

Relaxin is a hormone produced primarily by the placenta, so elevated serum relaxin is a very specific indicator of pregnancy. A test kit (Witness Relaxin) can detect relaxin in pregnant bitches 26 to 31 days after the LH surge. False-negative results occur if the test is performed too early during gestation; it is a more sensitive indicator of pregnancy when performed >30 days after breeding. A negative result could occur if the litter size is small. Relaxin disappears from the blood after abortion. Although pregnant cats also produce relaxin, this test has not yet been validated for accuracy in cats.

## Radiography and Ultrasonography

Radiology and ultrasonography are useful for evaluating the ovaries, uterine wall thickness, and uterine contents; for confirming pregnancy; and for assessing fetal viability. Ultrasonography may also help in identification of ovarian cysts in animals with persistent anestrus (nonfunctional or luteal cysts) or persistent estrus and hyperestrogenism (follicular cysts) and identification of ovarian neoplasia.

Vaginography can be considered if vaginoscopy fails to clearly identify strictures, anatomic defects, masses, or foreign material in the vagina. Positive-contrast vaginography using a Foley catheter and a water-soluble contrast agent (e.g., Renografin) is easily performed, but general anesthesia is necessary.

## Karyotyping

Some intersex conditions and developmental reproductive abnormalities are associated with chromosomal anomalies (e.g., XXX, XO). Affected animals usually have abnormal external genitalia, infertility, or persistent anestrus. Karyotype analysis can be considered when a congenital problem is suspected but routine diagnostic tests have failed to identify the cause of infertility.

### Laparoscopy and Celiotomy

Diagnostic laparoscopy or exploratory celiotomy should not be done until a non-invasive diagnostic evaluation has been completed. Laparoscopy and celiotomy allow visualization of the reproductive tract, bacterial culture of the uterine lumen, and full-thickness biopsy of the uterus. The patency of the uterine horn and possibly uterine tube lumina can be determined by infusion of sterile saline solution. Laparoscopy and celiotomy are best performed during anestrus.

## FEMALE INFERTILITY (TEXT PP 859-865)

### General Approach

A thorough history is critical in the evaluation of female infertility. History taking should investigate as many details as possible, including the present stage of the estrous cycle, a description of previous cycles, assessment of the male's fertility, events after breeding or unbred cycles, previous diagnosis and treatment, and non-reproductive problems and husbandry. The reproductive history often dictates the diagnostic approach. Most important are establishing the cycling behavior and interestrous interval of the female, identifying the criteria used to determine when the female is bred, and determining the female's behavior during mating.

#### Physical examination

A complete physical examination should be performed to identify (1) potential causes of infertility outside the reproductive tract; (2) other abnormalities that might affect the health of the female or the pregnancy itself should conception occur; and (3) congenital or heritable defects that should exclude this female from a breeding program.

*Reproductive tract.* The mammary glands are carefully palpated to assess size and consistency and the character of any secretions. The vulva, vestibular mucosa, and clitoris (bitches) are inspected for structural abnormalities and discharges. The uterus is then palpated transabdominally; vulvar discharge may be more apparent after abdominal palpation. The vestibule and posterior vagina should be palpated with a gloved finger in bitches of adequate size. Rectal palpation can also help determine the extent of abnormal vaginal structures.

#### Clinical pathology

Historic or physical abnormalities outside the reproductive tract should be investigated by evaluating a complete blood count (CBC), serum biochemistry panel, and urinalysis. All dogs should be tested for *B. canis* before breeding and before infertility is evaluated further.

### Failure to Cycle

Animals with persistent anestrus fall into two subcategories: primary anestrus, which affects females >24 months of age that have never cycled, and secondary anestrus, which affects females that have previously cycled but are no longer cycling. Gonadal dysfunction (e.g., intersex conditions, ovarian dysgenesis, progesterone-secreting luteal cysts, ovarian tumor), concurrent metabolic disorders or medications (e.g., hypothyroidism, glucocorticoid therapy), and advancing age should be considered in females that were cycling in the past.

#### Primary anestrus

An animal that has never cycled may be a normal prepubertal animal, may be experiencing "silent" heats, may have a congenital gonadal or chromosomal anomaly, or may have a concurrent disorder that is preventing estrous cycles. Exposure to light may be inadequate to initiate and maintain cyclicity in queens with persistent anestrus. Diagnostic tests for persistent anestrus are usually delayed until a female is 2 years of age because of the probability that she is a normal prepubertal animal.

*Silent heat.* Unobserved or silent heats may be detected retrospectively by measuring serum progesterone. If the concentration is >2 ng/ml (>6.4 nmol/L) in a bitch, a cycle has occurred within the last 60 to 90 days. The finding of high serum progesterone in a supposedly anestrous queen indicates that unobserved estrus has occurred and also that either unobserved mating or spontaneous ovulation occurred within the past 30 to 40 days. Clinical signs of false pregnancy (see p 557) would also indicate that an undetected cycle occurred approximately 45 days earlier in the queen or approximately 60 days earlier in the bitch. A silent cycle could be detected prospectively by examining vaginal cytology every 1 to 2 weeks.

*Gonadal dysfunction.* The functional status of the hypothalamic-pituitary-ovarian axis can be evaluated by measuring serum LH before and after GnRH administration. Serum progesterone can be measured to identify functional luteal cysts. Ultrasonographic evaluation of the ovaries may identify ovarian abnormalities such as cysts or neoplasia. Many phenotypically female intersex animals have detectable anatomic abnormalities of the clitoris, vestibule, and/or vagina. If these areas appear normal, measurement of serum testosterone after administration of human chorionic gonadotropin (hCG) or GnRH could be used to demonstrate the presence of testicular tissue. Karyotyping can also be performed, although intersex animals may have normal karyotypes. Abnormal karyotypes have been found in bitches and queens with ovarian dysgenesis.

*Other tests.* Induction of estrus may be tried if other diagnostic tests have failed to identify the cause of persistent anestrus. Exploratory celiotomy or laparoscopy, to assess the gross appearance of the reproductive tract and obtain biopsy specimens of the internal genitalia, should be considered only after all noninvasive diagnostic methods have been tried.

## Prolonged Interestrous Interval

Interestrous intervals of >12 months in bitches and >1 month in cycling queens usually are abnormal, although long interestrous intervals are normal in breeds of dogs that cycle only once a year (e.g., Basenjis, Tibetan Mastiffs, Dingoes). Pregnancy and pseudopregnancy lengthen the interestrous interval in queens but not in bitches. Prolonged interestrous intervals can also occur with increasing age.

### Diagnostic approach

Many of the causes of persistent anestrus, such as glucocorticoid administration in bitches and inadequate photoperiod in queens, can cause prolonged interestrous intervals. Silent heats could also be considered. The diagnostic approach should include (1) review of estrous identification techniques used by the owner and medications being administered, (2) assessment of overall metabolic health (CBC, serum biochemistry panel, urinalysis), and (3) in bitches, evaluation of thyroid gland and possibly adrenocortical function.

## Short Interestrous Interval

Interestrous intervals of <4 months are occasionally seen in bitches; many of these dogs are infertile, perhaps because the endometrium has not recovered from the previous cycle. In some breeds (e.g., German Shepherd Dogs) and in some individuals, an interestrous interval of 4 to 4 1/2 months is normal and may not interfere with fertility. Administration of gonadotropins, prostaglandin $F_{2a}$, prolactin antagonists, or estrogen can artificially shorten the interestrous interval. In most bitches, however, the cause of short interestrous interval is not discovered.

### Split heat

In bitches a short interestrous interval must be differentiated from a split heat cycle, in which proestrus stops without progressing to estrus then begins again 2 to 4 weeks later and progresses through normal, fertile estrus. Split heats are seen most often in pubertal bitches; normal proestrus and estrus usually occur during subsequent cycles. Rarely do split heats occur repeatedly. They do not cause infertility, other than misleading the kennel manager.

### Management

Diagnostic tests are usually not performed in bitches with confirmed short interestrous intervals. Administration of an androgen (e.g., methyltestosterone) to prevent estrus for at least 6 months can be considered; however, affected bitches usually remain subfertile. Breeding on the first estrus after therapy is important, as short interestrous intervals frequently resume. Use of progestins (e.g., megestrol acetate) to delay the next cycle is not recommended.

## Abnormal Proestrus and Estrus

The most common abnormalities of proestrus and estrus are refusal to allow mating, prolonged estrus, and abnormally short estrus.

### Refusal to mate

Females that are not in estrus refuse to mate. Inexperienced and timid females may also be reluctant to breed, and bitches with hypothyroidism may not exhibit normal behavior during estrus. Some females refuse to mate with one male but are willing with another. Vaginal cytology should be performed to identify the stage of the cycle.

*Genital abnormalities.* In bitches, abnormalities of the vulva or vagina are a common cause of refusal to mate. Abnormalities include vaginal strictures, congenital defects, vaginal hyperplasia or prolapse, and rarely, vaginal neoplasia. Digital palpation identifies vaginal prolapse and most strictures and congenital defects. Vaginoscopy can be performed when digital palpation fails to reveal a problem. Vaginal strictures that are identified during anestrus should always be palpated again during estrus to determine their significance. Similarly, normal findings during anestrus do not exclude vaginal hyperplasia or prolapse (which occurs only with estrogenic stimulation).

*Management.* Artificial insemination can be used to breed otherwise normal, estrual females that refuse to mate and those with vaginal hyperplasia or prolapse. Other physical abnormalities should be surgically corrected if the female is to remain in the breeding program. Surgery is best performed during anestrus.

### Prolonged estrus

In normal, fertile bitches, proestrus can last as long as 17 days and estrus as long as 21 days. A season (proestrus plus estrus) is not considered abnormally long in bitches until it exceeds 35 days. In queens, estrus lasting longer than 16 days is abnormal. Prolonged proestrus and estrus are usually caused by functional follicular cysts, although ovarian neoplasia and exogenous estrogen administration should also be considered.

*Diagnosis.* Vaginal cytology should be performed to confirm that estrogenic stimulation is a likely cause of the behavioral and physical signs. Abdominal ultrasonography, measurement of serum estrogen (increased), or exploratory celiotomy can be performed to identify follicular cysts.

*Treatment.* Spontaneous regression often occurs, so waiting 2 to 4 weeks is commonly recommended. Manual rupture via celiotomy can be performed in bitches with persistent or enlarging cysts. Alternatively, induction of ovulation can be attempted with GnRH (Cystorelin, 2.2 µg/kg intramuscularly [IM] once daily for 3 days), although results are variable. If mature follicles are present and can be induced to ovulate, signs of estrus usually resolve in 5 to 7 days. Ovariohysterectomy should be considered for females that fail to respond promptly to medical management.

### Short estrus

Abnormally short estrus (<3 days in bitches and <1 day in queens) is most often the result of an error in observation or recognition of estrus. Females >6 years of age may experience erratic cycles, including short estrus. Split heat cycles should also be considered in bitches. In some animals short estrus is normal.

Methods of proestrous and estrous detection should be changed in females with truly short estrus so that they can be bred at the appropriate time. Vaginal cytology or exposure to a male should begin well before the expected onset of the next estrus and continue until the first day of estrus is identified. Using measurement of serum progesterone or LH helps identify the optimal time for insemination.

## Infertility with Normal Cycles

Infertility in an otherwise normal female may result from male infertility, improper breeding management, reproductive tract lesions or infection, early embryonic death, or advancing age. Because of the age-related decrease in fertility after 6 years of age, an extensive diagnostic evaluation of older females may not be warranted.

### Male infertility

A common cause of apparent infertility in a normally cycling female is male infertility. The male should be evaluated (see Chapter 60) before an extensive diagnostic evaluation of the female is undertaken. Verification that the male successfully sired litters shortly before *and* shortly after breeding the bitch in question is good circumstantial evidence against male infertility.

### Breeding management

The most common causes of infertility in females with normal estrous cycles are improper timing of insemination and poor semen quality. A thorough breeding management history, particularly how the owner determines when to breed, is imperative.

*Identifying estrus.* The first day of estrus can be identified on the basis of behavioral or vaginal cytologic changes, but it cannot be recognized unless the bitch is first examined during proestrus. Cytologic examination should begin on the first or second day of proestrus and should be repeated every 2 to 3 days until 50% to 60% cornification occurs, at which time serum progesterone is measured for ovulation timing. Vaginal cytology performed in early proestrus may also allow identification of pathologic processes within the reproductive tract that could contribute to infertility.

*Number and timing of matings.* Allowing only one mating or restricting multiple matings to a short period (e.g., 24 hours) are common causes of infertility in bitches. Conception rates are improved by performing or allowing at least two inseminations, usually 24 to 48 hours apart, during the fertile period. Litter size may also increase when multiple breedings are made possible. In queens the frequency of mating is a more important determinant of ovulation, and therefore conception, than is the day of the cycle on which mating occurs.

### Ovulation failure and premature luteolysis

Ovarian pathology or, in queens, inadequate coital stimulation can prevent ovulation. Premature luteolysis or failure of the corpus luteum (CL) to maintain progesterone production is another cause of early embryonic loss (infertility) in normally cycling females.

*Differentiation.* There are two ways to differentiate ovulation failure from premature luteolysis. One is serial measurement of serum progesterone from proestrus through diestrus. Progesterone concentrations that never exceed 8 ng/ml (25 nmol/L) suggest ovulation failure; premature luteolysis is reflected by a more rapid decline than normal from high postovulatory concentrations.

The other way is to document early embryonic death with ultrasonography, beginning 10 days (cats) or 14 days (dogs) after breeding. However, pregnancy is very difficult to detect sonographically so early in gestation; negative findings are not conclusive before day 28. Detecting relaxin in an animal that was no longer pregnant would indicate very recent embryonic death.

### Other causes of infertility or early embryonic death

Lesions of the vagina, uterus, uterine tubes, placenta, or the conceptus itself can cause infertility or early embryonic death in a normally cycling female. Any condition that interferes with gamete or zygote transport or that creates an inhospitable environment can cause infertility. Abnormalities include developmental defects in the vagina (e.g., agenesis, vertical vaginal septa), cystic endometrial hyperplasia, bacterial endometritis, infectious placentitis, and congenital fetal anomalies that are incompatible with life.

Infectious agents are an important cause of early embryonic death and infertility. Although many agents are capable of causing placentitis or fetal death, *B. canis* in bitches and herpesvirus infection in queens are of most importance. Glucocorticoids and some antibiotics can also cause embryonic death.

*Diagnostic approach.* The diagnostic approach in a normally cycling female that has been appropriately bred to a fertile male and that is known to have ovulated should begin with a review of the history to identify potential causes of early embryonic death. Special attention should be paid to medications administered to the female and to signs of infectious disease in the colony. Serologic tests for herpesvirus and *B. canis* should be performed.

Vaginal lesions can easily be excluded by vaginoscopy and vaginal cytology. Anterior vaginal cultures should be performed in lieu of uterine cultures. Finally, exploratory celiotomy can be performed during anestrus to visualize the reproductive tract, assess the patency of the uterus and uterine tubes, obtain uterine specimens for culture, and obtain full-thickness uterine biopsy specimens for histologic assessment.

## ESTROUS SUPPRESSION AND POPULATION CONTROL (TEXT PP 865-867)

Ovariohysterectomy and castration are the most common methods of population control in dogs and cats. Other methods of sterilization are discussed in the text. The use of abortifacients to abort unwanted puppies and kittens is discussed in Chapter 59. Temporary suppression of estrus is sometimes desired and can be achieved by administering progestins (e.g., megestrol acetate), androgens, or GnRH analogs.

### Megestrol Acetate

Megestrol acetate (Ovaban) is the only progestin approved for estrous control in bitches in the United States; it is not approved for use in cats. Medroxyprogesterone acetate (MPA) and proligestone are commonly used for estrous suppression in other countries. The slow-release subdermal implant of levonorgestrel (Norplant) can be effective in suppressing estrus for 12 months in cats, with no adverse effects except the development of cystic endometrial hyperplasia. Progestins are most reliable in preventing estrus when treatment is initiated during anestrus; they are less reliable when administered during early proestrus.

#### Adverse effects

Progestins have many undesirable effects at therapeutic doses, including cystic endometrial hyperplasia with an increased potential for pyometra, mammary hyperplasia, and increased incidence of mammary tumors. When progestin therapy is discontinued, signs of false pregnancy can develop. Other adverse effects include diabetes mellitus, acromegaly, and adrenocortical suppression. In bitches, long-term treatment with high doses of some progestins (e.g., MPA, proligestone) may result in iatrogenic hyperadrenocorticism, including steroid hepatopathy. Alopecia, thinning of the skin, and hair discoloration at the site of injection have also been observed. For these reasons progestins are not recommended for estrous suppression.

### Androgens

Although not approved for this use, various forms of testosterone (e.g., testosterone propionate IM; methyltestosterone orally) are routinely administered to Greyhound bitches during training and racing. Prolonged anestrus occurs in some bitches after androgen therapy is discontinued.

#### Adverse effects

Adverse effects of androgens, including mibolerone, are clitoral hypertrophy (sometimes with permanent ossification), mucopurulent vulvar discharge, and vaginitis. Liver enzyme activity can also be increased. These effects are usually reversible after mibolerone is discontinued, but they can persist for months or years. Masculinization of female fetuses, which is irreversible, occurs if androgens are administered to pregnant females. Additional androgenic effects include an apparent increase in muscle mass and aggressiveness.

## GnRH Agonists

The GnRH agonist deslorelin effectively suppresses reproductive function for >1 year in male and female dogs and cats when administered as a slow-release subcutaneous implant. Depending on the stage of the cycle at which the drug is implanted, it can initially induce an estrous cycle. This unwanted effect can be overcome by the simultaneous administration of a progestin such as megestrol acetate. Another GnRH agonist, nafarelin, is also effective in estrous suppression in bitches.

## OVARIAN REMNANT SYNDROME (TEXT PP 867-868)

Occasionally queens and bitches resume or continue to exhibit signs of estrus after oophorectomy. The most common cause is remnant ovarian tissue that has regained folliculogenesis and estrogen production.

### Diagnosis

High concentrations of estrogen are indicated by cornified superficial epithelial cells on vaginal cytology. This finding justifies exploratory celiotomy to find and remove the ovarian remnants. If additional confirmation is desired before surgery, serum progesterone can be measured 5 to 7 days after expected ovulation. Serum progesterone >2 ng/ml (>6.4 nmol/L) is indicative of spontaneous ovulation and the presence of corpora lutea (CL). Alternatively, ovulation can be induced during estrus by administering hCG (10 U/kg IM in bitches; 250 IU/queen IM) or GnRH (0.5 µg/kg IM in bitches; 25 µg/queen IM). After 5 to 7 days, serum progesterone is >2 ng/ml if functional ovarian tissue is present.

### Treatment

Treatment consists of surgical removal of the ovarian remnants. Because these remnants often are small, they may be easier to identify during or shortly after estrus when follicles or CLs are present, rather than during anestrus.

## OVARIAN TUMORS (TEXT PP 867-868)

Granulosa cell tumors can occur in ovarian remnants as well as in intact females. Dogs with estrogen-producing ovarian tumors show signs of estrus, bone marrow toxicity, and/or dermatologic changes. These tumors do not respond to exogenous hCG or GnRH. Dogs with progesterone-producing granulosa cell tumors may show mammary gland development and may have cystic endometrial hyperplasia. Elevated serum progesterone confirms the presence of ovarian tissue.

## ESTROUS INDUCTION (TEXT PP 868-869)

Estrous induction can be attempted in bitches to shorten the normal interestrous interval; in bitches and queens to treat prolonged anestrus and to time pregnancy and parturition for the owners' convenience; and to synchronize estrus for embryo transfer. Of the many methods investigated for estrous induction in bitches, none is routinely effective in inducing fertile estrus (see text). Until a reliable, safe method of estrous induction is found and thoroughly investigated, estrous induction should probably be reserved for bitches with pathologic anestrus.

### Photoperiod in Queens

The photoperiod can be manipulated to induce estrus in queens. Continuous exposure to 12 to 14 hours of bright light and 10 to 12 hours of dark per day causes normal, mature queens to begin cycling within 4 to 8 weeks. Housing anestrous queens with cycling queens also helps to induce estrus. If hormonal induction of estrus is to be attempted, the queen should first be exposed to a minimum of 12 hours of light or day for several months. Protocols for hormonal induction of estrus in queens are discussed in the text.

## INDUCTION OF OVULATION (TEXT P 869)

Hormonal induction of ovulation succeeds only when mature ovarian follicles are present. It may be indicated in females with ovulation failure or with persistent estrus caused by follicular cysts.

### Queens

Ovulation in queens can be induced hormonally or mechanically (provided there exists sufficient vaginal stimulation to induce an LH surge). Administration of hCG (250 IU, IM) or GnRH (Cystorelin, 25 μg IM) on the first 2 days of estrus is recommended, although a single dose of GnRH causes an LH surge in normal cats. Brief (seconds) probing of the vagina with a smooth rod (e.g., thermometer) or cotton swab four to eight times at 5- to 20-minute intervals can also stimulate an LH surge. Repeated stimulation on several days is most likely to induce ovulation.

Successful stimulation of ovulation does not shorten that estrus but delays the onset of the next cycle. Estrus usually resumes 45 days (range, 35 to 70 days) after nonfertile induction of ovulation. Pseudopregnancy occurs if the queen ovulates but does not conceive.

### Bitches

Ovulation in bitches is induced with hCG (22 IU/kg IM) or GnRH (50 to 100 μg IM or Cystorelin at 2.2 μg/kg IM), given on the first day of estrus. Success can be confirmed by documenting serum progesterone >5 ng/ml in early diestrus. Treatment of follicular cysts using GnRH (2.2 μg/kg IM once daily for 3 days) has been disappointing.

# 57

# Disorders of the Vagina and Uterus

## (Text pp 870-881)

## VULVAR DISCHARGE (TEXT PP 870-872)

The source and significance of a vulvar discharge are determined by its cellular composition and by the stage of the reproductive cycle (Box 57-1). The diagnostic approach to vulvar discharge is discussed later.

### Etiology

*Hemorrhagic discharge.* Red blood cells (RBCs) are commonly found in both normal and abnormal vulvar discharges. Their significance is determined by the other types of cells present. RBCs are expected during proestrus and estrus. When RBCs predominate in the absence of cornified vaginal epithelial cells, a cause for hemorrhage (e.g., vaginal laceration, uterine or vaginal neoplasia subinvoluted placental sites, uterine torsion, coagulopathy) should be sought. When the number of white blood cells (WBCs) in the cytologic sample exceeds that expected in peripheral blood, a cause of inflammation rather than bleeding should be sought.

---

**Box 57-1**

## Differential Diagnoses for Vulvar Discharge Based on Predominant Cytologic Characteristics

**CORNIFIED (MATURE OR SUPERFICIAL) EPITHELIAL CELLS**
Normal proestrus
Normal estrus
Contamination with squamous epithelium
Skin or clitoris
Abnormal source of estrogen
  Exogenous
  Ovarian follicular cyst
  Ovarian neoplasia

**PERIPHERAL BLOOD**
Subinvoluted placental sites
Uterine or vaginal neoplasia
Trauma to reproductive tract
Uterine torsion
Coagulopathies

**MUCUS**
Normal late diestrus or late pregnancy
Normal lochia
Mucometra
Androgenic stimulation
(Idiopathic?)

**CELLULAR DEBRIS**
Normal lochia
Abortion

**NEUTROPHILS**
Nonseptic (no organisms seen)
  Normal first day of diestrus
  Vaginitis
  (Metritis or pyometra possible but
    unlikely)
Septic (organisms seen)
  Vaginitis
  Metritis
  Pyometra
  Abortion

---

*Neoplasia.* Leiomyoma, the most common neoplasm of the vagina and uterus in geriatric bitches and queens, often causes hemorrhagic vulvar discharge as the predominant clinical sign. Because leiomyomas do not exfoliate readily, neoplastic cells are usually not seen on cytologic preparations. Bitches with transmissible venereal tumors (TVTs) are more often examined because of a mass protruding from the vulva than for vulvar discharge. Neoplastic cells readily exfoliate from TVTs, so the diagnosis is easily made by cytology.

*Subinvolution of placental sites.* When placental sites do not involute properly, the lochia is more hemorrhagic and persists for longer than usual. Cytologically the discharge consists of RBCs with a mucoid background and some cellular debris.

*Other causes.* Uterine torsion is uncommon in bitches and queens. When it does occur, it almost always involves a near-term pregnancy. Bleeding from the vulva is uncommon in animals with coagulation defects, but it has been reported as the sole site of bleeding in some cases.

**Purulent discharge.** Purulent and mucopurulent vulvar discharges are characterized by a predominance of polymorphonuclear cells (PMNs). Large numbers of PMNs without signs of degeneration or sepsis are commonly found during the first 1 or 2 days of diestrus. This normal diestrual event can be differentiated from inflammation by the absence of clinical signs, the temporal correlation with estrus, and the prompt disappearance of WBCs within 48 hours. Nonseptic and septic vulvar discharges can also be caused by pyometra, metritis, abortion, and uterine stump granuloma or abscess (see Box 57-1).

*Vaginitis.* A nonseptic exudate is often found in prepubertal bitches with vaginitis. Androgenic stimulation (e.g., exogenous testosterone, intersex condition) can also cause nonseptic inflammation. Foreign material in the vagina (e.g., foxtail awns) may cause a hemorrhagic discharge, but more typically the discharge is predominantly purulent. If vulvitis or vaginitis is the cause of the discharge, hyperemia, edema, and other mucosal lesions of the vulva or vagina are found during physical and endoscopic examination. Note: The presence of vulvitis or vaginitis does not exclude the possibility of concurrent uterine pathology.

*Mucoid discharge.* Mucus is the predominant component of lochia. Mucus may also be present during normal late pregnancy and the nonpregnant luteal phase of the estrous cycle (small amounts). Cervicitis and mucometra can cause a mucoid vulvar discharge. In some bitches with slight mucous discharge, no abnormalities are found.

*Uteroverdin and cellular debris.* The presence of uteroverdin (dark green pigment) in a vulvar discharge indicates that placental separation has occurred. It is normal during stage II of parturition and during the first few hours postpartum. When seen before the onset of stage II labor, it indicates serious placental damage. When still present >12 hours postpartum, it may indicate retained placental tissue. Cellular debris is often the predominant component of the discharge that accompanies abortion or metritis associated with retained fetal or placental tissue.

### Diagnostic approach to vulvar discharge

The aim is to determine the origin of the discharge (vestibule, vagina, or uterus) and the cause. Initially the diagnostic approach includes a thorough history, physical examination, vaginal cytology, and vaginoscopy (see Chapter 56). Concurrent findings such as malaise, weight loss, vomiting, polyuria and polydipsia, fever, and dehydration are suggestive of systemic illness. Uterine disorders frequently result in systemic signs in addition to a vulvar discharge. Disorders confined to the vulva, vestibule, or vagina rarely cause signs other than vulvar discharge, licking of the vulva, or pollakiuria.

*Cytology.* The character of the vulvar discharge is determined by vaginal cytology (see Box 57-1). The presence of endometrial cells (columnar cells with basal nuclei and foamy cytoplasm) indicates uterine or cervical involvement; these cells may be a normal finding in lochia. Even in the absence of overt vulvar discharge, endometrial cells may be found in animals with cystic endometrial hyperplasia (CEH) or, less commonly, metritis.

*Other procedures.* The source of the discharge is confirmed by physical and endoscopic examination of the vestibule and vagina. When a uterine problem is suspected, abdominal radiography and/or ultrasonography should also be performed.

## CONGENITAL ANOMALIES OF THE VAGINA AND VULVA (TEXT PP 872-873)

Congenital anomalies of the vagina and vulva include a vertical band of tissue or annular fibrous stricture at the vestibulovaginal junction; elongated vertical septum that bisects the vagina; strictures within the vestibule and vagina; vaginal diverticulum (uncommon); complete duplication of parts of the urogenital tract, including a true double vagina (extremely rare); and hypoplasia or agenesis of parts of the reproductive tract. All of these anomalies have been reported in bitches, but they appear to be extremely rare in queens.

### Clinical features

These anomalies may cause no clinical signs, or they may result in chronic vaginitis. Occasionally they cause urinary incontinence from urine pooling cranial to the lesion. In breeding bitches, vulvar or vaginal anomalies may cause infertility, refusal to mate, or reluctance of the male to breed the bitch.

### Diagnosis

Vaginal and vulvar anomalies are easily identified by digital palpation. Because most are located just cranial to the urethral orifice, they are readily accessible to digital palpation and short endoscopic equipment (e.g., otoscope). Except for annular anomalies, they are almost always located on the midline. Vaginoscopy or vaginography can also be performed. Abdominal radiography or ultrasonography can be used to identify vaginal diverticula.

*Annular strictures.* Before treatment of annular strictures is considered, the bitch should be evaluated during proestrus and estrus. Especially in pubescent bitches, the vestibulovaginal junction is normally so narrow during anestrus that it may be mistaken for a stricture; this area relaxes during proestrus and estrus.

### Treatment

Treatment is unnecessary if the anomaly is causing no clinical signs. Those that are symptomatic should be surgically corrected during anestrus. Thin bands of persistent hymenal tissue can sometimes be broken using digital pressure alone, and some annular strictures are amenable to bougienage. Surgical correction is necessary for other annular strictures and vaginal septa.

### Prognosis

The prognosis for resolution of clinical signs after surgical correction of vaginal septa and hymenal remnants is excellent. Animals with annular strictures may, however, be prone to fibrosis and recurrent stricture.

## CLITORAL HYPERTROPHY (TEXT P 873)

The canine clitoris may enlarge and even ossify under the influence of androgens (e.g., exposure of female fetuses to androgens or progestins during gestation; exogenous androgen administration to female animals of any age; testicular tissue in intersex animals). Clitoral hypertrophy may go unnoticed; more commonly, however, the enlarged clitoris protrudes from the vulva.

### Clinical features

Clitoral hypertrophy is often first apparent when the female is near puberty or after administration of androgens. A mucoid discharge is common, as is licking of the area. There may also be a history of recurrent urinary tract infection. When present, ossification of the clitoris is usually palpable. The vulva may have a normal appearance and position, or it may be ventrally displaced. The vestibule-vagina may not be patent in females exposed in utero.

### Treatment

Treatment involves removal of the androgen source if it still exists. If the clitoris is ossified, it is not likely to regress, even in the absence of androgens. Unless it is clear that the female has been treated with androgens and was previously normal (e.g., racing greyhound bitches), affected animals should be evaluated for the presence of an intersex condition. Exploratory laparotomy with the intent of removing the gonads and internal genitalia may be the most cost-effective approach. Clitorectomy may also be performed if needed to eliminate the clinical signs.

## VAGINITIS (TEXT PP 874-875)

Vaginitis can occur in intact or neutered bitches of any age or breed, during any stage of the reproductive cycle. It is rare in queens. Vaginitis may result from bacterial or viral infection, reproductive tract immaturity, androgenic stimulation, chemical irritation (e.g., urine), or mechanical irritation (e.g., foreign material, neoplasia, anatomic abnormalities).

### Diagnosis

Diagnosis is primarily based on the historic and physical finding of a mucoid, mucopurulent, or purulent vulvar discharge; sanguineous discharge is rare. Licking of the vulva and pollakiuria are much less common (approximately 10% of cases). The diagnosis can be substantiated by vaginal cytology (nonseptic or septic inflammation without hemorrhage) and vaginoscopy. Vaginoscopy is especially useful for identification of anatomic abnormalities and other types of mechanical irritation that may predispose to vaginitis. Urinary tract disorders should be ruled out in animals with a history of pollakiuria (see Chapter 42).

*Bacterial culture.* The organisms isolated from bitches with vaginitis are usually those of the normal vaginal bacterial flora (see Table 56-1), so finding these potentially pathogenic organisms is not necessarily evidence of infection. The results of bacterial culture and sensitivity testing are used to formulate a therapeutic plan rather than to diagnose vaginitis.

### Treatment

*Prepubertal bitches.* In bitches <1 year of age, abnormalities are almost always limited to inflammation of the vulva and vagina, and vaginal cytology is most often nonseptic in nature. Systemic or topical antibiotics, douches, and perineal cleansing have been recommended, but in 90% of young bitches the vaginitis resolves with or without treatment; most recover spontaneously before their first estrous cycle. Young bitches with any additional historic or physical abnormalities should be evaluated further.

*Mature bitches.* Vaginitis is associated with identifiable predisposing abnormalities in approximately 70% of bitches >1 year old. The keys to successful therapy are the identification and elimination of concurrent abnormalities. Physical abnormalities of the genital tract are the most common (35%) and include vulvar anomalies, clitoral hypertrophy, vaginal strictures, vertical bands of tissue in the vagina, and vaginal neoplasia. Disorders of the urinary tract, including urinary tract infection and urinary incontinence, are the next most common (26%). Vaginoscopy, vaginal cytology, and analysis and culture of urine obtained by cystocentesis should always be included in the evaluation of mature animals with vaginitis.

*Antibiotics.* Systemic antibiotics are often beneficial, especially in animals with a known bacterial infection elsewhere (e.g., urinary tract). However, clinical signs of vaginitis recur when antibiotic therapy is stopped, unless the underlying abnormality is eliminated. Approximately 30% of mature bitches have no identifiable abnormalities other than vaginitis. Most recover spontaneously, although it may take months or years. Clinical signs can usually be lessened with intermittent systemic antibiotic therapy.

In animals with bacterial vaginitis, when a heavy growth (>100 colony-forming units) of a single organism is isolated from the vagina, it is usually considered to be a pathogen. Ampicillin, trimethoprim-sulfas, clavulanate-amoxicillin, enrofloxacin, and cephalosporins are usually effective against gram-positive and gram-negative organisms isolated from the urogenital tract. Tetracycline and chloramphenicol can also be considered for gram-negative infections. Several of these antibiotics are contraindicated during pregnancy (see Box 59-2).

*Ovariohysterectomy.* In most bitches ovariohysterectomy has no apparent effect on the outcome. Signs of vaginitis occur after ovariohysterectomy in some previously healthy bitches.

### Chronic, unresponsive vaginitis

Bacterial culture of the urine and cranial vagina should be repeated to identify resistant organisms. Vaginoscopy should also be repeated. Vaginal biopsy, preferably at the site of visible lesions or inflammation, is indicated to establish the character of the lesions (e.g., plasmacytic or lymphocytic inflammation, neoplasia, vesicular lesions with inclusion bodies suggestive of herpesvirus infection). A finding of plasmacytic or lymphocytic inflammation may support trial therapy with systemic glucocorticoids. Uterine stump abscess or pyometra should be considered in a spayed bitch with chronic vaginitis.

## VAGINAL HYPERPLASIA AND PROLAPSE (TEXT PP 875-877)

During proestrus and estrus the vaginal wall becomes edematous and hyperplastic. Sometimes the change is so severe that vaginal tissue protrudes from the vulva. This condition must not be confused with prolapse of the vagina or uterus that, although rare, occurs during parturition.

### Clinical features

Vaginal hyperplasia and prolapse occur in bitches only during times of estrogenic stimulation (proestrus and estrus). Prolapse recurs in a few bitches at the end of diestrus or at parturition, times when additional estrogen may be secreted. The amount of edema and hyperplasia is extremely variable. It may be identified only during vaginal palpation, or tissue from the vaginal floor may protrude from the vulva. Much less commonly, the prolapsed tissue involves the circumference of the vagina.

**Diagnosis**

Diagnosis is based on historic and physical findings. Bitches may be brought for treatment because they refuse to allow intromission or because a mass is protruding from the vulva. The history indicates whether they are in proestrus or estrus. If it does not, estrogenic stimulation can be confirmed by vaginal cytology. If doubt remains, the hyperplastic tissue can be differentiated from vaginal neoplasia by fine-needle aspiration cytology.

**Treatment**

Ovariohysterectomy is the recommended treatment. If it is not feasible, treatment is primarily supportive; the edema and hyperplasia resolve spontaneously during diestrus. Induction of ovulation using GnRH (see Chapter 56) could be attempted to hasten recovery. Artificial insemination can be performed if the condition prevents copulation. Cleansing and applying topical antibiotic or antibiotic-steroid creams to the exposed tissue as needed is recommended. Attention should also be paid to the underlying perineal and vulvar skin. Severely damaged or necrotic tissue should be surgically excised. Surgical resection of the edematous tissue may be considered for brood bitches with recurrent or persistent prolapse.

**Prognosis**

It is common for vaginal hyperplasia and prolapse to recur during each subsequent estrus; affected animals are not the best brood bitches. This condition appears to be at least familial in nature. Ovariohysterectomy is curative.

## DISORDERS OF THE UTERUS (TEXT PP 877-880)

Clinical signs of uterine disorders are variable and nonspecific and may even be absent. Many uterine disorders are manifest by the presence of an abnormal vulvar discharge. Uterine enlargement may cause abdominal distention and discomfort. Uterine disorders often cause signs of systemic illness, especially when infection exists. Specimens collected from the vagina, or less commonly from the uterus itself via transcervical catheterization, are useful in evaluation of uterine disease.

*Uterine cytology.* The presence of endometrial cells on vaginal cytology indicates uterine involvement. Specimens obtained from the uterus of normal bitches contain a few WBCs (neutrophils, lymphocytes, macrophages) throughout the cycle, but bacteria are observed only during proestrus and estrus. Spermatozoa are found during estrus and early pregnancy in mated animals.

**Neoplasia**

Uterine neoplasia is rare in dogs and cats. Specific neoplasms include leiomyoma (most common), adenocarcinoma (rare), and adenomyosis (geriatric bitches, but rare). Uterine neoplasia can be an incidental finding, or it can be associated with sanguineous vulvar discharge, anorexia, weight loss, and abdominal discomfort and enlargement. Diagnosis involves abdominal palpation (which may reveal uterine enlargement), abdominal radiography, and ultrasonography. Ovariohysterectomy is recommended. The prognosis for animals with uterine leiomyoma is good, except when its location precludes complete excision. The prognosis for animals with uterine carcinoma is poor, as metastasis is common.

**Uterine torsion**

Uterine torsion is a life-threatening condition that occurs most commonly in near-term pregnant bitches and queens. One or both horns may be involved, and dystocia results unless the torsion is corrected. (Torsion of the nongravid uterus has been reported in conjunction with other uterine disorders such as hematometra and pyometra.) Clinical signs include sanguineous vulvar discharge, abdominal distention, abdominal pain, lethargy, and fever. The diagnosis is suspected on the basis of physical examination and ultrasonographic findings. It is confirmed at surgery. Severe metabolic complications can be present, depending on the duration and severity of the torsion. Treatment involves ovariohysterectomy and intensive supportive therapy.

**CEH and pyometra.** CEH-pyometra complex is a potentially life-threatening uterine disorder. CEH develops during or shortly after diestrus, when progesterone production is high, and after administration of exogenous progestins. If the animal is examined before bacterial invasion occurs, CEH alone or in association with hydrometra or mucometra is found. Bacteria, presumably of vaginal origin, are able to colonize the abnormal uterus, resulting in pyometra. (Metritis is discussed in Chapter 59.)

**Bacterial infection.** *Escherichia coli* is the organism most commonly isolated from bitches and queens with pyometra. Although bacterial infection does not initiate CEH and pyometra, it is the primary cause of morbidity and mortality. No apparent correlation exists between the severity of clinical signs and the type of organisms isolated, but uteri infected with strains of *E. coli* that express cytotoxic necrotizing factor 1 have the most severe histologic lesions. Bitches with pyometra also are immunosuppressed.

**Other risk factors.** The risk of developing pyometra increases with age, presumably because of repeated hormonal stimulation of the uterus. Most affected bitches are 6.5 to 8.5 years of age; on average, approximately 25% of intact bitches develop pyometra by 10 years of age. There exists a sixfold increased risk in nulliparous bitches compared with primiparous or multiparous animals. Estrogen therapy (e.g., to prevent pregnancy after misalliance) also increases the risk for pyometra, particularly when given during diestrus (when progesterone is high).

### Clinical features

Pyometra is classified as open or closed, depending on whether vulvar discharge is present. A purulent, often bloody vulvar discharge is present in animals with open pyometra. Signs tend to be more severe in patients with closed pyometra, although inappetence or anorexia, lethargy, and vomiting occur with either presentation. Polyuria and polydipsia are common in bitches but not in queens.

**Physical examination.** A septic vulvar discharge is present in the majority of animals with pyometra. Dehydration is common, but fever is found in only 20% of bitches and queens with pyometra. The uterus usually is palpably abnormal. Untreated, pyometra can lead to septicemia and/or endotoxemia; affected animals may be moribund, hypothermic, and in shock.

### Diagnosis

Diagnosis is based on the presence of clinical signs in a sexually mature female during or shortly after diestrus or after exogenous progestin administration, presence of a septic vulvar discharge, and radiographic or ultrasonographic evidence of a fluid-filled uterus. Complete blood count, serum biochemistry profile, and urinalysis are necessary to confirm sepsis and evaluate renal function.

**Complete blood count.** Neutrophilia with a left shift, monocytosis, and WBC degeneration are the most common findings. Total WBC counts may be >100,000/ml, or sepsis may cause leukopenia with a degenerative left shift. Mild normocytic, normochromic, nonregenerative anemia usually is also evident.

**Biochemistry.** Abnormalities include hyperproteinemia, hyperglobulinemia, and azotemia. Occasionally, alanine aminotransferase and serum alkaline phosphatase are mildly to moderately increased. Findings on urinalysis include isosthenuria and/or proteinuria in approximately 33% of bitches with pyometra; bacteriuria is common. Renal abnormalities are potentially reversible once bacteria are eradicated.

**Cytology and microbiology.** Vaginal cytology reveals a septic exudate, sometimes containing endometrial cells. Findings usually are abnormal, even when no visible discharge is present. Bacterial culture and sensitivity testing of the exudate are used to identify the offending organism and determine the appropriate antibiotic(s) for therapy.

**Differentiating pregnancy.** Abdominal radiography and/or ultrasonography should always be performed to confirm pyometra and rule out pregnancy, because the goals of treatment of a pregnancy complicated by uterine infection may be quite different from those of treatment for pyometra. Radiographically, pyometra and a gravid uterus appear identical until fetal calcification is detectable (usually by day 42 to 45 of gestation). Ultrasonography can be used at any time to identify fetal structures, assess fetal viability, identify exudate in the uterine lumen, and assess uterine wall thickness.

### Treatment

Treatment of CEH and pyometra must be prompt and aggressive. Septicemia and/or endotoxemia can develop at any time, if not present already. Intravenous fluids are indicated to correct existing deficits, maintain adequate tissue perfusion, and improve renal function; aggressive fluid therapy is needed for animals in septic shock. Ovariohysterectomy is the treatment of choice and is recommended as soon as the fluid deficits are corrected and antibiotic therapy has been initiated.

*Glucocorticoids.* Large doses of a glucocorticoid (prednisolone sodium succinate, 15 to 30 mg/kg, or dexamethasone, 4 to 6 mg/kg intravenously given once or repeated q4-6h if shock persists) may be helpful for animals in septic or endotoxic shock. To be of benefit, they must be administered early (within 4 hours of development of shock) and in conjunction with other specific corrective measures (e.g., intravenous fluids, antibiotic therapy).

*Antibiotics.* Therapy should begin immediately with a broad-spectrum, bactericidal antibiotic that is effective against *E. coli* (e.g., trimethoprim-sulfonamides, ampicillin, or clavulanate-amoxicillin). Once culture and sensitivity results are available, the appropriate antibiotic is then continued for 2 to 3 weeks.

*Prostaglandins.* Medical management with prostaglandin $F_{2\alpha}$ ($PGF_{2\alpha}$) can be considered in valuable breeding animals with open pyometra that are not critically ill. Natural $PGF_{2\alpha}$ (Lutalyse, 0.1 to 0.25 mg/kg subcutaneously q12-24h) is administered until the uterus is completely empty, which takes 3 to 5 days and sometimes longer. The volume of vulvar discharge increases and the discharge becomes less purulent and more mucoid or sanguineous as the uterus empties. Uterine size should return toward normal, but CEH may persist. Ovariohysterectomy should be considered in animals that need prolonged treatment and in those that have recurrence of pyometra.

Undesirable effects of $PGF_{2\alpha}$ therapy include panting, salivation, emesis, defecation, urination, mydriasis, and nesting behavior. Intensive grooming and vocalization may also be seen in queens. Adverse reactions usually develop within 5 minutes of injection and last for 30 to 60 minutes. Severity is directly related to the dose administered and inversely related to the duration of therapy.

*Prognosis for fertility.* Bitches and queens should be bred on the next cycle using optimal breeding management. The interestrous interval after $PGF_{2\alpha}$ therapy in bitches may be shorter than usual. Pregnancy rates of 80% to 90% are reported in bitches that received $PGF_{2\alpha}$ therapy for open pyometra; younger bitches are more likely than older bitches to become pregnant. Pregnancy rates of 71% to 88% are reported for queens that received $PGF_{2\alpha}$ therapy for open pyometra. In both groups pyometra can recur after $PGF_{2\alpha}$ therapy. Recurrence rates of 77% (over 27 months) in bitches and 15% (over 24 months) in queens are reported.

# 58

## Disorders
## of the Mammary Gland

### (Text pp 882-885)

### MASTITIS (TEXT P 882)

Bacterial infection in one or more lactating mammary glands can occur postpartum in bitches; it is uncommon in bitches lactating because of false pregnancy and rare in queens. Affected glands are swollen, warm, firm, and painful. Fever, anorexia, dehydration, and neglect of the neonates (crying, unthrifty puppies) are often noted. In severe cases, abscess or gangrene of the glands can develop.

#### Diagnosis

Diagnosis is based on physical findings and the septic appearance of the mammary secretions. *Escherichia coli*, staphylococci, and β-hemolytic streptococci are the organisms most often isolated. Inflammatory carcinoma of a mammary gland may appear clinically similar to mastitis. However, inflammatory carcinoma is most likely to occur in geriatric animals, and there exists no association with lactation. Whenever inflammation and/or abnormal secretions are present in nonlactating glands, mammary neoplasia should be strongly suspected.

#### Treatment

Treatment of mastitis involves antibiotic therapy, fluid therapy, and supportive care. Therapy should be aggressive to enable the bitch to resume her maternal duties as soon as possible. Adequate water and caloric intake is crucial to ensure continued milk production. During lactation, food and water needs are often double what they were during gestation; this should be taken into account when one is planning fluid therapy. Intravenous fluids are indicated whenever even mild dehydration is present. Warm compresses applied to affected glands several times a day can reduce swelling and pain and should be included in the treatment of mastitis.

*Antibiotic therapy.* Amoxicillin and cephalosporins are good initial choices if culture results are not known. Penicillin is also a reasonable choice, but it is not likely to be effective against *E. coli*. Antibiotic therapy should continue only as long as necessary (usually 7 days). In addition to fluid and antibiotic therapy, surgical treatment of mammary abscesses and gangrene should be performed.

*Neonatal care.* It is recommended that puppies continue nursing as long as the dam is willing and able to provide adequate nutrition. Monitoring weight gain of the puppies (which should be approximately 10% of the birth weight per day) is a useful means of assessment. The puppies should also be watched closely for signs of illness; if present, supplemental feeding or hand-rearing should be considered.

### GALACTOSTASIS (TEXT PP 882-883)

Galactostasis is another cause of swollen, firm, warm, painful mammary glands, but the mammary secretions are not infected, and the dam is not ill. Galactostasis occurs most often at the time of weaning and occasionally during peak lactation. It may also occur with false pregnancy.

**Treatment**

Treatment is not indicated for the transient galactostasis that occasionally occurs early during lactation. If treatment is necessary for galactostasis at weaning, it is directed at reducing milk production and relieving discomfort. Reducing the caloric and water intake to amounts appropriate to maintain ideal body weight and normal hydration when the bitch is neither pregnant nor lactating is helpful in treating, as well as preventing, galactostasis at weaning. Gradual rather than abrupt weaning is also helpful. Massaging or expressing the mammary glands should be avoided, as it may stimulate prolactin release and promote continued lactation. Warm compresses may help relieve swelling and discomfort but may also stimulate prolactin release.

## GALACTORRHEA (TEXT P 883)

Galactorrhea (lactation not associated with pregnancy and parturition) is the most common clinical manifestation of false pregnancy in bitches (see Chapter 59). Galactorrhea of false pregnancy occurs in late diestrus, after the withdrawal of exogenous progestins, or after oophorectomy performed during diestrus. It is self-limiting and usually does not require treatment.

Any stimulation of the mammary glands, such as massage, application of warm or cold compresses, and licking by the bitch, should be avoided. Withholding food for 24 hours, followed by a gradual return to normal maintenance quantities, helps reduce lactation. Dopamine agonists (e.g., bromocriptine, cabergoline) are effective in reducing the galactorrhea of false pregnancy in bitches but are not approved for this use in the United States.

## FELINE MAMMARY HYPERPLASIA AND HYPERTROPHY (TEXT PP 883-884)

Feline mammary hyperplasia (fibroepithelial hyperplasia, fibroadenoma, fibroadenomatosis) is characterized by rapid, abnormal growth of mammary tissue, usually affecting all glands simultaneously. It is most common in young, cycling queens but has been reported in neutered cats (males and females) receiving exogenous progestins. Feline mammary hyperplasia is a benign condition, but its behavior and appearance may mimic those of mammary neoplasia. Histologic evaluation of a biopsy specimen is recommended if any doubt exists.

**Treatment**

Treatment consists of removing the progesterone source. Ovariohysterectomy is usually recommended, irrespective of pregnancy status, and is often performed through a flank incision. The hyperplastic tissue resolves over several weeks after oophorectomy. Mastectomy may be indicated if the abnormal mammary tissue becomes necrotic or when remission does not occur after progesterone withdrawal.

## MAMMARY NEOPLASIA (TEXT PP 884-885)

### Etiology

Mammary neoplasms account for approximately 50% of all tumors in bitches. Although less prevalent in queens, mammary neoplasms are the third most common tumor in cats. They primarily affect older animals (mean age, approximately 10 years); most are intact females or females spayed late in life. Mammary tumors are rare in males and in young animals.

*Contributing or protective factors.* The progestins used to suppress estrus promote hyperplastic and neoplastic changes in feline and canine mammary glands. Benign mammary tumors are found in >70% of bitches receiving long-term progestin therapy. Early ovariohysterectomy (before 2.5 years of age in bitches) is strongly protective against the development of mammary tumors.

**Tumor types.** Approximately 50% of mammary tumors in bitches are benign. Adenocarcinomas account for the majority of malignant mammary tumors; inflammatory carcinomas, sarcomas, and carcinosarcomas are much less common. In bitches some benign tumors show evidence of cellular atypia and are considered precancerous. Precancerous changes are associated with a ninefold increase in the risk of developing mammary adenocarcinoma at a later date. Benign mammary tumors are rare in cats; >80% of feline mammary tumors are malignant adenocarcinomas.

#### Clinical features

Mammary tumors are usually discrete, firm, and nodular. They may be found anywhere along the mammary chain; multiple glands are involved in >50% of cases. Their size is extremely variable, ranging from a few millimeters to several centimeters in diameter. The tumors may adhere to the overlying skin but usually are not attached to the body wall. Malignant tumors are more likely to be attached to the body wall and to be covered by ulcerated skin.

Abnormal secretions can often be expressed from the nipples of affected glands. The regional lymph nodes (axillary or inguinal) may be enlarged if metastasis has occurred. The remainder of the physical examination is often unremarkable. Animals with advanced neoplasia may have tumor cachexia.

#### Diagnosis

In older females, mammary neoplasia should be the primary consideration with any mammary nodule. Excisional biopsy is the method of choice to confirm the diagnosis; fine-needle aspiration cytology often yields equivocal results. Before excisional biopsy is performed, thoracic radiographs should be evaluated for evidence of pulmonary metastasis, which if found, justifies a grave prognosis.

Radiography and palpation are used to evaluate the tumor burden. Malignant mammary tumors frequently metastasize to regional lymph nodes and the lungs; hepatic metastasis is less common. Metastasis to distant sites is rare in the absence of local node or pulmonary involvement. The animal's overall health is assessed with a complete blood count, a biochemistry profile, and urinalysis.

#### Treatment

Treatment involves surgical excision of all abnormal tissue. If nodulectomy is performed, surrounding tissue should always be included and submitted for histopathologic evaluation. If evidence suggests extension beyond the nodule, mastectomy should be performed. Excised mammary tumors should always be submitted for histopathologic examination, because the prognosis is markedly affected by tumor type. Although no data support its beneficial effects, chemotherapy is often used as an adjunct.

#### Prognosis

Adenocarcinoma is the most common malignant mammary tumor in bitches and queens. If the neoplastic cells are confined to the duct epithelium, the prognosis after surgery is good. The prognosis is somewhat worse if neoplastic cells are found outside the duct system and even worse if they are found in blood or lymphatic vessels. If neoplastic cells are found in the regional lymph nodes, the disease-free interval is significantly shortened. Inflammatory carcinoma carries a grave prognosis in bitches and queens.

**Tumor size.** Tumor size is the single most important prognostic indicator for animals with mammary adenocarcinomas treated by surgery alone. In bitches, tumors <3 cm in diameter carry the best prognosis, with approximately 35% recurring after 2 years (compared with 80% recurrence for larger tumors). In queens, disease-free intervals after mastectomy are longest for tumors <2 cm in diameter (median survival, 4.5 years).

**Tumor differentiation.** In bitches, poorly differentiated (anaplastic) tumors have a 90% 2-year recurrence rate after mastectomy, compared with 68% and 24% for moderately and well-differentiated tumors, respectively.

# 59

# False Pregnancy, Disorders of Pregnancy, Parturition, and Postpartum Period

## (Text pp 886-904)

### FALSE PREGNANCY (TEXT PP 886-888)

False pregnancy is a condition in which a nonpregnant female exhibits maternal behavior and lactation at the end of diestrus. It is common in cycling bitches, and in fact is considered normal; it is uncommon in queens. False pregnancy in bitches also occurs after withdrawal of exogenous progestins and after oophorectomy performed during diestrus.

False pregnancy in bitches is not associated with any reproductive abnormalities, such as cycle irregularities, pyometra, or infertility. Why some bitches are more prone to developing clinical signs and why the severity of clinical signs varies from cycle to cycle are not known. Some individual predisposition apparently exists. Nutritional factors may also influence the occurrence of false pregnancy.

#### Clinical features

False pregnancy is characterized by display of maternal behavior, such as nesting, adoption of inanimate objects or other animals, mammary development, and galactorrhea. Additional signs can include restlessness, irritability, abdominal enlargement, anorexia, and vomiting.

#### Diagnosis

Diagnosis is based on the historical and physical findings in a nonpregnant female at the end of diestrus (or after oophorectomy during diestrus or withdrawal of exogenous progestins). Before medical treatment of false pregnancy is undertaken, it is essential that pregnancy be ruled out, because treatment is deleterious to pregnancy. Abdominal radiography or ultrasonography can be used to exclude pregnancy.

#### Treatment

Treatment is unnecessary in most cases; signs are self-limiting and usually resolve after 2 to 3 weeks. Self-nursing (licking the mammary glands) and application of warm or cold compresses or other stimuli to the mammary glands can promote lactation and should be avoided. Withholding food for 24 hours, followed by a gradual (3- to 5-day) increase back to usual quantities, helps to reduce lactation. Mild tranquilization can be considered for bitches showing aggressive behavior; however, phenothiazines should not be used, as they can increase prolactin secretion.

#### Prolactin inhibitors

When treatment is needed, drugs that inhibit prolactin release, such as dopamine agonists (e.g., bromocriptine, cabergoline) and serotonin antagonists (e.g., metergoline), are effective in ameliorating the manifestations of false pregnancy in bitches. However, these drugs are not marketed for veterinary use in the United States.

***Bromocriptine.*** The suggested dosage for bromocriptine (Parlodel) is 10 to 100 µg/kg orally (PO) q12h for 10 to 14 days. Vomiting is a very common side effect; reducing the dose and administering the drug after meals may help.

***Cabergoline.*** Cabergoline (Galastop) rarely causes vomiting and appears to be the drug of choice at this time. A daily dose of 5 µg/kg PO results in improvement in 3 to 4 days and resolution of signs within 7 days. Rarely, cabergoline causes increased aggression.

***Metergoline.*** The suggested dose of metergoline (Contralac) is 0.1 to 0.2 mg/kg PO q12h for 8 days. This drug does not cause vomiting, but it can cause hyperexcitability, aggression, and whining.

### Progestins and androgens

Progestins (e.g., megestrol acetate) and androgens suppress prolactin secretion and can thereby diminish the manifestations of false pregnancy. However, clinical signs often recur after progestins are withdrawn. Therefore progestins are not recommended for treatment of false pregnancy.

### Persistent signs

If severe signs of false pregnancy persist for >2 to 3 weeks, bitches should be evaluated for hypothyroidism (see Chapter 51). In some hypothyroid bitches, increased prolactin secretion may result in excessive galactorrhea if false pregnancy occurs. Thyroid hormone replacement therapy resolves the galactorrhea in these bitches.

### Ovariohysterectomy

False pregnancy may recur in subsequent estrous cycles. Ovariohysterectomy performed during late anestrus prevents recurrence. The bitch should not be spayed during diestrus, because false pregnancy can result. When false pregnancy does occur after ovariohysterectomy, it is likely to be more persistent than in intact bitches; and in bitches spayed during an episode of false pregnancy the condition may be prolonged, sometimes for years. Spaying during false pregnancy is therefore contraindicated. Cabergoline therapy is beneficial in the majority of these cases of prolonged false pregnancy. If signs of false pregnancy become recurrent in a spayed animal, the presence of an ovarian remnant should be considered.

## PREGNANCY CONFIRMATION (TEXT PP 888-890)

Pregnancy can be confirmed by abdominal palpation, ultrasonography, and/or radiography. Uterine enlargement caused by pregnancy cannot be differentiated by palpation alone from that caused by pyometra or another process. With use of ultrasonography, pregnancy is reliably detected 24 to 28 days after breeding in bitches and 20 to 24 days after breeding in queens, at which time fetal structures and cardiac activity are detectable within the gestational sacs.

Abdominal radiography can be used to confirm pregnancy once sufficient calcification of the fetal skeleton has occurred (40 to 45 days after breeding in bitches and 35 to 40 days in queens). Measurement of serum relaxin can also be used for pregnancy diagnosis in dogs (see Chapter 56).

## PREDICTING PARTURITION (TEXT PP 891-892)

In bitches, identification of the first day of diestrus based on vaginal cytology (see Chapter 56) can be used to predict when labor should occur. Most bitches whelp 57 ± 3 days after the first day of diestrus. In bitches, serum progesterone falls from >3 ng/ml (>9 nmol/L) to <1 ng/ml (<3 nmol/L) during the 24 hours before labor, so serial measurement of serum progesterone can be used to predict when parturition will occur.

### Physical changes

Most bitches experience a transient drop in rectal temperature of 1.1° to 1.7° C (2° to 3° F) 6 to 18 hours before parturition. In small breeds the temperature may drop as low as 35° C (95° F), in medium breeds as low as 36° C (96.8° F), and in large breeds to 37° C (98.6° F). Owners are instructed to monitor the bitch's rectal temperature two or three times per day during the last 2 weeks of pregnancy to establish a baseline and identify the expected drop that indicates impending labor.

A prepartum drop in rectal temperature is an inconsistent finding in queens. Many, but not all, queens refuse to eat during the last 24 to 48 hours of pregnancy, which is a good indicator of impending parturition. The bitch or queen should be examined if no obvious signs of labor have occurred within 24 hours of the rectal temperature drop (bitches) or loss of appetite (queens).

## DYSTOCIA (TEXT PP 892-895)

### Etiology

Dystocia may be caused by maternal factors, fetal factors, or ineffective uterine contractions (uterine inertia). Maternal factors include breed, age (more likely in older bitches), conformation of the pelvic canal (e.g., vertical diameter ≤ horizontal diameter), physical abnormalities of the birth canal (e.g., displaced acetabular fractures, vaginal anomalies), uterine torsion, and extreme anxiety. Fetal factors include malpresentation (most common), cephalopelvic disproportion (large fetal head and small maternal pelvic canal), relative fetal oversize (e.g., "litters" of one or two puppies), fetal death, and fetal monsters.

*Uterine inertia.* Uterine inertia is by far the most common cause of dystocia, accounting for 60% (queens) to 70% (bitches) of all cases. It has a variety of potential causes (genetic, age related, nutritional, metabolic). With the exception of mechanical obstruction that results in myometrial exhaustion and secondary uterine inertia, the cause is not usually identified.

### Evaluation

Early recognition and correction of dystocia is critical for neonatal survival. Indicators of dystocia are listed in Box 59-1. A common error is to delay intervention because the dam does not appear to be "in trouble." Any delay severely compromises fetal viability.

*History.* An accurate history is crucial. Information should include gestation length; predisposition to or history of dystocia; progression through the stages of labor; and any indication of maternal illness. The owner should be questioned regarding rectal temperature monitoring, dam's behavior, presence and character of vulvar discharge and contractions, presence of placental membranes or fetal parts at the vulva, any puppy or kitten born, the duration of each of these events, and whether any drugs have been given or obstetric procedures performed.

---

**Box 59-1**

### Indicators of Dystocia

Any sign of illness in full-term female
History of previous dystocia
Known predisposition to dystocia
More than 24 hr since rectal temperature drop in full-term bitch
More than 24 hr of anorexia in full-term queen
Abnormal vulvar discharge
Failure to progress from stage I to stage II after 12 hr
Partially delivered fetus for more than 10-15 min
More than 3 hr of stage II labor before birth of first neonate
More than 1 hr of active labor between births
Constant, unrelenting, unproductive straining of 20-30 min
Labor appears to have stopped before entire litter is delivered

*Physical examination.* In addition to routine physical examination, a vaginal exam should be performed in all dams of adequate size to determine if a fetus is lodged in the vagina and to stimulate the vagina ("feathering" with the fingertip) in hopes of initiating abdominal contractions.

Even if the dam shows no signs of discomfort or illness, if the expected due date has arrived and no signs of labor have occurred, the dam should be examined. A drop in rectal temperature to <99° F in a full-term bitch and anorexia in a full-term queen indicate stage I labor. If stage I has not progressed to stage II within 12 hours, the dam should be examined, even if no other signs of labor or maternal illness are present. Onset of stage II labor is recognized by the return of rectal temperature to normal, the presence of strong abdominal contractions, and the passage of amnionic fluid. The first puppy should be born within 2 to 3 hours of the passage of amnionic fluid.

*Discolored discharge.* A dark green (bitches) or red-brown (queens) discharge indicates that at least one placenta has begun to separate. If a puppy or kitten has not been delivered within 2 to 4 hours, the dam should be examined. A bright yellow vulvar discharge indicates passage of meconium and severe fetal stress. It is often associated with fetal aspiration of amnionic fluid, which carries a grave prognosis for neonatal survival. A purulent discharge may be found if uterine infection or fetal maceration exists.

*Diagnostic imaging.* Ultrasonography is ideal for assessing fetal well-being. Fetal movement and heart rates are decreased as a result of stress and hypoxemia. In fetal puppies, heart rates <160 bpm indicate fetal stress. Heart rates <130 bpm are associated with poor survival rates, unless the puppies are delivered within 1 to 2 hours. Presumably the situation is similar in cats if the normally faster feline heart rate is taken into account.

The number, size, shape, location, posture, and presentation of any remaining fetuses are often best determined by radiography. A cause for obstruction, such as large fetus or fetal monstrosity, an abnormal pelvic canal, or fetal malposition, may be identified. However, fetal viability is difficult to assess on radiographs.

*Further evaluation.* When it has been determined that an "overdue" dam is healthy and the fetuses are healthy, measurement of serum progesterone can be helpful when the gestation length is in question. If serum progesterone is >2 ng/ml (>6 nmol/L), the pregnancy has not yet reached full term. Intervention should be delayed, and watchful waiting should continue for several hours. If 24 hours pass with no progression of labor, all parameters should be reassessed.

Systemic illness in the dam should be investigated, starting with complete blood count (CBC) and serum biochemical profile. Mild anemia (packed cell volume approximately 35%) and a slight mature neutrophilia are normal in full-term bitches.

### Treatment

Treatment is dictated by the presence or absence of obstruction and by the health of the fetuses. If obstruction or serious fetal compromise exists, cesarean section is indicated without delay. If no obstruction exists, medical management may be attempted in healthy dams with no signs of fetal stress. Exercise often stimulates abdominal contractions; walking the bitch around for a few minutes is helpful in some cases.

*Oxytocin.* The goal of oxytocin therapy is simply to increase the frequency of uterine contractions to normal. Small doses (e.g., 0.25 U intramuscularly [IM] for dogs weighing 35 to 45 lb) are adequate. Labor should progress (i.e., straining should begin) within 30 minutes, and a puppy should be delivered soon after. Repeated doses can be used if necessary to perpetuate normal parturition. *Repeated doses should not be administered if a normal labor pattern is not established.*

If no response occurs within 30 to 45 minutes, it is unlikely that further administration will be beneficial. High doses and/or frequent administration of oxytocin are contraindicated, because they cause sustained uterine contractions that delay fetal expulsion and compromise placental blood flow. Placental separation can also occur.

*Calcium gluconate.* Generally, calcium administration increases the strength of uterine contractions even in the absence of hypocalcemia. For this reason some practitioners recommend routine administration of calcium gluconate to bitches with nonobstructive dystocia and weak, ineffective uterine contractions. One recommendation is to administer 10% calcium gluconate before oxytocin is given; if normal labor does not resume, oxytocin is added.

Calcium gluconate (up to 0.2 ml/kg, or 1 to 5 ml/dog) is given subcutaneously (SC) or intravenously (IV). High doses or bolus intravenous administration should be reserved for animals with clinical signs or laboratory evidence of hypocalcemia. The label directions must be followed precisely, because some preparations are too irritating to be administered SC.

If the intravenous route is chosen, calcium is administered slowly (1 ml/min) while the heart is auscultated. Administration should be immediately discontinued if brady-cardia or dysrhythmia occurs. If labor progresses (i.e., straining begins), calcium may be repeated as needed or continued with oxytocin. When medical management fails to initiate a normal labor pattern, cesarean section should be performed without further delay.

## POSTPARTUM DISORDERS (TEXT PP 895-898)

### Agalactia

Primary agalactia is a condition in which the gland is incapable of producing milk or the ducts are incapable of flow. More commonly the gland and ducts are normal but other factors diminish the capacity for production or inhibit milk letdown. Factors include poor body condition, inadequate caloric and/or water intake, and anxiety.

Phenothiazines increase prolactin secretion, so they may be useful sedatives for anxious dams. Metoclopramide (0.1 to 0.2 mg/kg PO or SC q6-8h) also stimulates prolactin secretion and has been used to enhance lactation. Oxytocin (0.5 to 2 U SC q2h) can be used to stimulate milk letdown. Treatment is usually needed for only a day or two. Meanwhile, nutritional and psychologic factors should be corrected.

### Puerperal Hypocalcemia (Puerperal Tetany, Eclampsia)

Puerperal hypocalcemia is an acute, life-threatening condition that occurs postpartum. Signs typically develop during peak lactation (1 to 3 weeks postpartum) in small bitches nursing large litters, although puerperal hypocalcemia can occur in cats, in any breed of dog, with any size litter, and at any time during lactation. Rarely it occurs during late gestation in bitches. Hypocalcemia may also be seen as a preparturient event in queens.

#### Clinical features

Initial clinical signs include panting, trembling, muscle fasciculations, weakness, and ataxia. If the condition is untreated, these early signs quickly progress (within hours) to tetany with tonic-clonic convulsions and opisthotonos. Heart rate, respiratory rate, and rectal temperature are increased, especially during convulsions, although hypothermia is common in queens with prepartum hypocalcemia. The dam is otherwise healthy, and the neonates are thriving.

#### Diagnosis

Diagnosis is based on appropriate clinical signs in a heavily lactating female. It can be confirmed by finding serum calcium below the reference range (see Chapter 55). Because the clinical signs in postpartum bitches are so suggestive, treatment is usually initiated before, or without, laboratory confirmation.

#### Treatment

Treatment consists of slow intravenous administration of 10% calcium gluconate until effective (usually 3 to 20 ml total, depending on the size of the dam). The heart must be closely monitored for dysrhythmias and bradycardia, and calcium admin-istration stopped immediately if any cardiac abnormalities are detected. If additional calcium is needed, it can be administered after the cardiac rhythm has normalized, at a much slower rate. Response to treatment is dramatic, and clinical signs resolve during intravenous calcium administration.

*Supportive care.* The same amount of calcium needed to control the signs can be mixed 50:50 with sterile saline and given SC before the dam is sent home. (Note:

Calcium chloride should not be given SC). Puppies or kittens should not be allowed to nurse for 12 to 24 hours. If hypocalcemia recurs, the puppies should be weaned. Feeding the dam on an ad libitum basis or at least three times per day with a nutritionally complete and balanced ration is recommended. Oral calcium (gluconate, carbonate, or lactate, 1 to 3 g/day) should be administered throughout the rest of lactation.

### Prevention
A high-quality, nutritionally complete and balanced diet should be fed during pregnancy and lactation. Oral calcium supplementation during gestation is contraindicated because it may worsen, rather than prevent, postpartum hypocalcemia. If necessary, the dam can be physically separated from the neonates for 30 to 60 minutes several times a day to encourage her to eat. Supplemental feeding of the litter with milk replacer and, after 3 to 4 weeks of age, with solid food may be helpful, especially for large litters.

## Metritis
Bacterial infection of the uterus can develop after abortion, dystocia, retention of placental or fetal tissues, obstetric procedures, or normal birth. Affected animals are febrile and have a fetid, septic uterine discharge. Dehydration, septicemia, endotoxemia, and/or shock can develop. Neglected, crying neonates are often one of the earliest signs.

### Diagnosis
Diagnosis is primarily based on historic and physical findings. The septic nature and uterine source of the exudate can be confirmed by cytologic and endoscopic examinations, if necessary. Bacterial culture and sensitivity testing of the discharge should be performed. Abdominal radiography and/or ultrasonography should also be performed to evaluate the uterine contents (e.g., fetal remnants) and to assess the integrity of the uterus.

### Treatment
Treatment must be prompt and aggressive. The decision to approach metritis medically or surgically is based on the health of the dam, the integrity of the uterus, and the animal's breeding future. Regardless of the approach, intravenous fluids should be given to correct existing deficits, maintain tissue perfusion, and provide for the additional demands of lactation. Broad-spectrum, bactericidal antibiotics should also be administered.

***Antibiotics.*** The choice of antibiotic(s) should be based on culture results and on safety in neonates. Penicillins, amoxicillins, and cephalosporins generally are considered safe for neonates (Box 59-2).

---

**Box 59-2**

#### Antimicrobial Therapy for Neonates

**DRUGS WITH KNOWN SAFETY**
Amoxicillin-clavulanate
Amoxicillin
Cephalosporins
Erythromycin
Penicillins
Tylosin

**SAFETY NOT ESTABLISHED**
Clindamycin
Lincomycin

**DRUGS KNOWN TO CAUSE UNDESIRABLE EFFECTS**
Aminoglycosides
Chloramphenicol
Ciprofloxacin
Enrofloxacin
Nalidixic acid
Nitrofurantoin
Norfloxacin
Polymyxin
Sulfonamides
Tetracyclines
Trimethoprim

***Surgery.*** Ovariohysterectomy is the treatment of choice for animals that will not be bred again and in those with evidence of uterine rupture (e.g., extreme abdominal discomfort, radiographic or ultrasonographic evidence of abdominal fluid accumulation). Ovariohysterectomy or hysterotomy with lavage is usually recommended if placental or fetal tissues remain in the uterus.

***Ecbolic agents.*** For breeding animals in which ovariohysterectomy is not feasible, oxytocin (5 to 20 IU, IM q12-24h for several days) or natural prostaglandin $F_{2\alpha}$ ($PGF_{2\alpha}$; Lutalyse, 0.1 to 0.25 mg/kg SC q12-24h) can be administered. Treatment should continue until the uterus is empty, which usually takes at least 2 days. Adverse reactions may be seen with $PGF_{2\alpha}$ therapy (see Chapter 57). Neither medication has deleterious effects on lactation or on the neonates.

## Subinvolution of Placental Sites

Subinvolution of placental sites (SIPS) causes persistent postpartum hemorrhage lasting at least 7 weeks, sometimes >12 weeks. Usually a fairly constant bloody vulvar discharge is present, although the volume is often very small. SIPS is most common in primiparous bitches <3 years of age, but it can occur in older, multiparous animals. It has not been reported in cats.

### Diagnosis

Diagnosis is based on historic, physical, and cytologic findings. Affected bitches are healthy and physically normal, except for a small amount of bloody vulvar discharge. Vaginal cytology can be used to differentiate the vulvar discharge associated with SIPS (cytology consistent with hemorrhage, ± multinucleated giant cells) from lochia and from the discharge associated with uterine infection (see Chapter 57).

### Treatment

Treatment is rarely necessary; recovery is spontaneous, and subsequent fertility is unaffected. Administration of ergonovine maleate or natural $PGF_{2\alpha}$ (Lutalyse) may diminish bleeding. Progestin therapy is not recommended, as its undesirable effects on the endometrium outweigh any potential benefit in this situation. If blood loss anemia is severe enough to require treatment, an alternative diagnosis should be considered. Ovariohysterectomy is curative.

## ABORTIFACIENTS (MISMATING) (TEXT PP 898-900)

When misalliance occurs, the safest approach for preservation of the health and fertility of the female may be to do nothing. In dogs approximately 60% of single mismatings fail to result in pregnancy. Ovariohysterectomy is an effective but permanent method of preventing an unwanted litter.

## Estrogens

Although estradiol cypionate (ECP; 44 µg/kg, up to 1 mg total, IM once) is reasonably effective in preventing pregnancy, *its use is strongly discouraged*. Pyometra develops in 25% of bitches given ECP during diestrus. Estrogens can also cause fatal aplastic anemia, prolong the duration of behavioral estrus, and predispose to cystic ovarian follicles. If ECP is used, it should not be administered during diestrus, the total dose should not exceed 1 mg, and the dose should never be repeated.

## Prostaglandins

Prostaglandins have been used to terminate unwanted pregnancy in dogs and cats, although these drugs are not approved for small animal use in the United States. One approach that avoids unnecessary treatment is to begin therapy 30 to 35 days (bitches) or 45 days (queens) after breeding, once pregnancy is confirmed. In bitches, natural $PGF_{2\alpha}$ (Lutalyse, 0.1 to 0.25 mg/kg SC q8-12h) is given daily until abortion is complete (typically 3 to 9 days). In queens, a dosage of 0.2 to 0.5 mg/kg SC q12h daily for up to 5 days may be tried. Adverse reactions to $PGF_{2\alpha}$ (see Chapter 57) can be worrisome, even though they usually become less severe as therapy progresses.

Abdominal ultrasonography should be performed once a vulvar discharge is seen, to confirm abortion and to identify any fetuses remaining in the uterus. If treatment is stopped when only part of the litter is aborted, the remaining fetuses may be carried to term. Because of the adverse reactions that can occur, the possibility that the entire litter may not be aborted, and the possibility of live puppies being born if abortion occurs near term, hospitalization is recommended.

**Early diestrous protocol.** Early diestrous protocol begins no sooner than day 8 and up to day 15 of cytologic diestrus. $PGF_{2\alpha}$ (Lutalyse, 0.25 mg/kg SC q12h) is given for 4 days. Serum progesterone is measured at the end of treatment and 15 to 20 days later. Fetal death is expected if serum progesterone declines and remains below 2 ng/ml (6.4 nmol/l). If progesterone is >2 ng/ml after treatment, pregnancy status should be assessed with ultrasonography or a second course of treatment given. Efficacy of early termination in bitches is approximately 85%. The advantage of early treatment is that fetuses are resorbed rather than expelled, and postabortion sequelae such as vulvar discharge are minimal. However, the interestrual interval may be shortened by 1 to 4 months.

### Antiprolactin drugs

Antiprolactin drugs such as bromocriptine and cabergoline can suppress serum progesterone and terminate pregnancy if used as single agents. When given after 7 weeks of gestation in bitches, cabergoline (5 µg/kg PO q24h) causes abortion in 3 to 5 days, with no side effects. However, at this late stage of gestation, recognizable fetal parts or live fetuses that die shortly thereafter may be passed.

### Combination therapy

Side effects of $PGF_{2\alpha}$ can be minimized by combining the drug with bromocriptine or cabergoline. One protocol involves treatment with $PGF_{2\alpha}$ (either Lutalyse at 0.1 to 0.2 mg/kg SC q24h or cloprostenol [Estrumate] at 1 µg/kg SC q48h) and bromocriptine (Parlodel, 15 to 30 µg/kg PO q12h) beginning 25 days after breeding, once pregnancy had been confirmed. Treatment is continued until abortion occurs (4 to 5 days on average). Fewer side effects may be noted with cloprostenol than with natural $PGF_{2\alpha}$.

When started 22 to 28 days after breeding, a single dose of cloprostenol (2.5 µg/kg SC) combined with cabergoline (5 µg/kg PO q24h for 10 days) may be effective in terminating canine pregnancy. Although fetuses are resorbed, a brown serosanguineous discharge that lasts for 4 to 21 days may develop. After the initial injection of cloprostenol, side effects are minimal, so treatment on an outpatient basis could be considered.

### Dexamethasone

Dexamethasone is an effective abortifacient in bitches; however, it is not recommended for this purpose. Treatment is associated with the development of a mucoid, red-brown vulvar discharge, polydipsia and polyuria, and anorexia. Because glucocorticoids are teratogenic, if they fail to cause abortion, puppies with facial or other deformities could be born.

## FETAL RESORPTION–ABORTION–STILLBIRTH COMPLEX (TEXT PP 900-901)

### Etiology

Embryonic death, abortion, and stillbirths can occur because of maternal, fetal, or placental abnormalities. Maternal factors include infection (Box 59-3), metabolic diseases, and abdominal trauma. Drugs known to be teratogenic or toxic to pregnant females (resulting in fetal death or abortion) are listed in Box 59-4. In many cases fetal death or stillbirth is an isolated event with no identifiable cause. Subsequent breedings often are uneventful.

### Clinical features

When embryonic death occurs early in gestation, usually no outward signs are present. Bitches may continue to appear pregnant for 60 days. With early pregnancy loss

---

**Box 59-3**

## Infectious Causes of Neonatal Morbidity and Mortality

### VIRAL CAUSES
Parvovirus
Feline leukemia virus
Herpesvirus
Canine adenovirus I
Canine distemper virus
(Role of coronavirus and rotavirus not
   established)

### BACTERIAL CAUSES
*Escherichia coli*
Hemolytic and nonhemolytic
   *Streptococcus* spp.
*Staphylococcus*
*Bordetella* spp.
*Pasteurella* spp.
*Salmonella* spp.
*Brucella* spp.
*Campylobacter* spp.

### PARASITIC CAUSES
*Toxocara* spp.
*Ancylostoma* spp.
*Giardia* spp.
*Coccidium* spp.
*Cryptosporidium* spp.

---

in queens, appearance of pregnancy subsides in 30 to 50 days; most queens resume cycling. When fetal death occurs in the last half of pregnancy, a vulvar discharge often occurs The later fetal death occurs, the more obvious it is that fetal parts are being expelled (abortion).

### Diagnosis

The diagnostic approach should begin with a thorough history, including changes in the dam's environment, recent addition of new animals, vaccination status, current drug therapy, and dietary supplements.

**Dam.** The dam should be thoroughly examined for signs of illness, and abdominal palpation, radiography, and/or ultrasonography should be performed to check for remaining fetuses. Ultrasonography is most useful for assessing fetal viability. CBC, serum biochemistry profile, and urinalysis should be performed. A sample of the uterine discharge should be submitted for cytologic examination and for bacterial culture and antibiotic sensitivity testing. Appropriate serologic tests (e.g., *Brucella*, feline leukemia virus, feline immunodeficiency virus) should also be performed.

**Abortus and placenta.** If available, the abortus and placenta should be submitted for gross, microscopic, and microbiologic examination. Complete postmortem examination of the abortus is the single most useful diagnostic procedure.

**Breeding history.** Hereditary causes of fetal anomalies can be difficult to prove. The breeding records of related animals should be scrutinized for similar occurrences. If any are found, hereditary causes should be strongly considered.

### Treatment

Therapy for the aborting female is supportive and symptomatic, unless a cause can be found. If viable fetuses remain, the pregnancy can be allowed to continue; if not, any remaining contents of the uterus should be removed by ovariohysterectomy or with ecbolic agents, such as oxytocin (1 to 10 U IM) or natural $PGF_{2a}$ (Lutalyse, 0.1 to 0.25 mg/kg SC). Antibiotic therapy should be initiated as soon as specimens for microbiology have been obtained.

---

**Box 59-4**

### Examples of Drugs with Probable or Known Risk to Pregnancy in Dogs and Cats

**HORMONES**
Androgens
Bromocriptine
Estrogens
Excessive thyroid hormone
  replacement
Glucocorticoids
Prostaglandins

**ANTIMICROBIALS**
Aminoglycosides
Amphotericin-B
Chloramphenicol
Ciprofloxacin
Doxycycline
Enrofloxacin
Griseofulvin
Metronidazole
Oxytetracycline
Tetracycline

**NONSTEROIDAL
ANTIINFLAMMATORY DRUGS**

**ANTICONVULSANTS**

**ANTICANCER DRUGS**

**ANESTHETICS OR PREANESTHETICS**
Barbiturates
Diazepam
Halothane
Methoxyfurane

**ANTIPARASITIC DRUGS**
Amitraz
Levamisole
Thiacetarsamide
Trichlorfon

**MISCELLANEOUS**
Captopril
Dantrolene
Dimethylsulfoxide (DMSO)
Diphenoxylate
Excessive vitamins
Isoproterenol
Loperamide
Methocarbamol
Methscopolamine
Mitotane (o,'p'-DDD)
Nitroglycerin
Nitroprusside
Propranolol
Thiazide diuretics

---

## NEONATAL MORBIDITY AND MORTALITY (TEXT PP 901-903)

The first 2 weeks of life, particularly the first 3 days, are the most precarious for puppies and kittens. Many of those early deaths are related to prolonged parturition and fetal stress. Early preweaning neonatal vulnerability is influenced most by the dam and by the environment into which the neonates are born.

A thorough history taking, including the events of parturition, is followed by examination of the affected neonate, its dam and littermates, and the environment; examination of only the affected neonate is insufficient. With any unexplained neonatal death a thorough postmortem examination should be performed. The findings determine how to treat or protect the remaining littermates and the dam, how to protect the rest of the colony, and how to prevent recurrence in future litters.

### Environmental Factors

The environmental factors of greatest concern are sanitation, control of infectious diseases, environmental temperature and humidity, and privacy. Puppies and kittens are incapable of thermoregulation until they are 2 weeks old. A room temperature of 29.4° C (85° F) with 55% to 65% humidity is often recommended for puppies and kittens, although some heavy-coated breeds may be uncomfortably warm and refuse to "cuddle" their young at this temperature. A quiet, familiar, private environment also is important.

### Dam

Ill or neglected puppies and kittens often are the first sign of maternal illness. Two common postpartum disorders often reflected by neonatal neglect are mastitis and metritis. When one neonate is ill, the entire litter and the dam should also be examined.

### Neonate

Newborn puppies and kittens should be round and sleek, with good muscle tone and pink mucous membranes. Respiratory rates are 15 to 35 breaths/min, and heart rates are >200 beats/min for the first 2 weeks. Normal rectal temperature at birth is 35.6° to 36.1° C (96° to 97° F); rectal temperature gradually increases to 37.8° C (100° F) by day 7.

#### Expected body weight

Normal birth weight for puppies varies with breed, ranging from 100 g to 750 g. Puppies should gain 5% to 10% of their birth weight per day, so that by 10 to 12 days of age they weigh twice their birth weight. Normal birth weight for kittens is 100 ± 10 g. Minimum expected weight gain is 7 to 10 g/day; by 6 weeks kittens should weigh at least 500 g. Weight loss in any puppy or kitten is not normal.

Supplemental bottle or tube feeding of milk replacer should be initiated for neonates that fail to gain weight at the expected rate. A foster mother can be considered, especially when poor weight gain is the result of inadequate lactation or maternal neglect. If the neonate loses >10% of its birth weight, the chances for survival are very poor.

#### Clinical features of neonatal illness

The most common signs of illness are persistent crying; decreased activity, including nursing; failure to gain weight; dry, rough haircoat; and decreased muscle tone. Crying for >20 minutes indicates that the neonate is cold, hungry, neglected, or ill. Eventually the ill neonate stops crying and becomes increasingly less active.

A dry, rough haircoat can be a sign of neonatal illness or maternal neglect. Decreased muscle tone, resulting in a limp or flat appearance, is a grave sign. Other signs of illness (e.g., dehydration, cyanosis, pale mucous membranes) are interpreted as for older animals.

### Common Causes of Neonatal Mortality

Noninfectious causes account for the majority of deaths in neonates 0 to 3 days old. They include hypothermia, hypoglycemia, anatomic abnormalities, and trauma. Trauma and infection are the more common causes of death in neonates older than 4 days.

#### Hypothermia

Hypothermia is a common cause of neonatal death. Immediately after birth, a neonate's temperature plummets unless the puppy or kitten is vigorously attended. The importance of appropriate environmental temperature and adequate maternal care to maintain body temperature cannot be overemphasized. Crying followed by decreasing activity is a sign of hypothermia. Dams may cull cold puppies and kittens as if they were already dead.

Hypothermic neonates should be warmed slowly until the rectal temperature is 36.1° to 36.7° C (97° to 98° F). Neonates that do not respond within a few hours are unlikely to do so and usually die. The cause of hypothermia must be found and eliminated.

#### Hypoglycemia

Anything that interferes with the quality or quantity of the dam's milk has the potential to cause neonatal hypoglycemia. Hypothermia <34.4° C (<94° F) can cause hypoglycemia, because digestive functions cease. Septicemia is another cause of hypoglycemia. Signs of hypothermia include weakness and decreased activity, crying, bradycardia, respiratory distress, convulsions, and coma.

Glucose solution should be administered orally while the cause is being investigated. Milk or milk replacer should be reinstituted as soon as possible. Note: Hypothermia must be corrected before milk or milk replacer can be digested and absorbed.

**Trauma**

Puncture wounds, umbilical herniation, or crushing can be accidentally caused by the dam. Deliberate bite wounds or cannibalism can occur with nervous or frightened dams, so every effort should be made to provide a stress-free environment. Tranquilization may be considered for very anxious dams.

**Infection**

Infectious agents known to cause neonatal mortality are listed in Box 59-3. The dam and other adults in the colony are usually the source. Poor environmental conditions, inadequate sanitation practices, and contact with older animals increase the neonate's exposure to infectious agents.

The diagnosis of infectious causes of neonatal illness and death is best established by thorough postmortem examination. Some infectious agents have characteristic gross pathology, but additional testing is usually necessary to establish the diagnosis. Samples of liver, spleen, lung, and gastrointestinal tract should be submitted for histopathologic examination, bacterial culture, and virus isolation. Lesions found during gross examination should also be submitted. With some infectious diseases (e.g., brucellosis), serologic tests or cultures may need to be performed on the dam or other colony members.

# 60

# Disorders of Male Fertility

## (Text pp 905-917)

### DIAGNOSTIC TECHNIQUES (TEXT PP 907-913)

#### Semen Evaluation

Collection techniques and sample handling are discussed in the text. The spermatozoal characteristics that best correlate with fertility are the total number per ejaculate, motility, and morphology. However, the presence of normal semen is not proof of normal fertility; the male must also have normal libido and normal mating ability. In addition, the presence of abnormal semen does not necessarily indicate sterility, unless azoospermia or complete, true necrozoospermia is present.

To help establish a prognosis or to resolve doubt about an unsatisfactory sample, the dog should be reevaluated several times over at least 60 days (the length of the canine spermatogenic cycle). Seminal quality may not improve for 3 to 5 months after testicular insult.

##### Color

Canine semen is normally white to opalescent, and opaque. A yellow color may indicate the presence of urine, which is not normal and is often associated with subfertility. A red or brownish color usually indicates the presence of blood, most often of prostatic origin or from damage to small surface vessels of the penis during collection. Large numbers of inflammatory cells in the semen may cause flocculation or a yellow-green color. Inflammatory cells can originate from anywhere in the urinary or genital tract, including the preputial cavity, and are an indication for culture (for bacteria and *Mycoplasma*) and testing for *Brucella canis* infection.

### Spermatozoa concentration

The number of sperm per ejaculate for normal dogs ranges from $250 \times 10^6$ to $2000 \times 10^6$. Breed of dog, testicular size, and frequency of ejaculation affect the number of sperm ejaculated. Smaller breeds often have fewer sperm per ejaculate than large-breed dogs, but, in general, a total sperm count $<200 \times 10^6$ in a mature dog should be considered abnormally low, regardless of breed or frequency of ejaculation.

### Motility

In normal dogs $>70\%$ of the sperm should have rapid, steady, forward motility. Decrease in the percentage of motile sperm is one of the first detectable changes following testicular injury. It may also be found with incomplete ejaculation or exposure of the sperm to excessive heat or cold, contaminated equipment, inflammatory cells, or bacteria. Spermatozoa that move in circles usually do so because of morphologic defects in the tail or midpiece.

### Morphology

In normal dogs, $<20\%$ of spermatozoa are morphologically abnormal. Abnormalities of the head, acrosome, midpiece, or proximal tail, and proximal droplets are usually considered the most severe. Loose or detached heads or acrosomes that are otherwise normal and distal droplets, as well as bent tails, are considered less severe, although they may be the first abnormalities noted after a testicular insult.

Normal motility in a sample with excessive numbers of bent tails suggests that the bent tails were caused by the stain. Abnormalities resulting from improper sample handling should not be found in subsequent, properly handled samples. Persistence of morphologic abnormalities is an indication for further diagnostic evaluation, including semen culture and possibly testicular biopsy.

### Cytology

When cells other than sperm are found, the sample should be examined cytologically with appropriate stains (e.g., Wright's stain). Cytologic examination of the third fraction of the ejaculate is helpful in evaluating prostatic disorders. The presence of red blood cells indicates hemorrhage, and a white blood cell (WBC) count $>2000/ml$ indicates inflammation somewhere in the urogenital tract. Dogs with leukospermia should be tested for *B. canis*. Some epithelial cells are normally present, and their numbers increase with sexual rest. Crystals may be found in samples contaminated with urine or with talc from collection equipment. When excessive numbers of cells other than sperm are found, further assessment of the urogenital tract may be warranted.

### Seminal alkaline phosphatase

In normal dogs, whole semen alkaline phosphatase (AP) is 4000 to 5000 U/L and indicates that epididymal fluid is present in the ejaculate. Azoospermic dogs with low seminal AP may have bilateral obstruction distal to the epididymides, or ejaculation could have been incomplete.

## Bacterial Culture of Semen

Semen culture is indicated (1) when inflammatory cells are found in the semen, (2) as part of the diagnostic evaluation of male infertility, and (3) in dogs with suspected bacterial prostatitis, epididymitis, or orchitis. Culture for *B. canis* should specifically be requested in dogs with epididymitis or orchitis. Culturing each seminal fraction separately aids in identification of the location of the infection: testes or epididymis (second fraction), or prostate gland (third fraction). Both fractions should yield $<100$ colony-forming units (CFUs)/ml in normal dogs. Normal feline semen may contain $>10,000$ CFUs.

Aerobes predominate in the normal bacterial flora of the prepuce and urethra (Table 60-1). The same organisms are most frequently isolated from animals with bacterial prostatitis, orchitis, or epididymitis. Urethral contamination may produce quantitative results of 100 to 10,000 CFU/ml. Separate culture of a urethral swab, obtained before ejaculation, can be used to identify urethral contamination. Anaerobic infection, although uncommon, should be considered when bacteria or inflammatory cells are seen but aerobic culture is negative.

Table 60-1

## Normal Preputial and/or Distal Urethral Flora

| Dogs | Cats |
|------|------|
| *Acinetobacter* spp. | *Bacillus* spp. |
| *Bacillus* spp. | *Enterococcus* spp. |
| *Corynebacterium* spp. | *Escherichia coli* |
| *Escherichia coli* | *Klebsiella oxytoca* |
| *Flavobacterium* spp. | *Proteus mirabilis* |
| *Haemophilus* spp. | *Pseudomonas aeruginosa* |
| *Klebsiella pneumoniae* | *Serratia odorifera* |
| *Moraxella* spp. | *Staphylococcus* spp. |
| *Mycoplasma* spp.* | *Streptococcus* spp. |
| *Proteus mirabilis* | *Yersinia intermedia* |
| *Pseudomonas aeruginosa* | |
| *Staphylococcus aureus* | |
| *Staphylococcus epidermidis* | |
| *Streptococcus canis* | |
| *Streptococcus equisimilis* | |
| *Viridans streptococci* | |

From Johnston SD: Disorders of the external genitalia of the male. In Ettinger SJ, ed: *Textbook of veterinary internal medicine*, ed 3, Philadelphia, 1989, WB Saunders, p 1882.
*See discussion in text.

### Radiography and Ultrasonography

Radiography is primarily used to assess the size of the prostate gland and to identify metastatic lesions in dogs with suspected prostatic adenocarcinoma. Ultrasonography can be used to identify and characterize lesions within the prostate, testis, and epididymis; to determine the cause of testicular or scrotal swelling; to assess the size of the vas deferens; and to establish the location of cryptorchid testes. Ultrasonography can also be used to guide biopsy of the prostate gland or focal lesions within the testis or epididymis.

### Testicular Aspiration and Biopsy

Testicular or epididymal aspiration and testicular biopsy are usually reserved for infertile animals that have been thoroughly but unsuccessfully investigated by less invasive means. These procedures may be performed earlier in animals with discrete, focal lesions or with marked changes in the consistency of the testis or epididymis.

Cytologic evaluation of testicular aspirates may reveal inflammatory or neoplastic cells and infectious agents, as well as sperm. Testicular biopsy also allows evaluation of the seminiferous tubules, progression of spermatogenesis, and interstitial and Sertoli cell numbers. Techniques are described in the text. Complications of fine-needle aspiration (swelling, hemorrhage, infection, sperm granuloma, local hyperthermia) are uncommon.

#### Handling of biopsy specimens

With testicular biopsy a portion of the tissue sample should be submitted for histopathology in Zenker's, Bouin's, glutaraldehyde, or Karnovsky's fixative; *formalin should not be used*. An unfixed portion of the sample should be submitted for bacterial culture.

### Hormonal Evaluation

#### Testosterone

Serum testosterone is most often measured to determine the presence and functional status of the testes. Serum testosterone in castrated males is usually <0.2 ng/ml;

in intact male dogs it ranges from 0.5 to 5 ng/ml, and in intact male cats from <0.05 to 3 ng/ml. However, a single measurement is seldom useful; provocative testing with human chorionic gonadotropin (hCG) or gonadotropin-releasing hormone (GnRH) is necessary for adequate assessment of testosterone production.

*Provocative testing.* Serum testosterone is measured before and 4 hours after administration of hCG (44 IU/kg in dogs, 250 IU/cat, intramuscularly [IM]) or 1 hour after administration of GnRH (2.2 mg/kg in dogs, 25 mg/cat, IM). A substantial increase in testosterone is expected in intact males. An increase in serum testosterone in a supposedly castrated male or intersex animal indicates the presence of testicular tissue. Animals with only one testis and intersex animals may have values between baseline and those typically found in normal males.

*Penile spines.* Because the development and maturation of penile spines in male cats are androgen dependent, they serve as a bioassay for testosterone. The finding of penile spines indicates the presence of testicular tissue.

### Luteinizing hormone

Serum luteinizing hormone (LH) in normal intact male dogs ranges from 0.2 to 20 ng/ml. Castrated males frequently have serum LH >30 ng/ml. LH is released in a pulsatile manner, so serial measurement (e.g., three samples q20min) is more likely to distinguish normal from abnormal animals. After GnRH administration, serum LH should increase; failure of this to occur is consistent with a pituitary lesion.

## DIAGNOSTIC APPROACH TO INFERTILITY (TEXT PP 913-915)

The diagnostic approach begins with a complete history and physical examination. The history should assess the male's past breeding performance, breeding management, fertility of the females, and current or previous health problems. Some common drugs and metabolic disorders known to affect male fertility are listed in Table 60-2.

### Physical Examination

A complete physical examination should be performed to assess the male's overall health, identify congenital or heritable anomalies, and reveal metabolic or physical abnormalities that may adversely affect spermatogenesis, libido, and/or mating ability (e.g., phimosis, persistent penile frenulum, abnormally short os penis in dogs, entanglement of the penis in preputial hair in cats).

#### Reproductive organs

The testes and epididymides are palpated to determine their size, shape, consistency, and location. The canine prostate is palpated per rectum and transabdominally. The penis and prepuce are palpated and inspected. Because the penis must be extruded from the prepuce for thorough examination, as well as for semen collection in dogs, the two procedures are often performed together. However, this approach is contraindicated if the history indicates the male may have a penile lesion that could be aggravated by sexual arousal.

#### Other body systems

A thorough neurologic and orthopedic examination, especially of the rear limbs, should also be performed. Various neurologic disorders can interfere with mounting, erection, intromission, and ejaculation.

### Semen Evaluation

Semen evaluation with culture and testing for *B. canis* should be performed in dogs. Abnormal spermatozoal motility and morphology are often the first indicators of gonadal damage. Causes include primary testicular disease, metabolic disorders, transient insults (e.g., fever), incomplete ejaculation, and improper sample handling (e.g., temperature shock; exposure to improper pH and osmolality; exposure to latex, rubber, plastic, or other spermicidal agents).

The semen should be reevaluated in 4 to 7 days (sooner if an iatrogenic cause is suspected). If abnormalities persist, semen culture and metabolic evaluation (complete

Table 60-2

## Common Drugs and Metabolic Disorders That Affect Male Reproduction

| Disorder | Cause |
|---|---|
| Decreased LH, testosterone, sperm output, seminal volume, and libido; increased sperm abnormalities | Glucocorticoids |
| | Hyperadrenocorticism |
| Decreased LH, testosterone, and spermatogenesis | Estrogens |
| | Androgens |
| | Anabolic steroids |
| Decreased testosterone, libido, and sperm count | Cimetidine |
| Decreased testosterone and libido | Spironolactone |
| | Anticholinergics |
| | Propranolol |
| | Digoxin |
| | Verapamil |
| | Thiazide diuretics |
| | Chlorpromazine |
| | Barbiturates |
| | Diazepam |
| | Phenytoin |
| | Primidone |
| Decreased testosterone | Progestogens |
| | Ketoconazole |
| Decreased spermatogenesis | Amphotericin B |
| | Many anticancer drugs |
| Decreased libido and sperm count; abnormal semen | Diabetes mellitus |
| Decreased libido and sperm count | Renal failure |
| | Stress |

*LH,* Luteinizing hormone.

blood count [CBC], serum biochemistry profile, urinalysis) of the animal are indicated. If a cause is not identified, semen should be reevaluated in 2 to 3 months before additional tests are performed.

## OLIGOZOOSPERMIA AND AZOOSPERMIA (TEXT PP 915-916)

A decrease in total sperm count may be present with or without abnormalities in sperm morphology or motility. The degree of arousal and frequency of ejaculation affect the number of sperm ejaculated. The number of sperm per ejaculate may decline because of abnormalities in spermatogenesis or ejaculation. It is important to exclude the possibility that the entire sperm-rich fraction was not collected by repeating semen collection.

### Diagnostic approach

Spermatogenesis can be affected by environmental factors (e.g., scrotal temperature), metabolic disorders (especially endocrinopathies), toxins, drugs, and infection. A thorough history, physical examination, routine laboratory tests, and semen culture help to identify the effects of these factors.

*Obstruction.* Oligozoospermia and azoospermia may also result from primary testicular failure, bilateral obstruction of the vas deferens or epididymides, or retrograde ejaculation. Obstruction could also occur at the level of the prostate gland, which should be carefully evaluated. Measurement of seminal AP helps determine whether epididymal fluid, which normally contains sperm, is present in the ejaculate.

***Retrograde ejaculation.*** Ejaculation of semen into the urinary bladder rather than out the urethra is probably neurogenic in origin (possibly, inadequate pressure in the proximal urethra or neck of the bladder). It is diagnosed by finding excessive numbers of sperm in the bladder after ejaculation. (Some sperm are normally found in urine, but large numbers, especially approaching those in discharged semen, are abnormal.) Treatment with α-adrenergic drugs (e.g., pseudoephedrine, 4 to 5 mg/kg orally q8h or twice, 3 hours and 1 hour before breeding) to increase urethral tone has been recommended.

### Treatment and prognosis

Treatment of oligozoospermia and azoospermia depends on the cause. In general, azoospermic males tend to remain azoospermic, especially when the testes are smaller than normal. The presence of small testes in an infertile male suggests either congenital hypoplasia or acquired testicular atrophy or fibrosis, conditions that generally are irreversible. Oligozoospermia may or may not progress to azoospermia. Reevaluation every 2 months for a year is reasonable before the male is pronounced irreversibly sterile.

***Managing subfertile males.*** Oligozoospermic males may be subfertile rather than infertile. Sperm reserves and spermatogenesis usually are poor in oligozoospermic males, so they should be bred judiciously with (1) infrequent ejaculation (e.g., every 4 to 7 days); (2) insemination based on vaginal cytology and ovulation timing with serum progesterone; and (3) breeding only to healthy, fertile females. Intrauterine, rather than intravaginal, insemination may also be considered.


## CONGENITAL INFERTILITY (TEXT P 916)

Congenital infertility should be considered in azoospermic animals that have never sired a litter. Abnormalities include hypogonadotropic hypogonadism, wolffian duct atresia, and disorders of sexual differentiation such as intersex. The phenotypic, gonadal, and chromosomal sex of the animal can be determined by evaluation of external and internal genitalia, measuring serum testosterone and LH, karyotyping, and gonadal biopsy. If the animal is found to be a genotypic and phenotypic male, the diagnostic approach is as for males with acquired infertility.


## ACQUIRED INFERTILITY (TEXT PP 916-917)

### Initial evaluation

In animals with acquired infertility a thorough history taking, physical examination, *B. canis* titer (dogs), and semen evaluation should be performed. Special attention should be paid to the possibility of toxin- or drug-induced infertility, excessive stress, or excessive frequency of ejaculation.

### Semen evaluation

When excessive numbers of WBCs are found in the semen, the site of contamination (urine, prepuce) or inflammatory process must be determined. In dogs, the third fraction of the ejaculate (prostatic fluid) should be submitted separately for cytology and culture. *B. canis* should be excluded with culture and serology. Ultrasonography plus fine-needle aspiration of the testis or prostate gland may also be helpful in localizing the lesion.

The semen should be cultured for aerobic and anaerobic bacteria and for *Mycoplasma*. Bacterial prostatitis is a common, potentially reversible cause of infertility. Appropriate antimicrobial therapy should continue for 2 to 4 weeks, or longer in cases of chronic bacterial prostatitis.

### Further evaluation

If the history, physical examination, prostate and testicular ultrasound, and semen evaluation and culture fail to establish the diagnosis, a thorough metabolic and endocrine evaluation should be conducted before more invasive procedures are performed. Diagnostic tests may include CBC, serum biochemistry profile, urinalysis, and adrenal function tests (see Chapter 53). Assessment of serum LH and testosterone may also be warranted.

### Testicular aspiration or biopsy

Testicular aspiration or biopsy should be considered when other noninvasive tests have failed to identify the cause and when the abnormalities in sperm morphology or concentration are still present after several months. Lesions include neoplasia, suppurative and nonsuppurative inflammation, mycotic orchitis, lymphocytic orchitis, granulomatous orchitis, spermatogenic arrest, testicular degeneration, and Sertoli cells only. Testicular biopsy may not be warranted in animals with testes that are already substantially smaller than normal.

# 61

# Disorders of the Penis, Prepuce, and Testes

## *(Text pp 918-926)*

## ACQUIRED PENILE DISORDERS (TEXT PP 918-919)

### Penile Trauma

Trauma to the penis can cause hematomas, lacerations, or fracture of the os penis. Penile injuries are usually very painful; other signs include swelling, bruising, and hemorrhage. The prepuce may also be affected. Fractures of the os penis are often associated with urinary outflow obstruction and/or urethral tears. Affected animals may have a distended bladder or postrenal uremia.

#### Diagnosis

Diagnosis is made by visual examination and radiographic evaluation of the penile urethra and os penis. The integrity of the urethra should be evaluated by retrograde urethrography whenever significant penile trauma is found. Ultrasonography and color-flow Doppler imaging can help differentiate penile hematoma from priapism.

#### Treatment

Treatment includes cleansing and débridement as necessary. Lacerations may require surgical closure with absorbable sutures. Antibiotic cream should be applied and the penis protruded twice daily until the lesions are healed. Sexual arousal must be avoided until the lesion is completely healed.

*Os penis fracture.* Treatment depends on the severity of urethral damage and fracture displacement. If necessary, the bladder is initially decompressed by cysto-centesis, then an indwelling urethral catheter is maintained while the urethra heals. Urethral tears may require suturing; temporary or permanent urethrostomy could be considered for severe tears. Displaced fractures can be immobilized with orthopedic wire. Penile amputation may be necessary if trauma is severe. Systemic antibiotics should be administered to prevent urinary tract infection.

## Priapism

Priapism is abnormal, persistent erection unassociated with sexual arousal. Possible causes include spinal cord lesions, general anesthesia, administration of phenothiazines, and thromboembolism, although in many cases a cause is not identified. Priapism must be differentiated from transient erections in excitable dogs, erection that persists for longer than expected after copulation or semen collection, and other causes of penile swelling (e.g., hematoma, edema). Visual inspection and palpation of the penis are usually sufficient to differentiate these conditions. Ultrasound examination (plus color-flow Doppler imaging) may help differentiate hematoma from priapism.

Fortunately, priapism is rare in dogs and cats. In every case it must be corrected promptly, because stagnated blood in the cavernous sinuses eventually clots, a situation that may not resolve even when venous drainage is reestablished. In addition, ischemic necrosis is common.

### Treatment

Nonischemic priapism may respond to treatment with anticholinergic agents or antihistamines, such as diphenhydramine and benztropine (0.015 mg/kg intravenously), if initiated early (within hours). Surgical drainage and intracorporeal lavage may also be successful when performed early.

The priapic penis must be protected from further damage or irritation that may perpetuate the problem or lead to sequelae such as edema, thrombosis, fibrosis, penile paralysis, or necrosis. Treatment includes cleansing the penis, application of antibiotic cream, and attempts to maintain the penis within the prepuce until the condition subsides.

Unfortunately, many cases of priapism are not presented until the condition has been present for days or weeks, by which time necrosis necessitates penile amputation or perineal urethrostomy.

## Miscellaneous Disorders

Vesicles, ulcers, pyogranulomatous lesions, warts, and neoplasia of the penis have been identified in dogs. Signs are similar and include preputial discharge, excessive licking of the prepuce or penis, or presence of a mass protruding from the prepuce. These lesions are differentiated by visual examination, cytology, bacterial and fungal culture, and biopsy. Lymphoid follicle hyperplasia may be confused with vesicles unless the tissues are examined microscopically. Penile warts often resolve spontaneously after biopsy of the lesion is performed.

## CONGENITAL PENILE DISORDERS (TEXT PP 919-920)

### Persistent Penile Frenulum

#### Dogs

Persistent penile frenulum in dogs is usually located on the ventral midline of the penis; it may cause the penis to deviate ventrally or laterally so that the dog is unable or unwilling to mate. No clinical signs may be present, or the dog may have a preputial discharge and/or lick the prepuce excessively. Diagnosis is made by visual examination. Treatment is surgical excision, which can often be accomplished with local anesthetic or sedation.

#### Cats

Persistence of the adhesions between the prepuce and penis may be seen in male cats that are castrated before 5 months of age. The clinical significance, if any, remains to be determined.

## PREPUTIAL DISORDERS (TEXT PP 920-921)

### Balanoposthitis

Inflammation of the preputial cavity is very common in dogs but rare in cats. The organisms involved usually are part of the normal preputial flora (see Table 60-1); infections with canine herpesvirus and *Blastomyces* have also been reported.

### Signs and diagnosis
Balanoposthitis usually causes no signs other than a purulent preputial discharge varying from scant white smegma to copious green pus. The discharge associated with uncomplicated balanoposthitis is not sanguineous. Diagnosis is based on physical examination. The penis should be thoroughly evaluated for foreign material, neoplasia, ulceration, and inflammatory nodules. Cultures and cytology are rarely performed unless herpesvirus or fungal infection is suspected.

### Treatment
Treatment is conservative: cleansing the preputial cavity with antiseptic solutions (e.g., chlorhexidine, povidone-iodine) and instilling topical antibacterial medications. Castration usually diminishes preputial secretions.

## Phimosis
Phimosis (entrapment of the penis within the prepuce) is usually caused by an abnormally small preputial opening. It is uncommon in cats and dogs. Phimosis may be recognized in young animals as a cause of urinary outflow obstruction or urine dribbling, or it may be identified when an affected male is unable to copulate. Treatment involves surgical enlargement of the preputial orifice. Entangled preputial hairs may cause similar signs in long-haired cats.

## Paraphimosis
Paraphimosis (inability to retract the penis into the prepuce) occurs most frequently after erection in dogs. It may occur in long-haired cats when the penis becomes entangled in preputial hairs; otherwise, paraphimosis is uncommon in cats.

### Signs
Initially the exposed penis appears normal and nonpainful. After several minutes it becomes edematous and increasingly painful; the surface becomes dry, and fissures may develop. Long-standing paraphimosis may result in gangrene or necrosis, but this is uncommon. Diagnosis is made by visual inspection.

### Treatment
Treatment involves gently sliding the prepuce back (i.e., in a caudal direction) until the cranial aspect "unfolds" and the preputial orifice is exposed. Circulation to the penis usually improves immediately after the prepuce is restored to its normal configuration; penile edema then begins to subside. The surface of the penis is cleansed or débrided as necessary; antibiotic or antibiotic-steroid cream can be applied if the penile mucosa is damaged. The penis is then replaced in the preputial cavity. If the edematous tissue is sufficiently thickened that the prepuce cannot slide over it, application of pressure with a cool water compress is usually effective in resolving the edema.

Rarely is it necessary to enlarge the preputial orifice. In such cases an incision is made on the ventral midline of the prepuce, and after the penis is in place the incision is closed in separate layers. Rarely does the still-swollen penis protrude from the prepuce. The preputial orifice may be temporarily (1 to 24 hours) sutured closed, but a risk exists that urine will accumulate in the preputial cavity during this time. If the penis has become necrotic or gangrenous, penile amputation is indicated.

# TESTICULAR DISORDERS (TEXT PP 921-926)
## Orchitis and Epididymitis
Infection of the testis or epididymis can occur hematogenously, by spread of pathogens from elsewhere in the urogenital tract or as a result of penetrating wounds. Extension or progression of infection from the epididymis to the testis, or vice versa, is common. Orchitis-epididymitis is more common in dogs than in cats. Aerobic bacteria are most often implicated. *Mycoplasma, Brucella canis, Blastomyces, Ehrlichia,* Rocky Mountain spotted fever, and feline infectious peritonitis can also infect the testes, epididymides, or scrotum.

### Clinical features

Acute infections usually cause scrotal swelling and pain. The affected epididymis or testis is enlarged, firm, and warm; the scrotal skin may be inflamed, and the dog may lick the scrotum excessively. Fever and lethargy may be present in animals with systemic infections. Some affected animals show minimal discomfort, and the acute phase may be unnoticed by the owner. With chronic orchitis and epididymitis the scrotum is usually normal; the testis becomes soft and atrophic, and the epididymis may seem firmer and more prominent than normal, especially if the testis is primarily affected. Infertility is common and may be the presenting complaint.

### Diagnosis

Diagnosis is based on physical examination, ultrasonography, and findings of cytology and culture (semen or fine-needle aspirate of the testis). Semen from dogs with active orchitis-epididymitis contains many inflammatory cells (leukospermia) and abnormal spermatozoa. Bacteria or other infectious agents, however, usually are not seen; they are more commonly observed in fine-needle aspirates. In animals with chronic infection and atrophy of the testes the number of inflammatory cells and spermatozoa decreases, eventually resulting in azoospermia. Serologic tests for *B. canis* should always be performed in dogs with these clinical and cytologic findings. Thorough evaluation of the prostate gland is also warranted.

***Semen culture.*** Semen culture from dogs with active bacterial infection usually yields >100,000 colony-forming units (CFU)/ml. Culture results must be interpreted in light of the normal urethral flora (see Table 60-1) and other clinical and cytologic findings. Culture may be negative in animals with chronic orchitis-epididymitis, especially in those with chronic *B. canis* infection.

### Treatment

Antimicrobial therapy should be initiated if semen culture is positive for significant bacterial growth. Antibiotics to consider before results are known include enrofloxacin, amoxicillin, clavulanate-amoxicillin, chloramphenicol, and trimethoprim-sulfonamide. Cephalosporins and tetracycline can also be considered. Antimicrobial therapy should continue for at least 2 weeks.

Soaking the scrotum in cool water may help minimize the damage caused by hyperthermia and swelling, but the prognosis for fertility is poor, regardless of the causal organism. Orchidectomy should be considered when fertility appears to be irreversibly lost. In cases of unilateral involvement, unilateral orchidectomy may be the best way to protect the apparently unaffected gonad. Antibiotics should be administered whether or not surgery is performed.

## Cryptorchidism

Cryptorchidism is hereditary (autosomal recessive), occurring more commonly in Toy and Miniature Poodles, Yorkshire Terriers, Chihuahuas, Boxers, Pomeranians, Miniature Schnauzers, Pekingese, Maltese, Shetland Sheepdogs, Cairn Terriers, and Persian cats. Both males and females carry the gene. Unilateral cryptorchidism is more common than bilateral cryptorchidism.

### Treatment

No known medical treatment reliably causes descent of cryptorchid testes. In dogs the cryptorchid testis is approximately 13 times more likely than the descended testis to develop neoplasia. Therefore castration of cryptorchid dogs while they are young is recommended. Ultrasonography may be helpful in locating the retained testis. Testicular neoplasia is rare in cats, regardless of the location of the testes.

## Testicular Torsion

Testicular torsion of an intraabdominal testis causes acute abdominal pain and is treated by castration. Torsion of a scrotal testis is less common. Pain is the major clinical sign, but scrotal and testicular swelling also occur and can be quite pronounced; often the spermatic cord is palpably thickened. Ultrasonography of the affected testis and spermatic cord usually reveals the abnormal course of the spermatic vessels. Treatment is unilateral orchidectomy, as spermatogenesis is irreparably damaged as a result of ischemia within 1 to 2 hours of testicular torsion.

## Testicular Neoplasia

Testicular tumors are very common in old dogs (mean age at diagnosis, approximately 10 years), but they are extremely rare in cats. In most dogs the tumor is benign, and often it is an incidental finding.

### Classification

Sertoli cell tumors, interstitial (Leydig) cell tumors, and seminomas occur with equal frequency. Nearly 100% of interstitial cell tumors and 75% of seminomas occur in descended testes, whereas 60% of Sertoli cell tumors occur in cryptorchid testes.

*Sertoli cell tumor.* Sertoli cell tumors are usually 1 mm to 5 cm in diameter, although they may be much larger; 10% to 20% metastasize, usually to lumbar or iliac lymph nodes. Affected dogs typically are presented because of inguinal or scrotal enlargement. Intraabdominal tumors may cause abdominal enlargement or signs of abdominal pain.

Some dogs with Sertoli cell tumors are brought for treatment because of the paraneoplastic syndromes associated with estrogen production: alopecia, hyperpigmentation, feminization (gynecomastia, pendulous scrotum and prepuce), squamous metaplasia of the prostate gland, bone marrow suppression (anemia, thrombocytopenia, leukopenia), depressed spermatogenesis, and/or testicular atrophy.

*Interstitial cell tumor.* Interstitial cell tumors usually are incidental findings; they tend to be fairly small (1 to 2 cm diameter) and rarely metastasize or cause clinical signs. They may, however, secrete hormones and cause paraneoplastic syndromes.

*Seminoma.* Seminomas are usually confined to one testis, although metastasis occurs in 6% to 11% of cases. They may be incidental findings or may grow to a size at which scrotal or inguinal enlargement is obvious. Estrogen-related paraneoplastic syndrome is rare with this type of tumor.

### Diagnosis

Diagnosis is usually straightforward. The index of suspicion is highest in old, cryptorchid males. Diagnosis is most challenging in animals (erroneously) assumed by owners to have been castrated because they do not have scrotal testes. Neoplasia is suspected when a mass is palpated in a testis or in the mid or caudal abdomen of a cryptorchid dog, or when signs of feminization are present. Less commonly, the dog may be brought for treatment of poor fertility, atrophy of the other testis, prostatic disease, or hematologic or dermatologic abnormalities.

*Diagnostic imaging.* Ultrasonography is helpful when testicular neoplasia is suspected but not palpable, and to differentiate intratesticular from extratesticular causes of scrotal enlargement. Testicular tumors have variable echotexture. Tumors <3 cm usually appear hypoechoic; larger tumors usually have mixed echogenicity. Ultrasonography and radiography can also be used to evaluate intraabdominal testes.

*Fine-needle aspiration.* Cytologic examination of aspirated material can be helpful in differentiating a testicular neoplasm from other masses such as abscess or granuloma. However, it is rarely necessary.

*Exfoliative cytology.* If preputial mucosal epithelial cells are cornified, it indicates the presence of an estrogen-secreting tumor (unless exogenous estrogens have been administered). The most likely source is a testis, but pathologic production of sex hormones by the adrenal gland has been reported in dogs with hyperadrenocorticism.

### Treatment and prognosis

Treatment for all testicular tumors is castration. When unilateral involvement occurs in a stud dog, hemicastration may be considered. Dogs with bone marrow suppression may need supportive care such as blood transfusion in anemic or thrombocytopenic animals and prophylactic systemic antibiotics in granulocytopenic animals. The prognosis for bone marrow recovery is guarded to poor, and improvement often takes months. Treatment of metastatic lesions with surgery and/or chemotherapy may be considered, but the prognosis is grave.

# 62

# Disorders
# of the Prostate Gland

## *(Text pp 927-933)*

Prostatic disorders are common in dogs but rare in cats. The most common signs are tenesmus, blood dripping from the urethra independent of urination, hematuria, and recurrent urinary tract infections. Nonspecific signs, such as fever, malaise, and caudal abdominal pain, are often present with bacterial infection or neoplasia. Less commonly, prostatic diseases cause urethral obstruction, infertility, or urinary incontinence.

## DIAGNOSTIC APPROACH (TEXT PP 927-928)

Physical examination (including abdominal and rectal palpation of the prostate gland) usually localizes the disease process to the prostate gland, but it is not possible to differentiate among the various prostatic conditions by physical examination alone. Abdominal radiography, ultrasonography, prostatic cytologic studies, bacterial culture, biopsy, or a combination of these studies is usually required to differentiate the specific prostatic disorders.

### Radiography

Abdominal radiographs help define the size, shape, and position of the prostate. Prostatomegaly is indicated by a prostatic length >70% of the distance from the sacral promontory to the pelvic brim on the lateral radiograph. Prostatic depth, however, is an unreliable indicator of prostatic size. The radiographic appearance of the sublumbar lymph nodes, lumbar vertebrae, and pelvis should be evaluated for evidence of metastasis. A positive-contrast cystourethrogram can be performed if it is difficult to differentiate an abnormal prostate from the urinary bladder, and to assess the prostatic urethra.

### Ultrasonography

Ultrasonography provides additional information about the dimensions of the prostate gland, homogeneity of the prostatic parenchyma, urethral diameter, and whether prostatic disease is diffuse or focal. Urethral invasion or destruction is highly suggestive of prostatic neoplasia. Other ultrasonographic findings do not differentiate cysts from abscesses or hyperplasia from metaplasia, prostatitis, or diffuse neoplasia.

### Cytology and microbiology

Prostatic material for cytologic and microbiologic examination can be obtained by prostatic massage, urethral brush, ejaculation, fine-needle aspiration, or biopsy. Techniques are described in the text. Prostatic massage is easily performed; however, there exists a risk of rupturing prostatic abscesses or liberating septic emboli during massage. When urinary tract infection is present (which is common with bacterial prostatitis), microbiologic examination of the prostatic portion (third fraction) of the ejaculate is more accurate for confirming bacterial prostatitis than is examination of specimens obtained by massage.

Fine-needle aspiration or biopsy of the prostate gland may be required to establish a diagnosis. Fine-needle aspiration is usually performed percutaneously, with or without ultrasound guidance. Despite the potential for peritoneal contamination or inadvertent penetration of surrounding structures, the risks are minimal with careful technique, especially when ultrasound guidance is used. Biopsy is the most definitive procedure for differentiation of prostatic diseases. It is performed through a celiotomy or percutaneously under ultrasound guidance.

## BENIGN PROSTATIC HYPERPLASIA (TEXT PP 928-930)

Benign prostatic hyperplasia (BPH) is the most common prostatic disorder in dogs. It occurs in most intact male dogs >6 years of age. BPH may be subclinical, or it may cause tenesmus, dripping of blood from the urethra in the absence of urination, or hematuria.

### Diagnosis

The diagnosis of BPH is suggested when tenesmus, a sanguineous urethral discharge, and/or hematuria is found in an otherwise healthy, middle-aged or older, intact dog with symmetric prostatomegaly. The prostate gland is not painful when palpated. Radiography confirms the presence of prostatomegaly, and ultrasonography reveals diffuse, relatively symmetric involvement throughout the prostate. Small, multiple, diffuse, cystic structures are commonly seen on ultrasound (cystic hyperplasia).

*Cytology and culture.* Cytologic examination of massage, ejaculate, or aspirate specimens reveals evidence of hemorrhage and perhaps mild inflammation but no evidence of sepsis or neoplasia. The diagnosis of BPH could be confirmed by prostatic biopsy, but biopsy is rarely necessary. In approximately 40% of cases bacterial culture of the cystic fluid is positive (most often *Escherichia coli, Streptococcus viridans,* or *Mycoplasma,* sometimes in mixed populations). In the majority of these cases urine culture is also positive for the same organisms. Asymptomatic urinary tract infection may be found in dogs in which prostatic culture is negative. Therefore urine culture should be a routine part of the diagnostic evaluation of dogs with BPH.

### Treatment

Treatment is not necessary for asymptomatic BPH. Castration is the treatment of choice in dogs showing clinical signs. Castration is curative, and complete involution of the gland is expected within 12 weeks; prostatic bleeding usually resolves within 4 weeks. In breeding males treatment with antiandrogen drugs can be considered, but it is not as effective as castration in resolving clinical signs, and results are only temporary; relapse occurs after such drugs are discontinued. *Estrogen therapy is not recommended.*

*Progestins.* In dogs megestrol acetate (0.5 mg/kg orally q24h for 10 days to 4 weeks) can resolve the signs without apparent effects on fertility. Delmadinone acetate (1.5 mg/kg subcutaneously [SC], repeated 1 week and 4 weeks later) can also be used to treat BPH. However, it causes adrenal suppression for up to 21 days after the last dose and is not as effective as castration in resolving prostatic bleeding. Medroxyprogesterone acetate (3 mg/kg SC once) relieves clinical signs in most dogs without affecting semen quality or libido; however, relapse occurs 10 to 24 months after treatment.

*Finasteride.* The most appropriate dose of finasteride (Proscar) for BPH in dogs remains to be determined. With oral daily doses of 0.1 to 0.2 mg/kg, clinical signs begin to improve after 1 week of treatment, and prostatic size is significantly decreased by 8 weeks. No adverse effects have been reported at this dose. Other than a decrease in prostatic fluid volume, the drug has no effect on semen quality, libido, or ejaculation, even after 4 to 6 months of treatment. Note: Finasteride is teratogenic, so pregnant women must not handle this drug.

## SQUAMOUS METAPLASIA (TEXT P 930)

Estrogen-secreting Sertoli cell tumors (see Chapter 61) or, rarely, adrenal tumors and estrogen therapy can each cause squamous metaplasia of the prostatic epithelium and prostatic fluid accumulation. The net effect is enlargement of the prostate gland. Clinical signs and physical findings may be identical to those of BPH; signs of hyperestrogenism (see Chapter 61) may also be present. A testicular mass or cryptorchidism may be identified on physical examination.

### Diagnosis and treatment

Diagnosis is tentatively based on the history and physical examination. Increased numbers of squamous epithelial cells are often found in ejaculated or aspirated prostatic specimens. If necessary, the diagnosis can be confirmed by fine-needle aspiration or biopsy. Treatment involves removal of the estrogen source by castration (testicular tumors) or discontinuation of estrogenic drugs. Unilateral castration might be considered in a breeding dog.

## BACTERIAL PROSTATITIS AND PROSTATIC ABSCESS (TEXT PP 930-932)

Bacterial infection of the prostate gland can be acute or chronic and can lead to prostatic abscess. Cystic hyperplasia, squamous metaplasia, and other prostatic disorders may increase the risk for infection. The most common source of infection is ascension of urethral flora (see Table 60-1); hematogenous spread is also possible. The organisms most commonly isolated are *E. coli, Staphylococcus, Streptococcus,* and *Mycoplasma.* Occasionally, *Proteus, Pseudomonas,* or anaerobes are found.

### Acute Bacterial Prostatitis or Abscess

Animals with acute bacterial prostatitis or prostatic abscess usually have a history of an acute onset of severe illness, with abdominal pain and perhaps a hemorrhagic preputial discharge. Fever, dehydration, and pain on palpation of the prostate gland are usually present. Septicemia and endotoxemia can develop.

#### Diagnosis

Diagnosis is based on physical findings, ultrasonography, culture of prostatic fluid or urine, and cytology of material obtained by prostatic aspiration. Prostatic size may not be markedly changed in dogs with prostatitis, whereas asymmetric prostatomegaly and fluctuant areas are usually palpable with prostatic abscesses. Ultrasonography of an abscessed prostate gland reveals intraparenchymal, fluid-filled spaces. Neutrophilic leukocytosis with variable left shift, signs of neutrophil toxicity, and monocytosis are typically found on complete blood count.

*Culture.* Prostatic fluid obtained by ejaculation is a good specimen for bacterial culture. Cultures from dogs with bacterial prostatitis usually yield >100,000 colony-forming units per milliliter. However, dogs with acute prostatitis or abscess usually are in too much pain and too ill to ejaculate. Fine-needle aspiration, preferably under ultrasound guidance, provides suitable samples for culture. Urine culture also is acceptable, as some prostatic fluid normally refluxes into the bladder. If urinalysis is abnormal (e.g., hematuria, pyuria, and/or bacteriuria), urine should always be submitted for culture. Prostatic massage for fluid collection is not advised if acute bacterial prostatitis or abscess is suspected.

*Cytology.* Cytologic evaluation of prostatic material should also be performed. It usually reveals inflammation with evidence of sepsis and hemorrhage; macrophages also are present with chronic infection.

#### Treatment

Acute bacterial prostatitis and prostatic abscess are serious, life-threatening disorders. Treatment must be prompt and aggressive. Antibiotic therapy is the principal mode of treatment. Erythromycin, clindamycin, oleandomycin, trimethoprim-sulfonamide, chloramphenicol, carbenicillin, enrofloxacin, and ciprofloxacin are the agents most capable of achieving therapeutic concentrations in the prostate gland. Antibiotic treatment should continue for 2 to 3 weeks. Urine and/or prostatic fluid should be recultured within a few days of discontinuation of therapy and again 2 to 4 weeks later.

In addition to antibiotics, fluid therapy is necessary to correct dehydration and shock. Large prostatic abscesses are most effectively treated by surgical drainage. The abscess may also be drained by fine-needle aspiration under ultrasound guidance. Castration should also be considered. It can be performed whenever the dog's condition is stable enough for general anesthesia. Prostatic abscesses recur in approximately 10% of dogs.

## Chronic Bacterial Prostatitis
Chronic bacterial prostatitis can be asymptomatic, except for recurrent urinary tract infection, and abnormalities can be limited to the urinary tract. Prostate size and shape can be normal, or the prostate can be asymmetric and firmer than normal; it may or may not be painful on palpation. Prostatic fluid and urine should be submitted for cytology and culture.

### Treatment
Chronic bacterial prostatitis can be difficult to resolve. Antibiotic therapy should continue for at least 4 weeks. Cultures should be repeated during and for several months after discontinuation of antibiotic therapy. Castration is often recommended because it hastens resolution of bacterial prostatitis.

## PARAPROSTATIC CYSTS (TEXT P 932)
Paraprostatic cysts are located outside the prostatic parenchyma but are attached to the gland by a stalk or adhesions. These cysts can become extremely large and cause signs, including tenesmus, referable to mechanical interference with abdominal viscera. Paraprostatic cyst should be considered in a male dog with a large, caudal abdominal mass. The mass may be difficult to differentiate from the bladder without a cystogram. Fine-needle aspiration of the cyst usually yields a sterile, yellow-to-serosanguineous fluid with minimal inflammation.

### Treatment
The treatment of choice is surgical excision of the cyst and castration. When the cyst cannot be completely excised, omentalization is recommended. If this approach fails to resolve the problem, marsupialization could be performed; however, it is a poor alternative because it is not curative and the permanent fistula may become infected.

## PROSTATIC NEOPLASIA (TEXT PP 932-933)
Adenocarcinoma is the most common prostatic neoplasm in dogs but is rarely reported in cats. It occurs in older dogs (mean age at diagnosis, 10 years). Transitional cell carcinoma of the urinary tract can invade the prostate. Signs and biologic behavior of these tumors in the prostate gland are similar. Prostatic adenocarcinoma is locally invasive and metastasizes to the sublumbar lymph nodes, pelvis, and lumbar vertebrae.

### Clinical features
Clinical signs include tenesmus and dyschezia, stranguria, pain, gait abnormalities, and weight loss. Palpation of the prostate gland usually elicits pain. In many cases the gland is not dramatically increased in size, although its shape may be irregular and its consistency firmer than normal.

### Diagnosis
Prostatic neoplasia is suggested by historic, physical, and radiographic findings. It should be the primary consideration for a "normal" or enlarged prostate gland in a castrated male. Urinary obstruction rarely occurs in dogs with prostatic diseases other than neoplasia, but it is fairly common in those with neoplasia. Ultrasonographically, prostatic adenocarcinomas usually are hyperechoic, but this is not pathognomonic. Urethral invasion demonstrated by contrast radiography or ultrasonography is highly suggestive of neoplasia.

The diagnosis is confirmed by fine-needle aspiration or biopsy. Neoplastic cells may be found in specimens aspirated through a urethral catheter, especially if the tumor has invaded the urethra. However, neoplastic cells are not usually found in massage or ejaculate specimens.

**Treatment and prognosis**

The prognosis for animals with prostatic adenocarcinoma is grave. To date, surgical (prostatectomy), chemotherapeutic, hormonal, and radiation therapy have been unsuccessful in improving the quality or length of life.

# 63

---

# Genital Infections and Transmissible Venereal Tumor

## *(Text pp 934-939)*

### HERPESVIRUS INFECTION (TEXT PP 934-935)

Mild respiratory disease is the most common sign of infection with canine or feline herpesvirus (CHV and FHV) in animals >12 weeks of age. CHV has been suggested as a cause of vesicular lesions on the vagina and prepuce. CHV has been recovered from semen and can be transmitted venereally, but venereal transmission of CHV and FHV is rare. Relative to respiratory infection in adults and neonatal herpesvirus infection, genital herpes is rare.

In neonates herpesvirus infection causes fulminant, multiple organ failure and death. Neonates become infected in utero or by postnatal exposure to infected secretions from the dam or to other infected adults. Adult carriers are often asymptomatic. Neonatal infection is one of the most common manifestations of CHV in a breeding colony. Abortion, stillbirths, and infertility have also been reported.

#### Diagnosis

Herpesvirus infection should be considered in cases of acute neonatal death and as a potential cause of abortion or vesicular lesions on the genital mucosa in adults. Suspicion is especially high in catteries with known respiratory infections with FHV. In this situation, FHV should also be considered in the evaluation of infertility. The diagnosis can be confirmed by finding intranuclear inclusions in tissue sections, by serology, and by virus isolation.

##### *Neonates or aborted materials.* The diagnosis is most easily established in cases of neonatal death; postmortem lesions are characteristic and include multifocal, diffuse hemorrhage and gray discoloration of parenchymal organs, especially kidney, liver, and lung. Samples of liver, kidney, and spleen should be submitted chilled (not frozen) for virus isolation, and formalin fixed for histopathology. The whole abortus or placenta can be submitted chilled for virus isolation. Although FHV causes abortion in cats, the virus usually is not recovered from aborted material; however, intranuclear inclusions

are found in histologic specimens from the uterus, placenta, and aborted fetuses of infected queens.

**Genital lesions.** In cases of suspected herpes-induced genital lesions, swabs (preferably Dacron-tipped applicators) from the affected area should be submitted on ice for virus isolation. Biopsy of the lesions can also be performed. Inclusions may be found but are less common than in nasal epithelium or kidney.

**Nasal and conjunctival swabs.** In cats, virus isolation can be attempted from nasal and conjunctival swabs collected during the first week of illness. Conjunctival smears may demonstrate intranuclear inclusions with fluorescent antibody techniques; however, the inclusions are transient and difficult to detect.

**Serology.** Serum antibody titers rise and fall quickly (within 4 to 8 weeks) after infection. Titers are relatively low for both FHV (1:8 to 1:64) and CHV (1:2 to 1:32). Detection of antibody indicates exposure to herpesvirus or, in animals <6 weeks old, the presence of maternal antibodies; it is not indicative of viral shedding. However, when seropositive animals also have typical signs, a positive serologic test is diagnostic for herpesvirus infection.

### Prevention and control

Transmission is by direct contact with infected animals and fomites, so prevention and control are accomplished by changing management practices to avoid overcrowding, improve sanitation and hygiene, and keep pregnant females and neonates separate from all other colony members. Commonly available disinfectants are effective against these viruses. Vaccines against FHV (i.e., against feline rhinotracheitis) are widely available.

## *MYCOPLASMA* AND *UREAPLASMA* (TEXT PP 935-936)

*Mycoplasma* and *Ureaplasma* are part of the normal genital flora in dogs and are isolated with equal frequency from normal dogs and those with reproductive disorders. Few species of *Mycoplasma* and *Ureaplasma* have been conclusively shown to be pathogenic. *Mycoplasma canis* has been recovered from bitches with endometritis and from infertile dogs with leukospermia, but its role is unclear.

### Diagnosis

*Mycoplasma* and *Ureaplasma* require a special medium such as Amies and should arrive at the laboratory within 24 hours, on ice. *Mycoplasma* or *Ureaplasma* infection should not be diagnosed on the basis of culture results alone; clinical signs and cytologic findings should be consistent with an infectious process.

### Treatment

These organisms usually are susceptible to tetracycline, chloramphenicol, and fluoroquinolones. Erythromycin, lincomycin, and aminoglycosides are less effective. However, many of these antibiotics are contraindicated during pregnancy and lactation (see Box 59-2). Antibiotic therapy should continue for 2 to 3 weeks, and longer if a bacteriostatic antibiotic is used.

## *BRUCELLA CANIS* (TEXT PP 936-938)

*Brucella canis* is a small, gram-negative coccobacillus. Bacteremia is present 1 to 4 weeks after infection and persists for 6 months to 5.5 years. Nonprotective antibody titers develop 4 to 12 weeks after infection and persist as long as bacteremia is present. Titers decline after bacteremia subsides, even though the organism is still present in tissues.

### Transmission

Oronasal and conjunctival exposure to infected material (especially aborted material) and contaminated fomites is the most important route of infection. Infected females transmit the organism in estrual discharge, transplacentally, and after abortion. The organism is also shed in lower numbers in milk, urine (females and males), and semen. Urinary excretion of the organisms coincides with the onset of bacteremia and persists for at least 3 months. Shedding of the organism in semen is greatest during the first 6 to 8 weeks of infection and may persist for 1 to 2 years.

### Clinical features

Abortion, especially late in gestation in an otherwise healthy, afebrile bitch, is the most common sign in females. However, abortion can occur at any time during gestation. Early embryonic death, conception failure, and early neonatal death are also reported. Occasionally, *B. canis* infects other tissues, potentially resulting in uveitis, diskospondylitis, osteomyelitis, or dermatitis.

The most common sign in males is infertility. Transient scrotal and epididymal enlargement may occur early in infection, but testicular swelling is uncommon. Reduction in semen quality occurs within 5 weeks of infection and is pronounced by 8 weeks. White blood cells, macrophages, sperm agglutination, and abnormal sperm morphology are found. Eventually, testicular atrophy and azoospermia develop.

### Diagnosis

The diagnosis is suggested by the history, relative lack of physical abnormalities, and, in males, semen abnormalities. Although serology is useful, confirmation requires identification of the organism by culture or polymerase chain reaction.

*Culture.* Aborted material and postabortion vulvar discharge are the preferred specimens for culture. Blood, urine, and semen are suitable alternatives. Blood culture is best for diagnosing early (2 to 8 weeks) infection; bacteremia subsides with chronic infection. Semen culture is most helpful during the first 3 months of infection in males. The organism may also be recovered from the spleen, liver, bone marrow, lymph nodes, prostate, epididymis, placenta, and uterine lumen.

*Serology.* Serologic testing is the most frequently used screening procedure. Antibodies to cell wall antigens are first detectable 3 to 10 weeks after infection. However, serum titers and the accuracy of results vary greatly among tests and laboratories. Results for rapid slide agglutination (RSAT), tube agglutination (TAT), and agar gel immunodiffusion (AGID) tests are not specific for *B. canis*, so false-positive results can occur.

*RSAT.* Despite its lack of specificity, RSAT (D-Tec CB) is easy, quick, and highly sensitive. False-negative results are rare (1%) in animals that have been infected long enough to develop antibodies to cell wall antigens. However, treatment with antibiotics may cause negative results despite persistence of the organism in tissues, and titers decline in animals with chronic infection.

*AGID.* The AGID tests using cytoplasmic antigen are highly specific for *Brucella* infection. Antibodies to these antigens are not detected for 8 to 12 weeks after infection, but they may persist up to 12 months after bacteremia has ceased—a time when other test results often are negative. However, the AGID test is complex, and it is less sensitive than RSAT or TAT.

### Treatment

*B. canis* is an intracellular organism, so antibiotic therapy rarely results in a cure; bacteremia often recurs days or months after treatment. Minocycline or gentamicin and doxycycline are sometimes prescribed; the fluoroquinolones are effective against *B. canis* in vitro. However, because the chance of successful treatment is so uncertain, and because infected animals remain a source of infection for other dogs and people, treatment is ill advised. If treatment is attempted, infected animals should be neutered.

### Prevention and control

RSAT is recommended for routine screening of asymptomatic animals; TAT and AGID can also be used. All animals should be tested before breeding, and new colony members quarantined for 8 to 12 weeks until at least two tests at 4-week intervals are negative. Animals with any symptoms of *B. canis* infection should never be admitted to the colony until *B. canis* is excluded as the cause (which can take as long as 3 months).

*Control in a breeding colony.* When results of RSAT or other screening test are positive, especially if the animal is showing signs compatible with *B. canis* infection, it should be isolated and the entire kennel quarantined until the results can be verified. When infection is confirmed, the animal with the infection should be culled, and the remaining colony members tested monthly until all animals are negative for 3 consecutive months.

**Control for pet dogs.** A different approach might be considered for a household pet. Antibiotic therapy plus neutering should essentially eliminate genital shedding of organisms, but that does not exclude the possibility that the animal might remain a source of infection for other dogs or humans. It is recommended that immunocompromised people avoid contact with infected dogs.

## CANINE TRANSMISSIBLE VENEREAL TUMOR (TEXT PP 938-939)

Transmissible venereal tumor (TVT) is a contagious round-cell tumor of dogs that primarily occurs on the mucosal surfaces of the external genitalia. Less often, primary TVTs are found on the skin or on oral or anal mucosae. TVTs can be transplanted to other sites and transmitted to other dogs by licking and by direct contact with the tumor; venereal transmission is most common. Some TVTs regress spontaneously, but most do not. Some metastasize to regional lymph nodes, the perineum, or the scrotum. Metastases are more likely with tumors that have been present for >1 month. Metastasis to distant sites (e.g., lungs, abdominal viscera, central nervous system) is rare.

### Clinical features

TVTs have a fleshy, hyperemic appearance; many are quite friable and bleed easily. Initially they appear as a raised area, and as they grow, they develop a cauliflower-like shape and may reach 5 cm in diameter. TVTs are most often found on the bulbus glandis of the penis, but they may appear anywhere on the penile or preputial mucosa. Affected animals are usually examined because of a mass on the external genitalia, but they may be brought for treatment because of a preputial or vulvar discharge.

### Diagnosis

The diagnosis is strongly suspected on the basis of the physical appearance and location of the tumor. Differential diagnoses, especially of nongenital lesions, include other round-cell tumors (e.g., mast cell tumor, histiocytoma, lymphoma); pyogranulomatous lesions of the genitalia can have a similar gross appearance. The diagnosis of genital TVT is easily confirmed by exfoliative cytology, fine-needle aspiration, or biopsy. Differentiation of TVT from other round-cell tumors is less confident when the lesion is not on the genitalia.

### Treatment

TVTs are responsive to several chemotherapeutic agents. Vincristine, administered once a week as a single agent, is very effective, has low toxicity, and is relatively cost effective. After the tumor has regressed, vincristine is continued for two more treatments; the total length of treatment is usually 4 to 6 weeks. Complete remission is achieved in >90% of cases, and treated dogs usually remain disease free. TVTs are also very sensitive to radiation therapy. Although surgical excision results in long-term control, relapse occurs in as many as 50% of cases.

# 64

# Artificial Insemination and Frozen Semen

## (Text pp 940-945)

### INSEMINATION TIMING

With artificial insemination (AI), timing is critical. In dogs, estrus should be identified using vaginal cytology, and ovulation estimated by measuring serum luteinizing hormone (LH) or progesterone (see Chapter 56). At least two inseminations should be planned for a particular estrous cycle, at least one of which is performed approximately 4 days after the preovulatory rise in progesterone (or LH). Alternatively, insemination is best performed when serum progesterone is 30 to 60 nmol/L (10 to 20 ng/ml). If measurement of serum progesterone is not possible, the second insemination should occur at least 48 hours after the first insemination during the fertile period, unless frozen-thawed semen is used.

Preparation and insemination techniques are discussed in the text. Vaginal insemination is acceptable for fresh and chilled semen, but intrauterine insemination should be used for frozen-thawed semen. A special canine AI catheter has been designed for transcervical intrauterine insemination (see text). Whether fresh, chilled, or frozen-thawed semen is used, documentation of adequate semen quality before insemination is important (see Chapter 60).

### CHILLED SEMEN

Properly extended and cooled semen of good quality can be stored at 5° C for 12 to 24 hours, and usually longer. Chilled semen is slowly warmed to room temperature before insemination. Pregnancy rates of 50% to 70% are reported for chilled semen and vaginal insemination. Motility should always be evaluated before insemination and, if possible, the dose adjusted to ensure adequate numbers of motile sperm. The American Kennel Club will register litters from chilled, extended semen.

Use of fresh and frozen-thawed semen and artificial insemination in cats are discussed in the text.

## Drugs Used in Reproductive Disorders

| Drug | Trade name | Use | Canine dosage | Feline dosage |
|---|---|---|---|---|
| Bromocriptine | Parlodel, Sandoz Lactafal, Eurovet BV | False pregnancy Abortifacient | 10 µg/kg PO q12h, 10-14 days Combined with cloprostenol, see below | |
| Cabergoline | Galastop, Boehringer-Ingeheim Dostinex, Pharmacia | False pregnancy Abortifacient | 5 µ/kg PO q24h, 4-7 days Combine with cloprostenol; see below | |
| | | Abortifacient, late gestation | 5 µg/kg PO q24h, 3-5 days beginning after gestation day 49 | |
| | | Estrus induction during anestrus | 5 µg/kg PO q24h, until 2 days after onset of proestrus | |
| Calcium gluconate, 10% solution | Various | Puerperal hypocalcemia | 10% slowly IV until effective (3-20 ml) | Same |
| Calcium gluconate, lactate, or carbonate | Example: Tums | Maintain eucalcemia during lactation | 1-3 g PO q24h | 500-600 mg PO q24h |
| Cloprostenol | Estrumate, Mallinckrodt | Abortifacient 25 days after LH surge | 1 µg/kg SC q48h, *plus* bromocriptine, 30 µg/kg PO q8h *or plus* Cabergoline, 5 µg/kg PO q24h | |
| Finasteride | Proscar, Merck Propecia, Merck | Benign prostatic hyperplasia | Preliminary recommendations: 0.1 mg/kg or 5 mg/dog PO q24h | |
| GnRH | Cystorelin, Abbott | Ovulation induction during estrus | 50-100 µg/dog IM, once | 25 µg/cat IM, once or twice, q24h |
| | | Follicular ovarian cysts Estrous induction | 2.2 µg/kg IM q24h, 3 days See text, Chapter 56 | |

| Drug | Source | Indication | Dose (dog) | Dose (cat) |
|---|---|---|---|---|
| hCG | Various | Ovulation induction during estrus | 10-20 U/kg IM, once | 250 U/cat IM, once or twice, q24h |
| Medroxyprogesterone | Depoprovera, Pharmacia | Benign prostatic hyperplasia | 3 mg/kg SC, once | |
| Megestrol acetate | Ovaban, Schering | Benign prostatic hyperplasia | 0.5 mg/kg PO q24h, 10 or more days | |
| Metergoline | Contralac, Virbac | False pregnancy | 0.1 mg/kg PO q12h, 8 days | |
| PGF$_{2\alpha}$ | Lutalyse, Pharmacia | Treatment of pyometra | 0.1-0.25 mg/kg SC q12-24h until uterus is empty | Same |
| | | Abortifacient, late gestation | 0.1-0.25 mg/kg SC q8-12h, begin ≥ gestation day 30, continue until abortion is complete | 0.25-0.5 mg/kg SC, q12h, begin ≥ gestation day 45, continue until abortion is complete |
| | | Abortifacient, early gestation | 0.25 mg/kg SC q12h, 4 days; begin during cytologic diestrus days 8-15; monitor progesterone | |

*GnRH*, Gonadotropin-releasing hormone; *hCG*, human chorionic gonadotropin; *IM*, intramuscularly; *IV*, intravenously; *LH*, luteinizing hormone; *PGF$_{2\alpha}$*, prostaglandin F$_{2\alpha}$; *PO*, orally; *SC*, subcutaneously.

# PART IX

# Neuromuscular Disorders

# 65

---

# Neurologic Examination

## (Text pp 946-960)

Systematic examination of the nervous system is the most important step in evaluation of a dog or cat with neurologic signs. In many cases the diagnosis depends on accurate localization of the lesion. The basic steps in neurologic diagnosis are as follows:

1. Describe the neurologic abnormalities.
2. Localize the lesion.
3. Describe any concurrent nonneurologic disease.
4. Characterize the onset and progression of the neurologic disease.
5. Generate a list of differential diagnoses.
6. Use ancillary tests, if needed, to make a diagnosis and gauge the prognosis (see Chapter 66).

Functional neuroanatomy and neurologic examination are described and discussed in the text. Tables 65-1 to 65-9 and Box 65-1 are provided as a quick reference.

## DIAGNOSTIC APPROACH (TEXT PP 957-959)

Once a neurologic lesion has been localized, it is necessary to generate a list of likely differential diagnoses. It is important to consider all of the possible mechanisms or causes of disease that may affect the nervous system (Box 65-2). If not all detected neurologic abnormalities can be explained on the basis of a single lesion, multifocal or diffuse disease may be present.

**Table 65-1**

### Essential Components of the Neurologic Examination

| Evaluation | More information |
|---|---|
| Mental state | Table 65-2 |
| Posture | Table 65-3 |
| Gait | Table 65-3 |
| Postural reactions | Table 65-3 |
| Muscle mass and tone | Table 65-4 |
| Spinal reflexes | Tables 65-5 and 65-6 |
| Sensation and pain perception | Limb withdrawal and behavioral response to superficial and deep pain (see text) |
| | Map out areas of local anesthesia or decreased sensation (see Table 73-1) |
| Neck pain | Box 65-1 |
| Urinary tract function | Table 65-4 (also see Table 41-2) |
| Cranial nerves | Tables 65-7 and 65-8 |

**Table 65-2**

## Possible Causes of Altered Mental State

| Alteration in mental state | Possible causes |
|---|---|
| Decreased level of consciousness (depression, stupor, coma) | Metabolic disturbance |
| | Cerebral cortical disease |
| | Compression or inflammation of the brainstem |
| | Disruption of pathways between brainstem and cerebral cortex |
| Agitation or delirium | Cerebral cortical disease |
| | Metabolic encephalopathy |
| Seizures | Primary brain lesion |
| | Metabolic or toxic condition |

**Table 65-3**

## Possible Causes of Postural and Gait Abnormalities

| Abnormality | Possible causes |
|---|---|
| **POSTURE** | |
| Head tilt (continuous, with resistance to straightening) | Vestibular disorder |
| Wide-based stance | Any cause of ataxia or generalized weakness |
| Extensor posturing | Any severe neurologic disease, particularly traumatic |
| **GAIT** | |
| Proprioceptive deficits (e.g., knuckling over while standing or walking, scuffing of the nails) | |
| Paresis or paralysis | Diseases of the cerebral cortex, brainstem, spinal cord, peripheral spinal nerves, or muscles |
| Compulsive circling with head tilt | Vestibular disease |
| Compulsive circling or pacing without head tilt, accompanied by delirium | Ipsilateral forebrain lesion (cerebral cortex, thalamus, hypothalamus) |
| Ataxia | Lesions of the cerebellum, vestibular system, or spinal cord proprioceptive pathways |
| Dysmetria—limb or head movements that are too long (hypermetria) or too short (hypometria) | Cerebellar or spinocerebellar pathway lesions |
| See Table 65-4 | |
| **POSTURAL REACTIONS** | |
| Proprioceptive positioning (knuckling) Hopping Wheelbarrowing Hemiwalking | Abnormalities of conscious proprioception are usually interpreted as UMN signs (see Table 65-4), which must then be confirmed with testing of the spinal reflexes (see Table 65-5) |
| Schiff-Sherrington posture—markedly increased muscle tone and hyperextension of the forelimbs in conjunction with normal forelimb proprioception and postural reactions | Most often seen with severe, acute mid to caudal thoracic spinal cord lesions causing UMN paralysis of the rear limbs |

*UMN,* Upper motor neuron.

Table 65-4

## Summary of Upper Motor Neuron and Lower Motor Neuron Signs

| Characteristic | Upper motor neuron | Lower motor neuron |
|---|---|---|
| Muscle tone | Normal or increased | Decreased |
| Spinal reflexes (see Table 65-5) | Normal or increased | Decreased |
| Motor function | Spastic paresis or paralysis caudal to lesion | Flaccid paresis or paralysis at site of lesion |
| Muscle atrophy* | Mild, gradual—disuse | Severe, rapid—neurogenic |
| Gait | Delayed protraction; long stride; stiff, spastic; ataxic; excessive abduction of limbs during turning | Weak, unable to support weight; short strides; appears lame; may "bunny-hop" |
| Urinary tract function | Large, tense bladder that is difficult to express | Large, flaccid, easily expressed bladder with absent or diminished perineal and bulbourethral reflexes (S1-S3 spinal cord segments, pudendal nerve, pelvic nerve) |

*Focal muscle atrophy is useful in localizing lesions of the peripheral nerves, nerve roots, or spinal cord. Mapping out areas of local anesthesia or decreased sensation also aids in localizing lower motor neuron deficits (see Table 73-1).

---

**Box 65-1**

## Causes of Neck Pain*

### MUSCLE
Myositis (immune, infectious)
Muscle injury

### BONE
Fracture or luxation
Diskospondylitis
Vertebral osteomyelitis
Neoplasia

### JOINT (FACETAL JOINTS)
Polyarthritis (immune, infectious)
Degenerative joint disease (osteoarthritis)

### INTERVERTEBRAL DISK
Disk degeneration or prolapse

### NERVE ROOT
Neoplasia
Compression (by disk, tumor, fibrous tissue)

### MENINGES
Neoplasia
Inflammation (immune, infectious)

### BRAIN
Mass lesion (neoplasia inflammatory)

*The presence or absence of cervical hyperesthesia (painful response to a normally nonpainful stimulus) should be assessed as part of every neurologic examination. Evaluation should include deep palpation of the vertebrae and cervical spinal epaxial muscles and assessment of resistance to flexion, hyperextension, and lateral flexion of the neck. Pain in other regions of the vertebral column may help to localize lesions caused by intervertebral disk disease, diskospondylitis, or neoplasia.

**Table 65-5**

## Spinal Reflexes

| Reflex | Stimulus | Normal response* | Spinal cord segments[†‡] |
|---|---|---|---|
| Thoracic limb withdrawal | Pinch foot of forelimb | Withdraw limb | C6, C7, C8, T1, (T2) |
| Patellar | Strike patellar ligament | Extension of stifle | L4, L5, L6 |
| Pelvic limb withdrawal | Pinch foot of rear limb | Withdraw limb | L6, L7, S1, (S2) |
| Sciatic | Strike sciatic nerve between greater trochanter and ischium | Flexion of stifle and hock | L6, L7, S1, (S2) |
| Cranial tibial | Strike belly of cranial tibial muscle just below proximal end of tibia | Flexion of hock | L6, L7 |
| Perineal | Stimulate perineum with pinch | Anal sphincter contraction, ventroflex tail | S1, S2, S3, pudendal nerve |
| Bulbourethral | Compress vulva or bulb of penis | Anal sphincter contraction | S1, S2, S3, pudendal nerve |
| Panniculus | Stimulate skin over dorsum just lateral to vertebral column | Twitch of cutaneous trunci muscle | Response is absent caudal to a spinal cord lesion that disrupts the superficial pain pathway; used to localize lesions between T3 and L3 |

*Each reflex is recorded as absent (0), decreased (1), normal (2), or increased (3).

[†]A depressed or absent reflex combined with lower motor neuron signs (Table 65-4) indicates a problem with the neuromuscular junction, peripheral nerve, or spinal cord segments responsible for mediating that reflex. Unilateral loss of a reflex strongly indicates that the lesion is in the peripheral nerve or nerve roots rather than in the spinal cord. An exaggerated reflex combined with upper motor neuron signs (Table 65-4) indicates a problem in the brain or spinal cord cranial to that reflex arc.

[‡]Parentheses indicate variable contribution.

Table 65-6

## Localization of Spinal Cord Disease

| Location of lesion | Neurologic findings |
|---|---|
| Cranial cervical spinal lesion (C1-C5) | Rear limbs—UMN signs |
| | Forelimbs—UMN signs |
| Caudal cervical spinal lesion (C6-T2) | Rear limbs—UMN signs |
| | Forelimbs—LMN signs |
| Thoracolumbar spinal cord lesion (T3-L3) | Rear limbs—UMN signs |
| | Forelimbs—normal |
| Lumbosacral spinal cord lesion (L4-S3) | Rear limbs—LMN signs; loss of perineal sensation and reflexes |
| | Forelimbs—normal |
| Sacral spinal cord lesion (S1-S3) | Rear limbs—loss of sciatic function; loss of perineal sensation and reflexes; normal patellar reflexes |
| | Forelimbs—normal |

*LMN*, Lower motor neuron; *UMN*, Upper motor neuron.

Table 65-7

## Cranial Nerve Function

| Cranial nerve | Signs of loss of function |
|---|---|
| I (olfactory) | Loss of ability to smell |
| II (optic) | Loss of vision, dilated pupil, loss of pupillary light reflex (direct and consensual when light shone in affected eye) |
| III (oculomotor) | Loss of pupillary light reflex on affected side (even if light shone in opposite eye), dilated pupil, ventrolateral strabismus |
| IV (trochlear) | Slight dorsomedial eye rotation |
| V (trigeminal) | Atrophy of temporalis and masseter muscles, loss of jaw tone and strength, dropped jaw (if bilateral), analgesia of innervated areas (face, eyelids, cornea, nasal mucosa) |
| VI (abducent) | Medial strabismus, impaired lateral gaze, poor retraction of globe |
| VII (facial) | Lip, eyelid, and ear droop; loss of ability to blink; loss of ability to retract lip; possibly decreased tear production |
| VIII (vestibulocochlear) | Ataxia, head tilt, nystagmus, deafness |
| IX (glossopharyngeal) | Loss of gag reflex, dysphagia |
| X (vagus) | Loss of gag reflex, laryngeal paralysis, dysphagia |
| XI (accessory) | Atrophy of trapezius, sternocephalicus, and brachiocephalicus muscles |
| XII (hypoglossal) | Loss of tongue strength |

### History

Age, gender, breed, and lifestyle may provide clues to the underlying disease process. For example, the incidence of congenital or hereditary disorders, intoxication, and infectious diseases is highest in young animals, whereas older animals are more susceptible to neoplastic diseases and degenerative disorders. Small brachycephalic breeds and some toy breeds are most commonly diagnosed with hydrocephalus. Dogs that engage in competitive or working activities may be at increased risk for activity-related injuries.

Table 65-8

## Quick Assessment of Cranial Nerve Function

| Physical examination finding | Cranial nerve(s) involved |
|---|---|
| Blind | II (brain, retina) |
| Loss of menace | II (VII, cerebellum) |
| Asymmetric pupils | II, III (sympathetic innervation, parasympathetic innervation) |
| Asymmetric eyes in palpebral fissure | III, IV, VI |
| Atrophy of temporal and masseter muscles | V (motor) |
| Dropped jaw, loss of jaw tone | V (motor) |
| Decreased facial sensation (inside ear, lip pinch, nasal mucosa, cornea) | V |
| Lip droop, ear droop | VII |
| Inability to blink | VII |
| Head tilt | VIII |
| Spontaneous resting nystagmus | VIII |
| Deafness | VIII |
| Difficulty swallowing | IX, X |
| Loss of gag reflex | IX, X |
| Laryngeal paralysis | IX, X |
| Weakness, asymmetry of tongue | XII |

Box 65-2

### DAMNIT-VP Scheme: Mechanisms of Disease

| | |
|---|---|
| *D* | Degenerative |
| *A* | Anomalous |
| *M* | Metabolic, malformation |
| *N* | Neoplastic, nutritional |
| *I* | Infectious, inflammatory, immune, iatrogenic, idiopathic |
| *T* | Traumatic, toxic |
| *V* | Vascular |
| *P* | Parasitic |

### Disease onset and progression

Onset and progression of neurologic signs is of primary importance in prioritizing the differential diagnoses (Box 65-3). Acute exacerbation of a more chronic disease may also result in an acute clinical presentation; a thorough history should identify these animals.

### Systemic signs

Identification of concurrent disease or systemic abnormalities aids in the diagnosis of neoplastic, metabolic, or inflammatory disorders. A complete physical examination and ophthalmologic evaluation, including funduscopic examination, should be performed on every patient with suspected neurologic disease. This step is important to facilitate diagnosis, exclude disorders that may mimic nervous system disease, and identify concurrent disorders that affect prognosis.

Table 65-9

## Characteristics That Aid in Localizing Brain Lesions

| Lesion location | Neurologic findings |
|---|---|
| Cerebral cortex | Altered behavior, mental status |
| | May pace or circle to side of lesion |
| | May head-press |
| | Gait usually relatively normal |
| | May have postural reaction, and proprioceptive deficits on side opposite lesion |
| | Cortical blindness (blind with normal pupils and pupillary light reflexes) on side opposite lesion |
| | Seizures |
| Diencephalon (thalamus and hypothalamus) | Altered mental status: aggression, disorientation, hyperexcitability, depression, coma |
| | Postural reaction and proprioceptive deficits on side opposite lesion |
| | Abnormalities of eating, drinking, sleeping, or temperature (hypothalamus) |
| | Diabetes insipidus |
| Brainstem (mesencephalon, pons, medulla oblongata) | Altered mental status: severe depression or coma |
| | Ipsilateral hemiparesis or quadriparesis and ataxia |
| | Multiple ipsilateral cranial nerve deficits |
| | Cerebellopontine angle lesion: V, VII, VIII |
| Vestibular system | Head tilt, asymmetric ataxia (incoordination), falling, rolling toward side of lesion |
| | Possibly spontaneous or positional abnormal nystagmus, with fast phase away from side of lesion |
| | Ipsilateral ventrolateral strabismus |
| | Important to differentiate central from peripheral vestibular disease (see Chapter 70) |
| Cerebellum | Normal mental status |
| | Ataxia, head tremor, intention tremor, dysmetria |
| | Normal strength |
| | Normal proprioceptive positioning |
| | Menace response may be lost on side of lesion |
| | Exaggerated limb responses (hypermetria), goose-stepping gait |

Box 65-3

## Characterization of Disease Processes Based on Onset and Progression

### PERACUTE, NONPROGRESSIVE
External trauma
Hemorrhage
Infarct
Internal trauma (disk, fracture)

### CHRONIC PROGRESSIVE
Most tumors
Degenerative disorders
Metabolic disorders

### SUBACUTE, PROGRESSIVE
Infectious inflammatory disease
Noninfectious inflammatory disease
Rapidly growing tumors (e.g., lymphoma, metastatic neoplasia)

# 66

# Diagnostic Tests for the Neuromuscular System

## *(Text pp 961-973)*

### HEMATOLOGY (TEXT P 961)

Routine complete blood count can be useful in patients with neurologic disease. Leukocytosis suggests inflammatory disease; severe inflammation and a left shift is expected with bacterial meningitis or encephalitis. Lymphopenia and inclusion bodies within red blood cells (RBCs) and lymphocytes may be seen in dogs with acute distemper. Occasionally, leukemia is detected in an animal with brain or spinal cord lymphoma. In most cases, however, hematologic findings are unremarkable when disease is confined to the central nervous system (CNS).

### SERUM BIOCHEMISTRY (TEXT P 961)

A serum biochemistry profile is most useful in detection of metabolic neuropathies and encephalopathies. Diabetes mellitus, hypoglycemia, hypocalcemia, hypokalemia, and uremia can be eliminated from the differential diagnosis list with a routine biochemistry panel. Greatly increased serum cholesterol may prompt further testing for hypothyroidism (see Chapter 51). High liver enzyme activities (alanine aminotransferase, alkaline phosphatase) or hypoalbuminemia may prompt consideration of liver disease and hepatic encephalopathy, necessitating liver function tests (see Chapter 36). Evidence of hepatocellular disease can also suggest multisystemic disease such as toxoplasmosis. High muscle enzyme activities (creatine kinase, aspartate aminotransferase) suggest muscle damage or inflammation.

### URINALYSIS (TEXT P 961)

When azotemia is present, measurement of urine specific gravity is important in differentiating renal from prerenal azotemia. Volume depletion with hypernatremia and prerenal azotemia is a common finding in animals that stop drinking because of intracranial disease. Ammonium biurate crystals are found in the urine of some patients with portosystemic shunts.

### RADIOGRAPHY (TEXT PP 961-962)

Thoracic and abdominal radiography can be useful as screening tests for infectious and neoplastic diseases, as well as to evaluate liver size. Spinal radiographs are necessary for the diagnosis of disk disease, diskospondylitis, and neoplastic diseases that affect the vertebrae. Rarely, a peripheral nerve tumor results in enlargement of its vertebral foramen.

   Although skull radiographs are a low-yield procedure, they should be performed in patients with disease above the foramen magnum. Occasionally, an area of lysis, tumor calcification, or an intranasal mass aids diagnosis of primary or secondary CNS neoplasia.

## CEREBROSPINAL FLUID ANALYSIS (TEXT PP 962-965)

Cerebrospinal fluid (CSF) analysis is indicated in every patient with suspected neurologic disease in which a diagnosis is not readily apparent. Techniques are discussed in the text.

### Contraindications and precautions

CSF analysis is not usually indicated in patients with metabolic abnormalities, obvious disk disease, CNS anomalies, or neurologic signs caused by trauma. The procedure is contraindicated in patients that are obvious anesthetic risks and animals with severe coagulopathies. Patients with high intracranial pressure (manifested by deteriorating mentation) are at increased risk for herniation. Endotracheal intubation, hyperventilation, and mannitol (1-3 g/kg intravenously [IV] over 30 min as a 20% solution) and dexamethasone (0.25-1 mg/kg IV) may reduce the risk of herniation in these patients.

### Analysis

Normal CSF is clear and colorless. A cell count and cytologic preparation should be made as soon as possible after collection. If the sample must be stored for >1 hour before analysis, the specimen should be refrigerated. Addition of autologous serum (10% by volume of the sample) preserves CSF cytology so that analysis up to 48 hours after collection will yield reliable results; a separate CSF sample must be saved for protein analysis, however. If the slide cannot reach the veterinary cytopathologist within a few hours, it should be fixed and stained with Diff-Quik, Wright's, or Giemsa stain.

*White blood cell count.* Normal ranges vary by laboratory, but in general the count should be <2 white blood cells (WBCs)/μl. Cytologic analysis is necessary even if the WBC count is normal, because abnormal cell types or organisms may be present.

*WBC differential.* Normally, most of the cells are monocytoid cells and lymphocytes. Macrophages may be seen in small numbers but are dramatically increased in some disease processes. Occasional neutrophils and eosinophils are present, but they normally make up <10% of the cell population. Typical CSF findings for some specific disorders are shown in Table 66-1. However, CSF cytology must always be interpreted in relation to the signalment, history, and clinical findings.

*Red blood cells.* Severe blood contamination can influence the cytologic findings, but even grossly apparent blood contamination has only a minor impact on WBC count and protein analysis. To approximate the maximum effect peripheral blood contamination will have, assume that one WBC can be expected for every 100 RBCs.

*Protein.* Increased CSF protein can occur with diseases that (1) disrupt the blood-brain barrier, (2) cause local necrosis, (3) interrupt normal CSF flow and absorption, or (4) result in intrathecal globulin production. Protein electrophoresis can be used to determine if the high CSF protein is caused by blood-brain barrier disruption, intrathecal immunoglobulin production, or both. Quantification of CSF immunoglobulins can also be performed using radial immunodiffusion, which helps differentiate inflammatory from noninflammatory disorders.

*Other analyses.* Cellular CSF should be submitted for Gram stain and culture. When canine distemper, Rocky Mountain spotted fever, borreliosis, ehrlichiosis, or toxoplasmosis is likely, CSF titers can be compared with serum titers. An increase in the CSF titer relative to that of the serum suggests active CNS infection.

## CONTRAST RADIOGRAPHY (TEXT PP 965-970)

### Myelography

In patients with clinical evidence of spinal cord disease or compression, a myelogram may be required to confirm, localize, and characterize the lesion. This procedure is particularly valuable for identification of herniated disks, spinal cord compression, and tumors. However, myelography should be reserved for patients in which surgery or radiotherapy is contemplated. Techniques are discussed in the text. Myelography should

**Table 66-1**

### Cerebrospinal Fluid in Various Neurologic Diseases

| Condition | WBC | WBC differential | Total protein |
|---|---|---|---|
| Normal | <2 cells/µl (dog) | Mononuclear cells | <25 mg/dl |
| Steroid-responsive suppurative meningitis | +++ | Neutrophils (mature, nontoxic) | +++ |
| Breed-associated meningeal vasculitis | +++ | Neutrophils (mature, nontoxic) | +++ |
| Granulomatous meningoencephalitis | ++ | Lymphocytes, monocytes, occasional plasma cells; occasional anaplastic mononuclear cell with lacy cytoplasm; neutrophils in 60% (<20% of cells) | ++ |
| Pug dog meningoencephalitis | +++ | Small lymphocytes | ++ |
| Bacterial meningitis | +++ | Neutrophils (toxic), bacteria | +++ |
| Canine distemper | + | Small lymphocytes | + |
| Rabies | + | Small lymphocytes | + |
| Toxoplasmosis | ++ | Lymphocytes, macrophages, occasional PMNs; may see organisms; may occasionally see eosinophils >50% | ++ |
| Neosporosis | ++ | Lymphocytes, monocytes, occasional PMNs; may see organisms; may occasionally see eosinophils >50% | ++ |
| Cryptococcosis | ++ | Neutrophils, mononuclear cells, occasionally eosinophils; organisms in 60% | ++ |
| Rocky Mountain spotted fever | + | Neutrophils | + |
| *Ehrlichiosis* infection | ++ | Lymphocytes | + |
| Feline infectious peritonitis | +++ | Mixed mononuclear cells and neutrophils | +++ |
| CNS parasite migration | + | Mononuclear cells, neutrophils, occasionally eosinophils | + |
| Brain or spinal cord infarct | N or + | Mononuclear cells, neutrophils | + |
| CNS neoplasia (except lymphoma, meningioma) | N or + | Mononuclear cells | + |
| Meningioma | N or ++ | Mononuclear cells, neutrophils | ++ |
| CNS lymphoma | ++ | Lymphocytes, neoplastic cells | + |

*Continued.*

**Table 66-1—cont'd**

## Cerebrospinal Fluid in Various Neurologic Diseases

| Condition | WBC | WBC differential | Total protein |
|---|---|---|---|
| Hydrocephalus | N | Normal | N |
| Lissencephaly | N | Normal | N |
| Degenerative myelopathy | N | Normal | N or + |
| Intervertebral disc prolapse | N | Normal | N or + |
| Polyradiculoneuritis | N | Normal | N or + |

*CNS,* Central nervous system; *PMN,* polymorphonuclear neutrophil; *WBC,* white blood cell.

*Table key:*

| | WBC count (WBC/µl) | Protein (mg/dl) |
|---|---|---|
| N = normal | <2 | <25 |
| + = mild increase | <50 | 25-50 |
| ++ = moderate increase | 50-100 | 50-100 |
| +++ = marked increase | 100 | <100 |

be performed after CSF analysis, because it increases total WBC and neutrophil counts and protein content in the CSF.

*Complications.* Seizures occasionally occur after recovery from anesthesia; this is more common in dogs >30 kg and when >2 injections of contrast were administered. The seizures can usually be controlled with diazepam (5 to 20 mg IV). Neurologic deterioration is occasionally seen after myelography. Large-breed dogs with cervical vertebral instability or malformation, dogs and cats with inflammatory CNS disease or extradural tumors, and dogs with degenerative myelopathy are most often affected. Fortunately, deterioration usually is transient.

### Epidurography
Epidurography can be used for evaluation of lumbosacral disease in dogs. (In most dogs the dural sac ends cranial to the lumbosacral junction, making myelography of limited value in evaluation of this region.) The technique is described in the text.

### Pneumoventriculography
Pneumoventriculography has been useful for confirming the presence of hydrocephalus in small animals (see text). This technique has largely been replaced by ultrasonography performed through open or incomplete fontanelles or, in neonates, through the temporal bones. Computed tomography (CT) and magnetic resonance imaging (MRI) are also used to evaluate the ventricular system in dogs and cats.

### CT and MRI
CT and MRI are noninvasive techniques that are valuable for localization, identification, and characterization of many brain and spinal cord lesions. CT is most useful for identification and characterization of bony abnormalities of the vertebral bodies and skull. MRI can be used to determine very small density differences in brain and spinal cord tissues. These techniques allow precise topographic mapping of lesions, making them very valuable tools in the evaluation of compressive lesions of the brain, spinal cord, or cauda equina when surgery is being considered.

## ELECTRODIAGNOSTIC TESTING (TEXT PP 970-972)

### Electromyography
Electromyography is used to identify disease that affects nerve roots or peripheral nerves, neuromuscular junctions, or muscle fibers. Severance, destruction, or demyelination of a peripheral nerve results in spontaneous fibrillations and positive sharp waves (denervation potentials) and prolonged insertional activity in affected muscles 5 to 7 days after denervation. These changes may also be seen with primary muscle disorders (e.g., myositis, myotonia).

### Nerve conduction velocities
Slow conduction times are seen in demyelinating disorders, allowing the diagnosis of peripheral neuropathy. Absence of conduction is seen in nerves that have been injured or avulsed and have undergone degeneration (typically 4 to 5 days after injury).

### Electroretinography
Electroretinography (ERG) is an objective method of evaluating retinal function. The ERG is abnormal with degenerative disorders of the retina but is normal if the lesion causing visual dysfunction is located caudal to the retina (in the optic nerves, optic chiasm, optic tract, or cerebral cortex).

### Brainstem-auditory evoked response
Brainstem-auditory evoked response (BAER) depicts the response of nervous tissues to an auditory stimulus. Lesions of the cochlea, peripheral vestibulocochlear nerve, or brainstem caudal to the midbrain cause characteristic changes in the response. BAER is used to detect unilateral and bilateral deafness and brainstem masses in dogs.

### Electroencephalography
Electroencephalography provides a graphic record of the electrical activity of the cerebral cortex. It can be useful in determining whether a cerebral disorder is focal or diffuse, although it rarely allows an etiologic diagnosis.

## MUSCLE OR NERVE BIOPSY (TEXT PP 972-973)

### Muscle biopsy

Muscle biopsies can confirm neuromuscular disease and may provide an etiologic diagnosis. Histology may reveal inflammatory or neoplastic changes and, if the disease is caused by infection, a causative agent. However, many muscle disorders cannot be diagnosed without histochemical staining and analysis of fiber types. Myofiber analysis requires special processing and immediate freezing of the biopsy specimens.

### Nerve biopsy

Nerve biopsies may be useful in evaluating peripheral nerve disorders. Fascicular nerve biopsies are performed whenever possible, leaving the majority of the nerve trunk intact. The common peroneal nerve and the ulnar nerve are the most often biopsied mixed (motor and sensory) nerves. As do muscle biopsy specimens, nerve biopsy specimens require special handling (see text).

## IMMUNOLOGIC AND SEROLOGIC TESTS (TEXT P 973)

### Canine distemper

Increased anti–canine distemper virus antibody in CSF relative to serum permits definitive diagnosis of distemper encephalitis or myelitis. Alternatively, immunofluorescence can be performed on cytologic smears of conjunctival, tonsillar, or respiratory epithelium or CSF. Antigen in extraneural tissues is most readily detectable early in infection, when clinical evidence of systemic disease is apparent. Distemper antigen may also be documented in CSF cells later in the disease.

### Toxoplasmosis

Approximately 30% of healthy dogs and cats have antibodies against *Toxoplasma gondii*, so increased immunoglobulin G (IgG) titers to *T. gondii* merely indicate prior infection. A fourfold rise in serum IgG over a 3-week period suggests active infection. Enzyme-linked immunosorbent assay detection of IgM and circulating *T. gondii* antigens improves the detection of recent or ongoing infection. However, many dogs and cats with CNS toxoplasmosis have negative antibody titers at the time of diagnosis. Comparison of *T. gondii* IgM in the CSF and serum provides the best means for diagnosis in some cases.

### *Neospora caninum* infection

A fourfold rise in serum IgG against *N. caninum* is diagnostic for infection. CSF antibody levels may also be increased in neurologic disease caused by this organism.

### Ehrlichiosis and Rocky Mountain spotted fever

Immunofluorescence for serum IgG is the traditional method of confirming *Ehrlichia canis* infection; a positive titer indicates infection. However, the test may be negative early in infection. Rocky Mountain spotted fever can be diagnosed by finding increased serum IgM or a rising IgG titer against *Rickettsia rickettsii*. Occasionally the diagnosis can be made by finding the organism in tissue biopsy specimens using direct immunofluorescence. Polymerase chain reaction may be more sensitive and specific for active infection.

### Other tests

Antinuclear antibody, lupus erythematosus cell, antiacetylcholine receptor antibody, and *Cryptococcus* latex agglutination tests are discussed in other chapters. Autoantibody directed against type IIM myofibers can be demonstrated in the serum of most dogs with masticatory muscle myositis (see Chapter 74).

# 67

# Disorders of Locomotion

## (Text pp 974-982)

### ATAXIA (TEXT P 974)

Ataxia, or incoordination, is seen whenever the sensory pathways responsible for proprioception are disrupted, which most commonly occurs with spinal cord disease but may also result from cerebellar or vestibular dysfunction. Diagnostic efforts must focus on localization of the disease as follows:

- Vestibular disease—incoordination and loss of balance, with a head tilt and nystagmus (see Chapter 70)
- Cerebellar disease—incoordination of the head, neck, and all four limbs, with normal strength; head, neck, and limb movements are jerky and lack control; overreaching and high-stepping gait (hypermetria)
- Spinal cord disease—ataxia of the limbs with some degree of weakness or paresis

Evaluation of spinal reflexes, muscle tone, and conscious proprioception facilitates lesion localization within the spinal cord (see Chapter 65).

### PARESIS AND PARALYSIS (TEXT PP 974-977)

Lesions in various locations can cause paresis or paralysis, sometimes with other localizing signs:

- Cerebral cortex (unilateral lesions)—generally very mild hemiparesis and slightly abnormal postural reactions in the limbs on the contralateral side
- Brainstem—obvious ipsilateral hemiparesis and postural reaction deficits; may also have cranial nerve deficits and/or altered mentation
- Spinal cord (focal cervical lesion or multifocal and diffuse lesions)—ataxia and paresis or paralysis of all four limbs with no evidence of brain or brainstem disease; muscle tone and spinal reflexes are increased in affected limbs
- Diffuse lower motor neuron (LMN) disease—paresis or paralysis without ataxia; normal conscious proprioception and postural reactions, but decreased muscle tone and spinal reflexes

Generalized weakness with normal postural reactions, normal reflexes, and no ataxia may also be seen in animals with metabolic, cardiorespiratory, or muscular system disorders.

### Localizing Spinal Cord Lesions

Spinal cord disorders may be caused by anomalies, degenerative conditions, neoplasia, inflammatory diseases, trauma, disk extrusion, and infarction. A complete neurologic examination allows localization of the spinal cord lesion (Table 67-1).

#### C1 to C5

Focal cranial cervical lesions may be mild or severe. Meningeal irritation or inflammation without cord compression or damage results in cervical pain without neurologic deficits. Mild compression results in quadrilateral ataxia and paresis, although rear limb signs usually are worse than forelimb signs. However, lesions that primarily affect the

Table 67-1

## Neurologic Findings in Dogs and Cats with Spinal Cord Lesions

| Site of lesion | Thoracic limbs | Pelvic limbs |
|---|---|---|
| C1-C5 | UMN | UMN |
| C6-T2 | LMN | UMN |
| T3-L3 | Normal | UMN |
| L4-S3 | Normal | LMN |

*LMN*, Lower motor neuron signs; *UMN*, upper motor neuron signs.

central C1 to C5 spinal cord (e.g., intramedullary neoplasia, infarcts, hydromyelia) sometimes cause quadrilateral UMN weakness that is most dramatic in the forelimbs (central cord syndrome).

Compressive lesions also cause postural reaction deficits, including decreased conscious proprioception. The animal is incoordinated and may stand knuckled over on all four paws. Muscle tone is normal or increased in all four limbs, and all spinal reflexes are normal or hyperactive. A unilateral lesion of the cervical cord results in signs only in the ipsilateral limbs.

### C6 to T2

Lesions at the level of C6 to T2 result in quadriparesis and ataxia that is most pronounced in the rear limbs. The forelimbs may appear to be more severely paretic because they lose muscle tone and strength as the muscles rapidly atrophy. Spinal reflexes in the forelimbs may be depressed or absent (LMN signs), whereas those in the rear limbs are normal or hyperactive (UMN signs). Proprioception in the rear limbs decreases, as the UMN tracts are disrupted. Unilateral lesions produce signs confined to the ipsilateral side.

Occasionally, forelimb signs are very subtle, even though the UMN signs in the rear limbs are remarkable, which makes it difficult to differentiate disease at this site from a T3 to L3 lesion. Atrophy of the muscles over the scapula may be the most prominent LMN sign in animals with a mild C6 to T2 lesion.

***Other signs.*** Horner's syndrome may be seen if the T1 to T2 region is involved (see Chapter 68), and the ipsilateral panniculus reflex may be lost if damage occurs to the C8 to T1 spinal cord segments, nerve roots, or peripheral nerve. A severe lesion at C5 to C7 could cause diaphragmatic paralysis.

### T3 to L3

Lesions at this level result in paresis and UMN signs (increased tone, hyperactive reflexes) in the rear limbs. Postural reactions and conscious proprioception are abnormal in the rear limbs, although the forelimbs are neurologically normal. As compressive lesions worsen, so do the neurologic deficits.

### L4 to S3

Lesions that affect the lumbar intumescence cause LMN paralysis (decreased tone, loss of reflexes) in the rear limbs only.

## Generalized LMN Paresis or Paralysis

Generalized paresis or paralysis with loss of reflexes is seen with various diffuse LMN disorders:

- Congenital and familial disorders of demyelination and axonal degeneration
- Inflammatory immune-mediated nerve disorders
- Polyneuropathies associated with metabolic, toxic, or neoplastic disease
- Neuromuscular junction toxicity, e.g., botulism and tick paralysis (see Chapter 73)

In many cases the rear limbs are affected more severely at first, with paralysis ascending until all four limbs are affected. Muscle tone is decreased, and spinal reflexes are decreased or absent. The gait is stiff, stilted, and choppy. Sensation may be normal or abnormal, depending on whether sensory nerves are affected. With peripheral neuropathies primarily affecting sensory axons, ataxia or self-mutilation without loss of reflexes may be seen.

## Episodic Weakness
Episodic weakness that worsens with exercise and improves with rest may be caused by a variety of conditions, only some of which directly involve the nervous system:
- Skeletal muscle disorders (e.g., polymyositis, other myopathies)
- Neuromuscular junction disorders (e.g., myasthenia gravis)
- Cardiac disease
- Respiratory disease
- Episodic hemorrhage (e.g., ruptured vascular neoplasm)
- Metabolic disturbances (e.g., hypoglycemia, hypoadrenocorticism)

Orthopedic and articular diseases may also manifest as apparent weakness if pain makes the animal reluctant to exercise. Physical examination and minimum database usually are sufficient for the differential diagnoses to be prioritized.

## DYSMETRIA AND HYPERMETRIA (TEXT PP 977-980)
Dysmetria and hypermetria are signs of cerebellar dysfunction. Damage to the very superficial spinocerebellar tracts in the cervical spinal cord results in quadrilateral ataxia, dysmetria, and hypermetria, but no head tremor or other "brain signs" are present.

### Neurologic signs of cerebellar dysfunction
Cerebellar dysfunction results in a broad-based stance, loss of balance, ataxia, tremor, hypermetria, and dysmetria without paresis. The animal is unable to judge distances or control the range of head movements; when it attempts to perform a certain movement, intention tremor occurs. A fine tremor of the head and body may be present at rest. The animal is strong but uncoordinated. Provided the body is supported, all postural reactions, spinal reflexes, and sensation are normal.

In most cases, cranial nerve examination is normal, although loss of the menace reflex may occur. Animals with a lesion in the flocculonodular lobe of the cerebellum may exhibit paradoxic central vestibular signs: head tilt and fast-phase nystagmus to the side opposite the lesion, and ipsilateral abnormal postural reactions.

### Causes of cerebellar dysfunction
Cerebellar dysfunction may occur at any age. Possible causes, based on onset and progression of signs, are listed in Box 67-1. In puppies and kittens that are alert and active, congenital hypoplasia, malformations, or abiotrophy should be suspected. No treatment for these conditions exists. Progressive disorders, such as abiotrophy, metabolic storage diseases, and degenerative disorders, become more severe with time, usually resulting in an inability to walk, necessitating euthanasia.

*Cerebellar hypoplasia.* Congenital cerebellar hypoplasia occurs in several breeds, including the Chow Chow, Irish Setter, Wire-Haired Fox Terrier, Boston Terrier, Labrador Retriever, Bull Terrier, Weimaraner, Dachshund, Miniature Poodle, Beagle, Silky Terrier, Siberian Husky, and Poodle. The cause is unknown; a genetic basis has not been documented. Clinical signs are present as soon as affected animals begin to walk. One or more animals in a litter may be affected.

Virus-induced cerebellar malformations in kittens (panleukopenia) and puppies (herpesvirus) also occur, causing cerebellar dysfunction that becomes apparent very early in life. Clinical signs do not progress, which helps differentiate these syndromes from cerebellar abiotrophy.

*Cerebellar abiotrophy.* Cerebellar neuronal abiotrophy is a syndrome of premature degeneration of cells within the cerebellum. Neonatal cerebellar abiotrophy has been reported in many different dog breeds (see text) and in cats. Clinical signs may be present at birth or may begin at a very young age and then worsen with time. Postnatal abiotrophy (onset ranging from a few weeks to several years of age) also has been reported in many dog breeds.

Progressive signs of cerebellar dysfunction may also be seen in animals affected by more generalized neurodegenerative conditions or metabolic storage diseases (see text).

---

**Box 67-1**

## Disorders Resulting in Signs of Cerebellar Disease

**ACUTE, NONPROGRESSIVE DISORDERS**
Trauma
Infarction

**SUBACUTE, PROGRESSIVE DISORDERS**
Infectious inflammatory diseases
Granulomatous meningoencephalitis (dogs)

**CHRONIC, SLOWLY PROGRESSIVE DISORDERS**
Neoplasia
Degeneration (see Box 72-1)

**YOUNG ANIMAL—PRESENT AT BIRTH, STATIC**
Panleukopenia (kittens)
Herpesvirus (puppies)
Cerebellar hypoplasia
Malformations

**YOUNG ANIMAL—PROGRESSIVE**
Cerebellar abiotrophy (neonatal or postnatal)
Metabolic storage diseases (see text)
Degeneration

---

Neurologic signs unrelated to the cerebellum enable differentiation of these conditions from cerebellar abiotrophy.

### Diagnostic approach

Cerebellar dysfunction can usually be identified during a neurologic examination. Age at onset, progression of cerebellar signs, and presence of other neurologic or systemic signs help differentiate the various causes of cerebellar dysfunction. In puppies and kittens that are otherwise healthy, congenital hypoplasia, malformations, or abiotrophy should be suspected. If other neurologic abnormalities are present, especially in an adult animal with cerebellar dysfunction, inflammatory or neoplastic diseases should be considered.

Complete physical and ophthalmologic examinations, minimum database (complete blood count, biochemistry profile, urinalysis), and thoracic and abdominal radiography may permit identification of an underlying disease. If no abnormalities are detected, cerebrospinal fluid (CSF) analysis should be performed. If available, computed tomography (CT) or magnetic resonance imaging (MRI) may be used to visualize the cerebellum and identify malformations, neoplasms, or granulomas. Degenerative disease is suspected if all test results are normal in an adult dog or cat.

Neuroaxonal dystrophy and other degenerative disorders that affect the cerebellum have been reported in cats and in Rottweilers, Chihuahuas, Jack Russell Terrier puppies, Scottish Terriers, and sporadically in other dog breeds. Definitive diagnosis requires cerebellar biopsy or postmortem examination.

## INVOLUNTARY ALTERATIONS IN MUSCLE TONE (TEXT PP 980-982)

### Dyskinesia

Dyskinesias are uncommon central nervous system (CNS) disorders that result in involuntary movements in a fully conscious individual. They may result from effects of structural disease on the basal ganglia. Episodes typically involve unpredictable, involuntary limb hyperextension or hyperflexion. No altered consciousness, preceding aura, or postictal phase is present. Anticonvulsant therapy is ineffective for prevention or termination of an episode.

### Tremors

Acute onset of severe, generalized tremors or tetany should raise the suspicion of a toxic cause, such as strychnine, metaldehyde, chlorinated hydrocarbons, mycotoxins, or organophosphates (see Box 69-1). Metabolic disturbances, such as hypoglycemia and hypocalcemia, can also cause tremors and tetany. Intention tremors of the head are usually associated with cerebellar disease.

#### "Shaker dogs"

Acute onset of head and body tremors unassociated with a metabolic or toxic disorder may be seen in young adult dogs (5 months to 3 years of age), predominantly white dogs of small breeds (Maltese, West Highland White Terrier, Beagle). The cause is unknown.

*Clinical features.* The tremors develop rapidly over 1 to 3 days and then occur continually, worsening with excitement and disappearing during sleep. No weakness is present, and neurologic examination usually is normal; nystagmus, dysconjugate eye movements, head tilt, and seizures are occasionally seen. Results of all laboratory tests are normal; occasionally, CSF analysis reveals mild lymphocytosis. Hydrocephalus of questionable significance may be found in a few dogs. In some dogs the tremors decrease and may subside 1 to 3 months after onset, but they persist for life in other dogs.

*Treatment.* Diazepam (0.5 mg/kg orally [PO] q8h) and prednisone (2 to 4 mg/kg/day PO) administered at initial onset may result in rapid clinical improvement, with most dogs dramatically improved within 4 to 5 days. Treatment should be gradually tapered over 4 to 5 months, with the drug doses titrated to control the clinical signs. A few dogs have a relapse months or years later, requiring retreatment. Some dogs need low-dose, life-long therapy.

#### Congenital tremors

Congenital tremor syndromes can occur as a result of metabolic storage diseases or congenital spongy degeneration of the CNS or in association with abnormal or deficient myelination (dysmyelinogenesis). A diffuse tremor syndrome associated with dysmyelinogenesis has been observed in puppies, especially male Springer Spaniels. Similar syndromes have been recognized in the Weimaraner, Bernese Mountain Dog, Samoyed, Dalmatian, Chow Chow, and sporadically in other breeds. In Springer Spaniels and Samoyeds, it is a sex-linked recessive trait.

*Clinical features.* Clinical signs usually begin within the first 4 weeks of life. Affected puppies stand with a wide-based stance and have whole-body tremors that worsen with exercise or excitement. The tremors are severe and progressive and usually result in death within 2 to 4 months. In Chow Chows and mildly affected dogs of other breeds, gradual clinical recovery may occur within 1 to 3 months. Diagnosis is based on signalment and absence of other neurologic deficits and clinicopathologic abnormalities.

#### Senile tremors

Trembling of the pelvic limbs may develop in old dogs that are weak but otherwise neurologically normal. Trembling disappears at rest but is apparent when the animal stands, and it worsens with exercise. It is important to rule out electrolyte disturbances, hypothyroidism, hypoadrenocorticism, hip dysplasia, and lumbosacral disease. Results of all tests are normal in these dogs. No effective treatment exists.

### Opisthotonos and Tetanus

Loss of consciousness in association with opisthotonos and tetanus (decerebrate rigidity) is seen in animals with severe brainstem disease caused by infection, trauma, or neoplasia. Brainstem disease is suspected after evaluation of the history, neurologic examination, and laboratory tests. CSF analysis and diagnostic imaging with CT or MRI can be used to make a diagnosis. Opisthotonos and tetanus in a conscious animal may be caused by mild strychnine poisoning, trauma to the rostral cerebellum, or *Clostridium tetani* infection (tetanus).

## Tetanus (*C. tetani* infection)

Clinical signs of tetanus occur 5 to 20 days after wound infection. Mild or early signs include a stiff gait, erect ears, elevated tail, and contraction of the facial muscles. Signs may be more severe in the area adjacent to where the toxin is being produced. Recumbency, quadrilateral extensor rigidity, opisthotonos, and, occasionally, seizures develop as the disease progresses. Death may occur from respiratory failure. Tetanus is diagnosed on the basis of clinical signs and history of a recent wound. Cats are more resistant to tetanus than are dogs.

### Treatment

Treatment consists of rest, wound débridement, antibiotics, neutralization of toxin, and intensive supportive care. Aqueous penicillin G (40,000 U/kg) is administered intravenously (IV), followed by intramuscular injections of procaine penicillin (40,000 U/kg q12h). Alternatively, metronidazole (10 to 15 mg/kg q8h) may be administered.

*Tetanus antitoxin.* A test dose of tetanus antitoxin (equine origin) should be injected intradermally 15 to 30 minutes before administration of a treatment dose. If no wheal develops, a single dose of antitoxin is administered IV (1000 U/kg, maximum 20,000 U). Injection of a small dose of antitoxin (1000 U) just proximal to the wound site may be beneficial in animals with localized tetanus.

*Sedation.* The animal is maintained in a quiet, dark environment. Muscle spasms are controlled with diazepam (0.5 to 1 mg/kg IV or PO, as needed), chlorpromazine (0.5 mg/kg IV q8h), or acepromazine (0.1 to 0.2 mg/kg intramuscularly [IM] q6h). Phenobarbital (2 mg/kg IV or IM q8h) or pentobarbital (5 to 15 mg/kg IV until effective) may be administered as needed.

*Supportive care.* Intravenous fluids are administered, and nutritional support is maintained using nasogastric or gastrotomy tube feeding. Handfeeding is begun as soon as the animal is able to eat. Urinary and fecal retention must be managed by repeated catheterization and enemas in some patients. Improvement is usually noticeable within 1 week, but signs may persist for 3 to 4 weeks.

### Prognosis

The prognosis is poor if signs progress rapidly; many severely affected animals die within 5 days from respiratory failure.

## Myoclonus

Myoclonus is a rhythmic, shocklike, repetitive contraction of a portion of a muscle, an individual muscle, or a group of muscles, occurring as often as 60 times per minute. Unlike tremors, these rhythmic contractions do not abate during sleep or general anesthesia. Limb and facial muscles are most often involved.

### Canine distemper

Myoclonus is most commonly associated with canine distemper meningoencephalomyelitis. Distemper-related myoclonus may appear alone or in association with other neurologic signs. Rarely, other focal inflammatory or neoplastic spinal cord lesions produce myoclonus. Evaluation is as for any CNS disorder. The prognosis for resolution is grave.

### Familial myoclonus

Familial reflex myoclonus occurs in 4- to 6-week-old Labrador Retriever puppies. Signs include intermittent spasms of the axial and appendicular muscles, with occasional episodes of opisthotonos resembling strychnine poisoning or tetanus. Signs worsen when an affected puppy is stressed or excited. Treatment with diazepam or clonazepam has been unsuccessful. The prognosis for recovery is grave.

# 68

## Abnormalities of Mentation, Loss of Vision, and Pupillary Abnormalities

### *(Text pp 983-990)*

#### MENTATION (TEXT P 983)

Abnormal behavior, delirium, and compulsions are seen in dogs and cats with cerebral cortex lesions, metabolic encephalopathies, and intoxications (Table 68-1). The history helps differentiate a behavioral problem from a neurologic disorder.

Severe depression, stupor, or coma, in conjunction with cranial nerve and postural reaction abnormalities, may be caused by disorders of the brainstem, thalamus, or cerebral cortex. Any animal with episodic or persistently abnormal mental status should be evaluated for a metabolic encephalopathy. Intoxication must be considered in any patient with acute neurologic signs. Anxiety and delirium may be observed early, with other neurologic and systemic signs seen concurrently or subsequently. A history of exposure is helpful for establishing the diagnosis but is rarely obtained.

#### HEAD TRAUMA (TEXT PP 983-984)

The outcome in patients with head trauma depends largely on the location and severity of the initial injury. Severe bilateral miosis (with normal responses to light) and diminished consciousness indicate acute, severe brain damage and increased intracranial

Table 68-1

| Possible Causes of Altered Mentation | |
|---|---|
| Cerebral cortical lesion | Anomalies (e.g., hydrocephalus, lissencephaly) |
| | Inflammatory diseases (e.g., meningitis, encephalitis) |
| | Degenerative disorders (see Box 72-1) |
| | Primary or metastatic brain tumors |
| | External trauma |
| | Vascular disorders (e.g., feline ischemic encephalopathy, canine vascular accident) |
| Metabolic encephalopathy | Hepatic disease |
| | Hypoglycemia |
| | Severe uremia |
| | Hyperosmolality caused by diabetes mellitus or hypernatremia |
| Intoxication | Household toxins, insecticides, rodenticides, drugs (see Box 69-1) |

pressure. Dilated pupils, lack of pupillary light reflex (PLR), stupor or coma, or an abnormal respiratory pattern usually indicates significant brainstem involvement and a grave prognosis.

Development of brainstem signs minutes or hours after the initial trauma usually indicates forebrain herniation from progressive edema or continuing hemorrhage. The primary goal of treatment is to prevent rising intracranial pressure, worsening neuronal edema and ischemia, and herniation. These complications usually develop over several hours, so patients with severe head trauma should be monitored closely for at least 48 hours before they are considered stable.

### Treatment

Treatment usually consists of supportive care and close observation (Box 68-1). Although overhydration-induced exacerbation of cerebral edema must be avoided, it is important to restore normal blood pressure as soon as possible. Hetastarch (6%) may be a better choice for volume replacement than large volumes of crystalloid fluids. Administration of high doses of methylprednisolone sodium succinate or dexamethasone in the first 6 hours after presentation may be beneficial.

*Severe brain injury.* In animals with very severe initial injury or in those in which neurologic signs worsen despite initial therapy, more intensive treatment is recommended (see Box 68-1). Administration of mannitol followed by furosemide produces a marked decrease in intracranial pressure within 10 minutes that generally lasts for 3 to 5 hours.

Continued administration of oxygen by mask or intranasally is indicated. Mechanical hyperventilation may be deleterious to patients whose increased intracranial pressure is not caused by hypercarbia-induced intracranial vasodilation. Hyperventilation in the first 24 hours after injury may decrease cerebral blood flow and worsen ischemic injury to the brain. Narcotic analgesics should not be administered, because they cause hypoventilation and increase intracranial pressure.

---

**Box 68-1**

### Management of Intracranial Injury

Establish patent airway, administer oxygen
Examine, assess, and treat concurrent injuries
Treat shock
   Intravenous fluids, colloids
   Glucocorticoids
Administer glucocorticoids
   Methylprednisolone sodium succinate: 30 mg/kg IV once, then q6h or administer
      constant infusion (5 mg/kg/hr) for 6 hr
   *or*
   Dexamethasone sodium phosphate: 1 mg/kg once
Administer antibiotics if open wound or craniotomy

#### IF SEVERE INITIAL INJURY OR DETERIORATION

Administer diuretics
   Mannitol 20%: 1 g/kg IV over 30 min (can repeat in 3 hr)
   Furosemide (Lasix): 1-2 mg/kg IV, 15 min after mannitol
Elevate head 30 degrees
Treat seizures with diazepam, barbiturates
±Dimethyl sulfoxide: 1 g/kg IV over 30 min
Consider craniotomy

---

*IV,* Intravenously.

Craniotomy can be performed if evidence suggests increasing intracranial pressure (e.g., progressive worsening of mentation) despite medical therapy. Ideally, the decision to operate is based on results of computed tomography (CT) or magnetic resonance imaging (MRI). Surgery can be beneficial to decompress the brain, evacuate hematomas, remove bone fragments, or lavage a penetrating wound.

## LOSS OF VISION AND PUPILLARY ABNORMALITIES (TEXT PP 984-990)

### Diagnostic approach

When a patient is presented for vision loss, it is important to determine whether or not the animal is actually blind. Lack of menace response could be because of poor vision, altered mental state, or cerebellar disease; or it could be normal in a puppy or kitten. It is often more useful to observe the animal's response to the environment, including the ability to negotiate doorways and stairs and awareness of rolling or falling objects.

Blindness can occur with or without systemic or other neurologic signs. Glaucoma, retinal detachment, and sudden acquired retinal degeneration (SARD) are common causes of acute blindness in dogs. When loss of vision is localized anterior to the optic chiasm, it is important to perform a thorough ophthalmologic examination of both eyes. The electroretinogram (ERG) can be used to further evaluate the retina. If the retina appears normal and the ERG is normal in a patient with blindness localized anterior to the chiasm, an optic nerve lesion must be suspected.

***Pupillary light reflexes.*** Evaluation of PLRs can help to localize the lesion within the visual pathway (Table 68-2). The direct response (constriction of the stimulated pupil) and consensual response (constriction of the unstimulated pupil) should be evaluated in a darkened room with a bright, focal light source. Lesions of the eye or optic nerve result in loss of vision in the affected eye and no direct or consensual PLR. If the opposite eye is normal, illumination of that visual eye results in normal pupillary responses in both eyes.

Note: Ocular or optic nerve disease must be very severe for the PLR to be abolished completely. Even animals that are functionally blind from progressive retinal atrophy or optic neuritis sometimes have intact PLRs to a bright light. The pupils may, however, be more dilated than normal in room light in these animals.

Lesions caudal to the optic chiasm result in normal pupil size and PLRs, but a consistent loss of vision occurs in the eye on the side opposite to the brain lesion.

***Anisocoria.*** When the pupils are asymmetric, it is necessary to decide which is abnormal: the more constricted or the dilated pupil. The most likely cause depends on whether unilateral miosis or mydriasis is present.

*Unilateral miosis.* Unilateral miosis is most often seen with primary ocular disease (e.g., uveitis, severe keratitis) and loss of sympathetic innervation to the eye (Horner's syndrome). In animals with Horner's syndrome, anisocoria becomes more pronounced when examination is performed in a darkened room, as the normal pupil dilates.

*Unilateral mydriasis.* Unilateral mydriasis that does not resolve when light is directed into either eye may be seen in patients with glaucoma, in geriatric animals with iris atrophy, and with lesions of the oculomotor nerve. Anisocoria in these patients is most pronounced when the animal is examined in ambient light. These animals warrant careful evaluation and observation, as some tumors that initially impinge on only the oculomotor nerve grow and eventually compress the midbrain, resulting in hemiparesis and other abnormalities.

Testing for feline leukemia virus (FeLV) is recommended in cats with unilateral mydriasis. Unilateral or bilateral mydriasis in cats and dogs has also been associated with dysautonomia (Key-Gaskell syndrome). Instilling one drop of pilocarpine (0.05% to 0.1%) in the affected eye results in pupillary constriction within 45 minutes in these patients (see Chapter 73).

**Table 68-2**

## Localization of Visual Pathway Lesions Based on Vision and Pupillary Light Reflexes

| Location of complete lesion | Vision in right eye | Vision in left eye | Light in right eye | Light in left eye |
|---|---|---|---|---|
| Right retina or eye* | Absent | Normal | No response in either eye | Both pupils constrict |
| Bilateral retina or eye* | Absent | Absent | No response in either eye | No response in either eye |
| Right optic nerve | Absent | Normal | No response in either eye | Both pupils constrict |
| Bilateral optic nerves | Absent | Absent | No response in either eye | No response in either eye |
| Optic chiasm (bilateral) | Absent | Absent | No response in either eye | No response in either eye |
| Lesion caudal to optic chiasm (right lateral geniculate nucleus, right optic radiation, or right occipital cortex) | Normal | Absent | Both pupils constrict | Both pupils constrict |
| Bilateral lesion caudal to optic chiasm | Absent | Absent | Both pupils constrict | Both pupils constrict |
| Right oculomotor nerve | Normal | Normal | Left pupil constricts; right is dilated, no response | Left pupil constricts; right is dilated, no response |

*Retinal or eye lesions must be very severe to cause loss of pupillary light reflexes.

## Specific Causes of Blindness
### Optic neuritis
Inflammation is the most common condition that affects the optic nerve. Causes of optic neuritis include the following:
- Infectious disease—canine distemper, toxoplasmosis, feline infectious peritonitis (FIP), cryptococcosis, blastomycosis, systemic aspergillosis, bacterial disease, FeLV
- Inflammatory disease—systemic lupus erythematosus, granulomatous meningoencephalitis (GME), steroid-responsive suppurative meningitis
- Neoplastic disease—systemic or intracranial neoplasia
- Idiopathic optic neuritis

*Diagnosis.* Swollen, out-of-focus optic disks, plus associated hemorrhage, typically are found on funduscopic examination. However, when optic neuritis occurs caudal to the globe, the funduscopic examination is normal. A normal ERG is needed to differentiate blindness caused by bilateral retrobulbar optic neuritis from that caused by SARD (in which there may exist very subtle retinal changes but an abnormal ERG).

In most cases of optic neuritis, no cause can be identified, and the diagnosis is made after elimination of infectious, inflammatory, and neoplastic disorders. The workup should include complete blood count, serum biochemistry profile, urinalysis, heartworm antigen test, serologic screening for infectious diseases, thoracic radiography, and cerebrospinal fluid (CSF) analysis. When all tests are negative, a tentative diagnosis of primary immune-mediated optic neuritis is made.

*Treatment.* When primary optic neuritis is diagnosed, oral corticosteroid therapy should be initiated. If response is favorable after 1 week (improved vision and PLRs), the dose should be gradually decreased over 2 to 3 weeks to alternate-day therapy. If no initial response occurs, the prognosis for return of vision is poor. Untreated optic neuritis leads to irreversible optic nerve atrophy and permanent blindness. Even with appropriate therapy, in many cases the condition progresses or recurs. The owner should always be warned of the possible existence of an undetected central nervous system (CNS) disorder that could result in development of other neurologic signs.

### Lesions of the optic chiasm and occipital cortex
Lesions of the optic chiasm cause blindness with abnormal PLRs (see Table 68-2). Bilateral lesions of the optic chiasm may be seen in animals with spontaneous infarcts, infectious inflammatory disease, pituitary tumors, or meningiomas.

*Central or cortical blindness.* Animals with lesions caudal to the optic chiasm have a normal fundic examination, normal ERG, normal PLRs (direct and consensual), and blindness in the eye opposite the side of the lesion (see Table 68-2). Causes include trauma-induced hemorrhage and edema, vascular infarcts, GME, infectious encephalitis (canine distemper, systemic mycoses, *Toxoplasma gondii,* FIP), and CNS neoplasia. Congenital disorders (e.g., hydrocephalus, lissencephaly, polymicrogyria, lysosomal storage disease), lead intoxication, and metabolic encephalopathies may cause diffuse or bilateral visual disturbances that are localized to the occipital cortex.

*Diagnostic approach.* Evaluation of intracranial blindness should include thorough physical, ophthalmologic, and neurologic examinations; laboratory database; CSF analysis; and CT or MRI evaluation.

## Horner's Syndrome
Horner's syndrome results from interruption of sympathetic innervation to the eye. The lesion can be found anywhere along the pathway (Box 68-2). Horner's syndrome has four clinical components:
- Anisocoria—miosis of the affected pupil; the other pupil is normal
- Ptosis—drooping of the upper eyelid
- Enophthalmos—inward sinking of the eyeball
- Prolapsed nictitans—partial protrusion of the third eyelid

### Lesion localization
Localization of the lesion is accomplished by physical and neurologic examinations and, if necessary, by pharmacologic testing.

---

**Box 68-2**

## Common Causes of Horner's Syndrome

### UMN CAUSES (RARE)
Intracranial neoplasia, trauma, infarct
Cervical spinal cord lesion
Intervertebral disk protrusion
Neoplasm
Fibrocartilaginous embolism
Trauma

### PREGANGLIONIC CAUSES (FIRST NEURON)
Spinal cord lesion T1-T4 (trauma, neoplasia, fibrocartilaginous embolism)
Brachial plexus avulsion
Thoracic spinal nerve root tumor
Cranial mediastinal mass
Cervical soft-tissue neoplasia, trauma
Skull base trauma

### POSTGANGLIONIC CAUSES (SECOND NEURON)
Otitis media or interna
Necplasia in middle ear
Retrobulbar injury, neoplasia

### UNKNOWN CAUSES
Idiopathic

---

*UMN,* Upper motor neuron.

*Central causes.* Brainstem or cervical spinal cord lesions are rare causes of Horner's syndrome. Ipsilateral hemiplegia and other neurologic abnormalities are expected in such patients.

*Preganglionic causes.* Injury to the thoracic spinal cord between T1 and T4 (especially T1) can result in mild forelimb paresis, ipsilateral UMN signs in the rear limb, and ipsilateral Horner's syndrome. Brachial plexus avulsion is common in dogs and cats injured by automobiles. Horner's syndrome is also commonly seen in dogs with nerve sheath tumors originating in the cranial thoracic spinal nerves (especially T1).

Thoracic inlet or cranial mediastinal tumors (e.g., lymphoma, thymoma) may cause Horner's syndrome without other neurologic deficits, as can bite wounds, neoplasia (e.g., thyroid adenocarcinoma), and surgery (e.g., thyroidectomy or intervertebral disk removal) in the cervical area.

*Postganglionic causes.* Otitis media or neoplasia (e.g., squamous cell carcinoma in cats) within the middle ear commonly results in Horner's syndrome, together with signs of peripheral vestibular disturbance and sometimes facial paralysis. Rarely, retrobulbar injury, neoplasia, or abscess can result in Horner's syndrome.

### Pharmacologic testing
Pharmacologic testing can be used to help determine whether a lesion is of the first (preganglionic) or second (postganglionic) neuron of the lower motor neuron portion of the pathway. However, results can be equivocal and may not always contribute practical information regarding cause or prognosis.

*Procedure.* Two drops of 0.1% phenylephrine (Neo-Synephrine 10% solution, diluted 1:100 with saline) are applied topically to each eye, and the size of each pupil is evaluated 20 minutes later. (Note: This dilute solution does not normally induce pupillary dilation.) If no dilation occurs after 20 minutes in either pupil, one drop of full strength (10%) phenylephrine should be applied to both eyes to confirm that dilation is possible.

*Interpretation.* Dilation of the abnormal (i.e., miotic) pupil within 20 minutes after the 0.1% solution and dilation of both pupils after the 10% solution suggests a postganglionic lesion (e.g., middle ear, retrobulbar).

**Other diagnostic procedures**

The diagnostic approach should include a complete physical examination and ophthalmologic, neurologic, and otoscopic examinations. Thoracic and cervical radiography should also be performed. Clinicopathologic testing, including CSF analysis and advanced diagnostic imaging (e.g., CT, MRI), should be considered if spinal or intracranial disease is suspected. When a postganglionic lesion is suspected, skull radiographs should be performed to evaluate the middle ear for signs of otitis media, neoplasia, or trauma.

The cause is not determined in approximately 50% of dogs and cats with Horner's syndrome that have no other neurologic deficits. The syndrome resolves spontaneously in some of these animals.

## PROTRUSION OF THE THIRD EYELID

The third eyelid may protrude over the corneal surface in the presence of corneal or conjunctival irritation, space-occupying orbital disease, decreased periorbital mass (e.g., dehydration, loss of retrobulbar fat), or loss of volume within the eye (e.g., microphthalmos, phthisis bulbi). Protrusion of the third eyelid is a conspicuous feature of Horner's syndrome (with miosis) and dysautonomia (with mydriasis). Systemic illness or tranquilization can also result in third eyelid protrusion.

In cats, Haw syndrome is dramatic bilateral third eyelid protrusion with no obvious cause. It is more common in cats <2 years old. Affected cats are usually in good health, although digestive disturbances or heavy intestinal parasite loads are occasionally found. Sympathomimetic drops result in rapid retraction of the membrane. The condition resolves spontaneously after several weeks.

# 69

# Seizures

## *(Text pp 991-1004)*

Seizure activity always indicates a functional or structural abnormality of the cerebrum, particularly of the frontal or temporal lobes. Seizure disorders are classified as intracranial, extracranial, or idiopathic (Table 69-1). Idiopathic, or primary, epilepsy is diagnosed in 25% to 30% of dogs having seizures. Another 35% of dogs with seizures have an identifiable abnormality within the brain (e.g., anomaly, inflammation, neoplasia); such dogs are said to have *secondary* epileptic seizures. Extracranial causes such as intoxication or metabolic derangements result in reactive epileptic seizures.

Table 69-1

| | |
|---|---|
| **Table 69-1** | |
| **Common Disorders Resulting in Seizures** | |

| INTRACRANIAL CAUSES (SECONDARY EPILEPTIC SEIZURES) | EXTRACRANIAL CAUSES (REACTIVE EPILEPTIC SEIZURES) |
|---|---|
| Congenital malformations | Toxins (see Box 69-1) |
| Hydrocephalus | Metabolic diseases |
| Lissencephaly | Hypoglycemia |
| Neoplasia | Liver disease |
| Primary brain tumors | Hypocalcemia |
| Metastatic tumors | Hyperlipoproteinemia |
| Inflammatory disease | Hyperviscosity |
| Infectious inflammatory disease | Electrolyte disturbances |
| Granulomatous meningoencephalitis | Hyperosmolality |
| Necrotizing encephalitis | Severe uremia |
| Vascular disease | |
| Hemorrhage | |
| Infarct | **IDIOPATHIC EPILEPSY** |
| Scar tissue | Primary epileptic seizures |
| Metabolic storage diseases (see text) | |
| Degenerative conditions (see Box 72-1) | |

## DIAGNOSTIC APPROACH (TEXT PP 991-993)

### Signalment and history

The signalment, history, and details of the onset, course, duration, and frequency of a seizure disorder are important in establishing a diagnosis. Congenital structural disorders and infectious brain diseases are more likely to occur in very young animals. Idiopathic epilepsy typically begins causing seizures in animals between 6 months and 3 years of age. In aged patients, cerebral neoplasia, vascular accidents, and acquired metabolic disturbances are more likely.

An acute onset of frequent, severe seizures, with or without concurrent neurologic abnormalities, most likely indicates a toxic, vascular, infectious, metabolic, or neoplastic process. A chronic, intermittent seizure disorder with no other clinical signs or neurologic deficits is most consistent with idiopathic epilepsy or a nonprogressive intracranial structural lesion (e.g., scar, anomaly).

### Examination

Complete physical, ophthalmologic, and neurologic examinations should be performed in all dogs and cats evaluated because of seizures. Results should be interpreted with caution if the animal is examined during the postictal phase, when transient neurologic abnormalities are common. Results of these examinations may be useful in determining whether the cause of the seizures is extracranial or intracranial and, if intracranial, where the lesion is located within the brain (see Table 65-9). The results may be completely normal, which is typical for idiopathic epilepsy and may also be the case in a variety of other disorders.

### Laboratory tests

Diagnostic evaluation may include screening tests (complete blood count [CBC], serum biochemistry panel, urinalysis) for metabolic and toxic disorders, and a more thorough workup for infectious diseases, neoplasia, and intracranial disease. The tests selected ultimately depend on the historical and physical examination findings, especially the age of the animal, the nature of any other neurologic abnormalities or clinical signs, and the frequency of the seizures. Dogs >5 years of age at the time of the first seizure, those with an initial interictal period of <4 weeks, and those with partial seizures are most likely to have an underlying intracranial or extracranial disease.

*Additional tests.* If indicated, a liver function test (e.g., serum bile acids) is performed to rule out portosystemic shunt and to obtain baseline information regarding liver function. Thoracic and abdominal radiography and abdominal ultrasonography are recommended in older animals seen after a single seizure, in any animal with severe or progressively worsening seizures, and in all animals with neurologic or systemic abnormalities detected interictally. Additional diagnostic tests for infectious diseases (feline leukemia virus antigen, feline immunodeficiency virus, *Neospora* and *Toxoplasma* serology) may be warranted in some cases.

### Evaluating intracranial disorders

Once metabolic and systemic diseases have been ruled out, intracranial disorders must be considered. In a young adult (<5 years old), neurologically normal dog with a nonprogressive, intermittent seizure disorder of >1 year's duration, idiopathic epilepsy is most likely, and an extensive intracranial workup may not be warranted. Evaluation for intracranial disease, including cerebrospinal fluid (CSF) analysis and computed tomography (CT) or magnetic resonance imaging (MRI), should be performed in all other cases. Because idiopathic epilepsy is uncommon in cats, evaluation for intracranial disease is warranted in every cat with an undiagnosed seizure disorder.

## DISORDERS RESULTING IN SEIZURES (TEXT PP 994-1001)

### Metabolic Disorders

Hypoglycemia, hepatic encephalopathy (HE), hypocalcemia, and primary hyperlipoproteinemia may each cause seizures. Other metabolic alterations, including hyperviscosity syndromes (e.g., multiple myeloma, polycythemia), severe electrolyte disturbances (e.g., hypernatremia), hyperosmolality (e.g., untreated diabetes mellitus), heat stroke, and prolonged severe uremia occasionally cause seizures.

For many of these disorders, other signs and physical findings indicate an extracranial cause. Most metabolic encephalopathies cause intermittent or persistent confusion, delirium, or depression. CBC, serum biochemistry panel, and urinalysis often provide direction for establishing a diagnosis. HE from portosystemic shunting occasionally causes seizures without other clinical or routine laboratory abnormalities, especially in cats, so evaluation of liver function is important in the initial evaluation for metabolic causes of seizures.

### Toxins

Common intoxications that result in seizures are listed in Box 69-1. Clinical signs usually are severe, rapid in onset, and progressive. Diagnosis is based on a history of ingestion or exposure to a toxin or characteristic clinical signs. Specific therapy, emergency treatment for persistent seizures (status epilepticus), and the general approach to removing the toxin, preventing its absorption, and speeding its elimination are summarized in Box 69-1, Box 69-2, and Box 69-3.

### Congenital Malformations

#### Hydrocephalus

Most cases of hydrocephalus are congenital. Dog breeds at risk include the Maltese, Yorkshire Terrier, English Bulldog, Chihuahua, Lhasa Apso, Pomeranian, Toy Poodle, Cairn Terrier, Boston Terrier, Pug, Chow Chow, and Pekingese. Cats are occasionally affected.

*Clinical features.* Many affected animals have an obviously enlarged head and palpably open fontanelles. Care must be taken, however, not to overinterpret these findings, as open fontanelles and mild, asymptomatic hydrocephalus are normal findings in some breeds.

Symptomatic hydrocephalic animals are slow learners and may seem dull or depressed. They may exhibit episodes of abnormal behavior or delirium and cortical blindness (normal pupillary light reflexes). Seizures occur with severe hydrocephalus or when previously asymptomatic animals are decompensated by mild trauma or

Box 69-1

## Intoxications Resulting in Acute Neurologic Dysfunction

### STRYCHNINE
**Common Use**

Rat, mole, gopher, and coyote poison

**Clinical Findings**

Stiff extension of legs and body, erect ears, tetanic spasms induced by auditory stimuli

**Diagnosis**

History of access or ingestion, characteristic signs, chemical analysis of stomach contents

**Treatment**

Vomiting (if no neurologic signs), gastric lavage, diazepam as needed, pentobarbital until effective, establishment of diuresis

### METALDEHYDE
**Common Use**

Snail, slug, and rat poison

**Clinical Findings**

Anxiety, hyperesthesia, tachycardia, hypersalivation, muscle fasciculations, and tremors; not worsened by auditory stimuli; nystagmus in cats; possible convulsions; depression, respiratory failure

**Diagnosis**

History of access or ingestion, characteristic signs, acetaldehyde odor on breath, analysis of stomach contents

**Treatment**

Gastric lavage, pentobarbital until effective, endotracheal tube and ventilation if necessary, establishment of diuresis

### CHLORINATED HYDROCARBONS
**Common Use**

Agricultural products and insecticides; lipid-soluble products are usually absorbed through skin

**Clinical Findings**

Apprehension, hypersensitivity, hypersalivation, exaggerated response to stimuli, muscle twitching of face and neck progressing to severe fasciculations and tremors; possible tonic-clonic seizures

**Diagnosis**

History of access, characteristic signs, insecticide smell to haircoat, analysis of stomach contents

**Treatment**

Wash with warm soapy water to prevent further exposure; if ingested (rare), gastric lavage and instillation of activated charcoal, pentobarbital until effective

### ORGANOPHOSPHATES AND CARBAMATES
**Common Use**

Insecticides

**Clinical Findings**

Excessive salivation, lacrimation, diarrhea, vomiting, and miosis; twitching of facial and tongue muscles, progressing to extreme depression and tonic-clonic seizures

**Diagnosis**

History of exposure, characteristic signs, analysis of stomach contents, low serum acetylcholinesterase activity

*Continued.*

---

**Box 69-1—cont'd**

## Intoxications Resulting in Acute Neurologic Dysfunction

**Treatment**

Prevent further exposure; wash if topical exposure; gastric lavage and activated charcoal if ingested; atropine (0.2 mg/kg IV initially and 0.2 mg/kg SC as needed q6-8h); pralidoxime (20 mg/kg IM q12h) if within 48 hr of exposure or if exposure was dermal

### LEAD
**Common Use**

Ubiquitous in environment in linoleum, rug padding, old lead-based paints (before 1950s), putty and caulking material, roofing materials, batteries, grease, used motor oil, golf balls, fishing sinkers, pellets, and lead shot

**Clinical Findings**

GI signs of anorexia, abdominal pain, vomiting and diarrhea, and megaesophagus; neurologic signs of hysteria, aggression, nervousness, barking, tremors, seizures, blindness, hypermetria and nystagmus (cats), and dementia

**Diagnosis**

History of exposure, characteristic signs, CBC changes (basophilic stippling of RBCs, increase in nucleated RBCs); blood lead level (heparinized tube: >0.5 ppm [50 µg/dl], diagnostic; >0.25 ppm, suggestive); radiographs may reveal radiopaque material in GI tract

**Treatment**

Emetics, gastric lavage, activated charcoal, enemas; surgery or endoscopy if lead in stomach; specific: calcium EDTA (10 mg/ml, give 25 mg/kg IV in dextrose q6h for 2-5 days) to chelate lead and hasten excretion; establish diuresis; alternative treatment: succimer (Chemet, 10 mg/kg PO for 10-14 days)

### ETHYLENE GLYCOL
**Common Use**

Automobile antifreeze, color film processing solutions

**Clinical Findings**

Ataxia, severe depression, polyuria-polydipsia, vomiting; seizures are rare

**Diagnosis**

History of exposure, characteristic signs, severe metabolic acidosis, calcium oxalate crystalluria; eventually, decreased urine production and acute renal failure; diagnosis and treatment of this disorder are discussed in detail in Chapter 44

*EDTA,* Ethylenediaminetetraacetic acid; *GI,* gastrointestinal; *IM,* intramuscularly; *IV,* intravenously; *PO,* orally; *RBCs,* red blood cells; *SC,* subcutaneously.

---

infection. Possible neurologic findings include tetraparesis, slow postural reactions, decreased proprioception, and hyperactive reflexes; bilateral divergent strabismus may also be seen.

*Diagnosis.* Suspicion of hydrocephalus is based on characteristic signs and physical findings in a young animal of a typical breed. If the fontanelles are open, ultrasonography can determine the size of the lateral ventricles. If the fontanelles are small or closed, ultrasonography may be attempted through the temporal bone in neonates. Alternatively, CT, MRI, or pneumoventriculogram (see Chapter 66) can be used. Note: In patients with mild or moderate hydrocephalus, very little correlation exists between ventricular size and clinical signs.

Box 69-2

## Status Epilepticus Treatment in Dogs and Cats

1. If possible, insert an intravenous catheter
2. Administer diazepam (2 mg/kg rectally if no intravenous access)
   If intravenous access is possible, administer 0.5-1 mg/kg; maximum, 20 mg
   Repeat this dose every 5 min if ineffective or if seizures recur
   Administer maximum of four doses if necessary, and proceed to steps 3 and 4
3. Administer if needed to stop the seizure activity
   SODIUM PENTOBARBITAL (3-15 mg/kg IV slowly until effective)
        *or*
   PROPOFOL (4-8 mg/kg IV slowly until effective)
4. Administer PHENOBARBITAL (2-4 mg/kg IV or IM) even if step 3 was not required
5. Maintain a patent airway and monitor respirations
6. Assess body temperature; if >41.4° C (>105° F), cool with cold water
   If patient is hyperthermic, if cerebral edema is suspected, or if seizure activity lasts
        for >15 min, administer:
   MANNITOL (1 g/kg IV over 15 min)
             *and*
   GLUCOCORTICOIDS
      methylprednisolone sodium succinate (30 mg/kg IV)
             *or*
      dexamethasone sodium phosphate (1 mg/kg IV)
             *and*
   THIAMINE (2 mg/kg IM)
7. Collect blood for analysis
   Determine blood glucose concentration; if low, administer 2 ml/kg of 50%
        dextrose IV
   If hypocalcemia is suspected, administer 0.5-1 ml/kg of 10% calcium gluconate
        IV slowly until effective
   Determine electrolyte and calcium concentrations and acid-base status; correct
        any abnormalities
   Initiate intravenous fluids (0.9% saline at 10 ml/kg/hr)
8. Question the owner regarding:
   Possible trauma, toxin exposure, previous seizures, medications, systemic or
        neurologic signs in past few weeks
9. If toxin is suspected, treat to decrease absorption and speed elimination (see
        Boxes 69-1 and 69-3)
10. If the cause of the seizures has not been determined and resolved, or if the animal
        has idiopathic epilepsy, maintain seizure control until the animal has recovered
        sufficiently to accept oral phenobarbital, using:
    DIAZEPAM as an intravenous drip (0.5 mg/kg/hr) in saline
             *or*
    PHENOBARBITAL (2-4 mg/kg IM q8h)
             *or*
    PENTOBARBITAL as an intravenous drip (2-5 mg/kg/hr until effective) in saline

*IM,* Intramuscularly; *IV,* intravenously.

---

**Box 69-3**

## Emergency Treatment of Intoxications

### PREVENT FURTHER ABSORPTION OF INTOXICANT
**Remove Intoxicant from Skin and Haircoat**

*If*

1. Toxin was cutaneously absorbed

*How*

1. Remove flea collar, if collar is source of toxin
2. Wash animal in warm, soapy water; rinse and repeat
3. Flush with warm water for 10 min

**Induce Emesis**

*If*

1. Ingestion of the intoxicant occurred <3 hr before presentation
2. Product ingested was not a petroleum distillate, strong acid, or base
3. Animal has a normal gag reflex and is not convulsing or very depressed (danger of aspiration)

*How*

1. At home—can recommend syrup of ipecac. 6.6 ml/kg; use this in cats
2. Administer apomorphine subcutaneously (0.08 mg/kg) or in conjunctival sac (one crushed tablet or one disk [6 mg]; rinse eye with saline solution after emesis)
3. Administer xylazine (cats, 0.44 mg/kg IM)
   Save vomitus for analysis

**Gastric Lavage**

*If*

1. Ingestion of the intoxicant occurred <3 hr before presentation
2. Attempts to produce emesis were unsuccessful or emesis was not recommended

*How*

1. Induce anesthesia, place cuffed endotracheal tube
2. Lower head relative to body
3. Pass a large-bore stomach tube to the level of stomach
4. Use water (5-10 ml/kg of body weight) for each washing; aspirate with syringe
5. Repeat 10 times
   Save stomach contents for analysis

**Gastrointestinal Adsorbents**

*How*

1. If gastric lavage has been performed, administer activated charcoal slurry (10 ml of a solution containing 1 g of activated charcoal per 5 ml of water per kg of body weight) as the last lavage; let this sit for 20 min, then administer a cathartic
2. If gastric lavage was not performed, administer slurry (dose as above) via stomach tube, or administer tablets of activated charcoal

**Cathartics**

*How*

1. Sodium sulfate 40% solution should be administered (1 g/kg PO) 30 min after activated charcoal is administered

**Diuresis**

*How*

1. Administer saline solution to effect diuresis
2. Mannitol (20% solution, 1-2 g/kg IV) or furosemide (2-4 mg/kg IV) may be added to enhance diuresis if needed

### ADMINISTER SPECIFIC ANTIDOTES
See Box 69-1

### SUPPORTIVE AND SYMPTOMATIC CARE
Administer as appropriate

---

*IM,* Intramuscularly; *IV,* intravenously; *PO,* orally.

*Treatment and prognosis.* Long-term management of neurologic signs can be attempted using prednisone, 0.5 mg/kg orally (PO) q48h. Seizures may be controlled with anticonvulsant therapy, as for epilepsy (see p 628). However, the prognosis for a normal life is poor if neurologic signs are present. Surgical drainage and placement of a permanent ventriculoperitoneal shunt has been successful in a few cases.

*Emergency care.* If acute, severe, progressive neurologic signs develop, it is important to rapidly lower intracranial pressure. If the fontanelles are open, a ventricular tap can be performed (see text), and a small volume of CSF (0.1 to 0.2 ml/kg) can be removed. Mannitol (20%, 1 g/kg intravenously [IV] over 30 minutes), furosemide (2 mg/kg subcutaneously [SC]), and corticosteroids (dexamethasone, 2 to 4 mg/kg, or methylprednisolone sodium succinate, 30 mg/kg, IV) are administered immediately after the tap, and long-term medical management is initiated.

### Lissencephaly

Lissencephaly is a rare condition in which sulci and gyri fail to develop normally; cerebellar hypoplasia may also be present. Lissencephaly is primarily recognized in Lhasa Apsos; Wire-Haired Fox Terriers and Irish Setters are occasionally affected. Behavioral abnormalities and visual deficits are common. These animals are very difficult to train and may not be housebroken. If seizures occur, they usually are not prominent until the dog is >1 year of age. Diagnosis may be suspected from electroencephalographic findings, but definitive diagnosis requires MRI, brain biopsy, or necropsy.

## Degenerative Diseases

Metabolic storage diseases are fatal neurodegenerative disorders that result from inherited enzyme deficiencies within the lysosomes of the nervous system cells (see text). Seizures are a prominent feature in affected animals; delirium and irritability are also common. Signs develop in young animals and are progressive and severe. Histopathologic examination of biopsy samples from affected organs may show characteristic changes, but enzyme assays are required for diagnosis. The prognosis is poor, and no treatment is currently available.

Leukodystrophies, hypomyelinating disorders, and spongy degeneration of the white matter occur as familial disorders in young dogs. Some of these degenerative disorders cause seizures. Diagnosis requires biopsy.

## Neoplasia

Neoplasms of the brain are common in dogs and cats. They usually result in a gradual onset of slowly progressive neurologic signs, but acute onset of signs may occur if the tumor causes hemorrhage or edema. With the exception of lymphoma, most primary and metastatic brain tumors occur in middle-aged and older animals. All breeds are affected; Boxers and Boston Terriers have a greatly increased incidence of glial tumors. Meningiomas are common in old cats.

### Clinical features

Seizures are a prominent clinical sign; circling, ataxia, and head tilt are less common. Increasing intracranial pressure causes progressive loss of consciousness and a change in mentation; the owner may report that the dog or cat has become dull, depressed, and "old." Progressive, subtle neurologic signs sometimes are present for weeks or months before the onset of seizures. In rare instances a small, slow-growing cerebral cortical tumor causes seizures without detectable interictal neurologic deficits. Acutely progressive behavioral changes, seizures, or motor deficits are seen in some dogs and cats with primary or metastatic brain neoplasms, presumably as a result of tumor-related intracranial hemorrhage.

*Neurologic examination.* Evidence of a focal neurologic abnormality is the most common finding. Compulsive circling toward the side of the lesion and abnormal postural reactions, vision, and proprioception on the contralateral side are common.

### Diagnosis

Intracranial neoplasia should be suspected in any older animal with insidious progression of clinical signs or neurologic deficits. Careful physical examination should be performed, looking for potential sites of primary neoplasia, especially lymph nodes, spleen, skin, mammary chain, and prostate gland. CBC, serum biochemistry panel, urinalysis, thoracic and abdominal radiographs, and abdominal ultrasound may reveal metabolic disorders or evidence of primary or metastatic tumors. Most dogs with seizures caused by metastatic brain tumors have detectable pulmonary metastatic lesions.

*Imaging.* Skull radiographs should be performed with the patient under general anesthesia. Although it is a low-yield procedure in patients with seizures, it occasionally reveals calcified superficial tumors (usually meningiomas) or nasal tumors invading the cribriform plate. CT and MRI are much more valuable for detection and characterization of intracranial tumors. In some cases granulomatous disease (granulomatous meningoencephalitis [GME]) is indistinguishable from neoplasia, making it necessary to rely on other tests for definitive diagnosis. Stereotactic CT-guided biopsy of brain tumors can result in a definitive diagnosis without invasive intracranial surgery.

*CSF analysis.* Although it is rarely diagnostic for neoplasia, CSF analysis should be performed to differentiate neoplastic from inflammatory central nervous system (CNS) disease. Patients with evidence of increased intracranial pressure (e.g., deteriorating mentation) should be treated aggressively to lower intracranial pressure before CSF collection (see Chapter 66).

The classic finding (seen in approximately 50% of dogs with brain tumors) is an increase in protein with a normal nucleated cell count (see Table 66-1). The cell count, when it is increased, usually is <50 white blood cells (WBCs) per microliter, although counts as high as 150 WBCs/µl may be seen, especially in animals with meningiomas. Mononuclear cells predominate in most cases, although a larger percentage of neutrophils is seen in a few patients with meningiomas. Neoplastic cells are rarely found, except with lymphoma, when CSF cell counts of >500/µl consisting entirely of neoplastic cells are common.

Quantitative CSF protein evaluation can help differentiate between inflammatory and neoplastic brain conditions. Albumin is increased with both processes, but dogs with brain tumors tend to have high α- and β-globulin concentrations, whereas those with inflammatory conditions such as GME have high γ-globulin concentrations.

### Treatment

Treatment depends on the tumor type, location, growth history, neurologic signs, and associated morbidity and mortality. Once identified with CT or MRI, some small, superficially located, well-encapsulated, benign cerebral tumors (especially meningiomas in cats), dorsal cerebellar tumors, and bony tumors of the skull are amenable to surgical removal.

*Chemotherapy.* Chemotherapy and radiotherapy for lymphoma are possible, but most of the available chemotherapeutic agents do not cross the blood-brain barrier. Intrathecal administration of cytosine arabinoside and methotrexate may be considered, but the prognosis for recovery is poor, and complications are common. Some nonlymphoid brain tumors respond to systemic chemotherapy with nitrosoureas (carmustine or lomustine).

*Radiation therapy.* Radiotherapy is often used as an adjunct to surgery for resectable tumors and as the sole therapy for nonresectable primary (nonmetastatic) brain tumors in dogs. Many dogs that are stable neurologically before therapy show some clinical improvement. Remissions after more than 1 year are common in dogs with certain brain tumors (e.g., meningioma) treated with radiotherapy or combined surgery and radiotherapy. Boron neutron capture therapy has been used to increase the radiation dose that can be administered to tumor cells while sparing normal brain cells. An important drawback of radiotherapy is that it requires multiple anesthesias and access to a referral center that offers this therapy.

*Supportive therapy.* Most intracranial neoplasms are not resectable, so treatment is primarily directed at improving the quality and length of life. In the event of an acute exacerbation of tumor-related clinical signs, a single large dose of dexamethasone (1 mg/kg IV) or methylprednisolone sodium succinate (20 to 40 mg/kg IV) should be administered. Maintenance doses of prednisone (0.5 mg/kg PO q48h) can be given later, as needed. Phenobarbital (PB) is the anticonvulsant of choice for animals with seizures. The initial dose is 2 mg/kg PO q12h. Subsequent changes in dose are based on response to therapy and blood PB levels (see p 628).

## Inflammatory Disorders

All of the infectious disorders discussed in Chapter 71 can cause seizures. Infectious diseases are progressive and nearly always associated with interictal neurologic abnormalities. GME, a noninfectious inflammatory disease in dogs, can also cause seizures, with or without concurrent interictal neurologic deficits. Pug Dog encephalomyelitis commonly causes seizures and other signs of cerebral cortical dysfunction. Feline polioencephalomyelitis may cause seizures in cats.

## Spontaneous Infarction and Hemorrhage

Spontaneous infarcts and hemorrhage occasionally occur in the CNS. Older dogs, dogs with renal failure or hypothyroidism, and cats with renal failure, hyperthyroidism, or primary hypertension may be predisposed. Intracranial hemorrhage or infarction may also occur secondary to septic emboli, neoplasia, coagulopathies, heartworm disease, or vasculitis.

### Signs and diagnosis

Onset of seizures or other neurologic abnormalities is peracute, and signs are non-progressive. Physical examination, laboratory tests, thoracic and skull radiographs, and CSF analysis may be unremarkable (aside from the neurologic abnormalities), or they may reflect the underlying disease process. Occasionally the CSF is xanthochromic, with erythrophagia apparent cytologically. MRI can be useful for antemortem diagnosis.

### Treatment and prognosis

Short-term corticosteroid therapy, as described for head trauma (see Box 68-1), may be indicated for the first 24 hours, once an infectious cause has been ruled out. Mannitol can be used to decrease edema and lower intracranial pressure. Surgical drainage of large, localized hematomas should be considered. Most mildly or moderately affected animals show dramatic improvement during the first 3 to 10 days, although some never return to normal.

## Feline Ischemic Encephalopathy

Feline ischemic encephalopathy (FIE) is a syndrome of acute cerebral cortical dysfunction in cats and is caused by cerebral infarction. Adult cats of any breed are affected. Most cases are diagnosed during the summer months in the northeastern United States in cats with access to the outdoors. Histopathologic features compatible with aberrant migration of *Cuterebra* fly larvae are present in many cases.

### Clinical features

Affected cats are presented because of a peracute onset of asymmetric neurologic abnormalities, including delirium, aggression, circling (to the side of the lesion), ataxia, and seizures. A loss of proprioception and hyperactive reflexes (upper motor neuron signs) may occur in the limbs opposite the side of the lesion, and the cat may be blind but have normal pupillary light reflexes (cortical blindness) on the side opposite the lesion.

### Diagnosis

FIE should be suspected in any cat with an acute onset of nonprogressive, unilateral cerebral cortical dysfunction and no history of trauma or systemic illness. Physical examination typically reveals no abnormalities other than the neurologic signs. Ophthalmologic examination, clinicopathologic evaluation, and skull radiography are also normal. CSF is normal cytologically, with a normal or only slightly increased protein content. MRI may be the best method of documenting the infarcted region.

### Treatment and prognosis

Corticosteroids and mannitol can be administered IV to decrease the edema associated with the vascular lesion (see Box 68-1). If seizures occur, anticonvulsants should be administered (see p 628). Specific treatment of the migrating parasite may be warranted in young and middle-aged cats from endemic areas with acute lateralizing cerebral cortical signs in the summer. Diphenhydramine (4 mg/kg intramuscularly) is given, followed 2 hours later by dexamethasone (0.1 mg/kg IV) and ivermectin (400 µg/kg SC); treatment is repeated 48 hours later.

Most cats show marked improvement in 2 to 7 days, whether or not ivermectin is given. Complete recovery occurs in approximately 50% of cats. Permanent neurologic sequelae may include aggressive behavior or recurrent seizures.

## Trauma- or Scar-Related Epilepsy

Trauma to the cerebral cortex may cause seizures at the time of severe damage (see Chapter 68), or seizures may begin weeks or months after the initial head injury, when a cerebral scar serves as an epileptogenic focus. Scar tissue–related acquired epilepsy can also occur after an inflammatory, toxic, metabolic, or vascular insult. The event usually precedes the onset of the seizure disorder by 6 months to 3 years.

Findings of physical and neurologic examinations, clinicopathologic tests, and CSF analysis are normal. The lesion is not always detectable using MRI or even at necropsy. Treatment is the same as for idiopathic epilepsy (i.e., anticonvulsant therapy). The prognosis for seizure control in some large-breed dogs may be better for those with scar-related acquired epilepsy than for those with idiopathic epilepsy.

## Thiamine Deficiency

Thiamine ($B_1$) deficiency occurs in cats fed uncooked, all-fish diets (which contain thiaminase). It may also occur after a period of illness and anorexia. Thiamine deficiency is almost never seen in dogs, except in racing sled dogs fed a diet high in raw fish. Clinical signs in cats include ataxia, weakness, and depression. Ventroflexion of the head and neck, delirium, head tilt, nystagmus, and seizures are also seen. Tentative diagnosis is based on history, signalment, and clinical signs and is further supported by remission within 24 hours of thiamine administration (2 mg/kg/day). Treatment is continued for 5 days or until the underlying disorder can be corrected.

## Idiopathic Epilepsy

Epilepsy is a syndrome of recurrent seizures unassociated with progressive intracranial disease. It can be caused by an inherited functional problem in the brain (primary, or idiopathic, epilepsy) or can result from a static cerebral anomaly or scar. Idiopathic epilepsy is the most common cause of seizures in dogs. It is characterized by repeated episodes of seizures with no demonstrable cause; affected dogs are normal between seizures. Idiopathic epilepsy is uncommon in cats; most seizure disorders in cats have an identifiable underlying cause, such as neoplasia or encephalitis.

### Breeds commonly affected

Idiopathic epilepsy is inherited in German Shepherd Dogs, Belgian Tervurens, Keeshonds, Beagles, and Dachshunds. A genetic basis is strongly suspected in Labrador Retrievers, Golden Retrievers, and Collies. Other breeds in which epilepsy is common include Saint Bernards, Cocker Spaniels, Irish Setters, Boxers, Siberian Huskies, Springer Spaniels, Alaskan Malamutes, Border Collies, Shelties, Miniature Poodles, and Wire-Haired Fox Terriers. It is seen sporadically in almost all breeds, in mixed-breed dogs, and in cats.

### Clinical features

Seizure episodes usually begin in animals between 6 months and 3 years of age; in some dogs, they do not occur until 5 years of age. In most breeds, the younger the age at onset, the more difficult the disorder is to control. Some purebred dogs develop difficult-to-control seizures at a very young age (e.g., 8 to 12 weeks in Cocker Spaniels) but may then "outgrow" the problem by 4 to 6 months of age. This condition is termed *juvenile epilepsy.*

***Seizure character.*** The seizures usually are generalized tonic-clonic seizures and last 1 to 2 minutes. Simple or complex focal seizures plus secondary generalization may also occur; some individuals exhibit more than one type of seizure. Some Miniature

Poodles and Labrador Retrievers initially exhibit a mild, generalized type of seizure in which they do not lose consciousness but appear anxious and are unable to walk (with either uncontrollable trembling or muscular rigidity); many of these dogs develop more classical generalized tonic-clonic seizures later in life.

*Seizure interval.* Seizures typically recur at regular intervals of weeks or months. With aging the frequency and severity of seizures may increase, especially in large-breed dogs. In some dogs, particularly large-breed dogs, the seizures eventually occur in clusters (multiple seizures during a 24-hour period). Clusters of seizures usually are not seen in association with the first seizure in dogs with idiopathic epilepsy, except in Border Collies, Dalmatians, and German Shepherd Dogs. If more than two seizures occur in the first week of a seizure disorder, a progressive intracranial or extracranial cause should be sought.

### Diagnosis

Physical, neurologic, and ophthalmologic examinations and routine laboratory tests are normal. In a young adult, neurologically normal patient with a nonprogressive, intermittent seizure disorder present for 1 year, idiopathic epilepsy is the most likely diagnosis. More extensive diagnostic testing may not be necessary unless the disorder progresses or changes. Metabolic and systemic evaluation, CSF analysis, and CT or MRI should be considered in the following circumstances: (1) if neurologic abnormalities are present between seizures; (2) in animals that are not of the typical age or breed to have idiopathic epilepsy; and (3) in animals that do not have the typical seizure pattern of idiopathic epilepsy.

### Treatment

Anticonvulsant medication is the only treatment for idiopathic epilepsy, but it may not be required in every case. Animals that have had only one seizure and animals that have very short, nonviolent, infrequent seizures probably do not require treatment unless their condition worsens. Dogs treated early in the course of their epilepsy may have better long-term control of seizures than dogs that are allowed to have many seizures before treatment is initiated. Each seizure may increase the likelihood of the development of more severe seizures, which may become unresponsive to medication or lead to status epilepticus (see p 632).

## ANTICONVULSANT THERAPY (TEXT PP 1001-1004)

Anticonvulsant therapy is indicated in dogs and cats with severe seizures, cluster seizures, individual seizures more often than once every 12 weeks, increasing frequency of seizures, or status epilepticus. Complete control or cure is rarely possible, but a decrease in frequency and severity can be accomplished in 70% to 80% of seizure patients.

### General approach

A minimum database (CBC, serum biochemistry profile, urinalysis) should always be compiled before anticonvulsant therapy is initiated; in many cases a liver function test is also recommended. PB and potassium bromide (KBr) are the initial drugs of choice. Whenever possible, animals should be treated with a single anticonvulsant drug to decrease the prevalence of adverse effects, optimize owner compliance, and decrease overall costs of drugs and monitoring. Clinical response and therapeutic drug concentrations should be monitored to determine the proper dose of anticonvulsant drug for the individual animal. If the initial drug is ineffective despite optimal serum drug levels, then another antiepileptic drug should be added or substituted (Box 69-4).

### Phenobarbital

PB is the drug of choice for both initial treatment and ongoing therapy in dogs and cats. The initial dose is 2 mg/kg PO q12h. Steady-state serum PB concentrations are achieved after 7 to 10 days of therapy. After 2 to 4 weeks of therapy, the animal should be examined and the trough serum PB concentration measured (ideally, just before the morning dose). The therapeutic range is 25 to 35 µg/ml (107 to 150 µmol/L) in dogs

---

**Box 69-4**

## Guidelines for Anticonvulsant Therapy in Dogs

1. Initiate treatment with phenobarbital (PB; 2 mg/kg PO q12h).
2. If seizures continue to occur after 48 hr of treatment, double the dose.
3. At least 10 days after initiating therapy, measure the trough (prepill) serum PB concentration.
   If <20 µg/ml (86 µmol/L), increase the PB dose by 25% and reevaluate 2 wk later. Repeat until the trough serum PB concentration is 20-30 µg/ml (86-130 µmol/L).
4. If seizures are adequately controlled, maintain the dose and monitor the serum PB concentration twice a year and the liver enzymes and function once a year.
5. If seizures continue to occur despite an adequate trough serum PB concentration, measure the serum PB peak (4 hr postpill) and trough (prepill) concentrations. If variation is >25%, increase PB administration to q8h.
6. If seizures continue to occur, increase the PB dose further to achieve a therapeutic concentration in the high range (30-35 µg/ml [130-150 µmol/L]).
7. If seizures continue to occur, add potassium bromide (KBr) therapy (15 mg/kg PO q12h with food).
8. If seizures are controlled but the dog is severely sedated, decrease the PB dose by 20%.
9. If seizures continue to occur, increase the dose of KBr to 20 mg/kg PO q12h.
10. Measure the trough KBr concentration in 3-4 mo. It should be 1-2 mg/ml (10-20 mmol/L).

---

*PO,* Orally.

and 10 to 30 µg/ml (45 to 129 µmol/L) in cats. Note: Serum separator tubes should not be used to collect serum for therapeutic drug monitoring.

### Adjusting the dose

If serum PB is below the therapeutic range, the dose should be increased by approximately 25%, and the trough measured again 2 to 4 weeks later. Any subsequent changes in dose should likewise be evaluated by measurement of serum PB 2 to 4 weeks after the dose change. The dose necessary to achieve therapeutic serum concentrations can vary dramatically among animals and even in an individual animal. If the measured PB concentration is adequate, the patient should be observed through two or three cycles of seizures. If control is acceptable, therapy is maintained at that dose.

Long-term use of PB can be complicated by the drug's induction of hepatic microsomal enzyme activity, which increases drug elimination. Dose increases, therefore, usually are required, especially during the first few months of therapy. Serum PB concentration should be reevaluated routinely every 6 months, 2 to 4 weeks after any change in dose, and whenever two or more seizures occur between scheduled evaluations.

### Drug failures

Most "drug failures" are the result of poor owner compliance or altered drug metabolism. Although twice-daily administration is sufficient in most dogs and cats, the drug's half-life may be shortened in some individuals, resulting in fluctuations in plasma concentration during the day. This effect can be identified by measuring peak (4-hour postpill) and trough (prepill) drug concentrations. If the serum concentration varies >25% during the day, then q8h administration is recommended.

If seizures are uncontrolled despite therapeutic serum concentrations, the dose should be gradually increased until the serum concentration reaches the high end of the therapeutic range. Peak and trough concentrations should be measured to avoid problems with toxicity. Severe hepatotoxicity has been documented in dogs, especially when serum PB is maintained >35 µg/ml (>150 µmol/L). Furthermore, increasing the serum PB beyond the therapeutic range rarely benefits seizure control. Additional or alternative drug therapy is a better alternative.

### Adverse effects

The most common adverse effects are polyuria, polydipsia, and polyphagia. During the first 7 to 10 days of PB therapy, sedation, depression, and ataxia may be pronounced; they usually resolve within 10 to 21 days. Hyperexcitability occurs as an idiosyncratic effect in up to 40% of dogs and cats. Many animals develop dependence on the drug, and sudden withdrawal precipitates seizures. Therefore it is important for owners to consistently administer the drug. Rarely, PB administration causes leukopenia, plus thrombocytopenia and anemia. These abnormalities may represent an idiosyncratic reaction rather than a dose-related effect, and they usually resolve after the drug is discontinued.

### Routine reevaluation

Reevaluation is recommended every 6 to 12 months to assess the effectiveness of the drug regimen, measure serum PB, and evaluate liver enzyme activities and liver function (e.g., serum bile acids). Mild to moderate elevations in the serum activities of alkaline phosphatase and alanine aminotransferase are seen in most dogs receiving PB. Significant hepatotoxicity is uncommon unless serum PB concentrations are high. If the serum PB increases while the animal is maintained on a stable dose of drug, diminished liver function must be suspected and liver function tests performed. If liver function deteriorates, then an alternate anticonvulsant must be administered.

### Drug and hormone interactions

PB increases the biotransformation of drugs metabolized by the liver, thereby decreasing the systemic effects of these drugs if administered concurrently. PB also increases the rate of thyroid hormone elimination, which decreases total and free thyroxine concentrations. However, thyroid hormone supplementation is recommended only if clinical signs of hypothyroidism develop (see Chapter 51).

Drugs that inhibit microsomal enzymes (e.g., chloramphenicol, tetracycline, cimetidine, ranitidine, enilconazole) may dramatically inhibit the hepatic metabolism of PB, resulting in increased serum concentrations of PB and potential toxicity.

### Refractory patients

Seizures are controlled in 70% to 80% of dogs and most cats treated with PB alone if serum PB is maintained within the therapeutic range. If seizures continue to occur at an unacceptable frequency or severity despite adequate serum concentrations, therapy with other drugs must be considered (see Box 69-4). Addition of a second drug (usually KBr) decreases the number of seizures by >50% in 70% to 80% of dogs.

## Potassium Bromide

Improved control of refractory seizures can be achieved with addition of KBr to PB therapy. KBr is also effective as a single agent in patients that do not tolerate PB and is considered by many to be the initial drug of choice (as monotherapy) for idiopathic epilepsy. The half-life of KBr is long (25 days in dogs, 11 days in cats), so a long lag period occurs between initiation of treatment and a therapeutic response.

### Protocol

When KBr is the only anticonvulsant used for a severe or progressive seizure disorder, or when PB toxicity makes it necessary to immediately switch drugs and rapidly achieve therapeutic serum concentrations of KBr, a loading dose of KBr should be administered. With this protocol, KBr is given at an initial dose of 60 to 80 mg/kg PO q12h with food for 5 days. The dose is then decreased to a maintenance dose of 15 mg/kg PO q12h with food, and therapeutic serum monitoring is performed.

When KBr is used as monotherapy for a less severe or less progressive seizure disorder, or when it is added to an existing PB regimen, KBr is initiated at the maintenance rate (15 mg/kg PO q12h with food). Whenever possible, PB is continued at the already-established dose. Serum KBr and PB should be measured 1 month and 4 months after initiation of therapy and every 6 to 9 months thereafter.

### Therapeutic monitoring

When used as monotherapy, a trough serum KBr concentration of 2 to 3 mg/ml (20 to 30 mmol/L) is desired. When KBr is used concurrently with PB, the target is a trough serum KBr concentration of 1 to 2 mg/ml (10 to 20 mmol/L).

### Adverse effects

Adverse effects of KBr include vomiting, polyuria, polydipsia, and polyphagia; sedation, incoordination, anorexia, and constipation may also occur. Limb stiffness, lameness, and muscle weakness can occur at high serum levels and generally resolve once the dose is decreased. Vomiting can be diminished by splitting the total daily dose into four equal doses (rather than two) and by feeding a small amount of food with each dose.

Dramatic sedation can occur in dogs concurrently treated with PB; this effect can be decreased by lowering the PB dose by 25%. If more serious neurotoxicity occurs, intravenous saline solution can be administered to increase renal excretion of bromide.

Biochemical abnormalities are uncommon with KBr monotherapy. KBr therapy does not cause hepatotoxicity, but pancreatitis occasionally develops. Chronic severe bronchitis has been documented in cats receiving KBr monotherapy. Increases in dietary chloride intake can dramatically increase bromide elimination and decrease seizure control.

## Diazepam

Diazepam (Valium) is of limited use as a primary anticonvulsant in dogs because of its expense and its very short half-life and the rapid development of tolerance to its anticonvulsant effects. The only common adverse effect is sedation. Idiosyncratic severe, life-threatening hepatotoxicity has been documented in cats receiving daily diazepam for >5 days. Therefore close observation of appetite and attitude and periodic monitoring of liver enzymes is warranted in all cats treated with diazepam. PB and KBr may be better choices for chronic anticonvulsant therapy.

### Dosage

Diazepam is administered orally at a dose of 0.3 to 0.8 mg/kg q8h to achieve trough blood concentrations of 200 to 500 ng/ml. When used as at-home therapy for dogs with idiopathic epilepsy and cluster seizures that show a recognizable preictal phase or a preceding aura, a dose of 10 to 30 mg PO may be used to decrease the severity of the impending seizure.

Alternatively, the injectable diazepam preparation (5 mg/ml) can be administered rectally (1 mg/kg) by the owner just after the seizure, to a maximum dose of 3 mg/kg in 24 hours. The dose can be doubled in dogs on long-term PB therapy (which increases diazepam clearance). Note: Diazepam dispensed for at-home rectal administration should be stored in a glass vial.

## Clonazepam and Clorazepate

Clonazepam and clorazepate have characteristics very similar to those of diazepam. They are highly effective anticonvulsants, but they have a very short duration of action, they are very expensive, and development of tolerance to their antiseizure effects is common. Cross-tolerance among benzodiazepines is common, so chronic use of one of these drugs for seizure control may limit the effectiveness of diazepam for emergency treatment.

Clonazepam (Klonopin) is given at a dose of 0.5 to 1.5 mg/kg PO q8-12h. When used for long-term seizure control with PB, serum clonazepam should be monitored (therapeutic target, 0.01 to 0.08 mg/ml). Clorazepate dipotassium (Traxene) is given at a dose of 1 to 2 mg/kg PO q12h. It is less likely to induce tolerance than clonazepam, but it is very expensive, and results in dogs refractory to PB have not been promising.

## Valproic Acid

Addition of sodium valproate improves seizure control in some large-breed dogs with idiopathic epilepsy that are refractory to PB monotherapy. This combination has not been evaluated in cats. The dose of valproic acid (Depakene) is 20 to 60 mg/kg PO q8-12h. Long-term adverse effects are uncommon, although alopecia and rapidly fulminating, fatal hepatic necrosis have been documented.

### Felbamate

Felbamate (Felbatol) can be beneficial in dogs refractory to anticonvulsant therapy with PB or KBr. The recommended starting dose is 15 mg/kg PO q8h. The dose can be increased in 15-mg/kg increments until the seizures are adequately controlled. Side effects have not been reported in dogs, but aplastic anemia and hepatotoxicity have been reported in humans.

### Other Options

Epilepsy is not well controlled using standard anticonvulsant therapy in 20% to 25% of dogs, despite therapeutic drug monitoring and appropriate dose adjustments. It is important to evaluate poorly controlled animals for underlying metabolic or intracranial disease that could be specifically treated. Alternative treatments could also be considered in these animals, including the feeding of hypoallergenic diets, acupuncture, surgical division of the corpus callosum, and vagus nerve stimulation.

## EMERGENCY THERAPY FOR STATUS EPILEPTICUS (TEXT P 1004)

Status epilepticus is a series of seizures without periods of intervening consciousness. It constitutes a medical emergency. Immediate seizure control is required, because continuous seizure activity of >20 minutes results in permanent neuronal damage. The goals of treatment are to stabilize the animal, stop the seizure activity, protect the brain from further damage, and allow recovery from the systemic effects of prolonged seizure activity. Specific therapy is outlined in Box 69-2.

# 70

# Head Tilt

## (Text pp 1005-1009)

Head tilt is a common neurologic abnormality in dogs and cats and indicates a lesion of the vestibular system (either central or peripheral). The head tilt is to the same side as the lesion. Vestibular problems also cause circling, ataxia, falling or rolling, and spontaneous nystagmus. As compensation occurs, spontaneous nystagmus often resolves within days in animals with acute vestibular dysfunction. Vomiting and salivation are other common presenting complaints in animals with vestibular disease.

## LOCALIZING THE LESION (TEXT PP 1005-1006)

Different disorders affect the central and peripheral vestibular systems, so localization of disease to one of these systems should always be attempted. The character of the

---

**Box 70-1**

### Clinical Findings in Vestibular Disease

#### CENTRAL AND PERIPHERAL VESTIBULAR DISEASE

Incoordination

Head tilt toward side of lesion

Falling or rolling toward side of lesion (a result of decreased extensor tone in limbs on ipsilateral side and increased extensor tone in limbs on contralateral side)

±Ventral strabismus on side of lesion

Vomiting, salivation

Spontaneous nystagmus (fast phase away from lesion)

Nystagmus may intensify with changes in body position

| PERIPHERAL VESTIBULAR DISEASE | CENTRAL VESTIBULAR DISEASE |
|---|---|
| Nystagmus is horizontal or rotatory | Nystagmus is horizontal, rotatory, or vertical |
| No change in nystagmus direction with changes in head position | Nystagmus may change direction with changes in head position |
| Normal postural reactions, proprioception, and strength | Abnormal postural reactions and proprioception may be seen on side of lesion |
| Concurrent Horner's syndrome, facial nerve paralysis with involvement of the middle and inner ear; other cranial nerves normal | Multiple cranial nerve deficits may be seen |

---

nystagmus, assessment of muscle tone, proprioception, and postural reactions and the presence of other neurologic abnormalities each help in localizing the lesion to either the central or peripheral vestibular system (Box 70-1).

**Paradoxic vestibular signs**

Central vestibular lesions primarily involving the caudal cerebellar peduncle or the flocculonodular lobe of the cerebellum can cause paradoxic vestibular signs: head tilt and fast phase of nystagmus toward the side *opposite* the lesion. Dysmetria, hypermetria, or proprioceptive abnormalities in the limbs on the *same side* as the lesion help localize the disease to the correct side. Head bobbing and intention tremor are occasionally seen in affected animals.

**Other neurologic signs**

The presence of concurrent neurologic abnormalities aids in localization of the lesions. Many diseases that affect the *peripheral* vestibular system within the inner ear also result in ipsilateral facial nerve paralysis or Horner's syndrome (see Chapter 68). Cranial nerve abnormalities other than facial nerve paralysis and Horner's syndrome in an animal with vestibular disease usually indicate *central* (i.e., brainstem) disease. Neoplasia or granulomas at the cerebellomedullary angle may result in simultaneous dysfunction of the vestibular, facial, and trigeminal nerves. The trigeminal nerve (i.e., facial sensation) should always be assessed during neurologic examination of any animal with vestibular signs. Other cranial nerve deficits, proprioceptive abnormalities, head tremor, or hypermetria all suggest central vestibular disease.

## PERIPHERAL VESTIBULAR DISEASE (TEXT PP 1006-1009)

Peripheral vestibular disease is much more common than central disease and generally has a better prognosis. The causes are many and varied: (1) congenital disorder;

(2) infection, neoplasia, polyps, or trauma affecting the vestibular nerve in the middle or inner ear; (3) neurotoxicity, e.g., aminoglycosides (rare), other drugs or chemicals, hypothyroidism-associated polyneuropathy; and (4) transient idiopathic syndrome in adult cats or geriatric dogs. Specific conditions that cause peripheral vestibular disease are discussed later in this section.

### General diagnostic approach

When peripheral vestibular disease is suspected, the external ear canal and tympanic membrane should be examined carefully. A ruptured, bulging, or cloudy tympanic membrane suggests disease of the middle and possibly the inner ear. The region of the osseous bullae and the temporomandibular joints should be palpated carefully for asymmetry or pain. If possible, the pharynx should be examined visually and by palpation. When idiopathic vestibular syndromes are suspected, waiting to assess reversibility of the signs may be warranted. Further diagnostic evaluation is indicated in patients that do not improve with rest and time (3 to 5 days) or in animals with other evidence of middle or inner ear disease.

### Diagnostic tests

Routine diagnostic tests (complete blood count, serum biochemistry panel, urinalysis) rarely contribute to the diagnosis, although test results occasionally suggest hypothyroidism. Radiographic examination of the tympanic bullae and bony labyrinth should be performed with the patient under anesthesia to check for evidence of chronic infection, trauma, inflammatory polyps, or neoplasia. Ventrodorsal, left and right lateral oblique, and open-mouth views are used. Computed tomography or magnetic resonance imaging (MRI) can also be used to evaluate the middle and inner ear. If no abnormalities are found, and the signalment, onset, or progression of signs does not support an idiopathic syndrome, cerebrospinal fluid (CSF) analysis should be performed. Brainstem auditory evoked response testing may help localize the lesion within the vestibular system (see Chapter 66).

### Congenital vestibular syndromes

Purebred dogs and cats that develop peripheral vestibular signs before 3 months of age most likely have a congenital vestibular disorder. Unilateral vestibular syndromes have been recognized in the German Shepherd Dog, Doberman Pinscher, Akita, English Cocker Spaniel, Beagle, Smooth Fox Terrier, and Tibetan Terrier, as well as in Siamese, Burmese, and Tonkinese cats.

Clinical signs may be present at birth or may develop during the first few months of life. Head tilt, circling, and ataxia may initially be severe, but, with time, compensation renders many affected animals acceptable pets. Diagnosis is based on the early onset of signs. If radiography and CSF analysis are performed, the results are normal. Deafness may accompany the vestibular signs, particularly in Dobermans, Akitas, and Siamese cats.

### Otitis media and interna

Extension of otitis externa to the middle or inner ear is a very common cause of peripheral vestibular disease in dogs and cats. Vestibular signs are consistent with a unilateral peripheral lesion (see Box 70-1). Ipsilateral facial nerve paralysis or Horner's syndrome may also be present. Obvious otitis externa, an abnormal or ruptured tympanic membrane, and pain on palpation of the bulla area may be found, but occasionally otoscopic examination is normal. Diagnosis and treatment of otitis media and interna are discussed in Chapter 73.

### Neoplasia

Tumors of the bullae or bony labyrinth may damage or involve the peripheral vestibular structures. Likewise, tumors within the ear canal (e.g., squamous cell carcinoma, ceruminous gland adenocarcinoma) may spread locally and result in vestibular disease. Less commonly, neurofibroma or neurofibrosarcoma of cranial nerve VIII may result in slowly progressive peripheral vestibular signs. Concurrent facial nerve paralysis or Horner's syndrome is common with tumors involving the middle or inner ear.

These tumors usually are evident on skull radiographs as areas of soft-tissue density within the bulla or bone lysis in the region of the bulla. Diagnosis can be confirmed by biopsy. Because of the invasive nature of most of these tumors, total resection is difficult. Radiotherapy or chemotherapy may be beneficial in some patients.

### Ototoxicity

Many drugs and chemicals are potentially toxic to the inner ear, but the prevalence of ototoxicity in dogs and cats is low. Whenever vestibular dysfunction becomes evident immediately after a substance is instilled in an ear canal, the product should be removed and the ear canal flushed with copious quantities of saline. Vestibular signs usually resolve within a few days or weeks.

### Aminoglycosides

Rarely, aminoglycoside antibiotics cause degeneration within the vestibular and auditory systems. Ototoxicity is usually associated with high doses or prolonged use, particularly in animals with impaired renal function. Vestibular degeneration may result in unilateral or bilateral peripheral vestibular signs and loss of hearing. In most cases the vestibular signs resolve if therapy is discontinued immediately, but deafness may persist.

### Hypothyroidism

Hypothyroidism is a possible cause of peripheral vestibular disease in adult dogs. Other signs of hypothyroidism may or may not be present. Laboratory tests may show abnormalities that suggest hypothyroidism, but the diagnosis is made with thyroid function testing (see Chapter 51). Response to replacement thyroid hormones is variable.

### Feline idiopathic vestibular syndrome

Feline idiopathic vestibular syndrome is an acute, nonprogressive disorder that is common in cats of all ages. The prevalence may be higher in the summer and early fall and in the northeastern United States, suggesting a possible role for an infectious or parasitic agent. The disorder is characterized by peracute onset of peripheral vestibular signs, with no abnormalities of proprioception or other cranial nerves. Diagnosis is based on clinical signs and absence of ear problems or other disease. Radiographs of the tympanic bullae and petrous temporal bone are normal, as is CSF analysis. Spontaneous improvement is usually seen in 2 to 3 days, with a complete return to normal in 2 to 3 weeks.

### Geriatric canine vestibular disease

Geriatric canine vestibular disease, an idiopathic syndrome, is the most common cause of unilateral peripheral vestibular disease in old dogs. Mean age at onset is 12.5 years. The disorder is characterized by a sudden onset of unilateral peripheral vestibular signs (see Box 70-1), which may be anywhere from mild to severe. No other neurologic abnormalities are found, and all other cranial nerves are normal. Transient nausea, vomiting, and anorexia occur in approximately 30% of patients.

*Diagnosis.* This condition should be suspected in any older dog with a peracute onset of unilateral peripheral vestibular signs and no other neurologic abnormalities. Thorough physical, neurologic, and otoscopic examinations should be performed. More extensive testing may be delayed for a few days. Diagnosis is based on exclusion of other causes of peripheral vestibular dysfunction and on improvement in clinical signs with time. Nystagmus usually resolves within a few days and is replaced by a transient positional nystagmus in the same direction. Ataxia gradually improves over 1 to 2 weeks, as does the head tilt, which is rarely permanent.

*Treatment and prognosis.* No therapy is recommended. Occasionally, vomiting is severe, and diphenhydramine (2 to 4 mg/kg subcutaneously q8h), chlorpromazine (1 to 2 mg/kg orally [PO] q8h), or meclizine (1 to 2 mg/kg PO q24h) is needed for 2 to 3 days. The prognosis for recovery is excellent. Recurrence is unusual but may occur, on the same side or on the opposite side.

## BILATERAL PERIPHERAL VESTIBULAR DISEASE (TEXT P 1009)

No head tilt may be discernible in animals with bilateral peripheral vestibular disease. Affected animals typically have a wide-based stance and are ataxic, although conscious proprioception is normal. The animal may fall or circle to either side and usually walks in a crouched position with a wide, side-to-side swinging of the head.

No spontaneous or positional nystagmus is present, and in most cases there exists loss of normal vestibular eye movements. Some affected animals are deaf. If the animal is held suspended by the pelvis and lowered toward the ground, there may be no normal extension of the thoracic limbs toward the floor. Instead, the affected animal may curl the head and neck toward the sternum.

Differential diagnoses include an idiopathic or congenital syndrome, trauma, ototoxicity, inner ear infections, and hypothyroidism. Diagnostic evaluation is as for unilateral peripheral vestibular disease.

## CENTRAL VESTIBULAR DISEASE (TEXT P 1009)

Central vestibular disease is much less common than peripheral vestibular disease and generally carries a poor prognosis. It can be caused by any inflammatory, neoplastic, vascular, or traumatic CNS disorder (Box 70-2). Granulomatous meningoencephalitis (dogs), Rocky Mountain spotted fever (dogs), and feline infectious peritonitis (cats) have a particular predilection for affecting this part of the brain.

### Diagnostic approach

A standard workup for intracranial disease is performed in animals that clearly have central vestibular disease. Complete physical, neurologic, and ophthalmologic examinations are essential to look for evidence of disease elsewhere in the body. Clinicopathologic testing and thoracic and abdominal radiography are warranted to search for neoplastic or infectious inflammatory systemic disease. Finally, diagnostic imaging (particularly MRI) and CSF analysis should be considered.

### Metronidazole toxicity

Toxicity can occur in dogs after administration of metronidazole at doses >60 mg/kg/day for >3 days. Signs develop acutely and include vertical nystagmus, ataxia (possibly severe), anorexia, and vomiting; seizures and head tilt occasionally occur. The prognosis for recovery is good once metronidazole administration is stopped.

## CONGENITAL NYSTAGMUS (TEXT P 1009)

A fine, oscillating or pendular nystagmus unassociated with other features of vestibular disease is occasionally seen as a congenital syndrome. The speed and force of nystagmus are equal in both directions of movement. This condition has been recognized in litters of puppies and may accompany other congenital abnormalities of the visual system, particularly in Belgian Sheepdogs and in Siamese and Himalayan cats.

---

**Box 70-2**

### Disorders Causing Head Tilt

| CENTRAL VESTIBULAR DISEASE | PERIPHERAL VESTIBULAR DISEASE |
|---|---|
| Trauma or hemorrhage | Otitis media and interna |
| Infectious inflammatory disorders | Middle ear tumors and feline |
| Granulomatous meningoencephalitis | nasopharyngeal polyps |
| (dogs) | Trauma |
| Neoplasia | Congenital vestibular syndromes |
| Vascular infarct | Geriatric canine vestibular disease |
| Thiamine deficiency | Feline idiopathic vestibular syndrome |
| | Aminoglycoside ototoxicity |
| | Hypothyroidism (?) |

# 71

# Encephalitis, Myelitis, Meningitis

## (Text pp 1010-1019)

### CLINICAL FEATURES (TEXT P 1010)

Bacterial, viral, protozoal, mycotic, rickettsial, and parasitic pathogens are all potential causes of inflammatory central nervous system (CNS) disease. In addition, several idiopathic (presumably immune-related) meningitis syndromes occur in dogs, including steroid-responsive suppurative meningitis of young dogs, meningeal vasculitis, granulomatous meningoencephalomyelitis, and Pug meningoencephalitis.

#### Clinical signs

Clinical signs of CNS inflammation vary with the anatomic location and with the severity of inflammation. Individual syndromes often have characteristic clinical signs. Cervical pain and rigidity are common in dogs with meningitis and may be manifested by reluctance to walk, a boardlike stance, an arched spine, and resistance to passive manipulation of the head, neck, and limbs; fever is common. Myelitis or encephalitis results in neurologic deficits localized to the particular region involved.

#### Analysis of cerebrospinal fluid

Analysis of cerebrospinal fluid (CSF) is necessary to confirm inflammatory CNS disease. CSF cytology, together with clinical and neurologic findings, aids in determination of the cause of the inflammation (see Table 66-1). CSF protein, culture, specific antibody titers, and other appropriate tests allow diagnosis of a specific disorder and initiation of appropriate treatment (Table 71-1).

### STEROID-RESPONSIVE SUPPURATIVE MENINGITIS (TEXT PP 1010-1011)

Suppurative meningitis that is responsive to corticosteroids is a common form of meningitis. Large dogs <2 years of age are most often affected; middle-aged and older dogs are occasionally affected. No causative agent has yet been identified. Clinical signs are probably caused by immune-mediated meningeal vasculitis. Signs include fever, cervical rigidity, and vertebral pain. Affected dogs are alert and systemically normal. Neurologic deficits are uncommon but may occur in untreated or inadequately treated dogs.

#### Diagnosis

Peripheral neutrophilia is usually present, although neutropenia is occasionally found. Analysis of CSF shows increased protein concentration and severe neutrophilic pleocytosis (usually >500 cells/µl; 75% to 100% neutrophils). High immunoglobulin A (IgA) concentrations are found in the CSF and serum. However, CSF may be normal early in the disease. CSF collected after corticosteroids are given may show nearly normal cell counts and a predominance of mononuclear cells within 24 to 48 hours of the beginning of therapy. Bacterial cultures of CSF and blood are negative. Some affected dogs also have immune-mediated polyarthritis.

Table 71-1

## Ancillary Tests in the Diagnosis of Infectious Inflammatory Central Nervous System Disease

| Disorder suspected | Ancillary diagnostics |
|---|---|
| Acute distemper (D) | Conjunctival scrapings |
| | Funduscopic examination |
| | Thoracic radiographs |
| | CSF antibody titer |
| | Skin biopsy immunohistochemistry |
| Bacterial infection (D, C) | Ear, throat, and eye exam |
| | Thoracic radiographs |
| | Cardiac ultrasound |
| | Skull and spinal radiographs |
| | Blood and urine cultures |
| | CSF culture |
| Toxoplasmosis (D, C) | Funduscopic exam |
| | ALT, AST, CK activities |
| | CSF, serum titers |
| Neosporosis (D) | Funduscopic exam |
| | AST, CK activities |
| | CSF, serum titers |
| Feline infectious peritonitis (C) | Funduscopic examination |
| | Ophthalmologic exam |
| | Serum globulin |
| | Abdominal palpation/ultrasound |
| | Coronavirus antibody in CSF and serum |
| | Coronavirus PCR on CSF |
| Cryptococcosis (D, C) | Funduscopic examination |
| | Thoracic radiographs |
| | Skull radiographs |
| | Nasal swab cytology |
| | Test for capsular antigen in serum |
| | CSF culture |
| Rocky Mountain spotted fever (D) | Thoracic radiographs |
| | CBC, platelet count |
| | Skin biopsy: IFA |
| | Serum titer (demonstrate rise) |
| Ehrlichiosis (D) | CBC, platelet count |
| | Serum titers |
| | Funduscopic exam |

*ALT,* Alanine aminotransferase; *AST,* aspartate aminotransferase; *C,* cats; *CBC,* complete blood count; *CK,* creatine kinase; *CSF,* cerebrospinal fluid; *D,* dogs; *IFA,* indirect fluorescent antibody; *PCR,* polymerase chain reaction.

### Treatment

The condition is not responsive to antibiotics, although initial fluctuation of signs may give the impression of antibiotic response. Fever and pain are rapidly alleviated when corticosteroids are instituted. Corticosteroids should initially be given at immunosuppressive doses (e.g., prednisone, 2 to 4 mg/kg/day). The dose is gradually decreased to alternate-day therapy over 1 to 2 months. The dose should be tapered more slowly in dogs that relapse. Dogs with aseptic meningitis that do not respond well to prednisone alone may benefit from addition of azathioprine (Imuran, 2.2 mg/kg/day) for 4 to 8 weeks. Long-term corticosteroid therapy is not necessary in most cases.

### Prognosis

Therapy may be necessary for 4 to 6 months, but the prognosis for survival and complete resolution generally is excellent. Dogs not appropriately treated early in the disease may develop neurologic deficits associated with spinal cord infarction and meningeal fibrosis; treatment may not resolve all signs in these dogs.

## MENINGEAL VASCULITIS (TEXT P 1012)

Severe, necrotizing vasculitis in the CNS occurs as a breed-associated syndrome in Beagles, Boxers, Bernese Mountain Dogs, and German Short-Haired Pointers. Multiple littermates are commonly affected, and many affected dogs are closely related, suggesting a hereditary basis. In affected beagles, similar pathologic changes occur in the coronary vessels, and if they experience repeated episodes, they may develop splenic, hepatic, and renal amyloidosis.

### Clinical features and diagnosis

Classic meningeal signs of fever, cervical rigidity, and spinal pain are seen. Progression to neurologic signs, including paralysis, blindness, and seizures, rarely occurs. Analysis of CSF reveals increased protein concentration and extreme neutrophilic pleocytosis. Some affected dogs have concurrent immune-mediated polyarthritis.

### Treatment and prognosis

Long-term treatment with prednisone (2 to 4 mg/kg/day orally [PO] initially, then 1 mg/kg q48h) is effective in most dogs. More aggressive immunosuppressive therapy with azathioprine (2 mg/kg PO q24-48h) is effective in some refractory cases. However, the prognosis is guarded in dogs that are severely affected and those that do not respond rapidly and completely to immunosuppressive therapy. Resolution after 4 to 6 months of treatment, without the need for continuing medication, occurs in some Bernese Mountain Dogs and most German Short-Haired Pointers.

## GRANULOMATOUS MENINGOENCEPHALITIS (TEXT PP 1012-1013)

Granulomatous meningoencephalitis (GME) is an idiopathic inflammatory disorder of the CNS in dogs. It occurs primarily in young adult dogs of small breeds, with Poodles and Terriers most commonly affected. Large-breed dogs are occasionally affected. Most dogs with GME are 2 to 6 years of age, although the disease may affect older or younger dogs.

### Clinical features

Focal and disseminated forms of the disease occur. An ocular form of GME also exists and can occur alone or, more often, in combination with focal or disseminated disease. Clinical signs reflect the location and nature of the lesion. The prominent feature may be cervical pain (suggesting meningeal involvement) or brainstem signs (e.g., nystagmus, head tilt, blindness, or facial and trigeminal paralysis). Ataxia, seizures, circling, and behavior change are common. Neurologic dysfunction and severe pain from meningeal involvement are common with both forms.

*Focal form.* Focal GME has a predilection to occur in the brainstem, cerebral cortex, cerebellum, or cervical spinal cord. It causes clinical signs suggestive of a single, enlarging, space-occupying mass in the brain or spinal cord. Signs have an insidious onset and are slowly progressive (3 to 6 months).

*Disseminated form.* The disseminated form most commonly affects the lower brainstem, cervical spinal cord, and meninges. Many affected dogs have a fever and peripheral neutrophilia but no other evidence of systemic disease. Onset is acute or subacute, and progression can be very rapid (1 to 8 weeks); 25% of cases progress to death within 1 week.

### Diagnosis

Analysis of CSF reveals an increase in protein concentration and mild to marked pleocytosis consisting primarily of lymphocytes, monocytes, and occasional plasma cells. Anaplastic mononuclear cells with abundant lacy cytoplasm (reticulum cells) are sometimes seen. Neutrophils are seen in approximately 66% of the samples, usually constituting <20% of cells but occasionally predominating. Sometimes a single CSF sample is normal. CSF electrophoresis typically shows evidence of blood-brain barrier disruption, and chronically affected dogs have dramatically increased levels of γ-globulins.

Evaluation for infectious causes via culture and appropriate serology should be performed before a diagnosis of GME is made. Computed tomography (CT) or magnetic resonance imaging (MRI) may show one or more masses in the brain or spinal cord. Definitive diagnosis requires biopsy or necropsy and histopathologic examination.

### Treatment and prognosis

Occasionally progression can be halted or reversed using corticosteroids. Prednisone (1 to 2 mg/kg/day) can cause a dramatic response in some patients, particularly those with slower progression. After signs stabilize, the prednisone dose may be gradually lowered.

More aggressive chemotherapy using cyclophosphamide or cytosine arabinoside is rarely effective. Leflunomide (Arava) has been used with some success. The drug is administered at an initial dose of 4 mg/kg/day, and the dose is adjusted to maintain a trough plasma level of 20 μg/ml (usual maintenance dose is 0.5 mg/kg/day).

Radiation therapy greatly benefits some dogs with focal intracranial masses resulting from GME. However, most affected dogs improve with treatment but relapse quickly, and the prognosis for permanent recovery is poor.

## PUG MENINGOENCEPHALITIS (TEXT P 1013)

A breed-specific necrotizing meningoencephalitis of the cerebral cortex is common in Pugs; a genetic predisposition is likely. Pathologic findings are suggestive of a viral cause, but no viral agents have been isolated. An autoantibody directed against brain tissue has been identified in the CSF of a few affected dogs. Recently a disorder with an identical clinical course and pathologic features was described in the Maltese. A pathologically similar disorder has also been described in the Yorkshire Terrier, but in that breed brainstem lesions predominate.

### Clinical features

Affected dogs first show signs between 9 months and 7 years of age. Acutely affected dogs are presented with sudden onset of seizures and neurologic signs referable to the cerebrum and meninges (see Chapter 65). They may have difficulty walking, be weak or uncoordinated, circle, head press, or have a head tilt, cortical blindness, or cervical rigidity and pain. Neurologic signs progress rapidly, and within 5 to 7 days the dog develops uncontrollable seizures or becomes recumbent, unable to walk, and comatose.

Generalized or partial motor seizures also are common in dogs with more slowly progressive disease. Initially such dogs may be neurologically normal between seizures, which recur at varying intervals from a few days to a few weeks. Other neurologic signs referable to the cerebral cortex then develop. Survival is generally only a few weeks (maximum, <6 months).

### Diagnosis

The diagnosis is suspected on the basis of signalment and clinical and laboratory features. Hematologic and serum biochemistry findings are unremarkable. Analysis of CSF reveals a high protein concentration and increased nucleated cell count (predominantly small lymphocytes). Definitive diagnosis requires brain biopsy or necropsy.

### Treatment and prognosis

The disorder has no specific treatment. Phenobarbital may decrease the severity and frequency of seizures for a short period of time. Corticosteroids do not significantly alter the course of this disease in most patients. As the disease progresses, treatment becomes ineffective or the interictal signs become too severe, and affected dogs are euthanized.

## FELINE POLIOENCEPHALOMYELITIS (TEXT PP 1013-1014)

A nonsuppurative encephalomyelitis, most likely viral, causes progressive seizures or spinal cord signs in young adult cats. Affected cats are 3 months to 6 years old; most are <2 years old. Neurologic signs have a subacute or chronic, progressive course. Hindlimb ataxia and paresis may be accompanied by hyporeflexia; seizures and intention tremors of the head may also occur. Seizures and behavior change are the only signs in some cats.

Laboratory findings are unremarkable in most cats. In some cases a mild increase occurs in CSF mononuclear cells, and CSF protein concentration is normal or slightly increased. Definitive diagnosis can be made only at necropsy. Lesions are found in the spinal cord, cerebral cortex, brainstem, and cerebellum. The prognosis is poor, although spontaneous recovery has been reported in a few cats.

## FELINE IMMUNODEFICIENCY VIRUS ENCEPHALOPATHY (TEXT P 1014)

Neurologic abnormalities associated with feline immunodeficiency virus (FIV) infection in cats include behavioral and mood changes, seizures, and twitching of the face and tongue. Depression, persistent staring, and inappropriate elimination also are common. Presumptive diagnosis is based on clinical signs, positive serology, and exclusion of other neurologic diseases. Analysis of CSF reveals an increase in lymphocytes and normal or slightly increased protein concentration. FIV antibodies can usually be demonstrated in the CSF, although care must be taken to avoid blood contamination during CSF collection. CSF culture may yield the virus. Zidovudine (20 mg/kg PO q12h) may reduce the severity of neurologic impairment in some cats.

## BACTERIAL MENINGITIS AND MYELITIS (TEXT PP 1014-1015)

Bacterial infection of the CNS is rare in dogs and cats. It may result from local extension of infection from adjacent structures (e.g., ears, eyes, sinuses, nasal passages) or areas of osteomyelitis. Hematogenous spread may also occur in animals with bacterial endocarditis, omphalophlebitis, prostatitis, metritis, diskospondylitis, pyoderma, or pneumonia. Bacterial CNS infection may be most common in immunocompromised animals. Bacteria most often implicated include *Staphylococcus aureus, Staphylococcus epidermidis, Staphylococcus albus, Pasteurella multocida, Actinomyces,* and *Nocardia*.

### Clinical features

Clinical signs can include cervical rigidity, hyperesthesia, pyrexia, vomiting, bradycardia, and seizures. Additional neurologic deficits, such as paresis, paralysis, hyperreflexia, blindness, nystagmus, and head tilt, are common and suggest parenchymal involvement. The clinical course is variable; however, once meningitis occurs, it can progress rapidly. Physical examination may reveal a focus of underlying infection. Affected animals are almost always systemically ill. Shock, hypotension, and disseminated intravascular coagulation may also be present.

### Diagnosis

The complete blood count (CBC) may be normal, may reveal leukocytosis, or may be indicative of sepsis. Definitive diagnosis requires analysis of CSF and bacterial culture. Analysis of CSF reveals increased protein concentration and a predominantly neutrophilic pleocytosis that may be severe (see Table 66-1). Bacterial infection should be suspected whenever degenerate neutrophils are observed in the CSF, although in many cases the neutrophils are mature and nontoxic. Treatment with antibiotics before CSF collection can lower the CSF cell count and cause a predominance of mononuclear cells. Intracellular bacteria are rarely identified in cytologic preparations.

*Further evaluation.* In addition to aerobic and anaerobic bacterial culture of CSF, blood and urine cultures, ophthalmologic and otic examinations, radiographs of the spine, skull, and thorax, and abdominal ultrasound should be performed in every case of suspected bacterial meningitis. Systemic illness or identification of a focus of infection in a dog or cat with inflammatory CSF should prompt immediate treatment for bacterial CNS infection.

### Treatment

Bacterial meningitis is a life-threatening infection and should be treated aggressively. Appropriate antibiotic therapy is based on culture and sensitivity results and on the ability of the selected drug to achieve therapeutic concentrations in the CNS. Antibiotics that achieve therapeutic concentrations in the CNS include trimethoprim-sulfadiazine, the quinolones, most third-generation cephalosporins (e.g., moxolactam, cefotaxime), and, in the presence of CNS inflammation, ampicillin, penicillin, and amoxicillin-clavulanic acid. Metronidazole is the drug of choice when anaerobic infection is likely. Chloramphenicol is not recommended.

When the causal organism is unknown, treatment is initiated with trimethoprim-sulfadiazine (15 mg/kg PO q12h) and either ampicillin (22 mg/kg intravenously [IV] q6h or PO q8h) or metronidazole (10 mg/kg PO q8h). Alternatively, an appropriate third-generation cephalosporin or quinolone can be used. Treatment response is monitored by resolution of clinical signs or reevaluation of CSF. Antibiotic therapy should continue for at least 2 weeks after resolution of clinical signs.

### Prognosis

Response to antibiotic therapy is variable, and relapses are common. The prognosis is guarded; even with appropriate therapy, many patients die. Treatment should be attempted, however, because some cases respond dramatically to therapy and recover completely.

## CANINE DISTEMPER VIRUS (TEXT PP 1015-1016)

Canine distemper virus (CDV) infection is usually seen as a multisystemic disease that may include multifocal, progressive CNS involvement. Clinical signs vary, depending on virulence, environmental conditions, and the dog's age and immune status. Widespread vaccination has substantially decreased the incidence of CDV infections, but outbreaks still occur among unvaccinated dogs (especially young dogs) and sporadically in vaccinated dogs.

### Clinical features

In many cases, mild to severe gastrointestinal (GI) and respiratory illness precedes the neurologic signs. Nonneurologic signs may include ocular and nasal discharge, coughing, dyspnea, vomiting, and diarrhea. Neurologic signs begin 1 to 3 weeks after dogs start to recover from systemic illness

*Neurologic signs.* Hyperesthesia, cervical rigidity, seizures, cerebellar or vestibular signs, tetraparesis, and ataxia may be seen. Seizures can be of any type, depending on the region of the brain affected, but "chewing gum fits" are common. Myoclonus ("distemper chorea") is most commonly associated with distemper encephalomyelitis. Older dogs may develop a more subacute or chronic encephalomyelitis with neurologic signs, including progressive tetraparesis or vestibular dysfunction, in the absence of systemic signs. (In dogs infected while their permanent teeth are developing, enamel hypoplasia [brown discoloration of the teeth] is noted.)

*Ocular manifestations.* Optic neuritis, chorioretinitis, and retinal detachment may be detected during an ophthalmologic examination. Irregular, ill-defined gray-pink densities in the fundus suggest acute or active chorioretinitis; well-defined hyperreflective regions are more indicative of chronic infection with scarring.

### Diagnosis

Diagnosis is based on historic, physical, and laboratory findings. The CBC may be normal or may reveal a persistent lymphopenia; distemper inclusions can sometimes be found in circulating lymphocytes and red blood cells.

*Immunofluorescence.* Immunofluorescent or immunocytochemical techniques may reveal CDV in smears from conjunctival or respiratory epithelium. However, CDV in conjunctival epithelium is usually detected only early in infection, before the development of neurologic signs. Virus may be detected for longer in epithelial cells and macrophages from the lower respiratory tract using transtracheal wash. Virus persists for up to 60 days in the skin, footpads, and CNS. Biopsy of the skin on the dorsum of the neck can be used for antemortem immunohistochemical testing to confirm acute or subacute infection with CDV.

***Analysis of CSF.*** Distemper meningoencephalitis causes an increase in CSF protein concentration and mild lymphocytic pleocytosis. Occasionally, the CSF is normal or more indicative of an inflammatory process (neutrophilia). CDV antibody titers in the CSF may be increased relative to serum titers. Using monoclonal antibody techniques, canine distemper antigen can be detected in cells from the CSF in many cases. Polymerase chain reaction (PCR) assay can also be used to detect CDV in the CSF, serum, or whole blood of affected dogs.

### Treatment and prognosis

Treatment is supportive and frequently unrewarding. Progressive neurologic dysfunction usually necessitates euthanasia. Anticonvulsant therapy and antiinflammatory doses of glucocorticoids are sometimes recommended in the absence of systemic disease. However, their beneficial effects are not well documented.

### Prevention

Prevention of CDV infection through routine vaccination is usually very effective. However, CDV infection can develop with exposure after stress, illness, or immunosuppression in a currently vaccinated dog. Meningoencephalitis has been reported in a few dogs 7 to 14 days after vaccination with modified-live CDV vaccines. Vaccination of immunosuppressed neonates, particularly those with known or suspected parvoviral infection, should be avoided.

## RABIES (TEXT P 1016)

Rabies virus infection usually produces fatal encephalomyelitis in dogs and cats. The source of infection generally is the bite of an infected animal (e.g., bat, raccoon, skunk, fox). Rabies can have a wide range of clinical signs, making it difficult to differentiate from other acute, progressive encephalomyelitis syndromes. Because of its public health significance, *rabies should be a differential diagnosis in every animal with rapidly progressing neurologic dysfunction.*

## Naturally Occurring Rabies

In naturally occurring rabies, initial signs may include behavior changes such as depression, dementia, or aggression. Excessive salivation, difficulty swallowing, and multiple cranial nerve deficits are usually seen. Ataxia and rear limb paresis that progresses to flaccid quadriparesis are common. There may exist a history of contact with a known rabid animal. The incubation period is extremely variable (1 week to 8 months). However, once neurologic signs are seen, the disease is rapidly progressive; death occurs within 7 days in most animals.

### Diagnosis

Any unvaccinated animal with acute, rapidly progressive neurologic signs should be considered a rabies suspect and handled with caution. CBC and serum biochemistry findings are normal. Analysis of CSF simply reveals increased mononuclear cells and protein concentration. Finding a positive IgG titer for rabies in the CSF is good evidence of rabies infection. Comparing CSF and serum antibody titers may aid diagnosis.

Fluorescent antibody tests may be performed on smears from the nasal mucosa or cornea, or on a skin biopsy sample from the sensory vibrissae in the maxillary region. However, a negative result does not eliminate the possibility of rabies, particularly in the early stages of disease. Diagnosis is usually made by examination of brain after death.

Note: *If rabies is a major concern, all ancillary testing should be performed with great caution, if at all. Gloves, masks, and protective clothing should be worn while the animal is examined and testing samples are collected.*

### Vaccine-Induced Problems

Vaccine-induced problems after rabies vaccination are rare in dogs and cats. Occasionally, rabies vaccination in dogs causes flaccid quadriparesis (without cranial nerve deficits) 10 to 21 days after vaccination. The prognosis for recovery from this syndrome is excellent. Less commonly, a rapidly progressive encephalomyelitis is seen in dogs after rabies vaccination. The prognosis for recovery from this disorder is poor.

Cats with vaccine-induced rabies typically develop rear limb paresis in the "vaccinated" leg, which progresses to flaccid paralysis of both rear limbs and finally to rigidity in all four limbs, cranial nerve deficits, and dementia. Euthanasia is recommended, as the prognosis for recovery is grave. Rarely, soft-tissue sarcomas develop at the site of injection in cats.

### Rabies Prophylaxis

Dogs and cats should receive their first rabies vaccine after 12 weeks of age and be revaccinated 1 year later. Subsequent boosters are administered every 1 to 3 years, depending on the vaccine used and local public health regulations.

## FELINE INFECTIOUS PERITONITIS (TEXT PP 1016-1017)

Progressive neurologic involvement is common in cats with the "dry" form of feline infectious peritonitis (FIP). Neurologic FIP is most common in cats <2 years of age and in those >9 years of age.

### Clinical features

Cerebellar signs may predominate, but rear limb paralysis and ataxia, central vestibular signs, seizures, and tetraparesis also are common. Most affected cats have systemic signs such as fever, anorexia, and depression. Concurrent anterior uveitis and chorioretinitis are common and should raise the suspicion for FIP. Careful abdominal palpation may reveal organ distortion caused by granulomas.

### Diagnosis

Typically the CBC reveals an inflammatory leukogram. Serum globulin concentrations may be very high. Tests for coronavirus antibody often are nondiagnostic. Although an extremely high serum titer with typical clinical findings suggests FIP, a negative titer does not rule it out. MRI and CT may reveal multifocal granulomatous lesions and secondary hydrocephalus.

*Analysis of CSF.* Analysis of CSF typically reveals nonseptic inflammation with many neutrophils, macrophages, and lymphocytes (>100 cells/μl; >70% polymorphonuclear neutrophil leukocytes) and an increase in protein concentration (>200 mg/dl). In a few cases, however, the CSF is normal or only mildly inflammatory. Coronavirus antibody can usually be detected in the CSF, and the virus itself can often be detected in the CSF and affected tissue using PCR.

### Prognosis

The prognosis is very poor. Some palliation may be achieved with immunosuppressive and antiinflammatory medications (see Chapter 102).

## TOXOPLASMOSIS (TEXT P 1017)

*Toxoplasma gondii* infection, although common in dogs and cats, rarely causes clinical disease. Clinical manifestations may be associated with young age or immunosuppression (e.g., FIV infection). Ocular lesions such as uveitis and chorioretinitis are common in cats. Neurologic signs are uncommon in dogs and cats.

### Clinical features

Clinical signs of neurologic involvement depend on the location of the lesion(s) in the cerebrum, cerebellum, brainstem, spinal cord, or muscles. A wide variety of signs may occur, including hyperexcitability, depression, tremor, paresis, paralysis, and seizures. Weakness, muscle pain, fever, and increased serum creatine kinase have been reported in cats with *Toxoplasma* myositis.

A syndrome of protozoal polyradiculoneuritis and myositis restricted to the rear limbs, causing neurogenic atrophy and progressive hind limb hyperextension, is recognized in young dogs. A rapidly progressive lower motor neuron (LMN) paralysis similar to acute idiopathic polyradiculoneuritis has also been seen in dogs infected with *T. gondii*. However, many dogs originally thought to have *Toxoplasma* myositis, neuritis, or meningoencephalitis have later been shown to have been affected by *Neospora caninum*.

### Diagnosis

Antemortem diagnosis of CNS toxoplasmosis may be difficult. If other organ systems are involved, biopsy of affected extraneural tissue may allow identification of the organism. A fourfold rise in IgG titer in two serum samples taken 3 weeks apart or a single elevated IgM titer supports a diagnosis of toxoplasmosis. However, subclinically infected dogs and cats occasionally have high antibody titers, and antibodies may be absent in animals with severe clinical disease (see Chapter 104). Affected cats should be tested for concurrent feline leukemia virus and FIV infections.

*Analysis of CSF.* Analysis of CSF often reveals increases in protein concentration and nucleated cell count. Lymphocytes and monocytes usually predominate, although neutrophils may be seen. Eosinophils predominate in a few infected dogs and cats. An increase in macrophages or monocytoid cells with abundant foamy cytoplasm is a characteristic finding. *T. gondii*-specific antibody is detectable in the CSF of some infected cats, but it does not necessarily indicate active CNS toxoplasmosis. Rarely, cytologic examination of the CSF reveals *T. gondii* organisms within host cells, allowing a definitive diagnosis of toxoplasmosis.

### Treatment and prognosis

The recommended treatment for CNS toxoplasmosis is clindamycin (10 mg/kg/day q8h for at least 4 weeks), or trimethoprim-sulfadiazine (15 mg/kg PO q12h) with pyrimethamine (1 mg/kg/day). Neurologic, ocular, and muscular manifestations of toxoplasmosis are not usually associated with patent infection and oocyte shedding, so isolation of affected animals is not necessary. The prognosis for recovery is grave in animals with profound neurologic dysfunction.

## NEOSPOROSIS (TEXT PP 1017-1018)

*N. caninum* is a protozoan species that can cause neuromuscular disease similar to that caused by *T. gondii*. Naturally occurring infections have been reported in dogs but not in cats.

### Clinical features

Adult dogs may have multifocal CNS involvement, polymyositis, and polyneuritis, usually in association with disseminated systemic disease that affects the liver and lung. Paraparesis, multifocal CNS disease, cerebellar signs, and seizures are reported. A rapidly progressive LMN paralysis similar to acute idiopathic polyradiculoneuritis has also been seen in adult dogs infected with *N. caninum*. Most affected puppies are evaluated for protozoal polyradiculoneuritis and myositis restricted to the rear limbs, causing neurogenic atrophy and progressive hind limb hyperextension and rigid contracture. Often, multiple puppies in a litter are affected.

### Diagnosis

Hematologic and biochemical findings vary with the organ systems involved. CSF findings may include mild increases in protein concentration and leukocyte count, with monocytes and lymphocytes predominating. Rarely the organism is seen in the CSF or tissues that undergo biopsy. Specific antibodies may be detected in the CSF, or a rising titer may be measured in the serum. Immunocytochemical staining can be used to differentiate *Neospora* from *Toxoplasma* in tissue biopsies.

### Treatment and prognosis

Treatment with clindamycin (10 mg/kg/day q8h for at least 4 weeks) is most effective in dogs without severe neurologic signs. Multifocal signs, rapid progression, pelvic limb rigid hyperextension, and delayed treatment are all associated with a poor prognosis for recovery.

## LYME DISEASE (TEXT P 1018)

CNS infection with *Borrelia burgdorferi* (Lyme neuroborreliosis) is occasionally reported in dogs. It should be a differential diagnosis for CNS disease in dogs from endemic regions. Most affected dogs have concurrent polyarthritis, lymphadenopathy, and fever. Neurologic signs include aggression, other behavior changes, and seizures. Analysis of CSF is normal or mildly inflammatory. An increase may occur in specific antibodies in CSF compared with serum. Early treatment with doxycycline or ceftriaxone may be effective (see Chapter 98).

## MYCOTIC INFECTIONS (TEXT P 1018)

Disseminated mycotic infections occasionally involve the CNS and eyes. Clinical signs depend on the fungus involved and may include GI, respiratory, skeletal, and neurologic signs. The most common neurologic signs are depression and seizures; fundic examination may reveal chorioretinitis. Typical CSF abnormalities include neutrophilic pleocytosis and increased protein content. Therapy may be attempted (see Chapter 103); however, the prognosis is poor when the nervous system is involved.

### Cryptococcosis

It is uncommon for systemic mycoses to manifest with only neurologic signs. The exception is *Cryptococcus neoformans*, which has a predilection for the CNS. Infection extends from the nose through the cribriform plate in cats or via the bloodstream in severely affected dogs and cats.

### Diagnosis

Analysis of CSF reveals increased protein concentration and cell count. Neutrophilic pleocytosis is most common, but eosinophilia has been reported. Organisms are seen in the CSF in approximately 60% of cases. Fungal CSF culture should be considered in dogs with inflammatory CSF in which no organisms are seen. Detection of capsular antigen in the CSF or serum using latex agglutination may also be useful. Cytologic examination of nasal exudate, draining tracts, enlarged lymph nodes, and granulomas may reveal the organisms, which are readily visible when Gram stain, India ink, or Wright's stain is used.

### Treatment and prognosis

Drugs commonly used include itraconazole, fluconazole, 5-flucytosine, and amphotericin B. The prognosis is poor, although some success has been reported in cats treated with itraconazole or fluconazole.

## RICKETTSIAL DISEASES (TEXT P 1018)

Rocky Mountain spotted fever (RMSF; caused by *Rickettsia rickettsii*) and ehrlichiosis (caused by *Ehrlichia canis*) commonly cause meningoencephalomyelitis. Neurologic signs are seen in approximately 30% of dogs with either disease, but signs are more acute, severe, and progressive in dogs with RMSF.

### Clinical features

Signs include hyperesthesia, cervical rigidity, mental changes, ataxia, vestibular signs, stupor, and seizures. Neurologic abnormalities are always accompanied by signs of concurrent systemic disease, which may include fever, anorexia, depression, vomiting, oculonasal discharge, cough, and lymphadenopathy.

### Diagnosis

Neutrophils predominate in the CSF of dogs with RMSF, whereas lymphocytes predominate in ehrlichiosis; however, the CSF is normal in some dogs. Serologic testing is essential to confirm the diagnosis and differentiate between these two diseases. CSF titers can be compared with serum titers, but titers may be negative in acutely infected dogs.

### Treatment and prognosis

Tetracycline (22 mg/kg PO q8h) is effective in most acute cases of ehrlichiosis and RMSF. Doxycycline (5 to 10 mg/kg PO or IV q12h) and chloramphenicol (25 to

50 mg/kg PO or IV q8h) may also be effective. Enrofloxacin is very effective in dogs with RMSF. Dramatic clinical improvement should be expected within 24 to 48 hours. The presence of neurologic signs may slow recovery, and in some cases neurologic damage is irreversible.

## PARASITIC MENINGITIS, MYELITIS, AND ENCEPHALITIS (TEXT PP 1018-1019)

Meningitis and meningoencephalitis caused by aberrant parasite migration have been reported in dogs and cats. An eosinophilic CSF pleocytosis should prompt consideration of parasitic migration through the CNS, although several more common neurologic disorders should also be considered, including intracranial neoplasia, toxoplasmosis, neosporosis, GME, and, in young Golden Retrievers, immune-mediated eosinophilic meningitis.

### Diagnostic evaluation

Diagnostic evaluation of animals with eosinophilic CSF should include a fundic examination, CBC, serum biochemistry profile, urinalysis, serum and CSF titers for *Toxoplasma* and *Neospora,* thoracic and abdominal radiographs, abdominal ultrasound, fecal flotation, and heartworm antigen testing. CT and MRI may document necrosis along the path of parasite migration within the CNS. Definitive diagnosis of parasitic CNS disease requires pathologic demonstration of the parasite in the CNS.

### Treatment

Empiric treatment with ivermectin (200 to 300 µg/kg PO or subcutaneously q2wk for three treatments) should be considered if parasite migration is likely. Antiinflammatory treatment with prednisone may also be indicated.

# 72

# Disorders of the Spinal Cord

## *(Text pp 1020-1048)*

## DIAGNOSTIC APPROACH (TEXT P 1020)

Spinal cord disorders can be caused by anomalies, degeneration, neoplasia, inflammatory conditions, trauma, disk extrusion, hemorrhage, or infarction. Clinical signs frequently include focal or generalized pain, paresis, or paralysis and, occasionally, inability to urinate. Examination of the signalment, history, onset, and progression of the disease can provide valuable clues regarding the likely cause.

Congenital malformations are present at birth, do not progress, and often are breed associated. Traumatic and vascular disorders are acute and nonprogressive. Acute spinal cord compression may result from trauma, atlantoaxial subluxation, or intervertebral disk disease. More progressive disease is expected in infectious or noninfectious inflammatory disease. Tumors and degenerative processes are usually slowly progressive.

Spinal cord lesions can often be localized with neurologic examination (see Table 65-6). Further diagnostic tests, including radiography, may be necessary to determine the cause.

### Diagnostic tests

If spinal radiographs are normal, analysis of cerebrospinal fluid (CSF) may be warranted to seek evidence of neoplasia or inflammation. Myelography, epidurography, or other imaging technique (e.g., computed tomography [CT] or magnetic resonance imaging [MRI]) may be necessary to identify compressive or expansive lesions in the spinal canal. In some cases surgical exploration is required for a diagnosis to be established. When analysis of CSF and diagnostic imaging results are normal, vascular or degenerative diseases should be suspected.

## ACUTE SPINAL CORD DYSFUNCTION (TEXT PP 1021-1031)

### Trauma

Traumatic injuries to the spinal canal are common; fractures, luxation, and traumatic disk protrusion are most common. Severe spinal cord bruising and edema can occur, even without disruption of the spinal canal. Note: Excessive manipulation or rotation during examination should be avoided until the vertebral column is determined to be stable. If vertebral instability is a concern, the animal should be restrained, examined, and transported in lateral recumbency on a stretcher or board.

#### Clinical features and diagnosis

Spinal trauma is readily diagnosed on the basis of history and physical findings. Clinical signs are acute and generally nonprogressive. Patients are often in pain, and other evidence of trauma (e.g., lacerations, abrasions, fractures) may be present. Neurologic findings depend on lesion location and severity. A thorough yet rapid physical examination is important to determine whether the animal has life-threatening, nonneurologic injuries that require immediate attention.

***Neurologic examination.*** Evaluation is limited to mental status, cranial nerves, posture, muscle tone, voluntary movement, spinal reflexes, panniculus reflex, and pain perception. Dogs with severe thoracic spinal cord lesions may exhibit the Schiff-Sherrington posture (see Chapter 65). The single most important prognostic indicator is the presence or absence of deep pain sensation. If deep pain is absent caudal to the lesion, the prognosis for return of neurologic function is very poor.

***Radiography.*** Neurologic examination allows localization of the lesion in most cases. Survey radiographs can then be used to identify the lesion, assess the degree of vertebral damage and displacement, and aid in prognosis. Note: Manipulation or twisting of unstable areas of the spine must be avoided during radiography.

The entire spine should be assessed radiographically; lower motor neuron (LMN) signs in a limb can mask an upper motor neuron (UMN) lesion located more cranially. Most spinal fractures and luxations occur at the lumbosacral junction or in the thoracolumbar (TL), cervicothoracic, atlantoaxial, or atlantooccipital region. Myelography or other advanced diagnostic imaging can be performed in potential surgical candidates.

***Pelvic and sacral fractures.*** Decompressive and exploratory spinal surgery must be considered whenever evidence of spinal nerve compression (i.e., severe pain plus neurologic deficits) is seen. Patients with sacral fractures and denervation of the tail nearly always have some denervation of the pelvic viscera. An intact perineal reflex, anal tone, and perineal sensation but an LMN bladder (i.e., large, easily expressed) indicates that the pudendal nerve is intact but the pelvic nerve has been damaged. Such animals have a much better chance of recovery than those with loss of anal tone and perineal sensation.

#### Treatment

Primary treatment involves immediate intravenous administration of highly soluble corticosteroids and treatment of other life-threatening injuries. Adverse effects of corticosteroids on the gastrointestinal (GI) tract (including bleeding) are common; they may be decreased by concurrent administration of a histamine-2–receptor blocker, proton pump inhibitor, or misoprostol and sucralfate (see Chapter 30). Controlled studies have not demonstrated efficacy for mannitol, dimethyl sulfoxide, naloxone, or other substances when administered after spinal cord injury. Narcotic analgesics (oxymorphone 0.05 mg/kg intramuscularly [IM] or butorphanol 0.2 mg/kg subcutaneously [SC] prn) may be administered for pain management.

*Surgery.* Surgery may be required to stabilize the vertebral column or decompress the spinal cord. Spinal cord contusion (i.e., no apparent compression) unassociated with bone damage rarely benefits from surgical decompression. Progression of clinical signs despite medical therapy may warrant further diagnostic imaging or surgical intervention. Because of the extremely poor prognosis for recovery, euthanasia generally is recommended in patients with complete loss of function (i.e., paralysis) and loss of deep pain sensation.

*Nursing care.* Intensive nursing care is critical whether the patient is managed conservatively or surgically. Splinting for stabilization and forced cage rest may be required. Thickly padded, clean, dry cages and frequent turning of the patient help prevent pressure sores. All impaired limbs should be moved repeatedly through a full range of motion many times each day. When an animal starts to regain voluntary motion in the limbs, physical therapy is increased; hydrotherapy or swimming also is useful.

*Urinary care.* Maintenance of an indwelling urinary catheter ensures a dry animal but may increase the risk of urinary tract infection, particularly when the catheter is kept in place for >3 days. When long-term care is necessary, the bladder should be gently expressed or catheterized and emptied four to six times per day, and urinary tract infections treated as they occur. In animals with UMN bladder (see Table 65-4) or with urethral spasm, medical therapy (phenoxybenzamine 1 mg/kg q8h and diazepam 1.25 to 2.5 mg/kg q8h) may help relax the urethral sphincter, making bladder expression easier and less traumatic.

### Prognosis

The prognosis for recovery depends on the site and severity of injury. Animals with intact voluntary motion have a good prognosis for return of full function. Animals that are paralyzed but retain deep pain and normal bladder function have a fair prognosis for recovery, although they may have residual neurologic deficits. Lesions of the white matter that produce strictly UMN signs have a better prognosis than those that affect clinically important LMNs.

Unstable cervical vertebral fractures are associated with very high mortality at the time of trauma and also in the perioperative period. Animals that have lost deep pain sensation have a very poor prognosis for recovery. If deep pain sensation is gone for at least 48 hours, the animal has virtually no chance of functional recovery (i.e., walking). In any animal with paralysis caused by a spinal cord injury, if no improvement is seen within 21 days after injury, the prognosis for recovery is poor.

## Nontraumatic Hemorrhage

Nontraumatic hemorrhage into the spinal canal that causes acute neurologic deficits and, in some cases, hyperesthesia has been recognized in young dogs with hemophilia A, dogs of any age with von Willebrand's disease, dogs and cats with acquired bleeding disorders (e.g., warfarin intoxication, thrombocytopenia), dogs with vascular anomalies (e.g., aneurysms, arteriovenous fistulas), and dogs and cats with primary or metastatic spinal neoplasia (e.g., lymphoma, hemangiosarcoma). Hemorrhage can be subdural or epidural.

Signs occur acutely and are minimally progressive, with neurologic signs reflecting the site and severity of spinal cord damage. Antemortem diagnosis usually requires advanced diagnostic imaging (e.g., MRI), although identification of a systemic bleeding disorder or neoplasia can suggest the diagnosis. In addition to treatment of the bleeding disorder, significant acute spinal cord compression should be treated with surgical decompression.

## Infarction

Spinal cord infarction is a rare cause of neurologic dysfunction in dogs and cats. Signs occur acutely and are referable to the site and severity of the vascular compromise.

Cardiomyopathy, hyperadrenocorticism, protein-losing nephropathy, immune-mediated hemolytic anemia, heartworm disease, and disseminated intravascular coagulation have all been associated with an increased risk of systemic thrombosis and occasionally result in regional spinal cord infarction. Treatment consists of general supportive care and medications to decrease the risk of further infarction; however, antemortem definitive diagnosis is difficult.

### Acute Intervertebral Disk Disease

Acute rupture of an intervertebral disk causes a large mass of disk material to enter the spinal canal and bruise or compress the spinal cord (Hansen type I protrusion). This injury is most common in small breeds of dog such as the Dachshund, Toy Poodle, Pekingese, Beagle, Welsh Corgi, Lhasa Apso, Shih Tzu, and Cocker Spaniel. In these breeds, disk degeneration, including mineralization of the nucleus, commonly occurs at a young age, predisposing to acute rupture in dogs 3 to 6 years old. Acute disk injuries are occasionally diagnosed in Basset Hounds, Doberman Pinschers with caudal cervical vertebral instability, and German Shepherd Dogs. Disk disease is a rare cause of clinically evident spinal cord compression in cats.

#### Clinical features

Pain is a prominent feature in most affected dogs. Some dogs have spinal pain and no accompanying neurologic deficits. Others suffer severe compressive spinal cord injury and have varying degrees of neurologic dysfunction (usually bilaterally symmetric). Clinical signs depend on the location and severity of the damage and the degree of spinal cord compression. Most disk extrusions in dogs occur in the caudal thoracic or lumbar spine; 65% occur between T11 and L2. Although rare, acute disk prolapse in cats occurs in older animals (mean, 10 years), most often in the lower thoracic and lumbar regions (especially L4 to L5).

The severity of initial signs and the speed of progression are related to the volume of disk material extruded, the degree of spinal cord compression, and the force of the extrusion. In some dogs evidence of pain and subtle weakness resulting from partial disk rupture and mild spinal cord compression may be present for days or weeks before mild trauma or movement results in extrusion of more disk material and paralysis.

*Cervical spine.* Cervical disk disease (C1 to C5) most commonly causes neck pain without neurologic deficits. Dogs with cervical disk extrusions commonly resist movement or manipulation of the neck and stand with the head and neck lowered. One forelimb may be lifted with caudal cervical disk prolapse. When significant spinal cord compression is present, UMN signs occur in all four legs. The C2/C3 disk is most frequently involved, with the prevalence decreasing from C3/C4 to C7/T1. The C6/C7 disk is more commonly affected in large-breed dogs as a component of cervical vertebral malformation-malarticulation syndrome (wobbler syndrome).

*TL spine.* Pain from TL disk disease characteristically results in arching of the back and tensing of the abdominal muscles, mimicking abdominal pain. Weakness and paralysis also are common; compression in this region results in UMN signs in the rear limbs only.

*Intumescences.* Disk extrusion at an intumescence (C6 to T2 or L4 to S2) results in LMN signs (lameness, occasionally muscle atrophy) in the corresponding limbs, even in the absence of significant cord compression.

#### Diagnosis

Disk disease should be suspected based on the signalment, history, physical examination, and neurologic findings. Trauma and fibrocartilaginous embolism (FCE) are the major differential diagnoses, but clinical and historical features generally differentiate these conditions. Neurologic examination and detection of a specific area of spinal pain are used to localize the lesion to a particular region of the spinal cord. Spinal radiographs are then taken to look for evidence of disk disease and rule out other diseases (e.g., diskospondylitis, lytic vertebral tumor, fracture).

*Radiography.* Not all herniated disks are apparent on survey radiographs, even with optimal positioning and technique. Observation of calcified disk spaces confirms the presence of generalized intervertebral disk disease but does not necessarily pinpoint the site of the extrusion causing neurologic dysfunction.

Radiographic changes consistent with herniation in the TL region include a narrowed or wedged disk space, a small or cloudy intervertebral foramen ("horse's head"), narrowing of the facetal joints, and a calcified density within the spinal canal above the involved disk space. Radiographs in dogs with cervical disk herniation usually demonstrate narrowing of the intervertebral space and dorsal displacement of mineralized disk material.

Careful positioning of the suspected disk space in the center of the beam, with the dog anesthetized, is usually necessary for diagnosis of subtle lesions. Radiographs under general anesthesia usually are recommended only in a potential surgical candidate, when preparations have been made for further diagnostic imaging and perhaps decompressive surgery during the same anesthetic episode.

*Advanced imaging.* Myelography, CT, or MRI usually is required to definitively locate an extruded disk when surgery is being considered. CT or MRI may be used as the sole technique for detection and characterization of a disk lesion, particularly in regions in which myelographic interpretation can be difficult and precise anatomic localization is important (e.g., caudal cervical and lumbosacral regions).

*Analysis of CSF.* Analysis of CSF should always be performed before myelography, even in dogs with classic signs of disk disease, as myelography can cause inflammatory CSF changes that last for several days. The clinical findings with inflammatory or neoplastic CNS lesions can be very similar to those of disk disease, so analysis of CSF may be important in differentiating these conditions. CSF in dogs with disk disease may have a very slight increase in protein concentration and cell count, or it may be normal.

### Nonsurgical treatment

Treatment may be nonsurgical or surgical. Surgical treatment and postoperative care are discussed in the text. Nonsurgical management is usually prescribed in an animal that has had a single acute episode of back or neck pain without neurologic deficits, and initially in dogs with mild neurologic deficits resulting from TL disk disease.

Dogs that have acute TL pain, proprioceptive abnormalities, and rear limb weakness but that can still support weight and walk are treated nonsurgically with strict in-hospital cage rest and monitored closely for up to 3 days. Decompressive surgery is recommended if neurologic signs deteriorate. In most cases these dogs deteriorate within 6 to 12 hours, and surgery is clearly indicated.

Dogs that are unable to move their limbs voluntarily should be assessed carefully for the presence of conscious perception of deep pain. In some dogs it is difficult to determine whether complete loss of sensation really is present. Whenever an animal has been truly analgesic for >48 hours, the prognosis for recovery, regardless of therapy, is poor, and euthanasia is often recommended. Dogs that have lost deep pain perception for a shorter time have a guarded prognosis for recovery, but up to 50% may recover and become ambulatory. Surgical exploration is recommended for decompression.

Even if cervical pain is the only clinical finding, most dogs with cervical intervertebral disk prolapse have a large amount of disk material within the spinal canal and will benefit from surgery. Dogs with repeated episodes of cervical pain, cervical pain that does not resolve with cage rest, and neurologic deficits caused by cervical disk disease should always be treated surgically.

*Initial management.* Strict cage confinement is the most important part of nonsurgical treatment. If pain is severe, nonsteroidal antiinflammatory drugs or narcotic analgesics (oxymorphone 0.05 mg/kg IM or butorphanol 0.2 mg/kg SC prn) may be administered for the first 3 days. Note: Whenever analgesics are administered, the animal should remain hospitalized to enforce cage rest and allow close observation for neurologic deterioration (precipitated by increased activity once pain is relieved). Animals being treated nonsurgically should be evaluated at least twice a day for deterioration in neurologic status. If the symptoms do not improve within 5 to 7 days or if even minor deterioration in neurologic status is seen, then surgery is indicated.

**Corticosteroids.** Corticosteroid therapy usually is not recommended in mildly affected dogs. Little evidence suggests that it influences the long-term outcome. In addition, prednisone can cause serious GI adverse effects, and it alters CSF cellularity, making definitive diagnosis of the actual problem (e.g., granulomatous meningoencephalitis [GME], neoplasia) difficult if the initial presumptive diagnosis of disk disease is incorrect.

Dogs with severe proprioceptive and motor deficits and an inability to support weight or walk and those whose condition deteriorates during medical management should immediately receive intensive intravenous corticosteroid therapy (e.g., methylprednisolone sodium succinate 30 mg/kg or dexamethasone 0.25 mg/kg) and undergo rapid surgical decompression. Any delay in decompression worsens the prognosis for recovery.

**At-home care.** After hospitalization, strict cage confinement should be continued at home for 3 to 4 weeks, followed by 3 weeks of house confinement and leash exercise. Dogs with cervical disk disease should wear a harness instead of a collar when walking. After the prescribed confinement period, monitored exercise should be increased gradually, and (if necessary) a weight reduction program instituted.

**Prognosis.** Most dogs (80% to 100%) with disk disease that are able to walk respond well to medical therapy. Recovery rates in nonambulatory dogs treated medically range from 43% to 50%, and recovery time may be quite prolonged. Dogs treated medically always face some risk that they may deteriorate markedly in the hours and days after presentation, which worsens their prognosis for recovery. Even if dogs recover from an acute episode, 30% to 40% of dogs treated nonsurgically experience recurrence weeks or months later. Persistent or recurrent pain is an indication for surgical intervention.

## Myelomalacia

Acute, forceful, intervertebral disk extrusions can cause considerable intramedullary hemorrhage and edema. In some dogs initially presented because of a rapid onset of complete paralysis resulting from TL disk disease, the associated hemorrhage, edema, and ischemia cause progressive myelomalacia of the cord cranial and caudal to the original lesion (ascending-descending myelomalacia).

This condition affects 3% to 6% of dogs with severe TL disk extrusions and becomes evident 24 to 36 hours after the initial paralysis. It should be suspected when the line demarcating the loss of panniculus reflex moves cranially or the patellar and withdrawal reflexes are lost in the rear limbs of a dog that previously had rear limb UMN signs. Most affected dogs also are very anxious and experience a great deal of pain. Euthanasia should be recommended, because no chance for recovery exists, and affected dogs die within a few days of respiratory paralysis.

## Fibrocartilaginous Embolism

Acute infarction and ischemic necrosis of the spinal cord can occur as a result of the lodging of fibrocartilage in the small vessels that supply the spinal cord and leptomeninges. This peracute, nonprogressive condition can affect any region of the spinal cord and result in paresis or paralysis. The cause is unknown. In approximately 50% of cases, embolism occurs immediately after minor trauma or during exertion. Concurrent, clinically significant disk degeneration is uncommon.

### Clinical features

FCE is most common in medium-sized and large-breed dogs. It has also been described in small-breed dogs (especially Miniature Schnauzers) and a few cats. Most affected dogs are 3 to 7 years old; a few dogs are <1 year old. Onset of neurologic signs is very sudden; signs usually do not progress, although occasionally they worsen for the first 2 to 6 hours.

**Neurologic findings.** Neurologic dysfunction may be mild or severe. Findings reflect a focal spinal cord lesion and depend on the region of the spinal cord affected and the severity of cord involvement. Asymmetry is common. The TL cord and lumbosacral intumescence are affected with equal frequency. The cervical cord is affected less frequently, but it is the site most often affected in small-breed dogs.

Affected dogs commonly cry out as though in pain at the onset of signs. Dogs evaluated within 6 hours of onset sometimes exhibit focal spinal hyperpathia (painfulness), but this resolves quickly so that most affected dogs are not in pain by the time they are brought to a veterinarian, even on manipulation of the spine. Lack of pain and asymmetry are very helpful in differentiating FCE from other disorders that cause acute, nonprogressive neurologic dysfunction, such as acute intervertebral disk protrusion, trauma, and diskospondylitis.

### Diagnosis

The diagnosis of FCE is made by exclusion of compressive and inflammatory acute spinal cord disorders. FCE is suspected on the basis of the signalment, history, and presence of acute, nonprogressive, nonpainful spinal cord dysfunction. Spinal radiographs, which are normal with FCE, help rule out diskospondylitis, fractures, lytic vertebral neoplasia, and intervertebral disk disease. CSF usually is normal, although increased protein (especially albumin) is found in up to 50% of cases, and for the first 24 hours a few dogs have a mild increase in neutrophils.

*Advanced imaging.* Myelography usually is normal, although subtle, focal cord swelling is seen in some patients. Myelography is most useful in ruling out compressive lesions for which surgery might be indicated. CT is not useful for diagnosis of FCE, but it does help in excluding a compressive myelopathy. MRI may reveal focal cord density changes in severely affected dogs, but mild lesions are not evident.

### Treatment

Treatment consists of supportive and nursing care. Corticosteroids are often used, but their effect on outcome has not been documented. In patients presented within the first 6 hours of paralysis, one dose of corticosteroids may be beneficial. Most improvement takes place within the first 7 to 10 days, although it may take 6 to 8 weeks for complete return to function. If no improvement is seen within 21 days, it is unlikely that the dog or cat will improve.

### Prognosis

Approximately 50% of patients recover sufficiently to be acceptable pets. The prognosis for recovery is best in dogs and cats with deep pain sensation and strictly UMN signs. Animals with severe LMN signs or loss of deep pain sensation have a very poor prognosis for satisfactory recovery.

## SUBACUTE PROGRESSIVE SPINAL CORD DYSFUNCTION (TEXT PP 1031-1034)

### Infectious Inflammatory Disease

All of the infectious inflammatory diseases discussed in Chapter 71 can result in myelitis (spinal cord inflammation), leading to progressive neurologic signs that suggest multifocal or focal spinal cord damage. Analysis of CSF is necessary to confirm that inflammatory disease is present. Additional diagnostic tests may be necessary to identify the cause (see Chapter 71).

### Noninfectious Inflammatory Disease

Noninfectious inflammatory diseases that can affect the spinal cord include GME, breed-associated meningeal vasculitis, steroid-responsive suppurative meningitis, and feline polioencephalomyelitis. Cervical pain is a constant feature of steroid-responsive meningitis and breed-associated meningeal vasculitis. Neurologic deficits are variable, being most common with GME and uncommon with steroid-responsive meningitis. Analysis of CSF is necessary to confirm noninfectious inflammatory myelitis, and additional tests are required to rule out infectious causes. See Chapter 71 for more information on these syndromes.

## Diskospondylitis

Diskospondylitis is infection of the intervertebral disks with concurrent osteomyelitis in the adjacent end plates and vertebral bodies. Introduction of organisms is thought to be hematogenous in nearly all cases. Other possible sources of infection include urinary tract infections, dermatitis, bacterial endocarditis, prostatitis, dental disease, orchitis, and extension from a local site or migration of an inhaled foreign body (e.g., a grass awn).

### Causal organisms

The most common organisms are coagulase-positive *Staphylococcus* spp., *Streptococcus* spp., *Escherichia coli,* and *Brucella canis* (in dogs). *Aspergillus terreus* and *Paecilomyces varioti* are isolated in a few cases. *Actinomyces* spp. have been implicated in diskospondylitis caused by grass awn migration.

### Clinical features

Diskospondylitis occurs most often in medium- to large-breed dogs, particularly German Shepherd Dogs and Labrador Retrievers. It is rare in cats. Males are affected more often than females in both species.

*Clinical signs.* The most common presenting complaint is spinal pain. Palpation of the affected region often allows localization of the lesion. Systemic signs such as fever, anorexia, depression, and weight loss occur in approximately 30% of affected dogs, but hematologic inflammatory changes are rarely found. Secondary (reactive) polyarthritis occurs in some dogs, resulting in a generally stiff, stilted gait.

*Neurologic findings.* Neurologic deficits are uncommon and do not correlate with the degree of spinal cord compression. Extension of infection to neurologic tissues is extremely rare, except in animals with diskospondylitis secondary to foreign body migration. Dogs with grass awn–associated diskospondylitis often have other evidence of infection, such as pyothorax, draining paralumbar tracts, or palpable sublumbar lymph nodes or abscesses.

### Diagnosis

Diskospondylitis is suspected after physical examination and confirmed by radiography. Radiographic changes typically involve the ventral parts of affected vertebrae and include erosion and lysis of one or both end plates, collapse of the disk space, bony proliferation, and sclerosis at the margins of bone loss. It is common for diskospondylitis to affect more than one disk space, so survey radiographs of the entire spine are recommended. Radiographic changes may not be apparent for several weeks after the onset of clinical signs. MRI may permit earlier identification of lesions.

*Culture and other tests.* Blood culture is the most rewarding noninvasive method of isolating the causal organism, yielding a positive result in approximately 50% of cases. Needle aspiration of the infected vertebrae may yield positive cultures when blood cultures are negative. Cardiac, urogenital, and hepatic systems should be evaluated as potential sources of infection. Although urine culture is sometimes positive (25%), it does not reliably yield the organism responsible for diskospondylitis. Brucella serology or polymerase chain reaction (PCR) should be considered in all affected dogs because of its public health significance.

### Treatment

Initial treatment usually consists of antibiotics, cage rest, and analgesics. If an organism is isolated, susceptibility testing should guide antibiotic therapy. If an organism is not found, initial treatment should be directed against *Staphylococcus* spp.

*Antibiotics.* First-generation cephalosporins (cefazolin, 25 mg/kg intravenously [IV] q8h or cephalexin, 22 mg/kg orally [PO] q8h) and amoxicillin with clavulanate (Clavamox 12.5 to 25 mg/kg PO q8h) are effective. Quinolones can be added if gram-negative organisms are suspected. Penicillin is the antibiotic of choice for *Actinomyces* infections associated with grass awn migration.

Antibiotics are administered parenterally for the first 3 days whenever fever, neurologic deficits, or rapidly progressing signs are present. Antibiotic therapy is continued orally for at least 8 weeks, up to 6 months if necessary. Most dogs show very rapid clinical improvement within the first week of treatment.

When grass awn migration and diskospondylitis resulting from *Actinomyces* spp. occurs, surgical removal of the grass awn followed by antibiotic treatment of the cultured organism is ideal, but it is rarely feasible. Instead, most cases are treated with ampicillin (22 mg/kg PO q8h), amoxicillin (20 mg/kg PO q8h), or Clavamox for a minimum of 6 months, and sometimes for life.

*Supportive care.* The patient's activity should be restricted to minimize discomfort and decrease the chance of pathologic fracture and luxation. Analgesics may be administered for 3 to 5 days if necessary, but their use will make it difficult to assess the efficacy of antibiotic therapy and may make it more difficult to enforce strict cage rest.

*Failure to respond.* Animals that worsen or do not improve after 5 days of antibiotic therapy must be reevaluated. Failure to respond could be the result of infection with *B. canis* (dogs), with another bacterium not sensitive to the antibiotic selected, or with a mycotic organism. If multiple sites of vertebral infection exist, changing to another broad-spectrum bactericidal antibiotic can be tried. If only one site is involved, vertebral body fine-needle aspiration or surgery to obtain a culture should be considered.

Patients with severe paresis or paralysis may not improve neurologically with conservative medical therapy. Analysis of CSF and myelography or MRI should be considered to rule out meningitis and determine the degree of spinal cord compression. Decompressive surgery and curettage followed by stabilization may be necessary if severe neurologic deficits are still present 5 to 10 days after initiation of antibiotic therapy and myelography reveals severe spinal cord compression.

*Monitoring.* Animals treated medically should be reevaluated clinically and radiographically every 3 weeks. With time, fusion of the affected vertebrae should occur. Ideally, blood cultures should be repeated 2 weeks and radiographs 2 months after antibiotics are discontinued.

### Prognosis

Most treated animals do not relapse, unless the diskospondylitis is caused by grass awn migration. The prognosis is guarded with severe neurologic dysfunction, regardless of treatment.

## CHRONIC PROGRESSIVE SPINAL CORD DYSFUNCTION (TEXT PP 1034-1043)

### Neoplasia

Tumors that compress or damage the spinal cord frequently cause chronic, progressively worsening signs of spinal cord dysfunction. Spinal tumors can be primary or metastatic. The most common in dogs are extradural tumors of the vertebral body (e.g., osteosarcoma, chondrosarcoma, fibrosarcoma, myeloma) and extradural soft-tissue tumors (e.g., metastatic hemangiosarcoma or carcinoma, liposarcoma, lymphoma). Intradural extramedullary tumors (e.g., meningioma, peripheral nerve sheath tumor) also are common. Intramedullary tumors (e.g., astrocytoma, ependymoma, metastatic tumors) are relatively rare in dogs, with the exception of metastatic hemangiosarcoma. Extradural lymphoma is the only common spinal tumor in cats.

#### Signalment

Spinal tumors occur with equal frequency in males and females and can occur in any breed of dog or cat, although large-breed dogs are most often affected. Most spinal cord tumors are found in middle-aged and older dogs (mean age at diagnosis, 5 to 6 years). Two exceptions are lymphoma, which can affect dogs of any age, and neuroepithelioma, which has a predilection for T1 to L1 in young dogs, particularly German Shepherd Dogs and Golden Retrievers. Vertebral osteomas can also occur in young dogs, as can benign cartilaginous exostoses. Spinal lymphoma is most common in young adult (mean, 4 years) feline leukemia virus (FeLV)–positive cats.

#### Clinical features

Clinical signs usually are insidious in onset and related to tumor location. Early diagnosis is difficult, because neurologic abnormalities are not clinically apparent until spinal cord compression is significant. Many patients have months of slowly progressive signs before a diagnosis is made. Highly malignant extradural tumors (e.g., lymphoma) and primary or metastatic intramedullary tumors can cause rapidly progressive neurologic signs. Rarely, rapidly growing intradural tumors cause hemorrhage into the cord and acute onset of paralysis. This situation is most common in dogs with metastatic spinal cord tumors (e.g., hemangiosarcoma, adenocarcinoma). Spontaneous fractures of diseased vertebrae may also result in acute onset of pain and neurologic dysfunction.

**Specific signs.** Pain may be a prominent feature in dogs and cats with invasive nerve root tumors, tumors involving the meninges, and aggressive tumors involving bone. Progressive lameness and pain on limb manipulation are common in dogs with peripheral nerve sheath tumors involving nerve roots in the cervical or lumbar intumescence. Ipsilateral Horner's syndrome and/or loss of panniculus reflex may be seen if the thoracic nerve roots are involved.

### Diagnosis

Neoplasia may be suspected after evaluation of the history, physical examination, screening blood tests, and plain radiographs. Definitive diagnosis frequently requires analysis of CSF, further diagnostic imaging (myelography, CT, MRI), and histopathologic evaluation of the lesion.

*Investigation of primary sites.* A thorough physical examination, including fundic examination, lymph node palpation, and rectal examination, should be performed, and thoracic and abdominal radiographs should be taken to look for a primary tumor site or metastatic lesions. Ultrasonography of the spleen, liver, and heart should be performed in dogs whenever metastatic hemangiosarcoma is suspected. Most dogs with spinal cord lymphoma have multicentric disease, so aspiration of the lymph nodes and examination of peripheral blood or bone marrow smears is warranted. Over 80% of cats with spinal lymphoma are FeLV-positive, and many have obvious systemic disease and hematologic evidence of bone marrow involvement.

*Spinal radiography.* Survey radiographs of the spine should be performed, although spinal tumors usually are not evident unless obvious osteolysis (e.g., myeloma) or bone proliferation (e.g., osteosarcoma) is present. Tumors within the vertebral canal sometimes cause loss of bone density (widening of the vertebral canal). Occasionally, pressure-induced enlargement of an intervertebral foramen is seen where a nerve root tumor enters the spinal canal.

*Analysis of CSF.* Analysis of CSF may reveal slight increases in protein concentration, plus increases in mononuclear cell numbers, but this finding is inconsistent and nonspecific. CSF from the lumbar region is more likely to be abnormal (>85%) than CSF from the cerebellomedullary cistern (>25%).

Neoplastic cells are rarely identified, although cats with intradural lymphoma often have diagnostic CSF (pleocytosis consisting almost entirely of neoplastic lymphocytes). Cats with the more common extradural lymphoma typically have normal CSF, whereas dogs with extradural lymphoma commonly have extensive meningeal infiltration and diagnostic CSF. Other tumors rarely exfoliate into the CSF sufficiently for diagnosis.

*Other tests.* Fine-needle aspiration of extradural lesions under fluoroscopic guidance can be used to diagnose lymphoma. Myelography is a fairly reliable method for identifying and localizing spinal tumors. (Note: Analysis of CSF should always be performed before myelography.) Where available, CT or MRI can add valuable information regarding precise tumor location and degree of spinal cord involvement, which may be important when one is considering surgical treatment and/or radiation therapy.

### Treatment and prognosis

Surgical decompression and attempts at tumor excision usually are limited to well-encapsulated intradural extramedullary tumors (e.g., noninvasive intradural extramedullary meningiomas in cats). Intramedullary tumors usually cannot be treated surgically because of their intimate involvement with neural tissue. Even with aggressive surgical treatment, local recurrence and metastases are common with vertebral tumors.

Corticosteroids, although they have little effect on most tumors, can decrease tumor-associated edema and result in remarkable temporary improvement. Chemotherapy and radiation therapy as primary or postoperative adjuvant therapies have met with limited success in the treatment of spinal tumors in dogs and cats. Radiation therapy may be of some benefit in dogs and cats with spinal lymphoma. Lymphoreticular tumors such as lymphoma and myeloma can be treated with traditional chemotherapy protocols, although only a few of the drugs used cross the blood-brain barrier, and the long-term prognosis is poor (see Chapter 82).

## Intraspinal Articular Cysts

Cysts arising from the joint capsule of spinal facetal joints can cause chronic, progressive, focal compression of the spinal cord or nerve roots. These cysts arise secondary to degenerative changes in the facetal joints, a consequence of congenital malformations, vertebral instability, or trauma. Signs are referable to the site and degree of resulting spinal cord or nerve root compression.

### Signalment

Young dogs of giant breeds such as Mastiffs and Great Danes most commonly develop single or multiple cysts in the cervical region, which cause a UMN myelopathy and occasionally cervical pain. Older dogs, particularly German Shepherd Dogs, have been identified with TL or lumbosacral articular cysts that cause spinal cord or cauda equina compression.

### Diagnosis and treatment

Radiographs reveal degenerative changes of the articular facets. Analysis of CSF reveals normal cytology and slightly increased protein consistent with a noninflammatory, chronic compressive myelopathy. Myelography reveals focal extradural compression. MRI is necessary to identify the facetal joints as the origin of the cysts and to precisely localize the cysts before surgical therapy. Treatment, which consists of spinal cord decompression, cyst drainage, and arthrodesis of the facetal joint, generally has excellent results.

## Type II Intervertebral Disk Disease

Fibroid degeneration of the intervertebral disk occurs with age in some dogs. Partial rupture of the disk annulus allows prolapse of a small amount of disk nucleus; this and the accompanying fibrotic reaction results in bulging of the disk into the spinal canal. Repetitive partial prolapse causes slowly progressive signs of spinal cord compression. This type of disk protrusion (Hansen's type II) is seen most commonly in aging large-breed dogs, particularly German Shepherd Dogs, Labrador Retrievers, and Doberman Pinschers.

### Clinical features

Clinical signs primarily result from spinal cord compression, although spinal discomfort is apparent in a few dogs. TL disk disease is most common, resulting in UMN signs in the rear limbs only. Cervical type II disk disease (as well as type I extrusion) may be seen in Doberman Pinschers in association with wobbler syndrome. In these dogs all limbs are affected, with neurologic signs most prominent in the rear limbs. Cervical pain is present if nerve roots are compressed or when concurrent type I disk herniation is present.

### Diagnosis

Neurologic examination should allow localization of the lesion. Spinal radiographs can help to identify type II disk disease, but they are normal in some dogs. Disk space narrowing, osteophyte production, and end-plate sclerosis are common at multiple sites. Myelography, CT, or MRI is necessary to determine the extent and location of the lesion and to distinguish disk protrusion from degenerative myelopathy (DM), spinal neoplasia, and diskospondylitis.

### Treatment and prognosis

Prednisone (0.2 mg/kg PO q24-48h) may result in neurologic improvement for a short time, but this treatment is not curative. Surgery is recommended as the definitive treatment. However, effective surgical decompression is often difficult to achieve because of the chronic nature of the lesion and the difficulty in removing the dorsal annulus. The goal of therapy is simply to stabilize the patient's neurologic status; full recovery should not be anticipated. A few dogs experience temporary or permanent worsening of clinical signs postoperatively.

## Degenerative Myelopathy

Degeneration of the spinal cord white matter occurs most often in aging German Shepherd Dogs. It has been recognized in dogs from 5 to 14 years of age and is occasionally seen in old dogs of other large breeds, and rarely in cats. A DM-like disorder has also been identified in Pembroke Welsh Corgis.

The cause of DM is uncertain. A deficiency of nutrients or vitamins is one possible cause. An inherited cause has also been proposed in German Shepherd Dogs. Whatever the initiating event, DM is generally considered to be an immune-mediated neurodegenerative disease. The thoracic and TL segments are most severely affected in all predisposed breeds.

### Clinical features

DM results in slowly progressive (6 months to 2 years) UMN paresis and ataxia of the rear limbs. Loss of conscious proprioception occurs, resulting in knuckling of the toes and wearing of the dorsal nail surfaces. Increased muscle tone and hyperactivity of rear limb reflexes allow localization of the problem to between T3 and L3. In <10% of cases a decrease or loss of rear limb reflexes is observed late in the disease. Neurologic deficits may be asymmetric. The thoracic limbs are normal, and urinary and fecal continence is maintained until very late.

### Diagnosis

DM should be suspected in any large-breed dog with slow progression of ataxia and weakness in the rear limbs. Affected dogs are systemically normal, and no localizable spinal pain is present. Differential diagnoses include neoplasia, type II disk disease, and musculoskeletal disorders (e.g., severe hip dysplasia, bilateral cruciate rupture).

Antemortem diagnosis is made by exclusion. Normal spinal radiographs, cytologically normal CSF (with normal or slightly increased protein content), and normal myelogram in an older dog with slowly progressive UMN signs in the rear limbs warrant a diagnosis of DM.

### Treatment

No effective treatment exists. Corticosteroids and other immunosuppressive agents have no long-term benefit. In fact, corticosteroids can cause muscle wasting and exacerbation of muscle weakness. Exercise may be helpful in slowing progression of the disease.

Supplementation with vitamins E, B complex, and C and with omega-3 fatty acids has been recommended. Some studies report success with aminocaproic acid (Amicar, 500 mg PO q8h). Drawbacks include GI irritation, high cost, and the need to treat for 2 to 3 months before response can be detected. Administration of Amicar in combination with the potent antioxidant acetylcysteine (5% solution, 25 mg/kg PO q8h for 14 days, then every other day) has also been recommended.

## Cauda Equina Syndrome

The sacral and caudal spinal nerves overlie the lumbosacral junction, so compression of the cauda equina nerves can occur with lumbosacral disk protrusion, tumors, diskospondylitis, vertebral or sacral osteochondrosis, congenital malformations, or degenerative lumbosacral stenosis. Type II disk prolapse with progressive lumbosacral stenosis is the most common cause in older, large-breed dogs.

German Shepherd Dogs, Labrador Retrievers, and Belgian Malinois, particularly those used as working dogs, are most often affected. Cauda equina syndrome is seen primarily in males >5 years old. Genetic predisposition, conformation, physical activity, and vertebral malformation are all proposed factors.

### Clinical features

Cauda equina compression results in characteristic clinical signs. Affected dogs are slow to rise and reluctant to run, sit up, jump, or climb stairs. Rear limb lameness and weakness worsen with exercise. Affected dogs may be reluctant to raise or wag their tails. Perineal hyperesthesia or paresthesia and self-inflicted moist dermatitis of the perineum and tail base may develop. Urinary and fecal incontinence rarely occur.

*Physical examination.* The most consistent finding is pain elicited by deep palpation of the sacrum, dorsiflexion of the tail, or hyperextension of the lumbosacral region. If no neurologic deficits are present, it can be difficult to distinguish this condition from diskospondylitis, prostatic disease, gracilis muscle contracture, or degenerative joint disease resulting from hip dysplasia or cruciate rupture.

Rear limb weakness, muscle atrophy in the caudal thigh, and decrease in limb (especially hock) flexion during the withdrawal reflex are seen when the cauda equina nerves are compressed. The patellar reflex is increased in some dogs because of loss of caudal thigh muscle tone. Urinary dysfunction, when it occurs, results in urine dribbling and a large, flaccid bladder that is easily expressed. A few dogs develop reflex dyssynergia (see Chapter 48).

### Diagnosis

Clinical findings are often the primary basis for reaching a diagnosis of cauda equina syndrome, as many of the routinely available diagnostic tests may be difficult to interpret. Spinal radiographs are useful to rule out causes of cauda equina compression (e.g., diskospondylitis, lytic vertebral neoplasia, fracture or luxation) and to identify predisposing factors for degenerative stenosis (e.g., sacral osteochondrosis, vertebral malformations).

*Radiography.* Radiographs most commonly reveal end plate sclerosis and spondylosis of the ventral and lateral margins of the L7 and S1 vertebral end plates. Narrowing or collapse of the L7-S1 intervertebral disk space or ventral displacement of the body of S1 relative to L7 may also be seen. Caution is critical when one is interpreting radiographs of this region, because these abnormalities are common in clinically normal dogs.

*Other tests.* Analysis of CSF to rule out inflammatory disease should be performed before myelography. Myelography is sometimes useful for documenting cauda equina compression, but it will not be diagnostic in the 20% of dogs in which the dural sac ends cranial to the lumbosacral junction or in dogs in which the primary lesion is lateral compression of the spinal nerves at the intervertebral foramen. Other tests that may be useful include epidurography or diskography, electromyography, and MRI (see text).

### Treatment and prognosis

Restriction of exercise and administration of analgesics or antiinflammatory drugs may result in temporary improvement in dogs with clinical signs limited to pain and lameness. More definitive treatment involves surgery: dorsal laminectomy, excision of compressing tissues, and possibly L7-S1 foraminotomy. Rapid pain relief occurs after surgery in most dogs, and the prognosis for resolution of lameness and mild neurologic deficits is excellent. Most dogs with mild to moderate deficits can return to working function. However, dogs with severe LMN deficits or incontinence are likely to have permanent deficits.

## Cervical Vertebral Instability or Malformation (Wobbler Syndrome)

Canine wobbler syndrome involves caudal cervical spinal cord and nerve root compression in large-breed dogs. It occurs secondary to developmental malformations, instability, or associated changes in the spinal canal. Vertebral body and end plate abnormalities can lead to type II disk protrusion, or, occasionally, type I disk herniation. Genetic predisposition, overnutrition, and conformation are all considered contributing factors.

### Signalment

Great Danes and Doberman Pinschers are most often affected, but the condition has been reported in many large-breed dogs. Males may be affected more often than females. Age at presentation varies from 7 weeks to 10 years. Cranial stenosis of C4, C5, or C6 and articular facet deformities are the most common abnormalities in young Great Danes. Vertebral instability plus malformation, usually of C5, C6, or C7, is more common in middle-aged and older Dobermans and in older dogs of other breeds.

### Clinical features
Slowly progressive paresis and an incoordinated or wobbly gait, particularly in the rear limbs, is characteristic. A broad-based stance is often noted in the rear limbs. Scuffing of the toenails or stiff gait in the forelimbs may also be seen. The rear limbs are always more severely affected than the forelimbs. Although increased muscle tone in the forelimbs is common, neurologic deficits can be subtle or undetectable. In some cases involving the caudal cervical spine, the only evidence of LMN disease in the forelimbs is pronounced muscle atrophy of the supraspinatus and infraspinatus muscles over the scapula.

Slow deterioration is common, but occasionally a traumatic episode results in acute exacerbation of signs. Affected dogs may be mildly ataxic with subtle loss of conscious proprioception, or they may be tetraparetic. Resistance to dorsal extension is common, but overt cervical pain is rare unless secondary disk prolapse has occurred. Lameness and muscle atrophy in one forelimb or pain when traction is applied to a limb suggests nerve root compression.

### Diagnosis
Diagnosis is suspected based on signalment, history, and clinical findings. Radiography, analysis of CSF (normal), and myelography or MRI allow definitive diagnosis and exclusion of other differential diagnoses, including neoplasia, disk disease, DM, GME, and infectious disease. Affected dogs should be evaluated for systemic disease; Dobermans, in particular, may have concurrent hypothyroidism, von Willebrand's disease, or cardiomyopathy.

*Radiography.* Radiologic diagnosis usually requires proper positioning with the animal under general anesthesia. Although radiographs are normal in some dogs with wobbler syndrome, most affected dogs have some radiographic changes, including ventral tipping of the craniodorsal aspect of the vertebral body, vertebral canal stenosis at the cranial aspect of the vertebra, collapsed disk spaces, and degenerative changes in the articular facets. In middle-aged Dobermans, chronic degenerative disk disease involving C5 to C6 or C6 to C7 is often seen. Cervical myelography or MRI should be performed whenever surgery is considered (see text).

### Treatment
Severe exercise restriction and corticosteroid therapy may result in temporary improvement. Dogs with minimal or mild neurologic signs can sometimes be managed long-term with corticosteroids alone: prednisone, 0.5 mg/kg PO q12h for 2 days; then0.5 mg/kg PO q24h for 2 days; then 0.5 mg/kg PO q48h for 2 weeks; then 0.25 mg/kg q48h for 2 months. Exercise should be restricted, and a chest harness used instead of a collar.

*Surgery.* Although initial improvement is common with medical therapy, the compression and instability persist and generally progress without more definitive treatment. Surgery is recommended in mildly affected dogs if the condition does not improve or continues to deteriorate during medical management and in all severely affected dogs. Surgical options are discussed in the text.

### Prognosis
The prognosis depends on the neurologic status, course of the disease, and specific abnormalities present. Surgical results in ambulatory patients with a short history and single lesion can be good (up to 80% success). Multiple lesions, chronic disease, and inability to walk are all associated with a poor prognosis.

## PROGRESSIVE SPINAL CORD DYSFUNCTION IN YOUNG ANIMALS (TEXT PP 1043-1047)

### Neuronal Abiotrophies and Degeneration
Neuronal abiotrophies and degenerative nervous system disorders occur in a few breeds of dog (Box 72-1). Progressive neurologic dysfunction usually begins early in life. In disorders that affect the spinal cord, signs involving the rear limbs are often noted early, but progression to tetraparesis may occur. Some disorders primarily affect the white matter and result in UMN signs; others result in LMN paralysis. Diagnosis is based

*Text continued on p 665.*

---

**Box 72-1**

## Congenital, Familial, and Idiopathic Degenerative Disorders of the Nervous System

### PREDOMINANTLY BRAIN OR SPINAL CORD UMN SIGNS
#### Hereditary Afghan Myelopathy
*Onset:* 3-13 mo of age

*Clinical signs:* Rapidly progressive rear limb paresis, ataxia, increased tone, hyperreflexia (initially); progresses to tetraplegia

*Pathology:* Extensive demyelination of spinal cord axons (especially thoracic)

#### Boxer Central-Peripheral Neuropathy
*Onset:* 6 mo of age

*Clinical signs:* Progressive severe ataxia and hypermetria; signs begin in rear limbs, progress to include forelimbs; loss of proprioception; weakness, patellar areflexia, normal flexor reflexes

*EMG:* Normal

*NCV:* Normal or slightly reduced

*Evoked muscle action potential:* Low amplitude

#### Spongiform Degeneration of the Gray Matter of Bull Mastiffs
*Onset:* 4-7 wk of age

*Clinical signs:* Ataxia, proprioceptive deficits, hypermetria, head tremors, visual deficits, dementia

#### Multisystem Neuronal Degeneration in Cocker Spaniels
*Onset:* 10-14 mo of age

*Clinical signs:* Progressive abnormal behavior, anxiety, cerebellar ataxia, intention tremor

*Pathology:* Neuronal degeneration in the brain and brainstem

#### Leukodystrophy of Dalmatians
*Onset:* 3-5 mo of age

*Clinical signs:* Visual deficits, progressive ataxia

*Pathology:* Brain atrophy; cavitation of white matter of cerebral hemispheres

#### Hereditary Ataxia in Jack Russell and Smooth-Coated Fox Terriers
*Onset:* 2-6 mo of age

*Clinical signs:* Weakness, rear limb incoordination, progressing to ataxia of all four limbs and hypermetria; signs may stabilize

*Pathology:* Bilaterally symmetric spinal cord degeneration predominantly involving the spinocerebellar tracts

#### Spongy Degeneration of the White Matter in Labrador Retrievers
*Onset:* 4-6 mo of age

*Clinical signs:* Progressive forelimb rigidity, opisthotonic posturing, cerebellar ataxia

*Pathology:* Spongiform degeneration in CNS cerebellar peduncles, cerebral white matter, and peripheral nerves

#### Labrador Retriever Axonopathy
*Onset:* 3-4 wk of age

*Clinical signs:* Rear limb gait short strided, adducted, and crouched; forelimbs wide based and stiff; hypermetria; progressive for 4-5 mo, then static, ± head tremor

*Pathology:* Spinal cord white matter degeneration

#### Leukoencephalomyelopathy in Rottweilers
*Onset:* 1.5-4 yr of age

*Clinical signs:* Very slow progression (years) of ataxia, tetraparesis, hypermetria, weakness, loss of proprioception; hyperactive reflexes

*Pathology:* Demyelination of spinal cord, caudal cerebellar peduncle, and lower brainstem

*Continued.*

**Box 72-1—cont'd**

## Congenital, Familial, and Idiopathic Degenerative Disorders of the Nervous System

### Neuroaxonal Dystrophy in Rottweilers
*Onset:* 3 mo to 6 yr of age

*Clinical signs:* Very slowly progressive disorder; initially clumsy gait, forelimb hypermetria progressing to obvious cerebellar ataxia, head intention tremor, and nystagmus; normal conscious proprioception, not weak

*Pathology:* Spheroids in granular level of cerebellum, vestibular nuclei, and spinal cord; similar syndromes in young Chihuahuas, Jack Russell Terriers, Collies, and tricolor cats

### Central Axonopathy of Scottish Terriers
*Onset:* 10-12 wk of age

*Clinical signs:* Generalized body tremors, ataxia, progress to paraparesis

*Pathology:* Neuroaxonal dystrophy, axonopathy

### Degenerative Myelopathy
*Affected:* Older (>5 yr of age) German Shepherd Dogs, Siberian Huskies, Chesapeake Bay Retrievers, other large-breed dogs; rarely seen in cats

*Clinical signs:* Slowly progressive loss of proprioception, UMN paralysis of the rear limbs

*Pathology:* Diffuse demyelination of all white matter tracts of spinal cord, particularly in thoracic region (focal areas of cerebellum, cerebrum, brainstem also involved)

### Metabolic Storage Diseases
See text p 979

### Cerebellar Atrophy and Abiotrophy
See text p 978

### Congenital Vestibular Disorders
See Chapter 70

## PREDOMINANTLY LMN SIGNS

### Hereditary Polyneuropathy of Alaskan Malamutes
*Onset:* 7-18 mo of age

*Clinical signs:* Slowly progressive weakness, exercise intolerance, muscle atrophy, hyporeflexia, megaesophagus, laryngeal paralysis

### Progressive Axonopathy of Boxers
*Onset:* 2-3 mo of age

*Clinical signs:* Rear limb ataxia, hypotonia, hyporeflexia progressing to tetraparesis ± cerebellar signs

*Pathology:* Axonal swellings in dorsal and ventral nerve roots, peripheral nerves, spinal cord

### Laryngeal Paralysis of Bouvier des Flandres
*Onset:* 4-8 mo of age

*Clinical signs:* Exercise intolerance, inspiratory stridor, dyspnea, laryngeal paralysis

*Pathology:* Axonal degeneration in recurrent laryngeal nerves, neuronal loss in nucleus ambiguous; autosomal dominant inheritance

### Spinal Muscular Atrophy of Brittany Spaniels
*Onset:* 1-6 mo of age

*Clinical signs:* Weakness and atrophy of proximal limb muscles; rapid or slow progression to tetraplegia, loss of reflexes, tendon contracture

*Pathology:* Neuronal degeneration of selected brainstem nuclei and ventral gray matter of spinal cord

*Continued.*

## Congenital, Familial, and Idiopathic Degenerative Disorders of the Nervous System

### Neuronal Chromatolysis of Cairn Terriers
*Onset:* 3-7 mo of age
*Clinical signs:* Initially episodic rear limb collapse with spontaneous resolution; rear limb weakness, loss of patellar reflexes, progress to tetraparesis; ataxia, hypermetria, head tremors
*Pathology:* Central and peripheral widespread chromatolytic degeneration and focal myelomalacia

### Motor Neuron Disease in Cats
*Onset:* >6 yr
*Clinical signs:* Progressive weakness, cervical ventroflexion, dysphagia, muscle atrophy, loss of reflexes (late)
*Pathology:* Degeneration of ventral horn of spinal cord and ventral nerve roots

### Dalmatian Laryngeal Paralysis and Polyneuropathy
*Onset:* 2-6 mo of age
*Clinical signs:* Acute respiratory distress, syncope, gagging, coughing, laryngeal paralysis, megaesophagus, muscle weakness, muscle atrophy, hyporeflexia
*Pathology:* Focal loss of myelinated fibers, distal polyneuropathy

### Distal Polyneuropathy of Doberman Pinschers
*Onset:* Adult (3-5 yr of age), slow progression
*Clinical signs:* Initial tendency to flex one or the other rear limb while standing ("dancing Doberman"); atrophy of gastrocnemius, semitendinosus, semimembranosus; rear limb weakness, one-half decrease in conscious proprioception, one-half normal hyperreflexia
*EMG:* Positive sharp waves and fibrillation potentials in gastrocnemius with advanced disease
*NCV:* Normal
*Pathology:* Type II muscle fiber atrophy in advanced disease; may be a primary muscle disorder

### Progressive Neurogenic Muscular Atrophy in English Pointers
*Onset:* 18-23 wk of age
*Clinical signs:* Trembling, rear limb weakness, hoarseness, progressing over 2-3 mo to stumbling, tetraplegia, extreme muscle atrophy (especially shoulder) and hyporeflexia
*EMG:* Denervation

### Giant Axonal Neuropathy in German Shepherd Dogs
*Onset:* 14-16 mo of age
*Clinical signs:* Progressive rear limb paresis, proprioceptive deficits, depressed patellar reflexes, atrophy of distal rear limb muscles, megaesophagus, hoarseness, fecal incontinence
*Pathology:* Axonal swellings containing neurofilaments

### Spinal Muscle Atrophy in German Shepherd Dogs
*Onset:* 12-14 wk of age
*Clinical signs:* Forelimb weakness, severe muscle atrophy
*Pathology:* Symmetric ventral horn degeneration confined to the cervical intumescence

### Hypomyelinating Polyneuropathy of Golden Retrievers
*Onset:* 7 wk of age
*Clinical signs:* Rear limb weakness, crouched stance, muscle atrophy, depressed postural reactions

*Continued.*

---

**Box 72-1—cont'd**

## Congenital, Familial, and Idiopathic Degenerative Disorders of the Nervous System

### Spinal Muscular Atrophy in Maine Coon Cats
*Onset:* 15-17 wk of age
*Clinical signs:* Progressive muscle weakness and atrophy, fasciculations
*Pathology:* Neurogenic muscle atrophy, loss of large motor neurons in ventral horns of spinal cord

### Distal Sensorimotor Polyneuropathy in Rottweilers
*Onset:* Adult (1-4 yr of age)
*Clinical signs:* Paraparesis slowly progressing to tetraparesis, hyporeflexia, hypotonia, muscle atrophy in distal limb muscles
*Pathology:* Degeneration of myelinated and unmyelinated peripheral axons

### Spinal Muscular Atrophy in Rottweilers
*Onset:* 4 wk of age
*Clinical signs:* Rapid progression of weakness, loss of proprioception, hyporeflexia, severe denervation atrophy, megaesophagus
*Pathology:* Degeneration of motor neurons in gray matter of spinal cord

### Laryngeal Paralysis in Siberian Husky Dogs, Crosses, and Alaskan Husky Dogs
*Onset:* 6 wk of age
*Clinical signs:* Inspiratory dyspnea, stridor, exercise intolerance, laryngeal paralysis

### Spinal Muscular Atrophy of Swedish Lapland Dogs
*Onset:* 5-7 wk of age
*Clinical signs:* Weakness, then rapid progression to flaccid tetraplegia with severe muscle atrophy; spinal reflexes are decreased
*EMG:* Denervation potentials
*Pathology:* Neuronal degeneration of spinal cord ventral gray matter and ventral nerve roots

### Inherited Hypertrophic Neuropathy In Tibetan Mastiffs
*Onset:* 7-10 wk of age
*Clinical signs:* Rapidly progressing weakness, loss of muscle tone, hyporeflexia, tetraplegia; cranial nerves normal
*NCV:* Slow because of extensive demyelination of peripheral nerves
*Pathology:* Extensive, chronic demyelination

### Metabolic Storage Diseases
See text p 979

## DISORDERS OF THE SENSORY NERVES
### Long-Haired Dachshund Sensory Neuropathy
*Onset:* 6 wk of age
*Clinical signs:* Rear limb ataxia, decreased superficial and deep sensation, loss of proprioception, urinary incontinence; no paresis, no muscle atrophy, normal tendon reflexes
*EMG:* Motor
*NCV:* Normal
*Sensory NCV:* Absent
*Pathology:* Loss of myelinated fibers, degeneration of unmyelinated sensory nerve fibers

### Sensory Neuropathy of English Pointers
*Onset:* 2-12 mo of age
*Clinical signs:* Loss of sensation, particularly distal limbs; self-mutilation; normal gait and reflexes

---

*CNS,* Central nervous system; *EMG,* electromyography; *LMN,* lower motor neuron; *NCV,* nervous condition velocity; *UMN,* upper motor neuron.

on the signalment, clinical course, and lack of any definable cause on screening blood tests, radiography, analysis of CSF, myelography, and other diagnostic tests. Diagnosis usually is confirmed at necropsy. No treatment is available.

### Atlantoaxial Luxation
Malformation or absence of the dens or loss of its ligamentous support is a congenital defect in many small breeds of dog including the Yorkshire Terrier, Miniature or Toy Poodle, Chihuahua, Pomeranian, and Pekingese and rarely in large-breed dogs and in cats. Malformation and resultant atlantoaxial instability can lead to acute atlantoaxial luxation as a consequence of minor trauma. Alternatively, congenital deformity of the dens may produce slowly progressive signs of spinal cord compression, as the supporting ligaments gradually stretch, causing instability and spinal cord compression before complete luxation occurs.

#### Clinical features
Clinical signs include neck pain, low head carriage, ataxia, and tetraparesis. Paralysis is rare. Some dogs have a persistent head tilt or turn. Physical examination reveals UMN signs in all four limbs and cervical pain. Dogs with atlantoaxial luxation typically keep their necks in extension and resist flexion of the cranial cervical region. Note: Manipulation of the spine should be avoided, as it can exacerbate motor dysfunction.

#### Diagnosis
Atlantoaxial luxation secondary to malformation should be suspected in any young (6- to 18-month-old) toy-breed dog with a history of cervical pain, tetraparesis, or tetraplegia. It should also be considered in any dog with evidence of cranial cervical spinal cord disease, particularly those with a history of trauma.

*Radiography.* Initial radiographs should be taken without anesthesia when atlantoaxial luxation is suspected, to prevent inadvertent overflexion or twisting of an unstable cervical spine. Instability with significant luxation is seen on a lateral view as widening of the space between the dorsal arch of the atlas and the dorsal spinous process of the axis, and dorsal displacement of the body of the axis. In cases of congenital luxation the dens may be obviously abnormal; fracture of the dens may be apparent with traumatic luxation.

If preliminary radiographs are not diagnostic, the patient should be anesthetized and the radiographs repeated with the dog's head *gently* flexed. Incidental radiographic findings in affected toy and miniature breeds may include occipitoatlantoaxial malformation and a larger-than-normal foramen magnum (occipital dysplasia), neither of which should alter the diagnostic or therapeutic plan or the prognosis.

#### Treatment and prognosis
Treatment as described for acute spinal cord trauma, followed by surgical stabilization, is recommended. The prognosis for recovery is good in dogs <2 years of age with voluntary motor function and pain perception.

## CONGENITAL SPINAL CORD DYSFUNCTION: NONPROGRESSIVE SIGNS (TEXT PP 1047-1048)

### Spina Bifida
Spina bifida can occur anywhere along the spinal canal, although the lumbosacral segment and the sacrococcygeal junction are most often affected. This malformation is most common in English Bulldogs and Manx cats. In Manxes the condition is an autosomal-recessive trait and may be associated with caudal agenesis (see next section). Development of neurologic signs is variable. Signs, when present, may include rear limb paresis, fecal and urinary incontinence, loss of perineal sensation, and decreased anal sphincter tone. No treatment is available.

### Caudal Agenesis of Manx Cats
Congenital malformations of the sacrococcygeal spinal cord and vertebrae are common in tailless Manx cats. Signs include a hopping or crouched rear limb gait, fecal and urinary incontinence, and chronic constipation.

## Spinal Dysraphism

Spinal dysraphism is an inherited congenital malformation of the spinal cord. It is most common in Weimaraners; other breeds are occasionally affected. Clinical signs are present at birth. Affected dogs have a symmetric, bunny-hopping rear limb gait, a wide-based stance, and depressed proprioception; patellar reflexes are normal. The flexor reflex stimulated in one rear limb usually elicits simultaneous flexion of both rear limbs. Signs do not progress, and mildly affected dogs can live a normal life.

## Syringomyelia and Hydromyelia

Cystic accumulations of fluid within the spinal cord that causes compression of adjacent parenchyma are recognized with increasing frequency with the use of advanced diagnostic imaging techniques (CT, MRI) for neurologic diagnosis. Syringomyelia is a CSF-filled cavity anywhere within the cord, and hydromyelia is the accumulation of excessive CSF within a dilated central canal. These disorders can develop as a result of altered CSF pressures within the spinal canal or a loss of spinal cord parenchyma or secondarily to obstructed CSF flow caused by congenital malformations or inflammatory or neoplastic obstruction.

### Clinical features

Clinical signs reflect the site and degree of spinal cord parenchymal destruction. Ataxia and paresis are common. With cervical lesions, UMN signs are more pronounced in the rear limbs if the dorsal and lateral portions of the cord are affected. When the spinal cord damage is more centrally located, ataxia and paresis often are more significant in the forelimbs than in the rear limbs (central cord syndrome).

Spinal pain may occur because of stretching of nerve roots or meninges. Scoliosis occasionally develops, as LMN cell body damage within the cord causes asymmetric denervation of the paraspinal muscles, resulting in vertebral deviation. Cervical paresthesia and scratching have been noted in Cavalier King Charles Spaniels with bony malformations that cause overcrowding of the foramen magnum, resulting in syringohydromyelia.

### Diagnosis and treatment

Diagnosis requires advanced diagnostic imaging. MRI is superior to CT for demonstration of the intraparenchymal spinal cord abnormalities. Treatment is controversial. Early surgical intervention to decompress the fluid accumulation and reestablish normal CSF flow or shunting is ideal but is rarely effective. Medical therapy consists of the administration of prednisone and acetazolamide to decrease CSF production.

# 73

# Disorders of Peripheral Nerves and the Neuromuscular Junction

## (Text pp 1049-1061)

### FOCAL NEUROPATHIES (TEXT PP 1049-1054)

#### Traumatic Neuropathies

Traumatic neuropathies are common and can result from mechanical blows, fractures, pressure, stretching, laceration, or injection into or around the nerve. Individual nerves or a group of nerves may be damaged. Traumatic radial nerve paralysis, brachial plexus avulsion, and sciatic nerve injury are most common.

##### Diagnosis

Diagnosis is based on history and clinical findings (Table 73-1). Cutaneous sensation and motor function should be mapped so that the precise location of the injury can be determined and progress monitored. Electromyogram (EMG) can be used to evaluate the extent of nerve damage. Denervation action potentials are detected 5 to 7 days after denervation of a muscle. Nerve conduction studies proximal and distal to the site of injury can also be used to assess nerve integrity.

##### Treatment and prognosis

Physical therapy (e.g., swimming, limb manipulation, massage) helps delay muscle atrophy and tendon contracture and speeds return of function in animals with incomplete lesions. Self-mutilation may become a problem 2 to 3 weeks after injury, as regeneration of sensory nerves can result in abnormal sensation lasting 7 to 10 days. If improvement in motor function is not seen after 1 month, amputation or arthrodesis should be considered.

If adequate perineural connective tissue remains, axonal regeneration can occur at a rate of 1 to 4 mm/day. The closer a nerve injury is to the innervated muscle, the better the chance of recovery. If a nerve is entirely disrupted, the prognosis for regeneration is poor.

#### Peripheral Nerve Tumors

Nerve sheath tumors (schwannoma, neurofibroma, neurofibrosarcoma) and sometimes lymphomas involve the nerve roots and peripheral nerves of dogs and (rarely) cats.

##### Clinical features

Clinical signs depend on tumor location and nerves involved. Tumors that involve the spinal nerve roots in the lower cervical and upper thoracic region and the peripheral nerves of the brachial plexus cause lameness (intermittent or persistent), muscle atrophy, and pain. Although the tumor may not be palpable, pain may be evident on palpation of the axillary region. With progression of the tumor, atrophy, weakness, and loss of reflexes may occur as the affected peripheral nerve is destroyed.

**Table 73-1**

## Traumatic Neuropathies

| Peripheral nerves damaged (spinal cord segments)* | Skin region of sensation loss | Motor dysfunction | Muscles affected |
|---|---|---|---|
| **LESIONS OF NERVES OF THE THORACIC LIMB** | | | |
| Peripheral radial nerve damage (at level of elbow) | Cranial and lateral forearm and dorsal forepaw | Loss of carpus and digit extension; may walk on dorsal paw or carry limb | Extensor carpi radialis, ulnaris lateralis, digital extensors |
| Brachial plexus avulsion (proximal damage) | | | |
| Suprascapular nerve ([C5], C6-C7) | None | Loss of shoulder extension; muscle atrophy over scapular spine | Supraspinatus, infraspinatus |
| Axillary nerve ([C6], C7, C8) | Small area dorsolateral brachium | Reduced shoulder flexion; deltoid muscle atrophy | Deltoideus, teres major, teres minor, subscapularis |
| Musculocutaneous nerve (C6, C7, C8) | Medial forearm | Reduced elbow flexion | Biceps brachii, brachialis, coracobrachialis |
| Radial nerve (C7, C8, T1, [T2]) | Cranial and lateral forearm, from toes to elbow | Reduced extension of elbow, carpus, and digits; cannot support weight | Triceps brachii, extensor carpi radialis, ulnaris lateralis, digital extensors |
| Median nerve (C8, T1, [T2]) | None | Reduced flexion of carpus and digits | Flexor carpi radialis, digital flexors |
| Ulnar nerve (C8, T1, [T2]) | Caudal forearm (toes to elbow), lateral digits | Reduced flexion of carpus and digits | Flexor carpi ulnaris, deep and digital flexor |
| **LESIONS OF NERVES OF THE PELVIC LIMB** | | | |
| Femoral nerve damage (L4, L5, L6) | Medial limb (toes to thigh) | Inability to extend stifle; cannot support weight; atrophy of quadriceps; loss of patellar reflex | Iliopsoas, quadriceps, sartorius |
| Sciatic nerve paralysis (L6, L7, S1, [S2]) | All regions below stifle except medial surface | Reduced flexion and extension of hip; loss of stifle flexion; loss of hock flexion and extension hock dropped; paw is knuckled, but weight bearing does occur; absent withdrawal reflex; atrophy of cranial, tibial, semimembranosus, and semitendinosus muscles | Biceps femoris, semimembranosus, semitendinosus |
| Tibial branch (L7, S1, [S2]) | Caudal plantar (stifle to paw) | Dropped hock | Gastrocnemius, popliteus, digital flexors |
| Peroneal branch (L6, L7, S1, S2) | Cranial and dorsal limb (stifle to paw) | Stands knuckled; no cranial tibial reflex | Peroneus longus, digital extensors, cranial tibial |

*Square brackets indicate variable contribution.

Tumors involving the T1 to T3 nerve roots may interrupt the sympathetic pathway and result in ipsilateral Horner's syndrome (see Chapter 68). Less commonly, trigeminal nerve sheath tumors result in ipsilateral atrophy of the temporalis and masseter muscles. Intradural nerve root tumors may eventually expand within the vertebral canal, causing spinal cord compression and upper motor neuron signs (see Table 65-4) caudal to the lesion site.

### Diagnosis

Spinal radiographs are indicated if a nerve root tumor is suspected. These tumors rarely cause bony changes, although expanding tumors may widen the surrounding intervertebral foramen. Myelography is useful to identify spinal cord compression. EMG and nerve conduction velocity studies can confirm the presence of a peripheral nerve lesion and aid localization. Computed tomography (CT) and magnetic resonance imaging (MRI) may be best to characterize the lesion once it has been localized and to determine treatment options.

### Treatment and prognosis

The treatment of choice for nerve sheath tumors is surgical removal, which sometimes results in cure. However, if neurologic damage is extensive, several spinal nerves or nerve roots are affected, or severe muscle atrophy has occurred, amputation may be required. Nerve root tumors that progress to cause spinal cord compression usually involve multiple nerve roots, are rarely resectable, and carry a poor prognosis. Postoperative irradiation may be indicated in an attempt to slow progression.

## Facial Nerve Paralysis

Facial nerve paralysis is common in dogs and cats. In 75% of dogs and 25% of cats with acute facial nerve paralysis, there are no associated neurologic or physical abnormalities, and no underlying cause can be found, prompting a diagnosis of idiopathic facial nerve paralysis. Causes in other cases include inflammation, infection, or neoplasia anywhere along the path of the facial nerve (brainstem, petrous temporal bone, middle ear, superficially) and, occasionally in dogs, hypothyroidism.

The most common identifiable cause is damage to branches of the facial nerve within the middle ear. Specific conditions include otitis media and interna, foreign bodies (e.g., grass awns), malignant tumors, and benign nasopharyngeal polyps (cats). Otitis media and interna usually occur from extension of bacterial otitis externa, particularly in breeds predisposed to chronic otitis externa (e.g., Cocker Spaniels, German Shepherd Dogs, and Setters).

### Clinical features

Drooping of the lip and ear on the affected side is common. Affected animals are unable to close the eyelid (or blink) or move the lip or ear. Keratoconjunctivitis sicca may develop from loss of lacrimal gland secretion. Many animals with facial nerve paralysis caused by middle ear disease also develop peripheral vestibular signs and/or Horner's syndrome. Rarely, a syndrome of hemifacial spasm with facial muscle contracture and lip retraction is seen, either acutely, as a result of facial nerve irritation, or chronically, resulting from muscle atrophy and contracture.

### Diagnosis

Idiopathic facial nerve paralysis can be diagnosed only after all other causes have been excluded. A complete neurologic examination should be performed to ensure that no other deficits suggestive of a brainstem lesion are present (see Table 65-9). Clinicopathologic testing (complete blood count [CBC], serum biochemistry profile, urinalysis) is required to check for systemic or metabolic disease. A suspicion of hypothyroidism warrants evaluation of thyroid function.

*Radiography.* Radiographs should be evaluated for changes in the tympanic bullae. Ventrolateral, oblique, lateral, and open-mouth radiographs of the skull should be taken. Radiographic evidence of otitis media or interna includes increased thickness of the tympanic bullae and petrous temporal bone and increased soft-tissue density within the bullae; however, radiographs often appear normal with acute infections. CT and MRI may be more sensitive techniques for detecting small amounts of fluid in the middle ear. Soft-tissue density within the bullae and bone lysis suggest a tumor. Nasopharyngeal polyps in cats cause soft-tissue bulla densities, but no bone lysis.

*Otoscopic examination.* After radiography, while the animal is still under general anesthesia, the external ear canal and tympanic membrane should be carefully examined using an otoscope or a small endoscope. The ear canal is flushed with warm 0.9% saline solution until the fluid obtained is clear and the tympanic membrane can be visualized. A sample is then obtained from the middle ear (via myringotomy, if the tympanic membrane is intact) for culture and cytology. Myringotomy is described in the text.

### Treatment and prognosis

No treatment for idiopathic facial nerve paralysis exists. If keratoconjunctivitis sicca is present, the eye should be medicated as needed. The paralysis may be permanent, or spontaneous recovery may occur in 2 to 6 weeks.

*Tumors and polyps.* If evaluation of the middle and inner ear reveals evidence of neoplasia (bony lysis or extensive soft-tissue proliferation), a biopsy should be performed, and surgery to debulk or remove the tumor considered. The prognosis for cure with benign nasopharyngeal polyps in this location in cats is excellent. Tumors of the bulla, bony labyrinth, ear canal, or peripheral nerve are less likely to be treated effectively with surgery alone. Radiotherapy or chemotherapy may be beneficial in some cases.

*Otitis media or interna.* Medical treatment for bacterial otitis media or interna can be attempted but is rarely effective. Systemic antibiotics are administered for 4 to 6 weeks. Pending culture results, treatment can be initiated using a broad-spectrum antibiotic such as a first-generation cephalosporin (cephalexin, 22 mg/kg orally [PO] q8h), a combination of amoxicillin and clavulanic acid (Clavamox, 12.5 to 25 mg/kg PO q8h), or enrofloxacin (5 mg/kg PO q12h).

If conservative treatment does not resolve the infection, or if radiographic evidence suggests fluid or tissue in the tympanic bulla or chronic bone changes in the bulla, ventral bulla osteotomy should be performed, followed by antibiotic therapy. Early recognition of inflammation and prompt initiation of appropriate therapy results in a good prognosis for recovery, although facial nerve paralysis may be permanent. Failure to treat otitis media or interna can result in ascent of the infection to the brainstem, progression of neurologic signs, and death.

## Trigeminal Nerve Paralysis

Idiopathic trigeminal nerve paralysis is seen in middle-aged and older dogs and rarely in cats. Nerve biopsy, if performed, reveals bilateral, nonsuppurative neuritis and demyelination of all motor branches. Bilateral paralysis of the motor component of cranial nerve V suddenly results in inability to close the jaw. The mouth hangs open, and food cannot be prehended; swallowing is normal. No obvious sensory deficit is present. Severe, rapid atrophy of the masticatory muscles may occur.

### Diagnosis and treatment

Diagnosis is based on signs and elimination of other possible causes. Rabies and inflammatory central nervous system diseases are unlikely in the absence of other signs; and neoplastic and traumatic disorders are not usually bilateral. Treatment consists of supportive care. Most dogs can drink and maintain their hydration if they are given water in a deep container. Handfeeding may be required. The prognosis is excellent; most patients recover completely in 2 to 4 weeks.

## HYPERCHYLOMICRONEMIA (TEXT P 1054)

Peripheral neuropathies occur in cats of all ages with defective lipoprotein lipase function and delayed clearance of chylomicrons. Most signs of hyperchylomicronemia are related to lipid deposition (xanthomas) in the skin and other tissues. Xanthomas can compress a nerve against bone, resulting in neuropathology. Horner's syndrome and tibial and radial nerve paralysis are most often seen. Blood samples are obviously lipemic, and laboratory tests reveal fasting hyperchylomicronemia. Diagnosis is by biopsy of the xanthomas or measurement of plasma lipoprotein lipase. Signs are reversible if hyperchylomicronemia is controlled by the feeding of a low-fat, high-fiber diet.

## ISCHEMIC NEUROMYOPATHY (TEXT P 1054)

Caudal aortic thromboembolism causing paralysis from ischemic damage to affected muscles and peripheral nerves is common in cats and rare in dogs. Acute onset of lower motor neuron (LMN) rear limb paralysis or paresis is seen. Femoral pulses are weak or absent; other nonneurologic signs are given in Chapter 7. Flaccidity and complete areflexia of the rear limbs are common, although sometimes the patellar reflex is maintained. With time (hours), contracture of ischemic muscle may cause rigid extension of the legs. A hypercoagulability disorder can usually be identified in dogs; endocarditis, neoplasia, nephrotic syndrome, hyperadrenocorticism, and heartworm disease should be considered. In cats cardiomyopathy is the most common underlying cause.

## POLYNEUROPATHY (TEXT PP 1055-1056)

Polyneuropathies affect more than one group of peripheral nerves, resulting in generalized LMN signs (flaccid muscle weakness or paralysis, marked muscle atrophy, decreased muscle tone, and reduced or absent reflexes). Proprioceptive deficits may be evident if the sensory portions of the nerves are severely affected.

Polyneuropathies may be any of the following:
- metabolic, associated with hypothyroidism, diabetes mellitus (especially cats), or insulinoma
- autoimmune, as a manifestation of systemic lupus erythematosus (SLE)
- paraneoplastic, with a variety of neoplasms (dogs)
- idiopathic, presumably immune mediated
- toxic, e.g., chronic organophosphate intoxication
- congenital or hereditary, as a breed-associated degenerative condition

### Diagnostic approach

Polyneuropathy should be suspected in any dog or cat with chronic, progressive LMN signs. EMG reveals evidence of denervation, and nerve conduction velocity is decreased in affected nerves. Peripheral nerve biopsy may be necessary to confirm the diagnosis. It is important to investigate known causes and attempt to reach a specific diagnosis.

Rarely, dogs with mononeuropathy or polyneuropathy have positive serology or polymerase chain reaction for *Ehrlichia canis* but no other signs of ehrlichiosis. In some dogs the neuropathy resolves after treatment with doxycycline (5 mg/kg PO q12h) or imidocarb dipropionate (5 mg/kg intramuscularly [IM] once).

### Metabolic Polyneuropathies
#### Diabetic polyneuropathy

All dogs and cats with confirmed peripheral neuropathy should be evaluated for diabetes mellitus. Signs of diabetic polyneuropathy usually are subtle or inapparent in dogs but can be dramatic in cats. Rear limb weakness, reluctance to jump, plantigrade rear limb stance, and tail weakness are characteristic. Physical findings may include rear limb hyporeflexia and marked muscle atrophy. Onset of signs generally is rapid (<1 week).

Diabetic polyneuropathy is likely when these neurologic signs are seen in a cat with diabetes mellitus. The diagnosis can be confirmed with biopsies of muscle and distal nerves. If the condition is diagnosed early, neurologic signs may improve once the diabetes is regulated.

#### Hypothyroid polyneuropathy

Dogs with polyneuropathy should also be evaluated for hypothyroidism. Hypothyroid polyneuropathy can cause diffuse LMN paralysis, unilateral peripheral vestibular disease, facial nerve paralysis, laryngeal paralysis, and megaesophagus in dogs. Nerve and muscle biopsy may show neuronal degeneration-regeneration and muscle fiber grouping indicative of neurogenic atrophy. In some dogs with mononeuropathy or polyneuropathy, neurologic signs resolve once thyroid hormone supplementation is initiated.

### Insulinoma and other tumors

Hypoglycemia in an older animal with polyneuropathy can indicate an insulin-secreting tumor. Other neoplastic processes (e.g., multicentric lymphoma, disseminated carcinoma) should also be considered in dogs and cats with polyneuropathies of no identifiable cause. Careful physical examination, thoracic and abdominal radiographs, abdominal ultrasonography, lymph node aspirates, and bone marrow examination may be warranted. In some cases removal of the offending neoplasm results in resolution of the clinical signs of polyneuropathy.

## Autoimmune Polyneuropathy

When systemic immune-mediated disease such as SLE is suspected, screening tests should include CBC, measurement of protein in the urine (i.e., protein/creatinine ratio), and analysis of synovial fluid. Skin lesions should undergo biopsy, and blood should be submitted for an antinuclear antibody titer. Immunosuppressive therapy should be initiated if evidence of immune-mediated disease is present (see Chapter 93).

## Idiopathic Polyneuropathy

A number of chronic, inflammatory, demyelinating polyneuropathies have been reported in dogs and cats. These disorders may resolve spontaneously or with corticosteroid therapy. Unfortunately, many idiopathic polyneuropathies in dogs and cats respond poorly to immunosuppressive therapy.

## Toxic Polyneuropathies

Toxins that can cause polyneuropathies include organophosphates, heavy metals, and industrial chemicals. Organophosphates, in particular, can have a delayed neurotoxic effect; demyelination may develop 1 to 6 weeks after most of the chemical has been excreted. Affected animals are weak but do not show classic autonomic signs of organophosphate intoxication (see Chapter 69). With chronic exposure, samples of hair, blood, fat, or liver may contain the toxin; and plasma acetylcholinesterase is low. Toxic neuropathy may be suspected from nerve biopsy findings. Improvement can be expected in 3 to 12 weeks once the substance is removed and reexposure is prevented.

# ACUTE POLYRADICULONEURITIS (TEXT PP 1056-1057)

Acute polyradiculoneuritis (Coonhound paralysis) is the most common acute poly-neuropathy in dogs. It affects dogs of any breed and gender; most affected dogs are adults. A similar disease is rare in cats. The disorder may result from an immune response to some component of raccoon saliva, but acute polyradiculoneuritis occurs in many dogs and cats with no possible exposure to raccoons. Previous systemic illness or vaccination (particularly rabies vaccination) has been implicated, but often no initiating factor can be identified.

### Clinical features

Weakness and hyporeflexia are sometimes preceded by a change in bark (e.g., hoarseness). Rear limb weakness ascends rapidly, resulting in flaccid, symmetric tetraplegia in most cases. Time from onset to complete paralysis may be as short as 12 hours or as long as 1 week. Paralyzed dogs maintain their appetite and are afebrile. In a few cases death results from respiratory paralysis.

*Neurologic examination.* Remarkably decreased muscle tone and rapid muscle atrophy are found. Motor impairment is more remarkable than sensory loss. Some dogs are hyperesthetic, reacting vigorously to mild stimulation. (Hyperesthesia does not occur with tick paralysis or botulism, the major differential diagnoses.) Spinal reflexes are diminished or absent; the perineal reflex is normal, as are bladder and rectal function. The cranial nerves generally are not involved, although a few severely affected dogs have bilateral facial nerve paralysis.

### Diagnosis

The diagnosis is suspected on the basis of clinical and neurologic findings. EMG reveals diffuse denervation after approximately 6 days of paralysis, and motor nerve conduction velocities are slow in affected nerves. Cerebrospinal fluid (CSF) is usually normal, although a mild increase in protein concentration may be seen.

### Treatment and prognosis

No specific treatment exists. Corticosteroids have not proved beneficial. Nursing care is very important; most dogs begin to improve after the first week, but full recovery may take months. The prognosis for recovery in dogs is good, although some dogs never recover completely. The prognosis for complete recovery in cats is poor. Recurrence can occur, particularly if the animal is reexposed to the inciting agent.

## TICK PARALYSIS (TEXT PP 1057-1058)

Flaccid, rapidly ascending motor paralysis occurs in dogs infested with toxin-producing strains of the common wood tick (*Dermacentor variabilis* and *Dermacentor andersoni*). Signs occur 5 to 9 days after tick attachment.

### Clinical features

Rear limb weakness rapidly progresses to recumbency over 24 to 72 hours, resulting in complete LMN paralysis. Loss of muscle tone and spinal reflexes occurs without significant muscle atrophy. Pain perception is normal, and no hyperesthesia is present. Usually the cranial nerves are not affected, although cough, altered voice, and dysphagia may occur, and mild jaw and facial weakness are sometimes seen. Without treatment, death from respiratory paralysis occurs in 1 to 5 days.

### Diagnosis and treatment

The diagnosis is based on the history (including geographic location) and clinical signs. Sometimes a tick is found on the patient and the diagnosis is confirmed by documenting rapid improvement after tick removal. EMG reveals absence of spontaneous activity (no denervation potentials). Removal of the tick or application of insecticide results in dramatic improvement within 24 to 72 hours. The prognosis for complete recovery is good.

## BOTULISM (TEXT P 1058)

Botulism is rare in dogs and cats. It results from ingestion of spoiled food or carrion containing preformed *Clostridium botulinum* toxin type C, which causes complete LMN paralysis. Signs occur hours or days after ingestion of the toxin.

### Clinical features

Progressive, ascending LMN paralysis affecting both spinal and cranial nerves is seen. Affected dogs are profoundly weak, with loss of muscle tone and absent spinal reflexes, but no muscle atrophy. Proprioception and pain perception are normal. Extensive cranial nerve involvement is common. Affected dogs may drool, cough, and have difficulty eating. Regurgitation from megaesophagus is common. Mydriasis and loss of the palpebral response may be seen in severely affected dogs.

### Diagnosis

The diagnosis is based on clinical findings and/or history of access to spoiled food. Botulism is especially likely if an outbreak of LMN paralysis is seen in a group of dogs. Rabies must be considered as a differential diagnosis in severely affected dogs, but it usually is rapidly progressive and associated with abnormal mentation. Muscle weakness in the face, jaw, and pharynx is much more pronounced with botulism than would be expected with acute polyradiculoneuritis or tick paralysis. Electrodiagnostic studies are as described for tick paralysis. Botulinum toxin (types C and D) may be demonstrated in the blood, vomitus, or feces.

### Treatment and prognosis

No specific treatment exists. Laxatives and enemas may help remove unabsorbed toxin from the gastrointestinal tract if ingestion was recent. Oral broad-spectrum antibiotics can reduce the intestinal population of clostridial organisms. Administration of commercially available trivalent antitoxin (types A, B, and E) is not likely to be effective. Type C antitoxin is recommended but is not readily available. Most dogs recover in 1 to 3 weeks with only supportive care.

## PROTOZOAL POLYRADICULONEURITIS (TEXT P 1058)

Rapidly progressive, flaccid paralysis with hyporeflexia and dysphagia (similar to tick paralysis or botulism) occasionally is seen in adult dogs or puppies infected with *Toxoplasma gondii* or *Neospora caninum*. EMG reveals denervation secondary to extensive involvement of the ventral nerve roots. *N. caninum* can also cause a syndrome of polyradiculoneuritis and myositis affecting only the rear limbs of young dogs. Progressive rear limb paresis occurs, with loss of patellar and (eventually) withdrawal reflexes and some pain on muscle palpation. Over time, quadriceps muscle contraction occurs, fixing the rear limbs in rigid extension.

### Diagnosis

Increases in serum creatine kinase and aspartate aminotransferase activities are common with either clinical presentation, because concurrent myositis is usually present. CSF analysis may reveal inflammatory changes and occasionally the presence of organisms. Evidence of systemic disease (especially liver or pulmonary involvement) may also be found, and cats with toxoplasmosis may have uveitis and chorioretinitis. Serology may be positive, but it can be difficult to interpret. Definitive diagnosis requires biopsy of the affected muscles and nerves. A mononuclear inflammatory reaction and many organisms are typical findings. Immunocytochemical stains can be performed to distinguish between *Toxoplasma* and *Neospora*.

### Treatment and prognosis

Some success is reported in dogs treated with clindamycin (5.5 to 11 mg/kg PO, subcutaneously [SC], or IM q12h), but severely affected animals are unlikely to respond.

## DYSAUTONOMIA (TEXT PP 1058-1059)

Dysautonomia is a disorder of the autonomic nervous system that has recently been recognized in dogs and a few cats in the United States, particularly in the Midwest. Lesions in the autonomic ganglia are consistent with a toxic etiology, but the cause is unknown. Signs reflect loss of neurons in the sympathetic and parasympathetic nervous systems, particularly involving the urinary, alimentary, and ocular systems.

### Clinical features

Young cats and dogs are most often affected. Clinical signs have a rapid onset and progression (48 hours). They include depression, anorexia, light-insensitive mydriasis, prolapse of the nictitating membrane, constipation, and regurgitation caused by megaesophagus. The mucous membranes of the eyes, mouth, and nose are dry. Other signs may include bradycardia, weakness, proprioceptive deficits, and loss of the anal reflex. Dysuria and urine retention resulting from bladder atony are reported in most dogs (80% to 100%) and some cats (17% to 40%).

### Diagnosis

The diagnosis is suspected on the basis of clinical signs. Thoracic and abdominal radiographs may reveal megaesophagus, aspiration pneumonia, and a distended bladder. The bladder is easily expressed.

*Pharmacologic testing.* Further support is gained by pharmacologic testing of the pupillary light reflex and bladder. Ocular administration of very dilute pilocarpine (Isoptocarpine 1%, diluted to 0.05% or 0.1% with saline) produces dramatic miosis within 30 to 45 minutes in affected animals. Administration of bethanechol (0.04 mg/kg SC) enables many affected animals to void urine normally and completely. Definitive diagnosis requires demonstration of lesions within the autonomic nervous system at necropsy.

### Treatment and prognosis

Treatment is supportive and includes fluid administration, forced feeding, lubricating eye ointments, enemas, and bladder emptying. Bethanechol administration may improve urinary function, and pilocarpine may be administered to stimulate tear production and relieve photophobia. Some animals recover spontaneously, but the prognosis is generally poor, with a mortality rate of >70%.

## MYASTHENIA GRAVIS (TEXT PP 1059-1061)

Myasthenia gravis (MG) is a neuromuscular disorder characterized by weakness that is exacerbated by exercise and alleviated by rest. Two forms have been described: congenital and acquired.

### Congenital form

The congenital form of MG results from an inherited deficiency of acetylcholine receptors (ACHRs) in skeletal muscle. Signs of impaired neuromuscular transmission first become evident at 3 to 8 weeks of age. The disorder has been recognized in English Springer Spaniels, Smooth-Haired Fox Terriers, Jack Russell Terriers, and a few cats. An unusual, poorly classified, transient congenital myasthenic syndrome has also been identified in Miniature Dachshunds; signs in these dogs resolve with maturity.

### Acquired MG

The acquired form of MG is a common immune-mediated disorder in which antibodies are directed against the ACHRs in skeletal muscle. It affects dogs of any breed. German Shepherd Dogs, Golden Retrievers, Labrador Retrievers, and Dachshunds are most commonly affected, but this may simply reflect the popularity of these breeds. Breeds that seem to be at increased risk relative to their popularity include Akitas, some terrier breeds, German Shorthaired Pointers, and Chihuahuas. Cats are rarely affected, but breed predispositions include the Abyssinian and Somali. A bimodal age distribution occurs in dogs, with young dogs (mean age, 2 to 3 years) and old dogs (mean age, 9 to 10 years) making up most of the affected population.

### Clinical features

The characteristic clinical abnormality in most animals with MG is appendicular muscle weakness that worsens with exercise and improves with rest. Mentation, postural reactions, and reflexes are normal, although reflexes may be fatiguable with repeated stimulation. Additional signs may include excessive salivation and regurgitation caused by megaesophagus. Megaesophagus is seen in 90% of dogs with acquired MG; it is found less consistently in cats and is less common with congenital MG. Dysphagia, hoarse character of the bark or meow, persistently dilated pupils, or facial muscle weakness may also be seen.

*Focal MG.* A focal form of MG, with signs attributable to megaesophagus but no appendicular weakness, has been reported in dogs. Dogs with focal MG exhibit weakness of the pharyngeal, laryngeal, and/or facial muscles, and they may have a fatiguable palpebral reflex. Up to 40% of all dogs with adult-onset megaesophagus actually suffer from acquired, focal MG. This disorder should always be considered in dogs with megaesophagus.

*Fulminant MG.* An acute, fulminating form of acquired MG, causing a rapid onset of severe appendicular muscle weakness, has also been recognized. Affected animals are often unable to stand and cannot even raise their heads. This form of MG is usually associated with severe megaesophagus and aspiration pneumonia. Profound muscle weakness and severe pneumonia may lead to respiratory failure and death.

### Diagnosis

MG should be considered in any dog with generalized muscular weakness and in all dogs with acquired megaesophagus. Definitive diagnosis of acquired MG is made by demonstrating circulating anti-ACHR antibodies. This test is positive in 90% of all dogs and cats with acquired MG and in 98% of those with generalized acquired MG.

---

**Box 73-1**

## Tensilon Test Protocol

1. Place an IV catheter.
2. Premedicate with IM atropine (0.04 mg/kg) to minimize muscarinic side effects.
3. Have equipment available for intubation and ventilation.
4. Exercise to the point of detectable weakness.
5. Administer IV edrophonium chloride (Tensilon):
   0.1-0.2 mg/kg (dogs)
   0.2 mg/kg (cats)

---

*IM*, Intramuscular; *IV*, intravenous.

False-positive results have not been documented. Rarely, dogs with acquired MG are negative for circulating ACHR antibodies, but immune complexes can be demonstrated at the neuromuscular junction using immunocytochemical methods.

*Tensilon test.* While results of the serum antibody test are pending, or in animals with suspected congenital MG, support for the diagnosis can be gained by a positive response to administration of edrophonium chloride (Tensilon; see Box 73-1). Most animals with MG show obvious improvement in clinical signs (e.g., resolution of weakness) within 30 to 60 seconds, with the effect lasting approximately 5 minutes. Some dogs with other myopathic or neuropathic disorders may show minor improvement, but a dramatic response is very suggestive of MG.

Failure to respond does not rule out MG, however. The response can be difficult to assess in dogs and cats with focal MG; also, many cats with generalized MG have an unpredictable response, and approximately 50% of dogs with acute fulminating MG do not respond because they have marked antibody-mediated destruction of ACHRs.

*Other tests.* EMG can aid in the diagnosis of MG. However, anesthesia should be avoided in animals with megaesophagus because of the risk of aspiration during recovery. Thoracic radiographs should be assessed for megaesophagus, aspiration pneumonia, and thymoma. If a cranial mediastinal mass is identified, fine-needle aspiration cytology should be used to check for thymoma—a tumor that has been identified in <5% of dogs and >25% of cats with acquired MG.

The patient should also be evaluated for underlying immune-mediated or neoplastic disorders. Concurrent immune-mediated disorders are common in dogs with MG and include hypothyroidism, thrombocytopenia, hemolytic anemia, hypoadrenocorticism, polymyositis, and SLE. MG may also develop as a paraneoplastic disorder in association with a wide variety of tumors, including hepatic carcinoma, anal sac adenocarcinoma, osteosarcoma, cutaneous lymphoma, and primary lung tumors. Drug-induced MG has also been documented in hyperthyroid cats treated with methimazole.

### Treatment

Treatment of acquired MG includes supportive care and administration of anticholinesterase drugs, and occasionally immunosuppressive agents. Surgical removal should be considered in animals with a thymoma, as it can result in dramatic resolution of MG signs. Management of megaesophagus is discussed in Chapter 31. Antibiotics that can impair neuromuscular transmission (ampicillin, aminoglycosides) should be avoided in dogs with MG that have aspiration pneumonia or other bacterial infections.

*Anticholinesterases.* Anticholinesterase drugs are commonly used to improve muscular strength. Pyridostigmine bromide (Mestinon, 1 to 2 mg/kg PO q8h) has been used in dogs. Pyridostigmine bromide syrup (5 mg/kg PO q12h, diluted 1:1 with water) is recommended for cats. In both dogs and cats the dose must be individualized on the basis of clinical response. Ideally, feeding should be timed to coincide with peak drug effect. In dogs initially unable to tolerate oral medication because of severe megaesophagus, neostigmine methylsulfate (Prostigmin, 0.01 to 0.04 mg/kg IM q6-8h) can be used. Note: Anticholinesterase drugs can effectively control appendicular muscle weakness in most animals, but their effect on esophageal function is variable.

If an animal appears to be responding to these drugs but then deteriorates, underdose (myasthenic crisis) or overdose (cholinergic crisis) should be suspected. Clinically, these problems are indistinguishable; a Tensilon test must be performed to distinguish between them. Patients in a myasthenic crisis improve with edrophonium, whereas those in a cholinergic crisis become transiently worse or show no change.

**Corticosteroids.** Administration of corticosteroids and other immunosuppressive drugs results in improvement in some dogs with acquired MG, but whenever possible their administration should be delayed until the animal is stable and aspiration pneumonia has resolved. When administered at high doses, corticosteroids commonly cause transient worsening of muscular weakness in dogs with MG. Therapy should always be initiated with a low dose (e.g., prednisone, 0.5 mg/kg/day) and the dosage gradually increased over 2 to 4 weeks to the level required for immunosuppression (2 to 4 mg/kg/day). Administration of azathioprine (Imuran, 2 mg/kg/day) alone or in combination with prednisone results in clinical improvement and a decrease in ACHR antibodies in many dogs.

### Prognosis

Response to medical management can be good if aspiration pneumonia is not severe and the complications of aspiration and anticholinesterase overdose are avoided. Severe aspiration pneumonia, persistent megaesophagus, acute fulminating MG, and the presence of a thymoma or other neoplasm are all associated with a poor prognosis for recovery. Most affected dogs die of aspiration pneumonia or are euthanized within 12 months.

It is important to recognize that many dogs with acquired MG go into spontaneous, permanent clinical remission approximately 6 months after diagnosis (range, 1 to 18 months), regardless of the treatment used. (Remission is unlikely to occur in animals with MG occurring secondary to a thymoma or other neoplasm.) Although no consistent relationship exists between disease severity and serum ACHR antibody concentration among animals, sequential antibody measurements in an individual animal can be correlated with disease progression or remission. Therefore it is recommended that ACHR antibody concentrations be monitored every 4 to 8 weeks in animals being treated for MG.

# 74

# Disorders of Muscle

## (Text pp 1062-1070)

### INFLAMMATORY MYOPATHIES (TEXT PP 1062-1065)

#### Masticatory Myositis

Masticatory muscle myositis (MMM) is a widely reported inflammatory disorder in dogs that involves primarily or exclusively the muscles of mastication, which are composed primarily of a unique myofiber (type 2M). Necrosis and phagocytosis are limited to these fibers, and circulating IgG is directed against the unique myosin component of these fibers. The cause is unknown, but the process suggests an immune-mediated mechanism. MMM can occur in any dog, but German Shepherd Dogs, retrieving breeds, Doberman Pinschers, and other large-breed dogs are most commonly affected. Young or middle-aged dogs are most often affected. The disorder occurs in two forms: acute and chronic.

#### Clinical features

The acute form is associated with recurrent, painful swelling of the masticatory muscles, particularly the temporalis and masseter muscles. The swelling may cause exophthalmus. Most dogs are presented for anorexia and depression; pyrexia, submandibular and prescapular lymphadenopathy, and tonsillitis are variably present. Affected dogs are reluctant to eat and may salivate profusely. Palpation of these muscles and attempts to open the mouth cause pain and resistance.

The chronic form is more common. Affected dogs have progressive, severe atrophy of the temporalis and masseter muscles. They may have difficulty opening their mouths to eat, but they are otherwise bright, alert, and systemically normal. The globes may sink deep into the orbits because of the dramatic loss of muscle mass. The chronic form may occur after repeated acute episodes or without any history of signs related to acute episodes.

#### Diagnosis

The diagnosis is suspected on the basis of clinical findings. In the acute form, various disorders that affect the teeth, eyes, mouth, and temporomandibular joints must be considered. Severe, nonpainful atrophy of the masticatory muscles with chronic MMM must be differentiated from atrophy caused by trigeminal neuropathy or widespread polymyositis.

*Routine tests.* Complete blood count (CBC) may reveal mild anemia and neutrophilic leukocytosis; occasionally a peripheral eosinophilia is found. Serum creatine kinase (CK), aspartate aminotransferase (AST), and globulin concentrations may be increased, particularly in the acute phase of the disease. Proteinuria sometimes occurs.

*Other tests.* Circulating antibodies against type 2M fibers can be detected in the serum of >80% of dogs with MMM. Electromyogram (EMG) can help confirm the presence of muscle disease restricted to the masticatory muscles, although it is normal in a few chronically affected dogs when most of the muscle has been replaced by fibrous connective tissue.

*Biopsy.* Muscle biopsy allows definitive diagnosis of MMM. In addition to submission of formalin-fixed samples, muscle tissue should be frozen or chemically fixed (e.g., using acetone) to permit histochemical and immunohistochemical stains that identify antibody bound to type 2M muscle fibers.

### Treatment and prognosis

Prednisone (1 to 2 mg/kg orally [PO] q12h) can result in rapid clinical remission. After 3 weeks the dose can be decreased (to 1 mg/kg q24h) and then gradually tapered over 4 to 6 months to the lowest effective alternate-day dose. An inadequate dose or treatment for an insufficient length of time is associated with a high rate of relapse. Dogs that do not respond adequately or that relapse each time the dose is decreased may benefit from azathioprine (Imuran, 2 mg/kg PO q24h, then q48h). Dogs treated aggressively have a good prognosis for recovery. They should be carefully monitored for relapse (using jaw mobility and discomfort and serum CK), particularly as the corticosteroid dose is tapered. Lifelong treatment may be required.

## Canine Idiopathic Polymyositis

Idiopathic polymyositis is a diffuse inflammation of skeletal muscle presumed to be an autoimmune process. Large-breed adult dogs are most commonly affected, with many reported cases in German Shepherd Dogs. A unique, focal form of polymyositis confined to the extraocular muscles and resulting in acute bilateral exophthalmus has recently been described in young dogs.

### Clinical features

Mild to severe weakness that may be exacerbated by exercise is the most common feature of idiopathic polymyositis. Lameness or a stiff, stilted gait may also be seen. Muscles are painful in some dogs, whereas nonpainful, severe atrophy occurs in others. Affected dogs may regurgitate as a result of megaesophagus. Occasionally, dysphagia, excessive salivation, and a weak bark are reported. Signs may be intermittent in mild or early cases. Some dogs with acute, severe disease are pyrexic and experience generalized pain. Neurologic examination reveals normal proprioception, mental status, and cranial nerves. Muscle atrophy is usually prominent, especially involving the temporalis and masseter muscles.

### Diagnosis

The diagnosis is based on clinical signs, serum CK concentration, EMG, and muscle biopsy. High serum CK (twofold to 100-fold increase) and AST activities are seen in most affected dogs at rest; even more dramatic increases are common after exercise. Gamma globulins may also be increased. EMG can be performed to document that multiple muscle groups are involved and to select a severely affected muscle for biopsy.

*Biopsy.* Definitive diagnosis requires muscle biopsy (see text). Occasionally a biopsy specimen is normal because of the multifocal, patchy nature of the disease, but this does not preclude a diagnosis of myositis if the clinical findings, EMG, and serum CK and AST activities suggest the diagnosis.

*Investigating the cause.* Generalized immune-mediated disease (e.g., systemic lupus erythematosus), neoplasia, and infectious myositis (e.g., *Toxoplasma, Neospora*) should be investigated as causes. CBC, synovial fluid analysis, urinalysis, serum ANA titer, serology, and/or immunohistochemical staining of muscle biopsies for protozoal antigens should be performed. Thoracic radiographs and abdominal ultrasound should be assessed for evidence of neoplasia, megaesophagus, and aspiration pneumonia. Lymph node aspirates and bone marrow biopsy may also be indicated. If the results of all these tests are normal, a diagnosis of idiopathic polymyositis is made.

### Treatment and prognosis

Prednisone (1 to 2 mg/kg q12h for 14 days, then q24h for 14 days, then q48h) results in dramatic clinical improvement and recovery in most dogs. Management of megaesophagus is discussed in Chapter 31. Aspiration pneumonia, if present, should be treated with antibiotics. Prednisone should be continued for at least 4 weeks at decreasing doses, with long-term treatment for 12 months or more occasionally required. Azathioprine should be administered if an inadequate response to prednisone is seen. The prognosis for recovery is good in dogs without severe megaesophagus or aspiration pneumonia if no underlying neoplastic cause is identified.

## Feline Idiopathic Polymyositis

An acquired inflammatory disorder of skeletal muscle similar to canine polymyositis has been described in cats. The cause is not known. Viral infection has been speculated; thymoma may be a contributing factor in some adult cats. An immune basis is likely in many cases.

### Clinical features

Age at onset is highly variable (from 6 months to 14 years). Affected cats have sudden onset of weakness with pronounced ventral neck flexion; they are unable to jump and have a tendency to sit or lie down after walking short distances. Muscle pain may be evident.

### Diagnosis

The diagnosis is suspected on the basis of clinical features, increased serum CK and AST activities, multifocal EMG abnormalities, and muscle biopsy findings (see text). Many affected cats are slightly hypokalemic, and some clinical features of this disease mimic mild thiamine deficiency. Therefore evaluation of the response to thiamine (10 to 20 mg/day intramuscularly) and correction of hypokalemia are recommended before one proceeds with extensive diagnostic testing.

*Investigating the cause.* Serum titers against *Toxoplasma gondii* should be evaluated, as should tests for feline leukemia virus antigen and feline immunodeficiency virus antibody. A complete drug history should be obtained to eliminate the possibility of drug-induced polymyositis. Thoracic and abdominal radiographs and abdominal ultrasound should be considered to look for an underlying neoplastic cause.

### Treatment and prognosis

Empiric treatment for *Toxoplasma* myositis (clindamycin 12.5 to 25 mg/kg PO q12h) is sometimes recommended. If the cat shows a dramatic response to clindamycin, treatment should be continued for at least 6 weeks. It is important to realize, however, that spontaneous recovery or remission is observed in at least 30% of cats with PM. Corticosteroid therapy (prednisone, 4 to 6 mg/kg/day initially, tapered over 2 months) aids recovery in some cats. Recurrence is common.

## Dermatomyositis

Dermatomyositis is an uncommon disease of dogs, characterized by dermatitis and polymyositis. Familial canine dermatomyositis has been reported in juvenile Rough-Coated and Smooth-Coated Collies and in Shetland Sheepdogs. Sporadic cases have been observed in Welsh Corgis, Australian Cattle Dogs, and Border Collies.

### Clinical features

Skin lesions appear during the first 3 months of life and may improve or resolve with time; the course often fluctuates. Lesions include erythema, ulcers, crusts, scales, and alopecia on the inner surfaces of the pinnae, and on the head and skin surfaces subjected to trauma (tail, elbows, hocks, sternum). Mild pruritus may be present.

Severely affected dogs may develop generalized muscle atrophy, facial palsy, decreased jaw tone, weakness, and stiff gait. Dysphagia is common, and regurgitation may result from megaesophagus. Some dogs with relatively severe skin lesions have no evidence of muscle disease.

### Diagnosis and treatment

Skin and muscle biopsies and EMG findings aid diagnosis (see text). Response to immunosuppressive doses of corticosteroids is variable. Dogs with confirmed dermatomyositis should not be bred.

## Protozoal Myositis

Myositis caused by *T. gondii* can occur alone or in conjunction with myelitis, meningitis, or polyradiculoneuritis in dogs and cats (see Chapters 71 and 73). Similar syndromes caused by *Neospora caninum* can occur in dogs. Lesions may be found in the lung, liver, eye, central nervous system, and muscle.

### Clinical features and diagnosis

Clinical signs referable to protozoal myositis typically include muscle pain, swelling or atrophy, and weakness. Increases in serum CK and AST activities are common, and serum titers for the offending organism may be positive. EMG may reveal spontaneous activity in affected muscles. Definitive diagnosis requires muscle biopsy; a mononuclear inflammatory reaction is present, and organisms are often seen. Immunohistochemical stains can be used to identify the organisms and to differentiate between *T. gondii* and *N. caninum* in affected dogs.

**Treatment**

Success has been reported with clindamycin (12.5 to 25 mg/kg PO q12h) for 14 days, but more prolonged treatment (4 to 6 weeks) may be advisable.

## METABOLIC MYOPATHIES (TEXT PP 1065-1066)

Myopathies may develop in association with hyperadrenocorticism, exogenous corticosteroid administration, and perhaps hypothyroidism. In cats a myopathy associated with hypokalemia has been reported.

### Glucocorticoid Excess

Spontaneous hyperadrenocorticism (Cushing's disease) or exogenous administration of glucocorticoids, especially in high doses, can result in a degenerative myopathy. Muscle weakness and atrophy are common. Rarely, affected dogs develop limb rigidity, stiff gait, and hyperextension of all four limbs.

**Diagnosis and treatment**

The diagnosis is suspected with a history of exogenous steroid administration or clinical findings consistent with steroid excess (polyuria [PU] and polydipsia [PD], hair loss, pendulous abdomen, thin skin). Diagnostic tests for hyperadrenocorticism (see Chapter 53) should be performed. Control of excess glucocorticoids may result in clinical improvement. However, in most dogs the prognosis is poor for complete resolution of the myopathy.

### Hypothyroidism

Hypothyroidism may be associated with a subclinical myopathy in dogs. The weakness and reduced exercise tolerance seen in hypothyroid dogs may be related to this myopathy. Electrodiagnostic findings are normal.

### Hypokalemic Polymyopathy

A polymyopathy linked to total body potassium (K) depletion has been recognized in cats. Cats with chronic renal failure and those consuming acidifying diets are most commonly affected, but cats with PU and PD secondary to hyperthyroidism and cats with anorexia from any cause may also be at risk. A similar syndrome has been reported in Burmese kittens, with a probable hereditary basis.

**Clinical features**

The predominant clinical feature is weakness characterized by persistent ventroflexion of the neck, a stiff and stilted gait, and reluctance to move. Some affected cats exhibit excessive scapular movement during walking. Muscle pain may be apparent, but neurologic examination is otherwise unremarkable, with normal postural reactions and spinal reflexes. Clinical signs may have an acute onset and be episodic.

**Diagnosis**

Serum CK activity is usually high (10 to 30 times normal) and serum K is decreased (<3.5 mEq/L); fractional urinary excretion of K may be increased. Many affected cats have renal disease, so serum urea and creatinine concentrations may be increased. However, interpretation of these indexes and the urine specific gravity can be difficult, because hypokalemia itself can decrease renal blood flow and interfere with urine-concentrating mechanisms. EMG and muscle biopsy help distinguish this condition from inflammatory polymyositis.

**Treatment and prognosis**

Signs usually resolve after parenteral or oral K supplementation. Oral treatment with K-gluconate is recommended for mildly affected cats (Kaon Elixir, 2.5 to 5 mEq/cat PO q12h for 2 days, then q24h). The dose is adjusted based on serum K levels. Cats with more dramatic hypokalemia (<2.5 mEq/L) or those with severe muscular weakness causing respiratory compromise initially require parenteral administration of lactated Ringer's solution, intravenously or subcutaneously, supplemented with at least 80 mEq/L of potassium chloride per liter of fluid. (Note: Intravenous supplementation of K should not exceed 0.5 mEq/kg/hr.) Oral supplementation with potassium gluconate may be beneficial long term. Monitoring of serum K concentration periodically is recommended.

## INHERITED MYOPATHIES (TEXT PP 1066-1068)

### Muscular Dystrophy

Muscular dystrophies (MDs) are a group of inherited myopathies characterized by progressive degeneration of skeletal muscle. Originally described in Golden Retrievers, dystrophic conditions have now been characterized in many breeds of dog including the Irish Terrier, Samoyed, Rottweiler, Belgian Shepherd, Miniature Schnauzer, Pembroke Welsh Corgi, Alaskan Malamute, Wire-Haired Fox Terrier, German Shorthaired Pointer, Brittany Spaniel, and Rat Terrier.

The clinical syndrome is similar in all affected breeds, although the clinical severity and precise genetic mutation may be different in each. In many breeds, including Golden Retrievers and Irish Terriers, an X-linked inheritance has been documented, causing the disease to be clinically apparent in male dogs and carried by female dogs. No effective treatment exists.

#### Clinical features

MD is well described in Golden Retrievers. All affected male dogs have the same genetic lesion, but the severity of clinical expression is variable. Puppies with MD are often stunted, even before weaning. Abduction of the elbows, a bunny-hopping gait, and difficulty opening the mouth may be noted. With time, affected puppies develop a progressively more stilted gait, exercise intolerance, a plantigrade stance, atrophy of the truncal, limb, and temporalis muscles, and muscle contractures. Muscle strength deteriorates until approximately 6 months of age, when the signs tend to stabilize. Proprioceptive positioning and spinal reflexes are normal, but spinal reflexes may be difficult to elicit if muscle fibrosis and joint contractures are present. Severely affected dogs may develop pharyngeal or esophageal dysfunction. Cardiac failure occurs occasionally.

#### Diagnosis

MD should be suspected when typical clinical signs are seen in a young male puppy of any predisposed breed. Serum CK levels are markedly increased as early as 1 week of age and peak at 6 to 8 weeks of age. Very dramatic increases in CK occur after exercise. EMG and muscle biopsy (histopathology and immunocytochemistry) are useful for diagnosis (see text).

#### Muscular dystrophy in cats

An X-linked MD has also been reported in cats. Clinical signs first appear at 5 to 6 months of age. Affected cats exhibit marked generalized muscular hypertrophy, protrusion of the tongue, excessive salivation, stiff gait, and bunny hopping. Megaesophagus is common. Serum CK is greatly elevated (often >30,000 U/L). Diagnosis requires muscle biopsy and dystrophin immunostaining.

### Hereditary Labrador Retriever Myopathy

Hereditary Labrador Retriever myopathy is a degenerative myopathy inherited as an autosomal recessive trait in both male and female Labrador Retrievers. It is also called *autosomal recessive MD.*

#### Clinical features

Age at onset of signs is variable (6 weeks to 6 months), but signs usually become evident by 3 to 4 months of age. A low head carriage (ventroflexion), muscular weakness, and a stiff, stilted gait are common. The back may be arched, and a bunny-hopping gait may develop with exercise. Activity, excitement, exercise, and cold temperatures exacerbate the clinical signs and may precipitate collapse. Affected dogs often have carpal overextension, carpal valgus deformity, and splaying of the toes. Muscle atrophy may be marked, especially in the proximal limbs and the muscles of mastication.

Affected dogs are bright and alert. Their muscles are not painful and, although the animals are weak, conscious proprioception is normal. Spinal reflexes are generally reduced or absent, even in mildly affected dogs. Megaesophagus causing regurgitation has been seen in a few affected dogs.

### Diagnosis and prognosis

Serum CK activity is usually normal. EMG and muscle biopsy are used for diagnosis (see text). In most cases the clinical signs stabilize between 6 and 12 months of age, so many affected dogs remain functional as pets.

## Myotonia

Myotonia is a rare muscle disorder that has been reported in Chow Chows, Staffordshire Bull Terriers, Labrador Retrievers, Rhodesian Ridgebacks, Great Danes, and individual dogs of a number of other breeds. It has also been reported in cats.

### Clinical features

Myotonia (continued active contraction and delayed relaxation of muscle) is characterized clinically by generalized muscle stiffness and hypertrophy that begins at a young age (2 to 6 months). Animals with myotonia are neurologically normal; no abnormalities of proprioception or mentation are present. Cold weather, excitement, and exercise exacerbate the clinical signs. Affected dogs may remain in rigid recumbency for up to 30 seconds if they are suddenly placed in lateral recumbency.

### Diagnosis and treatment

Serum CK and AST activities may be increased, indicating muscle fiber necrosis. EMG and muscle biopsy may be required for diagnosis, although muscle biopsy alone is rarely diagnostic. Treatment with procainamide (10 to 30 mg/kg PO q6h), phenytoin (20 to 35 mg/kg PO q12h), or mexiletine (Mexitil, 8 mg/kg PO q8h) is beneficial in some cases. Avoidance of cold temperatures is advised. Most dogs are euthanized because of the severity of signs.

## MISCELLANEOUS

A number of genetically based noninflammatory myopathies have been described in dogs and cats (see text). Common clinical signs include exercise intolerance; muscular weakness; a stiff, stilted gait; muscle tremors; and muscle atrophy. Establishing the precise cause of a metabolic myopathy can be difficult. Sometimes metabolic testing can be beneficial. Evaluation of plasma lactate and pyruvate before and after exercise and quantitative analysis of urinary organic acids and plasma, urinary, and muscular carnitine may also help to determine the affected biochemical pathway. This testing, although expensive, is recommended in all dogs with unexplained weakness and exercise-induced collapse. Histologic and ultrastructual examination of skeletal muscle also aids diagnosis.

## Malignant Hyperthermia

Malignant hyperthermia is a rare hypermetabolic disorder of skeletal muscle that results from a genetic defect of intracellular calcium homeostasis. In genetically susceptible dogs, various triggers (exertion, heat, anoxia, mechanical stress, administration of halothane anesthesia or succinylcholine) result in dramatic muscular contraction, lactic acidemia, and hyperthermia. Definitive diagnosis relies on physiologic testing on specially prepared muscle biopsies or identification of the defective gene in affected dogs.

## Drugs Used in Neurologic Disorders

| Drug name (trade name) | Purpose | Recommended dose | |
|---|---|---|---|
| | | Dog | Cat |
| Acetylpromazine (Acepromazine) | Restraint, sedation, relaxation | 0.1-0.2 mg/kg IM q6h | 0.1-0.2 mg/kg IM q6h |
| Activated charcoal (1 g/5 ml water) | Gastrointestinal adsorbent | 10 ml/kg | 10 ml/kg |
| Acetylsalicylic acid (Aspirin) | Analgesia, antiinflammatory | 25 mg/kg PO q8h | 10 mg/kg PO q48h |
| | Antithrombotic | 10 mg/kg PO q6h | 10 mg/kg PO q48h |
| Aminocaproic acid (Amicar) | Antiinflammatory for degenerative myelopathy | 500 mg PO q8h | Not evaluated |
| Ampicillin | Antibiotic | 22 mg/kg PO q8h or 22 mg/kg IV, SC, IM q6h | 22 mg/kg PO q8h or 22 mg/kg IV, SC, IM q6h |
| Apomorphine | Emetic | 0.08 mg/kg SC or 6 mg (1 crushed tablet) in conjunctival sac | Use alternative (xylazine) |
| Atropine | Antidote for cholinergic toxins | 0.5 mg/kg IV, then 1.5 mg/kg SC q6-8h | 0.5 mg/kg IV, then 1.5 mg/kg SC q6-8h |
| Azathioprine (Imuran) | Treatment of immune-mediated diseases | 50 mg/m$^2$ (approx. 2.2 mg/ kg) PO q24h | 0.2 mg/kg PO q48h |
| Bethanechol (Urecholine) | Treatment of bladder atony | 0.04 mg/kg PO, SC q8h | 0.04 mg/kg PO, SC q8h |
| Calcium EDTA (Versenate) (1 g/100 ml D$_5$W) | Lead poisoning antidote | 25 mg/kg SC q6h | 25 mg/kg SC q6h |
| Calcium gluconate (10%) | Treatment of hypocalcemia | 0.5-1 ml/kg IV | 0.5-1 ml/kg IV |
| Cefadroxil | Antibiotic | 22 mg/kg PO q12h | 22 mg/kg PO q24h |
| Cephalexin (Keflex) | Antibiotic | 20-40 mg/kg PO q8h | 20-40 mg/kg PO q8h |
| Cephalothin (Keflin) | Antibiotic | 25 mg/kg IV, IM, SC q6h | 25 mg/kg IV, IM, SC q6h |
| Chloramphenicol | Antibiotic | 25-50 mg/kg PO, IV q6-8h | 12.5-25 mg/kg PO, IV q12h |
| Chlorazepate dipotassium (Traxene) | Anticonvulsant | 1 mg/kg q12h | Unknown |
| Chlorpromazine (Thorazine) | Muscle relaxation | 0.5 mg/kg IV q8h | 0.5 mg/kg IV q8 |
| Cimetidine (Tagamet) | H$_2$-blocker antacid | 5 mg/kg PO, IM, IV q8h | 5 mg/kg PO, IM, IV q8h |
| Clonazepam (Clonapin) | Anticonvulsant | 0.5 mg/kg PO q8-12h | Not evaluated |
| Clindamycin (Cleocin) | Antibiotic | 10-15 mg/kg PO q12h | 10-15 mg/kg PO q12h |

| Drug | Indication | Dose | Dose |
|---|---|---|---|
| Cloxacillin (Tegopen) | Antibiotic | 10-15 mg/kg PO, IV q6h | 10-15 mg/kg PO, IV q6h |
| Dexamethasone | Treatment of acute spinal cord or brain edema | 2-4 mg/kg IV | 2-4 mg/kg IV |
|  | Antiinflammatory and antiedema agent | 0.1-1 mg/kg PO, IV, SC (see specific disorder) | 0.1-1 mg/kg PO, IV, SC (see specific disorder) |
| Dextrose (50%) | Treatment of hypoglycemia | 2 ml/kg | 2 ml/kg |
| Diazepam (Valium) | Anticonvulsant; treatment of status epilepticus | 5-20 mg IV (repeat if needed) | 5 mg IV (repeat if needed) |
|  | Chronic seizure management | 0.5-1 mg/kg PO q8h | 0.3-0.8 mg/kg PO q8h |
|  | Muscle relaxant | 0.5-1 mg/kg PO q8h | 0.3-0.8 mg/kg PO q8h |
| Dimethylsulfoxide (DMSO) | Treatment of cerebral edema | 1 g/kg IV/30 min | 1 g/kg IV/30 min |
| Diphenhydramine HCl (Benadryl) | Antiemetic (vestibular disease) | 2-4 mg/kg SC | 1-2 mg/kg SC |
| Doxycycline (Vibramycin) | Antibiotic | 5-10 mg/kg PO, IV q12h | 5-10 mg/kg PO, IV q12h |
| Edrophonium chloride (Tensilon) | Tension test—myasthenia gravis | 0.1-0.2 mg/kg IV | 0.2 mg/cat IV |
| Enrofloxacin (Baytril) | Antibiotic | 5 mg/kg PO, SC, IV q12h | 2-5 mg/kg PO, SC, IV q12h |
| Folinic acid | Treatment of pyrimethamine toxicity | 0.5-5 mg/day | 0.5-5 mg/day |
| Furosemide (Lasix) | Diuretic, antiedema agent | 2-4 mg/kg IV, IM, SC q6h | 2-4 mg/kg IV, IM, SC q6h |
| Ipecac syrup | Emetic | 6.6 ml/kg PO | 6.6 ml/kg PO |
| Mannitol (20% solution over 30 min) | Treatment of cerebral edema | 1-3 g/kg | 1-3 g/kg |
| Methocarbamol (Robaxin) | Muscle relaxant | 20 mg/kg PO q8-12h | None |
| Methylprednisolone sodium succinate (SoluMedrol) | Treatment of spinal, brain trauma | 20-40 mg/kg IV | 20-40 mg/kg IV |
| Metronidazole (Flagyl) | Antibiotic | 10-15 mg/kg PO q8h | 10-15 mg/kg PO q8h |
| Neostigmine bromide (Prostigmine) | Treatment of myasthenia gravis | 0.5 mg/kg q12h | None |
| Neostigmine methylsulfate (Stiglyn) | Treatment of myasthenia gravis | 0.01-0.04 mg/kg IM q6-8h | None |
| Penicillin G | Antibiotic |  |  |
|  | Aqueous (K or NA) | 40,000 U/kg IV q6h | 40,000 U/kg IV q6h |
|  | Procaine | 40,000 U/kg IM, SC q12h | 40,000 U/kg IM, SC q12h |
| Pentobarbital (Nembutal) | Anticonvulsant and anesthetic | 5-15 mg/kg IV to effect | 5-15 mg/kg IV to effect |
| Phenobarbital | Anticonvulsant | 0.5-2 mg/kg IV, IM, PO q8h | 0.5-2 mg/kg IV, IM, PO q8h |
| Phenoxybenzamine (Dibenzylin) | Adrenergic α-blocker | 0.25-0.5 mg/kg PO q8-12h | 2.5-7.5 mg/cat PO q8-12h |
| Phenylbutazone (Butazolidin) | Analgesia | 5-10 mg/kg PO q8h (max 800 mg/day) | None |

*Continued.*

## Drugs Used in Neurologic Disorders—cont'd

| Drug name (trade name) | Purpose | Recommended dose | |
|---|---|---|---|
| | | Dog | Cat |
| Potassium bromide | Anticonvulsant | 30-40 mg/kg PO q6h | 30 mg/kg PO q6h |
| Potassium gluconate (Kaon Elixir) | Treatment of hypokalemia | None | 2.5-5 mEq/cat PO q12h |
| Pralidoxime chloride (2-PAM, Protopam) | Organophosphate intoxication | 20 mg/kg IM q12h | 20 mg/kg IM q12h |
| Prednisone | Immunosuppression | 2-4 mg/kg/day PO | 2-6 mg/kg/day PO |
| | Antiinflammatory and antiedema agent | 0.5-0.75 mg/kg PO | 0.5-0.75 mg/kg PO |
| Primidone | Anticonvulsant | 10 mg/kg PO q8h—not recommended as first choice | None |
| Pyrimethamine | Treatment of toxoplasmosis | 0.25-0.5 mg/kg PO q12h | 0.25-0.5 mg/kg PO q12h |
| Pyridostigmine bromide (Mestinon) | Treatment of myasthenia gravis | 2 mg/kg PO q8-12h | 0.5 mg/kg PO q12h |
| Sodium sulfate (40%) | Cathartic | 1 g/kg PO | 1 g/kg PO |
| Tetracycline HCl | Antibiotic | 22 mg/kg PO q8h | 22 mg/kg PO q8h |
| Thiamine (vitamin B₁) | Thiamine deficiency | 10-100 mg IM, PO q6h | 10-50 mg IM, PO q6h |
| Trimethoprim sulfadiazine (Tribrissen) | Antibiotic | 15 mg/kg PO or SC q12h | 15 mg/kg PO or SC q12h |
| Valproic acid (Depakene) | Anticonvulsant | 20-60 mg/kg PO q8-12h | Not evaluated |
| Xylazine (Rompun) | Emetic (cats) | Not recommended | 0.44 mg/kg IM |

$D_5W$, 5% dextrose in water; *HCl*, hydrochloride; $H_2$, histamine 2; *IM*, intramuscularly; *IV*, intravenously; *K*, potassium; *Na*, sodium; *PO*, orally; *SC*, subcutaneously.

# PART X

# Joint Disorders

# 75

## Joint Disorders: Clinical Manifestations and Diagnostic Tests

### (Text pp 1071-1078)

Disorders that affect the joints can be divided into two major categories: noninflammatory and inflammatory. Noninflammatory joint diseases include developmental, degenerative, neoplastic, and traumatic processes. Inflammatory joint diseases include infectious and immune-mediated processes.

### CLINICAL MANIFESTATIONS (TEXT PP 1071-1073)

#### Lameness

Animals with joint disease are usually brought for treatment with a history of lameness or gait abnormality. Lameness typically involves only one joint in animals with traumatic or developmental joint disorders. When multiple joints are affected (polyarthritis), a shifting-leg lameness may be reported. With severe joint pain (e.g., polyarthritis), the animal may refuse to walk, or it may cry in pain when moved or touched, making it difficult to differentiate joint disease from other serious musculoskeletal and neurologic disorders.

#### Joint pain

Animals with joint disease may or may not have joint pain. Many animals with polyarthritis have joint pain. Affected joints should be flexed and extended to detect alterations in range of joint motion, degree of pain (discomfort), and crepitation, which suggests articular wear, osteophyte presence, or other periarticular changes. Joint stability should be evaluated to assess the integrity of the supporting ligaments.

#### Joint swelling

Some dogs with joint disease have dramatic joint swelling because of effusion, but many dogs with immune-mediated inflammatory polyarthritis do not have appreciable joint swelling. Therefore a joint that feels normal on palpation can still be severely affected by joint disease.

### Diagnostic Approach

#### Physical examination

It is important to maintain a high index of suspicion for polyarthritis when one is evaluating dogs and cats with nonspecific illness, as they may not exhibit obvious joint pain or have detectable joint swelling.

A complete physical examination should always be performed in animals with nonspecific pain, lameness, reluctance to exercise, or fever of unknown origin. Special attention should be given to the nervous system and anatomic localization of pain. The muscles, bones, and joints of each limb should be thoroughly palpated. Differential diagnoses for bone pain should include trauma, panosteitis, hypertrophic osteodystrophy, osteomyelitis, and bone neoplasia. Differential diagnoses for muscle pain should include conditions such as myositis and strain or sprain injuries. Pain on palpation or manipulation of the neck could indicate a variety of spinal cord or vertebral abnormalities, intracranial disease, meningitis, or polyarthritis; inflammation of the intervertebral facetal joints can manifest as neck or back pain.

Inflammatory joint disease is one of the most common causes of fever and nonspecific inflammation in dogs and cats. Signs of immune-mediated inflammatory joint disease can include cyclic fevers, stiffness, shifting-leg lameness, and reluctance to exercise. Many patients, particularly cats, have a vague history of decreased appetite, weakness, or fever, but no apparent lameness.

### Routine diagnostic tests

Initial diagnostic tests typically include radiographs (evaluate for degenerative, lytic, or erosive changes) and synovial fluid analysis (always required to make a diagnosis of inflammatory joint disease). When one is evaluating an animal with inflammatory joint disease, it is important to first eliminate infectious diseases (bacteria, *Mycoplasma* spp., bacterial L-forms, spirochetes, rickettsial agents, and fungi) as differential diagnoses. Diagnostic tests might include complete blood count (CBC), urinalysis, culture (urine, blood, and synovial fluid), and rickettsial and Lyme disease titers. Thoracic radiographs and fungal serology may also be warranted. Once infectious disorders have been ruled out, immune-mediated conditions should be considered.

### Immune-mediated arthritis

Noninfectious, immune-mediated arthritis is common in dogs and uncommon in cats. These polyarthritis syndromes are characterized as erosive or nonerosive on the basis of physical and radiographic findings.

*Nonerosive polyarthritis.* Immune-mediated, nonerosive polyarthritis is the most common form of inflammatory joint disease in dogs. It is most often an idiopathic syndrome but may also occur as a feature of systemic lupus erythematosus (SLE) or secondary to prolonged antigenic stimulation (reactive polyarthritis) caused by chronic infection, neoplasia, or drugs (e.g., penicillin, sulfas). Also, there exist a few breed-associated syndromes of polyarthritis or polyarthritis, meningitis, and myositis, possibly with a genetic basis (see Chapter 76).

Whenever noninfectious, nonerosive inflammatory joint disease is identified, a thorough history including recent drug administration should be obtained. In addition, tests must be performed to look for evidence of chronic infection or neoplasia (e.g., CBC, thoracic and abdominal radiographs, ophthalmologic examination, bacterial culture of urine and blood, cardiac ultrasonography, abdominal ultrasonography) or SLE (e.g., CBC, platelet count, urine protein/creatinine ratio, antinuclear antibody titer). If these are normal, a diagnosis of idiopathic immune-mediated polyarthritis is warranted.

*Erosive polyarthritis.* Rheumatoid arthritis is an uncommon immune-mediated, erosive polyarthritis characterized by progressive joint destruction. It should be considered if aseptic inflammatory joint disease is identified in a dog with radiographic evidence of joint destruction. Serologic testing for rheumatoid factor and synovial membrane biopsy should be performed to establish this rare diagnosis.

### Feline polyarthritis

Polyarthritis is uncommon in cats. Clinical signs may include fever, lethargy, reluctance to walk, and swollen, painful joints. In contrast to dogs, most cats with polyarthritis have erosive joint disease. This can result from septic arthritis, bacterial L-form infection, or a syndrome known as *chronic progressive polyarthritis,* which has been identified in male cats with feline leukemia virus and feline syncytium-forming virus infection.

Other infectious causes of feline arthritis are mycoplasma and calicivirus. Noninfectious, immune-mediated (nonerosive) polyarthritis resulting from SLE occurs rarely in cats.

A diagnosis of idiopathic immune-mediated nonerosive polyarthritis can be made only after infectious causes, SLE, and underlying neoplastic or inflammatory conditions have been ruled out. This rare condition seems to respond well to corticosteroids alone in most cats. Cyclophosphamide, chlorambucil, and gold salts have been used in some refractory cases with success.

## DIAGNOSTIC TESTS (TEXT PP 1073-1078)

### Clinical Pathology

Routine laboratory tests are indicated when polyarthritis is suspected. Depending on the underlying cause, abnormal findings may include anemia, leukocytosis, thrombocytopenia, hypoproteinemia, proteinuria, and urinary changes consistent with urinary tract infection. Normal test results do not rule out polyarthritis.

### Radiography

#### Views and regions

Physical examination usually identifies which joints should be radiographed. The hocks and carpi should be evaluated whenever erosive polyarthritis is suspected. Two views (lateral and anteroposterior) should always be obtained for each joint evaluated. Radiographs of the thorax and abdomen should also be considered when infectious or neoplastic disease is suspected. Spinal radiographs may be used to screen for diskospondylitis as a cause of immune-mediated or infectious polyarthritis (see Chapter 72).

#### Common findings

Radiographic findings aid in the diagnosis of degenerative joint disease (DJD), chronic septic arthritis, and rheumatoid arthritis. Nonbacterial infectious polyarthritis (e.g., rickettsial, Lyme disease, viral) and immune-mediated, nonerosive polyarthritis generally do not cause radiographic abnormalities other than mild joint capsule distention and soft-tissue swelling. Incidental radiographic evidence of DJD should not be confused with erosive or destructive articular changes. Radiographic features of erosive polyarthritis typically include periarticular osteoporosis, loss of articular cartilage, subchondral cyst formation, and joint luxation.

#### Interpretation

Many of the bony changes associated with degenerative and erosive joint diseases are not seen for weeks or months after the onset of disease. Although positive findings contribute a great deal to the diagnosis, negative findings should be interpreted with caution. Sequential radiographic studies may be warranted in patients in which a diagnosis of nonerosive polyarthritis is uncertain or in cases that do not respond to appropriate therapy.

### Synovial Fluid Analysis

Synovial fluid analysis is of value in confirming the presence of joint disease and differentiating inflammatory from noninflammatory disorders. It may also provide information for a specific diagnosis. Light tranquilization or sedation is usually used to prevent the animal from moving during sample collection and contaminating the sample. Collection procedures are described in the text.

#### Sites

Whenever polyarthritis is suspected, synovial fluid from at least six joints should be analyzed. Immune-mediated disease is most prominent in the distal small joints, such as the hock and carpus, whereas septic joint disease is more often detected in the larger proximal joints. Even if only one joint is clinically affected, synovial fluid should be collected from multiple joints.

#### Sample handling

Slides are made immediately, using one drop of fluid for each slide. A portion of the sample should be either saved in a sterile tube for culture and sensitivity or inoculated into enrichment media. When larger samples are obtained, the remaining fluid can be placed in a test tube containing EDTA for precise cell counts and further analysis.

### Gross appearance

Normal synovial fluid is clear and colorless. Cloudiness or turbidity is seen in any condition that causes red blood cells (RBCs) or white blood cells (WBCs) to enter the joint in high numbers. Hemorrhage from an earlier puncture attempt or an ongoing disease process results in diffuse discoloration, whereas blood from a traumatic tap is not homogeneously mixed with the joint fluid. Yellow-tinged fluid (xanthochromia) usually indicates previous hemorrhage into the joint and is occasionally seen in degenerative, traumatic, and inflammatory joint diseases.

*Viscosity.* Normal synovial fluid is very viscous, forming a long string when allowed to drop from the tip of the needle. Thin or watery consistency indicates that the synovial fluid is deficient in polymerized hyaluronic acid. This may occur after dilution by serum or through degradation by intense intraarticular inflammation.

*Mucin clot test.* The mucin clot test assesses the quantity and quality of mucin in the synovial fluid. Glacial acetic acid is added to the sample (if sufficient volume remains after other tests are performed). Normally, this results in formation of a firm, ropelike, nonfriable clot. In inflammatory joint diseases the quality of the mucin clot may be diminished. Particularly in patients with rheumatoid or septic arthritis, significant destruction of mucin results in formation of only loose, friable clots.

### Microscopic appearance

Cytologic evaluation is the most important aspect of synovial fluid analysis. Usually, estimates of cell numbers are made from a stained direct smear. Occasionally a sufficient volume of fluid is obtained to allow absolute cell counts with a hemocytometer. Smears of synovial fluid should also be submitted with any fluid preserved in EDTA, because synovial fluid cells degenerate with time.

*Cell count and differential.* Normal synovial fluid contains 100 to 3000 cells/μl. Mononuclear cells predominate; one to three mononuclear cells per high-power (100×) field may be seen on a smear of normal synovial fluid. Normally, a mixture of large and small mononuclear cells is present and frequently contains many vacuoles and granules. An occasional neutrophil may be seen, but these cells should represent <10% of the total. If blood contamination of normal synovial fluid has occurred, <1 neutrophil should be present for every 500 RBCs. When platelets are present, they indicate recent hemorrhage or blood contamination. Hemosiderin-laden macrophages and erythrophagia confirm prior hemorrhage.

*Mononuclear cytosis.* An increased nucleated cell count consisting primarily of mononuclear cells is seen in many chronically diseased joints and in joints that have been traumatized or undergone degenerative change (Table 75-1).

*Neutrophilia.* An increase in the number of neutrophils indicates inflammation of the synovial lining. The more inflamed the synovium, the greater the concentration of WBCs in the synovial fluid and the greater the percentage of neutrophils. Neutrophils in the synovial fluid of dogs and cats with immune-mediated disease have a normal appearance. In acute or severe cases of septic arthritis it is common to see bacteria within the cells, and the neutrophils may be toxic, ruptured, and degranulated.

**Table 75-1**

## Synovial Fluid Cytology in Common Joint Disorders

|  | WBCs/Fl | PMNs (%) |
| --- | --- | --- |
| Normal | 200-3000 | <10 |
| Degenerative | 1000-5000 | 0-12 |
| Traumatic | Variable | <25 |
| Septic | 40,000-280,000 | 90-99 |
| Rheumatoid arthritis (erosive) | 6000-80,000 | 20-80 |
| Immune-mediated (nonerosive) | 4000-370,000 | 15-95 |

*PMNs, Polymorphonuclear neutrophil leukocytes; WBCs, white blood cells.*

*Other abnormalities.* Intracellular organisms may be seen in patients with rickettsial polyarthritis. Occasionally, LE cells are seen in the synovial fluid of dogs with SLE-induced polyarthritis.

## Synovial Fluid Culture

Bacteria are the most common causes of joint infection. Septic arthritis can sometimes be diagnosed on the basis of toxic changes within neutrophils or identification of bacteria on stained smears of synovial fluid. However, some organisms such as *Mycoplasma* spp. do not induce characteristic cytologic abnormalities.

Any joint fluid with an increased nucleated cell count and high percentage of neutrophils should be cultured. Synovial fluid should be submitted for aerobic and anaerobic culture and for *Mycoplasma* culture. Bacterial culture is positive in approximately 50% of all cases of septic arthritis, so failure to grow bacteria does not rule out septic arthritis. The diagnostic yield can be improved by 85% to 100% by collecting synovial fluid, inoculating it into broth-enrichment media (such as thioglycolate blood culture bottles), incubating it for 24 hours, and then reculturing it. Culture of blood, urine, and synovial membrane biopsies is recommended to improve recovery of the offending organism.

## Synovial Membrane Biopsy

Synovial membrane biopsy is warranted whenever the cause of joint disease remains undetermined or routine therapy is ineffective. Examination of the synovial membrane is especially valuable for diagnosing neoplasia and differentiating infectious arthritis from immune-mediated disorders. It may also be used to collect a sample for culture in cases of suspected septic arthritis. Samples may be obtained by needle biopsy or surgical arthrotomy (see text).

## Immunologic and Serologic Tests

### Lyme disease titers

Infection with *Borrelia burgdorferi*, the cause of Lyme disease polyarthritis, results in an antibody response that can be detected using an indirect fluorescent antibody (IFA) test or enzyme-linked immunosorbent assay. Dogs with clinical signs of Lyme disease generally have high titers, but asymptomatic dogs in endemic areas may also have titers >1:8000. A positive titer, therefore, merely indicates exposure and cannot be used to diagnose active disease. Diagnosis of Lyme disease polyarthritis must rely on a combination of history (recent exposure to an enzootic area), clinical signs, elimination of other known causes of polyarthritis, serologic testing, and response to therapy.

### Rickettsial titers

Serologic testing plays an important role in the diagnosis of Rocky Mountain spotted fever (RMSF) and canine erlichiosis (see Chapter 101).

*Rocky Mountain spotted fever.* Immunofluorescence is the most commonly used serologic test for RMSF. Markedly increased immunoglobulin G (IgG) titers support the diagnosis. Titers may not increase for 2 to 3 weeks after exposure; therefore a negative or low titer does not rule out RMSF. A second sample obtained 3 weeks later should be evaluated if the initial titer is nondiagnostic. A fourfold increase between acute and convalescent titers is expected in active infections.

*Ehrlichiosis.* The IFA test is a reliable, highly sensitive, and specific serologic test for detecting *Ehrlichia canis* infection; any positive titer usually indicates active infection. Rarely, a dog with polyarthritis will be seronegative for *E. canis* but positive if polymerase chain reaction is used.

### Systemic lupus erythematosus

Tests used to help identify SLE include the LE cell test and the antinuclear antibody (ANA) test.

*LE cells.* The LE cell test requires identification of the LE cell, a WBC that has phagocytized nuclear material (amorphous purple material in the cytoplasm). This test is very laboratory dependent; reported incidence of a positive result of an LE cell test on blood from dogs with SLE varies from 30% to 90%. The test may also be positive in other immune or neoplastic disorders. Rarely, in dogs with SLE-induced polyarthritis, LE cells are detected in the synovial fluid and are convincing evidence of this disorder.

*Antinuclear antibody test.* The ANA test detects circulating antibodies to nuclear material, the most prominent autoantibodies associated with canine and feline SLE. The ANA test is a sensitive indicator of SLE and has a positive result (>1:10) in 90% of cases. However, a positive ANA test result is not specific for SLE. False-positive results may be seen in dogs and cats with many other systemic inflammatory or neoplastic diseases.

### Rheumatoid factor

The laboratory test for rheumatoid factor detects serum agglutinating antibody (RF) against IgG. Great variability exists in results among the different test systems currently in use. Nevertheless, a titer of 1:16 is generally considered positive, regardless of the test system used. A titer of 1:8 is considered suspect and should be repeated. Some normal dogs have positive test results of low titer (1:2, 1:4). The reliability of the test increases with the severity and chronicity of the disease; test results are positive in 20% to 70% of dogs with rheumatoid arthritis. Any disease associated with systemic inflammation and immune complex generation and deposition can result in weak false-positive results.

# 76

# Disorders of the Joints

## *(Text pp 1079-1092)*

## DEGENERATIVE JOINT DISEASE (TEXT PP 1079-1081)

### Etiology

Degenerative joint disease (DJD) is a chronic, progressive, noninflammatory joint disorder that results in articular cartilage damage and degenerative and proliferative changes. The initiating cartilage damage may be idiopathic or the result of abnormal mechanical stresses (e.g., congenital deformities, abnormal conformation, trauma).

DJD is the most common joint disorder in dogs. It is rarely diagnosed in cats, probably because mild-to-moderate DJD is usually subclinical in this species.

### Clinical signs

Signs are usually insidious and confined to the musculoskeletal system. Initially, lameness and stiffness may be prominent only with overexertion or in cold, damp weather. Mildly affected animals may "warm out" of the lameness with light exercise. As DJD progresses, fibrosis and pain lead to decreased exercise tolerance, constant lameness, and, in severe cases, muscle atrophy. One joint or multiple joints may be affected.

### Diagnosis

DJD is usually diagnosed on the basis of history, physical findings, and radiographic features. Clinical examination may reveal pain in the affected joint(s), decreased range of motion, crepitation on flexion and extension, and perhaps joint swelling. Unlike some inflammatory joint diseases, DJD does not cause fever, leukocytosis, or depression.

*Radiography.* Radiographic changes can include joint effusion, subchondral sclerosis and cyst formation, joint space narrowing, periarticular osteophytes and bone remodeling. Often a predisposing condition, such as trauma, rupture of supporting ligaments, poor conformation, or a congenital deformity, is evident.

*Synovial fluid analysis.* If synovial fluid is collected, it reveals minimal or no inflammation, although an increase in volume and a slight decrease in viscosity may be present. Total cell count may be normal or slightly increased, but it is rarely >5000 cells/μl; 70% to 80% are lymphocytes and <12% are neutrophils. Partial cruciate rupture in dogs is sometimes associated with increased total cell and neutrophil counts, suggesting an inflammatory reaction.

### Treatment

Goals are to alleviate discomfort and prevent further degeneration. Where possible, factors contributing to cartilage stress or joint laxity are eliminated. Surgery may be necessary to correct joint instability or deformity and to relieve discomfort. Medical treatment is symptomatic. Weight reduction may decrease stress on the joint. Rest often helps to decrease the discomfort associated with acute exacerbations of disease. High-impact exercise (e.g., running and jumping) should be discouraged, although some low-impact exercise (e.g., swimming and leash walking) is recommended to maintain strength and mobility. Other forms of physical therapy may include passive range-of-motion exercises, cold (acute) or heat (chronic) therapy, muscle and joint massage, acupuncture, ultrasound, and electrical stimulation.

*Corticosteroids.* Corticosteroids can decrease degradative enzyme release, but they are not widely recommended because they markedly inhibit synthesis of proteoglycans and collagen, resulting in progression of DJD.

*Nonsteroidal antiinflammatory drugs.* Nonsteroidal antiinflammatory drugs (NSAIDs) are often recommended for DJD because of their antiinflammatory and analgesic effects but can cause adverse gastrointestinal (GI) effects (nausea, vomiting, ulcers). Misoprostol (2.5 mg/kg orally [PO] q8h), a synthetic prostaglandin $E_1$ analog, can be administered concurrently to decrease the GI tract irritation. Buffered aspirin (10 to 20 mg/kg PO q8-12h), the NSAID most often administered to dogs, is an effective analgesic and antiinflammatory agent; however, chronically it may impair cartilage repair. Carprofen (Rimadyl) is very effective and is associated with fewer GI side effects than aspirin; however, duodenal ulceration has been documented in a few treated dogs, and, rarely, idiosyncratic hepatic necrosis can occur. Etodolac (10 to 15 mg/kg PO q24h), piroxicam (0.3 mg/kg PO q48h), and meloxicam (0.2 mg/kg once, then 0.1 mg/kg/day PO) have also been used to successfully treat dogs with DJD. Other NSAIDs can be used in dogs, but many are associated with a higher prevalence of GI adverse effects.

*Chondroprotective drugs.* Adequan (polysulfated glycosaminoglycan) can be used at 2 to 5 mg/kg intramuscularly (IM) every 4 days for four treatments, then every 30 days for six treatments. An oral combination of glucosamine hydrochloride, chondroitin sulfate, and manganese ascorbate has also been recommended (Cosequin RS: one or two tablets per day, cats or small dogs; Cosequin DS: two to four tablets per day, large dogs). Alternatively, oral glucosamine (15 to 20 mg/kg q12h) and chondroitin sulfate (15 to 20 mg/kg q12h) can be purchased separately and administered. For maximum theoretic benefit these products should be administered before DJD has occurred, such as in patients with traumatic or surgical cartilage damage.

## INFECTIOUS JOINT DISEASES (TEXT PP 1081-1085)

### Septic Arthritis

#### Etiology

Septic (bacterial) arthritis can occur as a blood-borne infection or by direct inoculation of a joint via surgery, foreign body penetration, or trauma. Infection of multiple joints suggests bacteremia originating from a distant site of infection (e.g., dermatitis, otitis externa, periodontal disease, metritis, omphalophlebitis, prostatitis, endocarditis, diskospondylitis), but such hematogenous spread is uncommon except in immunosuppressed animals or neonates. Polyarticular septic arthritis is most commonly seen in neonatal kittens secondary to omphalophlebitis because the queen has severed the umbilical cord too close to the abdominal wall.

The most common causal organisms are *Staphylococcus* spp., *Streptococcus* spp., and coliforms in dogs and *Pasteurella* spp. in cats. Regardless of the cause, septic arthritis is more common in dogs than in cats, is most common in large-breed dogs, and more frequently affects males.

### Clinical signs

Animals with septic polyarthritis are often systemically ill, febrile, and depressed. Affected joints are usually very painful, especially when manipulated, and may be distended. Inflammation and edema of the periarticular soft tissues may also be present. Septic arthritis resulting from bacteremia usually involves the larger proximal joints, whereas immune-mediated arthritis, the primary differential diagnosis, more commonly involves the smaller distal joints.

### Diagnosis

Diagnosis requires identification of bacteria in synovial fluid or a positive culture of synovial fluid, blood, or urine. Synovial fluid is often yellow, cloudy, or bloody; viscosity is decreased and the mucin clot test, if performed, results in a poor-quality clot. Rapid clotting of synovial fluid from infected joints is common, so a portion of the fluid should be immediately placed in EDTA for cytologic evaluation. Smears should also be made for Gram and differential staining.

*Cytology.* Nucleated cell count is markedly increased (40,000 to 280,000/µl), with neutrophils predominating (>90%). In acute or severe infections, it is common to see bacteria within the cells, and the neutrophils may be toxic, ruptured, and degranulated. Organisms that do not cause rapid destruction of articular cartilage (e.g., streptococci, *Mycoplasma*) may not cause remarkable toxic or degenerative neutrophil changes. In chronic infections, bacteria may no longer be evident, and neutrophils may appear healthy.

*Culture.* Synovial fluid should be cultured for aerobic and anaerobic bacteria. Synovial fluid culture is positive in approximately 50% of patients with septic arthritis; improved diagnostic yield may be obtained by inoculating synovial fluid into blood culture medium (9:1 ratio) and incubating it for 24 hours at 37° C before inoculation. Bacteria can also be recovered from cultures of synovial membrane biopsy, blood, or urine specimens.

*Radiography.* Radiographic changes may be minimal or nonspecific initially (thickened joint capsule, widened joint space, and irregular thickening of periarticular soft tissues). With chronic infection, cartilage degeneration, osteophytes, periosteal reaction, and subchondral bone lysis may be seen.

*Other tests.* When the inciting event is not known or more than one joint is involved, a search should be made for the primary site of infection. Radiographs of the thorax, abdomen, and spine and cardiac and abdominal ultrasonography are especially helpful. If possible, cultures should be obtained from any suspect site.

### Treatment and prognosis

Treatment is aimed at sterilizing the affected joints and, whenever possible, removing intraarticular accumulations of enzymes and fibrin debris. Identifiable sources of infection should also be eliminated.

*Antibiotics.* Antibiotics should be administered as soon as possible after all samples are collected. Until culture results are available, a broad-spectrum, β-lactamase–resistant antibiotic such as cephalexin (20 to 40 mg/kg q8h) or Clavamox (12 to 25 mg/kg q8h) is indicated. Quinolones should be used if Gram-negative organisms are suspected. Initially the antibiotic should be administered parenterally, followed by long-term therapy PO for a minimum of 6 weeks.

*Surgery.* Most animals with acute septic arthritis can be treated conservatively with joint drainage and systemic antibiotics for up to 3 days, after which surgery should be performed if dramatic improvement is not evident. Suspected intraarticular foreign bodies, postoperative joint infections, and chronic infections require immediate surgical débridement and lavage. Complete exploration of the affected joint is recommended if the underlying cause of the infection is unknown.

Prolonged rest is recommended after resolution of septic arthritis. Prognosis for return to normal function depends on the severity of cartilage damage. Secondary DJD is common.

*Cage Rest.* Cage rest is recommended to facilitate healing of articular cartilage.

### *Mycoplasma* Polyarthritis

Systemic mycoplasma infection occasionally occurs in debilitated or immunosuppressed animals. The prevalence of *Mycoplasma* arthritis is low. *Mycoplasma gateae* and *Mycoplasma felis* have caused clinical disease in cats (rare).

#### Clinical signs and diagnosis

*Mycoplasma* arthritis is a chronic polyarthritis indistinguishable from idiopathic immune-mediated, nonerosive polyarthritis. Signs include lameness, joint pain, depression, and fever. Synovial fluid has an increased nucleated cell count, predominantly consisting of nondegenerate neutrophils. Routine aerobic and anaerobic culture of joint fluid is negative. Diagnosis is made by isolation of organisms cultured in mycoplasma medium.

#### Treatment

Tetracycline (22 mg/kg PO q8h), doxycycline (5 mg/kg PO or intravenously [IV] q12h), tylosin (20 mg/kg PO q8h), and chloramphenicol (25 to 50 mg/kg PO q8h in dogs; 10 to 15 mg/kg q12h in cats) are each effective.

### Bacterial L-Form–Associated Arthritis

A rare syndrome of pyogenic subcutaneous abscesses with associated polyarthritis has been described in cats. This condition is infectious from one cat to another via bite wounds. Affected cats have swollen, painful joints and fever. Fistulating subcutaneous wounds develop over affected joints. Exudate from the joints or abscesses reveals degenerate and nondegenerate neutrophils and macrophages. Cultures for aerobic and anaerobic bacteria, *Mycoplasma*, and fungal organisms are negative. Growth of the organism requires specific L-form media. Treatment with doxycycline (5 mg/kg q12h) or chloramphenicol (10 to 15 mg/kg q12h) is effective within 48 hours and should continue for 10 to 14 days.

### Rickettsial Polyarthritis

Ehrlichiosis and Rocky Mountain spotted fever (RMSF) can occasionally cause nonerosive polyarthritis in dogs, but in most cases concurrent systemic signs are obvious. Joint pain and effusion are present. Increased numbers of nondegenerate neutrophils are found in the joint fluid; occasionally, *Ehrlichia* spp. morulae are seen.

In dogs with ehrlichiosis, fever and polyarthritis may be the only clinical abnormalities, although hematologic abnormalities such as mild thrombocytopenia and anemia are common. Serologic testing does not reliably identify affected dogs; polymerase chain reaction assay may be more sensitive.

Dogs with RMSF are more likely to show a variety of other signs, including fever, petechial hemorrhages, lymphadenopathy, neurologic signs, edema of the face or extremities, and pneumonitis. Hematologic abnormalities, including thrombocytopenia, are common. Diagnosis is established through serologic testing (see Chapter 101).

#### Treatment

Both disorders are treated with doxycycline (5 mg/kg PO q12h) or chloramphenicol (25 to 50 mg/kg PO or IV q8h). Empirical antibiotic treatment is warranted in dogs from endemic areas with confirmed polyarthritis and typical signs of rickettsial disease. Prednisone (0.5 to 2 mg/kg/day) may be necessary if antimicrobial therapy does not eliminate fever, lameness, and joint swelling.

## Lyme Disease

### Etiology

The tick-borne spirochete *Borrelia burgdorferi* can cause multisystemic illness (Lyme disease) in dogs that may include fever, lymphadenopathy, myocarditis, inflammatory joint disease, and glomerulonephritis. Lyme disease is prevalent throughout North America, but most confirmed cases have occurred in dogs from the northeastern and mid-Atlantic states. Lyme disease polyarthritis in pets is overdiagnosed, relative to its actual prevalence. The disease is poorly documented in cats, despite evidence of seropositivity.

### Clinical features

Most infected dogs never develop clinical signs. Immunodeficiency may play a role in the development of clinical disease. Acute polyarthritis is the most common form in dogs. Major clinical features are lameness, fever, lymphadenopathy, and anorexia. Signs occasionally resolve after a few days but may periodically recur. Acute signs of illness are most common in the summer months. Rarely, complete heart block, renal failure, and neurologic signs (seizures, behavioral changes) are found.

### Diagnosis

Lyme disease polyarthritis should be diagnosed only if the animal has a history of recent potential exposure, the synovial fluid is confirmed to be inflammatory and sterile, serologic testing is positive, and a prompt and permanent response to appropriate antibiotic therapy is seen. Complete blood count (CBC) and radiographs of the thorax, abdomen, and joints are usually normal during acute illness.

*Synovial fluid analysis.* Synovial fluid has an increased nucleated cell count (mean 46,300/µl); nondegenerate neutrophils predominate (43% to 85%). Although signs may wax and wane, synovial fluid analysis remains consistently abnormal.

*Serology.* Positive serum antibody titer is merely evidence of exposure and is not indicative of disease. Although most dogs presented with acute polyarthritis caused by Lyme disease have high antibody titers, some dogs are seronegative early in the disease.

*Other tests.* Attempts to culture *B. burgdorferi* from the blood, urine, and synovial fluid are usually unsuccessful. Identification of *Borrelia* organisms in biopsy specimens of diseased tissues (e.g., synovium, kidney) by direct immunofluorescence supports the diagnosis.

### Treatment

Antibiotic therapy for 3 to 4 weeks duration is advised. Doxycycline (5 mg/kg PO q12h), Amoxicillin (22 mg/kg PO bid), ampicillin (22 mg/ kg PO q8h), Clavamox (12.5 to 25 mg/kg PO q8-12h), and Cephalexin (20 to 40 mg/kg PO q8h) are all effective. Treatment during the acute stage of the disease should result in very rapid clinical improvement (i.e., within 2 to 3 days). Failure to recognize acute disease or inappropriate treatment can lead to chronic disease, including relapsing polyarthritis, glomerulonephritis, and cardiac abnormalities.

## Fungal Arthritis

Fungal arthritis is rare. When it does occur, it is usually as an extension of osteomyelitis of fungal cause (*Coccidioides immitis, Blastomyces dermatitidis*, or *Cryptococcus neoformans*). More often, reactive, immune-mediated, culture-negative polyarthritis occurs in dogs and cats with systemic fungal infections.

## Calicivirus Arthritis

Natural calicivirus infection and attenuated live calicivirus vaccination have been associated with transient polyarthritis in 6- to 12-week-old kittens. Signs, which include lameness, stiffness, and fever, usually resolve spontaneously after 2 to 4 days. Some kittens develop overt calicivirus infection, with glossal and palatine vesicles or ulcers and signs of upper respiratory tract disease. Synovial fluid analysis reveals a mildly to greatly increased nucleated cell count with small mononuclear cells and macrophages predominating, some of which contain phagocytosed neutrophils. Virus isolation from affected joints is unrewarding, although the virus can be found in the oropharynx of some infected cats.

## NONINFECTIOUS INFLAMMATORY (IMMUNE-MEDIATED) JOINT DISEASES—NONEROSIVE (TEXT PP 1085-1089)

Noninfectious inflammatory (immune-mediated) joint diseases are very common in dogs and rare in cats. Based on radiographic evidence of joint destruction, they are classified as erosive or nonerosive. Erosive (rheumatoid arthritis [RA]–like) conditions are very rare. Nonerosive conditions are thought to be mediated through immune-complex formation and deposition and can occur as a feature of systemic lupus erythematosus (SLE), secondary to chronic antigenic stimulation from chronic infection, neoplasia, or drugs (i.e., reactive polyarthritis), or as an idiopathic syndrome. Breed-associated syndromes of polyarthritis, polyarthritis and meningitis, or polyarthritis and myositis also exist and are thought to have a genetic basis.

### SLE-Induced Polyarthritis

SLE is an immune-complex disease of unknown cause that is well documented in dogs and, to a lesser extent, cats. Any breed of dog may be affected, but Spitzes, Shetland Sheepdogs, Collies, German Shepherd Dogs, Beagles, and sporting breeds may have an increased incidence. Most affected dogs are 2 to 4 years old. Familial clustering suggests a hereditary factor. Although SLE is an uncommon cause of polyarthritis, its effects on other organ systems can be devastating; accurate diagnosis is therefore important.

#### Clinical signs

Clinical manifestations vary with organ involvement and include intermittent fever, polyarthritis, glomerulonephritis, skin lesions, hemolytic anemia, thrombocytopenia, myositis, and polyneuritis. Polyarthritis is the most common manifestation, occurring in 70% to 90% of dogs with SLE. A sterile, nonerosive, inflammatory arthritis occurs, with distal joints (hocks, carpi) usually more severely affected than proximal joints. Some dogs show no signs of joint disease, and their polyarthritis is detected during workup for fever or after identification of other evidence of immune disease (e.g., anemia, proteinuria). More often, animals show generalized stiffness or shifting-leg lameness.

#### Diagnosis

SLE should be suspected in any dog or cat with noninfectious polyarthritis. Careful physical examination, CBC, platelet count, biochemistry profile, urinalysis, and urine protein/creatinine ratio should be performed in every such animal.

*Synovial fluid.* Analysis reveals an increased cell count (5000 to 350,000/µl) primarily consisting of nondegenerate neutrophils (>80%). In rare instances, LE cells are detected in the synovial fluid.

*Laboratory tests.* The LE cell test (positive in 30% to 90% of cases) and antinuclear antibody (ANA) test (positive in 55% to 90% of cases) can aid in diagnosis (see Chapter 75).

*SLE and SLE-like multisystemic, immune-mediated disease.* A patient may be said to have SLE if the animal has a positive result of an LE cell test or an ANA test and if two or more of the clinical abnormalities known to be associated with SLE (e.g., polyarthritis, glomerulonephritis, anemia, thrombocytopenia, dermatitis) are present. When two or more of the common clinical syndromes are recognized but none of the serologic tests are positive, the dog is determined to have an SLE-like multisystemic immune-mediated disease.

#### Treatment and prognosis

Treatment is as for idiopathic, immune-mediated polyarthritis. If the patient is clinically normal and synovial fluid is noninflammatory after 6 months, it may be worthwhile to discontinue medications, because long periods of drug-free remission can occur.

Prognosis is good for control of polyarthritis, but multisystemic involvement (particularly glomerulonephritis) may progress despite therapy, occasionally resulting in death.

## Reactive Polyarthritis

### Etiology

Reactive polyarthritis is a relatively common manifestation of immune-complex disease seen in association with chronic bacterial, fungal, or parasitic infections (bacterial endocarditis, pleuritis, diskospondylitis, and dirofilariasis), neoplasia (squamous cell carcinoma, mammary adenocarcinoma, and other tumors), drug administration (sulfadiazine-trimethoprim, phenobarbital, erythropoietin, penicillins, cephalexin, and routine vaccinations), or GI disease. It may develop with any chronic inflammatory disorder or persistent antigenic stimulus.

### Clinical signs and diagnosis

Signs may include cyclic fevers, stiffness, and lameness. Some signs attributable to the underlying disorder may also be present. Although the underlying condition is often obvious, occasionally patients are not presented until the polyarthritis makes them reluctant to walk. Therefore it is important that a thorough physical examination of every animal with polyarthritis be performed; that a complete history regarding the administration of medications and the presence or absence of systemic signs be obtained; and that the following screening tests be performed to detect underlying disease: CBC, thoracic and abdominal radiographs, abdominal ultrasound, culture of urine and blood, cardiac ultrasound, rickettsial and Lyme disease titers, heartworm test (dogs), and feline leukemia virus (FeLV) and feline immunodeficiency virus (FIV) tests (cats). Radiographically the only finding is joint swelling.

*Synovial fluid.* Analysis reveals an increase in white blood cell (WBC) count and percentage of neutrophils. Even when the primary inflammatory disease is infectious, culture of the synovial fluid is negative, suggesting an immune-mediated cause.

### Treatment

Treatment must be directed at eliminating the underlying disease or antigenic stimulus. If this can be accomplished, the polyarthritis usually resolves. Short-term, low-dose corticosteroid therapy (prednisone 0.25 to 1 mg/kg/day) may be needed to control the synovitis in severe cases.

## Idiopathic, Immune-Mediated, Nonerosive Polyarthritis

Nonerosive, noninfectious polyarthritis, in which an underlying disease process cannot be identified, is termed *idiopathic immune-mediated polyarthritis.* This disorder can be diagnosed only by ruling out the other causes of polyarthritis. It is the most common form of polyarthritis in dogs and is especially common in sporting and large breeds. Dogs of any age are affected, but the peak incidence is 2.5 to 4.5 years. This condition is uncommon in cats.

### Clinical signs

Signs may include cyclic fever, stiffness, and lameness that are unresponsive to antibiotics. Cervical pain and vertebral hypersensitivity may reflect intervertebral facetal joint involvement or concurrent meningitis. Signs may be subtle, and the diagnosis is easily missed. Often no palpable joint effusion or localizable pain is present. Many patients have a history of decreased appetite or fever of unknown origin. Multiple joints are usually involved, with the small distal joints (carpus and hock) affected most severely; disease affecting only the elbow joint has also been reported.

### Diagnosis

Diagnosis is based on synovial fluid analysis, radiography, failure to identify an infectious cause for the polyarthritis, the absence of evidence of SLE, and no identifiable cause to indicate reactive polyarthritis. CBC commonly reveals neutrophilia, although neutropenia is occasionally noted and some dogs have a normal CBC. Radiographic findings are normal or show only joint and periarticular swelling with no bone or cartilage abnormalities.

*Synovial fluid.* The fluid is thin and may be turbid, and the mucin clot test is normal or only slightly abnormal. Nucleated cell counts are increased (4000 to 370,000 cells/$\mu$l); nondegenerate neutrophils predominate (usually >80%). In less severe cases and cases in which corticosteroids have been administered, a lower WBC and neutrophil percentage (30% to 80%) may be present. Blood, urine, and synovial fluid cultures are negative for bacteria and mycoplasma.

*Investigating the cause.* Thorough evaluation for underlying immune-mediated disease should be performed. Dogs and cats with idiopathic polyarthritis are usually ANA negative and lack evidence of immune disease affecting other systems (unlike SLE). If synovial biopsies are performed, they reveal neutrophilic synovitis initially; but with chronicity, lymphocytes, plasma cells, and macrophages predominate, and villous hyperplasia may develop.

### Treatment

Glucocorticoids are the initial treatment of choice. Prednisone alone results in remission in 50% of cases; 2 to 4 mg/kg/day PO is given for 2 weeks and followed by 1 to 2 mg/kg/day for 2 weeks. If after that time the animal is clinically normal and the synovial fluid inflammation has subsided, the dose is decreased to 1 to 2 mg/kg q48h. This dose is administered for 4 weeks, and then the dose is further tapered if synovial fluid cytology is normal. If a dog can be maintained on a low, alternate-day dose of prednisone (<0.5 mg/kg every other day) for 2 months and the synovial fluid is not inflammatory, it may be possible to discontinue all therapy Management should initially include restricted exercise, followed by regular gentle exercise and weight control. Chondroprotective agents may also prove beneficial

*Monitoring.* Monthly synovial fluid evaluations are recommended during initial therapy. The fluid should be noninflammatory before each decrease in drug dose. If the joints remain noninflammatory, the drug dose may be tapered monthly. Rarely the drug can be discontinued, but most patients need lifelong therapy with at least alternate-day prednisone. In dogs on a stable dose of medication, synovial fluid should be evaluated every 4 to 6 months.

*Other immunosuppressive drugs.* Azathioprine (Imuran, 50 mg/m$^2$ q24h) should be used in dogs with persistent clinical signs or synovial inflammation despite prednisone therapy and in dogs that relapse when the prednisone dose is decreased. Azathioprine may also be used when a lower alternate-day dose of prednisone is desirable. Azathioprine (2.2 mg/kg) is given once daily for 4 to 6 weeks and then only on alternate days if the animal is doing well clinically and the synovial fluid is no longer inflammatory. The major toxic effect is myelosuppression; CBC and platelet count should initially be monitored every 2 weeks, and then every 6 to 8 weeks. Hepatic enzymes should also be monitored for evidence of hepatotoxicity. Dogs treated with azathioprine and prednisone may also be at increased risk for developing pancreatitis.

### Prognosis

Prognosis is good; one patient in 50 is difficult to treat and keep in remission. Additional therapies such as cyclophosphamide, leflunonamide, or chrysotherapy should be considered in these patients (see Chapter 93). Dogs on long-term (4 to 5 years) high-dose immunosuppressive drug therapy may develop symptomatic DJD secondary to chronic low-grade synovial inflammation or the detrimental effects of corticosteroids on cartilage synthesis and repair.

## Breed-Specific Polyarthritis Syndromes

Immune-mediated polyarthritis can occur as a breed-related problem with or without disease involving other organ systems. A heritable polyarthritis has been documented in Akitas <1 year of age and sporadically in Boxers and Weimaraners. Many of these dogs also have meningitis that resembles the meningeal vasculitis syndromes seen in other breeds (see Chapter 71). They are ANA negative and generally respond poorly to immunosuppressive therapy.

In contrast, polyarthritis that accompanies meningeal vasculitis in some Bernese Mountain Dogs, German Shorthair Pointers, and Beagles often responds completely to immunosuppressive therapy. Familial polyarthritis with concurrent myositis and poor response to therapy has been reported in a few Spaniel breeds.

### Shar Pei fever

Progressive renal amyloidosis and polyarthritis has been documented in the Shar Pei and is known as "Shar Pei fever" or "Shar Pei hock" syndrome. The disease affects growing puppies or adult dogs and is initially characterized by episodic fever and swelling of the hock or carpal joints. Over time, affected dogs develop renal or hepatic failure from amyloidosis. Monitoring severity of urinary protein loss using urine protein/creatinine ratios is recommended. Steroid treatment is of little value and may actually hasten the development of amyloidosis.

## Lymphoplasmacytic Synovitis

Lymphoplasmacytic synovitis is a rare syndrome that affects the stifle joints of dogs. Signs are limited to acute or chronic lameness involving one or both rear limbs. This immune-mediated synovitis can cause cruciate ligament degeneration and rupture, necessitating differentiation from more conventional causes of cruciate rupture such as trauma or instability.

### Clinical signs and diagnosis

Affected animals are in good body condition and are not systemically ill; CBC is normal. Synovial fluid is thin and turbid with an increased nucleated cell count (5000 to 20,000 cells/µl; occasionally >200,000/µl), and a predominance of lymphocytes and plasma cells in most affected dogs. Biopsy of ligament and synovium should be performed during surgical repair when dogs are presented for nontraumatic cruciate ligament rupture. Characteristic histopathologic changes seen in the synovial lining and cruciate ligaments include lymphocytic and plasmacytic infiltration and villous hyperplasia.

### Treatment

Treatment is as for idiopathic polyarthritis, together with surgical stabilization and synovectomy of diseased intraarticular tissue. Antiinflammatory therapy with colchicine (0.03 mg/kg PO q24h) is occasionally used.

## NONINFECTIOUS INFLAMMATORY JOINT DISEASES—EROSIVE (TEXT PP 1089-1092)

### Rheumatoid Arthritis

RA is a rare disease in dogs that results in erosive polyarthritis and progressive joint destruction. Small and toy breeds are most commonly affected. Age at onset is variable (9 months to 13 years), but most affected dogs are young or middle aged. Initially the disease is indistinguishable from idiopathic nonerosive polyarthritis, but the joints are destroyed over time (weeks or months). The precise cause is unknown, but extrapolation from human RA suggests an immune-mediated mechanism involving the formation of autoantibodies with immune-complex deposition in the synovium.

### Clinical signs

Initially signs are indistinguishable from other forms of polyarthritis. Joint pain and stiffness are prominent; the joints may appear normal or may be swollen and painful. In the early stages, signs may be sporadic, and stiffness is generally worse after rest and improves with mild exercise. Fever, depression, anorexia, and reluctance to exercise are common. As the disease progresses, clinical examination reveals crepitus, laxity, luxation, and deformity of affected joints. The joints most commonly affected are the carpi, hocks, and phalanges, although the elbows, shoulders, and stifles can also be affected.

### Diagnosis

RA should be suspected in any dog with noninfectious, erosive polyarthritis. Diagnosis depends on clinical and radiographic findings, characteristic synovial fluid, poor mucin clot test, positive rheumatoid factor (RF) test, and typical histopathologic changes seen in a synovial biopsy. Synovial fluid collection is best performed during a period when the dog is most symptomatic, as the cyclical nature of the disease could make diagnosis difficult.

*Radiography.* Early radiographic evaluation reveals periarticular swelling with minimal bony change. Later, radiographic features include periarticular osteoporosis, narrowing of the joint space, and focal, irregular, radiolucent cystlike areas of subchondral bone destruction. In long-standing cases, joint space collapse, marginal erosions, and subluxation or luxation are common.

*Synovial fluid.* The fluid is thin, cloudy, and hypercellular (6000 to 80,000/μl, average 30,000/μl), with a poor mucin clot. Neutrophils are usually the predominant cell (20% to 95%, average 74%), although in some animals mononuclear cells predominate. Synovial fluid culture is negative.

*Other tests.* Serologic tests detect circulating antibody (RF) against denatured or immune-complexed immunoglobulin G. A titer of 1:16 is considered positive and is found in 20% to 70% of affected dogs. Weak false-positive results may be seen in other systemic inflammatory diseases and DJD. Synovial biopsy often reveals thickening, hyperplasia, and proliferative synovitis with pannus formation. Culture of the biopsied tissue is typically negative.

### Treatment

Early treatment is important to prevent irreversible changes and progressive disease. Medical treatment usually includes immunosuppressive drugs, gold salts, and chondroprotective agents. Despite their antiinflammatory and immunosuppressive effects, systemic corticosteroids do not seem to have any effect on the long-term progression of RA in people, and the response in dogs is variable.

*Immunosuppressive drugs.* Initially, prednisone (2 to 4 mg/kg/day PO for 14 days, then 1 to 2 mg/kg/day for 14 days) and azathioprine (2.2 mg/kg/day) should be used as described for refractory idiopathic nonerosive polyarthritis. Cyclophosphamide (Cytoxan, 50 mg/m² PO) may be administered in addition to or instead of azathioprine on a 4-days-on and 3-days-off schedule or every other day. Chronic cyclophosphamide treatment (>2 months) increases the risk for sterile hemorrhagic cystitis.

*Chondroprotective agents.* Oral chondroprotective agents (Cosequin or glucosamine and chondroitin sulfate) are routinely administered. Subjective improvement has also been observed in dogs receiving injectable chondroprotective agents (e.g., Adequan).

*Monitoring.* After 1 month the dog is reexamined and synovial fluid reevaluated. If the fluid is still inflammatory, methotrexate (2.5 mg/m² PO [1 to 2 mg/kg]) may be added to the regimen of prednisone and azathioprine. If, however, the fluid is noninflammatory, the prednisone dose is decreased to 1 to 2 mg/kg PO q48h.

*Gold salts.* If synovial inflammation persists after 2 months, gold salts should be added to the therapy. Aurothioglucose (Solganol) is used at a dose of 1 mg/kg IM once weekly for 10 weeks or until remission occurs, followed by 1 mg/kg IM once a month. Toxicity is uncommon but may include fever, thrombocytopenia, leukopenia, dermatitis, glomerulonephritis, and stomatitis. Alternatively, the oral preparation, auranofin (Ridaura, 0.05 mg/kg PO q12h; maximum 9 mg/day) can be used, but it is less effective and very expensive.

*Other drugs.* Leflunomide has recently been used with some success when administered at an initial dose of 4 mg/kg/day, and the dose is adjusted to maintain a trough plasma level of 20 mg/ml (usual maintenance dose is 0.5 mg/kg/day).

*Analgesics.* Even in remission, many dogs require additional therapy to control joint pain. Aspirin (10 to 20 mg/kg PO q8-12h) and other NSAIDS (for doses, see the discussion of NSAIDS in the earlier section on DJD) have been recommended, but the additive GI toxicities of corticosteroids and NSAIDS must be considered. Concurrent administration of misoprostol can decrease GI adverse effects. Administration of these medications with food may also decrease GI adverse effects.

*Surgery.* Surgical procedures such as synovectomy, arthroplasty, joint replacement, and arthrodesis may decrease pain and improve function.

### Prognosis

RA is a progressive disorder, and even with appropriate therapy most dogs deteriorate with time. Some success may be expected if the treatment is initiated before the onset of severe joint damage. However, in most cases severe cartilage damage has already taken place.

## Erosive Polyarthritis of Greyhounds

An erosive, immune-mediated polyarthritis has been described in greyhounds 3 to 30 months of age, primarily in Australia. The proximal interphalangeal joints and other distal joints are most commonly affected. Cartilage erosions occur in the absence of pannus formation and subchondral bone lysis. Therapy as for idiopathic, immune-mediated, nonerosive polyarthritis is sometimes effective. The condition may be associated with infection with *Mycoplasma spumans;* antimycoplasma agents (Tylosin, 15 mg/kg PO q8h) should therefore be administered in affected animals.

## Feline Chronic Progressive Polyarthritis

Feline chronic progressive polyarthritis occurs exclusively in male cats. The pathogenesis is not well understood but may involve exposure to feline syncytium-forming virus (FeSFV) and FeLV (or occasionally FIV). Two clinical variants exist: proliferative periosteal arthritis, which occurs predominantly in young-adult cats (1 to 5 years), and a more severe, deforming erosive arthritis that primarily affects older cats.

Diagnosis is based on signalment, clinical and radiographic findings, and synovial fluid analysis. Tests for FeSFV and FeLV may be positive. Cultures of synovial fluid are negative, and there exists no evidence that an underlying disorder is causing reactive polyarthritis.

### Periosteal proliferative form

This form of the disease is characterized by acute onset of fever, joint pain, lymphadenopathy, and edema of the skin and soft tissues overlying the joint. Initial radiographic changes include soft-tissue swelling and mild periosteal proliferation. With time, periosteal proliferation worsens and periarticular osteophytes, subchondral cysts, and joint space collapse, with fibrosis and ankylosis, may be noted. Synovial fluid analysis reveals an increased WBC count, particularly neutrophils. With chronicity the numbers of lymphocytes and plasma cells increase.

### Deforming, erosive form

The deforming type is rare. Onset is insidious, with slow development of lameness and stiffness. Deformation of the carpal and distal joints is common. Radiographs reveal severe subchondral central and marginal erosions, and luxations or subluxations leading to joint instability and deformities. Cytologic findings in synovial fluid are limited to a mild-to-moderate increase in inflammatory cells (neutrophils, lymphocytes, and macrophages).

### Treatment and prognosis

Prednisone (4 to 6 mg/kg/day) may slow the progression of these diseases. If the cat's condition is clinically improved after 2 weeks, the dose is decreased to 2 mg/kg/day. In some cats alternate-day therapy (1 to 2 mg/kg q48h) is adequate. Combination therapy with cyclophosphamide (50 mg/m$^2$ PO, 4 days on, 3 days off) or chlorambucil (Leukeran, 20 mg/m$^2$ PO every 2 weeks) may aid long-term control.

Prognosis is good for temporary improvement but not for complete control. Lifetime therapy is required. FeLV-positive cats commonly develop other FeLV-related disorders.

## Drugs Used in Joint Disease

| Drug name (trade name) | Purpose | Recommended dose | |
|---|---|---|---|
| | | Dogs | Cats |
| Acetylsalicylic acid (aspirin) | Analgesic, antiinflammatory | 25 mg/kg PO q8h | 10 mg/kg PO q48h |
| | Antithrombotic | 10 mg/kg q12h | 10 mg/kg PO q12h |
| Amoxicillin | Antibiotic | 20 mg/kg PO, SC, IV q12h | 20 mg/kg PO, SC, IV q12h |
| Ampicillin | Antibiotic | 22 mg/kg PO q8h or | 22 mg/kg PO q8h or |
| | | 22 mg/kg IV, SC, IM q6h | 22 mg/kg IV, SC, IM q6h |
| Auranofin (Ridaura) | Treatment of immune-mediated diseases | 0.5-0.2 mg/kg PO q12h (max. 9 mg/day) | None |
| Aurothioglucose (Solganol) | Treatment of immune-mediated diseases | 1 mg/kg IM weekly for 10 wk, then q30days | 1 mg/kg IM weekly for 10 wk, then q30days |
| Azathioprine (Imuran) | Treatment of immune-mediated diseases | 50 mg/m$^2$ (approx. 2.2 mg/kg) q24h | 0.2 mg/kg PO q48h |
| Carprofen (Rimadyl) | Analgesic | | |
| | Antiinflammatory | 2.2 mg/kg PO q12h | Not evaluated |
| Ceftriaxone sodium | Antibiotic | 20 mg/kg IV q12h | 20 mg/kg IV q12h |
| Cephalexin (Keflex) | Antibiotic | 20-40 mg/kg PO q8h | 20-40 mg/kg PO q8h |
| Chloramphenicol | Antibiotic | 25-50 mg/kg PO, IV q6-8h | 25 mg/kg PO q12h |
| Chondroitin sulfate | Chondroprotective | 15 to 20 mg/kg q12h | Unknown |
| Cyclophosphamide (Cytoxan) | Treatment of immune-mediated diseases | 50 mg/m$^2$ (approx. 2.2 mg/kg), 4 days on, 3 off or q48h | 50 mg/m$^2$, 4 days on and 3 days off, or q48h |

| Drug | Classification | | |
|---|---|---|---|
| Doxycycline (Vibramycin) | Antibiotic | 5-10 mg/kg PO or IV q12h | 5-10 mg/kg PO or IV q12h |
| Erythromycin | Antibiotic | 10 mg/kg PO q8h | 10 mg/kg PO q8h |
| Etodolac (Etogesic) | Analgesic | 10-15 mg/kg PO q24h | Unknown |
| Glucosamine | Chondroprotective | 15 to 20 mg/kg q12h | Unknown |
| Ketoprofen (Anafen) | Analgesic Antiinflammatory | 1-2 mg/kg PO q24h | 1-2 mg/kg PO q24h |
| Meloxicam (Metacam) | Analgesic | 0.2 mg/kg once, then 0.1 mg/kg/day PO | Unknown |
| Minocycline (Minocin) | Antibiotic | 25 mg/kg PO q12h | None |
| Oxytetracycline | Antibiotic | 20 mg/kg PO q8h | 20 mg/kg PO q8h |
| Penicillin G | Antibiotic Aqueous (K or Na) Procaine | 40,000 U/kg IV q6h 40,000 U/kg IM, SC q12h | 40,000 U/kg IV q6h 40,000 U/kg IM, SC q12h |
| Phenylbutazone (Butazolidin) | Analgesia | 1-5 mg/kg PO q8h | None |
| Piroxicam (Feldene) | Analgesia | 0.3 mg/kg PO q48h | Unknown |
| Polysulfated glycosaminoglycan (Adequan) | Chondroprotective | 2-5 mg/kg IM q4days for four treatments, then q30days | None |
| Prednisone | Immunosuppression Antiinflammatory, antiedema agent | 2-4 mg/kg/day PO 0.5-0.75 mg/kg PO | 2-6 mg/kg/day PO 0.5-0.75 mg/kg PO |
| Sodium aurothiomalate (Myochrisine) | Treatment of immune-mediated diseases | 1 mg/kg IM weekly | None |
| Tetracycline hydrochloride | Antibiotic | 22 mg/kg q8h | 22 mg/kg PO q8h |
| Tylosin (Tylan) | Antibiotic | 20 mg/kg PO q8h | 20 mg/kg PO q8h |

*IM,* Intramuscularly; *IV,* intravenously; *K,* potassium; *Na,* sodium; *PO,* orally; *SC,* subcutaneously.

# PART XI

# Oncology

C. GUILLERMO COUTO

# 77

# Cytology

## (Text pp 1093-1099)

## SAMPLE COLLECTION AND PREPARATION (TEXT PP 1093-1094)

### Collection Techniques

#### Fine-needle aspiration

Fine-needle aspiration (FNA) of suspected neoplastic lesions is highly recommended; it can provide valuable information for definitive diagnosis, sometimes circumventing the need for surgical biopsy. Prognostic or therapeutic decisions should be based only on the evaluation of the cytologic specimen by a board-certified veterinary clinical pathologist.

*Procedure for FNA.* FNA is performed using a small-gauge (23- to 25-gauge) needle of appropriate length and a 12- or 20-ml sterile syringe. A needle without syringe can be used to obtain a cytologic specimen in some cases. Easily accessible tissues include the skin and subcutis, lymph nodes, spleen, liver, kidneys, lungs, thyroid, prostate, and mediastinal masses. The technique is described in the text. Clipping and sterile surgical preparation is not necessary for superficial masses but should always be used when organs or masses within body cavities are aspirated.

#### Scrapings and impression smears

Superficial ulcerated masses can easily be sampled by scraping their surface with a sterile scalpel blade, wooden tongue depressor, or gauze. Surgical specimens or open lesions can be sampled by making impression smears of the exposed surface. Surgical specimens should first be gently blotted onto a gauze pad or paper towel to remove any blood or debris; it is advisable to submit a different tissue specimen for histopathologic evaluation.

Smears are made by touching a glass slide onto the ulcerated lesion or scraping the surface with a tongue depressor and transferring the material onto the slide. "Pull" smears made using two glass slides are preferred over "push" smears. Once the smears are made, they are air-dried and stained.

### Staining

Practical staining techniques for in-office use include rapid Romanowsky's (e.g., Diff-Quik) and new methylene blue (NMB). Romanowsky's stains are more time consuming, but they offer better cellular detail and nucleus-cytoplasm contrast, and stained smears can be permanently archived. NMB staining is quick, but it is not permanent, and cellular details are not as sharp as with Romanowsky's stains; and because NMB stains nuclear ribonucleic acid very well, most cells appear "malignant." NMB can be used for initial assessment of the quality of the sample (and possibly a tentative diagnosis); the remaining slides should be stained with Diff-Quik or Wright's stain for final evaluation. Note: Rapid hematologic stains such as Diff-Quik do not stain the granules in some mast cell tumors (MCTs) and large granular lymphocytes (LGLs).

## INTERPRETING NONNEOPLASTIC SPECIMENS (TEXT PP 1094-1099)

The clinician should strive to be able to evaluate cytologic specimens proficiently; however, the ultimate cytologic diagnosis should be made by a board-certified veterinary clinical pathologist.

### Normal Tissues

Profiles of epithelial tissues, mesenchymal tissues, and hematopoietic tissues can be found in the text (p. 1094).

### Hyperplastic Processes

Hyperplastic changes may be difficult to recognize because they can mimic either normal or neoplastic tissues. Care should be taken when evaluating specimens from organs such as enlarged prostates or thickened urinary bladders; the high degree of hyperplasia and dysplasia may suggest malignancy (see later).

### Inflammatory Processes

Most inflammatory reactions are characterized by the presence of inflammatory cells and debris. The type of cell present depends on the causative agent and the duration of the inflammatory process. Acute processes are usually characterized by predominance of granulocytes, whereas macrophages and lymphocytes predominate in chronic processes. The following causative agents are frequently identified in cytologic specimens: *Histoplasma, Blastomyces, Cryptococcus, Coccidioides, Aspergillus* or *Penicillium, Toxoplasma, Leishmania*, other rickettsial agents, bacteria, and *Demodex*.

## MALIGNANCIES (TEXT PP 1095-1098)

Cells populating most normal organs and tissues (with the exception of bone marrow precursors) are well differentiated. Most of the cells are similar in size and shape, they have a normal nuclear/cytoplasmic ratio (N:C), the nuclei usually have condensed chromatin and no nucleoli, and the cytoplasm may exhibit differentiation (e.g., keratin formation in squamous epithelium).

### Criteria for Malignancy

Malignant cells exhibit one or more of the following features:
- low N:C (larger nucleus and smaller cytoplasm)
- fine chromatin pattern
- presence of nucleoli, usually multiple
- anisokaryosis (cells with nuclei of different sizes)
- nuclear molding (nuclei in multinucleated cells compressing each other)
- morphologic homogeneity (all cells look alike)
- pleomorphism (cells in different stages of development)
- cytoplasmic vacuolization, primarily in malignant epithelial tumors
- cytoplasmic basophilia
- anisocytosis (cells of different sizes)
- multinucleated giant cells
- phagocytosis

Another criterion of malignancy is heterotopia (presence of a given cell type where it is usually not found). In addition, malignant cells tend to be morphologically different from the progenitor cell population.

### Types of Malignancy

On the basis of the predominant cytologic features, malignancies can be classified as carcinomas (epithelial), sarcomas (mesenchymal), and round (or discrete) cell tumors.

### Carcinomas

Most carcinomas are composed of round or polygonal cells that tend to form clusters; cytoplasmic boundaries may be indistinct. The cytoplasm is usually deep blue and vacuolated in most adenocarcinomas (aCAs). In squamous cell carcinomas (SCCs), cells are usually individualized and have deep blue cytoplasm with an occasional eosinophilic fringe, but no vacuoles. Nuclei in both aCAs and SCCs are large, with a fine chromatin pattern and nucleoli.

### Sarcomas

Specific cytologic features vary with histologic type. However, most mesenchymal tumors have spindle-shaped, polygonal, polyhedral, or oval-shaped cells, with reddish-blue or dark blue cytoplasm and irregularly shaped nuclei. Most cells are individualized, although clumping may occur. The cells tend to form "tails," with the nuclei protruding from the cytoplasm. Spindle-shaped or polygonal cells with vacuolated, blue-gray cytoplasm are highly suggestive of hemangiosarcoma. Multinucleated giant cells are common in feline sarcomas. Osteosarcomas and chondrosarcomas usually have round or ovoid cells. Intercellular matrix (e.g., osteoid, chondroid) is occasionally found.

Because sarcoma cells do not exfoliate easily, aspirates of these masses may yield false-negative results. Therefore, when a sarcoma is suspected but FNA results are negative, a core biopsy should be obtained.

### Round (discrete) cell tumors

Tumors composed of a homogeneous population of round cells are referred to as *round* (or *discrete) cell tumors* (RCTs). They are common in dogs and cats and include lymphomas (LSAs), histiocytomas (HCTs), MCTs, transmissible venereal tumors (TVTs), plasma cell tumors (PCTs), and malignant melanomas; as discussed above, osteosarcomas and chondrosarcomas can be composed of round cells. RCTs are easily diagnosed on cytology; the presence or absence of cytoplasmic granules or vacuoles further aids their classification.

*Tumors with cytoplasmic granules.* Cells in MCTs, LGL LSAs, and melanomas usually have cytoplasmic granules; neuroendocrine tumors cells can also have granules. When hematologic stains are used, the granules are purple in MCTs; red in LGL LSAs; and black, green, brown, or yellow in melanomas. LSAs, HCTs, PCTs, and TVTs typically lack cytoplasmic granules, although cytoplasmic vacuoles are common in TVTs and HCTs.

*Lymphomas.* LSAs are characterized by a monomorphic population of individual, undifferentiated round cells with large nuclei, coarse chromatin, and one or two nucleoli.

*Histiocytomas.* HCTs are similar to LSAs, except that the cytoplasm is more abundant, the chromatin pattern is fine, and they are frequently vacuolated. Inflammation is an important component of HCTs, so inflammatory cells (mainly lymphocytes) are commonly found in these tumors.

*Mast cell tumors.* MCTs are characteristic in that the cytoplasm contains purple (metachromatic) granules; the granules can be so numerous as to obscure the nuclear features. Granules may be absent in poorly differentiated tumors or in those stained with Diff-Quik.

## INTERPRETING LYMPH NODE ASPIRATES (TEXT PP 1098-1099)

In approximately 90% of dogs and 60% to 75% of cats with lymphadenopathy, a definitive diagnosis can be made cytologically. If cytology of an enlarged lymph node is inconclusive, the node should be surgically excised and submitted for histopathologic examination.

### Cytologic Patterns

Lymph nodes react to a variety of stimuli. In general, four cytologic patterns are recognized: normal, reactive or hyperplastic lymphadenopathy, lymphadenitis, and neoplasia.

### Normal lymph node

Cytologic specimens from normal nodes are composed predominantly (75% to 90%) of small lymphocytes. These cells are 7 to 10 μm in diameter (1 to 1.5 times that of a red blood cell) and have dense chromatin and no nucleoli. The remaining cells are macrophages, lymphoblasts, plasma cells, and other immune cells.

### Reactive or hyperplastic lymphadenopathy

Lymphoid tissues reacting to different antigenic stimuli (e.g., bacterial, immunologic, neoplastic, fungal) are cytologically similar. The cell population is composed of a mixture of lymphocytes (small, intermediate, and large), lymphoblasts, plasma cells, and macrophages. Depending on the specific agent, other cell types may be present (e.g., eosinophils in parasitic or allergic reactions). The first impression when a reactive or hyperplastic node is evaluated cytologically is that of a heterogeneous population of cells. The presence of cells in different stages of development indicates that the lymphoid tissue is undergoing polyclonal expansion in response to multiple antigens.

### Lymphadenitis

Inflammatory processes affecting the lymph nodes result in cytologic changes similar to those in reactive lymphadenopathy, although there exists a profusion of inflammatory cells and, on occasion, degenerative changes (e.g., pyknosis, karyorrhexis) in most cell lines. The causative agent may be seen.

### Neoplasia

Neoplastic cells can appear in a lymph node either as a result of lymphatic or vascular dissemination (metastasis from a distant primary tumor) or as a primary process affecting the lymph node (e.g., lymphoma). Metastatic lesions are characterized by a reactive pattern and presence of neoplastic cells (morphology depends on the primary tumor type). It is usually difficult to identify normal lymphoid cells in advanced metastatic lesions. LSAs are characterized by a monomorphous population of large, immature lymphoid cells that have an abnormally low N:C, coarse chromatin, and nucleoli.

# 78

# Principles of Cancer Treatment

## *(Text pp 1100-1102)*

Several therapeutic modalities have been used in dogs and cats with cancer, including surgery, radiotherapy, chemotherapy, immunotherapy, hyperthermia, cryotherapy, phototherapy, photochemotherapy or thermochemotherapy, and unconventional (alternative) therapies. Although euthanasia is a reasonable alternative to cancer treatment, every effort should be made to investigate other treatment options. In addition to tumor-related factors such as tumor type, biologic behavior, and clinical staging, several factors influence treatment selection.

Table 78-1

## Modified Karnovsky's Performance Scheme for Dogs and Cats

| Grade | Activity and performance |
|---|---|
| 0—Normal | Fully active, able to perform at predisease level |
| 1—Restricted | Restricted activity compared with predisease level but able to function as an acceptable pet |
| 2—Compromised | Severely restricted activity level; ambulatory only to the point of eating but consistently defecating and urinating in acceptable areas |
| 3—Disabled | Completely disabled; must be force-fed; unable to confine urinations and defecations to acceptable areas |
| 4—Dead | |

Modified from International Histological Classification of Tumors of Domestic Animals, *Bull World Health Organ* 53:145-282, 1976.

## PATIENT-RELATED FACTORS (TEXT P 1100)

The best treatment for a particular tumor does not necessarily constitute the best treatment for a particular patient. The most important factor to be considered is the patient's general health and activity or performance status (Table 78-1). A cat or dog with markedly diminished activity and severe constitutional signs may not be a good candidate for aggressive chemotherapy or for the repeated anesthesia needed for radiotherapy. Age alone is not a factor that should be taken into consideration (i.e., "old age is not a disease"); rather, the emphasis should be on evaluation of the patient's health status (heart failure, renal disease, and so on).

Patient-related factors should be addressed (e.g., azotemia corrected; nutritional status improved with enteral feeding) before a specific cancer treatment is instituted.

## OWNER-RELATED FACTORS (TEXT PP 1100-1101)

Owner-related factors play an important role in small animal oncology. The owner-pet bond is so important that it often dictates the treatment approach. All potential treatment options should be discussed with the owner, including a thorough discussion of potential adverse effects and costs. The option of euthanasia should also be addressed at this time, as an immediate option or if treatment fails. Assigning owners tasks to perform at home, such as measuring the tumor(s) to monitor response to treatment, taking the pet's temperature daily, and monitoring performance status allows them to assume responsibility for the fate of their pet. As part of the medical team, they are usually quite cooperative.

## TREATMENT-RELATED FACTORS (TEXT PP 1101-1102)

Several treatment-related factors are important when planning cancer therapy. First, the specific indications of the treatment modalities should be considered. Surgery, radiotherapy, and hyperthermia are aimed at eradicating locally invasive tumors with low metastatic potential (potentially curative), although they can be used palliatively in patients with extensive or metastatic disease. In contrast, chemotherapy is not usually curative (except in dogs with transmissible venereal tumors treated with vincristine), although long-term palliation of advanced disease can easily be accomplished for several tumor types. Immunotherapy also constitutes an adjuvant or palliative approach.

### Combination therapies

For most tumors the highest success rates are obtained by combining two or more treatment modalities. For example, the combination of surgery and chemotherapy

**Table 78-2**

## Complications and Adverse Effects of Cancer Treatment

| Treatment | Common adverse effects and complications |
|---|---|
| Surgery | Bleeding |
| | Unacceptable appearance |
| | Functional abnormalities |
| Radiotherapy | Moist desquamation in irradiated site |
| | Permanent alopecia in irradiated site |
| | Necrosis (soft tissue or bone) |
| | Fistula or stricture formation |
| Chemotherapy | Myelosuppression |
| | Gastrointestinal |
| | Perivascular tissue necrosis |
| | Other (see Chapter 80) |

(with or without immunotherapy) can significantly prolong disease-free survival in dogs with osteosarcoma of the appendicular skeleton or splenic hemangiosarcoma.

**Adverse effects**

The complications and adverse effects of the treatment modalities also need to be considered when therapy is planned. Table 78-2 lists potential complications of different modalities. (Complications of chemotherapy are addressed in Chapter 80.) A good motto is, "The patient should feel better with the treatment than with the disease."

**Palliation versus cure**

Cancer treatment is intended to be either palliative (chemotherapy, immunotherapy) or curative (surgery, radiotherapy, and hyperthermia [potentially]), although these two approaches sometimes overlap. If possible, every effort should be made shortly after diagnosis to achieve a cure. In general, it is best to use an aggressive treatment when the tumor is first detected (because this is when the chances of eradicating every single tumor cell are the highest) rather than to wait until the tumor is at an advanced stage. With very few exceptions malignancies do not spontaneously regress; delay in treatment therefore only increases the probability that the tumor will disseminate locally or systemically, decreasing the likelihood of a cure.

If a cure cannot be achieved, the main goal of treatment is induction of remission (decrease in tumor mass) while achieving a good quality of life. When one objectively evaluates the effects of therapy, the tumor(s) should be measured, and the response assessed using the following criteria:

- complete remission (CR)—complete disappearance of all tumor masses
- partial remission (PR)—decrease in tumor size by more than 50%
- stable disease (SD)—less than 25% variation in tumor size
- progressive disease (PD)—increase in tumor size by more than 25%

If good quality of life cannot be maintained, treatment should be modified or discontinued.

***Palliative treatments.*** Palliative treatments, as the sole method of treatment for cancer, may provide prolonged, good-quality survival; palliation is an acceptable alternative to euthanasia in small animals with cancer and their owners.

***Surgery.*** In dogs or cats with ulcerated mammary carcinomas and small pulmonary metastases, mastectomy or lumpectomy (without chemotherapy) will likely result in several months of good-quality survival, until the metastatic lesions finally cause respiratory compromise. Surgery should also be considered when the removal of the lesion(s) will alleviate the patient's clinical signs, such as in cases of anal sac apocrine gland adenocarcinoma and metastatic sublumbar (or iliac) lymphadenopathy in which a mass is compressing the colon and rectum, causing the pet to strain to defecate. Sublumbar (or iliac) lymphadenectomies in combination with melphalan chemotherapy in dogs with metastatic apocrine gland adenocarcinoma of the anal sacs have resulted in survival times of 1 to 3 years.

**Paraneoplastic syndromes.** Paraneoplastic syndromes should be addressed even if specific antineoplastic therapy is not contemplated. Treatment of humoral hypercalcemia of malignancy with diphosphonates (bisphosphonates) greatly improves the quality of life of affected dogs. In my experience the serum calcium concentrations can be maintained within normal limits for most dogs, without the detection of any appreciable toxicity, using either etidronate (Didronel) at a dose of 10 to 20 mg/kg orally q12h or pamidronate (Aredia) at a dose of 1.3 to 1.5 mg/kg intravenously q6-8wk.

# 79

# Practical Chemotherapy

## *(Text pp 1103-1107)*

## PRINCIPLES OF CHEMOTHERAPY (TEXT PP 1103-1105)

Chemotherapeutic agents kill predominantly cells in rapidly dividing tissues. To exploit the effect of different chemotherapeutic drugs, it is common for three or more drugs to be combined to treat a given malignancy. Drugs used in combination chemotherapy protocols are selected on the basis of the following principles: (1) each should be active against the given tumor type, (2) each should act by a different mechanism of action, and (3) none should have superimposed toxicities.

### Single-agent chemotherapy

Combination chemotherapy generally results in more sustained remissions and prolonged survival times compared with the same malignancy treated with single-agent chemotherapy. Exceptions include the treatment of dogs with osteosarcoma using either cisplatin, carboplatin, or doxorubicin as single agents; dogs with chronic lymphocytic leukemia treated with chlorambucil alone; and dogs with transmissible venereal tumors treated with vincristine alone.

### Calculating dosage

The dosage of most chemotherapeutic agents is calculated on a surface-area basis, as follows:

$$\frac{\text{Weight (g)}^{2/3} \times \text{K (constant)}}{10^4} = \text{BSA (m}^2)$$

The constant is 10.1 for dogs and 10 for cats. Conversions of body weight into square meters of body surface area (BSA) are given in Tables 79-1 and 79-2. When drugs such as doxorubicin are used, calculation of dosage based on square meter of BSA usually causes adverse effects in small dogs (less than 10 kg) and in cats; a dose/kg is more appropriate in such patients.

## INDICATIONS (TEXT PP 1105-1106)

Chemotherapy is primarily indicated for patients with systemic (e.g., lymphoma, leukemias) or metastatic neoplasms, although it can be used for nonresectable,

Table 79-1

## Conversion of Body Weight to Body Surface Area in Dogs

| Body weight (kg) | Body surface area (m$^2$) |
| --- | --- |
| 0.5 | 0.06 |
| 1 | 0.10 |
| 2 | 0.15 |
| 3 | 0.20 |
| 4 | 0.25 |
| 5 | 0.29 |
| 6 | 0.33 |
| 7 | 0.36 |
| 8 | 0.40 |
| 9 | 0.43 |
| 10 | 0.46 |
| 11 | 0.49 |
| 12 | 0.52 |
| 13 | 0.55 |
| 14 | 0.58 |
| 15 | 0.60 |
| 16 | 0.63 |
| 17 | 0.66 |
| 18 | 0.69 |
| 19 | 0.71 |
| 20 | 0.74 |
| 21 | 0.76 |
| 22 | 0.78 |
| 23 | 0.81 |
| 24 | 0.83 |
| 25 | 0.85 |
| 26 | 0.88 |
| 27 | 0.90 |
| 28 | 0.92 |
| 29 | 0.94 |
| 30 | 0.96 |
| 31 | 0.99 |
| 32 | 1.01 |
| 33 | 1.03 |
| 34 | 1.05 |
| 35 | 1.07 |
| 36 | 1.09 |
| 37 | 1.11 |
| 38 | 1.13 |
| 39 | 1.15 |
| 40 | 1.17 |
| 41 | 1.19 |
| 42 | 1.21 |
| 43 | 1.23 |
| 44 | 1.25 |
| 45 | 1.26 |
| 46 | 1.28 |
| 47 | 1.30 |
| 48 | 1.32 |
| 49 | 1.34 |
| 50 | 1.36 |

Table 79-2

### Conversion of Body Weight to Body Surface Area in Cats

| Body weight (lb) | Body weight (kg) | Body surface area (m²) |
|---|---|---|
| 5 | 2.3 | 0.165 |
| 6 | 2.8 | 0.187 |
| 7 | 3.2 | 0.207 |
| 8 | 3.6 | 0.222 |
| 9 | 4.1 | 0.244 |
| 10 | 4.6 | 0.261 |
| 11 | 5.1 | 0.278 |
| 12 | 5.5 | 0.294 |
| 13 | 6 | 0.311 |
| 14 | 6.4 | 0.326 |
| 15 | 6.9 | 0.342 |
| 16 | 7.4 | 0.356 |
| 17 | 7.8 | 0.371 |
| 18 | 8.2 | 0.385 |
| 19 | 8.7 | 0.399 |
| 20 | 9.2 | 0.413 |

chemoresponsive neoplasms that are refractory to radiotherapy or hyperthermia. It can also be used as an adjuvant treatment after surgical debulking and is indicated for control of micrometastatic disease after surgical excision of a primary neoplasm (e.g., cisplatin, carboplatin, or doxorubicin therapy after limb amputation in dogs with osteosarcoma).

#### Intracavitary therapy
Intracavitary chemotherapy can be used in dogs and cats with malignant effusions or neoplastic involvement of the cavity or area in question (e.g., intrathecal cytosine arabinoside for central nervous system [CNS] lymphoma; intrapleural cisplatin or 5-fluorouracil for dogs with pleural carcinomatosis).

#### Neoadjuvant therapy
Neoadjuvant or primary chemotherapy refers to the use of anticancer drugs in patients with bulky tumors not amenable to surgical excision. After a decrease in size induced by the drugs, the tumor can be surgically excised and chemotherapy continued to eliminate any residual neoplastic cells (e.g., FAC for dogs with thyroid adenocarcinoma; VAC for dogs with subcutaneous hemangiosarcomas [see cancer chemotherapy protocol table]).

#### Contraindications
In general, chemotherapy should not be used as a substitute for surgery, radiotherapy, or hyperthermia. Nor should it be used in patients with severe underlying multiple organ dysfunction (or it should be used cautiously with dose modification).

## TYPES OF ANTICANCER DRUGS (TEXT PP 1106-1107)
Different types of anticancer drugs kill tumor cells by different mechanisms. Drugs that kill only dividing tumor cells by acting on several phases of the cycle are termed *cell cycle phase–nonspecific drugs;* alkylating agents belong to this group. Drugs that selectively kill tumor cells during a particular phase of the cell cycle are termed *phase-specific drugs;* most antimetabolites and plant alkaloids are phase specific. Drugs that kill both dividing and resting neoplastic cells are termed *cell cycle–nonspecific drugs.* These drugs (e.g., nitrosoureas) are extremely myelosuppressive. Most anticancer drugs are currently available as generic products.

### Alkylating agents

Alkylating agents cross-link DNA, preventing its duplication. They are phase-nonspecific drugs and are more active when given intermittently at high doses; they are also referred to as *radiomimetics*. The major toxic effects are myelosuppressive and gastrointestinal. Commonly used alkylating agents include cyclophosphamide (Cytoxan), chlorambucil (Leukeran), melphalan (Alkeran), cisplatin (Platinol, which should not be used in cats), and carboplatin (Paraplatin).

### Antimetabolites

Antimetabolites exert their effect during the S (synthesis) phase of the cell cycle and are more active when given repeatedly at low doses or as a continuous intravenous infusion. They are structural analogs of naturally occurring metabolites that substitute for normal purines or pyrimidines. The major toxic effects are myelosuppressive and gastrointestinal. Commonly used antimetabolites include cytosine arabinoside (Cytosar-U), methotrexate, 5-fluorouracil (5-FU, which should not be used in cats), and azathioprine (Imuran).

### Antitumor antibiotics

Antitumor antibiotics act by several mechanisms, the most important of which may be DNA damage by free radicals or a topoisomerase-II–dependent mechanism. The major toxic effects are myelosuppressive and gastrointestinal; doxorubicin is also extremely caustic if given perivascularly and has cumulative cardiotoxicity in dogs. Several natural, synthetic, or semisynthetic antitumor antibiotics are available, including doxorubicin (Adriamycin), bleomycin (Blenoxane), actinomycin D (Cosmegen), and mitoxantrone (Novantrone).

### Plant alkaloids

Plant alkaloids (or mitotic inhibitors) are derived from the periwinkle plant *(Vinca rosea)* and the May apple plant *(Podophyllum peltatum)*. *Vinca* derivatives disrupt the mitotic spindle and are therefore cell cycle phase specific. *Podophyllum* derivatives cross-link DNA. The major toxic effect is perivascular sloughing if the agent is extravasated; etoposide should not be used intravenously in dogs, because the vehicle (Tween 80) causes anaphylaxis. Commonly used plant alkaloids include vincristine (Oncovin), vinblastine (Velban), and etoposide or VP-16 (VePesid).

### Hormones

Hormones (e.g., glucocorticoids [prednisone]) are used for the treatment of hemolymphatic malignancies, CNS masses, and endocrine-related tumors. With the exception of corticosteroids the use of hormones is not recommended because of their related adverse effects.

### Miscellaneous agents

Miscellaneous agents, such as dacarbazine (DTIC) and L-asparaginase (Elspar), are drugs with a mechanism of action that is either unknown or different from those listed previously.

# 80

# Complications of Cancer Chemotherapy

## *(Text pp 1108-1116)*

Most anticancer agents are relatively nonselective in that they kill both rapidly dividing neoplastic tissues and some of the rapidly dividing host tissues (e.g., villus epithelium, bone marrow cells). In addition, most anticancer agents have low therapeutic indexes. Increasing the dose increases the proportion of neoplastic cells killed, but it also enhances the drug's toxicity.

Myelosuppression and gastrointestinal (GI) signs are the most common toxicities encountered in practice. Less common complications of chemotherapy are listed in Table 80-1.

### Contributing factors

Several factors can potentiate the effects of anticancer agents and therefore enhance their toxicity. Drugs that are primarily excreted via the kidneys (e.g., cisplatin, carboplatin, methotrexate) are more toxic to patients with renal disease; therefore dose reduction is usually recommended. In general, cats are more likely than dogs to develop anorexia and vomiting during chemotherapy but are less susceptible to myelosuppression. Also, certain breeds of dog, including Collies and Collie crosses, Old English Sheepdogs, Cocker Spaniels, and West Highland White Terriers, are more likely to develop GI signs and myelosuppression.

## HEMATOLOGIC TOXICITY (TEXT PP 1108-1111)

Hematologic toxicity is the most common complication of chemotherapy and often results in temporary or permanent discontinuation of the drug(s) because of severe and potentially life-threatening cytopenias. Agents commonly implicated are listed in Table 80-1.

Neutropenia occurs first, followed by thrombocytopenia. Anemia induced by chemotherapeutic agents is rare, and if it occurs it develops 3 to 4 months after initiation of therapy. Patient-related factors (e.g., malnutrition, concurrent organ dysfunction, prior extensive chemotherapy) and tumor-related factors (e.g., bone marrow infiltration, widespread metastases) can affect the degree of myelosuppression.

### Neutropenia

Neutropenia usually constitutes the dose-limiting cytopenia and occasionally leads to life-threatening sepsis primarily in dogs (extremely rarely in cats). For most drugs the nadir of neutropenia occurs 5 to 7 days after treatment, then the neutrophil count returns to normal within 36 to 72 hours. The nadir of neutropenia is delayed for certain drugs, such as carboplatin (approximately 3 weeks).

#### Patient monitoring

*Hematology.* Hematologic monitoring is the most effective way to prevent (or anticipate) severe, life-threatening sepsis or bleeding secondary to myelosuppression.

**Table 80-1**

## Toxicity of Anticancer Agents in Cats and Dogs

| Toxicity | DOX | BLEO | ACT | CTX | LEUK | CISP | MTX | araC | 5-FU | L-asp | VCR | VBL | DTIC |
|---|---|---|---|---|---|---|---|---|---|---|---|---|---|
| Myelosuppression | S | N | M | M/S | N/M | M | M/S | M/S | M | N/M | N/M | N/S | M/S |
| Vomiting, diarrhea | M/S | N | M | M | N/M | M/S | M/S | N/M | N/M | N | N/M | N/M | M/S |
| Cardiotoxicity | M/S | N | N | N/? | N | N | N | N | N | N | N | N | N |
| Neurotoxicity | N | N | N | N | N | N | N | N | M | N/M? | N/M | N | N |
| Hypersensitivity | M/S | N | N | N | N | N | N | N | N | M/S | N | N | N/M |
| Pancreatitis | M | N | N | N/M | N | N | N | N/M | N | M/S | N | N | N/M |
| Perivascular sloughing | S | N | M/S | N | NA | N/M | N | N | N/M | N | M/S | M/S | M/S |
| Urotoxicity | ? | N | N | M/S | N | M/S | M | N | N | N | N | N | N |

*ACT*, Actinomycin D; *araC*, cytosine arabinoside; *BLEO*, bleomycin; *CISP*, cisplatin; *CTX*, cyclophosphamide; *DOX*, doxorubicin; *DTIC*, dacarbazine; *5-FU*, 5-fluorouracil; *L-asp*, L-asparaginase; *LEUK*, chlorambucil; *M*, mild to moderate; *MTX*, methotrexate; *N*, none; *NA*, not applicable; *S*, severe; *VCR*, vincristine; *VBL*, vinblastine; *?*, questionable.

Complete blood count (CBC) should be obtained weekly or every other week (depending on the treatment protocol), and the drug(s) should be temporarily discontinued or the dose decreased if the neutrophil count is less than 2000 cells/μl or if the platelet count is less than 50,000 cells/μl. Discontinuing the drug(s) for two or three treatments is usually sufficient for cell counts to return to normal. When therapy is reinstituted, 75% of the initial dose should be given and gradually increased over 2 to 3 weeks until the recommended dose (or a dose that does not cause marked cytopenia) is reached.

**Sepsis.** It is important to monitor carefully for sepsis using laboratory means, because the cardinal signs of inflammation (i.e., redness, swelling, increased temperature, pain, abnormal function) may be absent as a result of insufficient neutrophils to participate in the inflammatory process. The same holds true for radiographic changes; dogs with neutropenia and bacterial pneumonia often have normal thoracic radiographs. Patients with neutrophil counts of less than 2000 cells/μl should be closely monitored for sepsis, although overwhelming sepsis rarely occurs with neutrophil counts of more than 1000/μl. As a rule, when a severely neutropenic patient (neutrophil count less than 500/μl) is pyretic (temperature higher than 104° F), the fever should be attributed to bacterial pyrogens until proved otherwise, and the patient should be treated aggressively with antimicrobial therapy.

### Vaccines

All dogs and cats undergoing chemotherapy should be up-to-date on their vaccines; it is best that patients be vaccinated before starting chemotherapy. In patients undergoing chemotherapy, it is controversial whether the use of modified-live vaccines should be avoided because of the potential for inducing illness in immunosuppressed animals. Recent evidence suggests that dogs with cancer undergoing chemotherapy have protective serum antibody titers for commonly used vaccines.

### Neutropenic, febrile patients

Neutropenic, febrile animals should be treated aggressively, as they generally are septic; fever in a neutropenic patient constitutes a medical emergency. Thorough physical examination should be performed to identify a septic focus, and intravenous fluids are administered as required. The anticancer agents should be discontinued at once (although corticosteroids should be discontinued gradually to avoid acute hypoadrenocorticism). Blood samples for CBC, serum electrolytes, blood glucose, and blood urea nitrogen or creatinine are obtained, along with a urine sample for urinalysis and bacterial culture. Aseptically collected blood samples can be obtained for aerobic and anaerobic bacterial cultures and antibiotic susceptibility tests, although this is usually not necessary, because the bacterial isolates are quite predictable.

**Treatment.** After the samples are collected for culture, bactericidal antibiotics are instituted. A combination of amikacin (5 to 10 mg/kg intravenously [IV] q8h or 15 to 20 mg/kg every 24 hours) and cephalothin (22 mg/kg IV q8h) or enrofloxacin (5 to 10 mg/kg IV q24h) and ampicillin (22 mg/kg IV q8h) is recommended. Most bacterial isolates in these patients are enterobacteria (mainly *Klebsiella* spp. and *Escherichia coli*) and staphylococci (less than 20% of patients), which commonly are susceptible to these agents. Once the neutrophil count returns to normal and the patient is clinically normal (which usually takes 3 to 4 days), the antibiotic combination is discontinued, and the patient is released on oral sulfa-trimethoprim (ST) at 13 to 15 mg/kg q12h or enrofloxacin (5 to 10 mg/kg orally [PO] q24h) for 5 to 7 days. When chemotherapy is reinstituted, the dose is reduced as described previously (see discussion of hematology).

### Neutropenic, afebrile patients

Asymptomatic patients can be treated as outpatients with discontinuation of the drug(s) and administration of ST (13 to 15 mg/kg q12h). If the patient is afebrile but has constitutional signs, its condition should be considered septic, and it should be treated as described previously. If the neutropenia is not severe (more than 2000 cells/μl), no therapy is needed. The patient should simply be monitored by the owner (take the pet's rectal temperature twice daily and call the veterinarian if pyrexia develops).

#### Drug therapy for myelosuppression

In some patients myelosuppression may be alleviated with lithium carbonate (10 mg/kg PO q12h) in dogs, or recombinant human granulocyte colony-stimulating factor (Neupogen, 5 µg/kg subcutaneously [SC] q12-24h) in dogs or cats.

### Thrombocytopenia

Although thrombocytopenia is probably as common as neutropenia, it is rarely severe enough to cause spontaneous bleeding (platelet counts usually less than 30,000/µl). In most dogs with chemotherapy-induced thrombocytopenia, the platelet count remains above 50,000 cells/µl. The protocols predictably associated with thrombocytopenia in dogs are doxorubicin and dacarbazine (ADIC) lomustine, and D-MAC; platelet counts are often less than 50,000/µl. Thrombocytosis is common in cats and dogs receiving vincristine.

## GASTROINTESTINAL TOXICITY (TEXT P 1111)

Although less common than myelosuppression in dogs, GI toxicity is a relatively common complication of chemotherapy. The two major GI complications are (1) anorexia, nausea, and vomiting, and (2) gastroenterocolitis.

#### Anorexia, nausea, and vomiting

Drugs associated with nausea and vomiting include dacarbazine (DTIC), cisplatin, doxorubicin (primarily in cats), methotrexate, actinomycin D, cyclophosphamide, and 5-fluorouracil (5-FU).

*Intravenous drugs.* Acute anorexia, nausea, and vomiting caused by injectable drugs are usually prevented by administering the drugs by slow intravenous infusion. If signs still develop, antiemetics such as metoclopramide (Reglan, 0.1 to 0.3 mg/kg IV, SC, or PO q8h) or prochlorperazine (Compazine, 0.5 mg/kg intramuscularly [IM] q8-12h) are indicated. Other antiemetics that may be effective in dogs are butorphanol (Torbugesic, 0.3 to 0.4 mg/kg IM q6h) or ondansetron (Zofran, 0.5 to 1 mg/kg IV immediately before chemotherapy and then q6h).

*Oral drugs.* Anorexia and vomiting often occur 2 to 3 weeks after oral methotrexate is initiated and can usually be controlled with metoclopramide. If signs persist, the agent may need to be discontinued. Oral cyclophosphamide tends to induce anorexia and/or vomiting in cats; cyproheptadine (Periactin, 1 to 2 mg total dose PO q8-12h) is effective as an appetite stimulant or nausea suppressant in cats.

#### Gastroenterocolitis

Gastroenterocolitis associated with anticancer agents is rare. Drugs that occasionally cause mucositis include methotrexate, 5-FU, actinomycin D, and doxorubicin. Collies and Collie crosses, Cocker Spaniels, Old English Sheepdogs, and West Highland White Terriers are extremely susceptible to doxorubicin-induced enterocolitis, which is characterized by hemorrhagic diarrhea (with or without vomiting), primarily of large bowel type, 3 to 7 days after administration.

*Management.* Supportive fluid therapy (if necessary) and treatment with bismuth subsalicylate (Pepto-Bismol, 3 to 15 ml PO q6-8h) are generally effective in controlling the signs in dogs within 3 to 5 days. If the patient is at risk for gastroenterocolitis, administering Pepto-Bismol from days 1 to 7 of treatment may alleviate or prevent these signs. The use of bismuth subsalicylate should be avoided in cats. Gastroenteritis associated with oral methotrexate usually occurs at least 2 weeks after the drug is received; treatment is as for doxorubicin-induced enterocolitis.

## HYPERSENSITIVITY REACTIONS (TEXT P 1112)

Acute type I hypersensitivity reactions occasionally occur in dogs receiving parenteral L-asparaginase or doxorubicin (the reaction to the latter is not a true hypersensitivity reaction) and are common in dogs treated with intravenous etoposide or Taxol. Etoposide can be safely administered orally to dogs. Hypersensitivity reactions to anticancer agents are extremely rare in cats.

### Signs

In dogs the signs are similar to those of other hypersensitivity reactions (primarily cutaneous and GI). Typical signs begin during or shortly after administration and include head shaking (ear pruritus), generalized urticaria and erythema, restlessness, occasional vomiting or diarrhea, and (rarely) collapse from hypotension.

### Treatment

Treatment includes immediate discontinuation of the agent, administration of $H_1$ antihistamines (e.g., diphenhydramine, 0.2 to 0.5 mg/kg, slowly IV), dexamethasone sodium phosphate (1 to 2 mg/kg IV), and fluids, if necessary. If the systemic reaction is severe, epinephrine (0.1 to 0.3 ml of a 1:1000 solution IM or IV) is indicated. Intravenous $H_1$ antihistamines should be used with caution in cats (if at all), as they can cause acute central nervous system depression, leading to apnea. Once the reaction subsides (and if it was mild), the administration of certain drugs, such as doxorubicin, may be continued.

### Prevention

Most anaphylactic reactions can be prevented by pretreatment with $H_1$ antihistamines (e.g., diphenhydramine, 1 to 2 mg/kg IM 20 to 30 minutes before drug administration) and by administering certain drugs (e.g., L-asparaginase) SC or IM, rather than IV. If the agent cannot be given by any other route (e.g., doxorubicin), it should be diluted and administered by slow intravenous infusion.

## DERMATOLOGIC TOXICITY (TEXT PP 1112-1113)

Dermatologic toxicity from anticancer agents is rare in small animals. Three types can occur: local tissue necrosis (caused by extravasation), delayed hair growth or alopecia, and hyperpigmentation.

### Local tissue necrosis

Extravasation of vincristine, vinblastine, actinomycin D, or doxorubicin occasionally causes local tissue necrosis in dogs (extremely rare in cats). Signs include pain, pruritus, erythema, moist dermatitis, and necrosis of the affected area; severe tissue sloughing may occur. These drugs are extremely caustic when given perivascularly, so every effort should be made to ensure that they are administered intravascularly.

*Retrievers.* Some retrievers (e.g., Labrador and Golden Retrievers) seem to experience pruritus or discomfort around the site of intravenous injection, even with careful injection. The pain or discomfort frequently leads to licking and pyotraumatic dermatitis ("hot spot") within hours of injection. Applying a bandage over the injection site or placing an Elizabethan collar prevents this type of reaction.

*Prevention.* Caustic drugs should be administered through a 22- or 23-gauge indwelling intravenous catheter (doxorubicin) or a 23- or 25-gauge butterfly catheter (*Vinca* alkaloids, actinomycin D). In addition, caustic drugs should be diluted before administration—vincristine to a final concentration of 0.1 mg/ml and doxorubicin to a concentration of 0.5 mg/ml. Further management recommendations are given in the text.

*Treatment.* If, despite these precautions, a local tissue reaction occurs, it develops 1 to 7 days after perivascular injection of *Vinca* alkaloids and 7 to 15 days after doxorubicin extravasation (which persists in the tissues for up to 16 weeks). Local tissue reactions can be treated with topical antibiotic ointment (with or without corticosteroids) and bandaging. An Elizabethan collar or muzzle may be necessary in some patients. If no bacterial contamination occurs, methylprednisolone acetate (Depo-Medrol, 10 to 20 mg) can be injected subcutaneously into the affected area. When severe necrosis or gangrene caused by anaerobic infection occurs, the area should be surgically débrided. With severe doxorubicin-induced soft-tissue necrosis, amputation may be required.

### Delayed hair growth

Delayed hair growth is more common than alopecia. Alopecia occurs predominantly in woolly or coarse-haired dogs such as Poodles, Schnauzers, and Kerry Blue Terriers. In short-haired dogs and cats, it primarily affects the tactile hairs. Drugs commonly associated with delayed hair growth and alopecia include cyclophosphamide, doxorubicin, 5-FU, 6-thioguanine, and hydroxyurea (Hydrea). Alopecia and delayed hair growth usually resolve shortly after discontinuation of the agent.

### Hyperpigmentation

Hyperpigmentation induced by anticancer agents is rare in dogs and extremely rare in cats. Cutaneous hyperpigmentation affecting the face, ventral abdomen, and flanks is more likely in dogs receiving doxorubicin or bleomycin.

## PANCREATITIS (TEXT PP 1113-1114)

Sporadic cases of pancreatitis have been reported in dogs (but not cats) receiving chemotherapeutic and immunosuppressive agents. Acute pancreatitis has occurred in dogs receiving L-asparaginase or combination chemotherapy such as COAP (cyclophosphamide, vincristine, cytosine arabinoside, and prednisone), ADIC (doxorubicin and DTIC), or VAC (vincristine, doxorubicin, and cyclophosphamide). Signs develop 1 to 5 days after chemotherapy is initiated and are characterized by anorexia, vomiting, and depression. Physical examination is unremarkable, and abdominal pain is rare. Serum lipase and amylase activities are high, and ultrasonographic evidence of pancreatitis is detected in approximately 50% of dogs. In most dogs signs resolve with intravenous fluid therapy within 3 to 10 days.

### Prevention

Prevention is difficult, as this problem is not predictable. As a precaution, L-asparaginase should be avoided in patients at high risk for pancreatitis (e.g., overweight, middle-aged or older female dogs). Also, dogs receiving drugs potentially associated with pancreatitis should be on a low-fat diet.

## CARDIOTOXICITY (TEXT P 1114)

Cardiotoxicity is a relatively uncommon complication of doxorubicin therapy in dogs; it is extremely rare in cats. Two types of cardiotoxicity are seen in dogs: an acute reaction during or shortly after administration, and chronic, cumulative toxicity.

### Acute cardiotoxicity

Acute doxorubicin toxicity is characterized by cardiac arrhythmias (mainly sinus tachycardia). Sinus tachycardia and hypotension can be prevented by pretreatment with $H_1$ and $H_2$ antihistamines.

### Chronic cardiotoxicity

Several weeks or months after repeated doxorubicin injections, persistent arrhythmias including ventricular premature contractions, atrial premature contractions, paroxysmal ventricular tachycardia, second-degree atrioventricular blocks, and intraventricular conduction defects may develop. These rhythm disturbances are usually associated with dilated cardiomyopathy, the hallmark of chronic doxorubicin toxicity (see Chapter 6).

Dilated cardiomyopathy can develop after a total cumulative dose of approximately 240 mg/m². The cumulative cardiotoxic dose in cats is unknown. Signs of toxicity in dogs and cats are those of congestive heart failure (usually left sided). Therapy involves discontinuing the drug and using cardiac drugs such as digitalis glycosides or other inotropic agents (see Chapters 3, 4, and 6). Once cardiomyopathy develops, prognosis is poor, as myocardial lesions are irreversible.

### Monitoring doxorubicin therapy

Monitoring of patients receiving doxorubicin is critical for prevention of cardiomyopathy. Dogs (and possibly cats) with underlying rhythm disturbances or impaired myocardial contractility should not receive doxorubicin. It is recommended that patients receiving this drug undergo echocardiography every three doxorubicin cycles (9 weeks) to assess myocardial contractility. Administration should be discontinued if fractional shortening decreases. Monitoring serum troponin concentrations to detect early myocardial damage from doxorubicin is currently being evaluated.

### Preventing doxorubicin cardiotoxicity

Weekly low-dose doxorubicin causes significantly fewer histologic changes than the conventional 3-week schedule. A total cumulative dose of 500 mg/m² is possible when dogs are given 10 mg/m$^2$ weekly. Recent reports describe a loss of antitumor activity when weekly low-dose doxorubicin is used in dogs with lymphoma. With the new compound dexrazoxane, doxorubicin doses of more than 500 mg/m$^2$ have been administered to dogs without causing significant cardiotoxicity.

## UROTOXICITY (TEXT P 1114)

The urinary tract is rarely affected by anticancer agents. The two complications of clinical importance are nephrotoxicity and sterile hemorrhagic cystitis. Transitional cell carcinomas of the bladder associated with chronic cyclophosphamide (CTX) therapy have also been reported in dogs.

### Nephrotoxicity

Nephrotoxicity is rare in dogs and cats undergoing chemotherapy. Several potentially nephrotoxic drugs are commonly used, but only doxorubicin (primarily in cats), cisplatin (dogs), and intermediate- and high-dose methotrexate (dogs) are of concern. In cats, the limiting cumulative toxicity of doxorubicin may be renal rather than cardiac, although nephrotoxicity is rare. Doxorubicin may also cause nephrotoxicosis in dogs with preexisting renal disease and in those also receiving other nephrotoxins such as aminoglycoside antibiotics or cisplatin. The administration of cisplatin using forced diuresis protocols minimizes the prevalence of nephrotoxicity in dogs.

### Cystitis

Sterile hemorrhagic cystitis is a relatively common complication of long-term CTX therapy in dogs. It develops in 5% to 25% of dogs, usually after an average of 18 weeks of therapy. Although rare, hemorrhagic cystitis may occur acutely after a single dose of CTX.

*Prevention.* Furosemide (Lasix, 2 mg/kg PO q12h) or prednisone administered with CTX decreases the prevalence of cystitis. Other recommendations include administering CTX in the morning, allowing the pet to urinate frequently (if an indoor dog), salting the food, and, if the protocol calls for prednisone, administering prednisone on the same day as the CTX.

*Signs.* Signs of sterile hemorrhagic cystitis are similar to those of other lower urinary tract disorders: pollakiuria, hematuria, and dysuria. Urinalysis typically reveals blood and a mild to moderate increase in white blood cell count, but no bacteria.

*Management.* Treatment involves (1) discontinuing the CTX, (2) forcing diuresis with furosemide (2 mg/kg PO q12h), (3) diminishing bladder wall inflammation with prednisone (0.5 to 1 mg/kg PO q24h), and (4) preventing secondary bacterial infections with sulfa-trimethoprim (13 to 15 mg/kg PO q12h). In most dogs this approach resolves the cystitis in 1 to 4 months; however, if signs worsen despite treatment, 1% formalin in water can be instilled into the bladder. Intravesical infusion of 25% to 50% dimethylsulfoxide solution may also alleviate signs of cystitis.

## HEPATOTOXICITY (TEXT P 1115)

With the exception of corticosteroids in dogs, only methotrexate, CTX, lomustine, and azathioprine are potential or confirmed hepatotoxins. In small animals, hepatotoxicity caused by anticancer drugs is extremely rare and of little or no clinical relevance, with the exception of lomustine. Hepatic changes associated with lomustine treatment include a low prevalence (10%) of hepatotoxicity, increased alanine aminotransferase (markedly, >1000 U/L) and AP (mild, <500 IU/L) activities, and potential development of end-stage liver disease.

## NEUROTOXICITY (TEXT P 1115)

Neurotoxicity from most anticancer agents is extremely rare. One exception is 5-FU, which causes neurotoxicosis commonly in cats and infrequently in dogs. Signs occur shortly (3 to 12 hours) after administration and primarily consist of excitation and cerebellar ataxia; death occurs in approximately 33% of dogs and most cats. Because of its high neurotoxic potential, this drug should not be used in cats.

Recently, neurotoxicity was reported in 25% of dogs receiving a combination of CTX, actinomycin D, and 5-FU (CDF) for metastatic or nonresectable carcinomas. This prevalence is considerably higher than that seen with 5-FU in combination with other drugs and may be a result of drug interactions.

## PULMONARY TOXICITY (TEXT P 1115)

Pulmonary toxicity is extremely rare in dogs and cats. Only cisplatin has been documented as a cause of pulmonary toxicity in cats. Acute signs of dyspnea leading to death occur within 48 to 96 hours of administration. Therefore cisplatin should not be used in cats. Carboplatin, a cisplatin derivative, does not cause this problem.

## ACUTE TUMOR LYSIS SYNDROME (TEXT PP 1115-1116)

Rapid lysis of certain tumor cells can lead to acute tumor lysis syndrome (ATLS). In dogs and cats ATLS has been reported only in association with lymphomas treated with chemotherapy and/or radiation therapy. It is characterized by hyperphosphatemia, with or without azotemia, hyperkalemia, hypocalcemia, metabolic acidosis, and hyperuricemia. Signs, which include depression, vomiting, and bloody diarrhea, develop within hours or days of initiation of chemotherapy. In most affected dogs the pretreatment serum creatinine concentration or tumor burden is high. Aggressive fluid therapy and correction of acid-base and electrolyte disturbances resolve the signs within 3 days, although the condition can be fatal. ATLS is rare in cats.

# 81

# Approach to the Patient with a Mass

## *(Text pp 1117-1121)*

## SOLITARY MASS (TEXT PP 1117-1118)

Several approaches are possible in a clinically healthy cat or dog with a solitary palpable mass: (1) do nothing and reevaluate later, (2) evaluate the mass cytologically, (3) evaluate the mass histopathologically, or (4) do a complete workup, including complete blood count (CBC), serum biochemistries, radiographs, abdominal ultrasonography, and urinalysis.

### Initial approach

Masses are abnormal and should always be evaluated; most masses, except inflammatory lesions, do not regress spontaneously. The first step is to perform a fine-needle aspiration (FNA) for cytologic evaluation (see Chapter 77); this allows a presumptive or definitive diagnosis in most patients. Once the type of mass has been defined (benign neoplastic, malignant neoplastic, inflammatory, or hyperplastic), additional evaluation can be recommended. An intensive workup of a cat or dog with a solitary mass may not be warranted, as additional information regarding the mass is rarely gained by these procedures. However, the presence of metastatic lesions on thoracic radiographs may suggest that the mass is a malignant tumor.

### Benign neoplasia

Two options exist when a cytologic diagnosis of benign neoplasia is made: (1) do nothing and reevaluate later, or (2) perform surgical excision. Benign neoplasms are rarely premalignant (except for solar dermatitis or carcinoma in situ preceding the development of squamous cell carcinomas in cats), so when a definitive diagnosis of benign neoplasia is made, a "wait-and-see" approach is reasonable. If the mass enlarges or becomes inflamed or ulcerated, surgical excision is recommended. However, most neoplasms are easier to excise when they are small, and many clients favor excision soon after diagnosis.

### Malignant neoplasia

When a cytologic diagnosis of malignancy is suggested or confirmed, additional workup is warranted. Depending on the cytologic diagnosis (carcinoma, sarcoma, or round cell tumor), different approaches are indicated.

*Radiography.* Thoracic radiographs should be obtained in most dogs and cats with malignant neoplasms (except mast cell tumors). Taking two lateral views and a ventrodorsal or dorsoventral view increases the detection rate for metastatic lesions. If available, computed tomography (CT) may be performed, as it can allow detection of masses smaller than those detectable on plain radiography. Radiographs of the affected area may also be indicated to evaluate for soft-tissue and bone involvement. With certain neoplasms, such as hemangiosarcoma, intestinal neoplasms, and mast cell tumors, abdominal ultrasonography or radiography may be indicated for further staging. CBC, serum biochemistry profile, and urinalysis may provide additional information, such as the presence of paraneoplastic syndromes or concurrent organ failure.

*Treatment.* If the mass is malignant and there is no evidence of metastatic disease, surgical excision is usually recommended. If metastatic lesions are present and the pathologist is confident with the cytologic diagnosis, chemotherapy is the best option. However, as discussed in Chapter 78, surgical resection of the primary mass (e.g., mammary carcinoma) in a patient with metastatic lesions may provide considerable palliation and prolong good-quality survival. If definitive diagnosis cannot be made on the basis of cytology, incisional or excisional biopsy is advisable. Euthanasia is not recommended in dogs and cats with metastatic lesions and good quality of life, because with certain tumors survival times commonly exceed 6 months (without chemotherapy).

## METASTATIC LESIONS (TEXT PP 1118-1119)

Often radiographic or ultrasonographic evidence of metastatic cancer is found during routine evaluation of a patient with a suspected or confirmed malignancy or a patient with obscure clinical signs. The metastatic behavior of the more common neoplasms is listed in Table 81-1.

### General approach

If a cytologic or histopathologic diagnosis of malignancy has already been obtained and the metastatic lesions are detected while the malignancy is being staged, treatment recommendations can be made at that point. If the metastases are detected during evaluation of a cat or dog with vague clinical signs and no previous history of neoplasia, a cytologic or histopathologic evaluation of one or more of these lesions should be performed.

### Lung metastases

A cytologic diagnosis of metastatic lung lesions can usually be made through blind or ultrasound-guided percutaneous FNA of the lungs over the area with the highest density of radiographic lesions. The technique is described in the text. Complications include pneumothorax (patients should be closely observed for 2 to 6 hours) and bleeding; FNA of the lungs should not be performed in cats or dogs with coagulopathies.

Table 81-1

## Metastatic Behavior of Some Common Neoplasms in Dogs and Cats

| Neoplasm | Species | Common metastatic sites |
|---|---|---|
| HSA | D | Liver, lungs, kidney, omentum, eye, CNS |
| OSA | D | Lungs, bone |
| SCC—oral | C, D | Lymph nodes, lung |
| aCA—mammary | C, D | Lymph nodes, lung, bone (?) |
| aCA—anal sac | D | Lymph nodes |
| aCA—prostate | D | Lymph nodes, bone, lungs |
| TCC—bladder | D | Lymph nodes, lung, bone |
| MCT | D | Lymph nodes, liver, spleen |
| MCT | C | Spleen, liver, bone marrow |

*aCA*, Adenocarcinoma; *C*, cat; *CNS*, central nervous system; *D*, dog; *HSA*, hemangiosarcoma; *MCT*, mast cell tumor; *OSA*, osteosarcoma; *SCC*, squamous cell carcinoma; *TCC*, transitional cell carcinoma.

*Lung biopsy.* If FNA fails to yield a diagnostic sample, lung biopsy performed with a biopsy needle (under ultrasonographic or CT guidance) or via a thoracotomy should be contemplated. This procedure has a low morbidity rate and should be recommended when owners are considering treatment.

*Liver and spleen.* Nodular lesions of the liver or spleen in dogs with a primary malignancy may not be metastatic. FNA or biopsies of such lesions frequently reveal normal hepatocytes (e.g., reactive hepatic nodule) or extramedullary hematopoiesis or lymphoreticular hyperplasia

### Other metastases

Metastatic lesions in other organs or tissues (e.g., liver, bone) can also be diagnosed with FNA, or in the case of bone metastases, by bone marrow aspiration (of the affected bone). If a cytologic diagnosis cannot be made, a core (needle) biopsy can be performed.

## MEDIASTINAL MASS (TEXT PP 1119-1121)

### Etiology

Several lesions can appear as anterior mediastinal masses (AMM) on physical examination or thoracic radiographs. Thymomas and lymphomas are the most common AMM in cats and dogs. Other neoplastic AMM include chemodectomas (heartbase tumors), ectopic thyroid carcinomas, and lipomas, among others. Nonneoplastic lesions of the mediastinum include mainly thymic or mediastinal hematomas and ultimobranchial cysts.

### Clinical and clinicopathologic features

In cats, age at presentation suggests a specific diagnosis: Anterior mediastinal lymphomas are more common in young cats (1 to 3 years old), and thymomas are more common in older cats (8 to 10 years old). Feline leukemia virus (FeLV) status is important; most cats with mediastinal lymphomas are FeLV-positive, whereas most cats with thymoma are not.

In dogs, most anterior mediastinal lymphomas and thymomas are diagnosed in older patients (more than 5 to 6 years old). A large proportion of dogs with mediastinal lymphoma and some dogs with thymoma are hypercalcemic. Peripheral lymphocytosis may be found in dogs and cats with either lymphoma or thymoma. Neuromuscular signs in either species suggest thymoma.

*Paraneoplastic syndromes.* Conditions such as generalized or focal myasthenia gravis, polymyositis, exfoliative dermatitis, and secondary neoplasms are well characterized in cats and dogs with thymoma. Hypercalcemia is a common paraneoplastic syndrome in dogs with mediastinal lymphoma, but it can also occur in those with thymoma.

#### Diagnosis

Thoracic radiographs are of little help in differentiating thymomas from lymphomas. Both neoplasms are similar in appearance, although lymphomas tend to originate in the dorsal anterior mediastinum, whereas thymomas originate more often in the ventral mediastinum. The prevalence of pleural effusion in both tumors is similar.

*Ultrasonography.* Ultrasonographic evaluation should be attempted before more invasive diagnostic techniques are used; it provides information regarding the resectability of the mass and can assist in obtaining a specimen for cytologic evaluation. Most thymomas have mixed echogenicity, with discrete hypoechoic or anechoic areas (cysts). In lymphomas the lack of supporting stroma can make the mass appear hypoechoic or anechoic, and diffusely "cystic."

*Fine-needle aspiration.* Transthoracic FNA is a relatively safe and reliable technique (see text). It can be performed blindly (for large masses against the thoracic wall) or guided by radiographs (three views), fluoroscopy, CT, or ultrasonography. Postaspiration bleeding is extremely rare if the patient remains still during the procedure. If the mass is large enough to come into contact with the thoracic wall, transthoracic needle biopsy for histopathologic evaluation can be performed.

*Lymphomas.* Cytologically, lymphomas are composed of a monomorphic population of lymphoid cells that are mostly immature (small nuclear/cytoplasmic ratio, dark blue cytoplasm, clumped chromatin, nucleoli). Occasionally, mediastinal lymphomas are composed primarily of large granular lymphocytes. In cats most anterior mediastinal lymphoma cells are heavily vacuolated.

*Thymomas.* Cytologically, thymomas are heterogeneous but primarily composed of small lymphocytes (although large blasts are sometimes present) and occasionally a distinct population of epithelial-like cells that are usually polygonal or spindle-shaped (individual cells or sheets). Hassal's corpuscles are rarely seen on Wright's-stained preparations. Plasma cells, eosinophils, neutrophils, mast cells, macrophages, and melanocytes are frequently seen.

#### Treatment

Treatment depends on the specific tumor type. Chemotherapy is indicated for lymphomas, whereas surgical excision may be curative for thymomas.

*Lymphomas.* Anterior mediastinal lymphomas are best treated with chemotherapy (see Chapter 82). Radiotherapy can be used in conjunction with chemotherapy to induce a more rapid remission, although this approach does not offer any advantages over chemotherapy alone and may in fact be detrimental. Many cats and dogs with anterior mediastinal lymphoma already have severe respiratory compromise; chemical restraint for radiotherapy may compound this problem.

*Thymomas.* Because most thymomas are benign, surgical excision is usually curative. Although there have been reports of high perioperative morbidity and mortality, in my experience most patients do well and are released from the hospital in 3 to 4 days. Radiotherapy can decrease the size of the mass, although complete, long-lasting remission is rarely achieved.

Chemotherapy may be beneficial in dogs and cats with nonresectable thymomas or in patients in which repeated anesthesia or a major surgical procedure poses a severe risk. Combination chemotherapy protocols commonly used for lymphoma, including COP (cyclophosphamide, vincristine, and prednisone), COAP (COP drugs plus cytosine arabinoside), and CHOP (COP drugs plus doxorubicin), have been used in a limited number of cats and dogs with thymomas. However, chemotherapy may eliminate only the lymphoid cell population; therefore it rarely results in complete or long-lasting remission.

*Other options.* If a definitive diagnosis cannot be made, two options exist: (1) perform a thoracotomy and excise the mass, or (2) start the patient on chemotherapy for lymphoma (COP, COAP, or CHOP). If no remission (or only partial remission) is observed 10 to 14 days after chemotherapy is initiated, the mass is most likely a thymoma, and surgical resection should be considered.

# 82

# Lymphoma in Cats and Dogs

## *(Text pp 1122-1132)*

Lymphoma (malignant lymphoma, lymphosarcoma, LSA) is a lymphoid malignancy that originates from solid organs such as the lymph nodes, liver, and spleen.

### Etiology and epidemiology

Approximately 70% of cats with lymphoma are feline leukemia virus (FeLV) positive—30% with the alimentary form, 90% with the mediastinal form, and 80% with multicentric lymphoma. Young cats with lymphoma are more likely to be FeLV-positive than are older cats. Feline immunodeficiency virus (FIV)–positive cats are almost six times more likely to develop lymphoma than noninfected cats, and cats coinfected with FeLV and FIV are more than 75 times more likely to develop lymphoma than noninfected cats.

The cause of lymphoma in dogs is multifactorial. A genetic component is evident in certain bloodlines. A distinct breed predisposition also exists; Golden Retrievers, Cocker Spaniels, Rottweilers, Boxers, Basset Hounds, St. Bernards, Scottish Terriers, Airedale Terriers, and English Bulldogs are at greater risk.

*Age.* Age at presentation is bimodal in cats, with the first peak occurring at approximately 2 years of age, and the second at 10 to 12 years. Mean age at presentation in FeLV-positive cats is 3 years, and in FeLV-negative cats 7 to 8 years. Most dogs with lymphoma are middle aged or older (6 to 12 years).

### Clinical features

Four anatomic forms are recognized:

1. Multicentric, characterized by generalized lymphadenopathy and hepatic, splenic, and/or bone marrow involvement
2. Mediastinal, characterized by mediastinal lymphadenopathy with or without bone marrow infiltration
3. Alimentary, characterized by solitary, diffuse, or multifocal gastrointestinal (GI) infiltration, with or without intraabdominal lymphadenopathy
4. Extranodal, affecting any organ or tissue (e.g., renal, neural, ocular, cutaneous)

The multicentric form is the most common in dogs, accounting for more than 80% of all canine lymphomas. In cats the mediastinal and alimentary forms are more common. Clinical findings are related to the anatomic form of presentation.

*Multicentric lymphoma.* Patients are usually presented with nonspecific signs such as weight loss, anorexia, and lethargy; frequently, owners detect one or more subcutaneous masses (enlarged lymph nodes) during grooming. Edema may develop from mechanical obstruction of lymph drainage, and coughing is a presenting complaint if enlarged lymph nodes cause airway compression.

Physical examination usually reveals massive, generalized lymphadenopathy, with or without hepatomegaly, splenomegaly, or extranodal lesions. Affected lymph nodes are markedly enlarged (5 to 15 times normal), painless, and freely movable. A syndrome of reactive (hyperplastic) lymphadenopathy can mimic multicentric lymphoma in cats (see Chapter 90).

*Mediastinal lymphoma.* Patients usually are presented for evaluation of dyspnea, coughing, or regurgitation (more common in cats) of recent onset. Polyuria and polydipsia are common complaints in dogs with mediastinal lymphoma and hypercalcemia; tumor-associated hypercalcemia is extremely rare in cats. Respiratory and esophageal signs are caused by compression from an enlarged anterior mediastinal lymph node, although malignant pleural effusion may contribute to the respiratory signs.

Physical examination findings are usually confined to the thoracic cavity and consist of decreased bronchovesicular sounds, dorsocaudal displacement of normal lung sounds, ventral dullness on percussion, and a noncompressible mediastinum (cats). Unilateral or bilateral Horner's syndrome may be found in cats (and occasionally in dogs). Some dogs with mediastinal lymphoma have marked head and neck edema resulting from compression from enlarged lymph nodes (anterior vena cava syndrome).

*Alimentary lymphoma.* GI signs such as vomiting, anorexia, diarrhea, and weight loss are common in dogs and cats with alimentary lymphoma. Occasionally, signs of intestinal obstruction or peritonitis (caused by rupture of a lymphomatous mass) develop. Physical examination findings include intraabdominal masses (enlarged mesenteric or ileocecocolic lymph nodes or intestinal masses) and thickened bowel loops (diffuse small intestinal lymphoma). Rarely, polypoid masses may protrude through the anus in cats and dogs with colorectal lymphoma.

*Extranodal lymphoma.* Signs and physical examination findings in cats and dogs with extranodal lymphomas are extremely variable and depend on the location of the mass(es). In general, signs are the result of compression or displacement of normal parenchymal cells in the affected organ (Table 82-1). Common extranodal forms in dogs are cutaneous and ocular, and in cats nasopharyngeal, ocular, renal, and neural.

*Cutaneous lymphoma.* Lesions are extremely variable and can mimic any skin lesion. Dogs with mycosis fungoides (an epidermotropic T-cell lymphoma) usually have a chronic history of alopecia, desquamation, pruritus, and erythema, eventually leading to plaque and tumor formation. Mucocutaneous and mucosal lesions are relatively common; generalized lymph node involvement may be absent on initial presentation. A characteristic lesion is a circular, raised, erythematous, donut-shaped dermoepidermal mass with normal skin in the center. Most cats with cutaneous lymphomas are FeLV negative.

*Renal lymphoma.* Renal lymphoma is relatively common in cats but rare in dogs. Cats are presented for vague signs, usually secondary to chronic renal failure. Physical examination reveals an emaciated, often anemic cat with large, irregular, firm kidneys. An association is purported to exist between renal and central nervous system (CNS) lymphoma in cats; some clinicians recommend using drugs that achieve high CNS concentrations (e.g., cytosine arabinoside, lomustine) in cats with renal involvement to prevent secondary CNS dissemination.

**Table 82-1**

## Clinical Signs and Physical Examination Findings in Dogs and Cats with Extranodal Lymphomas

| Organ involved | Clinical presentation | Physical examination finding(s) |
| --- | --- | --- |
| CNS | Solitary or multifocal CNS signs | Any neurologic |
| Eye | Blindness, infiltrates, photophobia | Infiltrates, uveitis, RD, glaucoma |
| Kidney | PU/PD, azotemia, erythrocytosis* | Renomegaly, renal masses |
| Lung | Coughing, dyspnea | None, radiographic changes |
| Skin | Any primary or secondary lesion | Any primary or secondary lesion |

*Only in dogs.

*CNS*, Central nervous system; *PU/PD*, polyuria and polydipsia; *RD*, retinal detachment.

*Ocular lymphoma.* Ocular lymphoma occurs in both dogs and cats. In dogs ocular involvement is often associated with the multicentric form, whereas in cats both primary ocular involvement and ocular involvement associated with the multicentric form are common. Abnormalities may include photophobia, blepharospasm, epiphora, hyphema, hypopyon, ocular masses, third eyelid infiltration, anterior uveitis, chorioretinal involvement, and retinal detachment.

*Nasopharyngeal lymphoma.* Nasopharyngeal lymphoma is a relatively common manifestation in cats and is one of the most common forms of extranodal lymphoma in this species; it is extremely rare in dogs. Signs are typical of any upper respiratory disorder and include sneezing, unilateral or bilateral nasal discharge (from mucopurulent to hemorrhagic), stertorous breathing, exophthalmus, and facial deformity.

*Neural lymphoma.* Three forms are recognized: solitary epidural (common in young, FeLV-positive cats), neuropil (intracranial or intraspinal; a true CNS lymphoma), and peripheral nerve. Neural lymphomas may be primary (e.g., epidural lymphoma) or secondary to the multicentric form (and possibly the renal form in cats). These patients are evaluated because of a variety of neurologic signs that reflect the location and extent of the neoplasms. CNS signs are more common than peripheral nerve signs (the latter are seen occasionally in cats). A relatively common presentation is that of a CNS relapse in dogs that have been receiving chemotherapy for multicentric lymphoma for months to years; these patients develop acute onset of neurologic signs, typically while the multicentric neoplasm is still in remission.

**Paraneoplastic Syndromes.** Occasionally, dogs with lymphoma are presented for evaluation of a paraneoplastic syndrome, such as hypercalcemia, monoclonal or polyclonal gammopathies, immune cytopenias, polyneuropathy, or hypoglycemia. Of all these syndromes, only humoral hypercalcemia of malignancy in dogs is of clinical relevance. Only hypercalcemia and gammopathies have been reported in cats with lymphoma, and with a much lower frequency than in dogs.

### Diagnosis

Signs and physical examination findings usually suggest lymphoma, but before therapy is instituted, a cytologic or histopathologic diagnosis should be made. Complete blood count (CBC), serum biochemistry profile, and urinalysis, and in cats FeLV and FIV tests, should also be obtained if owners are contemplating treatment. Once a decision to treat the patient has been made, clinicopathologic abnormalities usually dictate which treatment(s) to use. In an animal with pronounced cytopenias caused by lymphomatous bone marrow infiltration, highly myelosuppressive chemotherapy should be avoided.

**Radiography.** Radiographic abnormalities vary with the anatomic form and in general are secondary to lymphadenopathy or organomegaly; occasionally, infiltration of other organs (e.g., lungs) may cause additional radiographic abnormalities.

Radiographic changes in dogs and cats with multicentric lymphoma can include sternal and/or tracheobronchial lymphadenopathy; interstitial, bronchoalveolar, or mixed pulmonary infiltrates; pleural effusion (rare); intraabdominal lymphadenopathy; hepatomegaly; splenomegaly; renomegaly; and intraabdominal masses. Rarely, lytic or proliferative bone lesions are identified on abdominal or thoracic radiographs. With mediastinal lymphoma, radiographic changes are usually limited to a mediastinal mass, with or without pleural effusion.

In cats and dogs with alimentary lymphoma, abnormalities are not often detected on plain radiographs (less than 50%); when present, they variably include hepatomegaly, splenomegaly, and midabdominal mass(es). Contrast radiography reveals abnormalities in most patients, including mucosal irregularities, luminal filling defects, and irregular thickening of the wall, suggesting infiltrative mural disease.

*Ultrasonography.* Ultrasonographic abnormalities in dogs and cats with intraabdominal lymphoma include hepatomegaly, splenomegaly, changes in the echogenicity of liver and/or spleen (mixed echogenicity or multiple hypoechoic areas), intestinal thickening, lymphadenopathy, splenic masses, and effusion. Changes in the echogenicity of parenchymal organs usually indicate neoplastic infiltration. Cats with alimentary lymphoma may have hypoechoic masses in the gastric or intestinal wall, focal or diffuse gastric wall thickening, symmetric thickening of the intestinal wall, loss of the normal layered appearance of the gut wall, or abdominal lymphadenopathy. Ultrasound-guided fine-needle aspiration (FNA) or needle biopsies are easily obtained and are frequently diagnostic.

*Computed tomography and magnetic resonance imaging.*  Computed tomography or magnetic resonance imaging is advised in cats and dogs with suspected CNS lymphoma.

***Fine-needle aspiration.***  In most cats and dogs with multicentric, superficial extranodal, mediastinal, or alimentary lymphoma, diagnosis can easily be obtained by FNA cytology of the affected organs or lymph nodes (see Chapter 77). Lymphomas can be diagnosed cytologically in approximately 90% of dogs and 70% to 75% of cats. In only 10% of dogs and 25% to 30% of cats is histopathologic evaluation of a surgically excised lymph node or mass necessary for diagnosis. Two benefits of FNA over surgical excisional biopsies are reduced cost of the procedure and minimal or no morbidity.

***Cerebrospinal fluid analysis.***  In cats and dogs with suspected neuropil lymphoma, cerebrospinal fluid (CSF) analysis may be diagnostic, containing high numbers of neoplastic lymphoid cells and increased protein concentration. Diagnosis of extradural masses usually requires surgical biopsy for cytologic or histopathologic evaluation.

***Complete blood count.***  A variety of nonspecific hematologic and serum biochemical abnormalities may be detected, but in general, CBC and profile are rarely diagnostic. Common hematologic abnormalities include anemia, leukocytosis, neutrophilia (with or without left shift), monocytosis, presence of abnormal lymphoid cells (lymphosarcoma-cell leukemia), thrombocytopenia, isolated or combined cytopenias, and leukoerythroblastic reactions; lymphocytosis is rare, and when present is usually of low magnitude ($<$10,000 to 12,000/μl).

***Serum biochemistry.***  Biochemical abnormalities are more common in dogs than in cats and mainly include hypercalcemia and gammopathies. Hypercalcemia occurs in 20% to 40% of dogs with lymphoma and is more common in those with mediastinal lymphoma; it is extremely rare in cats. In most dogs with lymphoma and hypercalcemia, the tumor is of T-cell origin. Markedly increased serum 1,25 vitamin D concentration may be found in dogs, especially in Boxers with mediastinal lymphoma.

***Differential diagnoses.***  A variety of differential diagnoses should be considered when evaluating a cat or dog with suspected lymphoma. Lymphomas can mimic a large number of neoplastic and nonneoplastic disorders. Differential diagnoses are similar to those in patients with leukemia (see Chapter 83).

***Staging the disease.***  After a diagnosis of lymphoma is established, the disease is staged (Table 82-2). Dogs and cats with clinical signs are considered to be substage "b"; asymptomatic patients are substage "a." The only prognostic information of clinical relevance in the current staging system (devised by the World Health Organization) is that asymptomatic (substage a) dogs with lymphoma have a better prognosis than "sick"

Table 82-2

## "Tumor Node Metastasis" (TNM) Staging System for Dogs and Cats with Lymphoma

| Stage | Clinical features |
| --- | --- |
| I | Solitary lymph node involvement |
| II | More than one lymph node enlarged but on one side of the diaphragm (i.e., cranial or caudal) |
| III | Generalized lymph node involvement |
| IV | Stage III findings, plus hepatomegaly and/or splenomegaly |
| V | Any of the above, plus bone marrow or extranodal involvement |
| Substage a | Asymptomatic |
| Substage b | Sick |

(substage b) dogs. Also, staging based on a given chemotherapy protocol may be of limited prognostic value when a different drug combination is used. Until a new system is devised, prognosis should be based on the patient's clinical condition, FeLV and FIV status (cats), and presence or absence of constitutional signs and/or severe hematologic and biochemical abnormalities.

*Immunophenotyping.* Most oncologists routinely immunophenotype canine and feline lymphoma. Dogs with T-cell lymphoma treated with standard combination chemotherapy have a worse prognosis for remission and survival than dogs with B-cell tumors.

## Managing Lymphoma
### Expected survival times

Remission rates with chemotherapy are 65% to 75% in cats and 80% to 90% in dogs. Most cats with lymphoma live 6 to 9 months when treated with multiple-agent chemotherapy, with or without surgery and/or radiotherapy; approximately 20% live more than 1 year. Most dogs with lymphoma treated similarly live 12 to 16 months; approximately 20% to 30% are alive 2 years after diagnosis. Approximate survival times for untreated cats and dogs are 4 to 8 weeks. Remission is difficult to reinduce in cats once the tumor has relapsed; FeLV infection is a negative prognostic factor in cats.

### Treatment guidelines

The mainstay of treatment is chemotherapy, given the fact that lymphomas are (or will be) systemic neoplasms. Surgery and/or radiotherapy can be used to treat localized lymphomas before or during chemotherapy. Chemotherapy is usually divided into four phases: induction of remission, intensification, maintenance, and reinduction or "rescue" (Box 82-1).

*Summary.* Remission is induced with COAP; during this 6- to 8-week phase, patients are evaluated weekly with routine physical examination (with or without CBC) and receive an intravenous injection of vincristine. Once CR is achieved, treatment continues with oral LMP (chlorambucil [Leukeran], methotrexate, prednisone). The patient is monitored every 6 to 8 weeks until the tumor relapses, at which time the reinduction phase begins. Once remission is achieved, the patient is placed on a modified maintenance protocol (e.g., Cytosar, 200 to 300 mg/m$^2$ subcutaneously [SC] every other week, can be substituted for methotrexate). If the patient is not in CR at the end of the initial induction phase, intensification with L-asparaginase is recommended before the maintenance phase.

### Induction of remission

In most patients (more than 85% of dogs and 70% to 75% of cats), treatment with COAP results in CR within 1 to 4 days of initiating therapy; remission is usually maintained throughout the induction phase. Owners are instructed to monitor the pet's appetite and activity level, measure the lymph nodes (if superficial lymphadenopathy is present), and take the pet's rectal temperature daily.

*Adverse effects.* Toxicity is minimal during this phase. The dose-limiting toxicity is myelosuppression leading to neutropenia. The neutrophil nadir usually occurs around day 7 or 8 and typically is mild (2000 to 3500 cells/µl). Neutropenia can be severe in patients with neoplastic bone marrow infiltration, in patients with FeLV- or FIV-associated myelodysplasia, and in patients receiving cytosine arabinoside by constant-rate intravenous infusion (rather than SC). Cats receiving cyclophosphamide occasionally become anorectic, for which ciproheptadine (Periactin, 1 to 2 mg/cat PO q12h) is indicated. Hair loss is minimal and primarily occurs in woolly haired dogs (e.g., Poodle, Bichon Frise); cats (and some dogs) may shed their tactile hairs during treatment.

*Other protocols.* A more aggressive (and expensive) doxorubicin-containing protocol (CHOP; see Box 82-1) is used for dogs with diffuse alimentary lymphoma. In dogs and cats with neurologic signs, COAP is used, but the cytosine arabinoside is given as a continuous intravenous infusion (200 mg/m$^2$ intravenously [IV] over 24 hours for 1 to 4 days) to increase the concentration of this drug in the CNS. This protocol tends to cause marked myelosuppression in cats, so the cytosine arabinoside can be given as

---

**Box 82-1**

## Chemotherapy Protocols Used for the Treatment of Cats and Dogs* with Lymphoma at The Ohio State University Veterinary Teaching Hospital

---

### 1. INDUCTION OF REMISSION
**COAP Protocol[†]**

Cyclophosphamide (Cytoxan): 50 mg/m$^2$ PO q48h in dogs; in cats cyclophosphamide is given at a dose of 200-300 mg/m$^2$ PO every 3 weeks to decrease the likelihood of anorexia

Vincristine (Oncovin): 0.5 mg/m$^2$ IV weekly

Cytosine arabinoside (Cytosar-U): 100 mg/m$^2$ daily as an intravenous drip or SC for only 2 days in cats and 4 days in dogs

Prednisone: 50 mg/m$^2$ PO q24h for 1 week, then 20-25 mg/m$^2$ PO q48h

### 2. INTENSIFICATION
**Dogs**

L-Asparaginase (Elspar): 10,000-20,000 U/m$^2$ IM (one or two doses)
*or*
Vincristine (Oncovin): 0.5-0.75 mg/m$^2$ IV q1-2wk

**Cats**

Doxorubicin (Adriamycin): 1 mg/kg IV q3wk
*or*
Mitoxantrone (Novantrone): 4-6 mg/m$^2$ IV q3wk

### 3. MAINTENANCE[‡]
**LMP Protocol**

Chlorambucil (Leukeran): 20 mg/m$^2$ PO q2wk

Methotrexate (Methotrexate): 2.5 mg/m$^2$ PO two or three times per week

Prednisone: 20-25 mg/m$^2$ PO q48h

**COAP Protocol**

Use as above every other week for six treatments, then every third week for six additional treatments, then try to maintain the animal on one treatment every fourth week. Maintenance therapy is continued until the tumor relapses.

### 4. RESCUE
**Dogs**

*D-MAC protocol (14-day cycle)*

Dexamethasone: 0.5 mg/lb (1.1 mg/kg) PO or SC on days 1 and 8

Actinomycin D (Cosmegen): 0.75 mg/m$^2$ as intravenous push on day 1

Cytosine arabinoside (Cytosar): 200-300 mg/m$^2$ as intravenous drip over 4 hr *or* SC on day 1

Melphalan (Alkeran): 20 mg/m$^2$ PO on day 8[§]

*AC protocol (21-day cycle)*

Doxorubicin (Adriamycin): 30 mg/m$^2$ (or 1 mg/kg for dogs under 10 kg) IV on day 1

Cyclophosphamide (Cytoxan): 200-300 mg/m$^2$ on day 10 or 11

*ADIC protocol (cycle is repeated every 21 days)*

Doxorubicin (Adriamycin): 30 mg/m$^2$ (or 1 mg/kg for dogs under 10 kg) IV on day 1

Dacarbazine (DTIC): 700-1000 mg/m$^2$ as intravenous infusion (over 6-8 h) on day 1

*CHOP protocol (21-day cycle)*

Cyclophosphamide (Cytoxan): 200-300 mg/m$^2$ PO on day 10

Doxorubicin (Adriamycin): 30 mg/m$^2$ (or 1 mg/kg for dogs under 10 kg) IV on day 1

Vincristine (Oncovin): 0.75 mg/m$^2$ IV on days 8 and 15

Prednisone: 20-25 mg/m$^2$ PO q48h

**4. RESCUE—cont'd**

**Cats**

*MiC protocol (21-day cycle)*

  Mitoxantrone (Novantrone): 4-6 mg/m$^2$ as intravenous drip over 4-6 hr on day 1

  Cyclophosphamide (Cytoxan): 200-300 mg/m$^2$ PO on day 10 or 11

*AC protocol (21-day cycle)*

  Doxorubicin (Adriamycin): 1 mg/kg IV on day 1

  Cyclophosphamide (Cytoxan): 200-300 mg/m$^2$ PO on day 10 or 11

*MiCA protocol (21-day cycle)*

  Mitoxantrone (Novantrone): 4-6 mg/m$^2$ in intravenous drip over 4-6 hr on day 1

  Cyclophosphamide (Cytoxan): 200-300 mg/m$^2$ PO on day 10 or 11

  Cytosine arabinoside (Cytosar-U): 200 mg/m$^2$ in intravenous drip over 4-6 hr (mixed in the same bag with mitoxantrone) on day 1

*CHOP protocol (21-day cycle)*

  Cyclophosphamide (Cytoxan): 200-300 mg/m$^2$ PO on day 10

  Doxorubicin (Adriamycin): 1 mg/kg IV on day 1

  Vincristine (Oncovin): 0.5 mg/m$^2$ IV on days 8 and 15

  Prednisone: 20-25 mg/m$^2$ PO q48h

**5. "LOW BUDGET" PROTOCOLS**

  Prednisone: 50 mg/m$^2$ PO q24h for 1 week; then 25 mg/m$^2$ PO q48h

  Chlorambucil (Leukeran): 20 mg/m$^2$ PO q2wk

  Lomustine (CCNU; Ceenu): 60-90 mg/m$^2$ PO q3wk in dogs; 10 mg (total dose) q3wk in cats

  Prednisone and chlorambucil: doses as above

  Prednisone and lomustine: doses as above

*Unless otherwise specified, protocols can be used in both dogs and cats.

†Use for 6-10 weeks, then use LMP.

‡Use until relapse occurs, then go to "rescue."

§After four doses, substitute Leukeran (20 mg/m$^2$, PO, q2wk) for Alkeran.

*IM*, Intramuscularly; *IV*, intravenously; *PO*, orally; *SC*, subcutaneously.

a 12- to 24-hour infusion (200 mg/m$^2$) in this species. Lomustine (CCNU) has been shown to cause encouraging responses in dogs with epidermotropic lymphoma.

**Maintenance**

During this phase the patient is examined every 6 to 8 weeks, at which time complete physical examination and CBC are performed. Owners are instructed to continue monitoring the pet's activity, appetite, behavior, rectal temperature, and lymph node size. Most patients remain in remission for 3 to 6 months; when a relapse occurs, reinduction is instituted. After reinducing remission, the patient can be treated with a modified maintenance protocol (see later).

*Adverse effects.* Toxicities associated with LMP maintenance are minimal. Anorexia, vomiting, or diarrhea develops in approximately 25% of dogs and cats receiving methotrexate. Anorexia and vomiting are more common than diarrhea and usually occur after the patient has been receiving the drug for more than 2 weeks. Treatment with an antiemetic such as metoclopramide (Reglan, 0.1 to 0.3 mg/kg PO q8h) on the days methotrexate is given alleviates or corrects the upper GI signs. In cases of methotrexate-associated diarrhea, treatment with bismuth subsalicylate (Pepto-Bismol) may alleviate or correct the signs, although discontinuation of the drug may be required. In <5% of cats receiving chlorambucil for weeks to months, serum biochemical abnormalities consistent with cholestasis that resolve with the discontinuation of the drug may develop. Recently, seizures have been documented in cats receiving chlorambucil, but are extremely rare.

### Reinduction or "rescue"

Virtually every dog and cat treated with maintenance chemotherapy eventually relapses, generally 6 to 8 months after initiation of induction therapy, but relapse can occur within weeks of starting the maintenance phase or years after the original diagnosis is made. In most dogs remission can be reinduced one to four more times, but in most cats remission cannot be reinduced.

***D-MAC.*** The D-MAC protocol (see Box 82-1) is associated with an 80% remission rate in dogs, but chronic melphalan use can cause moderate-to-severe thrombocytopenia, so chlorambucil (Leukeran, 20 mg/m$^2$) is substituted for melphalan after four cycles. Once complete remission (CR) or partial remission (PR) is achieved after four to six cycles of D-MAC, the patient can again be placed on a maintenance protocol.

***ADIC.*** If the response to D-MAC is poor, ADIC or CHOP is recommended. Once CR is achieved, the patient is started on maintenance chemotherapy at the end of the second or third ADIC or CHOP cycle.

***Maintenance after relapse.*** Maintenance in these patients consists of LMP, with the possible addition of vincristine (0.5 to 0.75 mg/m$^2$ IV once weekly or every other week) or cytosine arabinoside (200 to 400 mg/m$^2$ SC every other week), alternating weeks with Leukeran.

***Further relapses.*** After a second relapse, D-MAC, ADIC, or CHOP is administered for two additional cycles. After two or three relapses, the percentage of patients in which remission can be easily reinduced decreases with each subsequent cycle. Other protocols that have been successfully used to reinduce remission in dogs with lymphoma are listed in Box 82-1. Doxorubicin- or mitoxantrone-containing protocols have been used with some degree of success in cats (see Box 82-1); asparaginase-containing protocols may not be as effective as in dogs.

### Intensification

If only PR is achieved with induction therapy, intensification with one or two doses of L-asparaginase (10,000 to 20,000 IU/m$^2$ intramuscularly, repeated once in 2 to 3 weeks) may be indicated; however, asparaginase should not be used in dogs with a history of pancreatitis or in patients at high risk for acute pancreatitis (e.g., obese, middle-aged, female dogs). L-Asparaginase seems to be less effective in cats; doxorubicin (1 mg/kg IV q3wk) or mitoxantrone (4 to 6 mg/m$^2$ IV q3wk) can be used as intensifying agents in this species.

### Solitary and extranodal lymphomas

Solitary lymphomas eventually become (or already are) systemic in most patients. Although cures have been obtained after surgical excision or irradiation of solitary lymphomas, this occurrence is extremely rare. The following guidelines can be used when dealing with affected patients:

1. If the tumor is easily resectable (e.g., cutaneous mass, superficial lymph node, intraocular mass), and the surgical procedure does not pose a high risk to the patient, the mass should be resected and evaluated histopathologically, and the patient treated with chemotherapy.
2. If the mass is difficult or impossible to resect or if a major surgical procedure would pose an undue risk, FNA or needle biopsy should be performed, and the patient treated with chemotherapy (with or without radiotherapy of the incompletely excised primary lesion).

***Radiotherapy.*** Radiotherapy is an excellent modality in patients with solitary lymphomas; marked responses (CR or PR) are seen within hours or days of initiation of treatment. In general, delivery of 3 to 5 Gy (300 to 500 rad) per fraction, for a total of 6 to 10 fractions (total dose of 30 to 50 Gy or 3000 to 5000 rad) is used. Specific situations in which radiotherapy is beneficial include CNS lymphomas (see later) and upper airway lymphomas.

***Chemotherapy.*** After surgical excision or irradiation, a standard induction protocol (COAP) is recommended for most cats and dogs with solitary lymphoma. The patient is then treated with a maintenance protocol (LMP), and remission is reinduced as necessary.

#### CNS lymphoma

The treatment of choice for primary or secondary epidural lymphoma is radiotherapy plus multiple-agent chemotherapy. If radiotherapy facilities are not available, multiple-agent chemotherapy (e.g., COAP) can be effective alone. When radiotherapy is available, three doses per week of 3.6 to 4 Gy, for a total of 25 to 30 Gy, is recommended. Surgical excision does not provide a significant advantage over chemotherapy or radiotherapy plus chemotherapy. The COAP protocol alone has been effective in inducing remission in cats with epidural lymphoma.

***Neuropil lymphoma.*** Chemotherapy with or without radiotherapy is recommended for patients with neuropil lymphoma. If neuroanatomic localization or imaging of the lesion is possible, radiotherapy should be used with chemotherapy. If localization is not possible, diffuse craniospinal irradiation can be used, at doses of 3.6 to 4 Gy three times per week, for a total of 25 to 30 Gy.

***Intrathecal chemotherapy.*** In cats and dogs with confirmed or highly suspected neuropil lymphoma, intrathecal chemotherapy can be used. The drug of choice is cytosine arabinoside, administered intrathecally at 20 to 40 mg/m$^2$ once or twice a week (after removal of an equivalent amount of CSF), for six to eight doses. Lactated Ringer's solution or CSF should be used as a diluent. Once diluted, the remaining drug should be discarded or used systemically within 24 hours; never reuse the vial for intrathecal injection. During administration strict asepsis should be followed.

Responses to intrathecal cytosine arabinoside are often spectacular. Within 6 to 48 hours of the first dose, normal neurologic status usually is regained, and neoplastic cells disappear from the CSF.

***Systemic chemotherapy.*** If radiotherapy or intrathecal chemotherapy cannot be used because anesthesia poses too great a risk, systemic chemotherapy can be used with success in most patients. Protocols should include cytosine arabinoside (administered as a slow intravenous drip), which attains high CSF concentration with minimal systemic toxicity. Doses range from 200 to 400 mg/m$^2$ for 1 to 4 days of continuous infusion. Intravenous cytosine arabinoside causes marked myelosuppression that may lead to neutropenia and sepsis; prophylactic antibiotics may therefore be indicated. Lomustine (see Box 82-1) also crosses the blood-brain barrier and is effective in eliminating lymphoma cells; treated dogs have shown marked improvement or disappearance of neurologic signs.

***Remission.*** Remission is easily attained in dogs and cats with CNS lymphoma, but the duration is relatively short. Most patients relapse within 2 to 4 months of diagnosis, although prolonged remission (6 to 12 months) can occur.

#### Ocular lymphoma

Cytosine arabinoside can be administered subconjunctivally; the doses and precautions are similar to those for intrathecal administration, including dilution with lactated Ringer's solution. Injections are given once or twice per week for 2 to 4 weeks. Responses are rapid and sustained, and ocular complications are minimal. Cytosine arabinoside intravenous drips or lomustine are also effective in dogs and cats with intraocular lymphoma.

#### Cutaneous lymphoma

In dogs with cutaneous involvement secondary to multicentric lymphoma a standard chemotherapy protocol (COAP) is used. In dogs with mycosis fungoides, "histiocytic" cutaneous lymphoma, or mucocutaneous epidermotropic lymphoma, doxorubicin-containing protocols (CHOP; see Box 82-1) or lomustine is used.

#### Alimentary lymphoma

In dogs and cats with solitary mural or nodal involvement, standard chemotherapy protocols (e.g., COAP) are used. Even though surgery may not be indicated, exploratory surgery and incisional or excisional biopsy are often performed for diagnosis. In general the response in these patients is good.

Dogs and cats with diffuse intestinal lymphoma usually respond poorly to chemotherapy. Responses to doxorubicin-containing protocols (e.g., CHOP) appear to be better than responses to COAP, although survival times are short (4 to 6 months).

Dogs with colorectal lymphoma and cats with gastric lymphoma tend to respond extremely well to COAP chemotherapy, with remission times in excess of 3 years.

**"Low-budget" lymphoma protocols**

Prednisone alone, prednisone and chlorambucil, chlorambucil alone, lomustine alone, or prednisone and lomustine can be used quite successfully when the owners do not wish to pursue treatment with standard multiagent chemotherapy. Although the duration of remission is shorter than when COP-based protocols are used, most of these patients (and their owners) enjoy prolonged (i.e., months), good-quality survival. These protocols are listed in Box 82-1.

# 83

# Leukemias

## *(Text pp 1133-1141)*

### CLASSIFICATION (TEXT P 1133)

Leukemias are malignant neoplasms that originate from hematopoietic precursor cells in the bone marrow. The neoplastic cells may or may not appear in peripheral circulation; the term *aleukemic* or *subleukemic leukemia* is used when the neoplastic cells are absent or scarce in circulation. Leukemias are classified according to the originating cell line as lymphoid or myeloid (nonlymphoid) (Table 83-1).

**Acute versus chronic**

Leukemias are also classified as acute or chronic. Acute leukemias are characterized by aggressive biologic behavior (death ensues shortly after diagnosis if the animal is untreated) and by the presence of immature (blast) cells in bone marrow and/or blood. Chronic leukemias have a protracted, often indolent course, and the predominant cell is a well-differentiated, late precursor (e.g., lymphocyte in chronic lymphocytic leukemia [CLL], neutrophil in chronic myeloid leukemia [CML]).

*Cytochemical staining.* Acute leukemias can be difficult to classify on Giemsa- or Wright's-stained blood or bone marrow smears. Cytochemical stains are needed to establish whether the blasts are lymphoid or myeloid and to subclassify myeloid leukemias as myeloid, monocytic, or myelomonocytic.

*Immunophenotyping.* Clinical correlations between immunophenotype and prognosis have not yet been established in animals.

*Blast crisis.* In dogs (and possibly in cats) CML can undergo blast transformation (blast crisis); the disease then behaves as an acute leukemia and is usually refractory to therapy. Blast crises do not appear to occur in dogs or cats with CLL.

*Myelodysplastic syndrome.*

Preleukemic or myelodysplastic syndrome (MDS or myelodysplasia) is a syndrome of hematopoietic dysfunction that precedes acute myelogenous leukemia by months or

Table 83-1

## Classification of Leukemias in Dogs and Cats

| Classification | Species |
|---|---|
| **ACUTE LEUKEMIAS** | |
| **Acute Myeloid (Myelogenous) Leukemia (AML)** | |
| Undifferentiated myeloid leukemia (AML-M$_0$) | D, C |
| Acute myelocytic leukemia (AML-M$_{1-2}$) | D, C |
| Acute progranulocytic leukemia (AML-M$_3$) | — |
| Acute myelomonocytic leukemia (AMML; AML-M$_4$) | D, C |
| Acute monoblastic or monocytic leukemia (AMoL; AML-M$_5$) | D, C |
| Acute erythroleukemia (AML-M$_6$) | C, D? |
| Acute megakaryoblastic leukemia (AML-M$_7$) | D, C |
| **Acute Lymphoblastic Leukemia (ALL)** | |
| ALL-L$_1$ | D, C |
| ALL-L$_2$ | D, C |
| ALL-L$_3$ | C, D? |
| Acute leukemia of large granular lymphocytes (LGL) | D, C? |
| **SUBACUTE AND CHRONIC LEUKEMIAS** | |
| Chronic myeloid (myelocytic) leukemia (CML) | D > C |
| Chronic (subacute) myelomonocytic leukemia (CMML) | D |
| Chronic lymphoid (lymphocytic) leukemia (CLL) | D > C |
| LGL variant of CLL | D |

*C*, Cats; *D*, dogs.

years. It is characterized by cytopenias and hypercellular bone marrow and is more common in cats than in dogs.

## LEUKEMIAS IN DOGS (TEXT PP 1133-1138)

Leukemias in dogs constitute less than 10% of all hemolymphatic neoplasms. Most canine leukemias are "spontaneous," although radiation exposure and viral particles are possible causative factors.

### Acute Leukemias

#### Prevalence

Acute myeloid leukemias (AMLs) are more common than acute lymphoid leukemias (ALLs), constituting approximately three fourths of the cases of acute leukemia. Most acute leukemias are initially classified as lymphoid. After performing cytochemical staining or immunophenotyping, however, one third to one half are reclassified as myeloid, approximately 50% of which are myelomonocytic.

#### Clinical features

Signs and physical examination findings are usually vague and nonspecific (Table 83-2). Neurologic signs are occasionally seen. Typically the spleen is markedly enlarged and has a smooth surface on palpation. Hepatomegaly, pallor, fever, and mild generalized lymphadenopathy are also commonly detected. Petechiae and/or ecchymoses are often found on the mucous membranes; icterus may also be detected if marked leukemic infiltration of the liver is present. The generalized lymphadenopathy is usually mild, in contrast to dogs with lymphoma; and most dogs with leukemia are clinically ill, whereas >50% of dogs with lymphoma are asymptomatic.

*AML versus ALL.* Although it is usually impossible to distinguish between AML and ALL on the basis of physical examination findings, some subtle differences exist.

Table 83-2

## Clinical Signs and Physical Examination Findings in Dogs and Cats with Acute Leukemias*

| Finding | Dogs | Cats |
|---|---|---|
| **CLINICAL SIGN** | | |
| Lethargy | >70 | >90 |
| Anorexia | >50 | >80 |
| Weight loss | 30-40 | 40-50 |
| Lameness | 20-30 | ? |
| Persistent fever | 30-50 | ? |
| Vomiting or diarrhea | 20-40 | ? |
| **PHYSICAL EXAMINATION FINDING** | | |
| Splenomegaly | >70 | >70 |
| Hepatomegaly | >50 | >50 |
| Lymphadenopathy | 40-50 | 20-30? |
| Pallor | 30-60 | 50-70? |
| Fever | 40-50 | 40-60? |

*Results are expressed as the approximate percent of animals showing the abnormality.
?, Unknown.

Shifting limb lameness, fever, and ocular lesions are more common in dogs with AML, whereas neurologic signs are more common in dogs with ALL.

### Hematologic features

Marked hematologic changes are usually present in dogs with acute leukemia. Abnormal (leukemic) cells are observed in the peripheral blood of most dogs with AML and ALL, although this is slightly more common in the latter (circulating blasts are absent in some dogs with AML). Isolated cytopenias, bicytopenias, or pancytopenia are present in almost all dogs with AML and ALL. Leukoerythroblastic reactions are detected in approximately 50% of dogs with AML but are rare in dogs with ALL.

*Complete blood count.* White blood cell (WBC) and blast counts are highest in dogs with ALL (median 298,200/μl; range 4000 to 628,000/μl); in general, only dogs with ALL have WBC counts greater than 150,000/μl. Most dogs with AML and ALL are anemic, but dogs with AML-M$_5$ (AMoL) have the least severe anemia (packed cell volume 30% versus 23% in all other groups). Thrombocytopenia is also common in dogs with acute leukemias, although it is less severe in those with AML-M$_5$ (median 102,000/μl; range 39,000 to 133,000/μl).

### Diagnosis

Presumptive diagnosis is often based on history and physical examination findings. Complete blood count (CBC) is usually confirmatory, although the hematologic changes with "aleukemic leukemia" may resemble those of ehrlichiosis or other bone marrow disorders.

*Cytology.* Bone marrow aspiration or biopsy is indicated to evaluate the extent of the disease. Splenic, hepatic, or lymph node aspirates for cytology are easily obtained, although they may not contribute significantly. When the neoplastic cells are poorly differentiated, cytochemical stains or immunophenotyping are required to establish a definitive diagnosis. This is important because the therapeutic approach and prognosis for AML are different than for ALL; survival times in dogs with AML are shorter than in those with ALL.

*Low circulating blasts.* Diagnosis can be difficult when a dog is presented with generalized lymphadenopathy, hepatosplenomegaly, and a low number of circulating blasts. The two main differential diagnoses are acute leukemia (ALL or AML) and lymphoma with circulating blasts (lymphosarcoma-cell leukemia). It is important to differentiate these disorders, as the prognosis for lymphoma is considerably better than for leukemia. Lymphoma is more likely if the lymphadenopathy is massive or if hypercalcemia is present. ALL or AML is more likely if the dog is systemically ill, bicytopenia or pancytopenia is present, or the percentage of blasts in the bone marrow is greater than 50%.

**Other differential diagnoses.** Other possibilities in patients with acute or chronic leukemias include malignant or systemic histiocytosis, systemic mast cell disease (mast cell leukemia), canine ehrlichiosis, hemobartonellosis, storage diseases, and tuberculosis.

**Summary.** The following principles of diagnosis apply to all patients with suspected leukemia:

1. If cytopenias or abnormal cells are present in peripheral blood, obtain a bone marrow aspirate or biopsy specimen.
2. If the spleen or liver is enlarged, obtain a fine-needle aspiration specimen for cytologic evaluation.
3. If blasts are present, submit blood and bone marrow specimens for cytochemical stains or immunophenotyping.
4. Perform other diagnostic tests (e.g., serology or polymerase chain reaction assay for *Ehrlichia* spp.) when appropriate.

**Treatment**

Chemotherapy protocols for acute leukemia are listed in Box 83-1. However, treatment is usually unrewarding; most dogs respond poorly, and prolonged remission is rarely achieved.

---

**Box 83-1**

**Chemotherapy Protocols for Dogs and Cats with Acute Leukemias**

**ACUTE LYMPHOBLASTIC LEUKEMIA**

1. Vincristine, 0.5 mg/m$^2$ IV once/wk
   Prednisone, 40-50 mg/m$^2$ PO q24h for 1 wk; then 20 mg/m$^2$ PO q48h
2. Vincristine, 0.5 mg/m$^2$ IV once/wk
   Prednisone, 40-50 mg/m$^2$ PO q24h for 1 wk; then 20 mg/m$^2$ PO q48h
   Cyclophosphamide, 50 mg/m$^2$ PO c48h in dogs or 200-300 mg/m$^2$ PO every 3 wk in cats
3. Vincristine, 0.5 mg/m$^2$ IV once/wk
   Prednisone, 40-50 mg/m$^2$ PO q24h for 1 wk; then 20 mg/m$^2$ PO q48h
   L-Asparaginase, 10,000-20,000 U/m$^2$ IM or SC once every 2-3 wk
4. Vincristine, 0.5 mg/m$^2$ IV once/wk
   Prednisone, 40-50 mg/m$^2$ PO q24h for 1 wk; then 20 mg/m$^2$ PO q48h
   Cyclophosphamide, 50 mg/m$^2$ PO q48h in dogs or 200-300 mg/m$^2$ PO every 3 wk in cats
   Cytosine arabinoside, 100 mg/m$^2$ SC or IV daily for 2 to 4 days*

**ACUTE MYELOID LEUKEMIAS**

1. Cytosine arabinoside, 5 to 10 mg/m$^2$ SC q12h for 2 to 3 wk; then on alternate weeks
2. Cytosine arabinoside, 100 mg/m$^2$ SC or IV caily for 2-6 days
   6-Thioguanine, 50 mg/m$^2$ PO q24-48h
3. Cytosine arabinoside, 100 mg/m$^2$ SC or IV daily for 2-6 days
   6-Thioguanine, 50 mg/m$^2$ PO q24-48h
   Doxorubicin, 10 mg/m$^2$ IV once/wk
4. Cytosine arabinoside, 100-200 mg/m$^2$ in IV drip over 4 hr
   Mitoxantrone, 4-6 mg/m$^2$ in IV drip cver 4 hr; repeat every 3 wk

*The daily dose should be divided into two to four daily administrations.
*IM,* Intramuscularly; *IV,* intravenously; *PO,* orally; *SC,* subcutaneously.

***Treatment failures.*** Poor response is usually because of one or more of the following factors:

1. Failure to induce remission (more common in AML than in ALL)
2. Failure to maintain remission
3. Organ failure from leukemic cell infiltration does not allow the use of aggressive combination chemotherapy because of enhanced toxicity
4. Development of fatal sepsis and/or bleeding caused by preexisting or treatment-induced cytopenias.

***Remission and survival.*** Prolonged remission in dogs with AML is extremely rare; survival rarely exceeds 3 months. Over 50% of dogs die from sepsis or bleeding during induction chemotherapy.

The outcome may be slightly better for dogs with ALL than AML, although responses and survival times are considerably lower than for those with lymphoma. Remission rates in dogs with acute leukemia are 20% to 40%, in contrast to those in dogs with lymphoma (up to 90%). Survival times are also shorter (average, 1 to 3 months with appropriate chemotherapy) than for lymphoma (average 12 to 18 months). Untreated dogs usually live less than 2 weeks.

## Chronic Leukemias
### Prevalence
CLL is far more common than CML in dogs and is one of the most commonly diagnosed canine leukemias.

### Clinical features
A history of chronic (i.e., months), vague clinical signs is present in only approximately half of the dogs with chronic leukemia. Therefore, many cases are diagnosed incidentally during routine physical and laboratory evaluation. Clinical signs are present in approximately 50% of dogs with CLL and include lethargy, anorexia, vomiting, polyuria and polydipsia, intermittent lameness, intermittent diarrhea and/or vomiting, and weight loss. Physical examination findings include mild generalized lymphadenopathy, splenomegaly, hepatomegaly, pallor, and pyrexia. Signs and physical examination findings in dogs with CML are similar.

***Richter's syndrome.*** A terminal event in dogs with CLL is the development of a diffuse, large-cell lymphoma (Richter's syndrome), characterized by massive generalized lymphadenopathy and hepatosplenomegaly. Once this multicentric lymphoma develops, long-lasting remission is difficult to attain, and survival times are short.

### Hematologic features
The most common hematologic abnormality in dogs with CLL is marked lymphocytosis resulting in leukocytosis. The lymphocytes usually appear normal, although large granular lymphocytes are occasionally present. Lymphocyte counts range from 8000/µl to more than 100,000/µl; counts of more than 500,000/µl are rare. In addition to the lymphocytosis, which may be diagnostic in itself, anemia is found in more than 80% of dogs, and thrombocytopenia in approximately 50%.

***Bone marrow aspirates.*** Cytologic evaluation of bone marrow aspirates in dogs with CLL usually reveals high numbers of morphologically normal lymphocytes, but occasionally, normal numbers of lymphocytes are found.

***Blast crises.*** Blast crisis, characterized by the appearance of immature blast cells in blood and bone marrow, can occur in dogs with CML months or years after the initial diagnosis. Hematologic findings during blast crisis are indistinguishable from those of dogs with AML and ALL. Blast crises do not appear to occur in dogs with CLL.

***Gammopathies and immune disorders.*** Monoclonal gammopathies (usually immunoglobulin M [IgM], but can be IgA or IgG) are present in approximately two thirds of dogs with CLL. This monoclonal gammopathy can lead to hyperviscosity. Rarely, dogs with CLL have paraneoplastic immune-mediated blood disorders (e.g., hemolytic anemia, thrombocytopenia, neutropenia).

***Chronic myeloid leukemia.*** Hematologic features in dogs with CML are poorly characterized but include leukocytosis with left shift down to myelocytes (or occasionally myeloblasts), anemia, and possibly thrombocytopenia, although thrombocytosis can occur.

### Diagnosis

Absolute lymphocytosis is the major diagnostic criterion for CLL. Canine ehrlichiosis, babesiosis, leishmaniasis, Chagas' disease, and Addison's disease should be considered as differential diagnoses in dogs with mild lymphocytosis (7000 to 20,000/µl), but marked lymphocytosis (>20,000/µl) is almost pathognomonic for CLL. Physical examination and hematologic abnormalities aid in establishing a diagnosis of CLL, although similar changes can be found in dogs with chronic ehrlichiosis.

*Chronic myeloid leukemia.* Diagnosis can be challenging because CML is poorly characterized in dogs. The diagnosis should be made only after careful evaluation of the clinical and hematologic findings and the ruling out of inflammatory and immune causes of neutrophilia.

### Treatment

If a dog with CLL is symptomatic or has organomegaly or concurrent hematologic abnormalities, treatment with an alkylator (with or without corticosteroids) is indicated. If paraneoplastic syndromes (e.g., immune hemolysis or thrombocytopenia, monoclonal gammopathies) are absent, single-agent chlorambucil (Leukeran) is recommended (Box 83-2). If paraneoplastic syndromes are present, addition of prednisone may be beneficial.

*Chronic lymphocytic leukemia.* A delayed response to therapy is common with CLL. In a high proportion of dogs treated with chlorambucil or chlorambucil and prednisone, resolution of the hematologic and physical examination abnormalities may take more than 1 month (and as long as 6 months). In contrast, remission is usually induced in 2 to 7 days in dogs with lymphoma or acute leukemias. Survival times for dogs with CLL are quite long; even without treatment, survival for more than 2 years is common. Most dogs with CLL die from other geriatric disorders.

*Chronic myeloid leukemia.* Treatment with hydroxyurea (Box 83-2) may result in prolonged remission, provided blast crisis does not occur. However, the prognosis is not as good as with CLL; dogs with CML survive for 4 to 15 months with treatment.

## LEUKEMIAS IN CATS (TEXT PP 1138-1140)

### Acute Leukemias

#### Prevalence

True leukemias are rare in cats (15% to 35% of all hemolymphatic neoplasms), although they are more common than in dogs. Approximately two thirds are myeloid and one third are lymphoid; myelomonocytic leukemias ($M_4$) are extremely rare.

---

**Box 83-2**

### Chemotherapy Protocols for Dogs and Cats with Chronic Leukemias

#### CHRONIC LYMPHOCYTIC LEUKEMIA

1. Chlorambucil, 20 mg/m$^2$ PO once every 2 wk
2. Chlorambucil as above, plus prednisone, 50 mg/m$^2$ PO q24h for 1 wk; then 20 mg/m$^2$ PO q48h
3. Cyclophosphamide, 200-300 mg/m$^2$ IV or PO once every 2 wk; vincristine, 0.5-0.75 mg/m$^2$ IV once every 2 wk (alternating weeks with the cyclophosphamide); prednisone as in 2, this treatment is continued for 6 to 8 wk, at which time protocols 1 or 2 can be used for maintenance

#### CHRONIC MYELOID LEUKEMIA

1. Hydroxyurea, 50 mg/kg PO q24h for 1 to 2 wk; then q48h

---

*IV,* Intravenously; *PO,* orally.

Feline leukemia virus (FeLV) is commonly implicated as a cause of leukemias in cats; the role of feline immunodeficiency virus (FIV) is unclear. Overall it is reported that approximately 90% of cats with leukemia are positive for FeLV p27 by enzyme-linked immunosorbent assay or immunofluorescence; however, the prevalence of FeLV infection appears to be decreasing, and cats with leukemia are now more often FeLV-negative.

### Clinical features

Signs and physical examination findings are similar to those in dogs (see Table 83-2). Shifting limb lameness and neurologic signs are not as common in cats as in dogs with myeloid leukemias.

### Hematologic features

More than three fourths of cats with AML or ALL have cytopenias; leuko-erythroblastic reactions are common in cats with AML but rare in those with ALL.

In cats with myeloid leukemias, cytomorphologic features can change from one cell type to another over time. Sequential diagnoses of erythremic myelosis, erythroleukemia, and acute myeloblastic leukemia are common. Therefore the term *myeloproliferative disorder* is preferred for cats.

### Diagnosis

Diagnosis follows the same general sequence as in dogs. If CBC changes are not diagnostic, a bone marrow aspirate is confirmatory. Cats with suspected or confirmed acute leukemias should be evaluated for circulating FeLV p27 and for serum antibodies against FIV.

### Treatment

Intensive chemotherapy does not appear to be beneficial in cats with acute leukemias. Survival times for cats with ALL treated with multichemotherapy range from 1 to 7 months, but survival times for cats with AML treated with single-agent chemotherapy usually range from 2 to 10 weeks (median approximately 3 weeks).

New alternatives for therapy for feline myeloproliferative disorder are currently being explored. Low-dose cytosine arabinoside (Cytosar-U, 10 mg/m$^2$ subcutaneously q12h) has been used to induce differentiation of the neoplastic clone. Complete or partial remission is achieved in most cats, with transient hematologic improvement. Although no major toxicities are seen, remission is short-lived (3 to 8 weeks).

## Chronic Leukemias

Chronic leukemias are extremely rare in cats. CLL is occasionally diagnosed incidentally during routine physical examination. More often, cats with CLL are presented because of a protracted history of vague signs of illness, including anorexia, lethargy, and gastrointestinal signs. Mature, well-differentiated lymphocytes predominate in peripheral blood and bone marrow, and response to therapy is good with chlorambucil and prednisone treatment. CML is poorly characterized in cats.

## MYELODYSPLASTIC SYNDROMES (TEXT PP 1140-1141)

MDS is recognized in both dogs and cats but is more common in retrovirus-infected cats. It causes a variety of hematologic abnormalities (cytopenias with normocellular or hypercellular bone marrow) and vague clinical signs that may precede the development of acute myelogenous leukemia by months or years. Functional abnormalities of granulocytes and platelets can also develop, leading to recurrent infections and/or spontaneous bleeding, even when neutrophil and platelet counts are normal.

### MDS in dogs

Affected dogs are lethargic, depressed, and anorectic; physical examination findings include hepatosplenomegaly, pallor, and pyrexia. Hematologic changes include pancytopenia or bicytopenia, macrocytosis, metarubricytosis, and reticulocytopenia. Some dogs subsequently develop AML months after initial diagnosis of MDS.

### MDS in cats

Most cats are presented for evaluation of nonspecific signs such as lethargy, weight loss, and anorexia; other signs such as dyspnea, recurrent infections, and spontaneous bleeding are occasionally observed. Physical examination reveals hepatosplenomegaly in more than 50% of cats; generalized lymphadenopathy and pyrexia are detected in approximately one third of affected cats.

*Hematologic features.* Hematologic abnormalities are similar to those of dogs, and include isolated or combined cytopenias, macrocytosis, reticulocytopenia, metarubricytosis, and presence of macrothrombocytes. Approximately one third of cats with MDS subsequently develop acute leukemia (often ALL) within weeks or months of diagnosis. More than 80% of affected cats are viremic with FeLV.

*Bone marrow.* Bone marrow changes include normal or increased cellularity, less than 30% blasts, increased myeloid:erythroid ratio, dyserythropoiesis, dysmyelopoiesis, and dysthrombo-poiesis. Megaloblastic red blood cell precursors are common, with occasional binucleated, trinucleated, or tetranucleated rubricytes or metarubricytes. Morphologic abnormalities in the myeloid cell line include giant metamyelocytes and asynchronous nuclear-cytoplasmic maturation.

### Management

A variety of treatment modalities have been tried, but none has proved effective. Supportive therapy (e.g., fluids, blood components, antibiotics) and low-dose cytosine arabinoside (see Box 83-1) are recommended. With this protocol, short-lived responses occur in a limited number of cats.

# 84

# Selected Neoplasms in Dogs and Cats

## (Text pp 1142-1155)

### HEMANGIOSARCOMA IN DOGS (TEXT PP 1142-1144)

Hemangiosarcomas (HSAs) are malignant neoplasms originating from the vascular endothelium. They predominantly occur in older dogs (8 to 10 years of age) and in males; German Shepherd Dogs and Golden Retrievers are at high risk.

### Characteristics

Common sites include the spleen (50%), right atrium (25%), and subcutis (13%). Five percent originate in the liver; 5% in the liver, spleen, and right atrium; and 1% to 2% simultaneously in other organs (e.g., kidney, bladder, bone, tongue, prostate). The last group is called *multiple tumor, undeterminable primary* (MTUP).

In general the biologic behavior of HSAs is highly aggressive, with both infiltration and metastases occurring early in the course of disease. The only exception is primary dermal HSAs, which have a lower metastatic potential than those originating in subcutaneous tissues.

### Clinical features
Presenting complaints and clinical signs are usually related to the site of origin of the primary tumor or to the presence of metastases, spontaneous tumor rupture, coagulopathies, or cardiac arrhythmias. More than 50% of patients are presented because of acute collapse after spontaneous rupture of the primary tumor or its metastases. Some episodes of collapse are a result of ventricular arrhythmias, which are relatively common in dogs with splenic or cardiac HSA.

*Specific presentations.* Dogs with splenic HSA are often presented because of abdominal distention (tumor growth or hemoabdomen). Dogs with cardiac HSAs usually are presented for evaluation of right-sided congestive heart failure (caused by cardiac tamponade or postcaval obstruction by a neoplastic mass) or cardiac arrhythmias. With cutaneous and subcutaneous HSAs, dogs usually are presented for evaluation of a lump.

*Anemia and bleeding.* Two common complaints, regardless of the primary location or stage, are anemia and spontaneous bleeding. Anemia is usually the result of intracavitary bleeding or microangiopathic hemolysis (MAHA). Bleeding is usually caused by disseminated intravascular coagulation (DIC) or thrombocytopenia secondary to MAHA. The association of HSA and DIC is so high that dogs with acute onset of DIC in which a primary cause is not obvious should be evaluated for HSA.

### Clinicopathologic findings
HSAs usually cause a wide variety of hematologic and hemostatic abnormalities, including anemia; thrombocytopenia; presence of nucleated red blood cells (RBCs), RBC fragments (schistocytes), and acanthocytes in the blood smear; and leukocytosis with neutrophilia, left shift, and monocytosis.

### Diagnosis
HSAs can be diagnosed cytologically in fine-needle aspiration (FNA) samples or impression smears. In general a presumptive clinical or cytologic diagnosis of HSA should be confirmed histopathologically. Because of the large size of some splenic HSAs, multiple samples from different areas should be submitted.

*Cytology.* The neoplastic cells are spindle shaped or polyhedral and have large nuclei with lacy chromatin and one or more nucleoli and bluish, usually vacuolated cytoplasm. These cells are easy to identify in tissue aspirates or impression smears but extremely difficult to identify in effusions. Reactive mesothelial cells may resemble neoplastic cells, leading to a misdiagnosis of HSA.

*Imaging.* Metastatic sites can be detected radiographically, ultrasonographically, or on computerized tomography (CT). Thoracic radiographs in dogs with metastatic HSA are typically characterized by interstitial or alveolar infiltrates. On ultrasound, neoplastic lesions appear as nodules of variable echogenicity, ranging from anechoic to hyperechoic; hepatic metastases can often be identified. However, "metastatic nodules" in the liver of a dog with a splenic mass may represent regenerative hyperplasia, rather than true metastatic lesions.

*Staging.* Routine staging requires complete blood count (CBC), serum biochemistry profile, hemostasis screen, urinalysis, thoracic and abdominal radiographs, abdominal ultrasonography, and echocardiography. Echocardiography is used to identify cardiac masses and measure fractional shortening before institution of doxorubicin-containing chemotherapy.

### Treatment and prognosis
Although surgery is the preferred therapeutic modality, survival times are extremely short. They vary with the location and stage, but with the exception of dermal HSAs, survival times average 20 to 60 days, with a 1-year survival rate of less than 10%. Postoperative chemotherapy with doxorubicin-containing protocols prolongs survival (median survival 140 to 202 days).

*Chemotherapy.* Median survival after VAC chemotherapy (vincristine, doxorubicin [Adriamycin], and cyclophosphamide) (see Chapter 79) is approximately 190 days, with a 30% 1-year survival rate. Adverse effects include myelosuppression, gastroenteritis, alopecia and hyperpigmentation, and cardiotoxicity. There is no apparent difference in survival times between dogs with bulky disease (no surgical cytoreduction) and those that undergo surgery. Similar results have been reported in dogs treated with either doxorubicin and cyclophosphamide or doxorubicin alone. Coagulopathies should be managed simultaneously, as discussed in Chapter 89. Dogs receiving liposome-encapsulated muramyl tripeptide (MTP) in combination with doxorubicin-containing chemotherapy after splenectomy for HSA have significantly longer survival times (277 days); however, liposomal MTP is not readily available to the practicing veterinarian.

## OSTEOSARCOMA IN DOGS AND CATS (TEXT PP 1144-1146)

### Characteristics

Primary bone neoplasms are relatively common in dogs and rare in cats. If untreated, most primary bone tumors in dogs result in death or euthanasia because of either local infiltration (pathologic fractures or extreme pain) or metastases (e.g., pulmonary metastases in osteosarcoma [OSA]). In contrast, most primary bone neoplasms in cats, although histologically malignant, are cured by wide surgical excision (i.e., amputation).

*Osteosarcomas.* OSAs are the most common primary bone neoplasms in dogs. They can affect either the appendicular or axial skeleton and occur primarily in large- and giant-breed, middle-aged or older dogs; OSA is the most common tumor in greyhounds. Their biologic behavior is characterized by aggressive local infiltration of the surrounding tissue and rapid hematogenous dissemination (usually to the lungs).

*Metastases to bone.* Neoplasms that metastasize to the bone are extremely rare in cats and dogs. Some malignancies that occasionally metastasize to bones in dogs are transitional cell carcinoma of the urinary tract, OSA of the appendicular skeleton, HSA, mammary adenocarcinoma, and prostatic adenocarcinoma.

### Clinical features

Appendicular OSAs predominantly occur in the metaphyses of the distal radius, distal femur, and proximal humerus, although other metaphyses can also be affected. The presenting complaint is lameness, swelling of the affected limb, or both. Physical examination usually reveals a painful swelling with or without soft-tissue involvement. Onset of pain and swelling can be acute, leading to a presumptive diagnosis of a nonneoplastic orthopedic problem.

### Diagnosis

Radiographically OSAs are characterized by a mixed lytic or proliferative pattern in the metaphyseal region of the affected bone. Adjacent periosteal bone formation leads to the development of Codman's triangle, composed of destroyed cortex and periosteal proliferation. OSAs typically do not cross the articular space, but occasionally they can infiltrate adjacent bone. Other primary bone neoplasms and some osteomyelitis lesions can mimic these changes, so every lytic or lytic and proliferative bone lesion should undergo biopsy before treatment is determined, unless the owner elects amputation of the limb as the initial treatment.

*Survey radiographs.* Once a presumptive radiographic diagnosis has been made, thoracic and/or bone (skeletal survey) radiographs (or radionuclide bone scan) should be used to determine the extent of the disease if treatment is contemplated. The presence of metastatic lesions considerably worsens the prognosis. However, only approximately 10% of dogs with OSA have radiographically detectable lung metastases on initial presentation.

*Cytology.* Confirmation of the diagnosis can be obtained before surgery by performing an FNA (if considerable cortical lysis is present) with a hypodermic or bone marrow needle, or a core biopsy (see text). OSA cells are usually round or oval and have distinct cytoplasmic borders, bright blue granular cytoplasm, and eccentric nuclei with or without nucleoli.

### Treatment and prognosis

The treatment of choice in dogs is amputation plus adjuvant single-agent or combination chemotherapy. Median survival time with amputation alone is approximately

---

**Box 84-1**

### Cisplatin Treatment Protocol for Dogs with Appendicular Osteosarcoma

1. Obtain a CBC, serum biochemistry profile, and urinalysis.
2. Place indwelling IV catheter and perform 0.9% saline diuresis (120-150 ml/kg/day) for 8 hr.
3. Initiate cisplatin (Platinol) treatment (70 mg/m$^2$); the dose of cisplatin is diluted in the volume of 0.9% saline solution to be administered over 8 hr, calculated on the basis of 120-150 ml/kg/24 hr (i.e., 40-50 ml/kg).
4. If vomiting occurs during cisplatin treatment, 0.3 mg/kg of metoclopramide (Reglan) or 0.1-0.3 mg/kg of ondansetron (Zofran) is administered SC or IV.
5. On completion of the cisplatin drip, 0.9% saline solution is administered for 8 additional hr as an IV drip.
6. The dog is discharged and readmitted every 3 wk for additional treatments.

---

*CBC,* Complete blood count; *IV,* intravenous; *SC,* subcutaneously.

4 months, whereas dogs treated with amputation plus cisplatin, carboplatin, or doxorubicin survive approximately 1 year.

*Chemotherapy.* Doses and recommendations for cisplatin chemotherapy are given in Box 84-1. If a diagnosis of OSA is made, we use either of the drugs mentioned above immediately after amputation for a total of four or five treatments. If diagnosis is not made until after surgery, chemotherapy is initiated as soon as the histopathologic diagnosis is available. Carboplatin and doxorubicin are also effective when used as single agents (see table at the end of this chapter—Cancer Chemotherapy Protocols Commonly Used at The Ohio State University Veterinary Teaching Hospital).

*Limb-sparing surgery.* In dogs with distal radial OSA a novel surgical approach spares the limb: the affected bone is resected and replaced with an allograft from a cadaver. The dogs are also treated with intravenous cisplatin, carboplatin, or doxorubicin and, in general, maintain almost normal limb function. Survival times are comparable to amputation plus chemotherapy, with the added benefit to the owners of having a four-legged pet. The main complication is the development of osteomyelitis in the allograft, which usually requires amputation of the limb.

*Radiotherapy.* If owners are reluctant to allow amputation, local radiotherapy plus cisplatin, carboplatin, or doxorubicin may be of some benefit (see Box 84-2). However, most dogs are euthanized within 3 to 4 months after diagnosis because of pathologic fractures, osteomyelitis, or metastases.

*Metastasectomy.* Chemotherapy appears to lower the prevalence of pulmonary metastases. Therefore in patients treated with chemotherapy after amputation and in which one to three pulmonary metastases are detected, surgical removal of the metastatic nodules may be recommended, followed by additional cisplatin or carboplatin.

*OSA in cats.* The treatment of choice is limb amputation alone. Long survival times (>2 years) are common. Cisplatin is extremely toxic in cats and should not be used; if necessary, carboplatin or doxorubicin can be used instead.

## MAST CELL TUMORS IN DOGS AND CATS (TEXT PP 1146-1149)

Mast cell tumors (MCTs) are one of the most common skin tumors in dogs and are relatively common in cats.

## MCTs in Dogs

### Epidemiology

MCTs constitute 20% to 25% of all canine skin or subcutaneous tumors. Brachiocephalic breeds (e.g., Boxer, Boston Terrier, Bull Mastiff, English Bulldog) are at high risk. These tumors are more common in middle-aged or older dogs (mean, 8.5 years); no gender predilection exists. MCTs have been reported in sites of chronic inflammation or injury, such as burn scars.

### Biologic behavior

The biologic behavior of canine MCTs is unpredictable. MCTs are classified as well differentiated (grade 1), moderately differentiated (grade 2), or poorly differentiated (grade 3). Dogs with grade 1 tumors have longer survival times than dogs with grade 3 tumors.

*Grade 1 MCTs.* Well-differentiated, solitary, cutaneous MCTs generally have a low potential for metastasis and systemic dissemination. However, it is relatively common for a dog to have several dozen well-differentiated cutaneous MCTs.

*Grades 2 and 3 MCTs.* Moderately or poorly differentiated MCTs have a higher potential for metastasis and systemic dissemination. These tumors commonly metastasize to regional lymph nodes (particularly in dogs with grade 3 tumors); pulmonary metastases are extremely rare. Distal limb, perineal, inguinal, and extracutaneous (e.g., oropharyngeal, intranasal) MCTs appear to have a higher metastatic potential than similarly graded tumors in other regions.

### Clinical and pathologic features

Dogs with MCTs commonly have diffuse swelling (edema and inflammation), erythema, or bruising of the affected area(s). These episodes can be acute and may occur during or shortly after exercise.

*Appearance.* MCTs appear either as dermoepidermal or subcutaneous masses. They can mimic any primary or secondary skin lesions, including macula, papule, nodule, tumor, and crust; 10% to 15% of MCTs are clinically indistinguishable from subcutaneous lipomas.

Most MCTs are solitary, although multifocal MCTs can occur. A "typical" MCT is a dermoepidermal, dome-shaped, alopecic, erythematous lesion. However, MCTs rarely appear typical. A clinical feature that may aid in diagnosis is the Darrier sign: erythema and wheal formation after the tumor is slightly traumatized (aspirated or compressed).

*Other signs.* Regional lymphadenopathy caused by metastatic disease is common in dogs with invasive MCTs. Gastrointestinal (GI) ulceration may occur as a result of hyperhistaminemia (approximately 80% of dogs with advanced MCTs have gastroduodenal ulceration), so every dog with MCT should undergo an occult fecal blood test. Also, profuse intraoperative and postoperative bleeding and delayed wound healing occur as a consequence of the release of bioactive substances from mast cells.

*Clinicopathologic features.* Most dogs with MCTs have a normal CBC, although eosinophilia (sometimes marked), basophilia, mastocythemia, neutrophilia, thrombocytosis, and/or anemia may be present. Serum biochemistry abnormalities are uncommon.

*Systemic mast cell disease.* Canine MCTs may become systemic, behaving like a hematopoietic malignancy. A history of a previously excised cutaneous MCT is usually present. Most dogs with systemic mast cell disease (SMCD) have lethargy, anorexia, vomiting, and weight loss in association with splenomegaly, hepatomegaly, pallor, and occasionally, detectable cutaneous masses. CBC commonly reveals cytopenias, with or without circulating mast cells.

### Diagnosis

Dogs presented with a suspected MCT or an unexplained subcutaneous swelling should be evaluated by FNA. As a rule, definitive diagnosis cannot be made until the lesion has been evaluated cytologically.

*Cytology.* MCTs are easily identified as a monomorphic population of round cells with prominent, purple intracytoplasmic granules; eosinophils are frequently present in the smear. In approximately one third of MCTs the granules do not stain with Diff-Quik, so when agranular, round cells are found in a dermal or subcutaneous mass that resembles an MCT, the slide should be stained with Giemsa or Wright's stain. Grading cells in a cytologic specimen does not correlate with the histopathologic grading system and therefore may not have the same prognostic implications.

*Further evaluation.* Clinical evaluation of a dog with a cytologically confirmed MCT should include careful palpation of the affected area and its draining lymph nodes; abdominal palpation, radiography, or ultrasonography to check for hepatosplenomegaly; CBC, serum biochemistry profile, and urinalysis; and thoracic radiographs (if the neoplasm is in the cranial half of the body). If lymphadenopathy, hepatomegaly, or splenomegaly is present, FNA of the enlarged lymph node or organ should be performed.

*Buffy coat smears.* Presence of mast cells in a buffy coat smear may not indicate systemic dissemination (and therefore a poor prognosis), as was previously thought. Dogs with a solitary, potentially curable MCT occasionally have low numbers of circulating mast cells that disappear from circulation after the primary tumor is excised or irradiated. Circulating mast cells are also more common in dogs with conditions other than MCTs (inflammatory disorders, regenerative anemia, tumors other than MCTs, and trauma).Cytologic evaluation of a bone marrow aspirate may therefore be more beneficial than buffy coat smears for staging purposes.

*Bone marrow aspirate.* Dogs with more than 5 mast cells/500 nucleated cells likely have SMCD. Disappearance of bone marrow mast cells has been documented after excision or irradiation of the primary tumor, making staging difficult. Bone marrow aspirates therefore are advised only if cytopenias or leukoerythroblastic reactions are present (not for normal CBCs).

*Staging.* MCT "staging" is outlined in Table 84-1.

**Treatment and prognosis**

Dogs with MCT can be treated with surgery, radiotherapy, and/or chemotherapy. The first two options are potentially curative, whereas chemotherapy is only palliative. Treatment guidelines are provided in Table 84-2. Blood in the stool suggests upper GI bleeding and, if repeatable, should be treated with $H_2$ antihistamines (e.g., famotidine, ranitidine) with or without sucralfate (see Chapter 30).

*Resectable tumors.* A solitary MCT in an area in which complete surgical excision is feasible should be treated with aggressive resection (3-cm margins around and beneath the tumor). If, on histopathologic evaluation, complete excision of a grade 1 or 2 MCT

**Table 84-1**

### Clinical Staging Scheme for Dogs with Mast Cell Tumors

| Stage | Description |
|---|---|
| I | One tumor confined to the dermis without regional lymph node involvement |
| | a. Without systemic signs |
| | b. With systemic signs |
| II | One tumor confined to the dermis with regional lymph node involvement |
| | a. Without systemic signs |
| | b. With systemic signs |
| III | Multiple dermal tumors or a large infiltrating tumor with or without regional lymph node involvement |
| | a. Without systemic signs |
| | b. With systemic signs |
| IV | Any tumor with distant metastases or recurrence with metastases |
| | a. Without systemic signs |
| | b. With systemic signs |

Table 84-2

## Treatment Guidelines for Dogs with Mast Cell Tumors

| Stage | Grade | Recommended treatment | Follow-up |
|---|---|---|---|
| I | 1, 2 | Surgical excision | Complete: observe<br>Incomplete: surgery or<br>radiotherapy |
| I | 3 | Chemotherapy* | Continue chemotherapy |
| II | 1, 2, 3 | Surgical excision or<br>radiotherapy | CCNU and prednisone<br>(see below)* |
| III, IV | 1, 2, 3 | Chemotherapy* | Continue chemotherapy |

*Prednisone, 50 mg/m$^2$ orally (PO) q24h for 1 wk; then 20-25 mg/m$^2$ PO q48h indefinitely plus lomustine (CCNU, CeeNU), 60-90 mg/m$^2$ PO q3wk.

is achieved and no metastatic lesions are present, usually no further treatment is required. If excision appears incomplete, two courses of action are possible: (1) perform a second surgery to excise the remaining tumor (with histopathologic evaluation to assess completeness of excision), or (2) irradiate the surgical site (35 to 40 Gy in 10 to 12 fractions). These options are equally effective, resulting in approximately 80% probability of long-term survival.

**Nonresectable tumors.** A solitary MCT in an area in which surgical excision is difficult or impossible or would have unacceptable cosmetic or functional results (e.g., prepuce, eyelid) can be successfully treated with radiotherapy. Approximately two thirds of dogs with localized grade 1 or 2 MCTs treated with radiotherapy alone are cured. Intralesional injections of triamcinolone (Vetalog, 1 mg/cm of tumor diameter, every 2 to 3 weeks) can be successful in reducing tumor size, although this is usually only palliative. Intralesional injections of deionized water may also be beneficial in management of local MCTs.

**Metastatic MCT or SMCD.** Once a patient develops metastatic or disseminated MCTs, a cure is rarely obtained. However, chemotherapy and supportive care provide long-term, good-quality survival times.

**Chemotherapy.** Three chemotherapy protocols are widely used in dogs with metastatic or nonresectable MCTs (see Table 84-2): (1) prednisone; (2) lomustine (CCNU); and (3) cyclophosphamide, vinblastine, and prednisone (CVP).

In dogs with metastatic or nonresectable MCTs, one approach is to begin with prednisone (see Table 84-2), with or without famotidine and/or sucralfate. In dogs with metastatic grade 2 or 3 MCTs, lomustine can be added to this treatment protocol (see Table 84-2) with extremely good results (>50% respond well, remissions in excess of 18 months). Lomustine is potentially myelosuppressive (but clinically relevant cytopenias rarely develop) and hepatotoxic (chemistry profiles must be monitored). CVP chemotherapy is reserved for patients that do not respond to the prednisone-lomustine combination. During CVP treatment, patients should be monitored for myelosuppression (see Chapter 80). Chemotherapy should be continued indefinitely (i.e., until death or relapse). Dogs receiving CVP may develop sterile hemorrhagic cystitis, so chlorambucil (Leukeran) should be substituted for cyclophosphamide after 8 to 12 weeks.

### MCTs in Cats

Most cats with MCTs are middle-aged or older (median, 10 years); no gender predilection exists, but Siamese cats may be at high risk.

#### Biologic behavior

Feline MCTs occur in two main forms: cutaneous and visceral. The cutaneous form may be more common than the visceral presentation; coexistence of both forms is extremely rare. Visceral MCTs involve either the hemolymphatic system or the intestinal tract.

*Classification.* Feline MCTs can be classified as either the mast cell (common) or the histiocytic (rare) type. Cats with mast cell–type MCTs are usually more than 4 years old and have solitary dermal masses; no apparent breed predilection exists. Histiocytic-type MCTs primarily occur in Siamese cats less than 4 years old and appear as multiple (miliary) subcutaneous masses; some of these neoplasms regress spontaneously. The subcutaneous MCTs commonly seen in dogs are extremely rare in cats. Histopathologic grading does not appear to correlate well with the biologic behavior of MCTs in cats.

### Clinical and pathologic features

Cutaneous MCTs usually manifest as solitary or multiple, small (2 to 15 mm), white-to-pink dermoepidermal masses. They primarily affect the head and neck, although solitary dermoepidermal or subcutaneous masses in other locations also occur.

*Hemolymphatic MCT.* Cats with hemolymphatic involvement are classified as having SMCD (or mast cell leukemia), because bone marrow, spleen, liver, and blood are commonly involved. Most cats are presented because of nonspecific signs such as anorexia and vomiting, although abdominal distention caused by massive splenomegaly is a consistent feature. Hematologic abnormalities are extremely variable and include cytopenias, mastocythemia, basophilia, and/or eosinophilia; however, a high percentage of cats have normal CBC.

*Intestinal MCT.* Cats with the intestinal form usually are presented for evaluation of GI signs such as anorexia, vomiting, or diarrhea; abdominal masses are palpated in approximately 50% of cases. Most tumors involve the small intestine and may be solitary or multiple. Metastatic disease affecting the mesenteric lymph nodes, liver, spleen, and lungs is common on initial presentation. Multiple intestinal masses in cats are most commonly associated with lymphoma or MCT, although both neoplasms can be present simultaneously. GI ulceration has also been documented in cats with MCT.

### Diagnosis

Diagnosis is similar to that for dogs with MCT. Some mast cells in cats are poorly granulated, and the granules may not be easily identified in routine cytologic or histopathologic evaluation.

### Treatment and prognosis

The treatment for cats with MCTs is controversial. As a general rule, surgery is indicated for cats with a solitary cutaneous mass, for cats with two to five skin masses, and for cats with intestinal or splenic involvement.

*Cutaneous MCT.* Cutaneous MCTs in cats are less aggressive than those in dogs. Surgical excision typically is curative in cats with solitary cutaneous MCTs and those with 3 to 5 dermoepidermal masses. Cats with multiple skin MCTs are best treated with prednisone. Although radiotherapy is effective, it is rarely necessary. Removal of a solitary dermoepidermal MCT using a biopsy punch is curative in most cats; the same applies to cats with fewer than five dermoepidermal MCTs.

*Visceral and metastatic MCT.* Splenectomy, prednisone, and chlorambucil (Leukeran) are recommended in cats with SMCD, in which survival times in excess of 1 year are common; splenectomy alone does not prolong survival. Surgical excision and prednisone are also recommended in cats with intestinal MCT. Prednisone alone at doses of 4 to 8 mg/kg orally [PO] q24 to 48h may be beneficial in cats with systemic or metastatic MCTs. Chlorambucil (Leukeran, 20 mg/m$^2$ PO q2wk) is quite effective and well tolerated when an additional chemotherapeutic agent is needed in cats.

## OROPHARYNGEAL NEOPLASMS IN DOGS AND CATS (TEXT PP 1149-1151)

Oropharyngeal neoplasms represent approximately 5% of all malignancies in dogs and cats. Most are malignant, and most patients are presented because of halitosis, dysphagia, drooling, or pain; facial swelling is occasionally seen.

## Oropharyngeal Neoplasms in Dogs

The four tumor types commonly found in dogs are malignant melanoma (MM), fibrosarcoma (FSA), squamous cell carcinoma (SCC), and epulis. MMs, FSAs, SCCs, and acanthomatous epulides (AEs) are malignant; fibromatous and ossifying epulides are benign. MM, FSA, and SCC each represents approximately 30% of all oropharyngeal tumors; male dogs appear to be at high risk. Most oropharyngeal tumors in dogs can be managed surgically, although radiotherapy is beneficial in some cases.

### Malignant melanoma

MM is more prevalent in middle-aged or older male dogs with pigmented oral mucous membranes. MMs typically manifest as pigmented, glistening, solitary masses, although they may be nonpigmented or only partially pigmented. They can be found anywhere in the oropharynx, although the gingiva and buccal or labial mucosae are more commonly affected. Bone invasion and metastatic lesions are common; bone invasion occurs in approximately two thirds of patients, and metastatic lesions to the regional lymph nodes and/or lungs are present in approximately 50% of patients. Most dogs with melanoma die as a result of recurrence or metastases.

### Fibrosarcoma

FSAs predominantly occur in younger male dogs (i.e., 2 to 6 years old); Golden Retrievers and Doberman Pinschers are at high risk. FSAs usually present as pink, sessile, fleshy, firm solitary masses in the gingiva or palate that deeply infiltrate the soft tissues and bone. Most FSAs are only locally invasive and have a low metastatic potential; less than 10% of dogs have metastases on initial presentation. Complete surgical excision is usually curative.

### Squamous cell carcinoma

Most SCCs occur in middle-aged or older dogs. Clinically, they manifest as either a sessile, fleshy, friable mass or, more commonly, as a progressive, ulcerative, and infiltrative lesion (usually invading bone). Regional lymphadenopathy is common, although it is frequently caused by hyperplasia rather than metastatic disease. Most tumors in the rostral oropharynx are locally invasive and have a low metastatic potential, whereas most tumors in the caudal oropharynx (e.g., tonsils, base of the tongue, soft palate, pharynx) are rapidly infiltrative and metastatic.

### Epulides

Epulides (singular, epulis) are fleshy, gingival tumors. Fibromatous and ossifying epulides are benign and can be cured by conservative surgery. AEs are locally invasive tumors that, if left untreated, result in severe facial distortion and mechanical interference with mastication. They are common in the rostral mandibular or premaxillary gingiva of middle-aged or older female dogs. They appear as pink, sessile, fleshy masses that are deeply invasive and often cause bone lysis.

## Oropharyngeal Neoplasms in Cats

Most oropharyngeal tumors in cats are malignant and primarily consist of SCCs (75%) and FSAs (<25%). Most SCCs are ulcerative, whereas most FSAs are proliferative. Bone invasion mimicking a primary bone tumor is common in cats with mandibular SCCs. Most cats with large oral tumors are presented in a state of malnutrition; therefore, in addition to tumor treatment, nutritional support via nasogastric, esophagostomy, or gastrostomy tube is vital.

## Diagnostic approach

Oropharyngeal masses or ulcers should undergo biopsy before treatment is instituted. FNA for cytology is not very reliable with these neoplasms, because they are frequently contaminated and some tumors do not yield cells easily. However, FNA of an enlarged regional lymph node should always be performed to rule out metastatic disease. Thoracic radiographs should also be obtained to check for pulmonary metastases. Radiographs or a CT scan of the affected area should be obtained to determine the extent of bone involvement; this can usually be done when the biopsy is performed.

Halitosis is usually caused by anaerobic bacterial infection of the neoplasm and can be successfully eliminated with clindamycin (5 mg/kg PO q12h) or metronidazole (20 to 25 mg/kg PO q12h) before definitive treatment is instituted.

## Treatment

### Surgery

The treatment of choice for localized tumors without metastases in dogs is aggressive surgical excision. Surgery is also indicated as palliative therapy for metastatic lesions. Given the high prevalence of bone invasion, these tumors can rarely be eliminated with conservative surgery. In general, aggressive surgery (maxillectomy or mandibulectomy) is curative if complete excision is achieved during the first surgery (provided no metastatic lesions are present). One-year survival rates with surgery alone are 25% to 40% in dogs with FSAs and 20% to 25% in dogs with MMs.

### Radiotherapy

Radiotherapy can be successful with some oropharyngeal SCCs (e.g., a small gingival mass). In dogs, survival times postradiotherapy for SCCs of the rostral oral cavity are considerably better than for those involving the tonsils or tongue. More than 50% of dogs in the former group may be cured with radiation therapy. Median survival in dogs with tonsillar or lingual SCCs treated with surgery or radiotherapy is 3 to 4 months. In cats, local control of SCCs is rarely achieved with either surgery or radiotherapy. Most cats die within 4 months of diagnosis; less than 10% are alive at 1 year.

FSAs and MMs are typically considered radioresistant. However, radiotherapy with hyperthermia provides long-term local control in more than 50% of dogs with FSA. Protocols of coarse fractionation result in a greater than 50% response in dogs with MM of the oropharynx. Radiotherapy is usually curative in dogs with AE, although up to 20% of dogs cured with orthovoltage irradiation develop a second tumor (usually SCC) in the irradiated site.

### Chemotherapy

Chemotherapy can be beneficial in some dogs and cats, although it is rarely of value in dogs with SCCs or MMs.

*Fibrosarcomas.* Dogs with incompletely excised, nonresectable, or metastatic FSAs may benefit from a combination of doxorubicin (Adriamycin, 30 mg/m$^2$ or 1 mg/kg for dogs <10 kg intravenously [IV] once every 3 weeks) and dacarbazine (DTIC, 1 g/m$^2$ intravenous drip over 8 hours, immediately after the doxorubicin). In cats a combination of mitoxantrone (Novantrone, 4 to 6 mg/m$^2$ IV every 3 weeks) and cyclophosphamide (Cytoxan, 200 to 300 mg/m$^2$ PO 10 days after the mitoxantrone), or single-agent carboplatin (Paraplatin, 240 to 280 mg/m$^2$ IV every 3 weeks) may be of benefit.

*Malignant melanomas.* Single-agent dacarbazine (DTIC, 1 g/m$^2$ IV drip over 8 hours, repeated every 3 weeks), cisplatin (Platinol, 70 mg/m$^2$ IV drip every 3 weeks), or carboplatin (Paraplatin, 300 mg/m$^2$ IV every 3 weeks) may be beneficial in up to 10% of dogs with nonresectable or metastatic MMs.

*Squamous cell carcinomas.* A combination of radiotherapy, doxorubicin (30 mg/m$^2$ or 1 mg/kg for dogs <10 kg) IV on day 1), and cisplatin (60 mg/m$^2$ on day 8), repeated every 3 weeks is promising in dogs with tonsillar SCCs.

## INJECTION SITE SARCOMAS IN CATS (TEXT PP 1151-1152)

With the syndrome of injection site sarcoma (ISS), cats develop FSA (or occasionally other types of sarcoma) in the subcutis and/or muscle at the injection or vaccination site (interscapular region or thigh). Approximately 1 to 3 in 10,000 cats that receive vaccines develop a sarcoma.

### Clinical features

Cats with ISS develop a rapidly growing soft-tissue mass at the injection site weeks or months after vaccination or injection. An inflammatory reaction usually precedes the development of this neoplasm.

### Diagnosis

Any cat with a superficial or deep mass in the interscapular region or thigh should be suspected of having ISS, and every effort should be made to establish a diagnosis immediately. Although FNA may provide a definitive answer, more often surgical biopsy is necessary. Pulmonary metastases are detected on presentation in many cats with ISS.

### Treatment and prognosis

ISS is quite aggressive and should be treated accordingly. The treatment of choice is aggressive surgical excision. An en block resection (including any biopsy tracts) should be performed immediately, provided that metastatic disease is not present. Cats treated with aggressive surgery have significantly longer disease-free survival than cats treated with conservative surgery (274 versus 66 days); also, cats with tumors in the limbs have significantly longer disease-free survival than cats with tumors in the trunk (325 versus 66 days). Cats with large or incompletely excised tumors may benefit from chemotherapy with either mitoxantrone and cyclophosphamide, doxorubicin and cyclophosphamide, or carboplatin. If metastatic disease is already present, chemotherapy is usually not effective, however, treatment with doxorubicin and cyclophosphamide combinations or with carboplatin alone may result in complete or partial responses in cats with nonresectable or metastatic ISS, with remission times of more than 1 year. Postoperative radiotherapy may also be effective.

# Cancer Chemotherapy Protocols Commonly Used at The Ohio State University Veterinary Teaching Hospital

I. Lymphoma
A. Induction of remission
  1. COAP protocol
    Cyclophosphamide (Cytoxan): 50 mg/m$^2$ PO 4 days/wk or q48h for 8 wk in dogs; 200-300 mg/m$^2$ PO every 3 wk in cats
    Vincristine (Oncovin): 0.5 mg/m$^2$ IV once/wk for 8 wk
    Cytosine arabinoside (Cytosar-U): 100 mg/m$^2$ IV or SC divided q12h for 4 days
    Prednisone: 40-50 mg/m$^2$ PO q24h for 1 wk; then 20-25 mg/m$^2$ PO q48h for 7 wk
    **In cats, cytosine arabinoside is administered for only 2 days and the remaining three drugs (cyclophosphamide, vincristine, prednisone) are administered for 6 wk rather than 8 wk.**
  2. COP protocol
    Cyclophosphamide (Cytoxan): 50 mg/m$^2$ PO 4 days/wk or q48h; or 300 mg/m$^2$ PO every 3 wk*
    Vincristine (Oncovin): 0.5 mg/m$^2$ IV once/wk
    Prednisone: 40-50 mg/m$^2$ PO q24h for 1 wk; then 20-25 mg/m$^2$ PO q48h
  3. CLOP protocol
    As in COP protocol, but with the addition of L-asparaginase (Elspar) at a dose of 10,000-20,000 IU/m$^2$ IM once every 4 to 6 wk
  4. CHOP protocol (21-day cycle)
    Cyclophosphamide (Cytoxan): 200-300 mg/m$^2$ PO on day 10
    Doxorubicin (Adriamycin): 30 mg/m$^2$ or 1 mg/kg IV if <10 kg IV on day 1
    Vincristine (Oncovin): 0.75 mg/m$^2$ IV on days 8, 15
    Prednisone: 40-50 mg/m$^2$ PO q24h on days 1-7; then 20-25 mg/m$^2$ PO q48h on days 8-21
    Sulfa-trimethoprim: 15 mg/kg PO q12h
B. Maintenance
  1. Chlorambucil (Leukeran): 20 mg/m$^2$ PO every other wk
    Prednisone: 20-25 mg/m$^2$ PO q48h
  2. LMP protocol: Chlorambucil (Leukeran) and prednisone, as above, plus methotrexate, 2.5-5 mg/m$^2$ PO two or three times per week
  3. Chlorambucil (Leukeran): 20 mg/m$^2$ PO every other wk
    Prednisone: 20-25 mg/m$^2$ PO q48h
    Cytosine arabinoside (Cytosar): 200-400 mg/m$^2$ SC every 2 wk, alternating with Leukeran
  4. COP protocol used every other week for six cycles; then every third week for six cycles; then once a month thereafter

C. "Rescue"

DOGS

1. D-MAC protocol (repeat continuously for 10-16 wk):

Dexamethasone: 0.5 mg/lb (1.1 mg/kg) PO or SC on days 1 and 8

Actinomycin D (Cosmegen): 0.75 mg/m$^2$ intravenous push on day 1

Cytosine arabinoside (Cytosar): 200-300 mg/m$^2$ intravenous drip over 4 hr on day 1

Melphalan (Alkeran): 20 mg/m$^2$ PO on day 8 (after four doses of melphalan, substitute Leukeran at the same dose)

2. ADIC protocol

Doxorubicin (Adriamycin): 30 mg/m$^2$ (or 1 mg/kg if <10 kg) IV q3wk

3. L-Asparaginase (Elspar): 10,000-30,000 IU/m$^2$ SC q2-3wk

4. CHOP protocol if second relapse in response to COAP protocol or if good response to Adriamycin was previously observed

CATS

1. Cytosine arabinoside (Cytosar-U): 100-200 mg/m$^2$/day intravenous drip for 1-2 days

Mitoxantrone (Novantrone): 4 mg/m$^2$ in intravenous drip, mixed in the bag with the Cytosar

Dexamethasone 0.5-1 mg/lb (1.1-2.2 mg/kg) PO once/wk; Repeat q3wk

II. Acute lymphoid leukemia (ALL)

COAP, CLOP, or COP protocol

III. Chronic lymphocytic leukemia (CLL)

1. Chlorambucil (Leukeran): 20 mg/m$^2$ PO every other wk (with or without prednisone, 20 mg/m$^2$ PO q48h)

2. Cyclophosphamide (Cytoxan): 50 mg/m$^2$ PO 4 days/wk

Prednisone: 20 mg/m$^2$ PO q48h

IV. Acute myelogenous leukemia

1. Cytosine arabinoside (Cytosar-U): 100 mg/m$^2$/day intravenous drip or SC (divided bid) for 4 days 6-thioguanine (6-TG): 40-50 mg/m$^2$ PO q24h or every other day

2. Cytosar and 6-TG plus Adriamycin (10 mg/m$^2$ IV on days 2 and 4 of the cycle)

3. Cytosine arabinoside (Cytosar-U): 100-200 mg/m$^2$/day intravenous drip for 1-2 days

Mitoxantrone (Novantrone): 4 mg/m$^2$ intravenous drip, mixed in the bag with the Cytosar; repeat q3wk

V. Chronic myelogenous leukemia

1. Hydroxyurea (Hydrea): 50 mg/kg PO divided q12h, q24h, or q48h until white blood count is normal

VI. Multiple myeloma

1. Melphalan (Alkeran): 2-4 mg/m$^2$ PO q24h for 1 wk; then q48h; can also be given at 6-8 mg/m$^2$ PO for 5 days, repeating every 21 days

Prednisone: 40-50 mg/m$^2$ PO q24h for 1 wk; then 20 mg/m$^2$ PO q48h

2. As in III.2

*Continued.*

## Cancer Chemotherapy Protocols Commonly Used at The Ohio State University Veterinary Teaching Hospital—cont'd

VII. Mast cell tumors (systemic)
  1. Prednisone: 40-50 mg/m$^2$ PO q24h for 1 wk; then 20-25 mg/m$^2$ PO q48h
  2. Lomustine (CCNU): 60-90 mg/m$^2$ PO q3wk (with or without prednisone as in 1)
  3. CVP protocol
      Vinblastine (Velban): 2 mg/m$^2$ IV once/wk
      Cyclophosphamide (Cytoxan): 50 mg/m$^2$ PO q48h or 4 days/wk
      Prednisone: 20-25 mg/m$^2$ PO q48h

VIII. Soft-tissue sarcomas—dogs
  1. ADIC protocol
      Doxorubicin (Adriamycin): 30 mg/m$^2$ (or 1 mg/kg if <10 kg) IV q3wk
      DTIC (Dacarbazine): 700-1000 mg/m$^2$ intravenous drip for 6-8 hr; repeat q21 days
      Sulfa-trimethoprim: 15 mg/kg PO q12h q3wk
  2. VAC protocol (21-day cycle)
      Vincristine (Oncovin): 0.75 mg/m$^2$ IV on days 8 and 15
      Doxorubicin (Adriamycin): 30 mg/m$^2$ (or 1 mg/kg if <10 kg) IV on day 1
      Cyclophosphamide (Cytoxan): 200-300 mg/m$^2$ PO on day 10
      Sulfa-trimethoprim: 15 mg/kg PO q12h

IX. Soft-tissue sarcomas—cats
  1. AC protocol (21-day cycle)
      Doxorubicin (Adriamycin): 1 mg/kg IV on day 1
      Cyclophosphamide (Cytoxan): 200-300 mg/m$^2$ on day 10
  2. VAC protocol (21-day cycle)
      Vincristine (Oncovin): 0.5 mg/m$^2$ IV on days 8 and 15
      Doxorubicin (Adriamycin): 1 mg/kg IV on day 1
      Cyclophosphamide (Cytoxan): 200-300 mg/m$^2$ on day 10

3. MiC protocol (21-day cycle)
   Mitoxantrone (Novantrone): 4-6 mg/m$^2$ in intravenous drip over 4 hr on day 1
   Cyclophosphamide (Cytoxan): 200-300 mg/m$^2$ PO on day 10
4. MiCO protocol (21-day cycle)
   Mitoxantrone (Novantrone): 4-6 mg/m$^2$ in intravenous drip over 4 hr on day 1
   Cyclophosphamide (Cytoxan): 200-300 mg/m$^2$ PO on day 10
   Vincristine (Oncovin): 0.5-0.6 mg/m$^2$ IV on days 8 and 15
5. Carboplatin (Paraplatin): 200-280 mg/m$^2$ IV q3wk

X. Osteosarcoma—dogs
1. Cisplatin (Platinol): 50-70 mg/m$^2$ in intravenous drip q3wk; prior intensive diuresis is required (see Box 84-2)
2. Carboplatin (Paraplatin): 300 mg/m$^2$ IV q3wk
3. Doxorubicin (Adriamycin): 30 mg/m$^2$ IV q2wk, for five doses
4. Doxorubicin and carboplatin as above, alternating drugs q3wk for two to three doses each

XI. Carcinomas—dogs
1. CMF protocol
   5-Fluorouracil (5-FU): 150 mg/m$^2$ IV once/wk
   Cyclophosphamide (Cytoxan): 50 mg/m$^2$ PO 4 days/wk or q48h
   Methotrexate: 2.5 mg/m$^2$ PO two or three times per week
2. FAC protocol (21-day cycle)
   5-FU: 150 mg/m$^2$ IV on days 8 and 15
   Doxorubicin (Adriamycin): 30 mg/m$^2$ (or 1 mg/kg if <10 kg) IV on day 1
   Cyclophosphamide (Cytoxan): 200-300 mg/m$^2$ PO on day 10
   Sulfa-trimethoprim: 15 mg/kg PO q12h
3. VAF protocol
   Vincristine (Oncovin): 0.75 mg/m$^2$ IV on days 8 and 15
   Doxorubicin (Adriamycin): 30 mg/m$^2$ (or 1 mg/kg if <10 kg) IV on day 1
   5-FU: 150 mg/m$^2$ IV on days 1, 8, and 15
4. VAC protocol
5. Cisplatin (Platinol): 70 mg/m$^2$ in intravenous drip q3wk; prior intensive diuresis is required (see Box 84-2)

Continued.

## Cancer Chemotherapy Protocols Commonly Used at The Ohio State University Veterinary Teaching Hospital—cont'd

XII. Carcinomas—cats

**5-Fluorouracil is toxic in cats, producing severe, and often fatal, CNS signs. Cisplatin is also extremely toxic, causing acute pulmonary toxicity in this species.**

1. Carboplatin (Paraplatin): 200-280 mg/m$^2$ IV q3wk
2. AC protocol (21-day cycle)
   Doxorubicin (Adriamycin): 1 mg/kg IV on day 1
   Cyclophosphamide (Cytoxan): 200-300 mg/m$^2$ PO on day 10
3. VAC protocol (21-day cycle)
   Vincristine (Oncovin): 0.5 mg/m$^2$ IV on days 8, 15, and 22
   Doxorubicin (Adriamycin): 1 mg/kg mg/m$^2$ IV on day 1
   Cyclophosphamide (Cytoxan): 200-300 mg/m$^2$ on day 10
4. MiC protocol (21-day cycle)
   Mitoxantrone (Novantrone): 4-6 mg/m$^2$ intravenous drip over 4 hr on day 1
   Cyclophosphamide (Cytoxan): 200-300 mg/m$^2$ PO on day 10
5. MiCO protocol (21-day cycle)
   Mitoxantrone (Novantrone): 4-6 mg/m$^2$ intravenous drip over 4 hr on day 1
   Cyclophosphamide (Cytoxan): 200-300 mg/m$^2$ PO on day 10
   Vincristine (Oncovin): 0.5-0.6 mg/m$^2$ IV on days 8 and 15

*The duration of chemotherapy using this protocol varies.

*CNS,* Central nervous system; *IV,* intravenously; *PO,* orally; *SC,* subcutaneously.

# PART XII

# Hematology and Immunology

C. GUILLERMO COUTO

# 85

# Anemia

*(Text pp 1156-1169)*

## CLINICAL AND CLINICOPATHOLOGIC EVALUATION (TEXT PP 1156-1160)

### Clinical Evaluation

The main presenting complaints for anemic animals include pale or icteric mucous membranes, lethargy, exercise intolerance, pica (mainly in cats), and decreased overall activity. These signs can be acute or chronic and of variable severity. Adaptive changes such as tachycardia or increased precordial beat may also be noticed by the owner.

#### History

It is important that the following questions be asked when the animal's history is taken:

- Is the pet currently taking any medication that could cause hemolysis, blood loss, or bone marrow hypoplasia? (Box 85-1)
- Have the owners detected any blood loss, dark stool, or discolored urine?
- Have the owners noticed any fleas? Severe flea infestation can cause iron-deficiency anemia (IDA).
- Has the cat recently been tested for feline leukemia virus (FeLV) or feline immunodeficiency virus (FIV) infection?
- Has the owner noticed any ticks on the dog? Ehrlichiosis and babesiosis can cause anemia.
- Has the pet been vaccinated recently? Modified-live vaccines can cause thrombocytopenia (bleeding) and hemolysis.
- Has the bitch recently received any estrogen derivatives because of mismating?

---

**Box 85-1**

### Drugs and Toxins That Can Cause Anemia in Cats and Dogs

| | |
|---|---|
| Acetaminophen | Methimazole |
| Antiarrhythmics | Methionine |
| Anticonvulsants | Methylene blue |
| Antiinflammatories (nonsteroidal) | Metronidazole |
| Benzocaine | Penicillins and cephalosporins |
| Chemotherapeutic agents | Phenothiazines |
| Chloramphenicol | Propylthiouracil |
| Cimetidine | Propylene glycol |
| Erythropoietin | Sulfa derivatives |
| Gold salts | Vitamin K |
| Griseofulvin | Zinc |
| Levamisole | |

---

## Physical examination

When a patient with pale mucous membranes is evaluated, it should be established whether the pallor is the result of hypoperfusion or anemia. Patients with anemia have low packed cell volume (PCV), whereas patients with hypoperfusion caused by cardiovascular disease usually have normal PCV and additional clinical signs; occasionally patients with congestive heart failure may have mild dilutional anemia caused by intravascular fluid retention. Patients with pallor should also be evaluated for petechiae, ecchymoses, and evidence of deep bleeding, which may suggest a platelet or clotting factor deficiency (e.g., Evan's syndrome, disseminated intravascular coagulation [DIC], acute leukemias).

*Lymph nodes and spleen.* Particular attention should be paid to the lymph nodes and spleen; several anemic disorders are associated with lymphadenopathy and/or hepatosplenomegaly. Common disorders include lymphoma, hemobartonellosis (in cats more often than dogs), acute leukemias, immune hemolytic anemia (IHA; in dogs more often than cats), and canine ehrlichiosis. Less common or rare disorders include systemic mast cell disease, bone marrow hypoplasia with extramedullary hematopoiesis, and hypersplenism.

## Hematology

### Grading anemias

Anemias are graded as follows:

| | | |
|---|---|---|
| *mild* | *PCV 30% to 36% (dogs)* | *20% to 24% (cats)* |
| *moderate* | *PCV 18% to 29% (dogs)* | *15% to 19% (cats)* |
| *severe* | *PCV <18% (dogs)* | *<14% (cats)* |

The severity of the anemia usually correlates with its pathogenesis. Severe anemia in association with mild to moderate clinical signs is likely a result of a chronic cause (bone marrow disease), whereas acute causes of severe anemia (e.g., hemolysis) result in clinical signs of marked severity. A PCV and total plasma protein should be performed, and the plasma examined for icterus or hemolysis. The microhematocrit tube should be carefully inspected for evidence of autoagglutination, and a slide agglutination test performed. It is also helpful to evaluate a blood smear to detect morphologic changes that may point the clinician toward the cause of the anemia.

### Regenerative versus nonregenerative anemias

Regenerative anemias are usually acute, whereas nonregenerative anemias are either peracute (e.g., blood loss or hemolysis of <48 hours' duration) or chronic. Determining whether the anemia is regenerative or nonregenerative involves obtaining a reticulocyte count during routine complete blood count (CBC) and calculating the reticulocyte index (RI) (Box 85-2). Examination of a blood smear for polychromasia can also be used

---

**Box 85-2**

## Calculation of the Reticulocyte Index in Dogs

1. $\dfrac{\text{Patient's PCV}}{45} \times \text{reticulocyte percentage} = A$

   where 45 is the average PCV in the dog; this corrects for the artifact caused by the anemia (i.e., with a low PCV, the percentage of reticulocytes exaggerates the absolute number of cells).

2. If polychromasia is found in the blood smear, divide A by 2 to correct for the maturation time in circulation.

3. If the results are >2.5, the anemia is regenerative.

From Couto CG, Hammer AS: Hematologic and oncologic emergencies. In Murtaugh R, Kaplan P, eds: *Veterinary emergency and critical care medicine*, St Louis, 1992, Mosby.

*PCV,* Packed cell volume.

Table 85-1

## Interpretation of Morphologic Red Blood Cell Abnormalities in Cats and Dogs

| Morphologic abnormality | Commonly associated disorders |
|---|---|
| Macrocytosis | Breed-related characteristic (Poodles); feline leukemia virus or immunodeficiency virus infection; regeneration; folate deficiency; dyserythropoiesis (bone marrow disease) |
| Microcytosis | Breed-related characteristic (Akitas, Shar Peis, Shiba Inu); iron deficiency; portosystemic shunt; polycythemia (erythrocytosis) |
| Hypochromia | Iron deficiency |
| Polychromasia | Regeneration |
| Poikilocytosis | Regeneration; iron deficiency, hyposplenism |
| Schistocytosis (fragments) | Microangiopathy; hemangiosarcoma; disseminated intravascular coagulation; hyposplenism |
| Spherocytosis | Immune hemolytic anemia; mononuclear phagocytic neoplasm |
| Acanthocytosis (spur cells) | Hemangiosarcoma; liver disease; hyposplenism |
| Ecchinocytosis (burr cells) | Artifact; renal disease; pyruvate kinase deficiency anemia |
| Elliptocytosis | Congenital elliptocytosis (dogs) |
| Heinz bodies | Oxidative insult to red blood cells |
| Howell-Jolly bodies | Hyposplenism; regeneration |
| Autoagglutination | Immune hemolytic anemia |
| Metarubricytosis | Breed-related characteristic (Schnauzers, Dachshunds); extramedullary hematopoiesis; regeneration; lead toxicity; hemangiosarcoma |
| Leukopenia | See text |
| Thrombocytopenia | See text |
| Pancytopenia | Bone marrow disorder; hypersplenism |

Modified from Couto CG, Hammer AS: Hematologic and oncologic emergencies. In Murtaugh R, Kaplan P, eds: *Veterinary emergency and critical care medicine*, St Louis, 1992, Mosby.

to determine whether the anemia is regenerative. Table 85-1 summarizes some of the abnormalities detectable on a blood smear.

*Regenerative anemias.* When the RI is at least 2.5, the anemia is a result of either hemolysis or blood loss (after 48 to 96 hours). When a patient with regenerative anemia is evaluated, it is useful to measure serum and plasma protein; blood loss usually results in hypoproteinemia, whereas hemolysis does not. Table 85-2 lists other physical examination and clinicopathologic findings that allow differentiation between blood loss and hemolytic anemias.

*Nonregenerative anemias.* Anemias in which the RI is less than 2.5 can be caused by bone marrow or extramarrow disorders, including erythroid hypoproliferation, chronic inflammatory disease, chronic renal disease, and acute hemorrhage or hemolysis (first 48 to 96 hours). IDAs are often classified as nonregenerative, even though most dogs with chronic blood loss leading to iron deficiency display mild (to moderate) regeneration and the red blood cell (RBC) indexes are different than in other nonregenerative anemias; therefore IDA is more appropriately classified as semiregenerative.

## REGENERATIVE ANEMIAS (TEXT PP 1160-1164)

### Blood Loss Anemia

Acute blood loss results in reticulocytosis (i.e., regeneration) within 48 to 96 hours in normal dogs and cats. The source of bleeding should be identified, and the bleeding

**Table 85-2**

## Criteria for Differentiating Blood Loss from Hemolytic Anemias

| Variable | Blood loss | Hemolysis |
|---|---|---|
| Serum (plasma) protein concentration | Normal-low | Normal-high |
| Evidence of bleeding | Common | Rare |
| Icterus | No | Common |
| Hemoglobinemia | No | Common |
| Spherocytosis | No | Common |
| Red blood cell inclusions | No | Occasional |
| Hemosiderinuria | No | Yes |
| Autoagglutination | No | Occasional |
| Direct Coombs' test | Negative | Usually positive (in IHA) |
| Splenomegaly | No | Common |

From Couto CG, Hammer AS: Hematologic and oncologic emergencies. In Murtaugh R, Kaplan P, eds: *Veterinary emergency and critical care medicine*, 1982, St Louis Mosby.

*IHA*, immune-mediated hemolytic anemia.

arrested. If the patient is bleeding because of a systemic hemostatic defect, specific treatment should be initiated (see Chapter 89). Aggressive intravenous fluid therapy with crystalloids or colloids or transfusion of blood or blood components may be required in cases of acute blood loss.

## Hemolytic Anemia

Hemolytic anemias can be classified as extravascular or intravascular and congenital or acquired (Table 85-3). Most dogs with hemolytic anemia have acquired extravascular hemolysis, whereas acquired extravascular and intravascular hemolysis are equally common in cats.

### Etiology

In extravascular hemolysis, RBCs are phagocytosed in the spleen, liver, and bone marrow. Stimuli include intracellular inclusions, such as RBC parasites or Heinz bodies (common in cats), and membrane coating with immunoglobulin (Ig) G or IgM (common in dogs). IHA (see text p 1162, text) is one of the most common causes of extravascular hemolytic anemia in dogs; in cats, drug-associated hemolysis (e.g., β-lactam antibiotics) and hemobartonellosis *(Mycoplasma hemofelis)* are the two most common causes.

Intravascular hemolysis can be caused by antibodies or complement (immune mediated), infectious agents (e.g., babesiosis), drugs or toxins (e.g., zinc), metabolic imbalances (e.g., hypophosphatemia in diabetes mellitus treated with insulin), or increased RBC shearing (microangiopathy, DIC). Intravascular hemolysis is considerably less common than extravascular hemolysis, with the exception of DIC in dogs with hemangiosarcoma, zinc toxicity, or hypophosphatemia.

### Clinical evaluation

Patients with congenital (frequently familial) hemolytic anemias may be presented with relatively prolonged clinical courses, with the exception of English Springer Spaniels with phosphofructokinase deficiency–induced hemolysis (acute hemolytic episodes after hyperventilation during exercise or excitement).

Patients with acquired hemolytic anemias usually are presented with acute signs of pallor, possibly icterus (approximately 50% of cases), and sometimes, prominent splenomegaly. If thrombocytopenia is also present (e.g., Evans' syndrome, DIC), petechiae and ecchymoses may be seen. Signs and physical examination findings associated with the primary disease can often be found in cases of secondary hemolytic anemias. Abdominal radiographs may show metallic foreign bodies in the stomach (zinc toxicosis).

Table 85-3

## Causes of Hemolytic Anemia in Dogs and Cats

| Disorder | Species | Breed |
|---|---|---|
| **CONGENITAL (INHERITED?)** | | |
| Pyruvate kinase deficiency | D | Basenji, Beagle, West Highland White Terrier, Abyssinian, Somali |
| Phosphofructokinase deficiency | D | English Springer Spaniel, Cocker Spaniel |
| Anemia and chondrodysplasia | D | Alaskan Malamute |
| Nonspherocytic hemolytic anemia | D | Poodle, Beagle |
| **ACQUIRED** | | |
| Immune hemolytic anemia | D > C | All |
| Neonatal isoerythrolysis | C | British breeds, Abyssinian, Somali (other type B cats) |
| Microangiopathic hemolytic anemia | D > C | All |
| Infectious | | |
|   Hemobartonellosis | C > D | All |
|   Babesiosis | D > C | All |
|   Cytauxoonosis | C | All |
|   Ehrlichiosis | D | All |
| Hypophosphatemia | D, C | All |
| Oxidants | | |
|   Acetaminophen | C | All |
|   Phenothiazines | D, C | All |
|   Benzocaine | C | All |
|   Vitamin K | D, C | All |
|   Methylene blue | C > D | All |
|   Methionine | C | All |
|   Propylene glycol | C | All |
| Drugs | | |
|   Sulfas | D > C | Doberman, Labrador Retriever |
|   Anticonvulsants | D | All |
|   Penicillins and cephalosporins | D > C | All |
|   Propylthiouracil | C | All |
|   Methimazole | C | All |
|   Antiarrhythmics? | D | All |
|   Zinc | D | All |

Modified from Couto CG, Hammer AS: Hematologic and oncologic emergencies. In Murtaugh R, Kaplan P, eds: *Veterinary emergency and critical care medicine*, St Louis, 1992, Mosby.
*C,* Cats; *D,* dogs.

***Autoagglutination.*** The blood sample should be evaluated for autoagglutination by placing a large drop of anticoagulated blood on a glass slide at both room temperature and 4° C. Agglutination can be distinguished from rouleaux formation by diluting the blood 5:1 with saline solution (i.e., autoagglutination persists after dilution with saline). Rouleaux formation is common in cats and extremely rare in dogs. Cryoagglutination (RBC agglutination when the blood sample is refrigerated for 6 to 8 hours) occurs in a large proportion of cats with hemobartonellosis.

***Direct Coombs' test.*** A direct Coombs' test to detect RBC-bound immunoglobulins should be submitted in dogs and cats with suspected hemolysis. A positive result should be interpreted with caution, however, as certain drugs and hemoparasites (e.g., *M. hemofelis* in cats) can cause secondary immune hemolysis and a positive result on Coombs' test. This test is not necessary in patients with autoagglutination.

## Approach to treatment

Hemolytic anemias not associated with immune destruction of RBCs are treated by removal of the cause (e.g., drug, infectious agent, zinc-containing gastric foreign body) and supportive therapy. Corticosteroids (see later) can be administered, although this is not always beneficial. In dogs and cats with hemobartonellosis, and in dogs with ehrlichiosis, doxycycline (5 to 10 mg/kg PO q12-24h for 2 to 3 weeks) usually resolves the signs. If the cause cannot be identified, the patient should be treated for primary or idiopathic IHA while further results (serology or polymerase chain reaction [PCR] assay for hemoparasites) are pending.

## Immune hemolytic anemia

IHA is the most common form of hemolysis in dogs. Most cases are primary or idiopathic. With the exception of immune hemolysis secondary to hemoparasites, IHA is rare in cats (although its prevalence appears to be increasing). Secondary causes of IHA include drug administration (e.g., β-lactam antibiotics) and vaccinations.

*Clinical signs.* Signs include acute or peracute onset of depression, exercise intolerance, and pallor or jaundice, occasionally accompanied by vomiting or abdominal pain. Additional physical examination findings usually consist of petechiae and ecchymoses (if immune thrombocytopenia is also present), splenomegaly, and a heart murmur.

In a subset of dogs with acute or peracute IHA (with icterus and autoagglutination), clinical deterioration caused by multifocal (liver, lungs, kidneys) thromboembolism or lack of response to conventional therapy occurs within hours or days. These dogs must be treated aggressively (see later).

*Hematology.* Findings typically include a strongly regenerative anemia, leukocytosis caused by neutrophilia with left shift and monocytosis, increased numbers of nucleated RBCs, polychromasia, and spherocytosis. Spherocytes are characteristic of IHA, although they can occasionally be seen in other disorders. Serum or plasma protein concentration is usually normal or increased, and hemoglobinemia or hyperbilirubinemia may be present. Autoagglutination is prominent in some dogs. Thrombocytopenia is also present in dogs with Evans' syndrome or secondary DIC.

*Direct Coombs' test.* Polychromasia with autoagglutination and spherocytosis in a dog with acute illness and anemia is virtually pathognomonic for IHA. In these cases a direct Coombs' test is usually not necessary to confirm the diagnosis; however, in patients in which some of these findings are absent, a direct Coombs' test should be performed. Approximately 10% to 20% of dogs with IHA have a negative direct Coombs' test, yet they respond to immunosuppressive therapy.

*Initial treatment.* Immunosuppressive doses of corticosteroids (equivalent to 2 to 4 mg/kg of prednisone q12-24h in dogs and up to 8 mg/kg q12-24h in cats) are the treatment of choice for primary IHA. A high percentage of dogs treated with corticosteroids markedly improve within 24 to 96 hours. Dexamethasone can be used initially, but it should not be used as maintenance therapy.

*Treatment for unresponsive cases.* Cyclophosphamide (Cytoxan) is recommended in dogs with acute or peracute IHA that have icterus, autoagglutination, and rapid clinical deterioration. The recommended dose is 200 to 300 mg/m$^2$ intravenously (IV) or PO as a single dose, administered over 5 to 10 minutes, in conjunction with a single intravenous dose of dexamethasone sodium phosphate (1 to 2 mg/kg). Chlorambucil (Leukeran, 20 mg/m$^2$ PO q2wk) is the best induction and maintenance agent in cats with IHA that is refractory to corticosteroids or in those in which corticosteroid-induced diabetes mellitus occurs.

Prophylactic heparin (50 to 75 IU/kg subcutaneously [SC] q8h) is also advisable in dogs. If clinical evidence of thromboembolism is present, high-dose heparin (700 to 1000 IU/kg SC q8h) or a dose that will prolong the activated clotting time up to 2.5 times normal is recommended. If excessive bleeding occurs, protamine sulfate can be administered by slow intravenous infusion (1 mg for each 100 IU of the last dose of heparin); 50% of the calculated dose is given 1 hour after the heparin, 25% 2 hours after the heparin, and the remainder as necessary. Frozen or fresh frozen plasma can also be used.

Aggressive fluid therapy should also be used, although hemodilution may be detrimental in anemic patients. Oxygen therapy should be used as necessary. Human IgG (Gammamune, 0.5 to 1.5 g/kg IV) has been used with success in dogs with refractory IHA; this product is extremely expensive. Other options include therapeutic plasmapheresis, danazol (Danocrine, 5 to 10 mg/kg PO q12h), cyclosporine (Neoral, 10 mg/kg PO q12 to 24h), and possibly splenectomy (may not be of much benefit).

*Blood transfusion.* Transfusion should not be withheld if it is a life-saving procedure (e.g., in the presence of tachypnea, dyspnea, orthopnea). However, patients with IHA may be more prone to destruction of transfused RBCs. Pretreatment with dexamethasone sodium phosphate (0.5 to 1 mg/kg IV), fluids administered through a separate intravenous catheter, and heparin therapy are recommended. If available, packed RBCs should be used instead of whole blood. Cross-matching is indicated, but because time is usually of the essence, non–cross-matched blood is frequently administered. Cross-matching results are difficult to interpret if the patient is autoagglutinating. If blood typing cards are used in dogs with autoagglutinating IHA, the results will be false positive for dog erythrocyte antigen (DEA) 1.1.

*Oxyglobin.* Administering Oxyglobin typically improves the clinical signs associated with anemia, but only for 2 or 3 days. Oxyglobin infusion may make it difficult to obtain some laboratory test results.

*Maintenance therapy.* Drugs used for maintenance therapy include prednisone (1 mg/kg PO q48h) and azathioprine (Imuran, 50 mg/m$^2$ PO q24-48h), used either singly or in combination. If myelosuppression or hepatotoxicity occurs, dose reduction is necessary; it may be necessary to discontinue azathioprine in dogs with hepatotoxicity (see Chapter 80). In general, dogs (and possibly cats) with IHA require prolonged, often lifelong immunosuppressive treatment. Decremental doses are used for 2 to 3 weeks, after which the patient is reevaluated. If the PCV has not decreased (or if it has increased) and the patient is clinically stable or has improved, the dose is further reduced. This procedure is repeated until the drug therapy is discontinued. More than two-thirds of dogs with IHA require lifelong treatment.

## NONREGENERATIVE ANEMIAS (TEXT PP 1164-1167)

### Etiology
Causes of nonregenerative anemia in cats and dogs include the following:
- anemia of chronic disease (ACD)
- hypoproliferative anemias—bone marrow (or erythroid) aplasia or hypoplasia; myelophthisis; myelodysplastic syndromes; myelofibrosis; osteosclerosis or osteopetrosis
- anemia of renal disease (ARD)
- acute blood loss or hemolysis (first 48 to 96 hours)
- anemia of endocrine disorders—hypoadrenocorticism; hypothyroidism (typically mild)

### Clinical evaluation
With the exception of ACD, clinically evident nonregenerative anemias are not as common as regenerative forms in dogs; the opposite is true in cats. Most nonregenerative anemias (and IDA) in cats and dogs are chronic, therefore allowing for physiologic adaptation. In many cases the anemia is mild and asymptomatic.

*Hematology.* In general, nonregenerative anemias are normocytic and normochromic, although in cats with FeLV- or FIV-related hypoproliferative anemias the RBCs are usually macrocytic and normochromic. Also, in cats and dogs with IDA, the indexes are typically microcytic and hypochromic.

*Bone marrow sampling.* Lack of regeneration usually reflects primary or secondary bone marrow abnormalities; therefore, after extramarrow causes have been ruled out, a bone marrow aspiration or biopsy is usually indicated.

*Acute onset anemias.* When dogs and cats with nonregenerative anemias of acute onset are evaluated, the following conditions should be considered: acute (<96 hours) blood loss or hemolysis; and acute leukemia, pure RBC aplasia, or chronic anemia that is now symptomatic because of intercurrent disease (e.g., heart failure, sepsis). In the absence of these conditions the patient may be treated symptomatically with a packed RBC transfusion. If possible, the precipitating factor should be eliminated (e.g., leukemia treated with chemotherapy).

## Anemia of Chronic Disease

ACD is the most common form of nonregenerative anemia in cats and dogs and is secondary to a variety of chronic inflammatory, degenerative, and neoplastic conditions. Given its mild degree, ACD usually does not cause signs of anemia. PCV values in most cats with ACD range from the high teens to the mid twenties, whereas in dogs they range from the mid twenties to the low thirties; therefore ACD can usually be excluded in dogs with PCVs of less than 20% and in cats with PCVs of less than 17% to 18%. The RBC indexes are normocytic and normochromic, and the CBC may reflect the nature of the primary problem. Some cats with ACD have microcytic hypochromic RBC indexes, which mimics IDA. Clinicopathologic features of ACD are listed in Table 85-4. It is frequently necessary to evaluate bone marrow iron stores by Prussian blue staining to conclusively differentiate ACD from IDA.

### Treatment

Patients with ACD usually do not require specific or supportive therapy; treatment of the primary disorder resolves the anemia. Anabolic steroids are sometimes advocated, although they are of little benefit. If used, dosages are as for dogs and cats with hypoproliferative anemias.

## Bone Marrow Disorders

Neoplastic, hypoplastic, or dysplastic bone marrow disorders can result in anemia and other cytopenias. Possible causes are listed in Box 85-3. With the exception of pure red cell aplasia (PRCA), these disorders typically affect more than one cell line, and the patients are bicytopenic or pancytopenic (see Chapter 88). In general, these disorders are chronic, and the clinical signs are those of anemia, with or without signs of the underlying disorder. Definitive diagnosis of anemia resulting from bone marrow disorders is usually obtained by the cytologic or histopathologic appearance of a bone marrow specimen and possibly results of serology or PCR assay for infectious agents (e.g., FeLV, FIV, canine ehrlichiosis).

### Bone marrow (or erythroid) aplasia-hypoplasia

Bone marrow aplasia-hypoplasia is characterized by aplasia or hypoplasia of all the bone marrow cell lines (bone marrow aplasia-hypoplasia or aplastic pancytopenia) or of only the erythroid precursor (RBC aplasia-hypoplasia or PRCA). This form of anemia (or combined cytopenias) can be caused by a variety of agents or disorders (see Box 85-3).

**Table 85-4**

### Distinguishing Features of Anemia of Chronic Disease versus Iron-Deficiency Anemia in Dogs

| Parameter | Anemia of chronic disease | Iron-deficiency anemia |
|---|---|---|
| Serum iron concentration | ↓ | ↓↓ |
| Total iron-binding capacity | N | N |
| Percentage saturation | ↓ | ↓↓ |
| Bone marrow iron stores | ↑ | ↓ |
| Platelet count | N, ↓, ↑ | ↑, ↑↑ |
| Fecal occult blood | — | ± |
| Ferritin | N | ↓ |

*N*, Normal; ↓, low; ↓↓, markedly low; ↑, high; ↑↑, markedly high; ±, positive or negative.

---

**Box 85-3**

## Disorders Associated with Hypoproliferative Anemias in Cats and Dogs

---

Marrow (or erythroid) aplasia-hypoplasia
    FeLV (C)
    Ehrlichiosis (D)
    Immune-mediated (D > C)
    Estrogen (D)
    Phenylbutazone (D)
    Other drugs (D, C)
    Idiopathic (D, C)
Myelophthisis
    Acute leukemias (D, C)
    Chronic leukemias (D > C)
    Multiple myeloma (D > C)
    Lymphoma (D, C)
    Systemic mast cell disease (C > D)
    Metastatic carcinoma (rare D, C)
    Histoplasmosis (rare D, C)
Myelodysplastic syndromes
    FeLV (C)
    FIV (C)
    Preleukemic syndrome (D, C)
    Idiopathic (D, C)
Myelofibrosis
    FeLV (C)
    Pyruvate kinase–deficiency anemia (D)
    Idiopathic (C, C)
Osteosclerosis or osteopetrosis
    FeLV (C)

---

*C*, Cats; *D*, dogs; *FeLV*, feline leukemia virus; *FIV*, feline immunodeficiency virus.

*Pure red cell aplasia.* Cats and dogs with PRCA usually have PCVs less than 15% and obvious clinical signs. Hematologically, severe (normocytic normochromic) non-regenerative anemia is usually the only abnormality; macrocytosis without reticulocytes is a consistent finding in cats with FeLV- or FIV-related PRCA, and mild microcytosis can occasionally be present in dogs with PRCA. PRCA of presumptive immune origin is relatively common in dogs and cats. Occasionally, dogs with PRCA have circulating spherocytes, suggesting an immune basis for the anemia; approximately 60% of these dogs also have a positive result on direct Coombs' test, and their anemia responds to immunosuppressive therapy. FeLV-negative cats with PRCA often have a positive result on direct Coombs' test and frequently benefit from immunosuppressive doses of corticosteroids (4 to 8 mg/kg of prednisone PO q24h); the use of human recombinant erythropoietin (Epo) is not indicated in these cats, and in fact may be harmful.

*Diagnostic tests.* FeLV and FIV testing should be done in cats with PRCA. Also, a bone marrow aspiration or biopsy should be performed to rule out other bone marrow disorders. Bone marrow aspirates in dogs and cats with PRCA reveal either erythroid hypoplasia, or hyperplasia of the early erythroid precursors and a "maturation arrest" at the rubricyte or metarubricyte stage.

*Treatment of FeLV-positive cats.* In FeLV-infected cats with PRCA the anemia is usually chronic and severe; PCVs of 5% to 6% are common, and despite therapy the condition deteriorates. Supportive treatment involves whole blood or packed RBC transfusions as needed (which eventually may be weekly). Oral interferon also may improve clinical signs (without resolution of the anemia) (see Chapter 102).

*Treatment in dogs.* The same treatment used during the maintenance phase of IHA is recommended for these dogs (see p. 1166, text). Lifelong treatment is usually required. Supportive therapy with blood or blood products is often necessary; packed RBC transfusions are preferred. It is recommended that cross-matching be performed before each transfusion.

## Anemia of Renal Disease

Anemia is common in patients with chronic renal failure. It is usually normocytic and normochromic, with few or no reticulocytes; PCVs in dogs and cats with ARD are usually in the 20% to low 30% range, although PCVs in the teens can also occur.

### Management

Improvement in renal function may result in marginal increases in RBC mass. Anabolic steroids have been advocated in cats and dogs with ARD. Nandrolone decanoate can be given at 1 to 4 mg/kg intramuscularly q2-3wk. Human recombinant Epo (Epogen) has been used successfully to treat anemia in cats and dogs with chronic renal failure. A dose of 100 to 150 IU/kg SC twice weekly is used until the PCV returns to a target value (usually 20% to 25%), then the interval between injections is lengthened for maintenance therapy. The PCV usually returns to normal within 3 to 4 weeks of the start of treatment. Anti-Epo antibodies (and resultant refractory anemia) may be produced by 6 to 8 weeks of therapy in up to 50% of patients.

## Acute and Peracute Blood Loss or Hemolysis

Blood loss and hemolytic anemias are nonregenerative during the initial phases of recovery (first 48 to 96 hours). In most patients with acute blood loss, there is either historic or clinical evidence of profound bleeding. If no obvious cause of bleeding is found or if the patient is bleeding from multiple sites, the hemostatic system should be evaluated for a coagulopathy. Initial management should include supportive therapy, as well as intravenous crystalloids or plasma expanders. If necessary, transfusion of blood or packed RBCs should be performed. Once the bleeding is arrested, resolution of the anemia occurs within days or weeks.

# SEMIREGENERATIVE ANEMIAS (TEXT PP 1167-1168)

## Iron-Deficiency Anemia

Iron-deficiency anemia is well characterized in dogs with chronic blood loss but is extremely rare in adult cats, where it is associated only with chronic gastrointestinal (GI) blood loss. In cats, IDA is well characterized only in weanling kittens, in which iron supplementation results in rapid improvement.

### Etiology

Chronic blood loss leading to iron depletion is common in dogs with GI bleeding caused by neoplasia (most common), gastroduodenal ulcers, or endoparasites (e.g., hookworms) and in those with heavy flea infestation. IDA from other causes of chronic blood loss, such as urogenital bleeding, is rare.

### Signs and diagnosis

Typically, dogs with IDA are presented because of signs associated with anemia or for evaluation of GI signs such as diarrhea, melena, or hematochezia. However, dogs with neoplasms in the jejunum may not exhibit any GI signs. Occasionally, mild IDA is recognized during routine evaluation of heavily parasitized dogs (mostly puppies).

*Hematology.* Most dogs with IDA have microcytic hypochromic indexes, mild reticulocytosis (1% to 5%), anisocytosis, thrombocytosis, low serum iron and total iron-binding capacity (transferrin) concentrations, extremely low saturation (usually <10%), low serum ferritin concentration, and low bone marrow iron stores (see Table 85-4). Microcytosis is normal in some dog breeds (e.g., Akita, Shiba Inu, Shar Pei) and also occurs with other disorders (e.g., portosystemic shunts).

***Fecal examination.*** Because the most common cause of IDA in adult dogs is chronic GI bleeding, the stools should be evaluated for occult blood using commercially available kits. If results are negative, this test should be repeated two or three times while the patient is not being fed canned dog food (which contains myoglobin). If occult blood is present in the stool, GI neoplasia should be ruled out. Tumors commonly associated with IDA in dogs include leiomyomas, leiomyosarcomas, and lymphomas, although chronic blood loss can also occur in dogs with GI carcinomas. Another condition that typically leads to IDA is gastroduodenal ulceration (see Chapter 32). Puppies should be evaluated for hookworms (fecal flotation or direct smear) and fleas, the two most common causes of IDA in young dogs.

### Treatment
IDA usually resolves within 6 to 8 weeks after the cause is eliminated. If the cause can be eliminated oral or intramuscular iron supplementation is usually not necessary to hasten resolution of the hematologic abnormalities; a balanced diet usually achieves the same effect. The dietary iron requirement for adult dogs and cats is 1.3 mg/kg/day.

## PRINCIPLES OF TRANSFUSION THERAPY (TEXT PP 1168-1169)

Whole blood can be used if the patient is hypovolemic and needs clotting factors, whereas packed RBCs are recommended for normovolemic dogs and cats with anemia (e.g., PRCA, ARD, hemolysis). Transfusion therapy should be used with extreme caution in patients with IHA, as massive transfusion reactions may occur; in those patients, hemoglobin derivatives may be a better alternative.

Clotting factor deficiencies resulting in hemorrhage can be corrected by administration of whole fresh blood or, ideally, fresh or fresh frozen plasma. Cryoprecipitate contains a high concentration of factor VIII (FVIII) and von Willebrand's factor (vWF), so it is typically used in dogs with hemophilia A or von Willebrand's disease. Cryo-poor plasma is a good source of clotting factors (except for FVIII and vWF) and albumin. Platelet-rich plasma or platelet transfusion, if available, can be used in dogs with severe thrombocytopenia resulting in spontaneous bleeding but is not usually effective in stopping the bleeding. Whole fresh blood, platelet-rich plasma, or fresh-frozen plasma is indicated in patients with DIC. Platelet-rich plasma and platelet transfusions are of no benefit in immune-mediated thrombocytopenic patients. Colloids or human albumin solutions are more effective in restoring plasma oncotic pressure than plasma.

### Blood Groups
#### Dogs
Several blood groups have been recognized in dogs, including DEA 1.1 and 1.2 (formerly blood group A), and DEA 3 through 8. Dogs do not have naturally occurring antibodies against blood group antigens; they can acquire them only after receiving a transfusion or after pregnancy. Transfused blood positive for DEA 1.1, 1.2, or 7 in a sensitized patient is likely to result in acute or delayed transfusion reactions (donors should be negative for those antigens); however, clinically relevant acute hemolytic transfusion reactions are quite rare in dogs.

#### Cats
Blood groups in cats include A, B, and AB. Cats in the United States are almost exclusively of type A. The prevalence of B-positive cats varies greatly from region to region and among different breeds. Breeds with 15% to 30% of type-B cats include Abyssinian, Birman, Himalayan, Persian, Scottish Fold, and Somali. Breeds with more than 30% of type-B cats include the British Shorthair and the Devon Rex. Because life-threatening transfusion reactions commonly occur in type-B cats receiving type-A blood, cats should always be typed or cross-matched before receiving a transfusion. Domestic Shorthair cats are typically type A. Blood typing is also vital for catteries to prevent neonatal isoerythrolysis (B- or AB-type kittens born to A-type queens).

---

**Box 85-4**

## Cross-Matching Procedure for Dogs and Cats

1. Collect 2 ml of blood from donor and recipient in EDTA tubes.
2. Centrifuge samples at 3000 g for 1 minute; remove and retain plasma.
3. Resuspend RBCs in saline, centrifuge, and discard supernate; repeat three times.
4. Prepare a 2% RBC suspension with 0.02 ml of washed RBCs and 0.98 ml of saline.
5. Major cross-match:
   Two drops of donor RBC suspension
   Two drops of recipient plasma
6. Minor cross-match:
   Two drops of recipient RBC suspension
   Two drops of donor plasma
7. Control:
   Two drops of donor RBC suspension
   Two drops of donor plasma
8. Incubate major, minor, and control specimens at 25° C for 30 minutes.
9. Centrifuge all tubes at 3000 g for 1 minute.
10. Agglutination is a positive result.

---

*EDTA*, Ethylenediaminetetraacetic acid; *RBC*, red blood cell.

## Cross-Matching and Blood Typing

Cross-matching is an alternative to blood typing in dogs that have a history of past transfusions or that will require multiple transfusions and in cats. Cross-matching detects many incompatibilities but does not guarantee complete compatibility. Box 85-4 describes the procedure for major and minor cross-matching. Blood-typing cards are currently available for dogs and cats (Rapid Vet-H, DMS Laboratories, Flemington, NJ).

## Blood Administration

Refrigerated blood may be warmed before or during administration, particularly in small dogs, but excessive heat must be avoided. Blood should not be exposed to room temperature for more than 6 hours. A blood administration set with a filter should be used. The recommended administration rate varies but should not exceed 22 ml/kg/day; up to 20 ml/kg/hr can be used in hypovolemic patients. Patients with heart failure may not be able to tolerate more than 5 ml/kg/day. A volume of 2.2 ml/kg (1 ml/lb) of transfused blood (PCV of donor approximately 40%) will raise the recipient's PCV by 1%.

## Complications of Transfusion Therapy

Complications can be divided into those that are immunologically mediated and those that are not. When signs of a transfusion reaction are noticed, the transfusion must be slowed or halted.

### Immune-mediated reactions

Immune-mediated reactions include urticaria, hemolysis, and fever. Signs of immediate immune-mediated hemolysis occur within minutes and include tremors, emesis, and fever; these are rare in dogs but common in cats receiving incompatible blood products. Delayed hemolytic reactions are more common and are primarily manifested as an unexpected decline in the PCV after transfusion, in association with hemoglobinemia, hemoglobinuria, and hyperbilirubinemia.

#### Non–immune-mediated reactions

Non–immune-mediated reactions include fever caused by improperly stored blood, circulatory overload, citrate intoxication, disease transmission, and the metabolic burden associated with transfusion of aged blood. Circulatory overload may be manifested as vomiting, dyspnea, or coughing. Signs of citrate intoxication are related to hypocalcemia and include tremors and cardiac arrhythmias.

# 86

# Erythrocytosis

## (Text pp 1170-1172)

### Etiology

Erythrocytosis is defined as a high (above reference values) packed cell volume (PCV) and is classified as either relative or absolute. Relative erythrocytosis is caused by hemoconcentration (dehydration); the red blood cell (RBC) mass is normal, and the total plasma protein is usually high. In absolute or true erythrocytosis, an increase in RBC mass is present. Certain dog breeds (e.g., sight hounds) have high PCVs.

*Primary erythrocytosis.* Primary erythrocytosis (polycythemia rubra vera [PRV]) results from proliferation of RBC precursors, independent of erythropoietin (Epo) production. Most patients have low-to-nondetectable serum Epo.

*Secondary erythrocytosis.* Secondary erythrocytosis results from increased orthotopic (i.e., produced by the kidneys) or heterotopic (i.e., produced in sites other than the kidneys) Epo production. Orthotopic Epo production occurs in response to tissue hypoxia, such as adaptation to high altitude, chronic cardiopulmonary disease, cardiovascular right-to-left shunts, and carboxyhemoglobinemia. Tumor-associated (heterotopic) erythrocytosis has been described in dogs with renal masses and in a dog with a nasal fibrosarcoma. Hyperadrenocorticism in dogs and hyperthyroidism in cats can also cause mild erythrocytosis. Secondary erythrocytosis is more common in dogs, whereas PRV is more common in cats. However, erythrocytosis is rare in both species.

### Clinical features

Although absolute erythrocytosis is a chronic process, signs may occur acutely and manifest primarily as functional central nervous system abnormalities (behavioral, motor, or sensory changes). Signs of transverse myelopathy are common in cats. A common manifestation in dogs is paroxysmal sneezing. Cardiopulmonary signs occasionally are present. Historical and physical examination findings may also include bright red mucous membranes (plethora), erythema, polyuria and polydipsia, splenomegaly, and presence of renal masses or neoplasia elsewhere.

*Hematology.* It is relatively common to find PCVs of 70% to 80% % in cats and dogs with absolute erythrocytosis. Abnormalities are usually limited to erythrocytosis, although thrombocytosis may be present in cats and dogs with PRV. Microcytosis caused by relative iron deficiency is common in dogs with erythrocytosis.

### Diagnosis

Relative erythrocytosis (dehydration) should be ruled out by measuring serum or plasma protein concentration, which is typically high in these patients. However, in certain circumstances, such as hemorrhagic gastroenteritis, dogs with relative erythrocytosis may have a high PCV with a relatively normal serum protein concentration.

### Initial treatment

The initial approach to the patient with absolute erythrocytosis is to decrease blood viscosity by reducing the number of circulating RBCs. This can be accomplished with therapeutic phlebotomy, in which 20 ml/kg of blood is collected from a central vein. Gradual phlebotomy (5 ml/kg, repeated as needed) is recommended for patients with right-to-left shunts. Sudden decreases in blood volume can result in marked hypotension, so a peripheral vein catheter should be used to simultaneously administer an equivalent volume of saline solution.

### Further investigation

Once the patient has been stabilized, the cause of erythrocytosis should be investigated:

1. Cardiopulmonary status should be evaluated and an arterial blood sample obtained for blood gas analysis. In some patients, blood viscosity is so high that the blood gas analyzer cannot generate results. Therapeutic phlebotomy should be performed before the sample is resubmitted in those patients.
2. If the $PO_2$ is normal, the kidneys should be evaluated for masses or infiltrative lesions with intravenous pyelography, ultrasonography, or computed tomography. If no lesions are found, the patient most likely does not have renal secondary erythrocytosis.
3. A search for an extrarenal neoplasm should then be conducted.
4. A serum sample for measurement of Epo activity should be submitted to a reliable laboratory (e.g., Dr Urs Giger, Department of Genetics, School of Veterinary Medicine, University of Pennsylvania).

### Subsequent treatment

If the patient proves to have PRV, hydroxyurea (Hydrea, 30 mg/kg orally q24h) is administered for 7 to 10 days. The dose is then gradually decreased and/or the interval lengthed. Because hydroxyurea is potentially myelosuppressive, complete blood counts should be obtained every 4 to 8 weeks, and the dose decreased according to the neutrophil count (see Chapter 80). Phlebotomy should be repeated as dictated by the patient's clinical status. If the final diagnosis is secondary erythrocytosis, the primary disorder should be treated (e.g., surgery for a renal mass).

### Prognosis

Most dogs and cats with PRV have extremely long survival times (>2 years) when treated with hydroxyurea (with or without phlebotomy). In dogs and cats with secondary erythrocytosis, the prognosis is related to the primary disease.

# 87

# Leukopenia and Leukocytosis

## (Text pp 1173-1180)

### GENERAL CONSIDERATIONS (TEXT P 1173)

Leukocytosis occurs when the white blood cell (WBC) count exceeds the upper limit of normal for the species; leukopenia occurs when the WBC count is below the reference range. The absolute leukocyte numbers (number of cells per microliter) should always be evaluated on the basis of the differential WBC count rather than percentages.

### NORMAL LEUKOCYTE MORPHOLOGY AND PHYSIOLOGY (TEXT PP 1173-1174)

Leukocytes are classified as either polymorphonuclear (neutrophils, eosinophils, and basophils) or mononuclear (monocytes and lymphocytes) cells.

#### Toxic neutrophils

Toxic neutrophils have characteristic cytoplasmic changes, including Döhle bodies (small, bluish cytoplasmic inclusions), basophilia or granulation, and vacuolation. Purplish cytoplasmic granules represent the most severe toxic change. Presence of giant neutrophils, bands, and metamyelocytes in circulation is another manifestation of toxic changes; they are more common in cats than in dogs.

#### Chédiak-Higashi syndrome

Chédiak-Higashi syndrome, a lethal autosomal recessive condition of Persian cats with smoke-colored haircoats and yellow eyes, is characterized by enlarged neutrophilic and eosinophilic granules in association with partial albinism, photophobia, increased susceptibility to infections, bleeding tendencies, and abnormal melanocytes.

#### Nuclear hypersegmentation

The finding of four or more distinct nuclear lobes may result from prolonged neutrophil transit time. It occurs in dogs with hyperadrenocorticism, cats and dogs undergoing corticosteroid therapy, and cats and dogs with chronic inflammatory disorders. It may also be noted in Poodles with macrocytosis.

### LEUKOCYTE CHANGES IN DISEASE (TEXT PP 1174-1180)

#### Neutropenia

Neutropenia, an absolute decrease in circulating neutrophil numbers, can occur as a consequence of decreased cell production within the bone marrow, or increased margination or destruction of circulating neutrophils (Box 87-1). Neutropenia is relatively common in cats and dogs; quite a few normal cats have neutrophil counts of 1800 to 2300/μl.

##### Clinical features

Frequently neutropenia is an incidental finding in an otherwise healthy animal. Signs in neutropenic patients are usually vague and nonspecific and include anorexia,

**Box 87-1**

## Causes of Neutropenia in Cats and Dogs

**DECREASED OR INEFFECTIVE PRODUCTION OF CELLS IN THE PROLIFERATING POOL**
Myelophthisis (neoplastic infiltration of the bone marrow)
   **Myeloproliferative disorders (D, C)**
   **Lymphoproliferative disorders (D, C)**
   Systemic mast cell disease (D, C)
   Malignant hystiocytosis (D, C)
   Myelofibrosis (D, C)
   Metastatic carcinoma (D?, C?)
Drug-induced
   **Anticancer and immunosuppressive agents (D, C)**
   *Chloramphenicol (C)*
   **Griseofulvin (C)**
   Sulfa-trimethoprim (D, C)
   *Estrogen (D)*
   *Phenylbutazone (D)*
   Phenobarbital (D)
   Other
Toxins
   Industrial chemical compounds (inorganic solvents, benzene) (D, C)
   *Fusarium sporotrichiella* toxin *(C)*
Infectious diseases
   **Parvovirus infection (D, C)**
   **Retrovirus infection** (feline leukemia virus, feline immunodeficiency virus) **(C)**
      Myelodysplastic or preleukemic syndromes (C)
      Cyclic neutropenia (C)
      Panleukopenia-like syndrome (C)
   Histoplasmosis (D, C)
   *Ehrlichiosis (D)*
   Toxoplasmosis (D, C)
   Early canine distemper virus infection (D)
   Early canine hepatitis virus infection (D)
Idiopathic bone marrow hypoplasia or aplasia (D, C)
Cyclic neutropenia of gray Collies (D)
Acquired cyclic neutropenia (D, C)
**Steroid-responsive or immune-mediated neutropenia (D, C)**

**SEQUESTRATION OF NEUTROPHILS IN MARGINATING POOL**
**Endotoxic shock (D, C)**
Anaphylactic shock (D, C)
Anesthesia (D?, C?)

**SUDDEN, EXCESSIVE TISSUE DEMAND, DESTRUCTION, OR CONSUMPTION**
Infectious diseases
   **Peracute, overwhelming bacterial infection** (e.g., peritonitis, aspiration pneumonia, salmonellosis, metritis, pyothorax) **(D, C)**
   Viral infection (e.g., canine distemper or hepatitis, preclinical stage) (D)
*Drug-induced (D, C)*
**Steroid-responsive or immune-mediated neutropenia (D, C)**
Paraneoplastic (D)
"Hypersplenism" (D?)

*C,* Cats; *D,* dogs; *?,* poorly documented.
Key: **Common**; *relatively common*; uncommon.

lethargy, pyrexia, and mild gastrointestinal (GI) signs. Dogs and cats with parvoviral enteritis have neutropenia in association with severe vomiting and/or diarrhea. Occasionally, neutropenic cats and dogs have septic shock on presentation.

### Evaluation

Evaluation should include (1) a detailed history of drug administration (e.g., estrogen or phenylbutazone in dogs, griseofulvin in cats) and vaccination (e.g., panleukopenia in cats, parvovirus in dogs); (2) a complete physical examination and imaging in search of a septic focus; (3) serology or virology for infectious diseases (e.g., feline leukemia virus [FeLV], feline immunodeficiency virus [FIV], canine ehrlichiosis, parvoviral enteritis); and if necessary (4) bone marrow cytology or histopathology. Evaluation of a complete blood count or blood smear may establish the pathogenesis of the neutropenia. Neutropenia in association with anemia (especially if nonregenerative) and/or thrombocytopenia is suggestive of a primary bone marrow disorder. Neutropenia in association with regenerative anemia and spherocytosis is suggestive of an immune-mediated disease. Toxic changes in neutrophils suggest infection.

*Reevaluation.* Sequential evaluation of the leukogram is helpful in excluding transient or cyclic neutropenia (or cyclic hematopoiesis). If the pathogenesis of neutropenia cannot be ascertained in an individual patient with no toxic WBC changes, sophisticated techniques such as leukocyte nuclear scanning or kinetic studies can be performed.

### Treatment approach

Corticosteroid-responsive neutropenia has been well characterized in cats and dogs, so if most infectious and neoplastic causes of neutropenia have been ruled out in an asymptomatic patient, immunosuppressive doses of prednisone (2 to 4 mg/kg/day for dogs and 4 to 8 mg/kg/day for cats) can be tried. Responses are usually observed within 24 to 96 hours. Treatment is continued as for dogs with immune hemolytic anemia and other immune-mediated disorders (see Chapters 85 and 93).

*Afebrile patients.* All asymptomatic, afebrile neutropenic patients should be treated with broad-spectrum bactericidal antibiotics. The drug of choice in dogs is trimethoprim-sulfa, 15 mg/kg orally (PO) q12h. An alternative is enrofloxacin (Baytril, 5 mg/kg PO q12-24h), which can be used in both dogs and cats. Antibiotics with an anaerobic spectrum should be avoided.

*Febrile patients.* Febrile (symptomatic) neutropenic patients should be treated with aggressive intravenous antibiotic therapy. The treatment of choice is cephalotin (20 mg/kg intravenously [IV] q8h) in combination with amikacin (15 mg/kg IV q24h); or a combination of ampicillin (20 mg/kg IV q8h) and enrofloxacin (5 to 10 mg/kg IV q12-24h).

*Colony-stimulating factor.* Neutrophil production can be stimulated by administration of human recombinant granulocyte colony-stimulating factor (G-CSF) (Neupogen, 5 µg/kg subcutaneously q24h). Although results are quite spectacular, responses are usually short-lived because of production of anti-CSF antibodies.

*Lithium.* Lithium carbonate (10 mg/kg PO q12h) is effective in increasing neutrophil counts in dogs, but it should be used with caution in dogs with decreased glomerular filtration rate. It does not appear to be effective (and may be toxic) in cats.

## Neutrophilia

Neutrophilia, an absolute increase in neutrophil numbers, is the most common cause of leukocytosis in dogs and cats. Although a high percentage of cats and dogs with neutrophilia have underlying infectious disorders, neutrophilia is not synonymous with infection. Rather, it often is the result of inflammatory or neoplastic processes.

### Etiology

Causes can be divided into the following three groups (the more common causes are in italics):

- physiologic or epinephrine-induced (e.g., *fear* [cats], excitement, exercise, seizures, parturition)

- stress- or corticosteroid-induced (e.g., *pain*, anesthesia, trauma, neoplasia, hyper-adrenocorticism [dogs], chronic disorders, metabolic disorders [uncommon])
- inflammation or increased tissue demand (e.g., *infection* [bacterial, viral, fungal, or parasitic], *tissue trauma or necrosis, immune-mediated disorders* [dogs], neoplasia, metabolic disorders [uremia, diabetic ketoacidosis], burns, neutrophil function abnormalities [dogs], and acute hemorrhage or *hemolysis*)

Degenerative left shifts (when the number of immature forms exceeds that of mature neutrophils) usually suggest an aggressive infectious process, such as pyothorax, septic peritonitis, bacterial pneumonia, pyometra, prostatitis, or acute pyelonephritis.

**Stress leukogram.** Stress- or corticosteroid-induced neutrophilia is associated with lymphopenia and eosinopenia, and with monocytosis in dogs. In cats, neutrophilia resulting from endogenous epinephrine release (physiologic neutrophilia) is often accompanied by erythrocytosis and lymphocytosis.

### Evaluation

Signs in cats and dogs with neutrophilia are usually secondary to the underlying disorder. Pyrexia may or may not be present. If the patient has persistent neutrophilia, if the neutrophils display toxic changes (text p 1173), or if a degenerative left shift is present, every effort should be made to identify a septic focus or infectious agent. This should be accomplished by (1) performance of a thorough physical examination; (2) evaluation of thoracic and abdominal radiographs; (3) performance of abdominal ultrasonography; and (4) submission of blood, urine, fluid, and/or tissue samples for bacterial and fungal cultures.

**Nuclear medicine.** Autologous or allogeneic neutrophils labeled with radionuclides (technetium 99m or indium 111) can be injected IV, and the septic focus or foci identified with gamma camera imaging.

### Treatment

Treatment is aimed at the primary cause. Empiric antibiotic therapy with a broad-spectrum bactericidal antibiotic (e.g., trimethoprim-sulfa, enrofloxacin) is an acceptable approach when the cause cannot be identified.

## Eosinopenia

Eosinopenia, an absolute decrease in circulating eosinophil numbers, is a common part of the stress leukogram and is usually of little clinical relevance. Acute inflammation or infection can also cause eosinopenia.

## Eosinophilia

Eosinophilia, an absolute increase in circulating eosinophil numbers, is relatively common and can have a variety of causes (Box 87-2). Eosinophilia is quite common in parasitic disorders, so parasitism should be ruled out before the eosinophilia is thoroughly investigated. Three other relatively common causes in cats are eosinophilic granuloma complex, bronchial asthma, and eosinophilic gastroenteritis. Eosinophilia can also occur (rarely) in dogs and cats with mast cell tumors.

### Evaluation and treatment

Signs are related to the primary disorder. Once parasitic causes have been excluded, other causes of eosinophilia should be pursued with appropriate procedures, such as tracheal wash for pulmonary eosinophilic infiltrates and endoscopic biopsy for eosinophilic gastroenteritis. Treatment is aimed at the primary disorder.

### Hypereosinophilic syndrome

A syndrome characterized by marked eosinophilia and tissue infiltration with eosinophils is well documented in cats and Rottweilers. It is usually indistinguishable from eosinophilic leukemia. Patients exhibit primary GI signs, although multisystemic signs are also common. In cats treatment with immunosuppressive doses of corticosteroids, 6-thioguanine, cytosine arabinoside, cyclophosphamide, and other anticancer agents (see Chapter 79) is unrewarding, and most cats die within weeks of diagnosis; Rottweilers, however, have shown clinical response to some of these drugs.

---

**Box 87-2**

### Causes of Eosinophilia in Cats and Dogs

**PARASITIC DISORDERS**
Ancylostomiasis (D)
Dirofilariasis (D, C)
Dipetalonemiasis (D)
**Ctenocephalidiasis (D, C)**
Filaroidiasis (C)
Aelurostrongylosis (C)
Ascariasis (D, C)
Paragonimiasis (D, C)
Demodicosis (D)

**HYPERSENSITIVITY DISORDERS**
Atopy (D, C)
**Flea allergy dermatitis (D, C)**
*Food allergy (D, C)*

**EOSINOPHILIC INFILTRATIVE DISORDERS**
Eosinophilic granuloma complex (D)
*Feline bronchial asthma (C)*
Pulmonary infiltrates with eosinophils (D)
*Eosinophilic gastroenteritis/colitis (D, C)*
Hypereosinophilic syndrome (D, C?)

**INFECTIOUS DISEASES**
Upper respiratory tract viral disorders (C?)
Feline panleukopenia (C?)
Feline infectious peritonitis (C?)
Toxoplasmosis (C)
Suppurative processes (D, C)

**NEOPLASIA**
Mast cell tumors **(D,** C)
Lymphomas (D, C)
Myeloproliferative disorders (C)
Solid tumors (D, C)

**MISCELLANEOUS**
Soft-tissue trauma (D?, C?)
Feline urologic syndrome (C?)
Cardiomyopathy (D?, C?)
Renal failure (D?, C?)
Hyperthyroidism (C?)
Estrus (?)

*C*, Cats; *D*, dogs; ?, poorly documented.
Key: **Common**; *relatively common*; uncommon.

---

### Basophilia

Basophilia, an absolute increase in basophil numbers, is commonly associated with eosinophilia. Causes include the following:

- disorders associated with excessive immunoglobulin E (IgE) production (e.g., heartworm disease, inhalant dermatitis)
- inflammatory disease (e.g., GI disease, respiratory disease, neoplasia [mast cell tumors, lymphomatoid granulomatosis, and in dogs, basophilic leukemia])
- hyperlipoproteinemia associated with hypothyroidism in dogs

### Monocytosis

Monocytosis, an absolute increase in monocyte numbers, can occur in response to inflammatory, neoplastic, or degenerative stimuli (Box 87-3). Traditionally, monocytosis is primarily associated with chronic inflammatory processes, but it is also common in acute disorders; in dogs, it is part of the stress leukogram. In the Midwest, systemic fungal disorders (e.g., histoplasmosis and blastomycosis) are relatively common causes of monocytosis.

#### Evaluation

Evaluation of patients with monocytosis is similar to that of patients with neutrophilia, in that infectious foci should be identified, if present. If an immune-mediated disorder is suspected, arthrocentesis for fluid analysis or immune tests should be performed (see Chapter 92). Treatment is aimed at the primary disorder.

---

**Box 87-3**

## Causes of Monocytosis in Cats and Dogs

Inflammation
  **Infectious disorders**
    **Bacteria**
      *Pyometra (D, C)*
      *Abscesses (D, C)*
      Peritonitis (D, C)
      *Pyothorax (D, C)*
      Osteomyelitis (D, C)
      *Prostatitis (D)*
    Higher bacteria
      Nocardia (D, C)
      Actinomyces (D, C)
      Mycobacteria (D, C)
    Intracellular organisms
      Ehrlichia (D)
      Hemobartonella
        (Mycoplasma spp.) (D, C)
    Fungi
      *Blastomyces (D, C)*
      *Histoplasma (D, C)*
      Cryptococcus (D, C)
      Coccidioides (D)
    Parasites
      Heartworms (D, C?)

Immune-mediated disorders
  **Hemolytic anemia (D, C)**
  Dermatitis (D, C)
  *Polyarthritis (D, C)*
Trauma with severe crushing injuries (D, C)
Hemorrhage into tissues or body cavities
  (D C)
**Stress or corticosteroid induced (D)**
*Neoplasia*
  Associated with tumor necrosis (D, C)
  Lymphoma *(D, C)*
  Myelodysplastic disorders (D, C)
  Leukemias
    Myelomonocytic leukemia (D, C)
    Monocytic leukemia (D, C)
    Myelogenous leukemia (D, C)

---

*C,* Cats; *D,* dogs; ?, poorly documented.
Key: **Common**; *relatively common*; uncommon.

## Lymphopenia
### Etiology
Lymphopenia, an absolute decrease in the lymphocyte count, is one of the most common hematologic abnormalities in hospitalized or sick dogs and cats, and is attributed to the effects of endogenous corticosteroids (stress leukogram) in these patients. Lymphopenia is common in dogs and cats with chronic loss of lymph (e.g., chylothorax, intestinal lymphangiectasia). It is also a common feature of certain acute viral diseases, including parvoviruses (cats and dogs), feline infectious peritonitis, FeLV, FIV, canine distemper, and canine infectious hepatitis. Chemotherapy and chronic corticosteroid use frequently result in lymphopenia. Lymphopenia does not appear to predispose to infections.

### Evaluation
In general, cats and dogs with lymphopenia have obvious clinical abnormalities. Lymphopenia should initially be disregarded in sick patients and in those receiving corticosteroids, and the lymphocyte count reevaluated after resolution of the clinical abnormalities or discontinuation of steroid therapy.

## Lymphocytosis
### Etiology
Lymphocytosis, an absolute increase in lymphocyte numbers, is found in several clinical situations. Fear is the most common cause in cats. Vaccination, chronic

ehrlichiosis, Addison's disease (hypoadrenocorticism), and chronic lymphocytic leukemia (CLL) are the most common causes in dogs. Other conditions that can cause lymphocytosis in cats and dogs include hypersensitivity reactions, immune-mediated diseases, and lymphoblastic leukemia, and in dogs, Chagas' disease, babesiosis, and leishmaniasis.

*Hematology.* In all these disorders (except for vaccination reactions), the lymphocytes are morphologically normal; reactive lymphocytes (see p. 731) are common after vaccination. High numbers of lymphoblasts are found in dogs and cats with acute lymphoblastic leukemia.

### Cats

In cats with marked lymphocytosis and neutrophilia, endogenous catecholamine release should be ruled out. If the cat is fractious and blood cannot be collected without a struggle, the sample should be collected with the patient under chemical restraint.

### Dogs

In dogs with lymphocytosis and reactive lymphocytes, recent vaccination should be ruled out. Most dogs with lymphocyte counts between 10,000 and 20,000 cells/μl have either chronic ehrlichiosis or CLL. Lymphocyte counts greater than 20,000 cells/μl are almost pathognomonic for CLL. A high proportion of these patients also have hyperproteinemia (monoclonal or polyclonal gammopathy). Clinical and hematologic features of CLL and ehrlichiosis are quite similar (cytopenias, hyperproteinemia, hepatosplenomegaly, lymphadenopathy).

Serology or polymerase chain reaction for *Ehrlichia* spp. and bone marrow aspiration may help differentiate these two disorders. Bone marrow cytology in dogs with chronic ehrlichiosis is usually characterized by generalized hematopoietic hypoplasia and plasmacytosis. In dogs with CLL, hypoplasia with lymphocytosis is more common.

# 88

# Combined Cytopenias and Leukoerythroblastosis

## *(Text pp 1181-1184)*

### Etiology

In general, bicytopenias (a decrease in the numbers of two circulating blood cell lines) and pancytopenias (all three cell lines are affected) result from primary bone marrow disorders (Box 88-1); less frequently, they may result from peripheral blood cell destruction (e.g., sepsis, disseminated intravascular coagulopathy [DIC], some immune-mediated disorders) or sequestration of circulating cells. In most cases, if anemia is present, it is nonregenerative. Regenerative anemia in association with other cytopenias usually suggests peripheral destruction of cells.

*Leukoerythroblastic reaction.* The presence of immature white blood cells (WBCs) and nucleated red blood cells in the circulation can result from a variety of mechanisms.

---

**Box 88-1**

### Causes of Bicytopenia and Pancytopenia in Dogs and Cats

**DECREASED CELL PRODUCTION**
Bone marrow hypoplasia-aplasia
  Idiopathic
  Chemicals (e.g., benzene derivatives)
  Hormones (endogenous or exogenous estrogen)
  Drugs (chemotherapeutic agents, antibiotics, griseofulvin, nonsteroidal anti-inflammatory agents)
  Radiation therapy
  Immune-mediated
  Infectious (parvovirus, FeLV, FIV, *Ehrlichia canis*, *Histoplasma capsulatum*)
Bone marrow necrosis
  Infectious disorders (sepsis, parvovirus)
  Toxins (mycotoxins)
  Neoplasms (acute and chronic leukemias, metastatic neoplasia)
  Other (hypoxia, DIC)
Bone marrow fibrosis-sclerosis
  Myelofibrosis
  Osteosclerosis
  Osteopetrosis
Myelophthisis
  Neoplasms
  Acute leukemias
    Chronic leukemias
    Lymphoma
    Multiple myeloma
    Systemic mast cell disease
    Malignant histiocytosis
    Metastatic neoplasms
  Granulomatous disorders
    *Histoplasma capsulatum*
    *Mycobacterium* spp.
    Storage diseases
Myelodysplasia

**INCREASED CELL DESTRUCTION AND SEQUESTRATION**
Immune-mediated disorders
  Evans' syndrome
  Steroid-responsive cytopenias
Infectious
  *B. canis*
  *B. gibsonii*
Sepsis
Microangiopathy
  DIC
  Hemangiosarcoma
Splenomegaly
  Congestive splenomegaly
  Hypersplenism
  Hemolymphatic neoplasia
  Other neoplasm

---

*DIC*, Disseminated intravascular coagulation; *FeLV*, feline leukemia virus; *FIV*, feline immunodeficiency virus.

In general, however, it is caused by premature cell release from the bone marrow or other hematopoietic organs (spleen, liver). Causes include the following:

- increased demand for blood cells (e.g., hemolytic anemia, blood loss, sepsis, peritonitis, DIC, chronic hypoxia from congestive heart failure)
- crowding out of normal precursors (e.g., leukemias, bone marrow lymphoma, multiple myeloma)
- extramedullary (spleen, liver) hematopoiesis with lack of normal feedback, hemangiosarcoma
- metabolic disorders (e.g., diabetes mellitus, hyperthyroidism, hyperadrenocorticism)

The WBC count is usually high, but it can be normal or, rarely, low.

### Clinical features

Signs and physical examination findings in dogs and cats with combined cytopenias and leukoerythroblastic reaction (LER) are usually related to the underlying disorder rather than to the hematologic abnormalities per se, with the exception of pallor and spontaneous bleeding (petechiae and ecchymoses) secondary to anemia and thrombocytopenia, respectively. Pyrexia may be present if a markedly neutropenic patient is septic. Several physical examination findings may help the clinician establish a more presumptive or definitive diagnosis in patients with cytopenias or LER. Feminization in a male dog (usually a cryptorchid) with pancytopenia suggests a Sertoli cell tumor or, less frequently, an interstitial cell tumor or seminoma with secondary hyperestrogenism. The finding of a cranial or midabdominal mass in a dog with anemia, thrombocytopenia, and LER is highly suggestive of splenic hemangiosarcoma.

### Evaluation

A detailed history should be obtained, particularly with regard to drugs given (e.g., estrogen or phenylbutazone in dogs; griseofulvin or chloramphenicol in cats), exposure to benzene derivatives, travel history, vaccination status, and exposure to other animals. Most drugs that cause anemia or neutropenia can also cause combined cytopenias (Boxes 85-1 and 87-1).

*Splenic cytology.* Cytologic evaluation of the spleen by percutaneous fine-needle aspiration is indicated in patients with cytopenias and diffuse splenomegaly.

*Serology.* Infectious diseases associated with bicytopenias and pancytopenias commonly diagnosed by serology or polymerase chain reaction (PCR) include ehrlichiosis in dogs and feline leukemia virus (FeLV) and feline immunodeficiency virus (FIV) in cats. When the clinical and hematologic features suggest immune-mediated disease (e.g., polyarthritis, proteinuria, spherocytosis), a direct Coombs' and an antinuclear antibody test should be performed. It is also helpful to submit fluid from one or more joints for cytology; suppurative nonseptic arthritis suggests an immune pathogenesis or a rickettsial disease.

Infectious diseases associated with bicytopenias and pancytopenias (e.g., ehrlichiosis in dogs and FeLV and FIV in cats) are commonly diagnosed on the basis of serology or PCR.

*Bone marrow evaluation.* Bone marrow aspiration and, ideally, core biopsy should be performed in all patients with combined cytopenias once peripheral blood cell destruction has been ruled out. Bone marrow should also be evaluated in patients with LER.

*Diagnostic imaging.* Abdominal radiography and ultrasonography should be used to search for hemangiosarcoma in dogs with LER.

### Bone marrow aplasia or hypoplasia

Bone marrow aplasia or hypoplasia is characterized by peripheral cytopenias and a paucity or absence of hematopoietic precursors in the bone marrow. It is commonly associated with administration of griseofulvin or chloramphenicol in cats and phenylbutazone or estrogen in dogs. It is also common with canine ehrlichiosis or FeLV infection. A corticosteroid-responsive syndrome of combined cytopenias or pancytopenia has been recognized in cats and dogs. Some patients with pancytopenia have hypercellular bone marrow, suggesting that the cells are destroyed peripherally.

***Bone marrow evaluation.*** Bone marrow aspirates typically are hypocellular or acellular, and histopathology on a core biopsy is frequently necessary for definitive diagnosis. After infectious diseases and drug exposure have been ruled out, a trial of immunosuppressive doses of corticosteroids (with or without other immunosuppressive drugs; see Chapter 93) is warranted. Anabolic steroids or erythropoietin is not beneficial in these patients.

### Myelophthisis

Infiltration of the bone marrow with neoplastic or inflammatory cells (see Box 88-1) can crowd out the normal hematopoietic precursors, leading to peripheral blood cytopenias. Often these patients are presented for evaluation of anemia, although fever and bleeding caused by neutropenia and thrombocytopenia, respectively, can also be presenting complaints. The presence of hepatomegaly, splenomegaly, and/or lymphadenopathy in a patient with anemia or combined cytopenias is highly suggestive of some of the neoplastic or infectious disorders listed in Box 88-1.

***Bone marrow evaluation.*** Definitive diagnosis is made by evaluating a bone marrow specimen; a bone marrow core biopsy may be more reliable than an aspirate.

***Treatment.*** Once a cytologic or histopathologic diagnosis is made, treatment is aimed at the primary neoplasm (chemotherapy) or infectious agent.

### Myelofibrosis, osteosclerosis, and osteopetrosis

Fibroblasts or osteoblasts within the bone marrow can proliferate in response to retroviral infections, chronic noxious stimuli, or unknown causes. This can lead to fibrous or osseous replacement of the bone marrow cavity and displacement of hematopoietic precursors (myelofibrosis and osteosclerosis or osteopetrosis, respectively). Although both syndromes are rare, they have been described in FeLV-infected cats and in dogs with chronic hemolytic disorders, such as pyruvate kinase deficiency anemia in Basenjis and Beagles.

Presumptive diagnosis of osteosclerosis or osteopetrosis is based on the finding of combined cytopenias with increased medullary radiographic density and can be confirmed with a bone marrow core biopsy. No effective treatment exists.

# 89

# Disorders of Hemostasis

## *(Text pp 1185-1199)*

Spontaneous bleeding resulting from hemostatic disorders is common in dogs but rare in cats; thromboembolic disorders are rare in both cats and dogs. The most common disorder leading to spontaneous bleeding in dogs is thrombocytopenia, usually immune mediated. Other common disorders include disseminated intravascular coagulation (DIC) and rodenticide poisoning; congenital clotting factor deficiencies are rare causes of spontaneous bleeding. Hemostatic abnormalities are frequently present in cats with liver disease, feline infectious peritonitis (FIP), or neoplasia, although spontaneous bleeding is rare in these patients. The key to diagnosing the patient's condition is to proceed in a logical and systematic fashion.

## CLINICAL MANIFESTATIONS OF SPONTANEOUS BLEEDING DISORDERS (TEXT PP 1186-1187)

### History

When evaluating a cat or dog with spontaneous or excessive bleeding, it is important to determine the animal's age and whether (1) this is the first bleeding episode; (2) the pet has had any previous surgeries, and if so, whether bleeding was excessive; (3) any littermates have or have had similar signs, and whether perinatal mortality in the litter was increased; (4) the pet has recently been vaccinated with modified-live vaccines (see Box 89-2); (5) the pet is currently taking any medication (including nonsteroidal antiinflammatory agents, sulfas, other antibiotics); and (6) the pet has access to rodenticides or roams freely.

### Clinical features

The manifestations of primary and secondary hemostatic abnormalities are clinically distinct (Table 89-1).

*Primary hemostatic defects.* Typical signs are those of superficial bleeding: petechiae, ecchymoses, bleeding from mucosal surfaces (e.g., melena, hematochezia, epistaxis, hematuria), and prolonged bleeding immediately after venipuncture. The vast majority of these disorders are caused by thrombocytopenia; occasionally, primary hemostatic defects result from platelet dysfunction (e.g., uremia, von Willebrand's disease [vWD], monoclonal gammopathies). Primary hemostatic defects caused by vascular disorders are rare.

*Secondary hemostatic defects (clotting factor deficiencies).* Signs are deep bleeding; bleeding into muscle, body cavities, and joints; and hematomas. Petechiation is rare. Most secondary bleeding disorders are caused by rodenticide poisoning or liver disease; occasionally, congenital clotting factor deficiencies lead to spontaneous bleeding. A combination of primary and secondary (mixed) bleeding disorders is almost exclusively seen in dogs and cats with DIC.

## CLINICOPATHOLOGIC EVALUATION OF THE BLEEDING PATIENT (TEXT PP 1187-1189)

Laboratory evaluation of the hemostatic system is indicated in the following two common situations: (1) in patients with spontaneous or prolonged bleeding, and (2) before surgery in cats and dogs with disorders commonly associated with bleeding (e.g., splenic hemangiosarcoma [HSA] in dogs) or in patients in which a congenital coagulopathy is suspected (e.g., Doberman Pinschers with suspected vWD). Confirmation of the clinical diagnosis can usually be obtained by performing some simple tests, described in the following sections and in Table 89-2.

### Interpreting blood smears

Examination of a well-prepared blood smear provides important clues regarding platelet numbers and morphology. First the smear should be scanned at low power to identify platelet clumps, which commonly result in pseudothrombocytopenia. With the oil immersion lens, several monolayer fields should then be examined and the

---

**Table 89-1**

### Clinical Manifestations of Primary and Secondary Hemostatic Defects

| Primary hemostatic defect | Secondary hemostatic defect |
|---|---|
| Petechiae common | Petechiae rare |
| Hematomas rare | Hematomas common |
| Bleeding at mucous membranes | Bleeding into muscles, joints, and body cavities |
| Bleeding from multiple sites | — |
| Bleeding immediately after venipuncture | Delayed bleeding after venipuncture |

**Table 89-2**

## Interpretation of Hemostasis Screens

| Disorder | BT | ACT | OSPT* | APTT | Platelets | Fibrinogen | FDPs |
|---|---|---|---|---|---|---|---|
| Thrombocytopenia | ↑ | N | N | N | ↓ | N | N |
| Thrombocytopathia | ↑ | N | N | N | N | N | N |
| Von Willebrand's disease | ↑ | N | N | N | N | N | N |
| Hemophilias | N | ↑ | N | ↑ | N | N | N |
| Rodenticide toxicity | N | ↑ | ↑ | ↑ | N↓ | N↓ | N↑ |
| Disseminated intravascular coagulation | ↑ | ↑ | ↑ | ↑ | ↓ | N↓ | ↑ |

*OSPT and APTT are considered prolonged if they are 25% or more than the concurrent controls.

ACT, Activated coagulation test; APTT, activated partial thromboplastin time; BT, Bleeding time; FDPs, fibrin degradation products; N, normal or negative; OSPT, one-stage prothrombin time; ↑, high or prolonged; ↓, decreased or shortened.

number of platelets in five fields averaged. In dogs 12 to 15 platelets should be present per oil immersion field, and 10 to 12 platelets per field should be seen in normal cats. The number of platelets per field times 15,000 roughly equals the number of platelets per microliter. The cause of bleeding is usually not thrombocytopenia if more than two or three platelets are seen in each oil immersion field.

### Activated coagulation time

Activated coagulation time (ACT), which uses 2 ml of fresh whole blood added to a tube containing diatomaceous earth, evaluates the integrity of the intrinsic and common pathways. If there exists a greater than 70% to 75% decrease in the activity of the clotting factors involved, the ACT, which normally is 60 to 90 seconds, is prolonged (see Table 89-2).

### Fibrin degradation products

The Thrombo Wellco Test, which detects circulating fibrin degradation products (FDPs), commonly has a positive result in dogs with DIC and occasionally in those with other disorders of fibrinolysis. The test also has a positive result in more than 50% of dogs with rodenticide poisoning.

### Buccal mucosa bleeding time

A template (Simplate-II) is used to make one or two incisions in the buccal mucosa, and the time for complete cessation of bleeding is measured (buccal mucosa bleeding time [BT]. Normal times are 2 to 3 minutes in dogs and 1.5 to 2.5 minutes in cats. This test is abnormal in dogs and cats with thrombocytopenia, platelet dysfunction, or, possibly, vasculitis. If a patient is presented with signs of a primary bleeding disorder (see p. 786 and Table 89-1) and the platelet count is normal, a prolonged BT indicates underlying platelet dysfunction (e.g., nonsteroidal antiinflammatory therapy, vWD), or possibly vasculitis.

### Further evaluation

A routine coagulation screen (or hemostasis profile) usually consists of the one-stage prothrombin time (OSPT), activated partial thromboplastin time (APTT), platelet count, fibrinogen concentration, and FDP concentration (or titer); in some laboratories, a D-dimer test (evaluates for systemic fibrinolysis) and antithrombin (AT) activity may be included. If further confirmation is required, plasma can be submitted to a referral laboratory or specialized coagulation laboratory (see text). Samples should be submitted in a purple-top tube (sodium EDTA) for platelet count, a blue-top tube (sodium citrate) for coagulation studies (OSPT, APTT, fibrinogen concentration, AT), and a special blue-top tube (Thrombo Wellco Test) for FDP.

*Clotting factor deficiencies.* If an unusual coagulopathy or a specific clotting factor deficiency is suspected, whole blood should be submitted to a veterinary coagulation laboratory for clotting factor analysis. Congenital and acquired clotting factor deficiencies are listed in Box 89-1.

### Other procedures

Because thrombocytopenia can result from decreased production or increased destruction, consumption, or sequestration of platelets, bone marrow aspiration is indicated in most cats and dogs with thrombocytopenia of unknown cause. Other tests in such patients may include titers or polymerase chain reaction (PCR) assay for tick-borne diseases or retroviral infection and antiplatelet antibody tests (see text p 1236).

## MANAGEMENT OF THE BLEEDING CAT OR DOG (TEXT PP 1189-1190)

A cat or dog with a spontaneous bleeding disorder should be managed aggressively, but iatrogenic bleeding should be minimized. Trauma should be avoided and the patient kept quiet, preferably confined to a cage, and only leash-walked. Venipuncture should be done with the smallest gauge needle possible, and pressure applied to the site for at least 5 minutes; a compressive bandage is applied once the pressure is released.

### Transfusions

Transfusion of blood or blood products is indicated in some patients. Fresh whole blood or a combination of packed red blood cells (RBCs) and fresh-frozen plasma

---

**Box 89-1**

## Congenital and Acquired Clotting Factor Defects

**CONGENITAL CLOTTING FACTOR DEFECTS**
Factor I or hypofibrinogenemia and dysfibrinogenemia (Saint Bernards and Borzois)
Factor II or hypoprothrombinemia (Boxers)
Factor VII or hypoproconvertinemia (Beagles and Malamutes)
Factor VIII or hemophilia A (many breeds)
Factor IX or hemophilia B (many breeds of dogs; Domestic Shorthair and British Shorthair cats)
Factor X or Stuart-Prower trait (Cocker Spaniels)
Factor XI or hemophilia C (English Springer Spaniels, Great Pyrenees, Kerry Blue Terrier)
Factor XII or Hageman factor (many breeds of dogs and cats)

**ACQUIRED CLOTTING FACTOR DEFECTS**
Liver disease
  Decreased production of factors
  Qualitative disorders
Cholestasis
Vitamin K antagonists
Autoimmune disease (lupus anticoagulant)
Disseminated intravascular coagulation

---

should be used if the patient is anemic and lacking one or more clotting factors; plasma transfusions are of no benefit in thrombocytopenic animals. Fresh-frozen plasma can be used to replenish clotting factors in patients with a normal or mildly decreased packed cell volume, although stored blood and frozen plasma are deficient in factors V and VIII. Fresh whole blood, platelet-rich plasma, and platelet transfusions rarely provide sufficient platelets to halt spontaneous bleeding in a cat or dog with thrombocytopenia, particularly if the bleeding is the result of platelet consumption. Cryoprecipitate is the component of choice in dogs with vWD or hemophilia.

## PRIMARY HEMOSTATIC DEFECTS (TEXT PP 1190-1194)

Primary hemostatic defects are the most common cause of spontaneous bleeding in dogs. They are characterized by the presence of superficial and mucosal bleeding (e.g., petechiae, ecchymoses, hematuria, epistaxis) and are usually caused by thrombocytopenia.

### Thrombocytopenia
#### Etiology
Decreased numbers of circulating platelets can be the result of either decreased production or increased destruction, consumption, or sequestration of platelets (Box 89-2).
*Decreased production.* Decreased production is the most common cause of thrombocytopenia in cats, particularly as a result of retrovirus-induced bone marrow disorders; it is rare in dogs.
*Increased destruction.* Increased destruction is the most common cause of thrombocytopenia in dogs; it is extremely rare in cats. The three most common mechanisms are immune-mediated, drug-related (see Box 85-1), and sepsis.
*Increased consumption or sequestration.* Platelet consumption occurs most commonly in DIC, and sequestration is usually caused by splenomegaly or, rarely, hepatomegaly.

---

**Box 89-2**

## Causes of Thrombocytopenia in Dogs and Cats

**DECREASED PLATELET PRODUCTION**
Immune-mediated megakaryocytic hypoplasia
Idiopathic bone marrow aplasia
Drug-induced megakaryocytic hypoplasia (estrogens, phenylbutazone, lomustine, melphalan, β-lactams)
Myelophthisis
Cyclic thrombocytopenia
Retroviral infection

**INCREASED PLATELET DESTRUCTION, SEQUESTRATION, OR USE**
Immune-mediated thrombocytopenia
Live viral vaccine-induced thrombocytopenia
Drug-induced thrombocytopenia
Microangiopathy
Disseminated intravascular coagulation
Hemolytic uremic syndrome
Vasculitis
Splenomegaly
Splenic torsion
Endotoxemia
Acute hepatic necrosis
Neoplasia (immune-mediated, microangiopathy)

---

### Diagnostic approach

Thrombocytopenia is confirmed by performing a platelet count or evaluating a blood smear. Platelet counts less than 25,000/μl are common in dogs with immune-mediated thrombocytopenia (IMT), whereas counts of 50,000 to 75,000/μl are more common in dogs with ehrlichiosis, lymphoma affecting the spleen, or rodenticide toxicity.

*History.* A drug history should be obtained; if the patient is receiving any medication, the thrombocytopenia should be considered drug related until proved otherwise. The drug should be discontinued (if possible), and the platelet count reevaluated in 2 to 6 days. If the platelet count returns to normal, a retrospective diagnosis of drug-induced thrombocytopenia is made.

*Bone marrow evaluation.* In thrombocytopenic cats, bone marrow aspiration should always be performed if there is no history of medication use. Feline leukemia virus and feline immunodeficiency virus tests should also be performed. Bone marrow evaluation is indicated in thrombocytopenic dogs that fail to respond to immunosuppressive drugs within 2 to 3 days. Infiltrative or dysplastic bone marrow disorders causing thrombocytopenia are usually obvious.

*Differential diagnoses.* IMT is a diagnosis of exclusion, so tick-borne diseases such as canine ehrlichiosis, Rocky Mountain spotted fever, cyclic thrombocytopenia, and babesiosis should be ruled out. If the patient does not have signs other than bleeding, sepsis and tick-borne diseases are unlikely. If sepsis is suspected on the basis of clinical signs and clinicopathologic findings, urine and blood should be obtained for bacterial cultures The presence of spherocytic hemolytic anemia or autoagglutination in a dog with thrombocytopenia highly suggests Evans's syndrome, a combination of IMT and immune hemolytic anemia (IHA). A direct Coombs' test is usually positive in these cases.

*Hemostasis screen.* A hemostasis screen should always be obtained to rule out DIC if a thrombocytopenic patient has RBC fragments in the blood smear or evidence of secondary bleeding. In dogs and cats with selective thrombocytopenia, the remainder of the hemostasis screen is usually normal.

*Diagnostic imaging.* Abdominal radiographs and/or ultrasonography may reveal an enlarged spleen not evident during physical examination. Diffuse splenomegaly may be the cause of the thrombocytopenia, or it may reflect "work hypertrophy" (mononuclear phagocytic system hyperplasia) and extramedullary hematopoiesis in a patient with IMT.

*Therapeutic approach.* Often a diagnosis of IMT is made only after a therapeutic trial with corticosteroids (see later) resolves the thrombocytopenia. If doubt exists as to whether the thrombocytopenia is caused by a rickettsial disease or IMT, doxycycline (5 to 10 mg/kg orally [PO] q12-24h) can be administered with the corticosteroids until serology or PCR results are available.

*Transfusion.* Currently no specific treatments exist for cats and dogs with thrombocytopenia. Transfusion of blood or blood products should be used when indicated. However, transfusion of fresh whole blood, platelet-rich plasma, or platelets rarely, if ever, normalizes the platelet count or even increases it to "safe" levels. Transfusion of packed RBCs tends to decrease the severity of bleeding in thrombocytopenic patients with blood-loss anemia.

### Immune-mediated thrombocytopenia

IMT is the most common cause of spontaneous bleeding in dogs but is extremely rare in cats. It primarily affects middle-aged female dogs; Cocker Spaniels and Old English Sheepdogs are overrepresented. Signs are those of a primary hemostatic defect; if bleeding is pronounced, acute collapse may occur. If the anemia is mild, most dogs are asymptomatic, although vomiting may be reported. In most dogs IMT is acute or peracute. Splenomegaly may be present.

*Clinicopathologic data.* Complete blood count is characterized by thrombocytopenia with or without anemia (depending on the degree of spontaneous bleeding and the presence or absence of IHA). Leukocytosis with a left shift may also be present. As a general rule, hematologic changes are limited to the thrombocytopenia. When IHA is associated with IMT (Evans's syndrome), a Coombs'-positive, regenerative anemia with spherocytosis or autoagglutination is usually found. However, in most dogs with IMT, thrombocytopenia is the only abnormality in the complete blood count.

*Other tests.* Bone marrow cytology typically is characterized by megakaryocytic hyperplasia, although in rare instances, megakaryocytic hypoplasia with free megakaryocyte nuclei is found. BT is the only other abnormal finding; usually an inverse relationship exists between the platelet count and the BT (longer BT with lower platelet count). Canine ehrlichiosis, drug-induced thrombocytopenia, and infectious thrombocytopenia (*Ehrlichia platys*) should be ruled out before a diagnosis of IMT is established.

*Corticosteroid therapy.* When the index of suspicion for IMT is high, a therapeutic trial with immunosuppressive doses of corticosteroids (e.g., 2 to 8 mg/kg/day of prednisone) should be instituted. Responses are usually seen within 24 to 96 hours. $H_2$-antihistamines, such as famotidine (0.5 mg/kg PO q24h), can be used in combination with the corticosteroids.

*Cytotoxic drugs.* Cyclophosphamide (Cytoxan, 200 to 300 mg/m$^2$ intravenously [IV] or PO once), in combination with corticosteroids, effectively induces remission, although it should not be used as a maintenance agent. Vincristine (Oncovin, 0.5 mg/m$^2$ IV) has been recommended for dogs with IMT; however, patients may experience further bleeding, as a result of platelet dysfunction despite a rising platelet count. Azathioprine (Imuran, 50 mg/m$^2$ PO q24-48h) is effective in maintaining remission but is not a good induction agent in dogs with IMT. In some dogs it is better tolerated than chronic corticosteroid therapy, although close hematologic monitoring is recommended.

*Other therapies.* Danazol (5-10 mg/kg PO q12h) may be beneficial, although it is usually cost prohibitive in large dogs. Fresh whole blood, stored blood, packed

RBCs, or hemoglobin solutions should be administered as needed for anemia. Dogs with refractory IMT can be successfully treated with Vinca-loaded platelets, pulse-dose cyclophosphamide, intravenous human immunoglobulin (0.5 to 1 g/kg, single dose), or splenectomy.

**Prognosis.** Most dogs with IMT have a good prognosis but usually require lifelong treatment. Cats with IMT may not respond as well as dogs, even when corticosteroids are used in combination with other drugs such as chlorambucil or cyclophosphamide; however, thrombocytopenic cats rarely bleed spontaneously.

## Platelet Dysfunction

Primary hemostatic bleeding in a patient with a normal platelet count is highly suggestive of a platelet dysfunction syndrome, although vasculopathies and enhanced fibrinolysis should also be considered. Platelet dysfunction syndromes can be congenital (e.g., vWD, canine thrombopathia, collagen disorders) or acquired (e.g., a result of prostaglandin inhibitors, antibiotics, phenothiazines, or vaccines; or secondary to myeloproliferative disorders, systemic lupus erythematosus, gammopathies, and renal or liver disease). They rarely result in spontaneous bleeding; more often, a prolonged BT is documented preoperatively in an otherwise healthy patient, or there is a history of pronounced bleeding during a previous surgery.

### von Willebrand's disease

vWD is the most common inherited bleeding disorder in dogs; it is rare in cats. vWD involves either low concentrations or absence of circulating von Willebrand factor (vWF) or low-to-normal concentrations of abnormal vWF. The result is mild (if any) spontaneous bleeding; more often, it is characterized by prolonged surgical bleeding. vWD is classified as follows:

- type I—low concentration of normal vWF; seen in Doberman Pinschers and other breeds
- type II—low concentration of abnormal vWF; seen in German Shorthaired Pointers
- type III—absence of vWF; seen in Scottish Terriers, Shetland Sheepdogs, and Chesapeake Bay Retrievers

**Heritability.** vWD has been reported in more than 50 breeds but is more common in Doberman Pinschers, German Shepherds, Poodles, Golden Retrievers, and Shetland Sheepdogs. In these breeds the defect is an autosomal dominant trait with incomplete penetrance. In Scottish Terriers and Shetland Sheepdogs, it can be an autosomal recessive trait; homozygous dogs have no detectable vWF and are usually severely affected.

**Acquired vWD.** Acquired vWD purportedly occurs in association with hypothyroidism in dogs; thyroxine supplementation may normalize or improve vWF concentrations, although clinical confirmation is lacking.

**Signs.** Most dogs with vWD do not bleed spontaneously, but rather bleed excessively during or after surgery or are presented for evaluation of diffuse oropharyngeal bleeding. Excessive bleeding during teething or estrus can also occur. Perinatal mortality or abortions and stillbirths are common in some litters.

**Hemostasis screen.** In most affected dogs the hemostasis screen is normal, with the possible exception of a mildly prolonged APTT if the patient also has partial factor VIII deficiency (although this is rare). The platelet count is usually normal. Typically the BT inversely correlates with the degree of vWF deficiency. Definitive diagnosis can be confirmed by quantifying vWF in specialized veterinary coagulation laboratories.

**Management.** Most dogs with type I vWD can be treated before surgery or during a bleeding episode with desmopressin acetate (DDAVP, 1 μg/kg subcutaneously [SC]), which shortens the BT within 30 minutes of a single subcutaneous dose of the intranasal preparation. DDAVP is not effective in dogs with types II or III vWD. Administration of fresh-frozen plasma, fresh whole blood, or cryoprecipitate increases circulating vWF concentration within minutes.

Use of topical hemostatic agents, such as fibrin, collagen, or methacrylate, is also indicated to control local bleeding. Dogs with vWD should not be bred.

### Other congenital platelet function defects

Platelet function defects leading to spontaneous bleeding have been described in Otterhounds, Foxhounds, and Basset Hounds. Signs and clinicopathologic findings are similar to those in dogs with vWD, but vWF concentrations are normal or high.

## SECONDARY HEMOSTATIC DEFECTS (TEXT PP 1194-1195)

Cats and dogs with secondary hemostatic defects usually are presented for evaluation of collapse, exercise intolerance, dyspnea, abdominal distention, lameness, or presence of masses (hematomas). Cats and dogs with secondary hemostatic disorders do not have petechiae or ecchymoses, although mucosal bleeding (e.g., melena, epistaxis) can rarely be seen. In general, the severity of the bleeding is directly related to the severity of the clotting factor deficiency.

### Congenital Clotting Factor Deficiencies

A list of congenital clotting factor deficiencies, as well as the breed affected, is presented in Box 89-1. Congenital factor deficiencies are relatively common in dogs and rare in cats. Hemophilia A and B are sex-linked; other coagulopathies have variable modes of inheritance. Signs usually include spontaneous hematoma formation and bleeding into body cavities, as well as "fading puppy syndrome" and protracted umbilical cord bleeding after birth; abortions or stillbirths in the litter are common.

Carriers may be asymptomatic but usually have prolonged clotting times. In dogs with factor XI deficiency, massive and often life-threatening postoperative bleeding (starting 24 to 36 hours after surgery) is common. Most patients with congenital coagulopathies are treated with supportive and transfusion therapies; no other treatments appear to be beneficial. Affected dogs should not be bred.

### Vitamin K Deficiency

Vitamin K deficiency is usually the result of ingestion of vitamin K antagonists such as warfarin, diphacinone, or their derivatives brodifacoum and bromadiolone. It can also occur in patients with obstructive cholestasis, infiltrative bowel disease, or liver disease as a result of vitamin K malabsorption.

#### Signs of rodenticide poisoning

Most patients present with acute collapse and a questionable history of rodenticide ingestion; coughing, thoracic pain, and dyspnea are common. These patients usually have signs compatible with secondary bleeding. The most common sites of bleeding are intrathoracic and intrapulmonary; some dogs have superficial bruising in areas of friction, such as the axilla or the groin. Other abnormalities include pale mucous membranes, anemia (usually regenerative if sufficient time has elapsed), and hypoproteinemia (which resolves shortly after internal hemorrhage). Sudden death may occur as a result of central nervous system or pericardial hemorrhage.

#### Emergency care

If ingestion occurred minutes or hours before presentation, induction of vomiting and administration of activated charcoal may eliminate or neutralize most of the rodenticide. If ingestion is questionable and no signs of coagulopathy are present, evaluation of the OSPT is recommended; prolonged OSPT usually occurs before spontaneous bleeding becomes evident.

#### Further evaluation

The typical hemostasis screen is characterized by marked prolongation of the OSPT and APTT; the FDP test is positive in more than 50% of affected dogs, and mild thrombocytopenia (70,000 to 125,000/µl) is also present.

#### Treatment

Treatment involves immediate transfusion with fresh whole blood, fresh-frozen plasma, stored plasma, or cryo-poor plasma. Packed RBCs are also indicated if the patient is anemic. It may take 12 hours before vitamin K therapy appreciably decreases bleeding. When severely affected animals are treated with vitamin K alone, it may take up to 48 hours for the OSPT to return to normal.

***Vitamin K.*** Subcutaneous administration of vitamin $K_1$ using a 25-gauge needle is preferred if the patient is properly hydrated; intravenous administration of vitamin K is not recommended. The loading dose is 5 mg/kg, followed in 8 hours by 2.5 mg/kg divided every 8 hours. Oral vitamin $K_1$ (5 mg/kg with a fatty meal, then 2.5 mg/kg divided every 8 to 12 hours) can also be used; animals with cholestatic or malabsorptive syndromes may require repeated subcutaneous injections. In critical cases the OSPT should be monitored every 8 hours until it normalizes.

***Maintenance therapy.*** If the anticoagulant is known to be warfarin or another first-generation hydroxycoumarin, oral vitamin $K_1$ administration for 1 week is usually sufficient. However, if the anticoagulant is indanedione or any of the second- or third-generation anticoagulants, oral vitamin $K_1$ must be given for at least 3 weeks (and possibly as long as 6 weeks). Most currently available rodenticides contain second- and third-generation anticoagulants. If the rodenticide ingested is unknown, it is recommended that the patient be treated for 1 week, and then treatment discontinued and the OSPT evaluated within 48 hours. If the OSPT is prolonged, therapy should be reinstituted for 2 more weeks and the OSPT reevaluated.

## DISSEMINATED INTRAVASCULAR COAGULATION (TEXT PP 1195-1199)

DIC is a mixed (combined) hemostatic abnormality. It is a complex syndrome in which excessive intravascular coagulation leads to multiple-organ microthrombosis (multiple organ failure [MOF]) and paradoxic bleeding. DIC is relatively common in dogs and cats.

### Etiology

Three basic mechanisms can lead to activation of intravascular coagulation: endothelial damage, platelet activation, and release of tissue procoagulants. Causes or contributing factors include sepsis, pancreatitis, FIP virus infection, trauma, hemolysis, bacterial infections, acute hepatitis, heartworm disease, certain neoplasms (e.g., HSA in dogs and lymphoma or carcinoma in cats), electrocution, and heat stroke.

In dogs symptomatic DIC is most commonly associated with neoplasia (primarily HSA), sepsis, pancreatitis, immune-mediated blood diseases, and liver disease. In cats symptomatic DIC is extremely rare, but hemostatic evidence of DIC is common in cats with liver disease (primarily hepatic lipidosis), malignant neoplasms (mainly lymphoma or carcinoma), or FIP. Symptomatic DIC has also occurred in some cats receiving methimazole.

### Clinical features

Several clinical presentations occur in dogs with DIC; the two common forms are chronic (subclinical) and acute (fulminant) DIC. Most patients with DIC are presented for evaluation of the primary problem rather than spontaneous bleeding, and DIC is diagnosed during the routine clinical evaluation.

***Chronic DIC.*** No spontaneous bleeding occurs, but a hemostatic profile reveals abnormalities compatible with DIC. Chronic DIC is common in dogs and cats with malignancy and in cats with liver disease.

***Acute DIC.*** Acute DIC may be a true acute phenomenon (e.g., after heatstroke, electrocution, or acute pancreatitis), but more commonly it represents acute decompensation of a chronic, silent process (e.g., HSA). Regardless of the pathogenesis, dogs with acute DIC are often presented for evaluation of profuse, spontaneous bleeding, in combination with signs secondary to anemia or parenchymal organ thrombosis (MOF). The signs suggest both primary (petechiae, ecchymoses, mucosal bleeding) and secondary (blood in body cavities) bleeding. Acute DIC is extremely rare in cats.

### Diagnosis

Several hematologic findings support a presumptive diagnosis of DIC: regenerative hemolytic anemia (although in patients with neoplasia, the anemia may be non-regenerative), hemoglobinemia, RBC fragments or schistocytes, thrombocytopenia, and neutrophilia with left shift (or rarely, neutropenia). Patients with MOF may develop ventricular premature contractions (VPCs).

***Biochemistry.*** Abnormalities can include hyperbilirubinemia, azotemia, and hyperphosphatemia (if severe renal microembolization has occurred), increased liver enzyme activities, decreased total carbon dioxide concentration, and, if bleeding is severe, panhypoproteinemia. Urinalysis usually reveals hemoglobinuria and bilirubinuria, with occasional proteinuria and cylindriuria.

***Hemostatic profile.*** Abnormalities may include thrombocytopenia, prolonged OSPT and/or APTT (>25% of control values), anemia, schistocytosis, hypofibrinogenemia, positive FDP or D-dimer test, and decreased AT. Enhanced fibrinolysis can also be documented in these patients (e.g., decreased plasminogen activity, enhanced clot lysis test). A diagnosis of DIC can be made if the patient exhibits at least four of these hemostatic abnormalities and/or schistocytosis.

### Treatment

Once the diagnosis has been established, or even in the presence of strong suspicion of DIC, treatment should be instituted immediately. Eliminating the precipitating cause is the first priority, although it is rarely possible. Treatment is therefore aimed at halting intravascular coagulation, maintaining good organ perfusion, and preventing secondary complications (especially pulmonary and renal dysfunction).

***Halting intravascular coagulation.*** Intravascular coagulation is halted by administration of heparin and blood or blood products. Sodium heparin can be used at a wide dose range, as follows:

- minidose—5 to 10 IU/kg SC q8h
- low dose—50 to 100 IU/kg SC q8h
- intermediate dose—300 to 500 IU/kg SC or IV q8h
- high dose—750 to 1000 IU/kg SC or IV q8h

Minidose or low-dose heparin, in combination with blood or blood products, is recommended. This dose of heparin is effective, and in normal dogs it does not prolong the ACT or APTT. If a dog with DIC is receiving intermediate-dose heparin, it is impossible to determine whether prolongation of the APTT is caused by the heparin or by progression of the DIC. However, if the ACT or APTT increases in a patient with DIC receiving minidose or low-dose heparin, deterioration is occurring and a treatment change is necessary.

If severe microthrombosis is evident (e.g., marked azotemia with isosthenuric urine, increased liver enzyme activities, VPCs), dyspnea, or hypoxemia, intermediate- or high-dose heparin can be used. The target is to prolong the ACT to 2 to 2.5 times normal. If overheparinization occurs, protamine sulfate or plasma products can be administered (see text). Once clinical and hemostatic improvement is achieved, the heparin dose should be tapered off gradually (over 2 to 4 days).

Aspirin can also be used to halt intravascular coagulation. Doses of 5 to 10 mg/kg PO, q12h in dogs and q72h in cats, have been recommended, although aspirin is rarely of clinical benefit. If it is used, the patient should be closely monitored for gastrointestinal bleeding. New recombinant anticoagulants, such as hirudin, may be beneficial in dogs and cats with DIC.

***Maintaining good organ perfusion.*** Good organ perfusion is best achieved by using aggressive fluid therapy with crystalloids or plasma expanders such as dextran. However, care should be taken not to overhydrate a patient with compromised renal or pulmonary function.

***Preventing secondary complications.*** Attention should be directed toward maintaining oxygenation (by oxygen mask or cage or nasopharyngeal catheter), correcting acidosis, correcting cardiac arrhythmias, and preventing secondary bacterial infections.

### Prognosis

The prognosis is grave. However, if the inciting cause can be controlled, most dogs recover with appropriate treatment. Marked prolongation of the APTT and marked thrombocytopenia are negative prognostic factors.

## THROMBOSIS (TEXT P 1199)

Several factors can result in thrombosis or thromboembolism, including blood stasis, activation of intravascular coagulation by abnormal or damaged endothelium, decreased activity of natural anticoagulants, and decreased or impaired fibrinolysis. Thrombosis can occur in association with cardiomyopathy (e.g., aortic or iliac thromboembolism secondary to hypertrophic cardiomyopathy in cats; see Chapter 7), hyperadrenocorticism, protein-losing enteropathy and nephropathy, and IHA.

### Management

Patients at high risk for thrombosis or thromboembolism should receive anticoagulants. The two commonly used drugs are aspirin and heparin (see above). Excessive bleeding has been documented in dogs and cats receiving coumarin derivatives.

# 90

# Lymphadenopathy and Splenomegaly

## *(Text pp 1200-1209)*

## LYMPHADENOPATHY (TEXT PP 1200-1204)

The various causes of lymphadenopathy are listed in Table 90-1. Table 90-2 lists the more common causes by clinical presentation: generalized, superficial, or intracavitary lymphadenopathy. Most cases of generalized lymphadenopathy are caused by systemic fungal or rickettsial infections (dogs), lymphoma (dogs), or nonspecific hyperplasia (mainly in cats).

### History

The history is important when patients with lymphadenopathy (or diffuse splenomegaly) are evaluated. Certain diseases have a defined geographic or seasonal presentation, such as salmon poisoning (Pacific Northwest) and histoplasmosis (Ohio River Valley).

### Clinical signs

Signs are often vague and nonspecific and are usually related to the primary disease. They may include anorexia, weight loss, weakness, abdominal distention, vomiting, diarrhea, and polyuria (PU) and polydipsia (PD) (in dogs with lymphoma-associated hypercalcemia). Occasionally, enlarged lymph nodes result in obstructive or compressive signs (e.g., dysphagia, cough). Systemic signs are usually present in dogs with systemic mycoses, salmon poisoning, Rocky Mountain spotted fever (RMSF), ehrlichiosis, leishmaniasis, or acute leukemia. Signs are rare or absent in patients with chronic leukemias, most lymphomas, and reactive lymphadenopathy after vaccination.

### Physical examination

The following lymph nodes are palpable in normal dogs and cats: mandibular, prescapular (or superficial cervical), axillary (in approximately 50% of patients), superficial inguinal, and popliteal. Lymph nodes that become palpable only when markedly enlarged include facial, retropharyngeal, mesenteric, and iliac (sublumbar).

Table 90-1

## Classification of Lymphadenopathies in Dogs and Cats

| Type | Species | Type | Species |
|---|---|---|---|
| **PROLIFERATIVE AND INFLAMMATORY LYMPHADENOPATHIES** | | *Viral* | |
| **Infectious** | | Canine viral enteritides | D |
| *Bacterial* | | Feline immunodeficiency virus | C |
| Actinomyces spp. | D, C | Feline infectious peritonitis | C |
| Bartonella spp. | D, C | *Unclassified* | |
| Borrelia burgdorferi | D | Pneumocystis carinii | D |
| Brucella canis | D | | |
| Corynebacterium spp. | C | **Noninfectious** | |
| Mycobacteria | D, C | Dermatopathic lymphadenopathy | D, C |
| Nocardia spp. | D, C | Drug reactions | D, C |
| Streptococci | D, C | Idiopathic | D, C |
| Contagious streptococcal lymphadenopathy | C | Distinctive peripheral lymph node hyperplasia | C |
| Yersinia pestis | C | Plexiform vascularization of lymph nodes | C |
| Localized bacterial infection | D, C | Immune-mediated disorders | |
| Septicemia | D, C | Systemic lupus erythematosus | D, C |
| | | Rheumatoid arthritis | D |
| *Rickettsial* | | Immune-mediated polyarthritides | D, C |
| Ehrlichiosis | D, C | Puppy strangles | D |
| Rocky Mountain spotted fever | D | Other immune-mediated disorders | D, C |
| Salmon poisoning | D | Localized inflammation | D, C |
| | | Postvaccinal | D, C |
| *Fungal* | | | |
| Aspergillosis | D, C | **INFILTRATIVE LYMPHADENOPATHIES** | |
| Blastomycosis | D, C | **Neoplastic** | |
| Coccidioidomycosis | D | *Primary hemolymphatic neoplasms* | |
| Cryptococcosis | D, C | Leukemias | D, C |
| Histoplasmosis | D, C | Lymphomas | D, C |
| Phaeohyphomycosis | D, C | Malignant histiocytosis | D, C |
| Phycomycosis | D, C | Multiple myeloma | D, C |
| Sporotrichosis | D, C | Systemic mast cell disease | D, C |
| Other mycoses | D, C | | |
| | | *Metastatic neoplasms* | |
| *Algal* | | Carcinomas | D, C |
| Protothecosis | D, C | Malignant melanomas | D |
| | | Mast cell tumors | D, C |
| *Parasitic* | | Sarcomas | D, C |
| Babesiosis | D | | |
| Cytauxzoonosis | C | **Nonneoplastic** | |
| Demodicosis | D, C | Eosinophilic granuloma complex | C, D? |
| Hepatozoonosis | D | Mast cell infiltration (nonneoplastic) | D, C |
| Leishmaniasis | D | | |
| Neospora caninum | D | | |
| Toxoplasmosis | D, C | | |
| Trypanosomiasis | D | | |

Modified from Hammer AS, Couto CG: Lymphadenopathy. In Fenner NR: *Quick reference to veterinary medicine*, ed 2, Philadelphia, 1991, Lippincott.

*C*, Cats; *D*, dogs.

Table 90-2

## Correlation between Clinical Presentation and Etiology in Dogs and Cats with Lymphadenopathy in the Midwestern United States (in Order of Relative Importance)

| Generalized | Solitary or regional | |
| --- | --- | --- |
| | Superficial | Intracavitary |
| Lymphoma | Abscess | Histoplasmosis (A, T) |
| Histoplasmosis | Periodontal disease | Blastomycosis (T) |
| Blastomycosis | Paronychia | Perianal gland aCA (A) |
| Postvaccinal | Deep pyoderma | Apocrine gland aCA (A) |
| Canine ehrlichiosis | Demodicosis | Primary lung tumors (T) |
| Leukemias | MCT | Lymphoma (A, T) |
| Brucellosis | Malignant melanoma | MCT (A, T) |
| SMCD | EGC | Prostatic aCA (A) |
| Multiple myeloma | Lymphoma | Malignant histiocytosis (A, T) |
| Malignant histiocytosis | | Tuberculosis (A, T) |
| SLE | | |
| Other | | |

*A*, Abdomen; *aCa*, adenocarcinoma; *EGC*, eosinophilic granuloma complex; *MCT*, mast cell tumor; *SLE*, systemic lupus erythematosus; *SMCD*, systemic mast cell disease; *T*, thorax.

***Palpable characteristics.*** In most patients with lymphadenopathy, the lymph nodes are firm, irregular, painless, and of normal temperature. In patients with lymphadenitis, the lymph nodes may be softer than usual, tender, and warmer than normal; and they may adhere to surrounding structures (fixed lymphadenopathy). Metastatic tumors and lymphomas with extracapsular invasion also may manifest as fixed lymphadenopathies.

***Size.*** In dogs massive lymphadenopathy (5 to 10 times normal size) occurs almost exclusively with lymphoma or lymph node abscessation, whereas in cats such enlargement usually is caused by lymph node hyperplasia. Rarely, this degree of enlargement occurs in metastatic lymph nodes. Dogs with salmon poisoning may be presented with marked generalized lymphadenopathy, preceded by or in conjunction with bloody diarrhea. Mild-to-moderate lymph node enlargement (two to four times normal size) mostly occurs in a variety of reactive and inflammatory lymphadenopathies (e.g., ehrlichiosis, RMSF, systemic mycoses, leishmaniasis, immune-mediated skin diseases) and with leukemias.

***Further examination.*** In patients with solitary or regional lymphadenopathy, the area drained by the lymph node(s) should be examined meticulously, as the primary lesion generally is found there. In patients with generalized lymphadenopathy, it is important to evaluate other hemolymphatic organs, including the spleen, liver, and bone marrow.

## SPLENOMEGALY (TEXT PP 1204-1206)

### Etiology

The various causes of splenomegaly are listed in Table 90-3.

***Hemolytic disorders.*** Splenomegaly occurs in dogs and cats with immune-mediated babesiosis, hemolytic anemia, drug-induced hemolysis, pyruvate kinase deficiency anemia, phosphofructokinase deficiency anemia, familial nonspherocytic hemolysis in Poodles and Beagles, Heinz body hemolysis, and hemobartonellosis.

***Extramedullary hematopoiesis.*** Nonneoplastic causes of infiltrative splenomegaly are uncommon, with the exception of extramedullary hematopoiesis (EMH), which is

Table 90-3

## Pathogenetic Classification of Splenomegaly in Dogs and Cats

| Type | Species | Type | Species |
|---|---|---|---|
| **INFLAMMATORY AND INFECTIOUS SPLENOMEGALY** | | **Pyogranulomatous Splenitis** | |
| **Suppurative Splenitis** | | Blastomycosis | D, C? |
| | | Sporotrichosis | D |
| Penetrating abdominal wounds | D, C | Feline infectious peritonitis | C |
| Migrating foreign bodies | D, C | Mycobacteriosis (i.e., tuberculosis) | D, C |
| Bacterial endocarditis | D, C? | Bartonellosis | D, C |
| Septicemia | D, C | | |
| Splenic torsion | D | **HYPERPLASTIC SPLENOMEGALY** | |
| Toxoplasmosis | D, C | Bacterial endocarditis | D |
| Infectious canine hepatitis (acute) | D | Brucellosis | D |
| | | Diskospondylitis | D |
| Mycobacteriosis (i.e., tuberculosis) | D, C | Systemic lupus erythematosus | D, C |
| | | Hemolytic disorders (see text) | D, C |
| **Necrotizing Splenitis** | | **CONGESTIVE SPLENOMEGALY** | |
| Splenic torsion | D | Pharmacologic (see text) | D, C |
| Splenic neoplasia | D | Portal hypertension | D, C |
| Infectious canine hepatitis (acute) | D | Splenic torsion | D |
| Salmonellosis | D, C | | |
| | | **INFILTRATIVE SPLENOMEGALY** | |
| **Eosinophilic Splenitis** | | **Neoplastic** | |
| Eosinophilic gastroenteritis | D, C? | Acute and chronic leukemias | D, C |
| Hypereosinophilic syndrome | C, D? | Systemic mastocytosis | D, C |
| | | Malignant histiocytosis | D, C |
| **Lymphoplasmacytic Splenitis** | | Lymphoma | D, C |
| | | Multiple myeloma | D, C |
| Infectious canine hepatitis (chronic) | D | Metastatic neoplasia | D, C (rare) |
| Ehrlichiosis (chronic) | D | | |
| Pyometra | D, C | **Nonneoplastic** | |
| Brucellosis | D | Extramedullary hematopoiesis | D, C? |
| Hemobartonellosis | D, C | Hypereosinophilic syndrome | C, D? |
| Leishmaniasis | D | Amyloidosis | D |
| **Granulomatous Splenitis** | | | |
| Histoplasmosis | D, C | | |
| Mycobacteriosis (i.e., tuberculosis) | D, C | | |
| Leishmaniasis | D | | |

Modified from Couto CG: Diseases of the lymph nodes and the spleen. In Ettinger S, ed: *Textbook of veterinary internal medicine*, ed 3, Philadelphia, 1989, WB Saunders.
*C*, Cats; *D*, dogs; *?*, poorly documented.

more common in dogs than in cats. A variety of stimuli, including anemia, severe splenic or extrasplenic inflammation, neoplastic infiltration, bone marrow hypoplasia, and splenic congestion, may cause the spleen to produce red blood cells (RBCs), white blood cells, and platelets. Splenic EMH can also occur in dogs with pyometra, immune-mediated hemolysis or thrombocytopenia, infectious diseases, and a variety of malignant neoplasms, as well as in seemingly healthy dogs.

*Hypereosinophilic syndrome.* In cats another disorder that commonly causes infiltrative splenomegaly is hypereosinophilic syndrome, a disease characterized by peripheral blood eosinophilia, bone marrow hyperplasia of eosinophil precursors, and multiple-organ infiltration with mature eosinophils (see Chapter 87).

*Drugs.* Congestive splenomegaly can be caused by tranquilizers, barbiturates, and anesthetics such as halothane.

*Portal hypertension.* Portal hypertension leading to congestive splenomegaly can result from right-sided congestive heart failure; obstruction of the caudal vena cava because of congenital malformations, neoplasia, or heartworm disease; and intrahepatic obstruction of the vena cava. Ultrasonography may reveal markedly distended splenic, portal, and/or hepatic veins.

*Splenic torsion.* Splenic torsion is a relatively common cause of congestive spleno- megaly in dogs. Torsion may be isolated, or it may occur in association with gastric dilatation-volvulus. Most affected dogs are of large, deep-chested breeds, primarily Great Danes and German Shepherd Dogs. Signs can be either acute or chronic. Dogs with acute splenic torsion usually are presented with acute abdominal pain and distention, vomiting, depression, and anorexia. Dogs with chronic splenic torsion display a variety of signs, including anorexia, weight loss, intermittent vomiting, abdominal distention, PU and PD, hemoglobinuria, and abdominal pain.

Physical examination usually reveals marked splenomegaly. Radiographs typically show a C-shaped spleen, and ultrasonography shows greatly distended splenic veins. Hematologic abnormalities usually include regenerative anemia, target cells, leukocytosis with regenerative left shift, and leukoerythroblastosis. Disseminated intravascular coagulation is a common complication. A high percentage of dogs with splenic torsion have hemoglobinuria. The treatment of choice is splenectomy.

*Splenic masses.* Focal splenomegaly is more common than diffuse splenomegaly in dogs; the opposite is true in cats. Neoplastic splenic masses can be benign or malignant, and in dogs mainly include hemangiomas (HAs) and hemangiosarcomas (HSAs). Other neoplasms that occasionally manifest as splenic masses are leiomyomas, leiomyosarcomas, fibrosarcomas, myelolipomas, and lymphomas. Nonneoplastic splenic masses primarily include hematomas and abscesses. Metastatic splenic neoplasms usually result in focal splenomegaly, but they are rare.

### Clinical features

The historical and physical examination findings in dogs with splenomegaly are similar to those in dogs with lymphadenopathy. Signs are vague and nonspecific and include anorexia, weight loss, weakness, abdominal distention, vomiting, diarrhea, and/or PU and PD (relatively common in dogs with marked splenomegaly, particularly in those with splenic torsion). Other signs result from the hematologic consequences of splenic enlargement and include spontaneous bleeding caused by thrombocytopenia, pallor caused by anemia, and fever caused by neutropenia or the primary disorder. In dogs, an enlarged spleen can be either smooth or irregular (i.e., "lumpy-bumpy"). In most cats with marked splenomegaly, the spleen usually has a smooth surface; a diffusely enlarged, "lumpy-bumpy" spleen in a cat suggests systemic mast cell disease.

## DIAGNOSTIC APPROACH TO THE PATIENT WITH LYMPHADENOPATHY OR SPLENOMEGALY (TEXT PP 1206-1208)

### Clinicopathologic Data

#### Hematology

Changes in the complete blood count may suggest a systemic inflammatory process or a diagnosis of hemolymphatic neoplasia (e.g., presence of circulating blasts in acute leukemia or lymphoma, or marked lymphocytosis with chronic lymphocytic leukemia). Occasionally the causative agent is identified by examining a blood smear (e.g., histoplasmosis, hemobartonellosis, trypanosomiasis, babesiosis).

*Anemia.* Anemia of chronic disease can be seen in association with inflammatory, infectious, or neoplastic disorders. Hemolytic anemia is usually present in patients with hemoparasitic lymphadenopathies or splenomegaly and in those with malignant histiocytosis. Severe, nonregenerative anemia may be seen in dogs with chronic ehrlichiosis, in cats with disorders related to feline leukemia virus or feline immuno-deficiency virus, and in dogs and cats with primary bone marrow neoplasms (e.g., leukemias, multiple myeloma).

***Thrombocytopenia.*** Thrombocytopenia is a common finding in patients with ehrlichiosis, RMSF, sepsis, lymphomas, leukemias, multiple myeloma, HSA, systemic mastocytosis, and some immune-mediated disorders.

***Pancytopenia.*** Pancytopenia is common in dogs with chronic ehrlichiosis, malignant histiocytosis, and systemic immune-mediated disorders; in dogs and cats with lymphoma and leukemia; and in cats with retroviral infections.

***Hypersplenism and hyposplenism.*** Hypersplenism is rare and is characterized by cytopenias in the presence of hypercellular bone marrow. These changes resolve after splenectomy. Hyposplenism is more common and results in hematologic changes similar to those seen in splenectomized patients: thrombocytosis, schistocytosis, acanthocytosis, Howell-Jolly bodies, and increased numbers of reticulocytes and nucleated RBCs.

### Serum biochemistry

Two major abnormalities are of diagnostic value in dogs and cats with lymphadenopathy: hypercalcemia and hyperglobulinemia.

***Hypercalcemia.*** Hypercalcemia is a paraneoplastic syndrome that occurs in 10% to 20% of dogs with lymphoma or multiple myeloma; it may also occur in dogs with blastomycosis. Hypercalcemia is extremely rare in cats with these diseases.

***Hyperglobulinemia.*** Monoclonal hyperglobulinemia commonly occurs in dogs and cats with multiple myeloma and occasionally in dogs with lymphoma, ehrlichiosis, or leishmaniasis. Polyclonal hyperglobulinemia commonly occurs in dogs and cats with systemic mycoses; in cats with feline infectious peritonitis; and in dogs with ehrlichiosis, lymphoma, or leishmaniasis (see Chapter 91).

### Serology and culture

Serology or polymerase chain reaction (PCR) assay for canine ehrlichiosis, RMSF, brucellosis, bartonellosis, babesiosis, and systemic mycoses may aid in the diagnosis of regional or systemic lymphadenopathies. Lymph node specimens for bacterial and fungal cultures or for PCR should be obtained when indicated.

## Diagnostic Imaging

### Radiography

Radiographic abnormalities in dogs and cats with lymphadenopathy either can be related to the primary disorder or can reflect the location and extent of the lymphadenopathy. Radiography or computed tomography (CT) is indicated for (1) evaluation of primary bone inflammation or neoplasia in patients with solitary lymphadenopathy, (2) detection of intrathoracic or intraabdominal lymphadenopathy in patients with generalized peripheral lymphadenopathy, and (3) evaluation of affected lymph nodes and changes in pulmonary parenchyma in patients with deep regional lymphadenopathy involving the thoracic cavity. Tranquilization or anesthesia may result in diffuse congestive splenomegaly, making radiographic interpretation of splenic size extremely difficult.

### Ultrasonography

Ultrasonography is the procedure of choice for evaluation of intraabdominal lymphadenopathy or splenomegaly. Ultrasound-guided fine-needle aspiration (FNA) or biopsies can be performed with minimal complications. In addition to lymphadenopathy, abdominal ultrasonography may reveal diffuse splenomegaly, splenic masses, splenic congestion, hepatic nodules (which may be neoplastic, nonneoplastic regenerative tissue, or normal), and other changes; in addition, color-flow Doppler imaging allows evaluation of the splenic blood supply.

### Other procedures

Radionuclide imaging using technetium 99m–labeled sulfur colloid permits evaluation of the spleen's ability to clear particulate matter. CT and magnetic resonance imaging can also be used to evaluate the spleen.

## Cytology and Histopathology
### Bone marrow aspirate or biopsy
Evaluation of bone marrow aspirates or core biopsies can be useful in patients with generalized lymphadenopathy or splenomegaly caused by hemolymphatic neoplasia or systemic infectious diseases. Bone marrow evaluation should always be conducted before splenectomy in patients with cytopenias. The spleen may take over hematopoiesis in patients with primary hypoplastic or aplastic bone marrow disorders; splenectomy in these patients removes the sole source of circulating blood cells and may lead to death.

### Lymph node and splenic aspirates
Cytologic evaluation of lymph node and splenic aspirates is often the definitive diagnostic procedure in patients with lymphadenopathy or diffuse splenomegaly. Mandibular lymph nodes should not be aspirated routinely in older dogs and cats, as these nodes are usually reactive, and that may obscure the primary diagnosis. Transabdominal splenic FNA is obtained with the animal in right lateral or dorsal recumbency using manual or mild chemical restraint. Phenothiazine tranquilizers and barbiturates should be avoided.

### Cytology
Normal lymph nodes are primarily composed of small lymphocytes (80% to 90% of all cells); a few macrophages, medium or large lymphocytes, plasma cells, and mast cells can also be found. Normal spleens are similar, except for the presence of a high concentration of RBCs.

*Reactive lymph nodes and hyperplastic spleens.* These tissues contain variable numbers of lymphoid cells in different stages of development (small, medium, and large lymphocytes; macrophages; and plasma cells).

*Lymphadenitis and splenitis.* The cytologic features vary with the cause and type of reaction. Causative agents can frequently be identified in cytologic specimens from nodes with lymphadenitis.

*Neoplasia.* Primary lymphoid neoplasms (lymphomas) are characterized by a monomorphic population of lymphoid cells, which are usually immature. The cytologic features of metastatic neoplasms depend on the degree of involvement and the cell type. Carcinomas, adenocarcinomas, melanomas, and mast cell tumors are easily diagnosed cytologically; cytologic diagnosis of sarcomas may be difficult, as the neoplastic cells do not exfoliate easily.

### Histopathology
When cytologic examination does not provide a definitive diagnosis, excision of the affected node or incisional (even excisional) splenic biopsy is indicated. It is preferable to excise the whole node, as core biopsies are difficult to interpret. The popliteal lymph nodes are usually chosen in dogs and cats with generalized lymphadenopathy.

*Tissue preparation.* Once a node is excised, it should be sectioned in half lengthwise, impression smears made for cytology, and the node fixed in 10% buffered formalin (1 part tissue to 9 parts fixative). Splenic samples should be similarly prepared.

## MANAGEMENT OF PATIENTS WITH LYMPHADENOPATHY OR SPLENOMEGALY (TEXT PP 1208-1209)
No specific treatment for lymphadenopathy or diffuse splenomegaly exists; treatment should be directed at the cause. Exploratory celiotomy provides considerable information regarding the gross morphology of an enlarged spleen and adjacent organs and tissues. However, visual evaluation of these structures can be misleading. It is impossible to differentiate some benign splenic masses (e.g., hematoma, HA) from a malignancy (e.g., HSA) on the basis of gross morphology alone.

### Splenectomy
Splenectomy is indicated in the following situations: (1) splenic torsion, (2) splenic rupture, (3) symptomatic splenomegaly, and (4) splenic masses. The value of splenectomy is questionable in (1) dogs with immune-mediated blood disorders, (2) dogs and cats

with splenomegaly caused by lymphoma in which chemotherapy failed to induce splenic remission, and (3) dogs and cats with leukemias. Splenectomy is generally contraindicated in patients with bone marrow hypoplasia in which the spleen is the main hematopoietic site.

*Complications.* A life-threatening syndrome of postsplenectomy sepsis occurs in approximately 3% of dogs. Most affected dogs are undergoing immunosuppressive therapy at the time of surgery or are having splenectomy for a neoplasm. The sepsis is usually rapid in onset, so prophylactic bactericidal antibiotic therapy is recommended postoperatively. Cephalothin (20 mg/kg intravenously q8h) is recommended for 2 to 3 days postoperatively.

### Lymph node excision

In patients in which an enlarged lymph node causes mechanical compression or occlusion of a viscus, airway, or vessel, surgical excision should be attempted. If the node is not resectable or if surgery or anesthesia poses a high risk for the patient, one or more of the following can be used:

1. In primary or metastatic neoplastic lesions, irradiation can reduce the size of the lymph node and ameliorate the signs.
2. In patients with fungal lesions, such as *Histoplasma*-induced tracheobronchial lymphadenopathy, antiinflammatory doses of corticosteroids can be effective.
3. In solitary lymphomas and metastatic mast cell tumors, if irradiation is not feasible, intralesional injections of prednisolone (50 to 60 mg/m$^2$) can be successful.
4. In patients with solitary suppurative lymphadenitis, systemic antibiotic therapy and surgical drainage may be beneficial.

# 91

# Hyperproteinemia

## *(Text pp 1210-1211)*

### Relative hyperproteinemia

Relative hyperproteinemia is caused by hemoconcentration (dehydration) and is usually accompanied by erythrocytosis (although in a dehydrated anemic patient, the packed cell volume may appear normal). With relative hyperproteinemia both the albumin and globulin concentrations are increased, whereas in cases of absolute hyperproteinemia (see later) increases in only the globulin concentration occur, usually in association with hypoalbuminemia.

The presence of "hyperalbuminemia" and hyperglobulinemia suggests either dehydration or laboratory error (a common cause of "hyperproteinemia"). Lipemia and hemolysis typically result in artifactual increases in plasma or serum protein concentration.

### Absolute hyperproteinemia

In most cats and dogs with absolute hyperproteinemia, an increase in serum globulin occurs, with a mild or marked decrease in serum albumin concentrations.

Increased globulin production occurs in a variety of clinical settings, but mainly in two groups of disorders: inflammatory or infectious, and neoplastic. Electrophoresis may reveal a polyclonal or monoclonal gammopathy.

***Polyclonal gammopathies.*** Inflammation and infection stimulate production of a variety of globulins, collectively termed *acute phase reactants,* which cause an increase in the alpha-1 and alpha-2 globulin fractions on protein electrophoresis. At the same time, production of immune proteins (mainly immunoglobulins) causes increases in the alpha-2, beta, and/or gamma regions. The result is a broad-based, irregular, "polyclonal" band.

Polyclonal gammopathies occur in several common disorders, including chronic pyoderma, pyometra, and other chronic suppurative processes; feline infectious peritonitis (FIP); hemobartonellosis, bartonellosis, babesiosis, and other hemoparasitic infections; canine ehrlichiosis and leishmaniasis; systemic mycoses; chronic immune-mediated disorders (e.g., systemic lupus erythematosus, immune polyarthritis); and some neoplasms (rare) (Box 91-1). Polyclonal gammopathies are also common in otherwise healthy old cats.

***Monoclonal gammopathies.*** In dogs, monoclonal (narrow-based) gammopathies occur with chronic lymphocytic leukemia, multiple myeloma, and lymphoma; they are also present in dogs with ehrlichiosis and occasionally in those with leishmaniasis. In most cats, monoclonal gammopathies are found in association with multiple myeloma or lymphoma; FIP is another possible cause. Occasionally, an M-component is detected in an otherwise asymptomatic cat or dog, and additional evaluation fails to reveal a cause. This "idiopathic monoclonal gammopathy" requires frequent reevaluation for a clinically emerging malignancy.

**Treatment**

Rehydration resolves relative hyperproteinemia. Treatment of patients with monoclonal or polyclonal gammopathies is aimed at the primary disease.

---

**Box 91-1**

**Diseases Associated with Polyclonal Gammopathies in Dogs and Cats**

**INFECTIOUS**
  **Chronic pyoderma**
  **Pyometra**
  Chronic pneumonia
  **Feline infectious peritonitis**
  Hemobartonellosis
  Bartonellosis
  **Ehrlichiosis**
  **Leishmaniasis**
  Chagas' disease
  Babesiosis
  **Systemic mycoses**

**IMMUNE-MEDIATED DISEASES**

**NEOPLASIA**
  Lymphomas
  Mast cell tumors
  **Necrotic or draining tumors**

Key: **Common;** uncommon.

# 92

# Immune-Mediated Diseases: Overview and Diagnosis

## (Text pp 1212-1215)

### Etiology

In most patients, immune-mediated diseases (IMDs) are idiopathic or primary (no underlying cause can be found); IMDs can also be secondary to infectious diseases. Occasionally, IMDs develop during or after drug therapy (e.g., propylthiouracil in cats) or shortly after vaccination. IMDs are considerably more common in dogs than in cats, and most are more common in females than in males.

### Clinical manifestations

IMDs can affect a solitary organ or tissue (e.g., immune hemolytic anemia, polyarthritis) or can be multisystemic (e.g., systemic lupus erythematosus). They are often associated with pyrexia or fever. Target organs and tissues commonly affected are listed in Table 92-1.

*Signs.* In addition to organ- or tissue-specific signs, such as proteinuria in a dog with glomerulonephritis or shifting-limb lameness in a dog with polyarthritis, dogs and cats with IMDs may be presented for evaluation of fever of unknown origin (see Chapter 95) or may have persistent neutrophilic leukocytosis and nonspecific signs.

## DIAGNOSTIC TESTS (TEXT PP 1213-1214)

A diagnosis of IMD is made after careful evaluation of the history and clinicopathologic data (Table 92-2). Most of these tests are species specific, so the laboratory must know if the specimen is from a dog or a cat. Except for the direct Coombs' test, most tests for IMD are nonspecific and have limited clinical application.

### Table 92-1

### Common Organ or Tissue Targets in Immune-Mediated Disorders

| Organ or tissue affected | Disorder |
|---|---|
| Red blood cells | Immune-mediated hemolytic anemia, pure red cell aplasia |
| Platelets | Immune-mediated thrombocytopenia |
| Neutrophils | Immune-mediated neutropenia |
| Bone marrow | Immune-mediated pancytopenia |
| Synovium | Polyarthritis |
| Glomeruli or tubules | Glomerulonephritis |
| Skin | Dermatitis |
| Muscle or end plate | Polymyositis, polyneuritis, myasthenia gravis |

Table 92-2

## Laboratory Diagnosis of Immune-Mediated Disease

| Test | Specimen | Interpretation* |
|------|----------|-----------------|
| Direct Coombs' test | Plasma[†] | IHA, RBC lysis in SLE |
| Antiplatelet antibodies | Serum | IMT |
| Antinuclear antibody | Serum | SLE, chronic antigen stimulation |
| Rheumatoid factor | Serum | Polyarthritis, SLE |
| Direct immunofluorescence or immunohistochemistry | Tissue | Antibody-complement deposition |

*For discussion, see text.

[†]Anticoagulated (EDTA) blood is commonly used as a source of RBCs.

*IHA,* Immune hemolytic anemia; *IMT,* immune-mediated thrombocytopenia; *RBC,* red blood cell; *SLE,* systemic lupus erythematosus.

### Direct Coombs' or Antiglobulin Test

The direct Coombs' test uses an antibody directed against canine (or feline) immunoglobulin (Ig) G, IgM, IgA, and complement; it is fairly sensitive and specific. The Coombs' reagent causes red blood cell (RBC) agglutination or lysis if IgG, IgM, IgA, or complement molecules are bound to the RBC surface. False-negative results can occur in patients with a small number of Ig molecules per RBC and in dogs receiving corticosteroids.

#### Interpretation

In most veterinary laboratories a direct antibody test (DAT) is considered positive if the titer is at least 1:32, but a positive DAT result indicates only that the patient has antibodies coating its RBCs, not that the patient has "autoimmune disease." A positive DAT result therefore should be interpreted with caution in patients with normal packed cell volumes. In dogs with IHA the titer does not correlate with either the severity of hemolysis or the response to treatment.

### Antinuclear Antibody Test

The antinuclear antibody (ANA) test detects circulating antibodies against the host's DNA. It is quite sensitive but not very specific. ANA test results are commonly positive in dogs and cats with a variety of infectious, inflammatory, and neoplastic diseases; certain drugs, such as propylthiouracil and procainamide, can also result in a positive ANA test. Unless the titer is extremely high, a positive ANA test result has little clinical relevance.

#### Interpretation

In most laboratories, titers greater than 1:10 are considered positive in dogs, and titers greater than 1:40 are considered positive in cats. Because chronic inflammatory, infectious, and degenerative processes can cause enough cell damage to release single strands of DNA (allowing production of antibodies against it), some laboratories are now evaluating ANA directed against double-stranded DNA, which may be more representative of true antibody-mediated nuclear damage.

### Direct Immunofluorescence or Immunohistochemistry

Direct immunofluorescence (DIF) or peroxidase-antiperoxidase (PAP) immunohistochemical stains detect Igs and complement in specially fixed tissue samples. DIF is also used in some laboratories for diagnosing IMT from a bone marrow sample. Fluorescence of the megakaryocytes suggests the presence of antimegakaryocyte (or antiplatelet) antibodies. However, this technique is not specific, and samples from dogs with malignancy or chronic inflammatory disease and normal platelet counts are often positive.

### Interpretation

In certain instances the pattern of antibody deposition suggests a specific pathologic process. In skin biopsies a positive DIF or PAP band in the basement membrane is suggestive of systemic lupus erythematosus (or discoid lupus), whereas intercellular epidermal fluorescence is compatible with pemphigus vulgaris, foliaceus, or vegetans; a combination of both is usually seen in pemphigus erythematosus.

## Other Tests

### Rheumatoid factor

The rheumatoid factor test detects the presence of IgM directed against Igs in the patient's serum and typically has a positive result in dogs with rheumatoid arthritis (see Chapter 76). However, this test is not very sensitive or specific. In most laboratories, titers greater than 1:40 are considered positive in dogs.

# 93

# Immunosuppressive Drugs

## *(Text pp 1216-1219)*

Immunosuppressive drugs are commonly used to induce or maintain remission in dogs and cats with immune-mediated diseases (IMDs). As with anticancer chemotherapy, the therapeutic approach with IMDs involves three (and possibly four) strategies or phases: (1) induction of remission, (2) maintenance, (3) reinduction of remission, or "rescue," and (4) intensification. In patients with mild IMDs the induction phase may not be necessary, and maintenance treatment can be initiated at the time of diagnosis.

Drugs commonly used for induction, intensification, maintenance, and rescue are listed in Box 93-1.

## CORTICOSTEROIDS (TEXT PP 1216-1217)

Corticosteroids are the most widely used immunosuppressants in dogs and cats. The two drugs most frequently used are prednisone and dexamethasone. Prednisone is used for both induction and maintenance, whereas dexamethasone is typically used only for induction, and only briefly. Prednisolone may be a better choice than prednisone in cats.

### Dosage

During induction, prednisone (or equivalent doses of dexamethasone) is used daily for 7 to 10 days at 2 to 4 mg/kg in dogs and 4 to 8 mg/kg in cats. The dose is then gradually decreased, and the administration interval lengthened to every other day.

### Adverse effects

Adverse effects in dogs include iatrogenic hyperadrenocorticism (see Chapter 53), gastrointestinal (GI) ulceration, recurrent urinary tract infections, and pancreatitis. Acute GI ulceration and pancreatitis are more likely to occur when dexamethasone is used. Adverse effects in cats are generally minimal or nonexistent, although diabetes mellitus (which usually resolves after the drugs are discontinued) may develop.

---

**Box 93-1**

## Immunosuppressive Drugs Used for Induction, Intensification, Maintenance, and Rescue in Dogs and Cats with Immune-Mediated Diseases

### INDUCTION OF REMISSION

Prednisone: 2-4 mg/kg PO q24h (dogs) or 4-8 mg/kg PO q24h (cats)
Dexamethasone sodium phosphate (Azium SP): 1-4 mg/kg IV single dose (dogs and cats)
Cyclophosphamide (Cytoxan): 200-300 mg/m$^2$ IV single dose (dogs) or 200-250 mg/m$^2$ PO single dose (cats)
Vincristine (Oncovin): 0.5 mg/m$^2$ IV single dose (dogs and cats)*
Human IV immunoglobulin: 0.5-1.5 g/kg IV, single dose (dogs)

### INTENSIFICATION

Cyclophosphamide (Cytoxan): 200-300 mg/m$^2$ IV single dose (dogs) or 200-250 mg/m$^2$ PO single dose (cats) *[used only if prednisone alone failed to induce remission]*

### MAINTENANCE

Prednisone: 1-2 mg/kg PO q48h (dogs) or 2-4 mg/kg PO q48h (cats)
Dexamethasone: 4 mg/cat PO every 1-2 week (cats)
Azathioprine (Imuran): 50-75 mg/m$^2$ PO q24-48h (dogs)
Chlorambucil (Leukeran): 20 mg/m$^2$ PO every 2 weeks or 2 mg/m$^2$ PO q48h (cats)

### RESCUE (REINDUCTION OF REMISSION)

Cyclophosphamide (Cytoxan): 200-300 mg/m$^2$ IV single dose (dogs) or 200-250 mg/m$^2$ PO single dose (cats)
Cyclophosphamide (Cytoxan): 50 mg/m$^2$ PO q48h for 4 days and off for 3 days (alternating) (dogs)
Danazol (Danocrine): 5 mg/kg PO q12h (dogs)(cats?)
Human IV immunoglobulin: 0.5-1.5 g/kg IV, single dose (dogs)

---

*Of questionable efficacy in immune-mediated thrombocytopenia (see text p 1191).
*IV,* Intravenously; *PO,* orally.

## CYCLOPHOSPHAMIDE (TEXT P 1217)

Cyclophosphamide (Cytoxan) is a very effective induction agent in dogs (and possibly cats) with IMDs. It is also effective in dogs with immune-mediated polyarthritis, dermatitis, and systemic lupus erythematosus (SLE).

### Dosage

At 200 to 300 mg/m$^2$ given once intravenously (IV), cyclophosphamide induces or consolidates remission in dogs with steroid nonresponsive or severe immune-mediated hemolytic anemia (IHA) and/or immune-mediated thrombocytopenia (IMT). In cats the same dose is given orally, because vomiting and anorexia are common with intravenous administration. The oral form can also be used every other day or 4 days on and 3 days off, continuously at a dose of 50 mg/m$^2$ in dogs.

### Adverse effects

A common adverse effect of chronic cyclophosphamide treatment in dogs is sterile hemorrhagic cystitis, which frequently develops after 8 to 10 weeks of continuous treatment. Female dogs are at increased risk and should be monitored by periodic urinalyses and physical examinations while receiving the drug. Concurrent administration of prednisone decreases the risk of cystitis. This problem is extremely rare in cats.

Two other common adverse effects are anorexia (mainly in cats) and myelosuppression (dogs and cats). A complete blood count (CBC) should be obtained every 2 to 4 weeks, and the dose adjusted accordingly (see Chapter 80).

## AZATHIOPRINE (TEXT PP 1217-1218)

Azathioprine (Imuran) is a very effective maintenance drug, but because it has a delayed onset of action (2 to 4 weeks), it is not the first drug of choice for induction. Azathioprine is an excellent drug for maintenance in dogs with immune-mediated cytopenias, dermatopathies, polyarthritis, and SLE.

### Dosage
Azathioprine (50 mg/m$^2$ orally [PO]) is usually given daily for 1 week and then every other day. It can be used routinely in dogs with IMDs and corticosteroid intolerance (e.g., polyuria and polydipsia, panting, psychosis) and in those in which corticosteroid therapy alone is not sufficient to induce or maintain remission. Myelosuppression is extremely common in dogs receiving azathioprine at doses of 2.2 mg/kg.

### Adverse effects
The most common adverse effect is myelosuppression, particularly in cats. Given its severe myelosuppressive effects, this drug should not be used in cats; chlorambucil is as effective and better tolerated. In dogs a CBC should be obtained every 2 to 4 weeks and the dose adjusted accordingly (see Chapter 80). A cholestatic hepatopathy can develop at high doses.

## CHLORAMBUCIL (TEXT P 1218)

Chlorambucil (Leukeran) is effective in maintenance protocols; like azathioprine, it appears to have a delayed action (2 to 4 weeks).

### Dosage
Chlorambucil is given at doses of 20 mg/m$^2$ PO every other week, or 2 to 4 mg/m$^2$ PO every other day. This drug is almost devoid of toxicity, although occasionally myelosuppression or anorexia occurs; cholestatic hepatopathy occurs in a few cats receiving chronic chlorambucil treatment. It is the drug of choice for maintenance in cats that do not tolerate or respond to corticosteroids. In cats it has been effective in lymphoplasmacytic gastroenteritis, stomatitis, pododermatitis, immune-mediated blood diseases, and SLE.

## GOLD SALTS (TEXT P 1218)

Gold salts are used for the management of steroid-refractory, immune-mediated dermatopathies and polyarthritis, as well as for other IMDs. Gold salts available for therapeutic use include gold sodium thiomalate (Myochrysine), aurothioglucose (Solganal), and thiethylphosphine gold or auranofin (Ridaura). The first two are administered intramuscularly, and the latter is given orally. Auranofin is effective in dogs with immune-mediated polyarthritis, pemphigus foliaceus, and pemphigus vulgaris.

### Dosage and adverse effects
Auranofin (Ridaura) is given at a dose of 0.05 to 0.2 mg/kg PO q12h, up to a total of 9 mg/day. Its major toxicity is reversible thrombocytopenia. Adverse effects of other gold salts include cutaneous and mucosal reactions, cytopenias, and reversible renal tubular damage.

## CYCLOSPORIN A (TEXT P 1218)

Cyclosporin A (CyA; Sandimmune; Atopica) is used extensively in dogs and cats undergoing bone marrow and kidney transplantation. No beneficial effects are apparent in dogs and cats with immune-mediated dermatitis, glomerulonephritis, or polyarthritis.

However, topical CyA is beneficial in dogs with keratoconjunctivitis sicca and pannus and in some immune-mediated dermatopathies. Some clinicians recommend CyA for dogs with refractory IHA or IMT.

#### Dosage and adverse effects

CyA is given at 7 to 15 mg/kg/day, doses that result in therapeutic serum concentrations of 200 to 400 ng/ml; toxicity usually occurs with serum concentrations greater than 600 ng/ml. CyA is usually cost prohibitive in large dogs, and it can cause anaphylaxis when administered IV to dogs. Other adverse effects in dogs include GI irritation, hirsutism, gingival hyperplasia, papillomatosis, and nephrotoxicosis.

## DANAZOL (TEXT PP 1218-1219)

Danazol (Danocrine) is an androgenic steroid with minimal masculinizing properties. It may be used in dogs with steroid-refractory IMT or IHA; beneficial responses have been reported in a limited number of patients. Danazol can also be used in patients with IMD in which conventional immunosuppressive treatment has failed; however, it may be cost prohibitive in large dogs. A dose of 5 mg/kg orally every 12 hours is used. At this dose, adverse effects are minimal.

# 94

# Systemic Lupus Erythematosus

## *(Text pp 1220-1221)*

#### Etiology

Systemic lupus erythematosus (SLE) is a chronic, multisystemic, immune-mediated disease in which immunity is directed against a variety of tissue components. Although its cause is unknown, SLE may be genetically transmitted or infectious in nature. This disease is well characterized in both dogs and cats.

#### Clinical features

SLE can mimic a variety of chronic inflammatory, infectious, and neoplastic disorders (Table 94-1). Typical findings include shifting limb lameness (polyarthritis), bullous or erythematosus skin lesions, petechiae and ecchymoses (thrombocytopenia and/or vasculitis), icterus (immune-mediated hemolysis), and edema or ascites (hypo-albuminemia secondary to immune-complex glomerulonephritis). In addition, patients with SLE usually display pyrexia, lymphadenopathy, splenomegaly, and/or polyclonal gammopathies.

*Hematology.* Complete blood count usually reveals hemolytic anemia, thrombocytopenia, neutropenia, and/or hyperproteinemia. If severe glomerulonephritis is present, the dog may become hypoproteinemic. Serum biochemistry changes variably

Table 94-1

## Organs and Tissues Affected in Dogs with Systemic Lupus Erythematosus

| Organ or tissue affected | Disorder |
| --- | --- |
| Red blood cells | Immune-mediated hemolytic anemia |
| Platelets | Immune-mediated thrombocytopenia |
| Neutrophils | Immune-mediated neutropenia |
| Clotting factors | Coagulopathy |
| Synovium | Nonerosive polyarthritis |
| Glomeruli (tubules) | Glomerulonephritis |
| Blood vessels | Vasculitis |
| Epidermis | Dermatitis |
| Central nervous system | Encephalitis |
| Skeletal muscle or end plate | Polymyositis, polyneuritis, myasthenia gravis |

include hypoalbuminemia, hyperglobulinemia, hyperbilirubinemia, azotemia, and high liver enzyme activities. Urinalysis may reveal proteinuria with or without bilirubinuria.

### Diagnosis

Diagnosis is based on careful evaluation of the clinical and clinicopathologic findings, as well as results of immunologic tests (see Chapter 92). If SLE is suspected, the following tests are indicated:

- radiography to rule out erosive (rheumatoid) polyarthritis
- joint tap for cytology
- direct Coombs' test (if the dog is anemic)
- bone marrow aspiration (if the dog has nonregenerative anemia, neutropenia, and/or thrombocytopenia)
- lymph node and/or splenic aspiration (if lymphadenopathy or splenomegaly is present)
- skin biopsy for histopathology and direct immunofluorescence or immuno-histochemistry (if cutaneous lesions are present)
- renal biopsy for histopathology and direct immunofluorescence or immuno-peroxidase (if glomerulonephritis is suspected)

A dog with two or more of the following should be considered to have SLE: cytopenia, oligoarthritis or polyarthritis, glomerulonephritis, focal or multifocal central nervous system signs, dermatitis, polymyositis, myasthenia gravis, or vasculitis, together with a positive antinuclear antibody test (>1:10).

*Differential diagnoses.* Canine ehrlichiosis, multiple myeloma, and bacterial endo-carditis are the most important differential diagnoses. Canine ehrlichiosis can be ruled out by serology or polymerase chain reaction assay for *Ehrlichia canis* (see Chapter 101); multiple myeloma by performance of bone marrow aspiration, radiography, and protein electrophoresis (see Chapter 91); and bacterial endocarditis by detection of a murmur, evaluation of an echocardiogram, and performance of bacterial blood culture.

### Treatment

Treatment is similar to that of dogs with other immune-mediated diseases (see Chapter 93).

# 95

# Fever of Undetermined Origin

## (Text pp 1222-1225)

In veterinary medicine, *fever of undetermined* (or *unknown*) *origin* (FUO) is the term used for fever that does not respond to antibacterial treatment and for which a diagnosis is not obvious after a minimum database has been obtained.

### Disorders Associated with FUO
The most common cause of FUO is infection, followed by immune-mediated, neoplastic, and miscellaneous disorders (Table 95-1). Despite aggressive evaluation, the cause of the fever cannot be found in 10% to 15% of patients.

### Diagnostic Approach
A three-stage approach is recommended. The first stage consists of a thorough history and physical examination and the compilation of a minimum database. The second stage involves additional diagnostic tests. The third stage, which consists of a therapeutic trial, is instituted when no diagnosis can be made.

#### Stage I
When a febrile patient fails to respond to antibacterial treatment, a thorough history should be obtained, a complete physical examination performed, and a minimum database collected.

*History.* The history rarely provides clues to the cause of the fever. However, a history of tick infestation suggests the possibility of a rickettsial or hemoparasitic disorder; tetracycline administration in a cat suggests the possibility of a drug-induced fever; and travel to areas in which systemic mycoses are endemic should prompt further investigation by means of cytology, serology, or fungal cultures.

*Physical examination.* It is important to evaluate the lymphoreticular organs. A number of infectious and neoplastic diseases affecting these organs (e.g., ehrlichiosis, Rocky Mountain spotted fever, bartonellosis, leukemia, systemic mycoses) can result in fever.

The oropharynx should be thoroughly inspected and palpated for signs of pharyngitis, stomatitis, or tooth root abscesses. The bones should also be thoroughly palpated, particularly in young dogs; metabolic bone disorders such as hypertrophic osteodystrophy can cause fever and bone pain. Palpation and passive motion of all joints are also indicated. A neurologic examination should be conducted to detect signs compatible with meningitis or other central nervous system lesions. In older cats the ventral cervical region should be palpated for thyroid enlargement or nodules.

The thorax should be carefully auscultated for a murmur, which could indicate bacterial endocarditis. A thorough ocular examination may reveal changes suggestive of a specific cause (e.g., chorioretinitis in cats with feline infectious peritonitis [FIP] or dogs with ehrlichiosis).

Table 95-1

## Causes of Fever of Undetermined Origin in Dogs and Cats

| Cause | Species affected | Cause | Species affected |
|---|---|---|---|
| **INFECTIOUS** | | Feline immunodeficiency | |
| **Bacterial** | | virus infection | C |
| Subacute bacterial | | **Protozoal** | |
| endocarditis | D | Babesiosis | D |
| Brucellosis | D | Hepatozoonosis | D |
| Tuberculosis | D, C | Cytauxzoonosis | C |
| Plague | C | Chagas' disease | D |
| Lyme disease | D | Leishmaniasis | D |
| Bartonellosis | D, C | | |
| Hemobartonellosis | D, C | **IMMUNE-MEDIATED** | |
| Suppurative infection | D, C | Polyarthritis | D, C |
| Abscesses (liver, pancreas, | | Vasculitis | D |
| stump pyometra) | | Meningitis | D |
| Prostatitis | | Systemic lupus erythematosus | D |
| Diskospondylitis | | Immune hemolytic anemia | D, C |
| Pyelonephritis | | Steroid-responsive fever | D |
| Peritonitis, pyothorax | | Steroid-responsive neutropenia | D, C |
| Septic arthritis | | | |
| | | **NEOPLASTIC** | |
| **Rickettsial** | | Acute leukemia | D, C |
| Ehrlichiosis | D | Chronic leukemia | D |
| Rocky Mountain spotted fever | D | Lymphoma | D, C |
| Salmon poisoning | D | Malignant histiocytosis | D, C |
| | | Multiple myeloma | D, C |
| **Mycotic** | | Necrotic solid tumors | D, C |
| Histoplasmosis | D, C | | |
| Blastomycosis | D, C | **MISCELLANEOUS** | |
| Coccidioidomycosis | D | Metabolic bone disorders | D |
| | | Drug-induced (tetracycline, | |
| **Viral** | | penicillins, sulfa) | C, D |
| Feline infectious peritonitis | C | Tissue necrosis | D, C |
| Feline leukemia virus infection | C | Hyperthyroidism | C, D |
| | | Idiopathic | D, C |

*C,* Cats; *D,* dogs.

*Clinicopathologic data.* A minimum database consisting of a complete blood count (CBC), serum biochemistry profile, urinalysis, and urine bacterial culture and susceptibility should be obtained. The CBC can provide important clues regarding the cause of the fever (Table 95-2). A serum biochemistry profile is rarely diagnostic in patients with FUO, although it provides indirect information regarding organ function. Hyperglobulinemia and hypoalbuminemia suggest an infectious, immune-mediated, or neoplastic disorder (see Chapter 91). A finding of pyuria or white blood cell casts on urinalysis may suggest a urinary tract infection such as pyelonephritis.

*Fine-needle aspiration.* An enlarged lymph node or spleen should be evaluated cytologically by means of fine-needle aspiration; a sample can also be obtained for bacterial or fungal culture, if indicated. Any palpable mass or swelling should also be aspirated to rule out neoplasia and granulomatous, pyogranulomatous, or suppurative inflammation.

Table 95-2

**Table 95-2**

## Hematologic Changes in Dogs and Cats with Fever of Undetermined Origin

| Hematologic change | Compatible condition |
|---|---|
| Regenerative anemia | Immune-mediated diseases, hemoparasites, drugs |
| Nonregenerative anemia | Infection, immune-mediated diseases, tissue necrosis, malignancy, endocarditis |
| Neutrophilia with left shift | Infection, immune-mediated diseases, tissue necrosis, malignancy, endocarditis |
| Neutropenia | Leukemia, immune-mediated diseases, pyogenic infection, bone marrow infiltrative disease, drugs |
| Monocytosis | Infection, immune-mediated diseases, tissue necrosis, lymphoma, endocarditis |
| Lymphocytosis | Ehrlichiosis, Chagas' disease, leishmaniasis, chronic lymphocytic leukemia |
| Eosinophilia | Hypereosinophilic syndrome, eosinophilic inflammation, lymphoma |
| Thrombocytopenia | Rickettsiae, leukemia, lymphoma, drugs, immune-mediated diseases |
| Thrombocytosis | Infections (chronic), immune-mediated diseases |

### Stage II

During a search for a silent septic focus or other source of persistent fever, the following diagnostic tests may be indicated:

- thoracic and abdominal radiography
- abdominal ultrasonography
- echocardiography (if the patient has a heart murmur)
- serial blood cultures (bacterial and fungal)
- immune tests (e.g., antinuclear antibody, rheumatoid factor; see Chapter 92)
- serum protein electrophoresis (see Chapter 91)
- serology or polymerase chain reaction assay (e.g., systemic mycoses, rickettsial diseases, bartonellosis, FIP, feline immunodeficiency virus, feline leukemia virus, brucellosis, babesiosis, Lyme disease)
- arthrocentesis for cytology and bacterial culture
- bone marrow aspiration for cytology and culture (bacterial and fungal)
- cerebrospinal fluid analysis (in patients with neurologic signs associated with fever)
- biopsy of any lesion or enlarged organ
- leukocyte scanning
- exploratory celiotomy

### Stage III

When a definitive diagnosis cannot be made, a therapeutic trial of antibacterial and antifungal agents, immunosuppressive doses of corticosteroids, or antipyretics can be initiated.

## Treatment Approach

If a definitive diagnosis is made, specific treatment should be initiated. A therapeutic trial is warranted in all other patients.

### Corticosteroids

If the patient has already been treated with broad-spectrum bactericidal antibiotics, immunosuppressive doses of corticosteroids can be tried (see Chapter 93). However, the owners should be informed of the potential consequences of this approach: if the dog or cat has an undiagnosed infectious disease, death can occur from systemic dissemination of the organism. The patient should be kept in the hospital and monitored frequently for worsening of clinical signs, in which case steroid therapy should be discontinued. In patients with immune-mediated (or steroid-responsive) FUO, the pyrexia and clinical signs usually resolve within 24 to 48 hours of initiation of treatment.

### Antipyretics or antibiotics

If no response to corticosteroids is observed, two courses of action remain. First, the patient can be released on antipyretic drugs, such as aspirin (10 to 25 mg/kg orally [PO] q12h in dogs, and 10 mg/kg PO q3d in cats), carprofen, or deracoxib, with instructions to return for complete reevaluation in 1 or 2 weeks. However, antipyretics should be used with caution. Fever is a protective mechanism, and suppressing it may be detrimental. Furthermore, most nonsteroidal antiinflammatory drugs have potential ulcerogenic effects and can cause cytopenias and tubular nephropathy (in patients that become dehydrated or receive other nephrotoxic drugs).

The second course of action is to continue antibiotic trials, using a combination of bactericidal drugs (e.g., ampicillin and enrofloxacin) for a minimum of 5 to 7 days.

# 96

---

# Recurrent Infections

## *(Text pp 1226-1228)*

Recurrent or persistent infections are usually the result of congenital or acquired abnormalities of the immune system.

### Congenital immunodeficiency syndromes

Congenital immunodeficiency syndromes can affect the humoral, cellular, or phagocytic systems, either singly or in combination (Table 96-1). They are more common in dogs than in cats.

*Humoral immunodeficiency.* Humoral immunodeficiency syndromes usually result in recurrent upper and lower respiratory tract infections, dermatitis, and enteritis. Some Beagles with selective immunoglobulin (Ig) A deficiency also experience grand mal seizures and may be more susceptible to immune-mediated diseases.

*Cellular immunodeficiency.* Cellular immunodeficiency disorders are less common; a T-cell abnormality has been documented in Weimaraners with pituitary dwarfism and in Bull Terriers with lethal acrodermatitis. The disease in Weimaraner puppies is characterized by retarded growth and recurrent respiratory and gastrointestinal infections. Necropsy findings include thymic hypoplasia with absence of thymic cortex. The disease in Bull Terriers causes growth retardation, progressive acrodermatitis, chronic pyoderma and paronychia, pneumonia, and diarrhea.

Other diseases with inconsistent cell-mediated immunologic abnormalities include *Pneumocystis carinii* infection in Dachshunds and systemic aspergillosis, generalized demodicosis, and prototothecosis in other breeds. Basset Hounds and Miniature Schnauzers have increased susceptibility to mycobacteriosis. Birman cats with congenital

Table 96-1

## Congenital Immunodeficiency Syndromes in Dogs and Cats

| Arm | Defect | Breed |
|---|---|---|
| Humoral | IgA deficiency | Beagle, Shar Pei, German Shepherd Dog? |
| | IgM deficiency | Doberman Pinscher? |
| | C3 deficiency | Brittany Spaniel |
| | Transient hypogammaglobulinemia | Samoyed |
| Cellular | | Weimaraner, Bull Terrier, Basset Hounds, Dachshunds? Birman cats |
| Phagocytic | Cyclic hematopoiesis | Gray Collie |
| | Abnormal granulation | Birman cat |
| | Chédiak-Higashi syndrome | Persian cat |
| | Mucopolysaccharidosis | Domestic Shorthair cat, Siamese cat. |
| | Defective neutrophil adhesion | Irish Setter |
| | Defective bactericidal capacity | Doberman Pinscher |
| | Abnormal chemiluminescence | Weimaraner |
| Combined | Severe combined immunodeficiency | Basset Hound |

*Ig,* Immunoglobulin.

hypotrichosis and thymic atrophy are born hairless and have severe cell-mediated immune deficiency.

***Phagocytic abnormalities.*** Specific disorders of phagocytic function are listed in Table 96-1. Irish Setters with defective neutrophil adhesion (leukocyte adhesion deficiency) have recurrent episodes of omphalophlebitis, gingivitis, lymphadenitis, pyoderma, respiratory infections, pyometra, and fulminant sepsis. Dobermans with defective bactericidal capacity exhibit recurrent episodes of rhinitis and pneumonia that respond transiently to antibiotic therapy.

***Combined immunodeficiency.*** Basset Hounds experience a syndrome that affects more than one arm of the immune system (SCIDS). It causes severe growth retardation and early death; low serum IgG and IgA concentrations are common in affected dogs.

### Acquired immunodeficiency

Acquired immunodeficiency syndromes include canine distemper virus, parvovirus, and ehrlichial infections, as well as generalized demodicosis in dogs and feline leukemia virus and feline immunodeficiency virus in cats. In addition, systemic anticancer agents can cause variable degrees of immunosuppression or little clinical consequence.

### Diagnosis

The type of infectious agent and the pattern of infection are usually determined by the nature of the defect. Defects in humoral immunity often result in infections with pyogenic organisms at one or more sites. Defects in T-cell function result in viral, fungal, or protozoal infections that are usually widespread. Abnormalities in the phagocytic system may result in skin, respiratory, meningeal, or systemic infections with pyogenic or enteric organisms.

***Specific tests.*** Several diagnostic tests can be used to evaluate dogs and cats with suspected immunodeficiency. Some of these tests (e.g., neutrophil function tests, lymphocyte blastogenesis) require fresh blood samples (within 4 hours of collection) and specialized laboratory equipment. Other tests can be performed on serum samples and mailed to referral laboratories. Table 96-2 lists tests that can be used to evaluate patients with recurrent infections.

Table 96-2

## Laboratory Diagnosis of Immunodeficiency Syndromes in Dogs and Cats

| Arm | Tests |
| --- | --- |
| Humoral | Serum protein electrophoresis, immunoelectrophoresis, radial immunodiffusion for Ig concentrations, complement activity, immunophenotyping |
| Cellular | Lymphocyte blastogenesis in response to concanavalin A, pokeweed mitogen, and phytohemagglutinin; enumeration of circulating T cells; NK cell assays; immunophenotyping |
| Phagocytic | Nylon-wool adhesion; migration under agarose; phagocytosis of bacteria, yeasts, or latex; phagocytosis of opsonized particles; chemiluminescence; nitroblue tetrazolium reduction test; bacterial killing assay; flow cytometry |

*Ig,* Immunoglobulin; *NK,* natural killer.

### Management

Management includes use of appropriate antimicrobial drugs based on results of bacterial or fungal culture and sensitivity. If an infectious agent cannot be isolated and the patient appears to have a bacterial infection, bactericidal antibiotics that attain high intraleukocyte concentrations (e.g., sulfa-trimethoprim, enrofloxacin) should be used. Dogs and cats with suspected or known immunodeficiencies should be kept current on their vaccinations, although modified-live vaccines should be avoided.

*Immunomodulators.* Nonspecific immunomodulators may be of benefit. Levamisole (3 mg/kg orally two to three times a week) is beneficial in some dogs with recurrent infections. This drug should be used with caution in cats.

# PART XIII

# Infectious Diseases

MICHAEL R. LAPPIN

# 97

# Laboratory Diagnosis of Infectious Diseases

## (Text pp 1229-1239)

### DEMONSTRATING THE ORGANISM (TEXT PP 1229-1237)

#### Fecal examination

Examination of feces can aid diagnosis of parasitic diseases of the gastrointestinal tract (Table 97-1) and respiratory tract (Table 97-2). Specific techniques are described in the text.

##### Direct smear.

Fresh, liquid feces or feces that contain large quantities of mucus should be examined for protozoal trophozoites, including *Giardia* spp., *Balantidium coli*, *Pentatrichomonas hominis*, and *Entamoeba histolytica*. The saline smear technique can improve detection of these motile organisms.

##### Stained smear.
A thin fecal smear should be made for all dogs and cats with diarrhea. Material should be collected by rectal swab, if possible. White blood cells and bacteria consistent with *Campylobacter* spp. or *Clostridium perfringens* can be observed after staining with Diff-Quik or Wright's-Giemsa stains. *Histoplasma capsulatum* or *Prototheca* may be observed in the cytoplasm of mononuclear cells. Methylene blue in acetate buffer (pH 3.6) stains trophozoites of the enteric protozoans. Iodine stains and acid methyl green are also used to demonstrate protozoans. Modified acid-fast staining of a thin fecal smear aids diagnosis of cryptosporidiosis: *Cryptosporidium* spp. are the only enteric organisms 4 to 6 μm in diameter that stain pink-to-red with acid-fast stain. Presence of neutrophils on rectal cytology suggests inflammation induced by *Salmonella* spp., *Campylobacter* spp., or *C. perfringens*; fecal culture is indicated in these cases.

##### Fecal flotation.
Most ova, oocysts, and cysts are easily identified after sodium salt flotation or zinc sulfate centrifugal flotation. Zinc sulfate centrifugal flotation is best for demonstrating protozoan cysts, particularly *Giardia* spp.

##### Fecal sedimentation.
Fecal sedimentation recovers most cysts and ova but also contains debris. It is superior to flotation procedures for identifying fluke eggs.

##### Baermann technique.
The Baermann technique is used to concentrate motile larvae (especially respiratory parasites) from feces. Eggs or larva from respiratory parasites can also be detected by cytologic evaluation of airway washings (see Chapter 20).

#### Cytology

Cytologic demonstration of some infectious agents constitutes a definitive diagnosis. Thin smears are preferred for demonstration of most organisms. Cells in airway or prostatic washings, urine, aqueous humor, and cerebrospinal fluid (CSF) should be pelleted by centrifugation at $2000 \times g$ for 5 minutes before staining. One drop of 22% albumin or normal canine serum should be added to CSF before centrifugation. Morphologic characteristics of selected bacterial and rickettsial agents are listed in Table 97-3.

**Table 97-1**

## Demonstration Techniques for Canine and Feline Gastrointestinal Parasites

| Organism | Form in stool | Species infested | Optimal fecal examination technique |
|---|---|---|---|
| **CESTODES** | | | |
| *Dipylidium caninum* | Ova | D, C | Identification of adult |
| *Echinococcus granulosus* | Ova | D | Identification of adult |
| *Echinococcus multilocularis* | Ova | D, C | Identification of adult |
| *Taenia* spp. | Ova | D, C | Identification of adult |
| **PROTOZOANS** | | | |
| *Balantidium coli* | Trophozoite | D | Direct or saline smear |
| | Cyst | D | Zinc sulfate centrifugal flotation |
| *Cryptosporidium parvum* | Oocyst | D, C | Acid-fast or monoclonal antibody stain |
| *Entamoeba histolytica* | Trophozoite | D, C | Direct or saline smear |
| | Cyst | D | Zinc sulfate centrifugal flotation |
| *Giardia* spp. | Trophozoite | D, C | Direct or saline smear |
| | Cyst | D | Zinc sulfate centrifugal flotation |
| *Isospora* spp. | Oocyst | D, C | Sugar or zinc sulfate centrifugal flotation |
| *Pentatrichomonas hominis* | Trophozoite | D, C | Direct or saline smear |
| | Cyst | D | Zinc sulfate centrifugation |
| *Toxoplasma gondii* | Oocyst | C | Sugar or zinc sulfate centrifugal flotation |
| **FLUKES** | | | |
| *Eurytrema procyonis* | Ova | C | Fecal sedimentation |
| *Nanophyetus salmincola* | Ova | D | Fecal sedimentation |
| *Platynosomum fastosum* | Ova | C | Fecal sedimentation |
| **HELMINTHS** | | | |
| *Ancylostoma* spp. | Ova | D, C | Sugar or zinc sulfate centrifugal flotation |
| *Ollulanus tricuspis* | Ova | C | Sugar or zinc sulfate centrifugal flotation |
| *Physaloptera* spp. | Ova | D, C | Sugar or zinc sulfate centrifugal flotation |
| *Spirocerca lupi* | Ova | D | Sugar or zinc sulfate centrifugal flotation |
| *Strongyloides stercoralis* | Larvae | D, C | Baermann technique |
| *Toxascaris* spp. | Ova | D, C | Sugar or zinc sulfate centrifugal flotation |
| *Toxocara* spp. | Ova | D, C | Sugar or zinc sulfate centrifugal flotation |
| *Trichuris vulpis* | Ova | D | Sugar or zinc sulfate centrifugal flotation |
| *Uncinaria stenocephala* | Ova | D, C | Sugar or zinc sulfate centrifugal flotation |

*C*, Cats; *D*, dogs.

Table 97-2

## Demonstration Techniques for Common Canine and Feline Respiratory Tract Parasites

| Organism | Form in stool | Species infected | Optimal fecal examination technique |
|---|---|---|---|
| *Aelurostrongylus abstrusus* (lungworm) | Larvae | C | Baermann technique |
| *Andersonstrongylus milksi* (lungworm) | Larvae | D | Baermann technique |
| *Capillaria aerophila* | Ova | D | Sugar or zinc sulfate centrifugal flotation |
| *Crenosoma vulpis* (lungworm) | Ova | D | Sugar or zinc sulfate centrifugal flotation |
| *Eucoleus boehmi* (nasal worm) | Ova | D | Sugar or zinc sulfate centrifugal flotation |
| *Filaroides hirthi* (lungworm) | Larvae | D | Baermann technique |
| *Oslerus osleri* (tracheal nodular worm) | Ova or larvae | D | Zinc sulfate centrifugal flotation and Baermann technique |
| *Paragonimus kellicotti* (lung fluke) | Ova | D, C | Fecal sedimentation |
| *Pneumonyssoides caninum* (nasal mite) | None | D | None; visualization of adults |

*C,* Cats; *D,* dogs.

***Bacterial diseases.*** If bacterial disease is suspected, materials are collected aseptically and prepared for culture; bacterial culture is recommended for all samples with increased numbers of macrophages or neutrophils. Some bacteria cannot be successfully cultured. Bacteria can be present in small numbers, so failure to document organisms cytologically does not totally exclude the diagnosis. One of the slides for cytology should be stained with Wright's-Giemsa or Diff-Quik. If bacteria are seen, Gram stain of another slide is performed to differentiate gram-positive and gram-negative agents; this information facilitates the empirical selection of antibiotics. If filamentous, gram-positive rods are noted, acid-fast staining helps differentiate between *Actinomyces* (non–acid fast) and *Nocardia* (generally acid fast). If macrophages or neutrophils are found, acid-fast staining is indicated for identification of *Mycobacterium* spp. within the cytoplasm.

*Helicobacter* spp. in specimens made from gastric brushings are easiest to see after staining with Warthin-Starry stain. Some organisms, such as *Mycoplasma,* are rarely documented cytologically.

***Haemobartonella.*** *Haemobartonella felis* (previously classified as *Rickettsia,* now classified as *Mycoplasma* spp.) and *Haemobartonella canis* can be detected on the surface of red blood cells (RBCs) but have never been successfully cultured. Documentation of infection is based on polymerase chain reaction (PCR) assay and/or cytology, but the latter is difficult because parasitemia is short-lived; also, if the blood is placed into ethylenediaminetetraacetic acid (EDTA), the organism commonly leaves the surface of the RBC. Collection of blood from an ear margin vessel, making thin blood smears immediately with blood that has not been placed into anticoagulant, or collecting blood into a heparinized syringe may aid in finding *Mycoplasma* spp. Wright's-Giemsa stain is the best stain to use in practice to detect these organisms.

***Rickettsial diseases.*** Occasionally, *Ehrlichia* spp. are found within the cytoplasm of cells in the peripheral blood, lymph node aspirates, bone marrow aspirates, and synovial

**Table 97-3**

## Cytomorphologic Characteristics of Small Animal Bacterial and Rickettsial Agents

| Agent | Morphologic characteristics |
|---|---|
| **BACTERIA** | |
| *Actinomyces* spp. | Gram-positive, non–acid-fast filamentous rod within sulfur granules |
| *Bacteroides fragilis* | Thin, filamentous, gram-negative rods |
| *Campylobacter jejuni* | Seagull-shaped spirochete in feces |
| *Chlamydia psittaci* | Large cytoplasmic inclusions in conjunctival cells or neutrophils |
| *Clostridium* spp. | Large gram-positive rods |
| *Clostridium perfringens* | Large spore-forming rods in feces |
| *Helicobacter* spp. | Tightly coiled spirochetes in gastric or duodenal brushings |
| *Mycobacterium* spp. | Intracytoplasmic acid-fast rods in macrophages or neutrophils |
| *Nocardia* spp. | Gram-positive, acid-fast filamentous rod within sulfur granules |
| *Leptospira* spp. | Spirochetes in urine; dark-field microscopy required |
| *Yersinia pestis* | Bipolar rods in cervical lymph nodes or airway fluids |
| *Haemobartonella felis* (*Mycoplasma haemofelis*) | Rod- or ring-shaped bacteria on the surface of red blood cells |
| *Haemobartonella canis* (*Mycoplasma haemocanis*) | Rod- or ring-shaped bacteria on the surface of red blood cells |
| **RICKETTSIA** | |
| *Ehrlichia canis* | Clusters of gram-negative bacteria (morulae) in mononuclear cells |
| *Ehrlichia ewingii* | Clusters of gram-negative bacteria (morulae) in neutrophils |
| *Ehrlichia equi* | Clusters of gram-negative bacteria (morulae) in neutrophils and eosinophils |
| *Ehrlichia platys* | Clusters of gram-negative bacteria (morulae) in platelets |
| *Ehrlichia risticii* | Clusters of gram-negative bacteria (morulae) in mononuclear cells |

fluid. *Ehrlichia* spp. morulae are found in different cell types (see Table 97-3). Wright's-Giemsa is superior to Wright's or Diff-Quik stain for demonstration of morulae.

*Fungal diseases.* Arthrospores and conidia of dermatophytes can be identified cytologically. Hairs plucked from the periphery of a lesion are covered with 10% to 20% potassium hydroxide (KOH) on a microscope slide, and the slide is heated and examined for dermatophytes. All cats with chronic, draining skin lesions should have imprints of the lesions made and stained with Wright's-Giemsa; microscopic examination may reveal the round, oval, or cigar-shaped yeast phase of *Sporothrix schenckii* within the cytoplasm of mononuclear cells. Periodic acid-Schiff (PAS) stain is superior to Wright's-Giemsa stain for demonstrating fungi. The cytologic appearance of systemic fungi is presented in Table 103-1.

*Cutaneous parasitic diseases. Cheyletiella* spp., *Demodex* spp., *Sarcoptes scabiei, Notoedres cati,* and *Otodectes cynotis* are the most common cutaneous parasites. *Cheyletiella* is found by pressing a piece of transparent tape against areas with crusts, placing the tape on a slide, and examining it microscopically. *Demodex* spp. are most commonly detected in deep skin scrapings and follicular exudates; *Cheyletiella* spp., *S. scabiei,* and *N. cati* are found in more superficial scrapings. *O. cynotis* or its eggs are detected in ceruminous exudates from the ear canals.

*Systemic protozoal diseases.* The cytologic appearance and location of the most common systemic protozoal diseases are summarized in Table 97-4. Wright's-Giemsa or Giemsa staining of thin blood films should be used to demonstrate *Leishmania* spp., *Trypanosoma cruzi*, *Babesia* spp., *Hepatozoon canis*, and *Cytauxzoon felis*. Collection of blood from an ear margin vessel may improve detection, particularly of *Babesia* spp. and *C. felis*. *Toxoplasma gondii* and *Neospora caninum* cause similar syndromes in dogs, and their tachyzoites cannot be distinguished morphologically; serology or immunocytochemical staining is required to differentiate these agents. Other systemic protozoans are rare and regionally defined (see Chapter 104).

*Viral diseases.* Rarely, viral inclusion bodies are detected cytologically after staining with Wright's-Giemsa. Distemper virus infection causes inclusions in circulating lymphocytes, neutrophils, and erythrocytes of some dogs. FIP virus can result in intracytoplasmic inclusions in circulating neutrophils. Feline herpesvirus 1 transiently causes intranuclear inclusion bodies in epithelial cells.

## Tissue techniques

Tissue samples should immediately be aseptically placed into appropriate transport media for culture or inoculation procedures (if indicated). Tissue impressions for cytology should be made before the sample is frozen or placed into either 10% buffered formalin or glutaraldehyde solution. Frozen specimens generally are superior for immunohistochemical staining and PCR. Glutaraldehyde-containing fixatives are best for electron microscopy (e.g., for demonstrating viral particles). Special stains may be needed for some infectious diseases; the histopathology laboratory should be notified of the suspected agent(s) for appropriate stain selection.

## Culture techniques

Successful culture depends on collecting the optimal materials without contamination and submitting them as quickly as possible in media that minimize organism

**Table 97-4**

## Cytomorphologic Characteristics of Small Animal Systemic Protozoal Agents

| Agent | Morphologic characteristics |
|---|---|
| *Babesia canis* | Paired piroplasms ($2.4 \times 5$ μm) in circulating red blood cells |
| *Babesia gibsoni* | Single piroplasms ($1 \times 3.2$ μm) in circulating red blood cells |
| *Cytauxzoon felis* | Piroplasms (1- $\times$ 1.5-μm "signet ring" form; 1- $\times$ 2-μm oval form; 1-μm round form) in circulating red blood cells or monocytes; macrophages of lymph node aspirates, splenic aspirates, or bone marrow |
| *Hepatozoon canis* | Gamonts in circulating neutrophils and monocytes |
| *Leishmania* spp. | Ovoid to round amastigotes (2.5-5 μm $\times$ 1.5-2 μm) in macrophages found on imprints of exudative skin lesions, lymph node aspirates, or bone marrow aspirates |
| *Neospora caninum* | Free or intracellular (macrophages or monocytes) tachyzoites (5-7 μm $\times$ 1-5 μm) in CSF, airway washings, or imprints of cutaneous lesions |
| *Toxoplasma gondii* | Free or intracellular (macrophages or monocytes) tachyzoites ($6 \times 2$ μm) in pleural effusions, peritoneal effusions, or airway washings |
| *Trypanosoma cruzi* | Flagellated trypomastigotes (one flagellum; 15-20 μm long) free in whole blood, lymph node aspirates, and peritoneal fluid |

*CSF*, Cerebrospinal fluid.

death and overgrowth of nonpathogens (see text). Culture results of body parts with normal bacterial and fungal flora (e.g., skin, ears, mouth, nasal cavity, trachea, feces, and vagina) are difficult to interpret. Positive culture results and the presence of inflammatory cells suggest that the organism is inducing disease. Culture of a single agent, particularly if the organism is relatively resistant to antimicrobials, is more consistent with a disease-inducing infection than if multiple, antibiotic-susceptible bacteria are cultured.

**Blood.** Samples for blood culture should be collected aseptically from a large vein after surgical preparation. In general, three 5-ml samples are collected over a 24-hour period in stable patients or every 1 to 3 hours in patients with sepsis. Culture for *Bartonella henselae* in cats is generally performed on 1.5 ml of whole blood collected aseptically and placed into EDTA.

**Feces.** Culture for *Salmonella* spp., *Campylobacter* spp., and *C. perfringens* requires 2 to 3 g of fresh feces. The samples should be submitted immediately, although *Salmonella* and *Campylobacter* are usually viable in refrigerated fecal specimens for 3 to 7 days; a transport medium should be used if a delay is expected. The laboratory should be notified of the suspected pathogen.

**Mycoplasma.** *Mycoplasma* and *Ureaplasma* cultures are performed on airway washings, synovial fluid, exudates from chronic draining tracts (cats), urine from animals with chronic urinary tract disease, and vaginal swabs from animals with genital tract disease. Samples should be submitted in Amies medium or modified Stuart bacterial transport medium. *Mycoplasma* spp. culture must be specifically requested.

**Mycobacterium.** Tissue samples or exudates from animals with suspected *Mycobacterium* spp. infection should be refrigerated immediately and transported to the laboratory as soon as possible. Exudates should be placed in transport media. The laboratory must be instructed to culture for *Mycobacterium* spp.

**Fungi.** Cutaneous fungal agents can be cultured in-house using routine culture media. Materials from animals with suspected systemic fungal infection should be transported to the laboratory as described for bacteria. The laboratory should be told specifically that fungal culture is needed. The yeast phase of systemic fungi is not zoonotic, but the mycelial phase of *Blastomyces*, *Coccidioides*, and *Histoplasma* can infect humans. In-house culture for these agents is therefore not recommended.

**Virus isolation.** Viral agents can sometimes be isolated from tissues or secretions. Samples should be collected aseptically as for bacteria, placed in transport media, immediately refrigerated, and transported to the laboratory on cold packs (but not frozen). The laboratory should be contacted before samples are submitted.

### Immunologic techniques

The laboratory should be contacted for details of specimen transport before collection. Immunocytochemistry and immunohistochemistry techniques are particularly valuable for detecting viral diseases and agents present in small numbers and for differentiating agents with similar morphologic features.

**Commercial assays.** Commercial assays for the detection of antigens in serum or plasma are routinely available for *Dirofilaria immitis*, *Cryptococcus neoformans*, and feline leukemia virus (Table 97-5). The *C. neoformans* latex agglutination procedure can also be performed on aqueous humor, vitreous humor, and CSF. Parvovirus, *Cryptosporidium parvum*, and *Giardia* spp. antigen detection procedures are available for use with feces. The parvovirus assay detects both canine and feline parvovirus antigen. Results of *C. parvum* and *Giardia* spp. assays should be interpreted in conjunction with results from fecal examination techniques.

**Immunocytochemistry and immunohistochemistry.** Immunocytochemistry and immunohistochemistry techniques are valuable for the detection of viral diseases, detection of agents present in small numbers, and for differentiation among agents with similar morphologic features. In general, these techniques are more sensitive and specific than histopathologic techniques and are comparable to culture. Focal feline infectious peritonitis granulomatous disease can be documented by immunohistochemical staining (see Chapter 102).

Table 97-5

## Immunodiagnostic Procedures for Common Infectious Agents in Small Animal Practice*

| Agent | Sample | Procedure[†] |
|---|---|---|
| **BACTERIAL or RICKETTSIAL** | | |
| *Chlamydophila felis* | Conjunctival scraping | DFA |
| *Leptospira* spp. | Tissues | DFA |
| *Rickettsia rickettsii* | Skin biopsy | DFA |
| *Yersinia pestis* | Exudate, airway washing | DFA |
| **FUNGAL** | | |
| *Cryptococcus neoformans* | Serum, plasma aqueous humor, vitreous humor, CSF | Latex agglutination |
| | Tissues | DFA |
| *Sporothrix schenckii* | Exudate or tissues | DFA |
| **HELMINTHS** | | |
| *Dirofilaria immitis* | Serum or plasma | ELISA |
| **PROTOZOAL** | | |
| *Cryptosporidium parvum* | Feces | ELISA |
| *Giardia* spp. | Feces | ELISA |
| *Neospora caninum* | Exudate, tissues | DFA |
| *Toxoplasma gondii* | Exudate, tissues | DFA |
| **VIRAL** | | |
| Feline calicivirus | Tissues | DFA |
| Feline coronavirus | Tissues | DFA |
| Feline herpesvirus I | Nasal swab, conjunctival scraping, oral-pharyngeal swab, tissues | DFA |
| Feline leukemia virus | Blood smear, bone marrow aspirate, tissues | DFA |
| | Blood, plasma, serum, tears, saliva | ELISA |
| Feline panleukopenia | Feces | ELISA |
| | Tissues | DFA |
| Canine coronavirus | Tissues | DFA |
| Canine distemper virus | Blood smear, buffy coat, conjunctival scraping, airway washings, CSF, tissues | DFA |
| Canine herpesvirus | Nasal swab, vaginal swab, tissues | DFA |
| Canine parvovirus | Feces | ELISA |
| | Tissues | DFA |
| Infectious canine hepatitis | Tissues | DFA |
| Rabies | Brain tissue | DFA |

*These procedures are available at most diagnostic laboratories, so specific references are not listed.

[†]Some organisms detected by DFA can also be detected by other immunohistochemical staining procedures or polymerase chain reaction.

*CSF,* Cerebrospinal fluid; *DFA,* direct fluorescent antibody staining; *ELISA,* enzyme-linked immunosorbent assay.

### Polymerase chain reaction

PCR assays are beneficial for documenting organisms that are either difficult to culture (e.g., *Ehrlichia* spp.) or cannot be cultured (e.g., *Mycoplasma* spp.). However, such assays can have false-positive results if sample contamination occurs. Specificity can be very high, but the test detects both live and dead organisms, so it may be posi-tive even if the infection has been controlled. When the organism being tested for commonly infects the background population of healthy pets (i.e., healthy pets are carriers, as in the case of FHV-1), interpretation of results for a single pet can be difficult. Therefore the predictive value of the PCR test must be carefully assessed. False-negative results can occur if the sample is handled inappropriately; results may also be affected by treatment. Currently no standardization exists among commercial PCR assays; in addition, no external quality control exists. PCR is commercially available for canine *Babesia* spp, canine and feline *Ehrlichia* spp. (blood), canine and feline *Bartonella* spp. (blood, aqueous humor), feline *Mycoplasma haemofelis* (blood), *T. gondii* (aqueous humor, CSF), feline coronavirus (tissues and body fluids), FHV-1 (conjunctival swabs, aqueous humor), feline calicivirus (conjunctival swabs), *Mycoplasma felis* (conjunctival swabs, joint fluid), and *Chlamydophila felis* (conjunctival swabs), and new tests are being developed almost daily. See specific chapters for a discussion of the use of PCR for the detection of the agents.

### Animal inoculation

*T. gondii* can be differentiated from *Hammondia hammondi* or *Besnoitia darlingi* by inoculation of sporulated oocysts into mice. However, because live animals are required, inoculation is rarely used in small animal practice.

### Electron microscopy

Electron microscopy is a very sensitive procedure for organism identification, especially detection of viral particles in feces. Approximately 1 to 3 g of feces without fixative should be transported overnight on cold packs to the diagnostic laboratory at which the procedure can be performed.

## ANTIBODY DETECTION (TEXT PP 1237-1238)

### Serum

Complement fixation, hemagglutination inhibition, serum neutralization, and agglutination assays generally detect all antibody classes in a serum sample. Western blot immunoassay, indirect fluorescent antibody assay, and enzyme-linked immunosorbent assay can be adapted to detect specific immunoglobulin (Ig) M, IgG, or IgA responses. Principles and methodology are discussed in the text.

Most infectious agents can induce disease within 3 to 10 days of initial exposure; but serum IgG antibodies are usually not detected until 2 to 3 weeks after exposure. Therefore false-negative results of serum antibody tests during acute disease probably are common. If results of specific serum IgG testing are negative in an animal with acute disease, repeat testing should be performed in 2 to 3 weeks; increasing antibody titers are consistent with recent or active infection. It is preferable to assess both the acute and convalescent sera in the same assay on the same day to avoid interassay variation. In general, serum antibody tests in puppies and kittens cannot be interpreted as specific responses until at least 8 to 12 weeks of age because of antibodies passed in colostrum.

Positive results should always be interpreted only as evidence of present or prior infection by the agent. Recent or active infection is suggested by the presence of IgM or by an increasing antibody titer or seroconversion over 2 to 3 weeks. However, failure to document recent or active infection based on serology does not exclude a diagnosis of clinical disease. Many cats with toxoplasmosis develop clinical signs after serum antibody titers have reached a plateau. Also, the magnitude of antibody titer does not always correlate with active or clinical disease. Many cats with clinical toxoplasmosis have IgM and IgG titers that are at the low end, and many healthy cats have IgG titers more than 1:16,384 for years after infection with *T. gondii*.

Diagnosis of an infectious disease usually requires the combination of (1) appropriate clinical signs, (2) serologic evidence of exposure to the agent, (3) exclusion of other possible causative agents, and (4) demonstration of the agent or response to treatment.

### Body fluids

Detection of locally produced antibodies in the eye (aqueous or vitreous humor) or CSF is used to aid diagnosis of canine distemper virus infection and feline toxoplasmosis. But ocular and CSF antibody titers are difficult to interpret, because inflammation allows leakage of serum antibodies into the eye or central nervous system (CNS). The following method can be used to determine local antibody production in the eye or CNS.

$$\frac{\text{Aqueous humor or CSF specific antibody}}{\text{Serum specific antibody}} \times \frac{\text{Serum total antibody}}{\text{Aqueous humor or CSF total antibody}}$$

A ratio of more than 1 suggests that the antibody in the aqueous humor or CSF was produced locally. This formula is used in cats with uveitis; approximately 60% of the cats have *T. gondii*–specific IgM, IgA, or IgG values more than 1.

# 98

# Practical Antimicrobial Chemotherapy

## *(Text pp 1240-1249)*

## GENERAL GUIDELINES (TEXT P 1240)

The antimicrobial selected must have an appropriate mechanism of action against the pathogen (confirmed or suspected) and must achieve an adequate concentration in infected tissues (Table 98-1). Bacteriostatic agents may be less effective for treatment of infections in immunosuppressed animals. Potential for toxicity is also an important consideration (Table 98-2).

### Selecting dosage and interval

In animals with simple, first-time infections or when drugs with potential for toxicity are used, the low-end dose and longest dosing interval should be used. For intracellular pathogens, anaerobic infections, and life-threatening infections (e.g., bacteremia, central nervous system [CNS] infections), the high-end dose and shortest interval should be used. In animals with life-threatening infections, antimicrobials should be administered parenterally for at least the first 5 to 7 days. Parenteral administration is also indicated in animals with vomiting or regurgitation.

### Duration

Most simple, first-time infections in immunocompetent animals respond adequately to 10 to 14 days of antimicrobial therapy. Chronic infections, bone infections, infections in immunosuppressed animals, infections resulting in granulomatous reactions,

**Table 98-1**

**Antibiotics Used for the Treatment of Bacterial Infections in Dogs and Cats**

| Drug | Mechanism | Bacteriostatic or bactericidal | Species | Dosage | Route of administration |
|---|---|---|---|---|---|
| **Aminoglycosides** | Protein synthesis inhibition | Bacteriostatic | | | |
| Amikacin | | | D, C | 5-10 mg/kg, q8h | IV, IM, SC |
| Gentamicin | | | D, C | 2-4 mg/kg, q8h | IV, IM, SC |
| Neomycin | | | D, C | 2.5-10 mg/kg, q8-12h | PO |
| Tobramycin | | | D, C | 2 mg/kg, q8h | IV, IM, SC |
| **Carbapenems** | Cell wall synthesis inhibition | Bactericidal | | | |
| Imipenem | | | D, C | 2-5 mg/kg, q6-8h | IV, SC |
| **Cephalosporins** | Cell wall synthesis inhibition | Bactericidal | | | |
| Cefadroxil (first generation) | | | D, C | 22 mg/kg, q12h | PO |
| Cephalexin (first generation) | | | D, C | 20-40 mg/kg, q8h | PO |
| Cefazolin (first generation) | | | D, C | 20-25 mg/kg, q8h | IM, IV |
| Cefoxitin (second generation) | | | D, C | 22 mg/kg, q8h | IM, IV |
| Cefotaxime (third generation) | | | D, C | 25-50 mg/kg, q8h | SC, IM, IV |
| Ceftiofur (third generation) | | | D | 2.2 mg/kg, q24h | SC |
| **Chloramphenicol** | Protein synthesis inhibition | Bacteriostatic | D | 25-50 mg/kg, q8h | PO, SC, IV |
| | | | C | 15-25 mg/kg, q12h | PO, IV |
| **Macrolides and lincosamides** | Protein synthesis inhibition | Bacteriostatic | | | |
| Azithromycin | | | D | 10-40 mg/kg, q24h | PO |
| | | | C | 5-10 mg/kg, q24h | PO |
| Clarithromycin | | | D, C | 5-10 mg/kg, q12h | PO |
| Clindamycin | | | D | 5.5-11 mg/kg, q12h | PO, SC, IM |
| | | | C | 5.5-11 mg/kg, q12-24h | PO, SC, IM |
| Erythromycin | | | D, C | 10-20 mg/kg, q8-12h | PO |
| Lincomycin | | | D, C | 15-25 mg/kg, q12h | PO, IM, IV |
| Tylosin | | | D, C | 10-40 mg/kg, q12h | PO |

*Continued.*

**Table 98-1**

## Antibiotics Used for the Treatment of Bacterial Infections in Dogs and Cats—cont'd

| Drug | Mechanism | Bacteriostatic or bactericidal | Species | Dosage | Route of administration |
|---|---|---|---|---|---|
| **Metronidazole** | Protein synthesis inhibition | Bactericidal | D | 10 mg/kg, q8h | PO |
|  |  |  | C | 10 mg/kg, q12h | PO |
| **Penicillins** |  |  |  |  |  |
| Amoxicillin | Cell wall synthesis inhibition | Bactericidal |  |  |  |
| Amoxicillin and clavulanate |  |  | D, C | 10-22 mg/kg, q8-12h | PO, SC |
|  |  |  | D | 12.5-25 mg/kg, q8-12h | PO |
|  |  |  | C | 62.5 mg, q8-12h | PO |
| Ampicillin sodium |  |  | D, C | 22 mg/kg, q8h | SC, IM, IV |
| Oxacillin |  |  | D, C | 22-40 mg/kg, q8h | PO |
| Penicillin G |  |  | D, C | 22,000 U/kg, q6-8h | IM, IV |
| Ticarcillin and clavulanate |  |  | D | 40-110 mg/kg, q6h | IM, IV |
| **Quinolones** |  |  |  |  |  |
| Ciprofloxacin | Nucleic acid inhibition | Bactericidal | D, C | 5-15 mg/kg, q12h | PO |
| Enrofloxacin |  |  | D, C | 2.5-10 mg/kg, q12h | PO, IM, SC, IV |
| Orbifloxacin |  |  | D | 2.5-7.5 mg/kg, q24h | PO |
| **Sulfonamide combinations** |  |  |  |  |  |
| Ormetoprim-sulfadimethoxine | Intermediary metabolism inhibition | Bactericidal | D, C | 55 mg/kg, q24h day 1, then 27 mg/kg q24h | PO |
| Trimethoprim-sulfonamide |  |  | D, C | 15-30 mg/kg, q12h | PO, SC |
| **Tetracyclines** |  |  |  |  |  |
| Doxycycline | Protein synthesis inhibition | Bacteriostatic | D, C | 5-10 mg/kg, q12h | PO, IV |
| Minocycline |  |  | D | 12.5 mg/kg, q12h | PO |
| Tetracycline |  |  | D, C | 22 mg/kg, q8-12h | PO |

*C, Cats; D, dogs; IM, intramuscularly; IV, intravenously; PO, orally; SC, subcutaneously.*

Table 98-2

## Common Antibiotic Toxicities

| Antibiotic examples | Toxicity |
|---|---|
| Aminoglycosides | Renal tubular disease |
| | Neuromuscular blockade |
| | Ototoxicity |
| Cephalosporins | Immune-mediated cytopenias |
| Chloramphenicol | Bone marrow–aplastic anemia (predominantly cats) |
| | Inhibition of drug metabolism |
| Macrolides and lincosamides | Vomiting or diarrhea |
| | Cholestasis |
| Penicillins | Immune-mediated cytopenias |
| Quinolones | Failure of cartilage development in young, growing puppies |
| Sulfonamides | Hepatic cholestasis or acute hepatic necrosis (rare) |
| | Macrocytic anemia (long-term administration in cats) |
| | Thrombocytopenia |
| | Suppurative, nonseptic polyarthritis (predominantly Doberman Pinschers) |
| | Keratoconjunctivitis sicca |
| | Renal crystalluria (rare) |
| Tetracyclines | Renal tubular disease |
| | Cholestasis |
| | Fever, particularly in cats |
| | Inhibition of drug metabolism |

and infections caused by intracellular pathogens are generally treated for a minimum 1 to 2 weeks beyond resolution of clinical or radiographic signs; the duration of therapy commonly exceeds 4 to 6 weeks. Conditions resulting in devitalized, granulomatous, or consolidated tissues (e.g., aspiration pneumonia) may not show radiographic improvement before 7 days. If possible, devitalized tissues should be débrided.

### Modifying treatment

When results of antimicrobial susceptibility tests become available, the antimicrobial choice is changed, if indicated. If therapeutic response in 72 hours is poor, and if an antibiotic-responsive infectious disease is likely, alternate treatment should be considered.

## SPECIFIC TYPES OF INFECTION (TEXT PP 1240-1249)

### Anaerobic Infections

The clinically relevant anaerobes in dogs and cats are *Bacteroides* spp., *Fusobacterium* spp., *Peptostreptococcus* spp., *Peptococcus* spp., *Clostridium* spp., *Actinomyces* spp. (facultative anaerobe), *Propionibacterium* spp., and *Eubacterium* spp. The origin of most anaerobic infections is the animal's own flora (e.g., oral cavity, vagina). Anaerobic infections are common in patients with aspiration pneumonia or consolidated lung lobes and in infections involving the oropharynx, CNS, subcutaneous space, musculoskeletal system, gastrointestinal (GI) tract, liver, and female genital tract. Clinical findings consistent with anaerobic infections are listed in Box 98-1. These infections are potentiated by poor blood supply, tissue necrosis, prior infection, or immunosuppression. Most usually have coexisting aerobic infections.

### Therapeutic approach

Improving the blood supply and oxygenation of the infected area is the primary goal of treatment; antimicrobial therapy should be used concurrently with drainage or

---

**Box 98-1**

## Clinical Findings Consistent with Anaerobic Infections in Dogs and Cats

### SIGNALMENT
All ages, breeds, or genders

### HISTORY
Fighting
Foreign body
Vomiting or regurgitation with aspiration
Recent surgery, open wound or fracture, or dentistry
History of immunosuppressive drugs or diseases
Infection resistant to sulfonamides or aminoglycosides
Neutrophilic inflammation with cytologically evident bacteria but negative aerobic culture

### PHYSICAL EXAMINATION
Flaccid paralysis *(Clostridium botulinum)*
Rigid paralysis and trismus *(Clostridium tetani)*
Subcutaneous gas production
Putrid odor from lesion
Serosanguineous discharge from a painful lesion
Necrotic tissue
Open wound or fracture
High fever
"Sulfur" granules
Abscesses
Blackish exudate

### CYTOLOGIC FINDINGS
Degenerate and nondegenerate neutrophils with mixed population of bacteria
Large gram-positive rods with minimal neutrophils
"Sulfur" granules
Branching filamentous rods *(Actinomyces* or *Nocardia* spp.)

---

débridement. Parenteral antimicrobials must be administered for several days in dogs or cats with pyothorax, pneumonia, peritonitis, or signs of bacteremia.

**Antimicrobial choices**

Penicillin derivatives, clindamycin, chloramphenicol, metronidazole, and cephalosporins (first and second generation) are commonly used (Table 98-3). If gram-negative coccobacilli suggestive of *Bacteroides* infection are detected in a neutrophilic exudate, particularly if associated with the oral cavity, metronidazole or clindamycin should be used instead of a penicillin. Combinations of aerobic and anaerobic antimicrobials are indicated, particularly if life-threatening signs of bacteremia exist (see next section).

## Bacteremia and Bacterial Endocarditis

Routine dentistry is a common cause of transient bacteremia. Intermittent bacteremia often develops in immunosuppressed or critically ill animals; the source of infection is commonly the urinary or GI systems. Continuous bacteremia occurs most frequently in association with bacterial endocarditis. Animals with bacteremia have intermittent fever, depression, and signs associated with the primary organ system infected. Sepsis is manifested by peripheral circulatory failure (septic shock).

**Table 98-3**

## Empiric Antibiotic Choices for Dogs and Cats with Cutaneous or Soft-Tissue Infections

| Infectious agent | Antibiotic choices |
|---|---|
| Staphylococcal pyoderma | 1. Cephalosporins (first generation) |
| | 2. Amoxicillin-clavulanate, cloxacillin, or oxacillin |
| | 3. Clindamycin, lincomycin, or erythromycin |
| | 4. Trimethoprim-sulfa or ormetoprim-sulfadimethoxine (superficial pyoderma) |
| Gram-negative pyoderma | 1. Quinolone |
| Abscesses (anaerobes) | 1. Penicillin derivatives |
| | 2. First-generation cephalosporins |
| | 3. Clindamycin |
| | 4. Chloramphenicol |
| | 5. Metronidazole |
| L-form bacteria | 1. Doxycycline |
| | 2. Chloramphenicol |
| | 3. Quinolone |
| Atypical *Mycobacterium* | 1. Doxycycline |
| | 2. Chloramphenicol |
| | 3. Quinolone |
| | 4. Trimethoprim-sulfa |
| | 5. Aminoglycosides |
| *Nocardia* or *Actinomyces* | 1. Penicillins (high dose) |
| | 2. Penicillins combined with trimethoprim-sulfa for penicillin-resistant *Nocardia* spp. |

### Common pathogens

*Staphylococcus, Streptococcus, Escherichia coli, Klebsiella, Enterobacter, Pseudomonas, Clostridium,* and *Bacteroides* are commonly isolated from the blood of animals with bacteremia. Bacterial endocarditis is usually a result of *Staphylococcus aureus, E. coli,* or β-hemolytic *Streptococcus.*

### Antimicrobial choices

If the source of infection is from an area with mixed flora (e.g., GI tract) or if the animal has signs of life-threatening disease, an antimicrobial or combination that is effective against gram-positive, gram-negative, aerobic, and anaerobic organisms (four-quadrant approach) should be used. Commonly prescribed combinations include an aminoglycoside or quinolone plus either ampicillin, a first-generation cephalosporin, or clindamycin (Table 98-4). Second- and third-generation cephalosporins, ticarcillin with clavulanate, and imipenem are some of the agents with a four-quadrant spectrum.

### Regimen

After parenteral treatment for 5 to 7 days, oral treatment is selected on the basis of culture and susceptibility results and continued for at least 4 to 6 weeks. Blood culture should be rechecked 1 and 4 weeks after discontinuation of therapy.

## Skin and Soft-Tissue Infections

*Staphylococcus intermedius* is the most common cause of pyoderma in dogs and cats, but deep pyoderma can be induced by any organism. Most soft-tissue infections, including open wounds and abscesses, are infected with a mixed population of bacteria; the aerobic and anaerobic flora from the mouth are often involved.

### Antimicrobial choices

Recommended empiric choices for routine cases of pyoderma and soft-tissue infections are listed in Table 98-3. Antimicrobials with a broad spectrum, such as first-

Table 98-4

**Empiric Antibiotic Choices for Dogs and Cats with Cardiorespiratory Infections**

| Organ system or infectious agent | Antibiotic choices |
|---|---|
| Sepsis, bacteremia, or bacterial endocarditis | 1. Quinolone plus penicillin, ampicillin, amoxicillin, clindamycin, or first-generation cephalosporin<br>2. Aminoglycoside plus penicillin, ampicillin, amoxicillin, clindamycin, or first-generation cephalosporin<br>3. Second- or third-generation cephalosporin<br>4. Imipenem<br>5. Ticarcillin-clavulanate |
| Upper respiratory infection | 1. Amoxicillin or amoxicillin-clavulanate<br>2. First-generation cephalosporins<br>3. Trimethoprim-sulfa<br>4. Clindamycin<br>5. Doxycycline*<br>6. Chloramphenicol*<br>7. Quinolone* |
| Bacterial pneumonia with bacteremia† | 1. Quinolone plus penicillin, ampicillin, amoxicillin, clindamycin, metronidazole, or first-generation cephalosporin<br>2. Imipenem |
| Bacterial pneumonia | 1. Amoxicillin-clavulanate<br>2. Trimethoprim-sulfa<br>3. First-generation cephalosporins<br>4. Chloramphenicol |
| Pyothorax† | 1. Penicillin derivatives<br>2. Clindamycin<br>3. Metronidazole<br>4. Chloramphenicol<br>5. First-generation cephalosporins |
| Toxoplasmosis | 1. Clindamycin<br>2. Trimethoprim-sulfa |

*Should be used if infection with *Bordetella*, *Mycoplasma*, or *Chlamydia* spp. is suspected.
†Generally mixed infections, often with gram-negative, gram-positive, aerobic, and anaerobic combinations. If signs of bacteremia or sepsis are present, use a four-quadrant antibiotic choice administered parenterally as discussed for sepsis until culture and antimicrobial susceptibility testing results return.

generation cephalosporins and amoxicillin-clavulanate, are common first choices. Other β-lactamase–resistant penicillins, such as oxacillin and cloxacillin, also can be used. Potentiated sulfas can be used, but resistance develops quickly; they should be avoided for long-term treatment.

### Resistant infections

Resistant infections may involve gram-negative bacteria, L-form bacteria, *Mycoplasma* organisms, atypical *Mycobacterium* spp., systemic fungi, or *Sporothrix schenckii*. Quinolones are the antibiotic class of choice for the treatment of gram-negative infections. Animals that do not respond to empiric antimicrobial treatment should undergo further diagnostic testing or should be treated with antimicrobials known to have an effect against the less common pathogens (see Table 98-3). Deep tissue samples should be obtained for aerobic, anaerobic, *Mycoplasma*, fungal, and atypical *Mycobacterium* spp.

culture. If not previously done, microscopic examination of tissue or pustule aspirates should be performed for *Sporothrix* organisms and *Mycobacterium* spp.

## GI Tract and Hepatic Infections

Oral antimicrobials are indicated for the treatment of small intestinal bacterial overgrowth, hepatic encephalopathy, cholangiohepatitis, hepatic abscessation, and infection by *Helicobacter felis*, *Campylobacter* spp., *Clostridium perfringens*, *Giardia* spp., *Cryptosporidium* spp., *Balantidium coli*, *Entamoeba histolytica*, *Tritrichomonas foetus*, *Toxoplasma gondii*, and *Cystoisospora* spp. (Table 98-5). Parenteral antimicrobials are indicated for bacteremia from enteric flora or *Salmonella* spp. infection.

### Protozoans

*Entamoeba*, *Giardia*, *Balantidium*, and *Pentatrichomonas* generally respond to metronidazole at 25 mg/kg orally [PO] q12h for 8 days. This is the maximum dose; lower doses should be used in large dogs to lessen the potential for toxicity. Albendazole, fenbendazole, and the combination of febantel, praziquantel, and pyrantel are also effective against giardiasis, the last two being less toxic.

***Cryptosporidiosis.*** Paromomycin (150 mg/kg PO q12-24h for 5 days) has been demonstrated to lessen the clinical signs of cryptosporidiosis in cats but should not be used if hemorrhagic diarrhea is present. Tylosin (10 to 15 mg/kg PO q12h for 21 days) lessens the clinical signs of cryptosporidiosis in some infected dogs and cats.

***Toxoplasmosis.*** *T. gondii* oocyst shedding can be shortened by administration of clindamycin at 12 mg/kg PO q12h for 10 days. *Cystoisospora* spp. generally respond to

**Table 98-5**

### Empiric Antibiotic Choices for Dogs and Cats with Hepatic or Gastrointestinal Infections

| Infectious agent | Antibiotic choices |
|---|---|
| Bacterial cholangiohepatitis | 1. Amoxicillin<br>2. First-generation cephalosporins<br>3. Chloramphenicol<br>4. Metronidazole<br>5. Quinolone |
| Bacterial overgrowth | 1. Penicillin derivative<br>2. Tetracycline derivative<br>3. Tylosin<br>4. Metronidazole |
| *Campylobacter jejuni* | 1. Erythromycin<br>2. Chloramphenicol<br>3. Quinolone<br>4. Tetracycline derivative |
| *Clostridium perfringens* | 1. Penicillin derivative<br>2. Tetracycline derivative<br>3. Tylosin<br>4. Metronidazole |
| Hepatic encephalopathy | 1. Neomycin<br>2. Ampicillin<br>3. Metronidazole |
| *Salmonella* spp. | 1. Trimethoprim-sulfa<br>2. Chloramphenicol<br>3. Amoxicillin<br>4. Aminoglycosides<br>5. Quinolone |

sulfadimethoxine at 25 mg/kg PO q24h for 7 days, with the treatment regimen repeated 7 days later.

### Bacteria

*C. perfringens* and bacterial overgrowth generally respond to treatment with tylosin, ampicillin, amoxicillin, tetracyclines, or metronidazole. Campylobacteriosis usually responds clinically to the oral administration of quinolones, erythromycin, chloramphenicol, or tetracyclines. Appropriate empiric antibiotics for the treatment of bacteremia from salmonellosis include quinolones, potentiated sulfonamides, and penicillins.

*Small intestinal bacterial overgrowth.* Bacterial overgrowth occurs secondary to many diseases of the GI tract and may also be induced by oral administration of broad-spectrum antimicrobials. It is managed by resolution of the primary problem and administration of tylosin or tetracyclines.

*Helicobacteriosis.* *H. felis* infection is usually treated with a combination of metronidazole and either tetracyclines or amoxicillin. Macrolide antibiotics such as azithromycin and clarithromycin may also be effective.

*Hepatic infections.* Hepatic infections generally respond to first-generation cephalosporins, amoxicillin, or chloramphenicol. Animals with apparent bacteremia resulting from enteric bacteria should be treated with parenteral antibiotics that have a spectrum against anaerobic and gram-negative organisms. Decreasing the number of enteric flora by oral administration of penicillins, metronidazole, or neomycin can lessen the signs of hepatic encephalopathy (see Chapters 37 and 38).

## Musculoskeletal Infections

### Osteomyelitis

Osteomyelitis and diskospondylitis are commonly associated with infections by *Staphylococcus*, *Streptococcus*, *Proteus*, *Pseudomonas* spp., *E. coli,* or anaerobes. First-generation cephalosporins, amoxicillin-clavulanate, and clindamycin are logical antimicrobials for empiric therapy (Table 98-6). Quinolones should be used if gram-negative organisms are suspected. Antimicrobial treatment should be continued for at least 2 weeks beyond resolution of radiographic changes.

### Infectious arthritis

Dogs and cats with septic polyarthritis should be treated as those with osteomyelitis. The source of infection should be removed, if possible. *Ehrlichia* spp., *Rickettsia rickettsii, Borrelia burgdorferi, Mycoplasma* organisms, and L-form bacteria can induce nonseptic, suppurative polyarthritis. Occasionally, morulae of *Ehrlichia* spp. are identified cytologically in the joint fluid, but in general, cytologic findings in joint fluid are similar to those in immune-mediated polyarthritis. Doxycycline is a logical empiric choice for dogs with nonseptic, suppurative polyarthritis, pending the results of further diagnostic tests. Amoxicillin is an alternative for treatment of *B. burgdorferi* infection. Enrofloxacin can also be used for *R. rickettsii, Mycoplasma,* and L-form bacteria infections but is not effective for *Ehrlichia* spp. infections.

### Myositis

Clindamycin hydrochloride often resolves muscle disease resulting from *T. gondii* infection. Trimethoprim-sulfadiazine combined with pyrimethamine, sequential treatment with clindamycin hydrochloride, trimethoprim-sulfadiazine, and pyrimethamine, and clindamycin alone have been effective in treatment of dogs with neosporosis. Acute *Hepatozoon americanum* infection is effectively treated with the combination of trimethoprim-sulfadiazine, pyrimethamine, and clindamycin for 14 days; use of decoquinate at 10 to 20 mg/kg given q12h with food lessens the likelihood of recurrence of clinical disease and prolongs survival time.

## CNS Infections

Chloramphenicol, sulfonamides-trimethoprim, metronidazole, and quinolones are choices for empiric treatment of bacterial infections (see Table 98-6). With anaerobic and rickettsial (e.g., *Ehrlichia canis* and *R. rickettsii*) infections of the CNS, chloramphenicol is a logical first choice. Clindamycin or potentiated sulfas should be used

Table 98-6

## Empiric Antibiotic Choices for Dogs and Cats with Central Nervous System or Musculoskeletal Infections

| Organ system or infectious agent | Antibiotic choices |
|---|---|
| **CENTRAL NERVOUS SYSTEM** | |
| Encephalitis | 1. Chloramphenicol |
| | 2. Amoxicillin |
| | 3. Trimethoprim-sulfa |
| | 4. Quinolone |
| Otitis media or interna | 1. Amoxicillin or amoxicillin-clavulanate |
| | 2. Chloramphenicol |
| | 3. Clindamycin |
| | 4. First-generation cephalosporins |
| | 5. Quinolone |
| Toxoplasmosis | 1. Clindamycin |
| | 2. Trimethoprim-sulfa |
| **MUSCULOSKELETAL** | |
| Diskospondylitis | 1. First-generation cephalosporins |
| | 2. Amoxicillin-clavulanate |
| | 3. Clindamycin |
| | 4. Chloramphenicol |
| | 5. Quinolone |
| Osteomyelitis | 1. Amoxicillin-clavulanate |
| | 2. Clindamycin |
| | 3. First-generation cephalosporins |
| | 4. Chloramphenicol |
| | 5. Quinolone |
| **POLYARTHRITIS** | |
| Bacterial polyarthritis | 1. First-generation cephalosporins |
| | 2. Quinolone |
| *Borrelia burgdorferi* | 1. Doxycycline |
| | 2. Amoxicillin |
| *Ehrlichia*, L-form bacteria, or *Mycoplasma* | 1. Doxycycline |
| | 2. Chloramphenicol |
| Rocky Mountain spotted fever | 1. Doxycycline |
| | 2. Chloramphenicol |
| | 3. Enrofloxacin |

if toxoplasmosis is suspected. Clindamycin is appropriate for toxoplasmosis in cats; potentiated sulfas are alternate antitoxoplasma drugs.

### Respiratory Tract Infections

#### Upper respiratory infections

The normal flora make it difficult to interpret culture and susceptibility results from the upper respiratory tract. Most bacterial upper respiratory infections (URIs) are secondary to primary diseases such as foreign bodies, viral infections, tooth root abscesses, neoplasms, trauma, and fungal infections. The primary insult should be resolved, if possible.

*Antimicrobial choices.* Broad-spectrum antimicrobials with an anaerobic spectrum, including amoxicillin, amoxicillin-clavulanate, potentiated sulfas, and first-generation cephalosporins, are commonly prescribed to treat URI secondary to normal flora overgrowth (see Table 98-4). Treatment duration is generally 1 to 2 weeks for acute, first-time infections.

***Chronic rhinitis.*** Chronic rhinitis often responds to treatment with macrolides like clindamycin. When it is suspected to involve the nasal septum, chronic rhinitis should be treated for at least 4 to 6 weeks or until signs have been resolved for 2 weeks.

***Resistant infections.*** *Bordetella bronchiseptica, Mycoplasma* spp., and *Chlamydophila felis* in cats are primary bacterial pathogens that infect the upper respiratory tissues. If the animal responds poorly to broad-spectrum antimicrobials, treatment with doxycycline, azithromycin, chloramphenicol, or quinolones generally is effective. Chloramphenicol is an excellent first choice in immunocompetent animals.

### Bronchitis
Canine kennel cough usually is effectively treated with doxycycline, chloramphenicol, quinolones, or amoxicillin-clavulanate. Bacterial bronchitis in cats generally responds to doxycycline or chloramphenicol. In dogs and cats with chronic bronchitis, doxycycline, chloramphenicol, quinolones, or amoxicillin-clavulanate are rational choices.

### Pneumonia
Common bacteria associated with pneumonia in dogs include *E. coli*; *Klebsiella*, *Pasteurella*, and *Pseudomonas* spp.; *B. bronchiseptica*, *Streptococcus*, *Staphylococcus*, and *Mycoplasma* spp. In cats *Bordetella*, *Pasteurella*, and *Mycoplasma* are common. Aspiration of GI contents is a common cause of pneumonia, often with a mixed population of bacteria. Multiple species of bacteria are also typically cultured from dogs and cats with bronchopneumonia. If consolidated lung lobes are detected radiographically, anaerobic infection should be suspected.

***Therapeutic approach.*** Culture and susceptibility tests should be performed on secretions collected by transtracheal wash or bronchoalveolar lavage. If the animal is showing signs of bacteremia or if radiographic evidence of lung consolidation is present, parenteral administration of a four-quadrant antimicrobial choice (as discussed for bacteremia) should be used initially.

***Antimicrobial choices.*** Quinolones combined with clindamycin or azithromycin, or chloramphenicol alone, are good choices for animals with consolidated lung lobes. In animals without signs of bacteremia or consolidation, broad-spectrum antimicrobials such as amoxicillin-clavulanate, potentiated sulfas, and first-generation cephalosporins may be effective (see Table 98-4). *B. bronchiseptica* and *Mycoplasma* may respond to nebulization with gentamicin (25 to 50 mg in 3 to 5 ml of saline or via nebulization). Treatment for bacterial pneumonia should be continued for at least 4 weeks or 1 to 2 weeks beyond resolution of clinical and radiographic signs.

***Yersinia pneumonia.*** *Yersinia pestis* causes pneumonia in cats in the western United States. It can be successfully treated with aminoglycosides, tetracycline derivatives, or quinolones.

***Toxoplasma and neospora pneumonia.*** *T. gondii* and *N. caninum* occasionally causes pneumonia in cats that are transplacentally or neonatally infected or immunosuppressed. Clindamycin or potentiated sulfas should be used if toxoplasmosis is suspected.

### Pyothorax
If pyothorax is a result of penetration of foreign material from an airway or the esophagus, thoracotomy is usually required for removal of devitalized tissue and the foreign body. Pleural lavage via chest tubes is the most effective treatment for patients with pyothorax and no obvious foreign material. Most dogs and cats with pyothorax have mixed aerobic and anaerobic bacterial infections. Animals with concurrent signs of bacteremia should initially receive parenteral four-quadrant antimicrobials, as discussed for bacteremia.

## Urogenital Tract Infections
### Urinary tract infections
Approximately 75% of urinary tract infections (UTIs) in dogs are caused by gram-negative organisms; *E. coli, Proteus, Klebsiella, Pseudomonas,* and *Enterobacter* are common.

In cats that have been previously catheterized, *E. coli* is most common; *Staphylococcus* and *Streptococcus* are common after urethrostomy.

*General recommendations.* Microscopic examination and Gram stain of urine sediment aids in the empiric choice of antimicrobial in animals with signs of UTI, although culture and susceptibility should be performed, if possible. Administration of antimicrobials for 10 to 14 days is generally sufficient for simple UTI. Urinalysis, culture, and susceptibility should be repeated 7 days after treatment is finished, if possible.

*Bitches.* In bitches with simple, first-time UTI, amoxicillin or amoxicillin-clavulanate should be used if cocci are observed; potentiated sulfas or first-generation cephalosporins should be used if rods are found. Quinolones are reserved for life-threatening or resistant infections.

*Male dogs.* It should be assumed that all male dogs with UTI have prostatitis, so antimicrobials that penetrate the prostate should be chosen (see below).

*Cats.* Most UTIs in cats respond to amoxicillin.

*Mycoplasma infections.* Poor response to penicillins, cephalosporins, or potentiated sulfas may be the result of *Mycoplasma* or *Ureaplasma* infection. If empiric therapy is necessary, chloramphenicol, doxycycline, or quinolones may be effective.

### Pyelonephritis

All dogs and cats with UTI and azotemia should be assumed to have pyelonephritis. Treatment should be based on susceptibility results, if possible, but potentiated sulfa combinations or quinolones are good initial choices. If renal insufficiency exists, tetracyclines (except doxycycline) and aminoglycosides should be avoided, and the dosage of quinolones and cephalosporins should be reduced or the administration interval extended. (See text for formula for reducing the dosage.)

*Duration.* Treatment for pyelonephritis and other chronic, complicated UTI should continue for at least 6 weeks. Urinalysis, culture, and susceptibility testing should be repeated 7 and 28 days after treatment ends. Some infections cannot be eliminated and require administration of pulse antibiotic therapy.

### Prostatic infections

Most bacterial prostatic infections are gram negative. During acute prostatitis almost all antimicrobials penetrate the prostate well. However, in dogs with chronic prostatitis, only basic antimicrobials (pKa <7) penetrate well (Table 98-7). Chloramphenicol also penetrates prostatic tissue. In acute prostatitis, penicillins or first-generation cephalosporins may lessen the signs of disease but do not eliminate the infection; this predisposes to chronic bacterial prostatitis and prostatic abscessation. Therefore penicillins and first-generation cephalosporins are contraindicated for treatment of UTI in male dogs. In dogs with chronic prostatitis, antimicrobial therapy should be continued for at least 6 weeks, and urine and prostatic fluid should be recultured 7 and 28 days after therapy.

### Brucellosis

*Brucella canis* causes a number of clinical syndromes in dogs including epididymitis, orchitis, endometritis, stillbirth, abortion, diskospondylitis, and uveitis. Long-term antimicrobial administration usually does not lead to a complete cure. Some dogs become antibody negative, but the organism can still be cultured from tissues. Several antimicrobial protocols have been suggested for dogs with brucellosis, but treatment is discouraged because of human health risks. (see Table 98-7).

### Vaginitis

Vaginitis generally results from normal flora overgrowth secondary to primary diseases, including herpesvirus infection, UTI, foreign bodies, vulvar or vaginal anomalies, vaginal or vulvar masses, and urinary incontinence. After resolution of the primary insult, broad-spectrum antimicrobials including amoxicillin, potentiated sulfas, first-generation cephalosporins, tetracyclines, and chloramphenicol are commonly successful. *Mycoplasma* and *Ureaplasma* are part of the normal vaginal flora, so a positive vaginal culture from an asymptomatic bitch is meaningless.

**Table 98-7**

## Empiric Antibiotic Choices for Dogs and Cats with Urogenital Infections

| Organ system or infectious agent | Antibiotic choices |
|---|---|
| Aerobic urinary tract infections | 1. Amoxicillin or amoxicillin-clavulanate<br>2. First-generation cephalosporins<br>3. Trimethoprim-sulfa<br>4. Quinolone |
| *Brucella canis* | 1. Streptomycin and tetracycline derivative<br>2. Enrofloxacin (high-dose)<br>3. Doxycycline or minocycline |
| *Leptospira* spp. | 1. Penicillin G or ampicillin intravenously during acute phase and oral amoxicillin during chronic phase<br>2. Dihydrostreptomycin or doxycycline to eliminate renal carriers |
| Mastitis | 1. First-generation cephalosporins<br>2. Amoxicillin or amoxicillin-clavulanate |
| *Mycoplasma or Ureaplasma* | 1. Doxycycline<br>2. Chloramphenicol<br>3. Quinolone |
| Prostatitis | 1. Trimethoprim-sulfa<br>2. Quinolone<br>3. Chloramphenicol<br>4. Erythromycin<br>5. Clindamycin |
| Pyometra | 1. Quinolone and amoxicillin<br>2. Chloramphenicol<br>3. Trimethoprim-sulfa<br>4. Amoxicillin-clavulanate |

### Pyometra

In all dogs and cats with pyometra, ovariohysterectomy or medical drainage of the uterus is imperative. Antimicrobial treatment is used for the often concurrent bacteremia (commonly *E. coli* and anaerobes; see Table 98-7). Animals with signs of bacteremia or sepsis should be treated with a four-quadrant antimicrobial regimen (as discussed for bacteremia). Potentiated sulfas or amoxicillin-clavulanate are appropriate empiric choices while results of culture and susceptibility tests are awaited. However, potentiated sulfas and quinolones are not effective for the treatment of anaerobic infections in vivo.

### Mastitis

Ampicillin, amoxicillin, and first-generation cephalosporins reach effective concentrations in milk and are relatively safe for neonates. Therefore they can be used in the empiric treatment of mastitis. Chloramphenicol, quinolones, and tetracyclines should be avoided.

# 99

---

# Prevention of Infectious Diseases

## *(Text pp 1250-1258)*

## BIOSECURITY PROCEDURES FOR SMALL ANIMAL HOSPITALS (TEXT PP 1250-1252)

Most hospital-borne (nosocomial) infections can be prevented by following the biosecurity guidelines listed in Box 99-1. Avoiding exposure is the most effective way to prevent infections. Hands should be washed before and after attending to each individual animal. Collect clean paper towels and use them to turn on water faucets, wash hands for 30 seconds with antiseptic soap (being sure to clean under the fingernails), rinse hands thoroughly, use the paper towels to dry the hands, and use the paper towels to turn off the water faucets.

---

**Box 99-1**

### General Hospital Biosecurity Guidelines

Wash hands before and after each animal contact.

Collect clean paper towels and use to turn on water faucets; wash hands for 30 seconds with antiseptic soap, being sure to clean under fingernails; rinse hands thoroughly; use the paper towels to dry hands; and use the paper towels to turn off the water faucets.

Wear gloves when handling animals when zoonotic diseases are on the list of differential diagnoses.

Minimize contact with hospital materials (e.g., instruments, records, door handles) while hands or gloves are contaminated.

Always wear an outer garment like a smock or scrub shirt when handling animals.

Change outer garments when soiled by feces, secretions, or exudates.

Clean and disinfect equipment (e.g., stethoscopes, thermometers, bandage scissors) with 0.5% chlorhexidine solution after each use.

Do not eat or drink in areas in which animal care is provided.

Examination tables, cages, and runs should be cleaned and disinfected after each use.

Litter pans and dishes should be cleaned and disinfected after each use.

Place animals with suspected infectious diseases immediately into an examination room or an isolation area on admission to the hospital.

Treat animals with suspected infectious diseases on an outpatient basis if possible.

Procedures using general hospital facilities (e.g., surgery, radiology) should be postponed until the end of the day if possible.

---

### Patient evaluation

Animals with GI or respiratory diseases are the most likely to be contagious. Infectious GI disease should be suspected in all dogs and cats with small or large bowel diarrhea, whether the syndrome is acute or chronic. Infectious respiratory disease should be suspected in all dogs and cats with sneezing (especially in those with purulent oculonasal discharge) or coughing (especially if productive). The index of suspicion for infectious diseases is increased for dogs or cats with acute disease and fever, particularly if the animal is from a crowded environment such as a breeding or boarding facility or humane society.

### Hospitalized patients

If possible, all animals with suspected infectious diseases such as *Salmonella* spp., *Campylobacter* spp., parvovirus, kennel cough syndrome, feline upper respiratory disease syndrome, or rabies should be housed in an isolated area of the hospital. Cats that are positive for feline leukemia virus (FeLV) or feline immunodeficiency virus (FIV) should not be placed in the isolation area, if possible, to avoid exposing them to other infectious diseases; nor should they be caged next to or above seronegative cats. There should be no direct contact between infected and naïve cats, as well as no sharing of litter boxes or food bowls.

*Personnel.* In addition to the protective clothing listed in Box 99-1, a surgical mask should be worn when attending to cats with plague. All biologic materials submitted to clinical pathology or diagnostic laboratories from animals with suspected or confirmed infectious diseases should be clearly marked as such.

### Basic disinfection protocols

The key to effective disinfection is cleanliness. Quaternary ammonium compounds or other disinfectants that can inactivate most viruses, including parvoviruses, as well as bacteria such as *Salmonella* should be used. Contaminated surfaces, including the cage or run floor, walls, ceiling, door, and door latch, should be wetted thoroughly with disinfectant. Surfaces should be in contact with the disinfectant for 10 minutes, particularly if known infectious agents are present.

*Parasite ova and oocysts.* Disinfectants are relatively effective against viral and bacterial agents but require high concentrations and long contact times to kill parasite eggs, cysts, and oocysts. Cleanliness is the key to lessening hospital-borne infection with these agents; detergent or steam cleaning inactivates most of these agents. Litter pans and dishes should be thoroughly cleaned with detergent and scalding water.

## Biosecurity Procedures for Clients

The optimal way to prevent infectious diseases is by housing animals indoors, in the home, away from other animals, fomites, and vectors. Clinical disease is often more severe in immunocompromised patients, including puppies and kittens, old or debilitated animals, animals with immunosuppressive diseases (e.g., hyperadrenocorticism, diabetes mellitus) or concurrent infections, and animals treated with glucocorticoids or cytotoxic agents. It is particularly important that exposure to infectious agents be avoided in these animals.

### Common sources of infection

Kennels, veterinary hospitals, dog and cat shows, and humane societies have an increased likelihood for infectious agent contact because of the concentration of potentially infected animals. Parks and other open areas are common sources of infectious agents that survive for long periods in the environment (e.g., parvoviruses). They should be avoided if possible until puppies and kittens have completed the vaccination series.

## VACCINATION PROTOCOLS (TEXT PP 1252-1256)

### General Considerations

Not all dogs and cats need all available vaccines. Vaccines are not innocuous and should be given only if indicated. The type of vaccine and route of administration for the disease in question should also be considered. A benefit, risk, and cost assessment should be discussed with the owner before the optimal vaccination protocol is determined.

### Vaccine failure
Before a vaccine is administered, the animal should be assessed for factors that may influence its ability to respond to the vaccine or that may have a detrimental effect. Potential causes of vaccine failure include the following:
- lack of protective immune response to the antigen in the vaccine
- exposure to a field strain of organism the vaccine fails to protect against
- waning or overwhelming of the vaccine-induced immune response by the time of exposure
- mishandling or improper administration of the vaccine (see next section)
- presence of the organism at the time of vaccination (the animal was incubating the disease)
- inability to respond to the vaccine because of immunosuppression, hypothermia, or fever
- presence of maternal antibodies
- induction of disease by a modified-live vaccine (more likely in immunosuppressed animals)

*Mishandling.* Vaccines can be rendered ineffective from mishandling. Proper handling includes: (1) storing vaccines at the recommended temperature and with protection from ultraviolet light, (2) reconstituting and thoroughly mixing immediately before use, (3) using a separate syringe for each product, (4) avoiding chemically sterilized syringes for modified-live products, and (5) discarding expired vaccines. Vaccines should not be administered while the animal is under anesthesia.

### Vaccine reactions
Adverse reactions can potentially occur with any vaccine. Modified-live vaccines can induce transient thrombocytopenia, so routine surgical procedures should be delayed for 3 weeks after immunization. These products may also cause the disease (e.g., canine distemper virus vaccines occasionally induce central nervous system signs in dogs with concurrent parvovirus infection). Bacterins are commonly associated with anaphylactoid or anaphylactic reactions, and vaccination has been associated with soft-tissue sarcomas in cats (see Chapter 84).

*Immune-mediated diseases.* Administration of any vaccine to animals with immune-mediated diseases (e.g., immune-mediated polyarthritis, hemolytic anemia, thrombocytopenia, glomerulonephritis, or polyradiculoneuritis) is questionable, because immune stimulation may exacerbate the condition.

## Vaccination Protocols for Cats
Healthy kittens and cats should be routinely vaccinated subcutaneously (SC) or intramuscularly (IM) for panleukopenia, rhinotracheitis, and calicivirus (FVRCP); intranasal products can also be used. Modified-live products should not be administered to clinically ill, debilitated, or pregnant animals but are preferred over killed products in healthy cats.

### Routine vaccination
Kittens presented at 6 to 12 weeks of age should receive modified live or killed FVRCP every 3 to 4 weeks until 12 weeks of age. Kittens presented after 12 weeks of age and adult cats with unknown vaccination history should receive two killed or two modified-live FVRCP 3 to 4 weeks apart. The FVRCP should be boosted at 1 year of age or 1 year later and then be administered no more frequently than every third year. The use of an arbitrary vaccine interval leads to unneeded vaccination in the majority of cats. Serology can be used in lieu of arbitrary vaccination with FVRCP.

*Rabies.* Rabies vaccine should be administered SC or IM in the right rear limb at 12 or 16 weeks of age, depending on local ordinances. Rabies vaccination should be repeated at 1 year of age. If a rabies product with known duration of immunity of 3 years is used, it should then be administered every 3 years or according to local ordinances.

### Optional vaccines
Optional vaccines currently available for use in cats include *Bordetella bronchiseptica, Chlamydophila felis* (previously *Chlamydia)*, FeLV, FIV, feline infectious peritonitis (FIP) virus, and ringworm. These vaccines should be used only under special circumstances.

***B. bronchiseptica.*** B. bronchiseptica vaccine is potentially indicated for use in young cats with a high risk of exposure (catteries and shelters).

***Chlamydophila.*** Use of the *Chlamyofelia* vaccine should be reserved for cats with a high risk of exposure (e.g., in catteries with endemic disease). Duration of immunity may be short, so high-risk cats should be immunized before potential exposure.

***Feline leukemia virus.*** Several FeLV vaccines are currently available. They are indicated in cats that are allowed to go outdoors or are otherwise exposed to cats of unknown FeLV status. FeLV vaccines are most helpful in kittens. Cats acquire resistance to FeLV infection as they age; this limits usefulness of vaccination. FeLV testing should be performed before vaccination. Cats should receive two vaccinations initially, followed by annual boosters. Adjuvanted products should be administered SC or IM in the *left* rear limb. FeLV vaccines are not effective (and therefore not indicated) in persistently viremic cats; however, the administration of the vaccine to viremic or latently infected cats does not increase the risk of vaccine reaction.

***Feline immunodeficiency virus.*** Currently a killed FIV vaccine is available; its efficacy and safety have not been assessed under field conditions. The vaccine induces antibodies detectable by the currently available antibody test; therefore a positive test could be indicative of FIV exposure and/or infection or vaccination for FIV. Polymerase chain reaction (PCR) assays are available for FIV, but no standardization and external quality control exist for the laboratories that provide PCR testing.

***Feline infectious peritonitis.*** An intranasal coronavirus vaccine protects some cats from developing FIP. Coronavirus vaccination is optional for pet cats because the incidence of disease is low, cats are commonly exposed to coronaviruses before vaccination, the duration of immunity is short, and the efficacy is less than 100%. The vaccine is indicated for seronegative cats entering a known FIP-infected household or cattery.

***Giardia.*** A *Giardia* spp. vaccine is available for use in cats but is not indicated for routine use in client-owned cats. The vaccine decreases the shedding of cysts and lessens clinical disease but may not be protective against strains other than the one used in challenge studies. The vaccine is adjuvanted and given SC and so may ultimately be proved to be associated with fibrosarcomas.

***Ringworm.*** A killed ringworm vaccine is available for use in cats. This vaccine is indicated for treatment of disease in some situations, but not as a preventative. Because the product is adjuvanted, granuloma formation occurs in some cats.

## Vaccination Protocols for Dogs
### Routine vaccination

Routine vaccines include canine distemper virus, parainfluenza, adenovirus 2, and parvovirus (DA2PP) (Table 99-1). Modified-live products should not be administered to clinically ill, debilitated, or pregnant animals. Puppies born to vaccinated bitches and presented at 6 to 12 weeks of age should be vaccinated every 3 to 4 weeks until 14 to 16 weeks of age. Puppies presented between 12 and 16 weeks of age and adult dogs with unknown vaccination history should be given two vaccines, 3 to 4 weeks apart. At 1 year of age or 1 year later the dog should return for a DA2PP and rabies booster vaccinations.

Puppies between 6 and 8 weeks of age should receive a distemper-measles vaccine at that time and then routine vaccines at 10, 13, and 16 weeks of age. High-antigen mass, low-passage parvovirus vaccines are not needed after 16 weeks of age and are likely to be effective in most puppies that are vaccinated to 12 weeks of age.

Dogs should be evaluated at least yearly for risk of infection by canine distemper virus, parainfluenza, adenovirus 2, and parvovirus. In low-risk dogs, DA2PP vaccines should be administered no more often than every third year. Positive serologic tests for canine distemper virus and canine parvovirus are predictive of resistance and can be used in lieu of arbitrary vaccination interval.

***Rabies.*** Rabies vaccine is administered at 12 or 16 weeks of age, depending on local ordinances. In areas in which rabies is endemic and exposure may occur before an animal is 16 weeks old, vaccination at 8, 10, or 12 weeks may be indicated. At 1 year

Table 99-1

## Routine Canine Vaccination Schedule*

| Age to vaccinate (wk) | Age at presentation (wk) | | | | | | | | |
|---|---|---|---|---|---|---|---|---|---|
| | 8 | 9 | 10 | 11 | 12 | 13 | 14 | 15 | 16 |
| 8 | VAC | | | | | | | | |
| 9 | | VAC | | | | | | | |
| 10 | | | VAC | | | | | | |
| 11 | | | | VAC | | | | | |
| 12 | VAC | VAC | | | VAC | | | | |
| 13 | | | VAC | VAC | | VAC | | | |
| 14 | | | | | | | VAC | | |
| 15 | | | | | | | | | |
| 16 | VAC | VAC | VAC | VAC | VAC | VAC | VAC | VAC | VAC |

*Rabies vaccines should be administered at 12 or 16 weeks of age depending on local ordinances.

VAC, Distemper, adenovirus 2, parainfluenza, and parvovirus.

of age or 1 year later the dog should return for a rabies booster. If a rabies product with known duration of immunity of 3 years is used, it should then be administered every 3 years.

### Optional vaccines

Optional vaccines for use in "high-risk" dogs include *B. bronchiseptica*, *Borrelia burgdorferi*, *Leptospira* spp., and coronavirus.

***Bordetella.*** *B. bronchiseptica* vaccines are optional, because the agent rarely causes life-threatening disease in otherwise healthy animals and it is not the only cause of kennel cough syndrome. Optimally, booster vaccines should be administered 5 days before potential exposure; concurrent use of an intranasal and parenteral product gives optimal protection in unvaccinated dogs, and parenteral product is superior to intranasal product in previously vaccinated dogs. Serum antibody titers persist for months, so most dogs need only one or two immunizations yearly.

***Borrelia and Leptospira.*** *Borrelia* and *Leptospira* vaccines can be administered to dogs in endemic areas, but efficacy is still in question. Vaccine reactions are more common with bacterins.

The potential for *B. burgdorferi* vaccine reactions approximates the potential for development of Lyme disease, even in endemic areas. Therefore in endemic areas vaccination is equally as harmful to dogs as it is helpful, and in nonendemic areas it is more harmful than helpful. Vaccination may be unnecessary in dogs previously infected with *B. burgdorferi*. Tick control plays a more important role in the prevention of this disease.

*Leptospira* vaccines do not contain all serovars and therefore are not 100% protective; products containing the most serovars should be used. Dogs in endemic areas should receive three vaccinations 2 to 3 weeks apart. Duration of immunity is more than 1 year in dogs receiving three vaccinations.

***Coronavirus.*** Coronavirus infection in dogs results in mild GI disease unless concurrent infection with parvovirus occurs. Vaccination against coronavirus is not indicated in adult dogs.

***Giardia.*** A *Giardia* spp. vaccine is available for dogs over 8 weeks of age. Two doses are given SC, 2 to 4 weeks apart. No adverse reactions were reported during a clinical study. The efficacy of this vaccine against all strains of *Giardia* is unknown. Routine use (as a preventative) in client-owned dogs is not advocated. Immunotherapy with the *Giardia* vaccine can aid in the elimination of cyst shedding and diarrhea in some infected dogs.

# 100

# Polysystemic Bacterial Diseases

## (Text pp 1259-1264)

### FELINE PLAGUE (TEXT PP 1259-1260)

#### Epidemiology

Plague is caused by *Yersinia pestis*, a facultatively anaerobic, gram-negative coccobacillus. Cats are susceptible and can die after infection; dogs are very resistant to infection. The organism has a life cycle involving rodent fleas and infected rodents (including rock squirrels, ground squirrels, and prairie dogs); most infected cats are housed outdoors and hunt. Clinical disease in cats and humans is recognized most often from spring through early fall in New Mexico, Arizona, and California.

The incubation period is 2 to 6 days after a flea bite and 1 to 3 days after ingestion or inhalation of the organism. A neutrophilic inflammatory response and abscess formation occur in infected tissues.

#### Clinical features

Bubonic, septicemic, and pneumonic plague can develop in infected cats (Box 100-1). Bubonic is the most common form, but individual cats can show clinical signs of all three syndromes. Anorexia, depression, cervical swelling, dyspnea, and cough are common presenting complaints; fever is detected in most cases. Unilateral or bilateral enlargement of the tonsils and the mandibular and anterior cervical lymph nodes is found in approximately 50% of infected cats. Those with pneumonic plague commonly have respiratory difficulty and may cough.

#### Diagnosis

Hematologic and serum biochemical abnormalities reflect bacteremia and are not specific for *Y. pestis* infection. Neutrophilic leukocytosis with a left shift and lymphopenia; and hypoalbuminemia, hyperglobulinemia, hyperglycemia, azotemia, hypokalemia, hypochloremia, hyperbilirubinemia, and increased alkaline phosphatase (AP) and alanine aminotransferase (ALT) activities are common. Pneumonic plague causes increased alveolar and diffuse interstitial densities on thoracic radiographs.

*Cytology.* Cytologic examination of lymph node aspirates reveals lymphoid hyperplasia, neutrophilic infiltrates, and bipolar rods; the organisms may also be found in exudates from draining abscesses and airway washings.

*Organism demonstration.* Cytologic demonstration of bipolar rods, combined with a history of potential exposure, presence of rodent fleas, and appropriate signs leads to a presumptive diagnosis of feline plague. Definitive diagnosis is made by culture or fluorescent antibody from smears of the tonsillar region, lymph node aspirates, exudates from draining abscesses, airway washings, or blood.

*Serology.* Because some cats survive infection, and antibodies can be detected in serum for at least 300 days, detection of antibodies alone indicates only exposure, not clinical infection. However, a fourfold increase in antibody titer is consistent with recent infection.

---

**Box 100-1**

## Clinical Findings in Cats with Plague

### SIGNALMENT
All ages and breeds and both genders

### HISTORY AND PHYSICAL EXAMINATION
Outdoor cats
Male cats
Hunting of rodents or exposure to rodent fleas
Depression
Cervical swellings, draining tracts, lymphadenopathy
Dyspnea or cough

### CLINICOPATHOLOGIC AND RADIOGRAPHIC EVALUATION
Neutrophilia with or without a left shift
Lymphopenia
Neutrophilic lymphadenitis or pneumonitis
Homogeneous population of bipolar rods cytologically (lymph node aspirate and airway washings)
Serum antibody titers either negative (peracute) or positive
Interstitial and alveolar lung disease

### DIAGNOSIS
Culture of blood, exudates, tonsillar region, respiratory secretions
Fluorescent antibody identification of organism in exudates
Fourfold increase in antibody titer and appropriate clinical signs

---

### Treatment and prognosis
Supportive care should be initiated as indicated for any bacteremic animal. Cervical lymph node abscesses should be drained and flushed while gloves, mask, and gown are worn.

*Antibiotic therapy.* Parenteral antibiotics should be administered until anorexia and fever resolve. Streptomycin (5 mg/kg intramuscularly [IM] q12h), gentamicin (2 to 4 mg/kg IM or intravenously [IV] q12-24h), or enrofloxacin (5 mg/kg IM or IV q12h) should be used initially. A combination of enrofloxacin and doxycycline can also be used. Chloramphenicol (15 mg/kg orally [PO] or IV q12h) can be used in animals with central nervous system signs. Antibiotics should be administered PO for 21 days after the bacteremic phase; tetracycline (20 mg/kg PO q8h) or doxycycline (5 mg/kg PO q12h) is an appropriate choice.

*Prognosis.* In one study 91% of cats treated with antibiotics survived, compared with only 24% survival in untreated cats. The prognosis is poor in cats with pneumonic or septicemic plague.

*Prevention.* Cats should be housed indoors and not allowed to hunt. Flea control should be used and rodents controlled, if possible. Tetracycline or doxycycline at the doses listed for therapy should be administered for 7 days to potentially exposed animals.

### Zoonotic aspects
Human infection occurs after contact with infected fleas and tissues or exudates from infected animals and after bites and scratches from infected cats. The organism can survive for weeks or months in infected carcasses and for up to 1 year in infected fleas. Between spring and early fall, cats from endemic areas showing signs of bacteremia, respiratory disease, or cervical draining areas or masses should immediately be treated

for fleas; gloves, mask, and gown should be worn while the cat is handled. While hospitalized, infected cats should be handled by as few people as possible, even though cats are not infectious to humans after 3 days of antibiotic therapy. Exposed people should see their physicians to discuss prophylactic antibiotic therapy. Areas in which infected cats are handled should be thoroughly cleaned with routine disinfectants.

## LEPTOSPIROSIS (TEXT PP 1260-1262)

Leptospires are 0.1- to 0.2-μm wide by 6- to 12-μm long, motile, filamentous spirochetes that infect animals and humans. *Leptospira interrogans* has multiple serovars that are infective to dogs (Table 100-1); cats are susceptible to *Leptospira* serovars *bratislava*, *canicola*, *grippotyphosa*, and *pomona* but appear to be resistant to clinical disease.

### Epidemiology

Infection occurs in both rural and suburban environments, in semitropical areas with alkaline soil. Clinical cases are most commonly diagnosed in the summer and early fall, and the prevalence is higher in years with heavy rainfall. The host acts as a reservoir, shedding the organism intermittently. Leptospires are passed in urine and enter the body through abraded skin or intact mucous membranes. Transmission also occurs by bite wounds; venereal contact; transplacentally; and by ingestion of contaminated tissues, soil, water, bedding, food, and other fomites. Hosts with preexisting antibody titers usually eliminate the organism quickly and remain subclinically infected. Leptospires replicate in multiple tissues; in dogs, the liver and kidneys have the highest levels of infection. Clinical signs develop approximately 7 days after exposure; animals that are treated or develop appropriate immune responses usually survive. Some untreated animals clear the infection 2 to 3 weeks after exposure but develop chronic active hepatitis or chronic renal disease. Cats generally are subclinically affected but may shed the organism for variable periods of time after exposure.

### Clinical features

Dogs of any age, breed, or gender can develop leptospirosis, if susceptible. Male, middle-aged, herding dogs; hounds; working dogs; and mixed breeds are at greater risk than companion dogs younger than 1 year of age. Most dogs have subclinical infection.

**Table 100-1**

### *Leptospira interrogans* Serovars That Infect Dogs

| Serovar | Primary reservoir | Clinical disease in dogs |
|---|---|---|
| *Leptospira bataviae* | Dog, rat, mouse | Acute hepatic and renal disease with hemorrhage |
| *Leptospira bratislava* | Rat, pig, horse, cow | Nephritis |
| *Leptospira canicola* | Dog | Acute interstitial nephritis<br>Chronic interstitial nephritis |
| *Leptospira grippotyphosa* | Vole | Chronic active hepatitis<br>Acute or subacute renal failure |
| *Leptospira harjo* | Cow | Subclinical interstitial nephritis |
| *Leptospira icterohaemorrhagiae* | Rat | Acute hemorrhagic disease with high fever and death<br>Acute hepatic syndrome with icterus, fever, and hemorrhage<br>Uremia and hemorrhagic enteritis |
| *Leptospira pomona* | Cow, pig | Acute or subacute renal failure |
| *Leptospira tarassovi* | Cow, pig | Acute hepatic syndrome with icterus and depression |

---

**Box 100-2**

## Clinical Findings in Dogs with Leptospirosis

**SIGNALMENT**

All ages and breeds and both genders

**HISTORY**

Exposure to appropriate reservoir host or contaminated environment
Anorexia, depression, lethargy

**PHYSICAL EXAMINATION**

Fever
Anterior uveitis
Hemorrhagic tendencies including melena, epistaxis, petechiae, and ecchymoses
Vomiting, diarrhea
Muscle or meningeal pain
Renomegaly with or without renal pain
Hepatomegaly
Polyuria and polydipsia
Icterus
Coughing or respiratory distress

**CLINICOPATHOLOGIC AND RADIOGRAPHIC EVALUATION**

Thrombocytopenia
Leukopenia (acute)
Leukocytosis (subacute)
Azotemia
Suboptimal urine concentrating ability
Pyuria and hematuria without obvious bacteriuria
Hyperbilirubinemia and bilirubinuria
Increased activities of ALT, AST AP, and CK
Interstitial to alveolar lung disease
Hepatomegaly or renomegaly

**DIAGNOSIS**

Culture of urine, blood, or tissues
Demonstration of the organism in urine by dark-field or phase-contrast microscopy
Combination of increasing antibody titer with clinical signs and response to therapy

*AP*, Alkaline phosphatase; *ALT*, alanine transaminase; *AST*, aspartate transaminase; *CK*, creatine kinase.

**Peracute infection.** Dogs with peracute leptospirosis are usually presented because of anorexia, depression, generalized muscle hyperesthesia, tachypnea, and vomiting (Box 100-2). Fever, pale mucous membranes, and tachycardia are usually present. Petechiae, ecchymoses, melena, and epistaxis frequently occur from thrombocytopenia and disseminated intravascular coagulation. Peracute infections may rapidly progress to death before marked renal or hepatic disease is recognized.

**Subacute infection.** Fever, depression, and signs or physical examination findings consistent with hemorrhagic syndromes, hepatic disease, renal disease, or a combination of hepatic and renal disease are common in subacutely infected dogs. Conjunctivitis, rhinitis, tonsillitis, cough, and dyspnea are seen occasionally. Oliguric or anuric renal failure can develop during the subacute phase.

***Chronic infection.*** Some dogs that survive peracute or subacute infection develop chronic interstitial nephritis or chronic active hepatitis. Polyuria and polydipsia, weight loss, ascites, and signs of hepatic encephalopathy resulting from hepatic insufficiency are the most common manifestations of chronic leptospirosis.

**Diagnosis**

Multiple nonspecific clinicopathologic and radiographic abnormalities occur in dogs with leptospirosis and vary with the host, serovar, and presentation (peracute, subacute, or chronic) (see Box 100-2).

***Hematology.*** Leukopenia (peracute leptospiremic phase), leukocytosis with or without left shift, thrombocytopenia, regenerative anemia (from blood loss), and non-regenerative anemia (from chronic renal or hepatic disease) are common abnormalities.

***Serum biochemistry.*** Hyponatremia, hypokalemia, hyperphosphatemia, hypo-albuminemia, hypocalcemia, azotemia, hyperbilirubinemia, decreased total carbon dioxide, and increased activities of ALT, AP, and aspartate transaminase are also common. Hyperglobulinemia is detected in some dogs with chronic leptospirosis. Dogs with myositis may have increased creatine kinase activity.

***Urinalysis.*** Abnormalities include bilirubinuria, granular casts, increased numbers of granulocytes and erythrocytes, and suboptimal urine specific gravity despite azotemia. The organism cannot be seen in urine sediment by light microscopy.

***Radiography.*** Renomegaly, hepatomegaly, and interstitial or alveolar pulmonary infiltrates are common radiographic abnormalities. Mineralization of the renal pelves and cortices can occur with chronic leptospirosis.

***Serology.*** Microscopic agglutination test (MAT) can be used to detect antibodies. In dogs, screening should be done for as many serovars as possible; *Leptospira bratislava, Leptospira canicola, Leptospira grippotyphosa, Leptospira harjo, Leptospira icterohaemorrhagiae,* and *Leptospira pomona* are the most common serovars. Positive titers can result from active infection, previous infection, or vaccination. Antibody titers can be negative in animals with peracute disease; seronegative dogs with classic clinical disease should be retested in 2 to 4 weeks. Documentation of seroconversion (negative result becoming positive over time), a single MAT titer greater than 1:3200, or a fourfold increase in antibody titers combined with appropriate clinicopathologic abnormalities and clinical findings is suggestive of clinical leptospirosis.

***Identification of the organism.*** Definitive diagnosis is made by demonstrating the organism in urine, blood, or tissues. The organisms can be seen in urine using darkfield or phase-contrast microscopy. However, because leptospiremia can be of short duration and only small numbers of organisms are shed intermittently, these procedures can be falsely negative. Polymerase chain reaction (PCR) may be used to demonstrate the organism in urine, blood, or tissues, but it is available only in research laboratories.

***Culture.*** The organism can be cultured from urine (collected by cystocentesis), blood, and renal or hepatic tissue. Materials for culture should be collected before treatment begins, immediately placed in transport media, and sent to the laboratory as quickly as possible.

**Treatment**

Fluid therapy is required for most dogs; intense diuresis may be needed for renal involvement. Hemodialysis or peritoneal dialysis may increase the probability of survival in dogs with oliguric or anuric renal failure. Dogs with severe disease should be treated with ampicillin (22 mg/kg IV q8h) or penicillin G (25,000 to 40,000 U/kg IM or IV q12h) during the initial treatment period. Some quinolones are effective against leptospires and can be used in combination with penicillins during the acute phase of infection. Penicillins should be given for 2 weeks. Doxycycline (2.5 to 5 mg/kg PO q12h) should then be used for 2 weeks to eliminate the renal carrier phase.

***Prevention.*** Vaccines available for some serovars can reduce the severity of disease but not the chronic carrier state. Vaccination against *L. canicola* and *L. icterohemorrhagiae* does not always cross-protect against other serovars. Bacterins are commonly associated with vaccine reactions; new subunit vaccines lessen these reactions. Dogs in endemic areas should receive three vaccinations, 2 to 3 weeks apart; duration of immunity is less than 1 year in vaccinated dogs.

### Zoonotic aspects
All serovars that infect mammals are potentially zoonotic to humans. Infected urine, contaminated water, and reservoir hosts should be avoided. Gloves should be worn when infected dogs are handled, and contaminated surfaces should be cleaned with detergents and disinfected.

## MYCOPLASMA AND UREAPLASMA (TEXT PP 1262-1264)

### Epidemiology
Some *Mycoplasma* spp. and *Ureaplasma* spp. are normal flora of mucous membranes (e.g., pharynx, vagina, prepuce). Their pathogenic potential is difficult to determine, because they can be cultured from both healthy and sick animals. In many cases *Mycoplasma* spp. or *Ureaplasma* spp. may be opportunists secondary to inflammation induced by other agents. Other bacteria are usually isolated concurrently, making it difficult to determine which agent is inducing disease. However, some species may be primary pathogens. Recently, *Haemobartonella felis* was reclassified as a *Mycoplasma* with two species, *Mycoplasma haemofelis* and *Mycoplasma haemominutum.*

### Clinical features
*Mycoplasma* spp. or *Ureaplasma* spp. infection should be considered a potential differential diagnosis in cats with conjunctivitis, sneezing, mucopurulent nasal discharge, coughing, dyspnea, fever, lameness (with or without swollen, painful joints), subcutaneous abscessation, or abortion (Table 100-2), but not in those with lower urinary tract inflammation. In dogs these organisms should be considered in patients with coughing, dyspnea, fever, pollakiuria, hematuria, lameness (with or without swollen, painful joints), mucopurulent vaginal discharge, or infertility. *M. haemofelis* and *M. haemominutum* infection can cause hemolytic anemia.

### Diagnosis
Clinicopathologic and radiographic abnormalities associated with *Mycoplasma* spp. or *Ureaplasma* spp. infections are similar to those induced by other bacterial infections. Neutrophilia and monocytosis are common in dogs with pneumonia; pyuria and proteinuria occur in dogs with urinary tract disease.

*Cytology.* Prepucial or vaginal discharges, chronically draining wounds, airway washings, and synovial fluid from animals with *Mycoplasma* spp. or *Ureaplasma* spp. infections have nondegenerate neutrophils as the most common cell type. These organisms generally are not recognized cytologically and do not grow on aerobic media; infection should be suspected in animals with neutrophilic inflammation without visible bacteria or negative aerobic culture. The index of suspicion is higher if the animal has neutrophilic inflammation and has been poorly responsive to cell wall–inhibiting antibiotics such as penicillins or cephalosporins.

**Table 100-2**

### Clinical Findings in Dogs and Cats with Mycoplasma or Ureaplasma Infections

| Cats | Dogs |
| --- | --- |
| Conjunctivitis | Pneumonia |
| Pneumonia | Nephritis, cystitis |
| Reproductive diseases or infertility | Reproductive diseases or infertility |
| Polyarthritis | Polyarthritis |
| Abscesses | |

**Radiography.** Dogs with lower respiratory tract disease and pure *Mycoplasma* cultures have alveolar lung patterns that cannot be differentiated from those in dogs with mixed bacterial and *Mycoplasma* cultures. Joint radiographs of animals with *Mycoplasma*-associated polyarthritis reveal nonerosive changes.

**Culture.** Specimens for *Mycoplasma* spp. or *Ureaplasma* spp. culture should be plated immediately or transported to the laboratory in Hayflicks broth medium, Amies medium without charcoal, or modified Stuart bacterial transport medium. Specimens should be shipped on ice packs if transit time is expected to be less than 24 hours and on dry ice if more than 24 hours. Because these organisms can be cultured from healthy animals, interpretation of positive culture results in sick animals is difficult. The disease association is strong if *Mycoplasma* spp. or *Ureaplasma* spp. are isolated in pure culture from tissues in which isolation is unusual (e.g., lower airways, uterus, joints). Response to treatment with drugs known to be effective against *Mycoplasma* spp. or *Ureaplasma* spp. supports the diagnosis.

**Polymerase chain reaction.** PCR assays for *Mycoplasma* are available but have the same diagnostic limitations as culture.

### Treatment

Tylosin, erythromycin, clindamycin, lincomycin, tetracyclines, chloramphenicol, aminoglycosides, and enrofloxacin are effective (see Chapter 98 for dosages). Doxycycline (5 mg/kg PO q12h) generally is effective in animals without life-threatening disease and may also be antiinflammatory. However, enrofloxacin may be more effective in cats with mycoplasmal polyarthritis. In animals with mixed infections or life-threatening disease, enrofloxacin (2.5 to 5 mg/kg PO q12h) is a good treatment choice. Erythromycin (20 mg/kg PO q8-12h) or lincomycin (22 mg/kg PO q12h) should be used in pregnant animals. Treatment for 4 to 6 weeks is usually required for lower airway, subcutaneous, or joint infections.

**Prevention.** Most *Mycoplasma* spp. or *Ureaplasma* spp. infections in dogs and cats are opportunistic and are not likely to be directly contagious from animal to animal. However, *Mycoplasma felis* may be transmitted from cat to cat by conjunctival discharges. *Mycoplasma* spp. have been associated with respiratory tract diseases in dogs and cats as primary pathogens and may be spread from animal to animal. Animals with conjunctivitis or respiratory tract disease should be isolated from other animals until signs of disease have resolved.

### Zoonotic aspects

Although risk of zoonotic transfer is minimal, bite wound transmission of *Mycoplasma* spp. from an infected cat has been reported. *Mycoplasma* spp. and *Ureaplasma* spp. are susceptible to routine disinfectants and rapidly die outside the host.

# 101

# Polysystemic Rickettsial Diseases

## (Text pp 1265-1272)

### ROCKY MOUNTAIN SPOTTED FEVER (TEXT PP 1265-1267)

#### Etiology and epidemiology

Rocky Mountain spotted fever (RMSF) is caused by *Rickettsia rickettsii* and transmitted by ticks, particularly *Dermacentor* spp. and *Amblyomma*. Canine RMSF is predominantly recognized in the southeastern states from April through September, when the tick vectors are most active. The organism is normally maintained in a cycle between ticks and small mammals such as voles, ground squirrels, and chipmunks. After infection, *R. rickettsii* replicates in endothelial tissues, causing vasculitis and diverse, sometimes severe clinical signs as early as 2 to 3 days after exposure. Cats are resistant to clinical infection.

#### Clinical features

Any dog not previously exposed to *R. rickettsii* can develop RMSF, although most infections in dogs are subclinical. Some develop acute disease with a clinical course of approximately 14 days. Frequently the tick has fed and left the dog before the development of clinical signs, and most owners were unaware of their dog's tick infestation.

Fever and depression are the most common signs. Body temperature of greater than 40° C is found in many dogs, although low-grade fever is more common. Other common signs, seen in more than 50% of cases, include anorexia, myalgia or arthralgia, lymphadenopathy, and vestibular signs; however, lymphadenopathy (and splenomegaly) is not as common as in dogs with ehrlichiosis. Less common signs (30% to 50% of cases) include dyspnea, cough, conjunctivitis and/or scleral injection, abdominal pain, and edema of the face and/or extremities.

Interstitial pulmonary disease, dyspnea, cough, and signs (e.g., nausea, vomiting, diarrhea) occur in some dogs. Petechiae, epistaxis, subconjunctival hemorrhage, hyphema, anterior uveitis, iris hemorrhage, retinal petechiae, and retinal edema are also common. Cutaneous manifestations include hyperemia, petechiae, and dermal necrosis. Hemorrhage results from vasculitis, thrombocytopenia (from platelet consumption at sites of vasculitis and from immune destruction), and disseminated intravascular coagulation (DIC). CNS manifestations include vestibular signs (nystagmus, ataxia, head tilt), seizures, and hyperesthesia. Fatal RMSF is generally secondary to cardiac arrhythmias and shock, pulmonary disease, acute renal failure, or severe central nervous system (CNS) disease.

#### Diagnosis

Clinicopathologic and radiographic abnormalities are common but do not definitively document RMSF. Presumptive diagnosis is based on the combination of appropriate historical, clinical, and clinicopathologic findings, serology, exclusion of other causes, and response to antirickettsial drugs.

*Hematology.* Neutrophilic leukocytosis, with or without left shift, is found in most patients. Platelet counts are variable. Anemia (resulting from blood loss) and coagulation abnormalities consistent with DIC occur in some dogs.

*Serum biochemistry.* Increased activities of alanine aminotransferase (ALT), aspartate aminotransferase, and alkaline phosphatase (AP), as well as hypoalbuminemia, frequently occur; hyperglobulinemia is rare. Renal insufficiency in some dogs causes azotemia and metabolic acidosis. Serum sodium, chloride, and potassium concentrations decrease in many dogs with GI signs or renal insufficiency. In contrast to dogs with chronic ehrlichiosis, chronic proteinuria from glomerulonephritis is rare. Results of the direct Coombs' test are positive in some dogs.

*Other tests.* CNS inflammation usually causes increased protein concentration and neutrophilic pleocytosis in CSF; some dogs have mononuclear cell pleocytosis or mixed inflammation. No pathognomonic radiographic abnormalities are associated with RMSF, but infected dogs commonly develop pulmonary interstitial patterns. Nonseptic, suppurative polyarthritis occurs in some dogs.

*Serology.* Most dogs with RMSF have positive immunoglobulin (Ig) M titers; IgG can be negative on initial evaluation, because positive titers do not develop until 20 to 25 days after infection. False-negative results may also occur with IgM testing because of the short duration of antibodies in serum. Seroconversion or an increasing titer over 2 to 3 weeks suggests recent infection. Positive serum antibody tests results alone do not prove infection by *R. rickettsii*; subclinical infection is common, and infection with nonpathogenic rickettsiae (e.g., *Rickettsia montana, Rickettsia belli, Rickettsia rhipicephali*) induces cross-reacting antibodies.

*Polymerase chain reaction.* Polymerase chain reaction (PCR) can be used to document the presence of rickettsial agents in blood, other fluids, and tissues.

### Treatment and prognosis

Supportive care for GI fluid and electrolyte losses, renal disease, DIC, and anemia is provided as indicated. Overzealous fluid therapy may worsen respiratory or CNS signs if vasculitis is severe.

*Antibiotics.* Tetracyclines, chloramphenicol, and enrofloxacin are the antirickettsial drugs used most frequently. Tetracycline (22 mg/kg orally [PO] q8h for 14 to 21 days) may be used; however, doxycycline (5 to 10 mg/kg PO q12h for 14 to 21 days) is an alternative with superior GI absorption and CNS penetration. Chloramphenicol (22 to 25 mg/kg PO q8h for 14 days) can be used in puppies less than 5 months of age to avoid dental staining caused by tetracyclines. Enrofloxacin (3 mg/kg PO q12h for 7 days) is as effective as tetracyclines or chloramphenicol. Antibiotics should be administered parenterally if GI signs are present. Administration of prednisolone at antiinflammatory or immunosuppressive doses in combination with doxycycline did not potentiate RMSF in experimentally infected dogs.

*Prognosis.* Fever, depression, and thrombocytopenia often begin to resolve within 24 to 48 hours after therapy is started. Prognosis for recovery is fair; death occurs in less than 5% of affected dogs.

### Zoonotic aspects and prevention

Because RMSF has not been reported twice in the same dog, permanent immunity is likely. Infection can be prevented by providing strict tick control. It is unlikely that people acquire RMSF from contact with dogs, but dogs may increase human exposure by bringing ticks into the human environment. People can also be infected when removing ticks with *R. rickettsii* from the dog by hand.


## CANINE EHRLICHIOSIS (TEXT PP 1267-1270)

### Epidemiology

*Ehrlichia* spp. are tick-borne *Rickettsia* that form intracellular clusters (morulae). The parasitized cells, vectors, and pathogenic potential for the species that can infect dogs are summarized in Table 101-1. *Ehrlichia canis* is the most common and causes the most severe disease. Dogs seropositive for *E. canis* have been identified in many regions of the

## Table 101-1

### *Ehrlichia* Species That Infect Dogs

| Species | Cells infected | Vector | Clinical disease |
|---|---|---|---|
| E. canis | Mononuclear | Rhipicephalus sanguineus | See text and Tables 101-2 and 101-3 |
| E. ewingii | Granulocytes | Amblyomma americanum? | Polyarthritis, fever, meningitis |
| E. platys | Platelets | Unknown | Fever, thrombocytopenia, uveitis |
| Anaplasma phagocytophila | Granulocytes | Ixodes pacificus | Fever, polyarthritis |
| E. risticii | Mononuclear | Unknown | Similar to E. canis |
| E. chaffeensis | Mononuclear | A. americanum; Dermacentor variabilis | Unclear in natural infections |

world and most parts of the United States, but the majority of cases occur in areas with a high concentration of brown dog ticks (*Rhipicephalus sanguineus*), such as the Southwest and Gulf Coast. *Ehrlichia risticii* var *atypicalis* has been detected only in the United States to date. *Ehrlichia platys* is most common in the southeastern United States, southern Europe, and South America. *Ehrlichia ewingii* is most common in the southern parts of the mideastern states. *Ehrlichia chaffeensis* infections are detected primarily in the southeastern United States. *Anaplasma phagocytophila* (formerly *Ehrlichia equi*) is most common in California, Wisconsin, Minnesota, and the northeastern states and is also found in Europe, Asia, and Africa. *Ehrlichia* spp. can be transmitted by blood transfusions, so blood donors should be serologically screened for evidence of infection.

*E. canis* infection causes acute, subclinical, and chronic phases of disease. The acute phase (vasculitis) begins 1 to 3 weeks after infection, lasts 2 to 4 weeks, and is recognized most frequently in the spring and summer when the tick vector is most active; most immunocompetent dogs survive. The subclinical phase lasts months to years. Although some dogs clear the organism during this phase, it persists intracellularly in others, leading to the chronic phase. Many of the clinical and clinicopathologic abnormalities during the chronic phase are from immune reactions against the intracellular organism. An individual dog can be infected by more than one ehrlichial agent.

### Clinical features

Clinical disease can occur in any dog, but severity varies with the organism, host factors, and presence of coinfections. Dogs with depressed cell-mediated immunity develop severe disease. Clinical findings are summarized in Table 101-2.

*Acute phase.* Signs of acute disease are very similar to those of RMSF. Fever is most common in dogs with acute ehrlichiosis. Petechiae or other evidence of bleeding is generally a result of mild thrombocytopenia (platelet consumption or immune-mediated destruction) and vasculitis. However, thrombocytopenia in the acute phase is usually not severe enough to cause spontaneous bleeding.

*Chronic phase.* Pale mucous membranes typically are seen only in the chronic phase. Evidence of hemorrhage is from thrombocytopenia (consumption, immune-mediated destruction, sequestration, decreased production), vasculitis, and/or platelet function abnormalities. Hepatomegaly, splenomegaly, and lymphadenopathy are common and result from chronic immune stimulation. Dyspnea or cough can be caused by interstitial or alveolar edema, pulmonary parenchymal hemorrhage, or secondary infections from neutropenia. Polydipsia, polyuria, and proteinuria are reported in dogs that develop renal insufficiency. Stiffness; exercise intolerance; and swollen, painful joints occur in some dogs with suppurative, nonseptic polyarthritis. Most dogs with polyarthritis are infected with *E. ewingii* or *A. phagocytophila* (previously *E. equi*).

Table 101-2

## Clinical Abnormalities Associated with *Ehrlichia canis* Infection in Dogs

| Stage of infection | Abnormalities |
|---|---|
| Acute | Fever |
| | Serous or purulent oculonasal discharge |
| | Anorexia |
| | Weight loss |
| | Dyspnea |
| | Lymphadenopathy |
| | Tick infestation often evident |
| Subclinical | No clinical abnormalities |
| | Ticks often not present |
| Chronic | Ticks often not present |
| | Depression |
| | Weight loss |
| | Pale mucous membranes |
| | Abdominal pain |
| | Evidence of hemorrhage; epistaxis, retinal hemorrhage, etc. |
| | Lymphadenopathy |
| | Splenomegaly |
| | Dyspnea, increased lung sounds, interstitial or alveolar lung infiltrates |
| | Ocular abnormalities: perivascular retinitis, hyphema, retinal detachment, anterior or posterior uveitis, corneal edema |
| | Central nervous system abnormalities: meningeal pain, paresis, cranial nerve deficits, seizures |
| | Hepatomegaly |
| | Arrhythmias and pulse deficits |
| | Polyuria and polydipsia |
| | Stiffness and swollen, painful joints |

Ophthalmic signs are common and include tortuous retinal vessels, perivascular retinal infiltrates, retinal hemorrhage, anterior uveitis, and exudative retinal detachment. CNS signs can include depression, pain, ataxia, paresis, nystagmus, and seizures.

### Diagnosis

Clinicopathologic abnormalities consistent with *E. canis* infection are summarized in Table 101-3. Presumptive diagnosis is based on the combination of appropriate clinical findings and positive results of serologic tests.

*Hematology.* Neutropenia is common during acute phase vasculitis and with bone marrow suppression in the chronic phase. Chronic immune stimulation causes monocytosis and lymphocytosis; lymphocytes often have cytoplasmic azurophilic granules (large granular lymphocytes). Regenerative anemia is from blood loss (acute and chronic phases); normocytic, normochromic, nonregenerative anemia is from bone marrow suppression or anemia of chronic disease (chronic phase). Thrombocytopenia can occur with either acute or chronic ehrlichiosis but is generally more severe with chronic phase disease. Thrombocytopathies from hyperglobulinemia potentiate bleeding in some dogs with chronic ehrlichiosis.

*Serum biochemistry.* Hypoalbuminemia in the acute phase results from vasculitis, whereas in chronic phase disease it results from glomerular loss from immune complex deposition or chronic immunostimulation (i.e., monoclonal or polyclonal gammopathy). Prerenal azotemia can occur with acute or chronic disease; renal azotemia develops in some dogs with severe glomerulonephritis.

**Table 101-3**

## Clinicopathologic Findings Associated with *Ehrlichia canis* Infection in Dogs

| Stage of infection | Clinicopathologic abnormalities |
| --- | --- |
| Acute | Thrombocytopenia |
| | Leukopenia followed by neutrophilic leukocytosis and monocytosis |
| | Morulae |
| | Low-grade, nonregenerative anemia, unless hemorrhage has occurred |
| | Variable *Ehrlichia* titer |
| Subclinical | Hyperglobulinemia |
| | Thrombocytopenia |
| | Neutropenia |
| | Lymphocytosis |
| | Monocytosis |
| | Positive *Ehrlichia* titer |
| Chronic | Monocytosis |
| | Lymphocytosis |
| | Thrombocytopenia |
| | Nonregenerative anemia |
| | Hyperglobulinemia |
| | Hypocellular bone marrow |
| | Bone marrow or spleen plasmacytosis |
| | Hypoalbuminemia |
| | Proteinuria |
| | Polyclonal or IgG monoclonal gammopathy |
| | CSF mononuclear cell pleocytosis |
| | Nonseptic, suppurative polyarthritis |
| | Rare azotemia |
| | Increased ALT and AP activities |
| | Positive *Ehrlichia* titer |

*ALT,* Alanine aminotransferase; *AP,* alkaline phosphatase; *CSF,* cerebrospinal fluid; *IgG,* immunoglobulin G.

Hyperglobulinemia with hypoalbuminemia is consistent with subclinical or chronic ehrlichiosis. Polyclonal gammopathies are most common, but monoclonal (IgG) gammopathies can also occur.

*Cytology.* Rarely, morulae from *E. canis* are detected in the cytoplasm of mononuclear cells. Identification of morulae in cells confirms *Ehrlichia* infection but is uncommon except with the granulocytic strains. Examination of buffy coat smears or blood smears made with blood collected from an ear margin vessel may increase the chances of finding morulae. Aspirates of enlarged lymph nodes and spleen reveal lymphoreticular and plasma cell hyperplasia. Nondegenerate neutrophils are the primary cells in synovial fluid from dogs with polyarthritis; *E. ewingii* and *A. phagocytophila* morulae can be identified in synovial neutrophils from some dogs. Bone marrow aspirates in dogs with chronic ehrlichiosis typically reveal myeloid, erythroid, and megakaryocytic hypoplasia, with lymphoid and plasma cell hyperplasia. Bone marrow plasmacytosis is common in dogs with subclinical and chronic ehrlichiosis and can be confused with multiple myeloma, particularly in dogs with monoclonal gammopathies.

*Radiography.* No pathognomonic radiographic signs are present in dogs with ehrlichiosis. The polyarthritis is nonerosive. Dogs with respiratory signs most commonly have increased pulmonary interstitial markings, but alveolar patterns can occur.

***Serology.*** Most commercial laboratories offer indirect immunofluorescent antibody assays (IFA) for detection of IgG against *E. canis* in serum. Positive antibody titers can be detected for up to 31 months after therapy in some dogs. Those with low titers (less than 1:1024) generally become negative within 1 year after therapy, whereas dogs with titers greater than 1:1024 often remain positive after therapy; it is unknown whether these dogs are carriers.

Negative *E. canis* serology does not exclude the possibility of infection by other *Ehrlichia* spp. or by *E. canis* (clinical disease can be detected before seroconversion). Likewise, positive *E. canis* serology is not diagnostic for *E. canis* because of the existence of cross-reactive antibodies between *Ehrlichia* spp. and also among *E. canis*, *Neorickettsia helminthoeca*, and *Cowdria ruminantium*. *E. canis* IFA antibody titers between 1:10 and 1:80 should be rechecked in 2 to 3 weeks because of the potential for false-positive results at these titer levels. A presumptive diagnosis of canine ehrlichiosis can be made in dogs with positive *E. canis* serology and clinical signs consistent with ehrlichiosis. IFA using *E. platys*, *A. phagocytophila*, and *E. risticii* are available commercially and may be indicated for the evaluation of dogs that are *E. canis* seronegative but still suspected of having ehrlichiosis.

***Other tests.*** PCR can be used to detect organism-specific DNA in peripheral blood leukocytes. It can be performed on joint fluid, aqueous humor, cerebrospinal fluid, and tissues. Blood PCR results can be positive before seroconversion, and positive results document infection, whereas positive serologic tests only document exposure. Lack of laboratory standardization and quality control can lead to both false-positive and false-negative results. PCR should be used along with serology, and not in lieu of it. Blood samples for PCR should be drawn before antibiotic therapy is initiated. *E. canis* can also be identified by inoculation of blood from infected dogs into susceptible dogs or by cell culture, but these procedures are impractical. Ehrlichiosis generally causes mononuclear pleocytosis and increased protein concentrations in CSF. Antinuclear antibody, Coombs', and rheumatoid factor tests and LE cell preparations are positive in some dogs with ehrlichiosis, leading to an inappropriate diagnosis of primary immune-mediated disease.

### Treatment and monitoring

Supportive care should be provided as indicated. Doxycycline (10 mg/kg PO q24h for 28 days) is recommended for treatment. Clinical signs and thrombocytopenia should rapidly resolve. If clinical abnormalities are not resolving within 7 days, other differential diagnoses should be considered. Tetracycline, doxycycline, or chloramphenicol have also been used. Imidocarb dipropionate (5 to 7 mg/kg subcutaneously [SC] repeated in 14 days) has also been used successfully, but some patients develop pain at the injection site, salivation, oculonasal discharge, diarrhea, tremors, and dyspnea. Quinolones are not effective for the treatment of ehrlichiosis.

It is currently unknown whether ehrlichial infections are cleared by treatment. Antibody titers are ineffective for monitoring response to therapy. The resolution of thrombocytopenia and hyperglobulinemia should be monitored as markers of therapeutic elimination of the organism. PCR can also be used to monitor treatment. The PCR test should be repeated 2 weeks after treatment is stopped; if results are still positive, treatment should be reinstituted for 4 weeks and retesting performed. If PCR results are still positive after two treatment cycles, an alternate antiehrlichial drug should be used. If PCR results are negative, the test should be repeated in 8 weeks, and if still negative it can be assumed therapeutic elimination is likely. Whether to treat seropositive, healthy dogs is controversial. The primary reason to treat a seropositive, healthy dog is to try to eliminate infection before development of chronic phase disease. (See text for counterarguments.)

Anabolic steroids and other bone marrow stimulants can be tried when bone marrow suppression occurs (chronic phase), but they are unlikely to be effective. Anti-inflammatory or immunosuppressive doses of glucocorticoids are recommended to counter immune-mediated destruction of red blood cells and platelets in acutely affected animals. Prednisone (2.2 mg/kg PO divided q12h) during the first 3 to 4 days after diagnosis may be beneficial in some cases.

***Prognosis.*** Prognosis is good for dogs with acute ehrlichiosis and variable to guarded for those with chronic ehrlichiosis. Fever, petechiation, vomiting, diarrhea, epistaxis, and thrombocytopenia often resolve within days after initiation of therapy in acute cases. Bone marrow suppression from chronic ehrlichiosis may not respond for weeks to months, if at all.

***Prevention.*** *E. canis* can be eliminated in the environment by tick control. If tick control is not feasible, tetracycline can be administered at a dosage of 6.6 mg/kg PO daily for 200 days. Blood donors should be screened serologically every year.

### Zoonotic aspects

Dogs and people are both infected by *E. canis*, *E. chaffeensis*, and *A. phagocytophila*. Although people cannot acquire ehrlichiosis from handling an infected dog, dogs may be reservoirs for these agents and may play a role in the human disease by bringing vectors into the human environment. Ticks should be removed and handled with care.

## FELINE EHRLICHIOSIS (TEXT P 1271)

### Epidemiology

*Ehrlichia*-like morulae have been detected in mononuclear cells and neutrophils of naturally exposed cats worldwide. A presumptive diagnosis of ehrlichiosis has been based on detection of morulae or DNA in clinically ill cats or by the combination of positive serology, clinical or clinicopathologic findings consistent with ehrlichial infection, exclusion of other causes, and response to an antirickettsial drug. Pathogenesis of disease associated with ehrlichiosis in cats is unknown; arthropod vectors have been associated with some cases.

### Clinical features

Anorexia, fever, inappetence, lethargy, weight loss, hyperesthesia or joint pain, pale mucous membranes, splenomegaly, dyspnea, and lymphadenomegaly are the most common historical and physical examination abnormalities. Concurrent diseases are rarely reported but have included *Haemobartonella felis* (i.e., *Mycoplasma*) infection and lymphoma.

### Diagnosis

PCR and gene sequencing can be used to confirm infection and should be considered the tests of choice at this time. However, as for dogs, no standardization exists among laboratories that provide *Ehrlichia* PCR. A tentative diagnosis of feline clinical ehrlichiosis can be based on the combination of positive serologic test results, clinical signs of disease consistent with *Ehrlichia* infection, exclusion of other causes of the disease syndrome, and response to antirickettsial drugs. Positive antibody titers are found in both healthy and ill cats, so a diagnosis of ehrlichiosis cannot be based on serology alone.

***Clinicopathologic findings.*** Anemia, usually nonregenerative, is common. Leukopenia is common, but leukocytosis (neutrophilia, lymphocytosis, monocytosis and intermittent thrombocytopenia) is also seen. Intermittent thrombocytopenia is sometimes reported. Hyperglobulinemia (often polyclonal gammopathy, but monoclonal gammopathy is possible) can also occur. Some cats with suspected clinical ehrlichiosis seroreact to *E. canis*, *E. risticii*, or *A. phagocytophila* morulae. Antibodies that seroreact to more than one *Ehrlichia* species are sometimes detected. Some cats infected with *E. canis* are seronegative. In contrast, most *A. phagocytophila*–infected cats have strongly positive antibody test results. Western blot immunoassay has been used to confirm some *E. risticii*–positive results. Positive serologic test results occur in both healthy and clinically ill cats, and so a diagnosis of clinical ehrlichiosis should not be based on serologic test results alone. *Ehrlichia* spp. have been cultured from some cats on monocyte cell cultures.

### Treatment

Treatment with doxycycline (10 mg/kg PO q24h for 28 days) is recommended. In cats with treatment failure or those intolerant of doxycycline, imidocarb dipropionate can be given safely (5 mg/kg SC twice, 14 days apart). Salivation and pain at the injection site are the common adverse effects. Tetracycline is an alternative treatment option. Most cats improve clinically after therapy with tetracycline, doxycycline, or imidocarb dipropionate.

### Zoonotic aspects and prevention

Cats are known to be infected by *E. canis* and *A. phagocytophila,* agents that also infect people. However, direct transmission of *Ehrlichia* organisms does not occur. Care should be taken when removing ticks, and arthropod control should be maintained at all times for cats, particularly if allowed outdoors.

## OTHER RICKETTSIAL INFECTIONS (TEXT P 1271)

Hemolytic anemia induced by *H. felis* (reclassified as a *Mycoplasma*) and *Haemobartonella canis* is discussed in Chapter 85. *N. helminthoeca* (salmon poisoning) causes enteric signs in dogs from the Pacific Northwest (see Chapter 33). *Coxiella burnetii* infection associated with parturient or aborting cats is primarily of zoonotic concern (see Chapter 105).

# 102

# Polysystemic Viral Diseases

## (Text pp 1273-1286)

### CANINE DISTEMPER VIRUS (TEXT PP 1273-1275)

Please see other chapters for a discussion of viral diseases more specific to one organ system.

#### Epidemiology

Canine distemper virus (CDV) induces disease predominantly in terrestrial carnivores, but seals, ferrets, porpoises, and exotic Felidae may also be infected. The virus replicates in lymphoid, nervous, and epithelial tissues and is shed in respiratory exudates, feces, saliva, urine, and conjunctival exudates for 60 to 90 days after infection. Disease severity and the tissues involved vary with the strain of virus and the host's immune status. Nonimmune dogs of any age are susceptible, but disease is most common in puppies 3 to 6 months old. Massive virus replication in epithelial cells of the respiratory, gastrointestinal (GI), and genitourinary tracts occurs in animals with poor immune responses by days 9 to 14 after infection; these dogs usually die from polysystemic disease. In dogs with moderate immune responses by day 9 to 14 after infection, the virus replicates in epithelial tissues and may cause clinical signs of disease. Most dogs with low or no antibody response develop clinical signs of central nervous system (CNS) disease. Dogs with good cell-mediated responses and virus-neutralizing antibody titers by day 14 after infection clear the virus from most tissues and may not be clinically affected.

#### Clinical features

Affected dogs generally are presented because of depression, malaise, oculonasal discharge, cough, vomiting, diarrhea, or CNS signs (Table 102-1). Dogs with poor immune responses generally have the most severe signs, which progress rapidly to life-

**Table 102-1**

## Clinical Manifestations of Canine Distemper Virus Infection

| | |
|---|---|
| In utero infection | Stillbirth |
| | Abortion |
| | Fading puppy syndrome in the neonatal period |
| | Central nervous system signs at birth |
| Gastrointestinal tract disease | Vomiting |
| | Small bowel diarrhea |
| Respiratory tract disease | Mucoid to mucopurulent nasal discharge |
| | Sneezing |
| | Coughing with increased bronchovesicular sounds or crackles on auscultation |
| | Dyspnea |
| Ocular disease | Chorioretinitis, medallion lesions, optic neuritis |
| | Keratoconjunctivitis sicca |
| | Mucopurulent ocular discharge |
| Neurologic disease | |
| Spinal cord disease | Paresis and ataxia |
| Central vestibular disease | Head tilt, nystagmus, conscious proprioception deficits |
| Cerebellar disease | Ataxia, head bobbing, hypermetria |
| Cerebral disease | Generalized or partial seizures (chewing gum fits) |
| | Depression |
| | Unilateral or bilateral blindness |
| Chorea myoclonus | Rhythmic jerking of single muscles or muscle groups |
| Miscellaneous | Fever |
| | Anorexia |
| | Tonsillar enlargement |
| | Dehydration |
| | Pustular dermatosis |
| | Hyperkeratosis of the nose and footpads |
| | Enamel hypoplasia in surviving puppies |

threatening disease. Some partially immune dogs have only mild respiratory disease, presumptively diagnosed as kennel cough. Tonsillar enlargement, fever, and mucopurulent ocular discharge are common. Increased bronchial sounds, crackles, and wheezes are usually ausculted in dogs with bronchopneumonia.

***CNS signs.*** Hyperesthesia, seizures, cerebellar or vestibular disease, paresis, and chorea myoclonus commonly develop within 21 days after recovery from systemic disease, although systemic signs are inapparent in approximately 30% of dogs with CNS signs. CNS involvement generally is progressive and carries a poor prognosis. "Old dog encephalitis" is a chronic, progressive panencephalitis in older dogs (more than 6 years of age) thought to be a result of CDV infection. Depression, circling, head-pressing, and visual deficits are common.

***Ocular signs.*** Abnormalities include anterior uveitis, optic neuritis with resulting blindness and mydriasis, and chorioretinitis. Encephalitis and chorioretinitis are found in approximately 40% of dogs with CDV infection. Keratoconjunctivitis sicca and hyperreflective retinal scars (medallion lesions) occur in some dogs with chronic infection.

***Other signs.*** Dogs infected before development of permanent dentition will usually have enamel hypoplasia. Hyperkeratosis of the nose and footpads and pustular dermatitis are the most common dermatologic abnormalities. Puppies infected transplacentally may be stillborn, aborted, or born with CNS disease.

### Diagnosis

Presumptive diagnosis is based on the combination of clinical findings and routine clinicopathologic and radiographic evaluation. Lymphopenia and mild thrombocytopenia are consistent hematologic abnormalities. Radiographically, interstitial and alveolar pulmonary infiltrates are common in dogs with respiratory signs. Although some dogs with CNS infection have normal cerebrospinal fluid (CSF) analyses, most have mononuclear cell pleocytosis and increased protein concentrations. The ratios of serum-to-CSF immunoglobulin (Ig) G and albumin commonly are high in dogs with CDV encephalitis.

*Serology.* Measurement of serum or CSF antibodies can aid diagnosis. Detection of IgM antibodies in serum or a fourfold increase in serum IgG over 2 to 3 weeks is consistent with recent infection or vaccination. CSF antibodies to CDV are increased in some dogs with encephalitis. False-positive results can occur in CSF samples contaminated with blood; but CSF antibody titers greater than those in serum are consistent with CNS infection with CDV. If increased protein, lymphocytic pleocytosis, and antibodies against CDV are detected in a CSF sample not contaminated with peripheral blood, a presumptive diagnosis of CDV encephalitis can be made.

*Virus detection.* Definitive diagnosis requires demonstration of viral inclusions by cytology, histopathology, or direct fluorescent antibody staining of cytologic or histopathologic specimens or polymerase chain reaction (PCR) documentation of CDV DNA in peripheral blood, CSF, or conjunctival scrapings. Viral inclusions can sometimes be found in erythrocytes, leukocytes, and leukocyte precursors, but they are generally present for only 2 to 9 days after infection and therefore are often absent when clinical signs occur. They may be easier to find in smears made from the buffy coat or bone marrow aspirates. Viral particles can be detected by immunofluorescence in cells from the tonsils, respiratory tree, urinary tract, conjunctival scrapings, and CSF for 5 to 21 days after infection.

### Treatment
Therapy is nonspecific and supportive. Secondary bacterial infections of the GI and respiratory systems are common and should be treated with appropriate antibiotics if indicated (see Chapter 98). Anticonvulsants are administered as needed to control seizures; there exists no known effective treatment for chorea myoclonus. Glucocorticoid administration may be beneficial in some dogs with CNS disease from chronic CDV infection, but it is contraindicated in acutely infected dogs. Prognosis for dogs with CNS distemper is poor.

### Prevention
The virus survives in exudates only for approximately 20 minutes and is susceptible to most routine hospital disinfectants. Dogs with GI or respiratory signs should be isolated, and care should be taken to avoid transmission by contaminated fomites. Dogs with only CNS signs generally are not shedding virus.

Puppies should be vaccinated with a modified-live vaccine at 6 to 8 weeks of age and receive boosters every 3 weeks until at least 14 weeks of age, with a booster given at 1 year of age. Recent data suggest that after the 1-year booster, repeat boosters are not needed again for a minimum of 3 years (see Chapter 99). In high-risk puppies, measles virus vaccines are used to induce heterologous antibodies that will protect puppies against CDV as maternal antibodies wane. Measles vaccine is given concurrently with modified-live distemper vaccine but should not be used before 6 weeks or after 12 weeks of age. At least two distemper boosters should be given after the initial measles vaccine. Vaccination is not as effective if body temperature is 39.9° C or more or if other systemic diseases are detected (see Chapter 99).

In some dogs coinfected with canine parvovirus, CDV encephalitis develops after vaccination with modified-live CDV vaccines. Mild, transient, thrombocytopenia can result from modified CDV vaccination but has not been associated with spontaneous bleeding.

## FELINE CORONAVIRUS (TEXT PP 1275-1278)

### Epidemiology
Coronaviruses that cause disease in cats include feline infectious peritonitis virus (FIPV) and feline enteric coronavirus (FECV). Enteric infection generally results in mild

GI signs, whereas systemic infection can induce a clinical syndrome with diverse manifestations (feline infectious peritonitis [FIP]). In cattery outbreaks, usually only one or two kittens in a litter are clinically affected.

**Transmission.** Enteric coronaviruses commonly are shed in feces and rarely in saliva and are very contagious. By use of reverse transcriptase PCR (RT-PCR) testing, coronaviruses can be detected in feces as early as 3 days after infection.

**Pathogenesis.** Disease resulting from FECV is related to inflammation associated with viral replication in the epithelial cells of the ileum and jejunum. Coronaviruses with the ability to infect monocytes can cause viremia and disseminate throughout the body, potentially resulting in FIP. The effusive form of FIP develops in cats with poor cell-mediated immunity; it is an immune-complex vasculitis characterized by leakage of protein-rich fluid into the pleural and pericardial spaces, peritoneal cavity, and subcapsular space of the kidneys. The noneffusive form develops in cats with partial cell-mediated immunity; pyogranulomatous or granulomatous lesions develop in multiple tissues, particularly in the eyes, brain, kidneys, omentum, and liver. Some cats have characteristics of both forms of FIP. Clinical disease may be influenced by the virulence of the strain, dose of the virus, route of infection, immune status of the host, genetically determined host factors, presence of concurrent infections, and previous exposure to a coronavirus. Inheritance of susceptibility appears to be polygenic. Feline leukemia virus (FeLV), feline immunodeficiency virus (FIV), and respiratory tract infections increase susceptibility to FIP.

### Clinical features

Enteric replication of coronaviruses commonly results in fever, vomiting, and mucoid diarrhea. With FECV infection, signs are self-limiting and generally respond within days to supportive care.

Fulminant FIP can occur in cats of any age but is generally seen in cats under 5 years of age; most affected cats are 1 year old. Intact males are overrepresented in some studies. Anorexia, weight loss, and general malaise are common presenting complaints (Box 102-1); fever and weight loss are often seen in both the effusive and the noneffusive forms. Icterus, ocular inflammation, abdominal distention, dyspnea, and CNS abnormalities are occasionally noted, and pale mucous membranes or petechiation is found in some cats. FIP is one of the most common causes of icterus in cats under 2 years of age.

The liver may be normal in size or enlarged; the margins generally are irregular. Abdominal distention is common; a fluid wave can often be balloted, and occasionally masses (pyogranulomas or lymphadenopathy) can be palpated in the omentum, mesentery, and intestines. A solitary ileocecocolic or colonic mass, resulting in obstruction leading to vomiting and diarrhea, occurs in some cats. The kidneys may be small (chronic disease) or large (acute disease or subcapsular effusion); renal margins are usually irregular. Sometimes, fluid accumulation causes scrotal enlargement in male cats. Pleural effusion can result in dyspnea and a restrictive breathing pattern (shallow and rapid), as well as muffled heart and lung sounds.

Anterior uveitis and chorioretinitis occur most often with the noneffusive form and can be its only manifestation. Pyogranulomatous disease can develop anywhere in the CNS, leading to a variety of neurologic signs including seizures, posterior paresis, and nystagmus.

### Diagnosis

Multiple clinicopathologic and diagnostic imaging abnormalities develop in cats with FIP, but none are pathognomonic. Presumptive diagnosis is usually based on the combination of clinical and laboratory findings.

**Clinicopathologic findings.** Normocytic, normochromic, nonregenerative anemia; neutrophilic leukocytosis; and lymphopenia are common. Disseminated intravascular coagulation resulting in thrombocytopenia develops in some cats. Hyperproteinemia with or without hypoalbuminemia can occur; polyclonal gammopathies resulting from increases in alpha-2 globulins and gamma globulins are most often found; monoclonal gammopathies are rare. Hyperbilirubinemia with variable increases in alanine aminotransferase and alkaline phosphatase (AP) activities occur in some cats with hepatic

---

**Box 102-1**

## Clinical Findings Suggestive of Feline Infectious Peritonitis

### SIGNALMENT AND HISTORY

Cats younger than 5 years of age or older than 10 years of age
Purebred cat
Purchase from a cattery or living in multicat household
Previous history of a mild, self-limiting gastrointestinal or respiratory disease
Serologic evidence of infection by feline leukemia virus
Nonspecific signs of anorexia, weight loss, or depression
Seizures, nystagmus, or ataxia
Acute, fulminant course in cats with effusive disease
Chronic, intermittent course in cats with noneffusive disease
Reproductive failure or kitten mortality complex rarely

### PHYSICAL EXAMINATION

Fever
Weight loss
Pale mucous membranes with or without petechiae
Dyspnea with a restrictive breathing pattern
Muffled heart or lung sounds
Abdominal distention with a fluid wave with or without scrotal swelling
Icterus with or without hepatomegaly
Chorioretinitis or iridocyclitis
Multifocal neurologic abnormalities
Irregularly marginated kidneys with or without renomegaly
Mesenteric lymphadenopathy
Splenomegaly

### CLINICOPATHOLOGIC ABNORMALITIES

Nonregenerative anemia
Neutrophilic leukocytosis with or without a left shift
Lymphopenia
Hyperglobulinemia characterized as a polyclonal gammopathy with increases in $alpha_2$ and gamma globulins; rare monoclonal gammopathies
Nonseptic, pyogranulomatous exudate in pleural space, peritoneal cavity, or pericardial space
Increased protein concentrations and neutrophilic pleocytosis in cerebrospinal fluid
Positive coronavirus antibody titer
Pyogranulomatous or granulomatous inflammation in perivascular location on histologic examination of tissues
Positive results of immunofluorescence or PCR performed on pleural or peritoneal exudate

---

disease. Increases in lipase and amylase activities in serum or peritoneal effusions can be detected in cats with pancreatic involvement. Prerenal or renal azotemia and proteinuria are the most common.

*Diagnostic imaging.* Radiographs may reveal pleural, pericardial, or peritoneal effusions; hepatomegaly; or renomegaly. Mesenteric lymphadenopathy results in mass lesions in some cats. Ultrasonography can be used to confirm the presence of abdominal fluid in cats with minimal fluid volumes and to evaluate the pancreas, liver, lymph nodes, and kidneys. Magnetic resonance imaging showed periventricular contrast enhancement, ventricular dilation, and hydrocephalus in one group of cats with neurologic FIP.

*Fluid analysis.* Effusions from cats with FIP are sterile, colorless, or straw colored; may contain fibrin strands; and may clot when exposed to air. The protein concentration commonly ranges from 3.5 g/dl to 12 g/dl. If the albumin/globulin ratio of the effusion is more than 0.81 or the albumin component is greater than 48% of the total protein, FIP is unlikely. But if the gamma-globulin concentration is more than 32% of the total protein or if the total protein is more than 3.5 g/dl and the globulin component is more than 50%, FIP is likely. Mixed populations of lymphocytes, macrophages, and neutrophils are seen most often; neutrophils predominate in most cases, but in some cats macrophages are the primary cell type. In some cats coronavirus antibody titers are greater in the effusion than in serum.

*Cerebrospinal fluid.* Increased protein concentration (more than 30 mg/dl) and nucleated cell counts (40 to 1600 cells/$\mu$l; predominantly neutrophils) are common in cats with CNS involvement. High coronavirus antibody titers are common in the CSF of cats with neurologic FIP. The presence of coronavirus antibodies in the CNS can aid in the diagnosis of neurologic FIP.

*Serology.* Detection of serum antibodies is of limited benefit. Infection by any coronavirus can cause cross-reacting antibodies, so a positive titer does not diagnose FIP, protect against disease, or predict when a cat may develop FIP. Occasionally cats with FIP are seronegative because of rapidly progressive disease, disappearance of antibody in the terminal stages, or immune complex formation. Kittens infected postnatally become seropositive at 8 to 14 weeks of age, so serologic testing of kittens can be used to prevent spread of coronaviruses. Serologic testing is also indicated as a screening procedure in antibody-negative breeding colonies.

*Other tests.* Coronavirus antigens are commonly detected by direct immuno-fluorescent antibody (IFA) in the effusions of cats with FIP but not in the effusions of cats with other disease. Viral RNA can be detected by RT-PCR in effusions with approximately 90% sensitivity and specificity.

*Definitive diagnosis.* Characteristic histopathologic findings, virus isolation (impractical), or demonstration of the virus in effusions or tissue by use of immuno-cytochemical or immunhistochemical staining, or RT-PCR allows definitive diagnosis. RT-PCR is used most frequently to detect coronaviruses in feces. Detection of coronavirus by RT-PCR in whole blood does not always correlate with the development of FIP.

### Treatment and prognosis

Supportive care, including correction of fluid and electrolyte imbalances, should be provided as needed.

*Antiviral drugs and immunotherapy.* To date there exists no uniformly successful antiviral treatment.

*Antiinflammatory therapy.* Modulation of the inflammatory reaction is the principal goal of palliative therapy. Low-dose prednisolone (1 to 2 mg/kg orally [PO] q24h) may lessen clinical manifestations of noneffusive FIP. However, the use of immune-suppressive drugs is controversial.

*Other medications.* Antibiotics may be indicated for the treatment of secondary bacterial infection. Anabolic steroids (e.g., stanozolol, 1 mg PO q12h), aspirin (10 mg/kg PO q48-72h), and ascorbic acid (125 mg PO q12h) have also been used.

*Prognosis.* The effusive form carries a grave prognosis. Most cats with systemic signs of FIP die or require euthanasia within days or months of diagnosis. Depending on the organ system involved and the severity of polysystemic signs, cats with non-effusive disease have a variable survival time. Cats with ocular FIP may respond to antiinflammatory treatment or enucleation and have a better prognosis than those with systemic FIP.

### Prevention and zoonotic aspects

Prevention is best accomplished by avoiding exposure to the virus. Although viral particles can survive in dried secretions for up to 7 weeks, routine disinfectants inactivate the virus. There exists no known transfer of FIPV or FECV to humans.

Kittens are most likely to become infected by contact with cats other than their queens after maternal antibodies wane (4 to 6 weeks of age). Kittens born in a breeding situation with seropositive cats should be separated from adult cats from weaning until the time they are sold; they should be serologically tested at 14 to 16 weeks of age and sold only if seronegative. Ideally, a seronegative household should be maintained. Cats can eliminate coronavirus infections; previously infected cats should be seronegative and have a negative fecal RT-PCR for 5 months in order to be considered coronavirus naïve.

An intranasal vaccine is available and is effective in at least some cats. Whether it protects against all field strains, mutations, or recombinants is unknown. The only indication for the vaccine is seronegative cats with risk of exposure to coronaviruses. It is unlikely that the vaccine is effective in previously infected cats. Vaccination induces serum antibody titers, making interpretation of serologic tests difficult in vaccinated cats that show clinical signs of FIP.

## FELINE IMMUNODEFICIENCY VIRUS (TEXT PP 1278-1281)

### Epidemiology

FIV infection has worldwide distribution in cats; prevalence rates vary greatly by region and the lifestyle of the cats. Biting is likely the primary route of transmission; therefore older, male, outdoor cats are most often infected. FIV is present in semen and can be transmitted by artificial insemination. Transplacental and perinatal transmission also occurs. The primary phase of infection occurs as the virus spreads throughout the body, initially causing low-grade fever, neutropenia, and generalized reactive lymphadenopathy. A subclinical, latent period of variable duration then develops. The median ages of infected, healthy cats and clinically ill cats are approximately 3 years and 10 years, respectively, suggesting a long latent period in most strains of FIV. After months or years, an immunodeficiency stage, similar to acquired immunodeficiency syndrome in humans, develops. Co-infection with FeLV potentiates the primary and immunodeficiency phases of FIV.

### Clinical features

Signs can be caused by direct viral effects or secondary infections that develop immunodeficiency. Primary (acute) FIV is characterized by fever and generalized lymphadenopathy.

FIV-infected cats in the immunodeficiency stage are commonly presented because of nonspecific signs such as anorexia, weight loss, and depression or because of abnormalities associated with specific organ systems (Table 102-2). In addition to those listed, lymphadenopathy and hyperglobulinemia are common findings. FIV-infected cats are also at higher risk for the development of lymphoma. Behavioral abnormalities commonly associated with neurologic involvement include dementia, hiding, rage, inappropriate elimination, and roaming. Occasionally seizures, nystagmus, ataxia, and peripheral nerve abnormalities are seen.

### Diagnosis

Neutropenia, thrombocytopenia, and nonregenerative anemia are the most common hematologic abnormalities. Monocytosis and lymphocytosis occur in some cats. Cytologic examination of bone marrow aspirates may reveal maturation arrest (myelodysplasia), lymphoma, or leukemia. The presence of a multitude of serum biochemical abnormalities is possible, depending on which syndrome is occurring. Renal azotemia and polyclonal gammopathy are the changes most likely to be caused by direct viral effects. There exist no pathognomonic radiographic abnormalities.

*Serology.* Serum antibodies against FIV are detected by enzyme-linked immunosorbent assay (ELISA). Clinical signs can occur before seroconversion in some cats, and some infected cats never seroconvert; therefore false-negative reactions can occur. False-positive reactions are common using ELISA. In addition, the currently available FIV vaccine induces antibodies indistinguishable from antibodies in FIV-exposed or FIV-positive cats. Positive ELISA results in healthy cats, low-risk cats, or cats vaccinated

**Table 102-2**

## Clinical Syndromes Associated with FIV Infection and Possible Opportunistic Agents

| Clinical syndrome | Primary viral effect | Opportunistic agents |
|---|---|---|
| Dermatologic or otitis externa | None | Bacteria; atypical *Mycobacterium*; *Otodectes cynotis*; *Demodex cati*; *Notoedres cati*; dermatophytosis; *Cryptococcus neoformans*; cowpox |
| Gastrointestinal | Small bowel diarrhea | *Cryptosporidium* spp.; *Isospora* spp.; *Giardia* spp.; *Salmonella* spp.; *Campylobacter jejuni* |
| Glomerulonephritis | Yes | Bacteria; FeLV; FIP |
| Hematologic | Nonregenerative anemia; neutropenia; thrombocytopenia | *Mycoplasma haemofelis*; FeLV |
| Neoplasia | Myeloproliferative disorders; lymphoma; carcinomas; sarcomas | FeLV |
| Neurologic | Behavioral abnormalities | *Toxoplasma gondii*; *Crytococcus neoformans*; FIP; FeLV |
| Ocular | Pars planitis | *T. gondii*; FIP; *C. neoformans* |
|  | Anterior uveitis | *T. gondii*; *C. neoformans*; FIP; FeLV |
| Pneumonia or pneumonitis | None | Bacteria; *T. gondii*; *C. neoformans* |
| Pyothorax | None | Bacteria |
| Renal failure | Yes | Bacteria; FIP; FeLV |
| Stomatitis | None | Calicivirus; overgrowth of bacterial flora; candidiasis |
| Upper respiratory tract | None | Feline herpesvirus 1; overgrowth of bacterial flora; *C. neoformans* |
| Urinary tract infection | None | Bacteria |

*FeLV*, Feline leukemia virus; *FIP*, feline infectious peritonitis.

with the currently available FIV vaccine should be confirmed using Western blot immunoassay or PCR. Kittens can have detectable, colostrum-derived antibodies for several months. Kittens less than 6 months of age that are FIV seropositive should be tested every 60 days until the result is negative. If antibodies persist at 6 months of age, the kitten is likely infected. Detection of serum antibodies against FIV correlates well with persistent infection but not with disease induced by the virus.

***Virus detection.*** FIV infection can be confirmed by virus isolation or PCR, but these procedures are available only in some laboratories. Results of virus isolation or PCR on blood are positive in some antibody-negative cats.

### Treatment

Because FIV-seropositive cats are not necessarily immunosuppressed or sick, they should be evaluated and treated for other potential causes of the clinical syndrome.

If infectious diseases are identified, bactericidal drugs administered at the upper end of the dose range should be chosen. Long-term antibiotic therapy or multiple treatment periods may be required. The only way to accurately determine whether an FIV-seropositive cat with a concurrent infectious disease has a poor prognosis is to treat the concurrent infection.

***Antiviral drugs and immunotherapy.*** Antiviral agents such as AZT (Retrovir; see Table 102-3) have had mixed success in the treatment of FIV. AZT (5 mg/kg given PO or subcutaneously q12h) improves overall quality of life and stomatitis and aids in the treatment of neurologic signs. Cats treated with AZT should be monitored for anemia. Owners have reported positive responses to immunomodulators such as interferon-γ, but scientific information is not available.

Bovine lactoferrin (given PO) is beneficial in the treatment of intractable stomatitis. Removal of all premolar and molar teeth is also an effective treatment for intractable stomatitis in some cats (see Chapter 31). Erythropoietin administration increases red blood cell (RBC) counts in FIV-infected cats without adverse effects. Granulocyte-macrophage colony stimulating factor is contraindicated for the treatment of FIV in cats because of adverse effects.

### Prevention and zoonotic aspects

Housing of cats indoors, to avoid fighting, and testing of new cats before introduction to an FIV-seronegative household prevents most cases. FIV-positive cats should be housed indoors at all times to avoid exposing FIV-naïve cats in the environment and to lessen the chance that an opportunistic infection will be acquired. Cleaning shared litterboxes and dishes with scalding water and detergent inactivates the virus. Kittens queened by FIV-infected cats should not be allowed to nurse, and they should be shown to be serologically negative at 6 months of age before being sold. A killed vaccine is currently available, however, the efficacy and safety have not been assessed under field conditions in large numbers of cats (see Chapter 99). Antibodies against FIV have not been documented in the serum of human beings even after exposure to virus-containing material. However, cats with FIV-associated immunodeficiency may be more likely to spread zoonotic agents into the human environment.

## FELINE LEUKEMIA VIRUS (TEXT PP 1281-1284)

### Epidemiology

FeLV is spread by prolonged contact with infected cat saliva and nasal secretions (e.g., grooming, sharing common water or food sources). The organism does not survive in the environment, feces, or urine. Transplacental, lactational, and venereal transmission are less important than casual contact. FeLV infection has worldwide distribution; seroprevalence of infection varies geographically and by the population of cats tested. Infection is most common in outdoor male cats 1 to 6 years of age.

The virus replicates in the oropharynx, then spreads to the bone marrow (Table 102-4). If persistent bone marrow infection occurs, infected white blood cells and platelets leave the bone marrow, and epithelial structures including salivary and lacrimal glands are ultimately infected. Approximately 30% of exposed cats become persistently

**Table 102-3**

## Drug Treatment Regimens for Viremic, Clinically Ill Cats with Feline Leukemia Virus Infection

| Therapeutic agent* | Proposed mechanism of action | Administration |
|---|---|---|
| **ANTIVIRAL DRUG** | | |
| AZT | Reverse transcriptase inhibition | 20 mg/kg by mouth three times daily for 7 days and then 10 mg/kg by mouth three times daily; cats should be monitored for development of anemia |
| | | 5 mg/kg by mouth or subcutaneously twice daily |
| **IMMUNOTHERAPY** | | |
| Interferon-α | Prevents release of budding virions | Dilute $1.5 \times 10^6$ units of interferon-α into 500 ml of sterile saline and freeze in 1 ml aliquots; solution is stable for years if frozen |
| | | Dilute 1 ml with 100 ml of saline to make a concentration of 30 units/ml; solution is stable for several months if refrigerated |
| | | Administer 30 units (1 ml) by mouth once daily for 7 days, every other week until the cat is clinically normal |
| *Staphylococcus* A | B-lymphocyte and T-lymphocyte activation, immune-complex binding, interferon induction, and immunoglobulin Fc binding | Dissolve contents of a 5-mg vial in 3 ml of sterile water and add to 500 ml of sterile saline to give 10 µg/ml |
| | | Freeze in 5-ml aliquots |
| | | 1 ml/kg intraperitoneally twice weekly for 10 weeks followed by 1 ml/kg intraperitoneally twice weekly every fourth week for life |
| *Propionibacterium acnes* | Activation of macrophages and natural killer cells; increased production of interferon, tumor necrosis factor, and interleukin-1 | 0.5 ml intravenously twice weekly for 2 weeks followed by 0.5 ml intravenously weekly for 20 weeks or until p27 antigen is no longer detected in serum |
| Acemannan | Enhanced release of tumor necrosis factor, prostaglandin $E_2$, and interleukin-1α by macrophages | 2 mg/kg intraperitoneally once weekly for 6 weeks |

Modified from McCaw DL: In August JR, ed: *Consultations in feline internal medicine*, ed 2, Philadelphia, 1994, WB Saunders, p 21; Hartmann K, Donath A, Kraft W: *Fel Pract* 23:16,1995; and Hartmann K, Donath A, Kraft W: *Fel Pract* 23:13,1995.

*AZT. Retrovir, GlaxoSmithKline, Research Triangle Park, NC.
Interferon-α, Roferon, Hoffman LaRoche, Nutley, NJ.
*Staphylococcus* A, Pharmacia, Piscataway, NJ.
*Propionibacterium acnes*, Immunoregalin-Immunostimulant, ImmunoVet, Tampa, Fla.
Acemannan, Carrington Laboratories, Irving, Tex.

Table 102-4

## Stages of Feline Leukemia Virus Infection with Corresponding Test Results

| Stage | Organism localization | Timing | IFA result | ELISA result |
|-------|----------------------|--------|------------|--------------|
| I | Replication in local lymphoid tissues (tonsillar and pharyngeal with oronasal exposure) | 2-12 days | Negative | Negative |
| II | Dissemination in circulating lymphocytes and monocytes | 2-12 days | Negative | Positive |
| III | Replication in the spleen, distant lymph nodes, and gut-associated lymphoid tissue | 2-12 days | Negative | Positive |
| IV | Replication in bone marrow cells and intestinal epithelial crypts | 2-6 weeks | Negative | Positive |
| V | Peripheral viremia, dissemination via infected bone marrow–derived neutrophils and platelets | 4-6 weeks | Positive | Positive |
| VI | Disseminated epithelial cell infection with virus secretion in saliva and tears | 4-6 weeks | Positive | Positive |

Modified from Rojko JL, Kociba GJ: *J Am Vet Med Assoc* 199:1305-1310, 1991.

*ELISA,* Enzyme-linked immunosorbent assay; *IFA,* immunofluorescent antibody.

viremic; 30% are transiently viremic, developing neutralizing antibodies and clearing the infection within 4 to 6 weeks, and the remainder develop latent or sequestered (virus found in bone marrow, spleen, lymph node, and small intestine but not blood) infection. Latent and sequestered infections can be activated by glucocorticoids or other immunosuppressive drugs. Cats with persistent viremia usually die of an FeLV-related illness within 2 to 3 years.

### Clinical features

Owners generally present FeLV-infected cats for evaluation of nonspecific signs such as anorexia, weight loss, and depression or because of abnormalities associated with specific organ systems. Various clinical syndromes can result from specific effects of the virus or from immunosuppression and opportunistic infections (as for FIV; see Table 102-2).

*GI and hepatic signs.* Bacterial or calicivirus-induced stomatitis occurs in some FeLV-infected cats. FeLV infection can result in vomiting or diarrhea from (1) enteritis that clinically and histopathologically resembles panleukopenia, (2) alimentary lymphoma, or (3) secondary infections. Icterus can be (1) prehepatic, from immune-mediated hemolysis induced by FeLV or secondary infection by *Haemobartonella felis* (*Mycoplasma haemofelis* and *Mycoplasma haemominutum*); (2) hepatic, from hepatic lymphoma, hepatic lipidosis, or focal liver necrosis; or (3) posthepatic, from alimentary lymphoma. Some FeLV-infected cats with icterus are concurrently infected with FIPV or *Toxoplasma gondii.*

*Respiratory signs.* Secondary infections cause rhinitis or pneumonia in some FeLV-infected cats. Dyspnea from mediastinal lymphoma is seen in some cases. These cats generally are under 3 years of age and may have decreased cranial chest compliance on palpation; pleural effusion, if present, causes muffled heart and lung sounds.

*Lymphoma.* Mediastinal, multicentric, and alimentary lymphoma are the most common neoplasms associated with FeLV; lymphoid hyperplasia also occurs. Alimentary lymphoma most commonly involves the small intestines, mesenteric lymph nodes, kidneys, and liver of older cats. Renal lymphoma can involve one or both kidneys, which are usually enlarged and irregularly marginated on physical examination. Approximately 25% of infected cats have evidence of neoplasia (96% lymphoma or leukemia) at necropsy; the remainder die from other nonneoplastic diseases.

***Other neoplasms.*** Lymphocytic, myelogenous, erythroid, and megakaryocytic leukemia have all been reported secondary to FeLV infection; erythroid and myelomonocytic leukemias are most common. Fibrosarcomas occasionally develop in young cats co-infected with feline sarcoma virus.

***Urinary tract signs.*** Renal lymphoma or glomerulonephritis causes renal failure in some cases. Affected cats are presented for evaluation of polyuria and polydipsia, weight loss, and inappetence during the last stages of disease. Urinary incontinence resulting from either sphincter incompetence or detrusor hyperactivity occurs in some cats; small-bladder, nocturnal incontinence is reported most often.

***Ocular signs.*** Some FeLV-infected cats are presented because of miosis, blepharospasm, or cloudy eyes from ocular lymphoma. Aqueous flare, mass lesions, keratic precipitates, lens luxations, and glaucoma are often found on ocular examination.

***Neurologic signs.*** Nervous system disease is likely to develop as a result of polyneuropathy or lymphoma. Abnormalities can include anisocoria, ataxia, weakness, tetraparesis, paraparesis, behavioral change, and urinary incontinence. Intraocular and nervous system disease in FeLV-infected cats can also result from infection with other agents, including FIPV, *Cryptococcus neoformans*, and *T. gondii*.

***Reproductive signs.*** Abortion, stillbirth, or infertility occurs in some FeLV-infected queens. Kittens infected in utero that survive to parturition generally develop accelerated FeLV syndromes or die as part of the kitten mortality complex.

***Musculoskeletal signs.*** Some FeLV-seropositive cats are presented because of lameness or weakness resulting from neutrophilic polyarthritis attributed to immune complex deposition. Multiple cartilaginous exostoses occur in some cats and may be FeLV related.

### Diagnosis

A variety of nonspecific laboratory and radiographic abnormalities occur. When a clinical syndrome is diagnosed in an FeLV-seropositive cat, the workup should include diagnostic tests for other potential causes. The opportunistic agents discussed for FIV also are common in FeLV-infected cats (see Table 102-2).

***Hematology.*** Nonregenerative anemia alone or with decreases in lymphocytes, neutrophils, and platelets is common. Increased numbers of circulating nucleated RBCs or macrocytosis without appropriate reticulocytosis occurs frequently; examination of bone marrow often reveals maturation arrest in the erythroid line (erythrodysplasia). Immune-mediated hemolysis can be induced by FeLV and also occurs in cats co-infected with *M. haemofelis;* regenerative anemia, RBC microagglutination or macroagglutination, and positive direct Coombs' test are common in these cats. FeLV-infected cats with the panleukopenia-like syndrome have GI signs and neutropenia and are difficult to differentiate from cats with panleukopenia virus infection. The FeLV-infected cats usually have anemia and thrombocytopenia, abnormalities rarely associated with panleukopenia virus infection.

***Serum biochemistry.*** Azotemia, hyperbilirubinemia, bilirubinuria, and increased activities of liver enzymes are common. Proteinuria occurs in some cats with glomerulonephritis.

***Imaging.*** Cats with lymphoma have mass lesions that vary with the organ system affected. Mediastinal lymphoma can result in pleural effusion. Alimentary lymphoma can cause obstructive intestinal patterns.

***Cytology.*** Lymphoma can be diagnosed by cytologic or histopathologic evaluation of affected tissues. Cats with mediastinal masses, lymphadenopathy, renomegaly, hepatomegaly, splenomegaly, or intestinal masses should be evaluated cytologically before surgical intervention. Malignant lymphocytes are also occasionally identified in peripheral blood smears, effusions, or CSF.

***Virus detection.*** Most cats with suspected FeLV infection are screened for FeLV p27 antigen in neutrophils and platelets by IFA, or in whole blood, plasma, serum, saliva, or tears by ELISA. IFA is not positive until the bone marrow has been infected (see Table 102-3), but results are accurate more than 95% of the time. False-negative reactions may occur when leukopenia or thrombocytopenia prevents evaluation of an adequate number of cells. False-positive reactions can occur if the blood smears are too thick. A positive IFA indicates that the cat is viremic and contagious; approximately 90% of cats with positive IFA results will be viremic for life.

***Enzyme-linked immunosorbent assay.*** When used with blood, serum, or plasma, ELISA results are positive in some cats during early stages of infection or with self-limiting infection, even though IFA results may be negative. Cats with positive ELISA and negative IFA results are probably not contagious, but they should be isolated and retested in 4 to 6 weeks. Generally a delay of 1 to 2 weeks occurs after the onset of viremia before ELISA tear and saliva test results become positive, so these tests can have negative results even when results using serum are positive. They are also more likely than results of tests on blood, serum, or plasma to be false positive. Negative serum, plasma, or blood ELISA results correlate well with negative IFA results and an inability to isolate the virus.

***Latent infection.*** ELISA-positive cats that revert to negative have developed neutralizing antibodies, latent infection, or localized infection. Virus isolation, IFA on bone marrow cells, immunohistochemical staining of tissues, and PCR can be used to confirm localized or latent infection. Affected cats probably are not contagious to other cats, but infected queens may pass the virus to kittens during gestation, parturition, or lactation. Cats with localized or latent infection can be immunodeficient and may become viremic (IFA- and ELISA-positive) after receiving corticosteroids or after extreme stress.

### Treatment
A number of antiviral agents have been tried; AZT (see Table 102-3) has been studied the most, but it does not appear to clear viremia in most persistently viremic cats, and it had minimal benefits for clinically ill cats in a recent study. Immunotherapy with the other drugs listed can improve clinical signs in some cats. Chemotherapy should be used in cats with FeLV-associated neoplasia (see Chapter 82). Opportunistic organisms should be managed as indicated; the upper dose range and duration of antibiotic therapy are generally required. Supportive therapies such as hematinics, vitamin $B_{12}$, folic acid, anabolic steroids, and erythropoietin generally are unsuccessful for treatment of nonregenerative anemia; blood transfusion is required in many cases. Cats with autoagglutinating, hemolytic anemia require immunosuppressive therapy, but this potentially activates virus replication.

***Prognosis.*** Prognosis for persistently viremic cats is guarded; most die within 2 to 3 years.

### Prevention and zoonotic aspects
Avoiding contact with the virus by housing cats indoors is the best form of prevention. Potential fomites like water bowls and litterpans should not be shared between seropositive and seronegative cats. Removal of seropositive cats can result in FeLV-free catteries and multiple-cat households.

***Infected cats.*** FeLV-infected cats should be housed indoors to prevent infection of other cats and to avoid exposure to opportunistic agents. Flea control should be maintained to avoid exposure to *M. haemofelis* and *Bartonella henselae*. To avoid infection by *T. gondii, Cryptosporidium parvum, Giardia* spp., and other infectious agents carried by transport hosts, FeLV-infected cats should not be allowed to hunt and should not be fed undercooked meats.

Vaccination of cats not previously exposed to FeLV should be considered in those at high risk (e.g., contact with other cats), but owners should be warned that efficacy is less than 100%. Cats with persistent viremia do not benefit from vaccination. Vaccination is related to the development of fibrosarcoma in some cats, particularly if adjuvanted products are used.

***Zoonotic potential.*** FeLV antigens have not been documented in the serum of human beings, so zoonotic risk is minimal. However, FeLV-infected cats may be more likely to pass other zoonotic agents such as *C. parvum* and *Salmonella* spp. into the human environment.

# 103

# Polysystemic Mycotic Infections

## (Text pp 1287-1295)

### CRYPTOCOCCOSIS (TEXT PP 1287-1290)

#### Epidemiology

*Cryptococcus neoformans* is a yeastlike organism (Table 103-1). Many human and animal infections are reported in southern California. Environmental associations include bird excrement and *Eucalyptus* trees. Transmission is by inhalation. Nasal and pulmonary manifestations are common; however, an inapparent carrier state also occurs. The organism probably spreads to extrapulmonary sites hematogenously; the central nervous system (CNS) may also be infected by direct extension across the cribriform plate. Individuals with incomplete immune responses fail to completely eliminate the organism, which results in granulomatous lesions. Preexisting immunosuppressive conditions have been documented in some cats and a few (less than 10%) dogs with cryptococcosis. Examples include feline immunodeficiency virus and feline leukemia virus (FeLV) in cats; and corticosteroid administration, ehrlichiosis, heartworm disease, and neoplasia in dogs.

**Table 103-1**

## Morphologic Appearance of Systemic Canine and Feline Fungal Agents

| Agent | Cytologic appearance |
|---|---|
| *Blastomyces dermatitidis* | Extracellular yeast; 5 to 20 μm in diameter; thick, refractile double-contoured wall; broad-based bud; routine stains are adequate |
| *Cryptococcus neoformans* | Extracellular yeast; 3.5 to 7 μm in diameter; thick, unstained capsule; thin-based bud; violet color with light red capsule on Gram stain; unstained capsule with India ink |
| *Coccidioides immitis* | Extracellular spherules (20 to 200 μm in diameter) containing endospores; deep red to purple double outer wall with bright red endospores with PAS stain |
| *Histoplasma capsulatum* | Intracellular yeast in mononuclear phagocytes; 2 to 4 μm in diameter, basophilic center with lighter body on Wright's stain |
| *Sporothrix schenckii* | Round, oval, or cigar-shaped intracellular yeast; 2 to 3 μm × 3 to 6 μm |

*PAS*, Periodic acid–Schiff.

### Clinical features

Cryptococcosis is the most common systemic fungal infection in cats and should be a differential diagnosis in cats of all ages with respiratory tract disease, subcutaneous nodules, lymphadenopathy, intraocular inflammation, fever, or CNS disease; male cats are overrepresented. Snoring and stertor are common in cats and dogs with nasopharyngeal involvement.

*Cats.* Infection of the nasal cavity frequently results in sneezing and nasal discharge. The discharge can be unilateral or bilateral, ranges from serous to mucopurulent, and often contains blood. Granulomatous lesions protruding from the external nares, facial deformity over the bridge of the nose, and ulcerative lesions on the nasal planum are also common. Mandibular lymphadenopathy is found in most cats with cryptococcal rhinitis.

Single or multiple, small (less than 1 cm), cutaneous or subcutaneous masses have been commonly reported in infected cats. The masses can be either firm or fluctuant and have a serous discharge if ulcerated. Anterior uveitis, chorioretinitis, or optic neuritis occurs with ocular infection; lens luxations and glaucoma are common sequelae. Chorioretinitis lesions can be punctate or large; suppurative retinal detachment occurs in some infected cats. CNS signs result from diffuse or focal meningoencephalitis or focal granuloma formation. Manifestations may include depression, behavioral changes, seizures, blindness, circling, ataxia, loss of the sense of smell, and paresis; peripheral vestibular disease can also occur. Nonspecific signs of anorexia, weight loss, and fever are seen in some infected cats.

*Dogs.* Cryptococcosis is diagnosed most commonly in young purebred dogs; Doberman Pinschers and Great Danes are overrepresented. Manifestations include respiratory tract infection, disseminated disease including intraabdominal masses, CNS disease, ocular lesions, skin lesions, nasal cavity disease, and lymph node involvement. Seizures, ataxia, central vestibular syndrome, cranial nerve deficits, and signs of cerebellar disease are the most common CNS manifestations.

### Diagnosis

Nonregenerative anemia and monocytosis are the most common clinicopathologic abnormalities; neutrophil counts and biochemical panels are generally normal. In dogs with CNS involvement, cerebrospinal fluid (CSF) protein varies from normal to 500 mg/dl, and cell counts vary from normal to 4500/$\mu$l. Neutrophils and monocytes are often found in increased numbers; eosinophils are present in some cases. Radiographic changes include increased soft-tissue density in the nasal cavity (fungal granuloma), nasal bone deformity and lysis, hilar lymphadenopathy, and diffuse or miliary pulmonary interstitial patterns.

*Serology.* Cryptococcal antigen is detected in serum, aqueous humor, or CSF using latex agglutination (LA); serum antigen test results are positive in most animals with cryptococcosis. Measurement of antibodies against this organism does not document clinical disease, because antibodies can be detected in both healthy and diseased animals. Animals with acute disease, chronic low-grade infections, drug-induced remission, or nondisseminated disease can be LA-negative. The LA performed on CSF has a positive result in almost all animals with CNS cryptococcosis.

*Definitive Diagnosis.* Definitive diagnosis is based on cytologic, histopathologic, or culture demonstration of the organism (see Table 103-1). The organism is usually found during cytologic evaluation of nasal lesions, cutaneous lesions, lymph node aspirates, CSF, and bronchoalveolar lavage fluid. The organism can be cultured from the nasal cavity of some asymptomatic animals; therefore positive results do not always correlate to disease in this region of the body. It can be cultured from CSF in animals with neurologic involvement.

### Treatment and prognosis

Dogs and cats may be treated with amphotericin B, ketoconazole, itraconazole, fluconazole, or 5-flucytosine, alone or in various combinations (Table 103-2). Ketoconazole, itraconazole, or fluconazole is used as a single agent in dogs or cats without life-threatening disease.

**Table 103-2**

**Antifungal Drugs Used in the Management of the Systemic Canine and Feline Fungal Diseases**

| Drug | Species* | Dosage | Organism[†] |
|------|----------|--------|-------------|
| Amphotericin B | D | 0.5 mg/kg intravenously three times weekly[‡] | B, H, Cr, Co |
|  | C | 0.25 mg/kg intravenously three times weekly[§] | B, H, Cr, Co |
| Amphotericin B (liposomal) | D | 0.5 mg/kg intravenously as test dose, then 1-3 mg/kg intravenously three times weekly[‖] | B, H, Cr, Co |
| Fluconazole | C | 1.25-2.5 mg/kg by mouth twice a day | Cr |
| Flucytosine | D, C | 50 mg/kg by mouth four times a day | Cr |
| Ketoconazole | D, C | 10 mg/kg by mouth once a day | B, H, Cr, Co, Sp |
| Itraconazole | D | 5 mg/kg by mouth twice a day for 4 days and then 5 mg/kg by mouth once a day | B, Cr, H, Sp |
|  | C | 5 mg/kg by mouth twice a day | B, Cr, H, Sp |

C, Cats; D, dogs.

[†]*B, Blastomyces; Co, Coccidioides; Cr, Cryptococcus; H, Histoplasma; Sp, Sporothrix.*

[‡]In dogs with normal renal function, dilute in 60 to 120 ml of 5% dextrose and administer intravenously over 15 min; in dogs with renal insufficiency but blood urea nitrogen <50 mg/dl, dilute in 500 ml to 1 L of 5% dextrose and administer intravenously over 3 to 6 hr. Cumulative dose of 8 to 10 mg/kg if used alone or 4 to 6 mg/kg if combined with another antifungal drug.

[§]In cats with normal renal function, dilute in 50 to 100 ml 5% dextrose and administer intravenously over 3 to 6 hr.

[‖]Dilute the contents of a vial with 5% dextrose to a final concentration of 1 mg/ml and shake for 30 sec. Draw up needed volume and filter through an 18-gauge Monoject filter needle into 100 ml of 5% dextrose. Infuse intravenously over 15 minutes. Abelcet, Liposome Co., Princeton, NJ.

***Amphotericin B.*** Amphotericin B is usually not indicated except for life-threatening, disseminated disease. Intravenous administration of lipid or liposomal encapsulated amphotericin is optimal in this situation; however, a less expensive subcutaneous protocol for administration of regular amphotericin B has been used successfully. If amphotericin B is used, the animal should be well hydrated with 0.9% saline, and treatment should be discontinued if blood urea nitrogen (BUN) exceeds 50 mg/dl.

***Ketoconazole.*** Ketoconazole is reportedly effective in some cats, but it often causes inappetence, vomiting, diarrhea, weight loss, and increases in liver enzyme activities in both dogs and cats. Chronic use of ketoconazole in dogs suppresses testosterone and cortisol production and has been associated with cataracts. Itraconazole and fluconazole are better treatment options.

***Itraconazole and fluconazole.*** Itraconazole administration to cats at 100 mg/day can induce anorexia, depression, and increased serum alanine aminotransferase (ALT) activity; reducing the dose to 50 mg/day all but eliminates these problems. Itraconazole and flucytosine can induce drug eruptions in some dogs. If toxicity develops, drug therapy should be stopped and then reinstituted at 50% of the original dose after signs of toxicity abate. Inappetence in a few cats is the only adverse effect attributed to fluconazole. Fluconazole and itraconazole are effective for the treatment of CNS disease.

***Flucytosine.*** Flucytosine is used primarily for the treatment of CNS cryptococcosis. It must be used in combination with other antifungal drugs and has many adverse effects, including vomiting, diarrhea, hepatotoxicity, cutaneous reactions, and bone marrow suppression.

***Prognosis.*** Nasal and cutaneous cryptococcosis generally resolve with treatment; CNS and ocular disease are less likely to respond. Clinically ill animals should be treated until they are normal and the LA titer is less than 1 or the titer has decreased thirty-two-fold or more. Antigen titers fail to decrease in some asymptomatic animals, suggesting persistence of the organism in tissues or false-positive results.

### Zoonotic aspects and prevention

People and animals can have the same environmental exposure to *C. neoformans,* but zoonotic transfer from contact with infected animals is unlikely. The disease can be prevented by limiting the risk of exposure, especially avoiding areas with high concentrations of pigeon droppings. Application of hydrated lime solution (40 g/L of water) at 1.36 $L/m^2$ can reduce the number of organisms in contaminated areas.

## BLASTOMYCOSIS (TEXT PP 1290-1291)

### Epidemiology

*Blastomyces dermatitidis* is a saprophytic yeast found primarily in the Mississippi, Missouri, and Ohio River valleys, the mid-Atlantic states, southern Canada, and recently Colorado. Its characteristics are outlined in Table 103-1. The infectious mycelial phase is found in soil and in culture.

Blastomycosis develops most frequently in areas exposed to high humidity and fog; excavation sites; and sandy, acid soils near bodies of water. Most cases are diagnosed in the fall. Transmission is by inhalation or contamination of open wounds. The organism probably replicates in the lungs and then spreads hematogenously to other tissues. The organism can be swallowed and passed in feces. Incomplete clearance by individuals with poor cell-mediated immunity results in pyogranulomatous inflammation in affected organs. Subclinical infection is uncommon in dogs.

### Clinical features

***Dogs.*** Large-breed, young, male sporting dogs are infected most often. Anorexia, cough, dyspnea, exercise intolerance, weight loss, ocular disease, skin disease, depression, and lameness are the most common presenting complaints.

Fever occurs in approximately 40% of affected dogs, and lymphadenopathy and cutaneous or subcutaneous nodules, abscesses, plaques, or ulcers occur in 20% to 40%;

splenomegaly is also common. Interstitial lung disease and hilar lymphadenopathy result in cough, dry harsh lung sounds, and dyspnea. Dyspnea from chylothorax caused by cranial vena cava syndrome has also been described. Hypertrophic osteopathy occurs in some dogs, and lameness from fungal osteomyelitis of the spine or limbs is found in approximately 30% of cases. Ocular manifestations are seen in approximately 30% of dogs and include anterior uveitis, enophthalmitis, posterior segment disease, and optic neuritis. Depression and seizures from diffuse or multifocal CNS involvement occur in some dogs. Infection of the testes, prostate, urinary bladder, and kidneys is rare.

**Cats.** Blastomycosis can occur in any cat but is most common in young males. Infected cats may develop respiratory, CNS, skin, ocular, gastrointestinal (GI), and urinary tract disease and regional lymphadenopathy. Ocular disease usually involves the posterior segment. Pleural or peritoneal effusion resulting in dyspnea or abdominal distention occurs in some cats.

### Diagnosis

Common hematologic abnormalities are normocytic, normochromic, non-regenerative anemia; lymphopenia; and neutrophilic leukocytosis with or without left shift. Hypoalbuminemia and hyperglobulinemia (polyclonal gammopathy) are common serum biochemical abnormalities. Hypercalcemia occurs rarely. Most dogs and cats with respiratory disease have diffuse, miliary, or nodular interstitial lung patterns and intrathoracic lymphadenopathy on thoracic radiographs; a single mass or pleural effusion from chylothorax is sometimes found. Bone lesions are lytic with secondary periosteal reaction and soft-tissue swelling.

**Serology.** Many infected cats are negative for serum antibodies by agar gel immuno-diffusion (AGID). False-negative results can occur in animals with peracute infection, immunosuppression, or advanced, overwhelming infection. Antibody titers do not always revert to negative after successful treatment. Because blastomycosis rarely causes subclinical infection, positive serologic results combined with appropriate signs and radiographic abnormalities allow presumptive diagnosis.

**Cytology.** Definitive diagnosis is based on cytologic, histopathologic, or culture demonstration of the organism (see Table 103-1). Impression smears from skin lesions and aspirates from enlarged lymph nodes and focal lung lesions usually reveal pyogranulomatous inflammation and organisms that can usually be seen at low power; recovery of organisms from urine is less consistent. Bronchoalveolar lavage is more sensitive than transtracheal wash for organism demonstration. Growth in culture requires 10 to 14 days and is of lower yield than cytology or biopsy.

### Treatment

Amphotericin B, ketoconazole, both drugs combined, and itraconazole alone are used most frequently (see Table 103-2). Amphotericin B is generally used only in animals with life-threatening disease; the liposomal encapsulated product is less likely to cause toxicity. If amphotericin B is used, the animal should be well hydrated with 0.9% saline, and treatment should be discontinued if BUN exceeds 50 mg/dl. Itraconazole is as effective as amphotericin B and ketoconazole and has fewer adverse effects, so it is the drug of choice. A dose of 5 mg/kg/day is as effective as 10 mg/kg/day. Treatment should continue for 60 to 90 days or for 2 to 4 weeks beyond resolution of measurable disease (e.g., radiographic abnormalities, skin lesions).

Relapse occurs in 20% to 25% of treated dogs; when it occurs, a complete course of therapy should be reinstituted. Posterior segment ocular disease responds well to itraconazole, but anterior uveitis and enophthalmitis often necessitate enucleation.

### Zoonotic aspects and prevention

Direct zoonotic transmission from infected animals is unlikely, although contaminated biologic materials are potentially infectious, and the disease has reportedly been contracted via a dog bite. There exist multiple reports of canine and human blastomycosis developing from the same environmental exposure. Avoiding lakes and creeks in endemic areas is the only way to prevent the disease.

## HISTOPLASMOSIS (TEXT PP 1291-1293)

### Epidemiology

*Histoplasma capsulatum* is a saprophytic fungus found in the soil in tropical and subtropical regions; it is concentrated most heavily in soil contaminated with bird or bat excrement. Histoplasmosis is diagnosed most frequently in the Mississippi, Missouri, and Ohio River valleys and in the mid-Atlantic states and has also been diagnosed in Japan and Australia.

Infection is by ingestion or inhalation; the organism is engulfed by mononuclear phagocytes and transported throughout the body in blood and lymph. Granulomatous inflammation develops in persistently infected organs; disseminated disease is common in cats. Subclinical infections are common in dogs. Dogs in endemic areas are commonly exposed, but the incidence of disease is low. Immunosuppression may predispose to clinical infection in dogs and cats.

### Clinical features

*Dogs.* Most affected dogs are members of sporting breeds under 7 years of age. Subclinical, pulmonary, and disseminated infections are recognized most frequently. Most dogs are presented for evaluation of anorexia, fever, depression, weight loss, cough, dyspnea, or diarrhea. Large bowel diarrhea is most common, but small bowel diarrhea, mixed diarrhea, and protein-losing enteropathy can also occur. Physical examination findings often include increased lung sounds, respiratory wheezes, pale mucous membranes, hepatomegaly, splenomegaly, icterus, ascites, and intraabdominal lymphadenopathy. Airway obstruction from massive hilar lymphadenopathy occurs in some dogs. Lameness (from bone infection or polyarthritis), peripheral lymphadenopathy, chorioretinitis, CNS disease, and skin disease are occasionally seen. Subcutaneous nodules rarely drain or ulcerate and are less common than in dogs with cryptococcosis or blastomycosis.

*Cats.* Infected cats either are normal or develop disseminated disease. Most clinically affected cats are under 4 years of age, and some are co-infected with FeLV. Depression, anorexia, weight loss (can be severe and rapid), lameness, and dyspnea are common presenting complaints. Fever (103.5° F to 105° F), pale mucous membranes, abnormal lung sounds, oral erosions or ulcers, peripheral or visceral lymphadenopathy, icterus, soft-tissue swelling around osseous lesions, hepatomegaly, skin nodules, and, rarely, splenomegaly are physical findings consistent with histoplasmosis. Disseminated disease has a grave prognosis in cats. Osseous histoplasmosis is most common in one or more limbs, distal to the stifle or elbow. Feline ocular histoplasmosis manifests with conjunctivitis, chorioretinitis, retinal detachment, or optic neuritis and may cause glaucoma and blindness. CNS signs are uncommon.

### Diagnosis

A variety of nonspecific clinicopathologic and radiographic abnormalities exist. Normocytic, normochromic, nonregenerative anemia is the most common hematologic abnormality in both dogs and cats. Neutrophil counts can be normal, increased, or decreased. Unlike other systemic fungi, *H. capsulatum* is occasionally seen in circulating cells, particularly on examination of a buffy coat smear (mononuclear cells most often, followed by eosinophils). Thrombocytopenia from disseminated intravascular coagulation (DIC) occurs in some dogs and cats. Some affected cats develop pancytopenia from bone marrow infection, and some have co-infection with FeLV. Hypoproteinemia and increased activities of alkaline phosphatase and alanine aminotransferase are found in some patients.

*Diagnostic imaging.* Lysis predominates in animals with bone infection; periosteal and endosteal new bone production occurs in some cases. In dogs with pulmonary infection, radiographic abnormalities include diffuse, miliary, or nodular interstitial disease; hilar lymphadenopathy; pleural effusion; and calcified pulmonary parenchyma (chronic disease); in some dogs massive hilar lymphadenopathy is the only radiographic finding. Alveolar lung disease, tracheobronchial lymphadenopathy, and calcified lymph nodes are uncommon in cats. Colonoscopy in dogs or cats with GI infection may reveal increased mucosal granularity, friability, ulceration, and thickness.

***Serology.*** Several tests have been evaluated for detection of circulating antibodies, but sensitivity and specificity are poor for all. Serologic diagnosis is unreliable and should be used only to establish a presumptive diagnosis when the organism cannot be demonstrated by cytology, histopathology, or culture but signs are suggestive of the disease.

***Cytology.*** Definitive diagnosis requires demonstration of the organism by cytology, biopsy, or culture (see Table 103-1). The organism is found most frequently in (1) rectal scrapings or biopsies from dogs with large bowel diarrhea; (2) bone marrow or buffy coat cells from cats with disseminated disease; and (3) lymph nodes, lung, spleen, liver, skin nodules, and other locations. The organism has also been identified in pleural and peritoneal effusions and in CSF.

### Treatment and prognosis

Itraconazole is the initial drug of choice in both dogs and cats (see Table 103-2). Treatment should continue for 60 to 90 days or until clinical evidence of disease has been resolved for at least 1 month. Amphotericin B can be used in animals with life-threatening disease or in those unable to absorb oral medications because of intestinal disease. Ketoconazole and fluconazole are also effective in some animals.

Glucocorticoids with or without antifungal drugs lessen clinical signs associated with chronic hilar lymphadenopathy much more quickly than antifungal drugs alone, without resulting in disseminated histoplasmosis. However, if the infection is active, glucocorticoids may exacerbate clinical disease.

***Prognosis.*** Pulmonary disease in dogs carries a fair to good prognosis; disseminated disease carries a poor prognosis. The overall success rate in cats was 33% in one study; in another study, all eight cats treated with itraconazole at 5 mg/kg q12h were eventually cured.

### Zoonotic aspects and prevention

Like blastomycosis, direct zoonotic transmission from infected animals is unlikely, although care should be taken when the organism is cultured. Prevention entails avoiding potentially contaminated soil. Organism numbers in contaminated areas can be decreased with 3% formalin solution.

## COCCIDIOIDOMYCOSIS (TEXT PP 1293-1294)

### Epidemiology

*Coccidioides immitis* is a dimorphic fungus found deep in sandy, alkaline soils in regions with low elevation, low rainfall, and high environmental temperatures (e.g., California, Arizona, New Mexico, Utah, Nevada, and southwest Texas). Large numbers of arthrospores return to the surface after periods of rainfall and are dispersed by the wind; the prevalence of coccidioidomycosis increases in years after high rainfall. Most cases of feline coccidioidomycosis are diagnosed between December and May.

Infection occurs by inhalation or wound contamination. Most people, dogs, and cats exposed to the organism are subclinically affected. In some individuals, the organism disseminates to sites including mediastinal and tracheobronchial lymph nodes, bones and joints, viscera (liver, spleen, kidneys), heart and pericardium, testicles, eyes, brain, and spinal cord. Signs of respiratory and disseminated disease occur 1 to 3 weeks and 4 months after exposure, respectively.

### Clinical features

***Dogs.*** Clinical disease in dogs is most common in young males. Approximately 90% have lameness with swollen, painful bones or joints. Cough, dyspnea, anorexia, weakness, weight loss, lymphadenopathy, ocular inflammation, and diarrhea are other presenting complaints. Crackles, wheezes, and muffled lung sounds (pleural effusion) are common. If subcutaneous abscesses, nodules, ulcers, and draining tracts are present, they are usually associated with infected bones. Evidence of myocarditis, icterus, renomegaly, splenomegaly, hepatomegaly, orchitis, epididymitis, keratitis, iritis, granulomatous uveitis, and glaucoma are other possible findings. Depression, seizures, ataxia, central vestibular disease, cranial nerve deficits, and behavioral changes are the most common signs of CNS infection.

**Cats.** The median age of infected cats is 5 years; no obvious gender or breed predilection exists. The most common manifestations are skin, respiratory, musculoskeletal, and ophthalmic or neurologic disease.

### Diagnosis

The combination of skin disease, radiographic signs of interstitial lung disease or osteomyelitis, and positive serologic tests in animals from endemic areas can be used to make a presumptive diagnosis if the organism cannot be demonstrated.

*Clinicopathologic findings.* Normocytic, normochromic, nonregenerative anemia; leukocytosis or leukopenia; and monocytosis are the most common hematologic abnormalities. Hyperglobulinemia (polyclonal gammopathy), hypoalbuminemia, renal azotemia, and proteinuria are found in some patients.

*Imaging.* Diffuse interstitial lung patterns are more common than bronchial, miliary, or nodular interstitial, or alveolar patterns in animals with pulmonary coccidioidomycosis.

Pleural effusion secondary to pleuritis, right-sided heart failure, or constrictive pericarditis may also be found. Hilar lymphadenopathy is common, but sternal lymphadenopathy and lymph node calcification are not. Bone lesions usually involve the distal diaphysis, epiphysis, and metaphysis of one or more long bones. They are more proliferative than lytic.

*Serology.* Serum antibodies are detected by complement fixation, AGID, and tube precipitin tests. The first two detect immunoglobulin (Ig) G, and the latter detects IgM. False-negative results can occur in dogs and cats with early infections (<2 weeks), chronic infection, rapidly progressive acute infection, and primary cutaneous coccidioidomycosis. The assays can cross-react with *H. capsulatum* and *B. dermatitidis*. Titers may persist for months or years after resolution of clinical disease.

*Cytology.* Definitive diagnosis requires demonstration of the organism by cytology, biopsy, or culture (see Table 103-1). The organism is often difficult to demonstrate cytologically; transtracheal aspiration or bronchoalveolar lavage is commonly negative. Extracellular spherules are most often found in lymph node aspirates, draining masses, and pericardial fluid; wet-mount examination of unstained or periodic acid–Schiff–stained smears is more suitable than dry mounts.

### Treatment

Ketoconazole is the drug of choice in dogs (see Table 103-2). The adverse effects are the same as those listed above for cryptococcosis. Amphotericin B should be used if life-threatening disease is present or if response to ketoconazole is poor. Itraconazole can be used in animals with toxicity from ketoconazole; fluconazole should be used for those with meningoencephalitis. Cats and dogs should be treated for 60 to 90 days or until clinical illness has been resolved for at least 1 month. Bone infections are often incurable, and repeated treatments are often required.

### Zoonotic aspects and prevention

People exposed to *C. immitis* develop asymptomatic infection or mild, transient respiratory signs. The organism is not transmitted from infected animals to people; however, fomites such as used bandage materials and cultures should be handled carefully. Avoiding endemic areas is the only way to prevent disease.

# 104

# Polysystemic Protozoal Infections

## (Text pp 1296-1306)

## FELINE TOXOPLASMOSIS (TEXT PP 1296-1299)

### Epidemiology

*Toxoplasma gondii* is an important parasite of cats; approximately 30% to 40% of cats and people in the United States are seropositive and presumed to be infected. Infection in cats occurs via ingestion or transplacentally. Most cats are infected by ingesting bradyzoites during carnivorous feeding; oocysts are then shed in feces for 3 to 21 days. Sporulated oocysts can survive in the environment for months or years and are resistant to most disinfectants. Tachyzoites disseminate in blood or lymph during active infection and rapidly replicate intracellularly until the cell is destroyed. Bradyzoites are the slowly dividing, persistent tissue stage, and form in extraintestinal tissues; tissue cysts form readily in the central nervous system (CNS), muscles, and viscera. Bradyzoites may persist in tissues for the life of the host.

### Clinical features

Experimentally, 10% to 20% of cats develop self-limiting, small bowel diarrhea for 1 to 2 weeks after oral inoculation with tissue cysts. However, detection of *T. gondii* oocysts in feces is rarely reported in naturally exposed cats with diarrhea, although toxoplasmosis may occasionally induce inflammatory bowel disease.

***Disseminated infection.*** Fatal extraintestinal toxoplasmosis can develop after primary infection; hepatic, pulmonary, CNS, and pancreatic tissues are most often affected. Transplacentally or lactationally infected kittens develop the most severe signs and generally die of pulmonary or hepatic disease. Common findings include depression, anorexia, and fever followed by hypothermia, peritoneal effusion, icterus, and dyspnea. If an animal with chronic toxoplasmosis is immunosuppressed, bradyzoites in tissue cysts can replicate rapidly and disseminate again as tachyzoites; disseminated toxoplasmosis has been documented in cats co-infected with feline leukemia virus (FeLV), feline immunodeficiency virus (FIV), or feline infectious peritonitis virus, as well as after renal transplantation.

***Chronic infection.*** Sublethal, chronic toxoplasmosis occurs in some cats. It should be a differential diagnosis in cats with anterior or posterior uveitis, fever, muscle hyperesthesia, weight loss, anorexia, seizures, ataxia, icterus, diarrhea, or pancreatitis. Toxoplasmosis is a common cause of uveitis in cats. Kittens infected transplacentally or lactationally commonly develop ocular disease. Because none of the anti-*Toxoplasma* drugs totally clears the organism, recurrence of disease is common.

### Diagnosis

Cats with clinical toxoplasmosis can have a variety of laboratory and radiographic abnormalities, but none documents the disease. Antemortem diagnosis can be tentatively based on the combination of (1) appropriate clinical signs; (2) antibodies in serum, which document exposure to *T. gondii;* (3) an immunoglobulin (Ig) M titer above 1:64

or a fourfold or greater increase in IgG titer, which suggests recent or active infection; (4) exclusion of other common causes; and (5) positive response to drugs.

*Clinicopathologic findings.* Abnormalities include nonregenerative anemia; neutrophilic leukocytosis or neutropenia; lymphocytosis; monocytosis; eosinophilia; proteinuria; bilirubinuria; hyperproteinemia; hyperbilirubinemia; and increased activities of creatine kinase (CK), alanine aminotransferase, alkaline phosphatase (AP), or lipase.

*Other clinical tests.* Radiographically, diffuse interstitial or alveolar patterns and pleural effusion are common with pulmonary toxoplasmosis. Cerebrospinal fluid (CSF) protein and cell counts are often higher than normal. The predominant white blood cells are small mononuclear cells, but neutrophils also are commonly found.

*Serology.* *T. gondii*–specific antibodies (IgM, IgG, IgA), antigens, and immune complexes can be detected in the serum of normal cats, as well as in those with signs of disease, so it is impossible to make an antemortem diagnosis based on these tests alone. In serum, the presence of IgM correlates best with clinical toxoplasmosis (IgM is rarely detected in healthy cats). Some clinically affected cats will have reached their maximal IgG titer or will have undergone a shift from IgM to IgG by the time they are evaluated, so failure to document an increasing IgG titer or a positive IgM titer does not exclude the diagnosis. Because some healthy cats have extremely high titers and some ill cats have low titers, the titer magnitude is relatively unimportant. It is not necessary to repeat serum antibody titers after the clinical disease has resolved, because the organism cannot be cleared from the body, and most cats remain antibody-positive for life.

*Organ-specific serology.* The combination of aqueous humor or CSF serology and polymerase chain reaction (PCR) is the most accurate way to diagnose ocular or CNS toxoplasmosis (Diagnostic Laboratory, College of Veterinary Medicine and Biomedical Sciences, Colorado State University). Although *T. gondii*–specific IgA, IgG, and organism DNA can be detected in aqueous humor and CSF of both normal and ill cats, *T. gondii*–specific IgM has been detected only in the aqueous humor or CSF of ill cats and may be the best indicator of clinical disease. Because *T. gondii* DNA can be detected in blood of healthy cats, positive PCR results do not correlate with clinical disease.

*Organism identification.* Definitive diagnosis can be made antemortem if the organism is demonstrated; however, this is uncommon, particularly with fatal disease. Bradyzoites or tachyzoites are rarely detected in tissues, effusions, bronchoalveolar lavage fluids, aqueous humor, or CSF. Identification of $10 \times 12$ μm oocysts in the feces of cats with diarrhea suggests toxoplasmosis but is not definitive; *Besnoitia* and *Hammondia* infections produce similar oocysts.

**Treatment and prognosis**

Supportive care should be instituted as needed. Clindamycin hydrochloride (Antirobe, 10 to 12 mg/kg orally [PO] q12h for 4 weeks) or trimethoprim-sulfonamide combination (15 mg/kg PO q12h for 4 weeks) is often used in cats. Azithromycin (7.5 mg/kg PO q12h) has been used successfully in a limited number of cats, but the optimal duration of therapy is unknown. Doxycycline at 5 mg/kg PO q12h for 4 weeks may be effective. Pyrimethamine combined with sulfa drugs commonly causes toxicity in cats. Cats with systemic clinical signs of toxoplasmosis (fever or muscle pain) combined with uveitis should be treated with anti-*Toxoplasma* drugs in combination with topical, oral, or parenteral corticosteroids to avoid secondary lens luxations and glaucoma. Cats with uveitis that are otherwise normal can be treated with topical glucocorticoids alone, unless the uveitis is recurrent or persistent, in which case anti-*Toxoplasma* drugs may be beneficial. Chorioretinitis may respond to clindamycin alone.

*Clinical course.* Signs not involving the eyes or CNS usually resolve within 2 to 3 days of clindamycin or trimethoprim-sulfa administration; ocular and CNS toxoplasmosis respond more slowly. If fever or muscle hyperesthesia is not decreasing after 3 days of treatment, other causes should be considered. No evidence suggests that any drug totally clears the body of the organism, so recurrence is common, especially in cats treated for less than 4 weeks; infected cats will always be seropositive.

*Prognosis.* Prognosis is poor for cats with hepatic or pulmonary disease, particularly immunocompromised patients. Clindamycin has been used successfully in a limited number of cases with suspected CNS toxoplasmosis.

### Zoonotic aspects and prevention

*T. gondii* is a significant zoonosis. Primary infection of pregnant women can lead to clinical toxoplasmosis in the fetus; stillbirth, CNS disease, and ocular disease are common. Primary infection in immunocompetent individuals results in self-limiting fever, malaise, and lymphadenopathy.

*Preventing zoonotic spread.* People most commonly acquire toxoplasmosis by ingesting sporulated oocysts or tissue cysts, or transplacentally. Although owning a pet cat was epidemiologically associated with acquiring toxoplasmosis in one study of pregnant women, touching individual cats is probably not a common way to acquire toxoplasmosis. Cats generally shed oocysts only for days or weeks after primary inoculation. Repeat oocyst shedding is rare, even in cats receiving glucocorticoids or coinfected with FIV or FeLV. However, because some cats repeat oocyst shedding when exposed a second time, feces should always be handled carefully. Prevention of toxoplasmosis is summarized in Box 104-1.

*Monitoring shedding.* Fecal oocysts measuring $10 \times 12$ μm should be assumed to be *T. gondii*. The cat's feces should be collected daily until oocyst shedding is finished. Oral administration of clindamycin (25 to 50 mg/kg divided q12h) or sulfonamides (100 mg/kg/day) can reduce oocyst shedding.

*Serologic screening.* Testing healthy cats for toxoplasmosis is not recommended, because people are usually not infected by handling individual cats. Fecal examination is adequate to determine when cats are actively shedding oocysts, but most cats that are shedding oocysts are seronegative. Most seropositive cats have completed the oocyst shedding period and are unlikely to repeat shedding.

---

**Box 104-1**

### Prevention of Human Toxoplasmosis

**PREVENTION OF OOCYST INGESTION**

Avoid feeding cats undercooked meats.
Do not allow cats to hunt.
Clean the litterbox daily and incinerate or flush the feces.
Clean the litterbox daily with scalding water or use a litterbox liner.
Wear gloves when working with soil.
Wash hands thoroughly with soap and hot water after gardening.
Wash fresh vegetables well before ingestion.
Keep children's sandboxes covered.
Boil water for drinking that has been obtained from the general environment.
Control potential transport hosts.
Treat oocyst-shedding cats with anti-*Toxoplasma* drugs.

**PREVENTION OF TISSUE CYST INGESTION**

Cook all meat products to 66° C (151° F).
Wear gloves when handling meats.
Wash hands thoroughly with soap and hot water after handling meats.
Freeze all meat for a minimum of 3 days before cooking.

## CANINE TOXOPLASMOSIS (TEXT P 1299)

### Epidemiology

Dogs do not produce *T. gondii* oocysts, but they can mechanically transmit oocysts after ingesting feline feces. The tissue phases of *T. gondii* infection occur in dogs and can induce clinical disease; seroprevalence is approximately 20%. Many dogs diagnosed with toxoplasmosis before 1988 were actually infected with *Neospora caninum*.

### Clinical features

Generalized toxoplasmosis affects the respiratory, gastrointestinal (GI), and neuromuscular systems, commonly resulting in fever, vomiting, diarrhea, dyspnea, and icterus. Generalized toxoplasmosis is most common in immunosuppressed dogs. Neurologic signs depend on the location of the primary lesions and include ataxia, seizures, tremors, cranial nerve deficits, paresis, and paralysis. Rapid progression to tetraparesis and paralysis with lower motor neuron dysfunction can occur, although some dogs with suspected neuromuscular toxoplasmosis probably have neosporosis. Dogs with myositis present with weakness, stiff gait, or muscle wasting. Myocardial infection resulting in ventricular arrhythmias occurs in some dogs. Retinitis, anterior uveitis, iridocyclitis, and optic neuritis can occur but are less common than in cats.

### Diagnosis

As in cats, clinicopathologic and radiographic abnormalities are nonspecific. Increased CSF protein concentrations and mixed inflammatory cell infiltrates occur in dogs with CNS toxoplasmosis. Demonstration of the organism in tissues or exudates allows definitive diagnosis. More commonly, antemortem diagnosis is based on the combination of appropriate clinical signs, exclusion of other likely causes, positive serum antibody tests, exclusion of *N. caninum* infection by serologic testing, and response to therapy. Interpretation of serum, aqueous humor, and CSF antibody and PCR tests is as described for feline toxoplasmosis.

### Treatment

Clindamycin hydrochloride (10 to 12 mg/kg PO q12h) is the drug of choice; trimethoprim-sulfa (15 mg/kg PO q12h) is an alternative protocol. Treatment should be continued for a minimum of 4 weeks. If uveitis occurs, topical glucocorticoid treatment should also be used.

### Zoonotic aspects and prevention

Dogs do not complete the enteroepithelial phase of *T. gondii* but can mechanically transmit oocysts after ingesting feline feces. Toxoplasmosis in this species can be prevented by not allowing coprophagia and feeding only cooked meat and meat by-products.

## NEOSPOROSIS (TEXT PP 1299-1300)

### Epidemiology

*N. caninum* is a coccidian previously confused with *T. gondii* because of similar morphology. In dogs, infection has been documented after ingestion of infected bovine placental tissue. Transplacental infection is well documented and may be repeated during subsequent pregnancies; this increases the risk for puppies from a bitch that previously birthed infected puppies. Pathogenesis of disease is primarily related to the intracellular replication of tachyzoites. Although organism replication occurs in many tissues, including the lungs, in dogs clinical illness is primarily neuromuscular. Administration of glucocorticoids may activate bradyzoites in tissue cysts, resulting in clinical illness. Clinical disease in naturally infected cats has not been reported.

### Clinical features

Ascending paralysis with hyperextension of the hindlimbs in congenitally infected puppies is the most common manifestation. Muscle atrophy occurs in many cases. Polymyositis and multifocal CNS disease can occur alone or in combination. Signs may be evident soon after birth or may be delayed several weeks. Neonatal death is common. Although the disease tends to be most severe in congenitally infected puppies, dogs as old as 15 years have been affected; exacerbation of chronic infection is a possible cause in these patients. Myocarditis, dysphagia, ulcerative dermatitis, pneumonia, and hepatitis occur in some dogs. Cough may also be a principal sign. If left untreated, the disease generally results in death.

### Diagnosis

Clinicopathologic findings are nonspecific; myositis commonly results in increased activities of CK and aspartate aminotransferase. CSF abnormalities include increased protein concentration (20 to 50 mg/µl) and mild, mixed inflammatory cell pleocytosis (10 to 50 cells/µl) consisting of monocytes, lymphocytes, neutrophils, and rarely, eosinophils. Interstitial and alveolar patterns can be noted on thoracic radiographs. Mixed inflammation with neutrophils, lymphocytes, eosinophils, plasma cells, macrophages, and tachyzoites was noted on transthoracic aspirate of one dog with lung disease.

*Serology.* Presumptive diagnosis can be made by combining appropriate clinical signs and positive serology or presence of antibodies in CSF with exclusion of other causes that induce similar clinical syndromes (in particular, *T. gondii*). IgG titers greater than or equal to 1:200 are detected in most dogs with clinical neosporosis; serologic cross-reactivity with *T. gondii* is minimal at titers 1:50 or higher.

*Organism identification.* Definitive diagnosis is based on demonstration of the organism in CSF or tissues. Tachyzoites are rarely identified in CSF, imprints of skin lesions, or bronchoalveolar lavage fluid. *N. caninum* tissue cysts have a wall more than 1 µm (whereas *T. gondii* tissue cysts have a wall less than 1 µm). Oocysts can be detected in feces by microscopic examination after flotation or by PCR. The organism can be differentiated from *T. gondii* by electron microscopy, immunohistochemistry, and PCR.

### Treatment and prognosis

Most dogs die, but several have survived after treatment with trimethoprim-sulfadiazine plus pyrimethamine; sequential treatment with clindamycin hydrochloride, trimethoprim-sulfadiazine, and pyrimethamine; or clindamycin alone. Trimethoprim-sulfadiazine (15 mg/kg PO q12h for 4 weeks) with pyrimethamine (1 mg/kg PO q24h for 4 weeks) or clindamycin (10 mg/kg PO q8h for 4 weeks) is currently recommended. Treatment should be started before extensor rigidity develops, if possible. Prognosis for dogs with severe neurologic involvement is grave.

### Zoonotic aspects and prevention

*N. caninum* antibodies have been detected in people; however, no known zoonotic risk exists. Bitches that whelp clinically affected puppies should not be rebred. Glucocorticoids should not be administered to seropositive animals, if possible. Contamination of livestock feed with dog fecal matter should be prevented, and dogs should not be allowed to ingest bovine placentas. Dogs should not be allowed to roam freely, as it is possible that wildlife intermediate hosts play a role in canine infection.

## BABESIOSIS (TEXT PP 1300-1301)

### Epidemiology

*Babesia* organisms are protozoans that parasitize red blood cells (RBCs), leading to progressive anemia. Babesiosis in dogs is most commonly associated with *Babesia canis* and *Babesia gibsoni*. *Babesia* organisms are transmitted by various species of ticks and can also be transmitted by blood transfusion. None of the *Babesia* species that infect cats are found in the United States. The incubation period varies from 10 to 21 days. Parasitemia can be detected transiently from day 1; recurrent parasitemia is detected by day 14, with peak organism levels occurring on day 20. Severity of disease depends on the species and strain of *Babesia* and the host's immune status; chronic, subclinical infection can be common with some. Administration of glucocorticoids or splenectomy may activate chronic disease. The organism replicates in RBCs and causes intravascular hemolytic anemia. Immune-mediated reactions worsen the hemolysis and commonly result in a positive direct Coombs' test. Macrophage stimulation leads to fever and hepatosplenomegaly. Disseminated intravascular coagulation (DIC) occurs in some infected dogs during acute infection.

### Clinical features

Peracute or acute infections cause anemia and fever, leading to pale mucous membranes, tachycardia, tachypnea, depression, anorexia, and weakness. Icterus, petechiae, and hepatosplenomegaly are found in some dogs. Severe anemia, DIC, metabolic acidosis, and renal disease are most common during acute infection. Chronically infected dogs commonly have weight loss and anorexia. Ascites, GI signs, CNS disease, edema, and clinical evidence of cardiopulmonary disease occur in some dogs with atypical infection. Subclinical infection occurs as well.

### Diagnosis

Regenerative anemia, hyperbilirubinemia, bilirubinuria, hemoglobinuria, thrombocytopenia, metabolic acidosis, azotemia, polyclonal gammopathy, and renal casts are common but nonspecific findings. The main differential diagnosis for acute babesiosis is primary immune-mediated hemolytic anemia.

*Serology.* Presumptive diagnosis can be based on historical and physical examination findings, clinicopathologic data, and positive serology. IFA tests for *B. canis* and *B. gibsoni* are available; however, cross-reactivity exists between these two *Babesia* species. Increasing titers over 2 to 3 weeks is consistent with recent or active infection. Currently no standardization exists among laboratories, and so suggested positive cutoff titers vary. False-negative results can occur in peracute cases and in immunosuppressed dogs. Many clinically normal dogs are seropositive, so serology alone cannot be used for definitive diagnosis.

*Organism identification.*
Definitive diagnosis is made when the organisms are found in RBCs using Wright's or Giemsa stains on thin blood smears. *B. canis* is typically found as paired, piriform bodies measuring $2.4 \times 5$ μm. *B. gibsoni* is typically identified as singular, annular bodies measuring $1 \times 3.2$ μm.

### Treatment

Supportive care including blood transfusion, bicarbonate for acidosis, and fluid therapy should be administered as indicated. No currently available drugs are known to eliminate infection, and so it is unknown whether it is beneficial to treat healthy, seropositive dogs. Phenamidine isethionate (15 mg of a 5% solution per kilogram subcutaneously [SC] q24h for 2 days) reportedly is effective for lessening clinical disease associated with *Babesia* spp. infections. Imidocarb dipropionate (5 to 6.6 mg/kg SC or intramuscularly [IM] twice, 14 days apart, or 7.5 mg/kg SC or IM once) is effective for *B. canis,* but adverse effects include transient salivation, diarrhea, dyspnea, lacrimation, and depression. Metronidazole (25 mg/kg PO q8-12h for 2 to 3 weeks) or clindamycin hydrochloride (12.5 mg/kg PO q12h for 2 to 3 weeks) may lessen clinical disease if other drugs are not available. Diminazene aceturate, pentamidine isethionate, parvaquone, and niridazone have also been used.

### Zoonotic aspects and prevention

No current evidence suggests that the *Babesia* species that infect dogs and cats cause human disease. Tick control is important. Administration of immunosuppressive drugs and splenectomy should be avoided in previously infected dogs. Blood donors should be assessed for infection by PCR or serologic screening.

## CYTAUXZOONOSIS (TEXT PP 1301-1302)

### Epidemiology

*Cytauxzoon felis* is a protozoal disease of cats in the southeastern and south central United States. Bobcats are usually subclinically affected and may be the natural host. The organism is transmitted by *Dermacentor* ticks. After infection, schizonts and macroschizonts form in mononuclear phagocytes. Clinical disease results from obstruction of blood flow through affected veins and from hemolytic anemia.

### Clinical features

Most cases occur in cats allowed to go outdoors. Fever, anorexia, dyspnea, depression, icterus, pale mucous membranes, and death are the most common findings;

sublethal cytauxzoonosis has been recently documented, suggesting that less virulent variants exist. Ticks are generally not identified on affected cats. A primary differential diagnosis is haemobartonellosis.

### Diagnosis

Regenerative anemia and neutrophilic leukocytosis are the most common hematologic findings; thrombocytopenia occurs in some cats. Hemoglobinemia, hemoglobinuria, hyperbilirubinemia, and bilirubinuria are uncommon. Antemortem diagnosis is based on demonstration of the erythrocytic phase on thin blood smears stained with Wright's or Giemsa stain. Infected macrophages can be detected in bone marrow, spleen, liver, or lymph node aspirates. The organism is easily identified on histopathologic evaluation of most organs. Serologic testing is not commercially available. PCR can be used to amplify organism DNA from blood.

### Treatment

Supportive care including fluid therapy and blood transfusion should be administered as indicated. Treatment with diminazene or imidocarb (2 mg/kg IM) twice, 14 days apart, has been effective. Historically, treatment with parvaquone (10 to 30 mg/kg IM or SC q24h for 2 to 3 days), buparvaquone (10 mg/kg IM or SC q24h for 2 to 3 days), and thiacetarsamide (0.1 mg/kg intravenously [IV] q12h for 2 days) has been attempted. Parvaquone and buparvaquone are not routinely available, and thiacetarsamide is toxic in cats and probably should not be used.

### Zoonotic aspects and prevention

*C. felis* is not known to be zoonotic. The disease can be prevented only by avoiding exposure. Ticks should be controlled, and cats in endemic areas should be housed during periods of peak tick activity.

## HEPATOZOONOSIS (TEXT PP 1302-1303)

### Epidemiology

Hepatozoonosis in dogs is caused by the protozoal agents, *Hepatozoon canis* and *Hepatozoon americanum*. In North America *H. americanum* predominates; it is transmitted by *Amblyomma maculatum* (Gulf Coast tick) and is most common in the Texas Gulf Coast, Mississippi, Alabama, Georgia, Florida, Louisiana, and Oklahoma. In Africa, southern Europe, and Asia, *H. canis* predominates and is transmitted by *Rhipicephalus sanguineus* (brown dog tick). A *Hepatozoon* species is occasionally found in the blood of cats in Europe. Clinical disease associations are currently unclear, but the cats are commonly coinfected with FeLV or FIV. After a dog ingests an infected tick, sporozoites infect mononuclear phagocytes and endothelial cells of the spleen, liver, muscle, lungs, and bone marrow. Ultimately, cysts containing macromeronts and micromeronts (which develop into micromerozoites and infect leukocytes) form. Tissue phases induce pyogranulomatous inflammation. Glomerulonephritis or amyloidosis may occur secondary to chronic inflammation and immune complex disease.

### Clinical features

*H. americanum* can be a primary pathogen, resulting in clinical illness without concurrent immune deficiency. Dogs of all age groups are at risk, but disease is most commonly recognized in puppies. Fever, weight loss, and severe paraspinal hyperesthesia are common findings. Anorexia, pale mucous membranes (anemia), depression, oculonasal discharge, and bloody diarrhea occur in some dogs. Clinical signs can be intermittent or recurrent.

### Diagnosis

Neutrophilic leukocytosis (20,000 to 200,000 cells/µl) with a left shift is the most common hematologic finding; normocytic normochromic nonregenerative anemia is common. Increased SAP activity occurs in some *H. americanum*–infected dogs. Hypoalbuminemia, hypoglycemia, and rarely, polyclonal gammopathy occur in some dogs. Periosteal reactions from the inflammatory reaction in muscle can occur in any bone (except the skull) and are most common in young dogs but are not pathognomonic for hepatozoonosis. Definitive diagnosis is based on identification of the organism in neutrophils or monocytes in Giemsa- or Leishman-stained blood smears or in muscle biopsy sections. An indirect enzyme-linked immunosorbent assay for detection of serum antibodies against *H. americanum* is available; the sensitivity and specificity are 93% and 96%, respectively.

### Treatment
No therapeutic regimen has been shown to eliminate *H. canis* or *H. americanum* infection from tissues. However, clinical disease resolves rapidly with several drug protocols. For treatment of *H. americanum,* the combination of trimethoprim-sulfadiazine (15 mg/kg PO q12h), pyrimethamine (0.25 mg/kg PO q24h), and clindamycin (10 mg/kg PO q8h) for 14 days is very successful in the acute stage. Use of decoquinate (10 to 20 mg/kg q12h) with food lessens the likelihood of recurrence of clinical disease and prolongs survival time. Imidocarb dipropionate (5 to 6 mg/kg IM or SC) administered once or twice 14 days apart is the drug of choice for treatment of *H. canis* infection and may also be effective against *H. americanum.* Nonsteroidal antiinflammatory drugs may lessen discomfort in some dogs.

### Zoonotic potential and prevention
There exists no evidence for transfer of *H. canis* from infected dogs to people. Tick control is the best form of prevention. Glucocorticoid administration should be avoided, because it may exacerbate clinical disease.

## LEISHMANIASIS (TEXT P 1303)

### Epidemiology
*Leishmania* organisms are flagellates that cause cutaneous, mucocutaneous, and visceral disease in dogs, humans, and other mammals. Rodents and dogs are primary reservoirs; people and cats are probably incidental hosts, and sandflies are the vectors. Leishmaniasis has recently been documented in 20 states in the United States and also in Canada. After a sandfly bite, promastigotes are engulfed by macrophages and disseminate through the body. After an incubation period of 1 month to 7 years, amastigotes (nonflagellate) form, and cutaneous lesions develop. Infection induces extreme immune responses, commonly resulting in glomerulonephritis and polyarthritis.

### Clinical features
Dogs generally develop visceral leishmaniasis. A subclinical phase may persist for months or years. Weight loss despite a normal or increased appetite, polyuria and polydipsia, muscle wasting, depression, vomiting, diarrhea, cough, epistaxis, sneezing, and melena are common presenting complaints. Splenomegaly, lymphadenopathy, facial alopecia, fever, rhinitis, increased lung sounds, icterus, swollen painful joints, uveitis, and conjunctivitis are common findings. Cutaneous lesions are characterized by hyperkeratosis, scaling, thickening, mucocutaneous ulcers, and intradermal nodules on the muzzle, pinnae, ears, and foot pads. Bone lesions are detected in some dogs. Cats usually are subclinically infected, but dermatologic disease has been reported.

### Diagnosis
Common clinicopathologic abnormalities include leukocytosis with left shift, lymphopenia, thrombocytopenia, hyperglobulinemia, hypoalbuminemia, increased liver enzyme activities, azotemia, and proteinuria. The hyperglobulinemia is usually polyclonal, but IgG monoclonal gammopathy has been reported. Neutrophilic polyarthritis occurs in some dogs.

*Serology.* Antibodies can be detected in serum; IgG titers develop 14 to 28 days after infection and decline 45 to 80 days after treatment. Serologic cross-reactivity occurs between *Trypanosoma cruzi* and *Leishmania.* Because dogs are unlikely to eliminate infection spontaneously, a true-positive antibody test indicates infection.

*Organism identification.* Demonstration of amastigotes (2.5 to 5 μm × 1.5 to 2 μm) in lymph node or bone marrow aspirates, or skin imprints stained with Wright's or Giemsa stain, allows definitive diagnosis. The organism can also be identified by histopathologic or immunoperoxidase evaluation of skin or organ biopsy, culture, inoculation of hamsters, or PCR. PCR can be performed on ethylenediaminetetraacetic acid (EDTA)– anticoagulated blood, bone marrow, or lymph node aspirates.

### Treatment and prognosis

No drug or drug combination has been used to successfully eliminate *Leishmania* from the body. The combination of antimony and allopurinol (15 mg/kg PO q12h) may be superior to treatment with either drug alone; however, antimony drugs are not available in the United States. Liposomal amphotericin B (3 to 3.3 mg/kg IV q48h) for three to five treatments has also been used. Prognosis is variable; most cases are recurrent. Dogs with renal insufficiency have a poor prognosis.

### Zoonotic aspects and prevention

The primary zoonotic risk is from dogs acting as reservoir hosts; direct contact with amastigotes in draining lesions is unlikely to result in human infection. Avoidance of infected sandflies is the only means of prevention. In endemic areas, animals should be housed during night hours and sandfly breeding places destroyed.

## AMERICAN TRYPANOSOMIASIS (TEXT P 1304)

### Epidemiology

*T. cruzi* is a flagellate that infects many mammals; the disease is diagnosed primarily in South America, but several cases have been detected in dogs of North America, primarily in Fox Hounds. Infected reservoir mammals (dogs, cats, raccoons, opossums, armadillos) and vectors (reduviid [kissing] bugs) are found in the United States, but infection in dogs or people is rare. Transmission can occur by ingestion of the vector, blood transfusions, and ingestion of infected tissues or milk and transplacentally. Peak parasitemia and acute disease occur 2 to 3 weeks after infection. The disease in dogs is primarily a cardiomyopathy that develops from parasite-induced or immune-mediated damage to myocardial cells.

### Clinical features

Exercise intolerance and weakness are nonspecific presenting complaints related to myocarditis or heart failure during acute infection. Generalized lymphadenopathy, pale mucous membranes, tachycardia, pulse deficits, hepatomegaly, and abdominal distention can be detected on physical examination. Anorexia, diarrhea, and neurologic signs occasionally occur. Dogs that survive acute infection can be presented for evaluation of chronic dilative cardiomyopathy; right-sided cardiac disease, conduction disturbances, ventricular arrhythmias, and supraventricular arrhythmias are common.

### Diagnosis

Common clinicopathologic abnormalities include lymphocytosis and increased activities of liver enzymes and CK. Thoracic and abdominal radiographic and echocardiographic findings are consistent with cardiac disease and failure but are not specific for trypanosomiasis. The primary ECG findings are ventricular premature complexes, heart block, and T-wave inversion. PCR can also be used to detect infection.

*Serology.* In North American cases, positive serologic test results correlate with infection.

*Organism identification.* Tryptomastigotes (1 flagellum, 15 to 20 μm long) can be identified during acute disease on thick blood film or buffy coat smears stained with Giemsa or Wright's stain. The organism can sometimes be detected in lymph node aspirates or abdominal effusions, and tryptomastigotes can also be cultured from blood or grown by bioassay in mice. Histopathologic evaluation of cardiac tissue may reveal amastigotes (1.5 to 4 μm).

### Treatment

Nifurtimox (2 to 7 mg/kg PO q6h for 3 to 5 months) is prescribed most often but is not routinely available. Glucocorticoid therapy may improve survival. Therapy for arrhythmias or heart failure should be instituted as needed; most dogs that survive acute infection develop dilative cardiomyopathy.

### Zoonotic aspects and prevention

Infected dogs can serve as a reservoir for *T. cruzi*, and blood from infected dogs can be infectious to humans. Vector control is the primary means of prevention. Dogs should be kept from other reservoir hosts such as opossums and should not be fed raw meat. Potential blood donors from endemic areas should be serologically screened.

# 105

# Zoonoses

## (Text pp 1307-1321)

### ENTERIC ZOONOSES (TEXT PP 1307-1312)

The minimum diagnostic plan to assess for enteric zoonoses includes a fecal flotation, *Cryptosporidium* spp. screening procedure, fecal wet mount, and rectal cytology. Fecal culture should be considered if infection with *Salmonella* spp. or *Campylobacter* spp. is on the list of differential diagnoses.

### Helminths

#### Roundworms

Visceral larval migrans can be due to infestation with *Toxocara cati, Toxocara canis,* or *Baylisascaris procyonis* (Table 105-1). Humans are infested after ingesting the eggs, which are passed in cat or dog feces and can survive in the environment for months. Because the eggs are not immediately infectious, human infestation through direct contact with dogs or cats is extremely unlikely.

*Clinical signs.* Dogs and cats can be subclinically affected or may develop a poor coat, poor weight gain, vomiting, and rarely, diarrhea. Eosinophilic granulomatous reactions involving the skin, lungs, central nervous system (CNS), and eyes can occur, potentially leading to clinical disease. Signs and physical examination findings in humans include skin rash, fever, failure to thrive, CNS signs, cough, pulmonary infiltrates, and hepatosplenomegaly; peripheral eosinophilia is common. Ocular larva migrans most often involves the retina and can cause reduced vision; uveitis and enophthalmitis can also occur.

*Management.* Prevention is achieved by control of animal excrement in human environments. All puppies and kittens should have a fecal flotation performed and should be routinely treated with an anthelmintic (e.g., pyrantel pamoate twice, 3 weeks apart) during their initial vaccination period, whether or not ova are detected on fecal examination. In puppies with high worm burdens, deworming with pyrantel pamoate can be started at 1 to 2 weeks of age and repeated at 2-week intervals. In heavily infested kittens, deworming with pyrantel should be done at 6, 8, and 10 weeks of age. Heartworm preventatives that also control roundworms are indicated in areas with a high prevalence of roundworms.

#### Hookworms

*Ancylostoma caninum, Ancylostoma braziliense, Ancylostoma tubaeforme, Uncinaria stenocephala,* and *Strongyloides stercoralis* have been associated with cutaneous larva migrans in the United States. Humans are infested by skin penetration.

*Clinical signs.* Animals are either subclinically affected or have nonspecific signs such as poor haircoat, failure to gain weight, vomiting, and diarrhea. Heavily infested puppies and kittens may have pale mucous membranes from blood loss anemia. In humans signs are related to cutaneous larval migration that results in erythematous, pruritic tunnels in the skin. Abdominal pain can occur in humans with intestinal *A. caninum* infection.

Table 105-1

## Common Enteric Zoonoses Associated with Contact with Dogs or Cats or Their Excrement

| Organism | Species | Incubation |
|---|---|---|
| **BACTERIAL** | | |
| *Campylobacter jejuni* | D, C | Immediately infectious |
| *Escherichia coli* | D, C | Immediately infectious |
| *Salmonella* spp. | D, C | Immediately infectious |
| *Shigella* spp. | D | Immediately infectious |
| *Yersinia enterocolitica* | D, C | Immediately infectious |
| **PARASITIC** | | |
| **Amoeba** | | |
| *Entamoeba histolytica* | D | Cysts are immediately infectious |
| **Cestodes** | | |
| *Echinococcus multilocularis* | D, C | Ova are immediately infectious |
| *Echinococcus granulosus* | D | Ova are immediately infectious |
| *Multiceps multiceps* | D | Ova are immediately infectious |
| **Ciliate** | | |
| *Balantidium coli* | D | Cysts are immediately infectious |
| **Coccidians** | | |
| *Cryptosporidium parvum* | D, C | Oocysts are immediately infectious |
| *Toxoplasma gondii* | C | Oocysts are infectious after 1 to 5 days incubation; exposure from environment |
| **Flagellates** | | |
| *Giardia* spp. | D, C | Cysts are immediately infectious |
| *Pentatrichomonas hominis** | D, C | Cysts are immediately infectious but are rare in cats |
| **Helminths** | | |
| *Ancylostoma caninum* | D | Larva infectious after more than 3-day incubation; skin penetration from larva in environment |
| *Strongyloides stercoralis* | D, C | Larva immediately infectious |
| *Toxocara canis* | D | Larvated ova infectious after 1- to 3-week incubation; exposure from environment |
| *Toxocara felis* | C | As for T. canis |

*May be only a commensal organism.
C, Cats; D, dogs.

***Management.*** Skin irritation usually resolves after several weeks. Prevention and treatment of infested dogs and cats is as described for roundworms. Fenbendazole administered orally at 50 mg/kg for 5 days is an effective treatment for *S. stercoralis* infection.

### Cestodes

*Dipylidium caninum, Echinococcus granulosus,* and *Echinococcus multilocularis* are cestodes that can infest humans. *E. granulosus* ova can be transmitted in dog feces; *E. granulosus* eggs can be transmitted in feces of dogs after ingestion of infected sheep tissues.

*E. multilocularis*, which is most common in the northern and central parts of North America, can be transmitted in dog or cat feces after ingestion of an infected vole. Transmission to humans occurs after ingestion of infested fleas (*Dipylidium*) or by ingestion of ova (*Echinococcus* spp.).

Infestation in dogs and cats is generally subclinical. *Dipylidium* spp. infestation is most common in children and can lead to diarrhea and pruritus ani. In people, *Echinococcus* spp. organisms enter the portal circulation and spread throughout the liver and other tissues. Prevention or control of cestodes is based on sanitation procedures and use of taeniacides. Praziquantel is effective against *Echinococcus* spp. and *D. caninum*. Dogs and cats should not be allowed to hunt and should be fed only cooked meat and meat by-products.

## Coccidians

### Cryptosporidiosis

*Cryptosporidium parvum* is a coccidian parasite that inhabits the respiratory and intestinal epithelium of birds, mammals, reptiles, and fish. It causes gastrointestinal (GI) disease in mammalian species including rodents, dogs, cats, calves, and humans. In the United States the prevalence of immunoglobulin (Ig) G in serum is 8.6% in cats and up to 58% in humans. Human infection associated with contact with infected dogs and cats has been reported but is thought to be unusual, even in people infected with the human immunodeficiency virus (HIV). Fecal-oral contamination and ingestion of contaminated water are the most likely routes of exposure. Multiple species of *Cryptosporidium* exist, including *Cryptosporidium felis* and *Cryptosporidium canis*; some isolates infect multiple species, but others have a limited host range. Strains that infect pets and people cannot be differentiated by light microscopy from those that infect only pets, so all *Cryptosporidium* spp. should be considered potentially zoonotic.

*Clinical signs.* Infection in dogs and cats is usually subclinical, but small bowel diarrhea occurs in some cases. Immunosuppression (e.g., concurrent feline leukemia virus [FeLV] or canine distemper virus infection or intestinal lymphoma) may potentiate disease. In humans cryptosporidiosis is characterized by small bowel diarrhea and is generally self-limiting in immunocompetent individuals; it is often fatal in those with acquired immunodeficiency syndrome (AIDS).

*Diagnosis.* The small size (4 to 6 μm) of *C. parvum* oocysts makes diagnosis difficult. Routine salt solution flotation and microscopic examination at 100× often yield false-negative results. The combination of concentration techniques with fluorescent antibody staining or acid-fast staining is even more sensitive. An enzyme-linked immunosorbent assay for detection of *C. parvum* antigen in feces is commercially available, but whether this assay detects *C. felis* or *C. canis* is unknown. Polymerase chain reaction (PCR) is the most sensitive test to date, but assays are not routinely available and are not standardized among laboratories.

*Prevention.* Feces from all dogs and cats with diarrhea should be evaluated for *C. parvum* oocysts, particularly if the animal resides in the home of an immunodeficient person. No drug has been shown to eliminate *Cryptosporidium* spp. from the GI tract. Paromomycin (150 mg/kg orally [PO] q24h for 5 days) in dogs or cats or tylosin (10 to 15 mg/kg PO q12h for 14 to 21 days) in cats is effective in resolving clinical signs. Avoiding exposure is the most effective preventative measure. Routine disinfectants require extremely long contact time to be effective, but drying, freeze-thawing, and steam-cleaning can inactivate the organism. Water collected in the field for drinking should be boiled or filtered.

### Toxoplasmosis

*Toxoplasma gondii* is a ubiquitous coccidian. Seroprevalence studies suggest that at least 30% of cats and humans have been exposed. Infection occurs transplacentally or after sporulated oocysts or tissue cysts are ingested. Transplacental infection in humans and cats usually occurs only if the mother is infected for the first time during gestation.

*Clinical signs.* In dogs and cats clinical disease occurs occasionally and is manifested most often by fever, uveitis, and pulmonary, hepatic, and CNS disease (see

Chapter 104). Infected immunocompetent humans are generally asymptomatic; self-limiting fever, lymphadenopathy, and malaise occasionally occur. Transplacental infection can result in stillbirth, hydrocephalus, hepatosplenomegaly, and chorioretinitis. Chronic tissue infection in humans can be reactivated by immunosuppression, leading to dissemination and severe illness.

**Diagnosis.** Oocysts are most effectively demonstrated in cat feces after sugar solution centrifugation. Clinical toxoplasmosis is difficult to diagnose in humans, dogs, and cats; it usually involves the combination of clinical signs, serologic tests, organism demonstration techniques, and response to anti-*Toxoplasma* drugs (see Chapter 104).

**Prevention.** Because oocysts are passed only for approximately 7 to 14 days and are unsporulated (noninfectious), humans are not usually infected by direct contact with cats. Care should be taken to avoid ingesting tissue cysts in undercooked meats. No association was present between cat ownership and *T. gondii* seroprevalence in a group of HIV-infected humans. Prevention is discussed further in Chapter 104.

## Flagellates, Amoebae, and Ciliates

*Giardia* spp. (flagellate), *Entamoeba histolytica* (amoeba), and *Balantidium coli* (ciliate) are enteric protozoans that can be transmitted to humans by contact with feces. Multiple *Giardia* species exist. Some *Giardia* species infect humans, dogs, and cats, but this does not appear to be the case with all *Giardia* species; species-specific strains have been documented. Zoonotic strains of *Giardia* spp. cannot be identified by microscopic examination, so feces from all dogs and cats infected with *Giardia* spp. should be treated as a potential human health risk. *Giardia* organisms are immediately infectious when passed as cysts in stool. *E. histolytica* infection is extremely rare in dogs and cats. *B. coli* infection is rare in dogs and has not been reported in cats.

### Signs and diagnosis

*Giardia* spp. can be detected in feces of normal dogs and cats and in those with small bowel diarrhea (and occasionally mixed bowel diarrhea in cats). *Pentatrichomonas hominus*, *E. histolytica*, and *B. coli* infect the large bowel and cause signs of colitis. Signs of disease are generally more severe in immunodeficient individuals. Fecal examination should be performed on all dogs and cats at least yearly. Zinc sulfate centrifugation is the optimal fecal flotation technique to demonstrate cysts. Examination of a wet mount (from fresh feces) to detect the motile trophozoites improves sensitivity. Monoclonal antibody–based IFA tests and fecal antigen tests are available but have not been validated for detection of dog and cat strains; these techniques should be used in addition to fecal flotation.

### Treatment and prevention

Treatment with drugs with anti-*Giardia* activity, such as fenbendazole, metronidazole, or febantel, praziquantel, and pyrantel, should be instituted if indicated (see Chapter 30).

*Giardia* vaccines for subcutaneous administration are now available for both dogs and cats (see Chapter 99). The feline *Giardia* vaccine is not currently recommended for routine prophylactic use in cats, but vaccination against *Giardia* could be considered in cats or dogs with recurrent infection and is being evaluated as a therapeutic agent. Prevention of zoonotic giardiasis includes boiling or filtering surface water for drinking and washing hands that have handled fecally contaminated material, even if gloves were worn. It is unknown whether treated dogs and cats are cured, and it is likely that if a treated dog or cat is exposed again, it will be reinfected.

## Bacteria

*Salmonella* spp., *Campylobacter* spp., *Escherichia coli*, *Yersinia enterocolitica*, and *Helicobacter* spp. infect dogs and cats and cause disease in humans. Transmission from animals to humans is by fecal-oral contact. Dogs can also be subclinical carriers of *Shigella* spp., but humans are the natural hosts. *Salmonella* spp. and *Campylobacter* spp. infections are uncommon in pet dogs and cats and therefore an unlikely source of infection in humans; however, the prevalence of *Salmonella* and *Campylobacter* infections is greater in animals housed in unsanitary or crowded environments.

#### Clinical signs

Infection by *Salmonella* spp., *Campylobacter* spp., or *E. coli* can cause gastroenteritis in dogs or cats. *Y. enterocolitica* and *Shigella* spp. are probably commensal agents in animals but cause fever, abdominal pain, and bacteremia in humans. *Helicobacter* infections cause gastritis, which is commonly manifested as vomiting, belching, and pica. *Helicobacter pylori*, the primary cause of disease in people, was isolated from a colony of cats. *Salmonella* infection in dogs and cats is often subclinical. Approximately 50% of clinically affected cats have gastroenteritis, and many are presented with signs of bacteremia alone. Abortion, stillbirth, and neonatal death can result from in utero infection.

#### Diagnosis

Diagnosis of *Salmonella* spp., *C. jejuni*, *E. coli*, and *Y. enterocolitica* is based on fecal culture. A single negative culture may not rule out infection. Rectal cytology should be performed on all animals with diarrhea. If neutrophils are noted, culture for enteric bacteria is indicated, particularly if the animal is owned by an immunodeficient individual.

#### Management

Antibiotic therapy can control clinical signs of disease from infection by *Salmonella* spp. or *Campylobacter* spp. (see Chapter 30) but should not be administered orally to animals that are subclinical carriers of *Salmonella* because of the risk for antibiotic resistance; strains of *Salmonella* that were resistant to most antibiotics have been detected in several cats. Prevention of enteric bacterial zoonoses is based on sanitation and control of exposure to feces. Immunodeficient humans should avoid young animals and animals from crowded or unsanitary housing, particularly if signs of GI disease are present. Salmonellosis of cats and humans has been associated with songbirds (songbird fever).

## BITE, SCRATCH, OR EXUDATE EXPOSURE ZOONOSES (TEXT PP 1312-1315)

### Bacteria

#### *Bartonella henselae*

*Bartonella henselae* is the most common cause of cat scratch disease, as well as bacillary angiomatosis and bacillary peliosis—common disorders in humans with AIDS (Table 105-2). Cats can also be infected with *Bartonella clarridgeiae, Bartonella koehlerae,* and *Bartonella weissii*. *B. henselae* has been isolated from the blood of subclinical, seropositive cats and also from some cats with a variety of clinical manifestations such as fever, lethargy, lymphadenopathy, uveitis, gingivitis, and neurologic diseases. The organism is transmitted among cats by fleas, so the prevalence is greatest in cats from states in which fleas are common; 55% to 81% of cats in some geographic areas of the United States are *Bartonella* spp. seropositive. Transmission to humans commonly occurs with cat bites or scratches, most commonly from kittens.

*Signs and diagnosis.* Humans with cat scratch disease develop a variety of clinical signs such as lymphadenopathy, fever, malaise, weight loss, myalgia, headache, conjunctivitis, skin eruptions, and arthralgia. Bacillary angiomatosis is a diffuse disease that results in vascular cutaneous eruptions. Bacillary peliosis is a diffuse systemic vasculitis of parenchymal organs, particularly the liver. The incubation period for cat scratch disease is approximately 3 weeks. Most cases are self-limiting but may take several months to completely resolve. Blood culture, serologic testing, and PCR can be used to determine risk in individual cats. Serologic testing can determine exposure, but both seropositive and seronegative cats can be bacteremic. False-negative culture or PCR results may also occur because of intermittent bacteremia. False-positive results can occur with PCR, and positive results do not necessarily indicate that the organism is alive. Testing is currently recommended only in cats with suspected clinical bartonellosis, and not for healthy cats. Cats that are culture-negative or PCR-negative, regardless of whether they are antibody-negative or antibody-positive, are probably not shedding.

Table 105-2

## Common Canine and Feline Bite, Scratch, or Exudate Contact-Associated Zoonoses

| Organism | Species | Clinical disease |
|---|---|---|
| **BACTERIAL** | | |
| *Bartonella henselae* | C | Cat—subclinical |
| | | Human—fever, malaise, lymphadenopathy, bacillary angiomatosis, bacillary peliosis |
| *Capnocytophaga canimorsus* | D, C | Dog and cat—subclinical oral carriage |
| | | Human—bacteremia |
| *Francisella tularensis* | C | Cat—septicemia, pneumonia |
| | | Human—ulceroglandular, oculoglandular, glandular, pneumonic, or typhoidal (depending on route of infection) |
| L-form bacteria | C | Cat—chronic draining tracts |
| | | Human—chronic draining tracts |
| *Yersinia pestis* | C | Cat—bubonic, bacteremic, or pneumonic |
| | | Human—bubonic, bacteremic, or pneumonic |
| **FUNGAL** | | |
| *Blastomyces dermatitidis* | D | Dog—chronic draining cutaneous tracts, interstitial pulmonary disease, uveitis, central nervous system disease |
| | | Human—chronic draining cutaneous tract at bite wound |
| Dermatophytes | D, C | Dog, cat, and human—superficial dermatologic disease |
| *Sporothrix schenkii* | C | Cat—chronic draining cutaneous tracts |
| | | Human—chronic draining cutaneous tracts |
| **VIRAL** | | |
| Rabies | D, C | Dog and cat—progressive central nervous system disease |
| | | Human—progressive central nervous system disease |

*C,* Cats; *D,* dogs.

***Treatment and prevention.*** Administration of doxycycline, tetracycline, erythromycin, amoxicillin-clavulanate, or enrofloxacin can limit bacteremia but does not cure infection in all cats and has not been shown to lessen the risk of cat scratch disease. Therefore antibiotic treatment of healthy bacteremic cats is controversial. Treatment should be reserved for cats with suspected clinical bartonellosis.

Cat-induced wounds should immediately be cleansed, and medical advice sought. Strict flea control should be maintained. Kittens should be avoided by immunodeficient people. Cat claws should be kept clipped, and cats should never be teased.

### Feline plague

Feline plague is caused by *Yersinia pestis* (see Chapter 100). Rodents are the natural hosts. Dogs are more resistant to infection and have not been associated with zoonotic transfer. Humans are most commonly infected by rodent flea bites, but many cases of transmission by exposure to wild animals and infected domestic cats have been documented. Infection can be induced by inhalation of respiratory secretions of cats with pneumonic plague, through bite wounds, or by contamination of mucous membranes or abraded skin with secretions or exudates.

*Signs and diagnosis.* Bubonic, septicemic, and pneumonic plague can develop in cats and humans; each form has accompanying fever, headache, weakness, and malaise. In cats, suppurative lymphadenitis (buboes) of the cervical and submandibular lymph nodes is the most common manifestation. Exudates from these cats should be examined cytologically for the characteristic bipolar rods (see Chapter 100). Diagnosis is confirmed by fluorescent antibody staining of exudates; culture of exudates, tonsillar area, and saliva; and by documentation of increasing antibody titers.

*Treatment and prevention.* Doxycycline, chloramphenicol, and aminoglycosides are each potentially effective. Parenteral antibiotics should be used during the bacteremic phase. Drainage of lymph nodes may be required. Cats with suppurative lymphadenitis should be considered plague suspects, and extreme caution should be exercised when exudates are handled or draining wounds are treated. Suspect animals should be treated for fleas and housed in isolation. People who are exposed to infected cats should be urgently referred to physicians for antimicrobial therapy, and public health officials alerted, although cats are not infectious to humans after 3 days of antibiotic treatment.

### Tularemia

*Francisella tularensis* is the gram-negative bacillus that causes tularemia. *Dermacentor variabilis* (American dog tick), *Dermacentor andersoni* (American wood tick), and *Amblyomma americanum* (Lone Star tick) are known vectors. Human tularemia occurs most commonly after exposure to ticks and less commonly from contact with infected animals, including cats. Dogs are not considered a source of human tularemia but may facilitate human exposure by bringing infected ticks into the environment. Most cases of feline tularemia have been documented in the midwestern states, particularly Oklahoma.

*Signs and diagnosis.* Infected cats exhibit generalized lymphadenopathy and abscess formation in organs such as the liver and spleen. This causes fever, anorexia, icterus, and death. Ulceroglandular, oculoglandular, glandular, oropharyngeal, pneumonic, and typhoidal forms have been described in humans. Unlike plague, the organism is not often recognized in exudates or lymph node aspirates from infected cats. Culture and increasing antibody titers can be used to confirm the diagnosis in cats and humans.

*Treatment and prevention.* Most cases in cats are diagnosed at necropsy, so optimal treatment is unknown. Streptomycin and gentamicin are the drugs used most commonly to treat humans. The disease is prevented by avoiding exposure to lagomorphs, ticks, and infected cats. All cats dying with bacteremia should be handled carefully.

### Oral bacteria

The majority of bacteria associated with dog or cat bite or scratch wounds lead only to local infection in immunocompetent individuals. However, 28% to 80% of cat bites become infected, and severe sequelae, including meningitis, endocarditis, septic arthritis, osteoarthritis, and septic shock, can occur. Immunodeficient humans or those exposed to *Pasteurella* spp., *Capnocytophaga canimorsus* (DF-2), or *Capnocytophaga cynodegmi* more consistently develop systemic clinical illness. Splenectomized humans are at increased risk for development of bacteremia.

Bacteremia and associated fever, malaise, and weakness are common, and death can occur within hours of infection with *Capnocytophaga* spp. in immunodeficient humans. Diagnosis is confirmed by culture. Treatment of carrier animals is not needed; treatment of clinically affected humans includes local wound management and parenteral antibiotic therapy. Penicillin derivatives are very effective against most *Pasteurella* infections, and penicillins and cephalosporins are effective against *Capnocytophaga* spp. in vitro.

### Mycoplasma and L-form bacteria

*Mycoplasma* spp. infection resulting in cellulitis and septic arthritis has been reported in humans secondary to cat bites. L-form bacteria are associated with chronic, draining skin wounds in cats and are commonly resistant to cell wall–inhibiting antibiotics like penicillins and cephalosporins; infection in a human after a cat bite has been documented. Diagnosis can be confirmed only by histologic examination of tissue. Doxycycline has been used to successfully treat cats and people. Gloves should be worn when attending to cats with draining tracts. Hands should be cleaned thoroughly.

### Fungal agents

Of the many fungal agents that infect both humans and animals, only *Sporothrix schenckii* and the dermatophytes infect humans on direct exposure. *Histoplasma, Blastomyces, Coccidioides, Aspergillus,* and *Cryptococcus* infections of humans and animals can occur in the same household, but they generally result from a common environmental exposure (see Chapter 103).

#### Sporothrix

*Sporothrix* is cosmopolitan in distribution. Soil is likely the natural reservoir. Cats are thought to be infected by scratches from contaminated claws of other cats; infection is most common in outdoor males. Humans can be infected by contamination of cutaneous wounds with exudates from infected cats. Dogs generally do not produce large numbers of *Sporothrix* in exudates and therefore are less of a zoonotic risk.

*Signs.* Infection in cats can be cutaneolymphatic, cutaneous, or disseminated. Chronic draining cutaneous tracts are common. Cats often produce large numbers of the organism in feces, tissues, and exudates; veterinary personnel are therefore at high risk when treating infected cats. The clinical disease in humans is similar to that in cats.

*Diagnosis and treatment.* The organism can be demonstrated by cytologic examination of exudates or culture. Fluconazole, itraconazole, and ketoconazole are effective treatments. Gloves should be worn when attending to cats with draining tracts. Hands should be cleansed thoroughly.

### Viral agents

#### Rabies and pseudorabies

Rabies is the only relevant small animal viral zoonosis in the United States (see Chapter 71). Pseudorabies is a herpesvirus that infects pigs. Dogs and humans can develop self-limiting pruritic skin disease after exposure. Dogs occasionally develop severe CNS disease, characterized by depression and seizures. Diagnosis is suspected based on exposure history, and infection is prevented by avoiding exposure.

#### Feline retroviruses

Concern exists regarding whether FeLV, feline immunodeficiency virus (FIV), and feline foamy virus (FeFV) can infect humans, because FeLV subtypes B and C can replicate in human cell lines. Although to date no documentation of human infection from these viruses exists, FeLV- and FIV-infected cats are more likely than retrovirus-naïve cats to be carriers of other potential zoonotic agents, particularly if GI tract signs are occurring.

## RESPIRATORY AND OCULAR ZOONOSES (TEXT PP 1315-1316)

### Bordetella

*Bordetella bronchiseptica* is a species of bacteria that induces respiratory tract infections in dogs and cats. The classic manifestation is tracheobronchitis, but the organism can also cause pneumonia, sneezing, and nasal discharge. Humans rarely develop clinical disease unless they are immunologically compromised. Amoxicillin-clavulanate, chloramphenicol, enrofloxacin, and tetracycline derivatives are all effective treatments. Animals with upper or lower respiratory tract inflammatory disease should be isolated from immunodeficient people until clinically normal. However, treated animals can still shed the organism.

### Chlamydia

*Chlamydophila felis* (formerly *Chlamydia psittaci*) causes mild conjunctival disease and rhinitis in cats (Table 105-3) and can also cause conjunctivitis in humans after direct contact with ocular discharges. Occasionally the organism is associated with systemic disease in humans. Diagnosis is based on organism demonstration by culture, cytologic documentation of characteristic inclusion bodies, or fluorescent antibody staining of conjunctival scrapings. Tetracycline or chloramphenicol-containing eye ointments generally are effective for treatment. Care should be taken to avoid direct conjunctival contact with discharges from the respiratory or ocular secretions of cats, especially by immunosuppressed persons. Employees should be directed to wear gloves or wash hands carefully when attending to cats with conjunctivitis.

### Streptococci

Humans are the principal natural hosts for the *Streptococcus* group A bacteria, *Streptococcus pyogenes* and *Streptococcus pneumoniae,* which cause "strep throat" in humans. Dogs and cats in close contact with infected humans can develop transient, subclinical colonization of pharyngeal tissues and can transmit the infection to other humans, but this is poorly documented and thought to be unusual. The organism can be cultured from the tonsillar crypts. Culture-positive animals should be treated with penicillin derivatives. If animals are to be treated in a household with recurrent "strep throat," all humans should also be treated, because they may be chronic, subclinical carriers.

### Feline plague and tularemia

*Y. pestis* and *F. tularensis* can be transmitted from cats to people in respiratory secretions (see discussion of bite, scratch, or exudate exposure zoonoses). In endemic areas cats with clinical signs or radiographic abnormalities consistent with pneumonia should be handled as plague or tularemia suspects. Gloves, mask, gown, and eye protection should be worn while transoral airway washings are performed in suspect cats.

## GENITAL AND URINARY TRACT ZOONOSES (TEXT PP 1316-1317)

### Q fever

*Coxiella burnetii* is a rickettsial agent found throughout the world, including North America. Many ticks, including *Rhipicephalus sanguineus*, are naturally infected with *C. burnetii.* Cattle, sheep, and goats are commonly subclinically infected and pass the organism into the environment in urine, feces, milk, and parturient discharges. Seropositive dogs have been detected, but zoonotic transfer to humans from dogs has not been documented. Infection of cats appears to be common; infection most commonly occurs with tick exposure, ingestion of contaminated carcasses, or aerosolization from a contaminated environment.

***Signs.*** Fever, anorexia, and lethargy develop in some experimentally infected cats. Infection has been associated with abortion, but the organism can also be isolated

**Table 105-3**

### Common Zoonoses Associated with Direct Contact with Respiratory or Ocular Secretions of Dogs or Cats

| Organism | Species | Clinical signs |
|---|---|---|
| *Bordetella bronchiseptica* | D, C | Dog and cat—upper respiratory, rarely, pneumonia<br>Immunosuppressed humans—pneumonia |
| *Chlamydophila felis* | C | Cat—conjunctivitis, mild upper respiratory<br>Human—conjunctivitis |
| *Francisella tularensis* | C | Cat—septicemia, pneumonia<br>Human—ulceroglandular, oculoglandular, glandular, pneumonic, or typhoidal (depending on route of infection) |
| *Streptococcus* group A | D, C | Dog and cat—subclinical, transient carrier<br>Human—"strep throat," septicemia |
| *Yersinia pestis* | C | Cat—bubonic, bacteremic, or pneumonic<br>Human—bubonic, bacteremic, or pneumonic |

*C,* Cats; *D,* dogs.

## Table 105-4

### Common Canine and Feline Urinary and Genital Tract Zoonoses

| Organism | Species | Clinical disease |
|---|---|---|
| **BACTERIAL** | | |
| *Brucella canis* | D | Dog—orchitis, epididymitis, abortion, stillbirth, vaginal discharge, uveitis, diskospondylitis, fever, malaise<br>Human—fever, malaise |
| *Leptospira* spp. | D, C | Dog and cat—fever, malaise, inflammatory urinary tract or hepatic disease, uveitis, central nervous system disease<br>Human—fever, malaise, inflammatory urinary tract or hepatic disease, uveitis, central nervous system disease |
| **RICKETTSIAL** | | |
| *Coxiella burnetii* | C | Cat—subclinical, abortion, or stillbirth<br>Human—fever, lymphadenopathy, myalgia, arthritis |

C, Cats; D, dogs.

from normal parturient cats (Table 105-4). Human illness associated with cats primarily occurs after aerosol exposure to the organism passed by parturient or aborting cats; clinical signs develop 4 to 30 days after contact. Humans commonly develop acute clinical signs similar to those of other rickettsial diseases: fever, malaise, headache, interstitial pneumonitis, myalgia, and arthralgia. Chronic Q fever develops in approximately 1% of infections and can manifest as hepatic inflammation or valvular endocarditis.

***Treatment and prevention.*** Administration of tetracyclines, chloramphenicol, or quinolones is usually effective in people. Gloves and masks should be worn when attending to parturient or aborting cats. People that develop fever or respiratory disease after exposure to parturient or aborting cats should seek medical attention.

### Leptospirosis

*Leptospira* spp. can be transmitted in urine from infected dogs and cats to humans. Infection by non–host adapted species commonly causes clinical illness. The organisms enter the body through abraded skin or intact mucous membranes. Human clinical syndromes vary with the serovar but are similar to those in dogs (see Chapter 100). Gloves should be worn when handling animals with suspected leptospirosis. Contaminated surfaces should be cleaned with detergents and disinfected with iodine-containing products.

### Brucellosis

*Brucella canis* is a bacterium that preferentially infects the testicles, prostate, uterus, and vagina of dogs. Humans can be infected by direct contact with vaginal and preputial discharges from dogs. Clinical syndromes in dogs are diverse but commonly include abortion, stillbirth, failure to conceive, orchitis, epididymitis, vaginal discharge, uveitis, diskospondylitis, and bacteremia. Intermittent fever, depression, and malaise are common in infected people.

***Diagnosis.*** Diagnosis is based on serologic testing or culture. Dogs with any clinical sign of brucellosis should be evaluated serologically using the 2-mercaptoethanol rapid slide agglutination test. Seropositive dogs should have results confirmed by tube agglutination or agar gel immunodiffusion. Seronegative dogs are unlikely to be harboring *Brucella* unless the clinical syndrome was peracute.

***Treatment.*** Long-term antibiotic treatment (tetracyclines, aminoglycosides, quinolones) usually does not clear the infection. Ovariohysterectomy or castration lessens contamination of the human environment.

## Drugs Used in Dogs and Cats with Infectious Diseases

| Generic name | Trade name | Dogs | Cats |
|---|---|---|---|
| **ANTIBIOTICS** | | | |
| **Aminoglycosides** | | | |
| Amikacin | Amiglyde-V | 5-10 mg/kg, q8h, IV, IM, SC | 5-10 mg/kg, q8h, IV, IM, SC |
| Gentamicin | Gentocin | 2-4 mg/kg, q8h, IV, IM, SC | 2-4 mg/kg, q8h, IV, IM, SC |
| Neomycin | | 2.5-10 mg/kg, q8-12h, PO | 2.5-10 mg/kg, q8-12h, PO |
| Tobramycin | Nebcin | 2 mg/kg, q8h, IV, IM, SC | 2 mg/kg, q8h, IV, IM, SC |
| | | | |
| **Carbapenems** | | | |
| Imipenem | Primaxin | 2-5 mg/kg, q6-8h, IV, SC | 3-10 mg/kg, q6-8h, IV, SC |
| | | | |
| **Cephalosporins** | | | |
| Cefadroxil | Cefa-Tabs | 22 mg/kg, q12h, PO | 22 mg/kg, q12h, PO |
| Cephalexin | | 20-40 mg/kg, q8h, PO | 20-40 mg/kg, q8h, PO |
| Cefazolin | | 20-25 mg/kg, q8h, IM, IV | 20-25 mg/kg, q8h, IM, IV |
| Cefoxitin | Mefoxin | 22 mg/kg, q8h, IM, IV | 22 mg/kg, q8h, IM, IV |
| Cefotaxime | Claforan | 6-40 mg/kg, q8h, SC, IM, IV | 6-40 mg/kg, q8h, SC, IM, IV |
| Ceftiofur | Naxcel | 2.2 mg/kg, q24h, SC | |
| Chloramphenicol | | 25-50 mg/kg, q8h, PO, SC, IV | 15-25 mg/kg, q12h, PO, IV |
| | | | |
| **Macrolides and lincosamides** | | | |
| Azithromycin | Zithromax | 10-40 mg/kg, q24h, PO | 5-10 mg/kg, q24h, PO |
| Clarithromycin | Biaxin | 5-10 mg/kg, q12h, PO | 5-10 mg/kg, q12h, PO |
| Clindamycin | Antirobe | 5.5-11 mg/kg, q12h, PO, SC, IM | 5.5-11 mg/kg, q12-24h, PO, SC, IM |
| Erythromycin | | 10-20 mg/kg, q8-12h, PO | 10-20 mg/kg, q8-12h, PO |
| Lincomycin | | 15-25 mg/kg, q12h, PO, IM, IV | 15-25 mg/kg, q12h, PO, IM, IV |
| Tylosin | | 10-40 mg/kg, q12h, PO | 10-40 mg/kg, q12h, PO |
| | | | |
| **Metronidazole** | | 10 mg/kg, q8h, PO | 10 mg/kg, q12h, PO |

| Drug | Brand | Dose | Dose |
|---|---|---|---|
| **Penicillins** | | | |
| Amoxicillin | | 10-22 mg/kg, q8-12h, PO, SC | 10-22 mg/kg, q8-12h, PO, SC |
| Amoxicillin and clavulanate | Clavamox | 12.5-25 mg/kg, q8-12h, PO | 62.5 mg, q8-12h, PO |
| Ampicillin sodium | | 22 mg/kg, q8h, SC, IM, IV | 22 mg/kg, q8h, SC, IM, IV |
| Oxacillin | | 22-40 mg/kg, q8h, PO | 22-40 mg/kg, q8h, PO |
| Penicillin G | | 22,000 U/kg, q6-8h, IM, IV | 22,000 U/kg, q6-8h, IM, IV |
| Ticarcillin and clavulanate | Timentin | 40-110 mg/kg, q6h, IM, IV | |
| **Quinolones** | | | |
| Ciprofloxacin | Cipro | 5-15 mg/kg, q12h, PO | 5-15 mg/kg, q12h, PO |
| Enrofloxacin | Baytril | 2.5-10 mg/kg, q12h, PO, IM, SC, IV | 2.5-10 mg/kg, q12h, PO, IM, SC, IV |
| Orbifloxacin | Orbax | 2.5-7.5 mg/kg, q24h, PO | |
| **Sulfonamide-combos** | | | |
| Ormetoprim-sulfadimethoxine | Primor | 55 mg/kg, q24h day 1, PO, then 27 mg/kg, q24h | 55 mg/kg, q24h day 1, PO, then 27 mg/kg, q24h |
| Trimethoprim-sulfonamide | Tribrissen (sulfadiazine) | 15-30 mg/kg, q12h, PO, SC | 15-30 mg/kg, q12h, PO, SC |
| **Tetracyclines** | | | |
| Doxycycline | | 5-10 mg/kg, q12h, PO, IV | 2.5-5 mg/kg, q12h, PO, IV |
| Minocycline | Minocin | 12.5 mg/kg, q12h, PO | |
| Tetracycline | | 22 mg/kg, q8-12h, PO | 22 mg/kg, q8-12h, PO |
| **ANTIVIRAL OR IMMUNE MODULATION** | | | |
| Acemannan | | | 1-2 mg/kg, q7days, for 6 weeks, IP |
| Alpha-interferon (FeLV) | Intron A | | 30 U, q24h, PO |
| AZT | Retrovir | | 20 mg/kg, q8h, for 7 days, then 5-10 mg/kg, q8h, PO |
| *Propionibacterium acnes* | Immunoreglan | | 0.5 ml twice weekly for 2 weeks, then 0.5 ml weekly for 20 weeks, IV |
| *Staphylococcus* A | | | 10 μg/kg twice weekly for 10 weeks, then 10 μg/kg twice weekly every fourth week for life, IP |

*Continued.*

## Drugs Used in Dogs and Cats with Infectious Diseases—cont'd

| Generic name | Trade name | Dogs | Cats |
|---|---|---|---|
| **ANTIPROTOZOAL** | | | |
| ***Babesia* spp.** | | | |
| Diminazene aceturate | | 3.5 mg/kg, once, IM | |
| Imidocarb dipropionate | | 5-7 mg/kg, q7-14 days, IM | |
| Phenamidine isethionate | | 15 mg/kg, q24h, SC | |
| Primaquine phosphate | | 0.5 mg/kg, once, SC | |
| ***Cryptosporidium*** | | | |
| Paromomycin | | 165 mg/kg, q12h, PO | 165 mg/kg, q12h, PO |
| Tylosin | | 10-15 mg/kg, q8-12h, PO | 10-15 mg/kg, q8-12h, PO |
| ***Cytauxzoon felis*** | | | |
| Buparvaquone | | | 10 mg/kg, q24h, IM, SC |
| Diminazene aceturate | | | 2 mg/kg, q7days IM |
| Imidocarb dipropionate | | | 5 mg/kg, 14 days, IM |
| Parvaquone | | | 10-30 mg/kg, q24h, IM, SC |
| ***Giardia*** | | | |
| Albendazole | | 25 mg/kg, q12h, for 2-5 days, PO | 25 mg/kg, q12h, for 2-5 days, PO |
| Fenbendazole | | 25 mg/kg, q12h, for 3-7 days, PO | 25 mg/kg, q12h, for 3-7 days, PO |
| Metronidazole | Flagyl | 25 mg/kg, q12h, PO | 25 mg/kg, q12h, PO |
| ***Hepatozoon canis*** | | | |
| Toltrazuril | | 5-10 mg/kg, q24h, PO | |

*Leishmania*

| | | |
|---|---|---|
| Allopurinol | | 15 mg/kg, q12h, PO |
| Meglumine antimonate | | 100 mg/kg, q24h, IV, IM, SC |
| Sodium stibogluconate | | 30-50 mg/kg, q24h, IV, SC |

***Toxoplasma gondii***

| | | |
|---|---|---|
| Clindamycin hydrochloride | | 12.5 mg/kg, q12h, PO |
| Pyrimethamine | Daraprim | 1 mg/kg, q24h, PO |
| Trimethoprim-sulfadiazine | | 15 mg/kg, q12h, PO |

**ANTIFUNGAL**

| | | |
|---|---|---|
| Amphotericin B | | 0.5 mg/kg, three times weekly, IV |
| Amphotericin B (liposomal) | Abelcet | 0.5 mg/kg, to test, then 1 mg/kg three times weekly, IV |
| Fluconazole | Diflucan | 1.25-2.5 mg/kg, q12h, PO |
| Flucytosine | Ancobon | 50 mg/kg, q6h, PO |
| Itraconazole | Sporanox | 5 mg/kg, q12h, for 4 days, then 5 mg/kg, q12h, PO |
| Ketoconazole | Nizoral | 10 mg/kg, q12-24h, PO |

*IM,* Intramuscularly; *IP,* intraperitoneal; *IV,* intravenously; *PO,* orally; *SC,* subcutaneously.

## Conversion to Système International (SI) Units for Hormone Assays

| Measurement | SI Unit | Common Unit | Common→SI* | SI→Common* |
|---|---|---|---|---|
| Aldosterone | pmol/L | ng/dl | 27.7 | 0.036 |
| Corticotropin (ACTH) | pmol/L | pg/ml | 0.220 | 4.51 |
| Cortisol | nmol/L | µg/dl | 27.59 | 0.036 |
| C-peptide | nmol/L | ng/ml | 0.331 | 3.02 |
| β-Endorphin | pmol/L | pg/ml | 0.292 | 3.43 |
| Epinephrine | pmol/L | pg/ml | 5.46 | 0.183 |
| Estrogen (estradiol) | pmol/L | pg/ml | 3.67 | 0.273 |
| Gastrin | ng/L | pg/ml | 1 | 1 |
| Gastrointestinal polypeptide | pmol/L | pg/ml | 0.201 | 4.98 |
| Glucagon | ng/L | pg/ml | 1 | 1 |
| Growth hormone | µg/L | ng/ml | 1 | 1 |
| Insulin | pmol/L | µU/ml | 7.18 | 0.139 |
| α-MSH | pmol/L | pg/ml | 0.601 | 1.66 |
| Norepinephrine | nmol/L | pg/ml | 0.006 | 169 |
| Pancreatic polypeptide | mmol/L | mg/dl | 0.239 | 4.18 |
| Progesterone | nmol/L | ng/ml | 3.18 | 0.315 |
| Prolactin | µg/L | ng/ml | 1 | 1 |
| Renin | ng/L/s | ng/ml/hr | 0.278 | 3.60 |
| Somatostatin | pmol/L | pg/ml | 0.611 | 1.64 |
| Testosterone | nmol/L | ng/ml | 3.47 | 0.288 |
| Thyroxine ($T_4$) | nmol/L | µg/dl | 12.87 | 0.078 |
| Triiodothyronine ($T_3$) | Nmol/L | µg/dl | 0.0154 | 64.9 |
| Vasoactive intestinal polypeptide | pmol/L | pg/ml | 0.301 | 3.33 |

*Factor to multiply to convert from one unit to another.

# BIBLIOGRAPHY

## PART I: CARDIOVASCULAR SYSTEM DISORDERS

Belanger MC et al: Usefulness of the indexed effective orifice area in the assessment of subaortic stenosis in the dog, *J Vet Intern Med* 15:307, 2001 (abstract).

Biondo AW et al: Genomic sequence and cardiac expression of atrial natriuretic peptide in cats, *Am J Vet Res* 63:236, 2002.

Calvert CA et al: Evaluation of stability over time for measures of heart-rate variability in overtly healthy Doberman Pinschers, *Am J Vet Res* 63:53, 2002.

Davidow EB et al: Syncope: pathophysiology and differential diagnosis, *Compend Contin Educ* 23:608, 2001.

DeFrancesco TC et al: Prospective clinical evaluation of serum cardiac troponin T in dogs admitted to a veterinary teaching hospital, *J Vet Intern Med* 16:553, 2002.

Eisenberg MS et al: Cardiac resuscitation, *N Engl J Med* 344:1304, 2001.

Fox PR: Feline cardiopathy. I. Hypertrophic cardiomyopathy, *Proceedings of the Nineteenth ACVIM Forum*, Denver, 2001, p 145.

Herndon WE et al: Cardiac troponin I in feline hypertrophic cardiomyopathy, *J Vet Intern Med* 16:558, 2002.

Knight DH et al: 1999 Guidelines for the diagnosis, treatment and prevention of heartworm (*Dirofilaria immitis*) infection in cats, *Vet Ther* 2:78, 2001. Available at: http://www.heartwormsociety.org.

Maggio F et al: Ocular lesions associated with systemic hypertension in cats: 69 cases (1985-1998), *J Am Vet Med Assoc* 217:695, 2000.

Miller MW et al: Pericardial disorders. In Ettinger SJ et al, eds: *Textbook of veterinary internal medicine*, ed 5, Philadelphia, 2000, WB Saunders, p 923.

Miyamoto M et al: Acute cardiovascular effects of diltiazem in anesthetized dogs with induced atrial fibrillation, *J Vet Intern Med* 15:559, 2001

Rush JE et al: Clinical, echocardiographic and neurohormonal effects of a sodium-restricted diet in dogs with heart failure, *J Vet Intern Med* 14:512, 2000.

Sleeper MM et al: Vertebral scale system to measure heart size in growing puppies, *J Am Vet Med Assoc* 219:57, 2001.

Straeter-Knowlen IM et al: ACE inhibitors in heart failure restore canine pulmonary endothelial function and ANG II vasoconstriction, *Am J Physiol* 277:H1924, 1999.

## PART II: RESPIRATORY SYSTEM DISORDERS

Allen HS et al: Nasopharyngeal diseases in cats: a retrospective study of 53 cases (1991-1998), *J Am Anim Hosp Assoc* 35:457, 1999.

Bach JF et al: *Proceedings of the Twentieth Symposium of the Veterinary Comparative Respiratory Society*, Boston, 2002.

Bauer TG: Lung biopsy, *Vet Clin North Am Small Anim Pract* 30: 1207, 2000.

Fossum TW, ed: *Small animal surgery*, ed 2, St Louis, 2002, Mosby.

Hamlin RL: Physical examination of the pulmonary system, *Vet Clin North Am Small Anim Pract* 30:1175, 2000.

Lappin MR et al: Use of serologic tests to predict resistance to feline herpesvirus 1, feline calcivirus, and feline parvovirus infection in cats, *J Am Vet Med Assoc* 220:38, 2002.

MacPhail CM et al: Outcome of and postoperative complications in dogs undergoing surgical treatment of laryngeal paralysis: 140 cases (1985-1998), *J Am Vet Med Assoc* 218:1949, 2001.

Norris CR et al: Pulmonary thromboembolism in cats: 29 cases (1987-1997), *J Am Vet Med Assoc* 215:1650, 1999.

Puerto DA et al: Surgical and nonsurgical management of and selected risk factors for spontaneous pneumothorax in dogs: 64 cases (1986-1999), *J Am Vet Med Assoc* 220:1670, 2002.

Rudorf H et al: The role of ultrasound in the assessment of laryngeal paralysis in the dog, *Vet Radiol Ultrasound* 42:338, 2001.

## PART III: DIGESTIVE SYSTEM DISORDERS

Boothe DM: Gastrointestinal pharmacology. In Boothe DM, ed: *Small animal clinical pharmacology and therapeutics*, Philadelphia, 2001, WB Saunders.

DiBartola SP, ed: *Fluid therapy in small animal practice*, ed 2, Philadelphia, 2000, WB Saunders.

Easton S: A retrospective study into the effects of operator experience on the accuracy of ultrasound in the diagnosis of gastric neoplasia in dogs, *Vet Radiol Ultrasound* 42:47, 2001.

Ettinger SJ, Feldman EC, eds: *Textbook of veterinary internal medicine,* ed 6, Philadelphia, 2005, WB Saunders.

Guilford WG et al: *Small animal gastroenterology,* ed 3, Philadelphia, 1996, WB Saunders.

Hill SL et al: Prevalence of enteric zoonotic organisms in cats, *J Am Vet Med Assoc* 216:687, 2000.

Lanz OI et al: Surgical treatment of septic peritonitis without abdominal drainage in 28 dogs, *J Am Anim Hosp Assoc* 37:87, 2001.

Rewerts JM et al: CVT update: diagnosis and treatment of parvovirus. In Bonagura JD, ed: *Current veterinary therapy XIII,* ed 13, Philadelphia, 2000 WB Saunders.

Willard MD et al: Gastrointestinal, pancreatic, and hepatic disorders. In Willard MD et al, eds: *Small animal clinical diagnosis by laboratory methods,* ed 3, Philadelphia, 1999, WB Saunders.

## PART IV: HEPATOBILIARY AND EXOCRINE PANCREATIC DISORDERS

Bennett PF et al: Ultrasonographic and cytopathological diagnosis of exocrine pancreatic carcinoma in the dog and cat, *J Am Anim Hosp Assoc* 37:466, 2001.

Bigge LA et al: Correlation between coagulation profile findings and bleeding complications after ultrasound-guided biopsies: 434 cases (1993-1996), *J Am Anim Hosp Assoc* 37:228, 2001.

Bunch SE et al: Idiopathic noncirrhotic portal hypertension in dogs: 33 cases (1982-1998), *J Am Vet Med Assoc* 218:392, 2001.

Cole T et al: Diagnostic comparison of needle biopsy and wedge biopsy specimens of the liver in dogs and cats, *J Am Vet Med Assoc* 220:1483, 2002.

Cornelius LM et al: CVT Update: therapy for hepatic lipidosis. In Bonagura JD et al, eds: *Kirk's current veterinary therapy XIII,* ed 13, Philadelphia, 2000, WB Saunders, p 686.

Harkin KR et al: Hepatotoxicity of stanozolol in cats, *J Am Vet Med Assoc* 217:681, 2000.

Howe LM et al: Detection of portal blood and systemic bacteremia in dogs with severe induced hepatic disease and multiple portosystemic shunts, *Am J Vet Res* 60:181, 1999.

Maddison JE: Newest insights into hepatic encephalopathy, *Eur J Comp Gastroenterol* 5:17, 2000.

Seguin MA et al: Iatrogenic copper deficiency in Bedlington terrier associated with long-term copper chelation treatment for copper storage disease, *J Am Vet Med Assoc* 218:1593, 2001.

Taboada J et al: Hepatic encephalopathy: clinical signs, pathogenesis, and treatment, *Vet Clin North Am Small Anim Pract* 25:337, 1995.

Washabau RK: Feline acute pancreatitis—important species differences. Proceedings of the European Society of Feline Medicine Symposium, *J Feline Med Surg* 3:95, 2001.

Wright KN et al: Peritoneal effusion in cats: 65 cases (1981-1997), *J Am Vet Med Assoc* 214:375, 1999.

## PART V: URINARY DISORDERS

Brown SA et al: Effects of the angiotensin-converting enzyme inhibitor benazepril in cats with induced renal insufficiency, *Am J Vet Res* 62:375, 2001.

Buffington CAT et al: CVT update: idiopathic (interstitial) cystitis in cats. In Bonagura JD, ed: *Current veterinary therapy XIII,* ed 13, Philadelphia, 2000, WB Saunders, p 894.

Ettinger SJ, Feldman EC, eds: *Textbook of veterinary internal medicine,* ed 6, Philadelphia, 2005, WB Saunders.

Hess RS et al: Concurrent disorders in dogs with diabetes mellitus: 221 cases (1993-1998), *J Am Vet Med Assoc* 217:1166, 2000.

Hoppe A et al: Cystinuria in the dog: clinical studies during 14 years of medical treatment, *J Vet Intern Med* 15:361, 2001.

Lane IF: Functional urethral obstruction in 3 dogs: clinical and urethral pressure profile findings, *J Vet Intern Med* 14:43, 2000.

Lees GE et al: Persistent albuminuria precedes onset of overt proteinuria in male dogs with X-linked hereditary nephropathy, *J Vet Intern Med* 16:353, 2002 (abstract).

Oluch AO et al: Nonenteric *Escheria coli* isolates from dogs: 674 cases (1990-1998), *J Am Vet Med Assoc* 218:381, 2001.

Osborne CA: Techniques of urine collection and preservation. In Osborne CA et al, eds: *Canine and feline nephrology and urology,* Philadelphia, 1995, Williams & Wilkins, p 100.

Seaman R et al: Canine struvite urolithiasis, *Compend Contin Educ Pract Vet* 23:407, 2001.

Vaden SL et al: Longitudinal study of microalbuminuria in Soft-Coated Wheaten Terriers, *J Vet Intern Med* 15:300, 2001.

## PART VI: ENDOCRINE DISORDERS

Appleton DJ et al: Dietary chromium tripicolinate supplementation reduces glucose concentrations and improves glucose tolerance in normal-weight cats. *J Feline Med Surg* 4:13, 2002.

Bojrab MJ: *Current techniques in small animal surgery,* ed 4, Philadelphia, 1998, Williams & Wilkins.
Feldman EC, Nelson RW: *Canine and feline endocrinology and reproduction,* ed 3, Philadelphia, 2004, WB Saunders.
Fossum TW, ed: *Small animal surgery,* ed 2, St Louis, 2002, Mosby.
Hoffman SB et al: Bioavailability of transdermal methimazole in a pluronic lecithin organogel (PLO) in healthy cats, *J Vet Intern Med* 16:259, 2002.
Meij BP et al: Transsphenoidal hypophysectomy for treatment of pituitary-dependent hyperadrenocorticism in 7 cats, *Vet Surg* 30:72, 2001.
Peterson ME et al: Measurement of serum concentrations of free thyroxine, total thyroxine, and total triiodothyronine in cats with hyperthyroidism and cats with nonthyroidal disease, *J Am Vet Med Assoc* 218:529, 2001.
Pollard RE et al: Percutaneous ultrasonographically guided radiofrequency heat ablation for treatment of primary hyperparathyroidism in dogs, *J Am Vet Med Assoc* 218:1106, 2001.
Ruckstuhl NS et al: Results of clinical examinations, laboratory tests, and ultrasonography in dogs with pituitary-dependent hyperadrenocorticism treated with trilostane, *Am J Vet Res* 63:506, 2002.
Syme HM et al: Hyperadrenocorticism associated with excessive sex hormone production by an adrenocortical tumor in two dogs, *J Am Vet Med Assoc* 219:1725, 2001.

## PART VII: METABOLIC AND ELECTROLYTE DISORDERS

Bhatnagar D: Lipid-lowering drugs in the management of hyperlipidemia in dogs, *Pharmacol Ther* 79:205, 1998.
Bissette SA et al: Hyponatremia and hyperkalemia associated with peritoneal effusion in four cats, *J Am Vet Med Assoc* 218:1590, 2001.
Burkholder WJ et al: Foods and techniques for managing obesity in companion animals, *J Am Vet Med Assoc* 212:658, 1998.
Center SA et al: The clinical and metabolic effects of rapid weight loss in obese pet cats and the influence of supplemental oral L-carnitine, *J Vet Intern Med* 14:598, 2000.
DiBartola SP, ed: *Fluid therapy in small animal practice,* ed 2, Philadelphia, 2000, WB Saunders.
Feldman EC, Nelson RW: *Canine and feline endocrinology and reproduction,* ed 3, Philadelphia, 2004, WB Saunders.
Hawthorne AJ et al: Predicting the body composition of cats: development of a zoometric measurement for estimation of percentage body fat in cats, *J Vet Intern Med* 14:365, 2000.
Kimmel SE, Nelson RW: Incidence and prognostic value of low plasma ionized calcium concentration in cats with acute pancreatitis: 46 cases (1996-1998), *J Am Vet Med Assoc* 219:1105, 2001.
Scarlett JM et al: Associations between body condition and disease in cats, *J Am Vet Med Assoc* 212:1725, 1998.
Toll J et al: Prevalence and incidence of serum magnesium abnormalities in hospitalized cats, *J Vet Intern Med* 16:217, 2002.

## PART VIII: REPRODUCTIVE SYSTEM DISORDERS

Atalan G et al: Comparison of ultrasonographic and radiographic measurements of canine prostate measurements, *Vet Radiol Ultrasound* 40:408, 1999.
Concannon PW et al, eds: Advances in reproduction of dogs and cats and exotic carnivores, *J Reprod Fertil Suppl* 57, 2001.
Davidson AP, ed: Clinical theriogenology, *Vet Clin North Am Small Anim Pract* 31:2, 2001.
Drobatz KJ et al: Eclampsia in dogs: 31 cases (1995-1998), *J Am Vet Med Assoc* 217:216, 2000.
Gobello C et al: Dioestrous ovariectomy: a model to study the role of progesterone in the onset of canine pseudopregnancy, *J Reprod Fertil Suppl* 57:55, 2001.
Goodman M: Ovulation timing: concepts and controversies, *Vet Clin North Am* 31:219, 2001.
Linde-Forsberg C: Hints on semen freezing, cryoextenders and frozen semen artificial insemination, *Proceedings of the Annual Conference of the Society of Theriogenology and the American College of Theriogenology,* Colorado Springs, 2002, p 303.
Moe L: Population-based incidence of mammary tumours in some dog breeds, *J Reprod Fertil Suppl* 57:439, 2001.
Root-Kustritz MV: Theriogenology question of the month (priapism), *J Am Vet Med Assoc* 202:633, 1993.
Scott KC et al: Characteristics of free-roaming cats evaluated in a trap-neuter-release program, *J Am Vet Med Assoc* 221:1136, 2002.
Sirinarumitr K: Effects of finasteride on size of the prostate gland and semen quality in dogs with benign prostatic hypertrophy, *J Am Vet Med Assoc* 218:1275, 2001.

Verstegen JP et al: The ovarian cycle and oestrus induction in the bitch, prostate diseases in the male dog, *Proceedings of the Annual Conference of the Society for Theriogenology and American College of Theriogenology;* Colorado Springs, 2002, p 321.

Wilson MS: Transcervical insemination techniques in the bitch, *Vet Clin North Am* 31:291, 2001.


## PART IX: NEUROMUSCULAR DISORDERS

Bagley RS: Spinal fracture or luxation, *Vet Clin North Am Small Anim Pract* 30:133, 2000.

Coates JR et al: Congenital and inherited neurologic disorders of dogs and cats. In Bonagura JD, ed: *Current veterinary therapy XIII,* ed 13, Philadelphia, 2000, WB Saunders, p 1111.

Dewey CW et al: Primary brain tumors in dogs and cats, *Compend Contin Educ Pract Vet* 22:756, 2000.

Hamilton HL et al: Diagnosis of blindness. In Bonagura JD, ed: *Current veterinary therapy XIII,* ed 13, Philadelphia, 2000, WB Saunders, p 1038.

Hawthorne JC et al: Fibrocartilaginous embolic myelopathy in Miniature Schnauzers, *J Am Anim Hosp Assoc* 37:374, 2001.

Klopp LS et al: Autosomal recessive muscular dystrophy in Labrador Retrievers, *Compend Contin Educ Pract Vet* 22:121, 2000.

Munana KR et al: Intervertebral disk disease in cats, *J Am Anim Hosp Assoc* 37:384, 2001.

Shelton GD: Myasthenia gravis and other disorders of neuromuscular transmission, *Vet Clin North Am Small Anim Pract* 32:188, 2002.

Taylor SM: Selected disorders of muscle and the neuromuscular junction, *Vet Clin North Am Small Anim Pract* 30:59, 2000.

Thomas WB: Initial assessment of patients with neurologic dysfunction, *Vet Clin North Am Small Anim Pract* 30:1, 2000.


## PART X: JOINT DISORDERS

Bennett D: Treatment of the immune-based inflammatory arthropathies of the dog and cat. In Bonagura JD, Kirk RW, eds: *Kirk's current veterinary therapy XII,* Philadelphia, 1995, WB Saunders, pp 1188-1195.

Carro T: Polyarthritis in cats, *Compend Contin Educ Pract Vet* 16:57-67, 1994.

Lewis RM: Rheumatoid arthritis, *Vet Clin North Am Small Anim Pract* 24:697-701, 1994.

Schrader SC: The use of the laboratory in the diagnosis of joint disorders in dogs and cats. In Bonagura JD, Kirk RW, eds: *Kirk's current veterinary therapy XII,* Philadelphia, 1995, WB Saunders, pp 1166-1171.


## PART XI: ONCOLOGY

Baker R et al: *Color atlas of cytology of the dog and cat,* St Louis, 2000, Mosby.

Baskin CR et al: Factors influencing first remission and survival in 143 dogs with lymphoma: a retrospective study, *J Am Anim Hosp Assoc* 36:404, 2000.

Clifford CA et al: Treatment of canine hemangiosarcoma: 2000 and beyond, *J Vet Intern Med* 14:479, 2000.

Cowell RL et al: *Diagnostic cytology and hematology of the dog and cat,* ed 2, St Louis, 1999, Mosby.

LaRue SM et al: Recent advances in radiation oncology, *Compend Contin Educ Pract Vet* 15:795, 1993.

Madewell BRL: Diagnosis, assessment of prognosis, and treatment of dogs with lymphoma: sentinel changes (1973-1999), *J Vet Intern Med* 13:393, 1999.

Moore AS et al: Lomustine (CCNU) for the treatment of resistant lymphoma in dogs, *J Vet Intern Med* 13:395, 1999.

Radin MJ et al: *Interpretation of canine and feline cytology,* Wilmington, Del, 2001, the Gloyd Group.

Raskin RE et al: *Atlas of canine and feline cytology,* Philadelphia, 2001, WB Saunders.

Weiss DJL: Flow cytometric and immunophenotypic evaluation of acute lymphocytic leukemia in dog bone marrow, *J Vet Intern Med* 15:589, 2001.


## PART XII: HEMATOLOGY AND IMMUNOLOGY

Bateman SW et al: Diagnosis of disseminated intravascular coagulation in dogs admitted to an intensive care unit, *J Am Vet Med Assoc* 215:805, 1999.

Carothers M et al: Disorders of leukocytes. In Fenner WR, ed: *Quick reference to veterinary medicine,* ed 3, New York, Lippincott, 2000, p 149.

Feldman BF et al, eds: *Schalm's veterinary hematology,* ed 5, Philadelphia, 2000, Lippincott Williams & Wilkins.

Peterson ME et al: Diagnosis and treatment of polycythemic cats, *J Am Anim Hosp Assoc* 32:294, 1996.

Scott-Moncrieff JCR et al: Treatment of nonregenerative anemia with human gamma-globulin in dogs, *J Am Vet Med Assoc* 206:1895, 1995.

Spangler WL et al: Pathologic factors affecting patient survival after splenectomy in dogs, *J Vet Intern Med* 11:166, 1997.

Stokol T et al: Idiopathic pure red cell aplasia and nonregenerative immune-mediated anemia in dogs: 43 cases (1988-1999), *J Am Vet Med Assoc* 216:1429, 2000.

## PART XIII: INFECTIOUS DISEASES

Ano H et al: Detection of *Babesia* species from infected dog blood by polymerase chain reaction, *J Vet Med Sci* 63:111, 2001.

Buttera ST et al: Survey of veterinary conference attendees for evidence of zoonotic infection by feline retroviruses, *J Am Vet Med Assoc* 217:1475, 2000.

Chandler JC et al: Mycoplasmal respiratory infections in small animals: 17 cases (1988-1999), *J Am Anim Hosp Assoc* 38:111, 2002.

Dodds WJ: Vaccination protocols for dogs predisposed to vaccine reactions, *J Am Anim Hosp Assoc* 37:211, 2001.

Gage KL et al: Cases of cat-associated human plague in the Western US, 1977-1998, *Clin Infect Dis* 30:893, 2000.

Greene CE et al: Canine vaccination, *Vet Clin North Am Small Anim Pract* 31:473, 2001.

Hill DE et al: Specific detection of *Neospora caninum* oocysts in fecal samples from experimentally infected dogs using the polymerase chain reaction, *J Parasitol* 87:395, 2001.

Jensen WA et al: Prevalence of *Haemobartonella felis* infection in cats, *Am J Vet Res* 62:604, 2001.

Kano R et al: PCR detection of the *Cryptococcus neoformans* of *CAPS9* gene from a biopsy specimen from a case of feline cryptococcosis, *J Vet Diagn Invest* 13:439, 2001.

Lappin MR et al: Use of serologic tests to predict resistance to feline herpesvirus 1, feline calcivirus, and feline parvovirus infection in cats, *J Am Vet Med Assoc* 220:38, 2002.

Meier HT et al: Feline cytauxzoonosis: a case report and literature review, *J Am Anim Hosp Assoc* 36:493, 2000.

Neer TM et al: Consensus statement on ehrlichial disease of small animals from the Infectious Disease Study Group of the ACVIM, *J Vet Intern Med* 16(3):309, 2002.

Paltrinieri S et al: Laboratory profiles in cats with different pathological and immunohistochemical findings due to feline infectious peritonitis (FIP), *J Feline Med Surg* 3:149, 2001.

Schulman RL et al: Use of corticosteroids for treating dogs with airway obstruction secondary to hilar lymphadenopathy caused by chronic histoplasmosis: 16 cases (1979-1997), *J Am Vet Med Assoc* 214:1345, 1999.

Spain CV et al: Prevalence of enteric zoonotic agents in cats less than 1 year old in central New York State, *J Vet Intern Med* 15:33, 2001.

Stubbs CJ et al: Feline ehrlichiosis; literature review and serologic survey, *Compend Contin Educ Pract Vet* 22:307, 2000.

Wolf AM: Feline leukemia virus. In Bonagura J, ed: *Current veterinary therapy XIII*, ed 13, Philadelphia, 2000, WB Saunders, p 280.

# Index

Arrhythmias—cont'd
  magnesium imbalances and, 532, 533
  potassium imbalances and, 524, 526
Arrhythmogenic right ventricular
  cardiomyopathy, 68, 78-79
Arsenicals, antidote for, 336, 364
Arterial blood gas analysis, 157, 167-168
Arterial thromboembolism, 79-82
Arterioportal fistula, 343
Arteriovenous shunts, extracardiac, 90-93
Arthritis. *See also* Joint disorders;
    Polyarthritis.
  bacterial L-form–associated, 696
  calcivirus, 697-698
  fungal, 697
  immune-mediated, 689
  rheumatoid, 689, 691, 693, 701-702
  septic, 691, 692, 694-696, 836, 837
Artifacts, electrocardiographic, 8
Artificial insemination (AI), 587
  female infertility and, 542, 543
  hormone measurement for, 538, 539
Ascites, 309, 352
L-Asparaginase test for hypercalcemia,
    528-529
Aspartate aminotransferase (AST), serum,
    316, 317
Aspergillosis, nasal, 136, 143-144
Aspiration pneumonia, 183-185
Aspirin for thromboembolism, 81, 82, 189
Asthma, feline, 172-173
Ataxia, 593, 605, 661
Atelectasis, 160
Atenolol, 41, 42, 52
Atlantoaxial luxation, 665
Atrial conduction disturbances, 16
Atrial enlargement, 11, 22, 23
Atrial fibrillation, 15, 16, 45-46
Atrial flutter, 15
Atrial premature complexes, 14-15, 43
Atrial septal defect (ASD), 91, 92, 96
Atrial standstill, 47-48
Atrial tachycardia, 14, 15, 43-44
Atrioventricular (AV) block
  electrocardiographic evaluation of, 17, 18
  treatment of, 47, 48
Atrioventricular (AV) valves
  degenerative diseases of, 82-86
  malformations of, 97
Atrophic gastritis, 266
Atrophic myositis, 259
Atropine, 41, 43, 54
Atropine challenge test, 48, 54
Auscultation, thoracic
  for atrioventricular valve disease, 83-84
  for cardiovascular disorders, 5-7
  for respiratory disorders, 156
Autoagglutination in hemolytic anemia,
    765-766

Autoantibodies, thyroid hormone, 452, 456,
    458
Autoimmune polyneuropathy, 672
Autonomic bladder, 418
Axonopathy, breed-specific, 661, 662, 663
Azathioprine
  for chronic hepatitis, 344
  for gastrointestinal disorders, 252
  for immune-mediated diseases, 808, 809
Azoospermia, 572-573
Azotemia, 375-376
  acute renal failure and, 387, 389
  urethral obstruction with, 413

**B**
Babesiosis, 885-886, 902
Bacteremia
  antibiotics for, 832-833, 834
  *B. canis*, 584-585
Bacteria
  canine vaginal, 537
  intestinal, diarrhea related to, 279-281
  preputial and urethral, 569, 570
  tracheal wash for, 163
  urinary
    antibiotic sensitivities for, 381, 399, 400
    infection-causing, 398
Bacterial cultures
  for estrous cycle disorders, 537
  fecal, 234-235
  for lower respiratory disorders, 164-165
  of semen, 569, 577
  vaginal, 537, 549-550
Bacterial endocarditis, 87-90, 832-833, 834
Bacterial infections. *See also* Infectious
    diseases; *specific infection*.
  antibiotics for, 828-840, 829-830, 900-901
  central nervous system, 638, 641-642,
    644-646
  diagnostic tests for, 822, 823, 825-827
  neonatal morbidity/mortality and, 565
  polysystemic, 846-852
  uterine, 552-553
  zoonotic
    bite, scratch, or exudate, 894-897
    enteric, 891, 893-894
    respiratory and ocular, 897-898
    urogenital, 899
Bacterial L-form–associated arthritis, 696
Bacterial meningitis and myelitis, 641-642
Bacterial myocarditis, 68, 79
Bacterial overgrowth, small intestinal, 835,
    836
Bacterial pneumonia, 179-180, 834, 838
Bacterial prostatitis, 581-582, 839, 840
Bacterial pyelonephritis, 399, 839
Bacterial rhinitis, 138, 144
Baermann technique for fecal examination,
    820, 821, 822

Lymphoma—cont'd
  alimentary, 294
  chemotherapy protocols for, 733-738,
    756-757
  cytologic evaluation of, 710
  diagnosis of, 731-733
  etiology and features of, 729-731
  feline leukemia virus-associated, 870
  large-cell, 742
  mediastinal, 194, 195, 727-728
  spinal, 655-657
Lymphomatoid granulomatosis, 186-187
Lymphopenia, 781
Lymphoplasmacytic rhinitis, 136, 145
Lymphoplasmacytic splenitis, 799
Lymphoplasmacytic synovitis, 701
Lypressin, 432
Lysine for herpesvirus infection, 140

**M**
"Machinery" murmurs, 7
Macrolides, 829, 831, 900
Macrophages, bronchoalveolar, 164
Macrophagic inflammation, 163
Magnesium
  dietary, urolithiasis and, 408
  for hypomagnesemia, 533
  serum, imbalances of, 532-533
Magnetic resonance imaging
  for hyperadrenocorticism, 494
  for lower respiratory disorders, 161
  for lymphoma, 732
  for neuromuscular disorders, 603
Maintenance phase
  of immunosuppressive therapy, 807, 808
  of lymphoma chemotherapy, 734, 735-736
Malabsorptive diseases, 222-223, 285-289
Maldigestion, 222-223, 234, 238
Male fertility, disorders of, 543, 568-574, 585
Malignancies. *See also* Neoplasms.
  criteria for, 709
  hypercalcemia with, 527, 528, 714, 731
  treatment options for, 711-714, 726
  types of, 709-710
Malignant hyperthermia, 683
Malignant melanoma, oropharyngeal, 753,
    754, 755
Mammary gland, disorders of, 554-556
Manx cats, caudal agenesis of, 665
Masses. *See also* Neoplasms.
  approach to patient with, 725-728
  mediastinal, 195, 727-728
  metastatic, 726-727
  oropharyngeal, 256-258
  solitary, 725-726
  splenic, 800
Mast cell tumors (MCTs), 749-753
  in cats, 752-753
  chemotherapy for, 758

cytologic evaluation of, 710
  in dogs, 749-752
Masticatory myositis, 259, 678-679
Mastitis, 554, 840
Matings
  abortifacients for unwanted, 563-564
  frequency and timing of, 543
  refusals of, 542
Mean electrical axis (MEA)
  estimating, 7, 8
  normal, 9, 10
Measles vaccine, canine, 844, 862
Mediastinal disease
  clinical manifestations of, 192-196
  diagnostic tests for, 196-198
Mediastinal lymphoma, 729, 730
Mediastinal masses, 195, 727-728
Medications. *See* Chemotherapy; Drugs.
Megacolon, idiopathic, 300
Megaesophagus, 260-261
Megestrol acetate, 544
Melanoma, malignant oropharyngeal, 753,
    754, 755
Melarsomine, 103, 105-106
Melena, 225
Meningeal vasculitis, 601, 639
Meningitis, 637-647
  bacterial, 641-642
  diagnostic tests for, 601, 638
  parasitic, 647
  steroid-responsive suppurative, 637-639
Meningoencephalitis
  cerebrospinal fluid in, 601
  granulomatous, 601, 639-640
  pug, 640
Mentation, altered
  causes of, 593, 611
  head trauma and, 611-613
Mesenteric torsion and volvulus, 291
Metabolic acidosis, 168
  cardiac arrest with, 58-59
  cardiogenic shock with, 70
  diabetic ketoacidosis with, 485
  renal failure with, 390-391, 394
Metabolic alkalosis, 168
Metabolic disorders, 514-519
  drugs for, 534
  encephalopathy in, 611
  male infertility in, 572
  myopathies in, 681-682, 683
  polyneuropathies in, 671-672
  seizures in, 619
Metabolic storage diseases, 624
Metaldehyde intoxication, 620
Metastasectomy for osteosarcoma, 748
Metastases, 726-727
  mast cell tumor, 749, 751-752, 753
  to/from bone, 747
Metered-dose inhaler therapy, 175